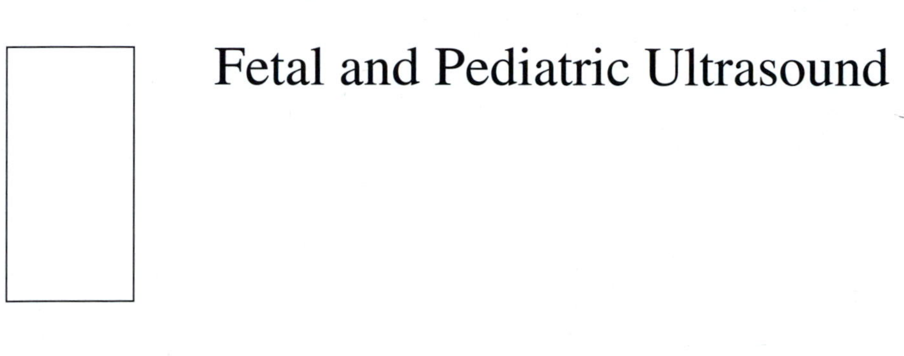

Fetal and Pediatric Ultrasound

Notice

Medicine is an ever-changing science. As new research and clinical experience broaden our knowledge, changes in treatment and drug therapy are required. The editors and the publisher of this work have checked with sources believed to be reliable in their efforts to provide information that is complete and generally in accord with the standards accepted at the time of publication. However, in view of the possibility of human error or changes in medical sciences, neither the editors nor the publisher nor any other party who has been involved in the preparation or publication of this work warrants that the information contained herein is in every respect accurate or complete, and they disclaim all responsibility for any errors or omissions or for the results obtained from use of the information contained in this work. Readers are encouraged to confirm the information contained herein with other sources. For example and in particular, readers are advised to check the product information sheet included in the package of each drug they plan to administer to be certain that the information contained in this work is accurate and that changes have not been made in the recommended dose or in the contraindications for administration. This recommendation is of particular importance in connection with new or infrequently used drugs.

Fetal and Pediatric Ultrasound

A CASEBOOK APPROACH

Editors

HARRIS L. COHEN, MD, FACR

Visiting Professor of Radiology
Director, Division of Pediatric Imaging
The Russell H. Morgan Department
of Radiology and Radiological Science
Johns Hopkins Medical Institutions
Baltimore, Maryland

Professor of Radiology
SUNY–Downstate Medical Center
Until recently: Director, Division of Ultrasound
Co-Director, Division of Pediatric Radiology
Brooklyn, New York

CARLOS J. SIVIT, MD

Director, Division of Pediatric Radiology
Rainbow Babies and Children's Hospital
Professor of Radiology and Pediatrics
Case Western Reserve University
School of Medicine
Cleveland, Ohio

McGRAW-HILL

Medical Publishing Division

New York St. Louis San Francisco Auckland Bogotá Caracas Lisbon London Madrid Mexico City Milan Montreal New Delhi San Juan Singapore Sydney Tokyo Toronto

McGraw-Hill
A Division of The McGraw-Hill Companies

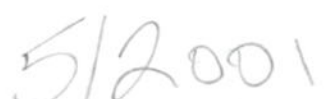

Fetal and Pediatric Ultrasound

1234567890 KGPKGP 09876543210

ISBN 0–8385–8864–6

The book was set in Times Roman by Pine Tree Composition, Inc.
The photoprep was completed by Jay's Publishers Services, Inc.
The editors were Martin Wonsiewicz, Susan R. Noujaim, and Muza Navrozov.
The production supervisor was Richard Ruzycka.
The design was done by Joan O'Connor.
Quebecor World/Kingsport was printer and binder.

This book is printed on acid-free paper.

Library of Congress Cataloging in Publication Data

Cohen, Harris L.
Fetal and pediatric ultrasound : a casebook approach / authors, Harris L. Cohen, Carlos J. Sivit.
p.; cm.
Includes bibliographical references and index.
ISBN 0–8385–8864–6
1. Children—Diseases—Diagnosis. 2. Diagnosis, Ultrasonic. 3.
Fetus—Diseases—Diagnosis. 4. Diagnosis, Ultrasonic. I. Sivit, Carlos J. II. Title.
[DNLM: 1. Ultrasonography, Prenatal—Case Report. 2. Ultrasonography—Infant,
Newborn—Case Report. WQ 209 C678F2001]
RJ51.U45 C64 2001
618.92′007543—dc21
99–088758

To

—my wife, Sandra W. Cohen, M.D., and my children, David, Lauren, and Ben, who put up with the inordinate commitment necessary to create a text in a world with less and less academic time and forgave my sins of holing up in my computer room, leaving piles of teaching files around the house and being generally frenetic when something (and it's always something) could not be found;

—my ultrasound, pediatric radiology, general radiology and clinical pediatric and obstetric mentors and colleagues, including sonographers, residents and fellows, who have reinforced my view that the best imagers are those with an open and inquisitive mind, who plan their approach to their exams based on proper communication with the requesting physicians and the patients themselves, and who are nimble enough to *not* do everything by rote or a cookbook approach and who are willing to look, hear, and listen;

—my patients and their families whose travels and travails through the current health care system can be arduous, a fact of life we must always consider and hopefully improve, but most of all…

—the memory of my mother, Lola (Esther Leah bas Elazar Hertz) Cohen neé Altman, who survived the Radom ghetto and Auschwitz concentration camp and was allowed to build a new, if not easy or long, life in America along Emma Lazarus's welcoming shores. She was exacting in detail and would have made a great radiologist; and…

—the memory of my recently departed father, Samuel (Ben Ben Zion Ha) Cohen né Gozanski of Druzginiki, Poland (now Lithuania), who went from the white collar world of bookkeeping and bank secretary to the no collar world of an internment camp, resistance in the Polish/Lithuanian woods, internment in Siberia, messing officer work in a DP camp in Ulm, Germany, and finally to 50 years of blue collar work (always dressed in a white shirt and tie), selling appetizing in America, mostly at Zabar's. He adored the United States of America. He was incredibly honest and hard-working and loved playing to the crowds of lox and caviar purchasers who were his audience. He, hopefully, passed those qualities down to his children. Whereas I may not be able to slice lox as thin as he did, spiral CT and ultrasound certainly allow me to carry on his tradition of working with fine slices.

They both are missed.

HLC

To

—my wife, Julie, for her patience and understanding
—my children, Margaret and Alexander, for sharing their dad
—my parents, Olga and Rosendo, for their sacrifices and inspiration

CJS

How to Use This Book

The goal of this book is to present most, if not all, of what one has to know in fetal and pediatric ultrasound in a format that also allows self-testing for board examination preparation. In order to do this, the book has been divided into 120 chapters, which begin with an unknown case on a right-sided page. The first page of the chapter, therefore, has a number but no title. On the turned page, a left-sided one, there is a chapter title, which is the answer to the unknown image(s) as well as interpretation of the unknown images and the case's diagnosis. The remainder of each chapter consists of information related to the disease or finding of the unknown images and expanded information on that ultrasound topic, including information and images on an associated larger topic. This may include, e.g., a discussion of pelvic inflammatory disease after introductory unknown images of a tuboovarian abscess, differential diagnostic possibilities for an unknown image or ultrasound techniques used in obtaining those images.

In order to avoid prematurely informing the reader of the answers to the unknowns, the Abbreviated Table of Contents, in the front of the book, has just chapter numbers and pages. A complete Table of Contents, with chapter titles and authors' names, is available at the back of the book. Color Doppler images presented as black and white in individual chapters appear as color plates.

We want this book to be authoritative in its information, educational in its casebook method as well as fun to use. We hope we succeeded. Only you, the reader, can tell.

Abbreviated Table of Contents

Section D. Genital Cyst

Section E. Musculoskeletal System

Section F. General Obstetrics and Miscellaneous

PART II THE PEDIATRIC PATIENT

Section A. Central Nervous System

Section B. Hepatobiliary System

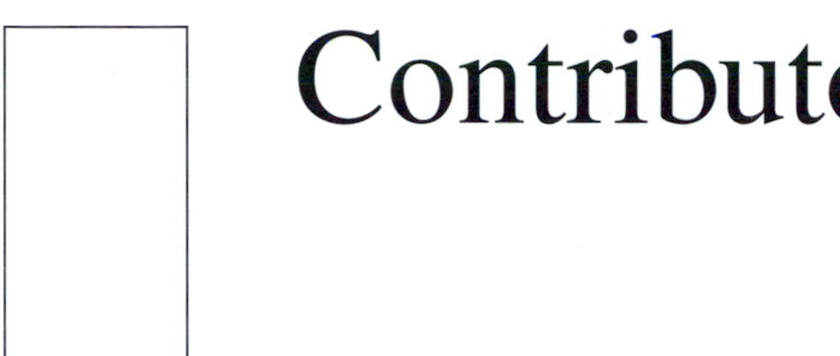

Contributors*

JANICE W. ALLISON, MD [32, 33]
Department of Radiology, Arkansas Children's Hospital, University of Arkansas for Medical Sciences, Little Rock, Arkansas

KAREN E. BASILE, MD [75]
Fellow in Pediatric Radiology, Division of Pediatric Radiology, Rainbow Babies and Childrens Hospital, Cleveland, Ohio

SHEILA C. BERLIN, MD [38, 109, 110]
Assistant Professor of Radiology, Division of Pediatric Radiology, Rainbow Babies and Children's Hospital, Cleveland, Ohio

ELLEN C. BENYA, MD [47, 50, 54]
Assistant Professor of Radiology, Department of Radiology, University of Chicago, 5841 S. Maryland Ave., Chicago, Illinois

DOROTHY BULAS, MD [22, 65]
Professor of Radiology and Pediatrics, The George Washington University Medical Center; Staff Radiologist, Children's National Medical Center, Washington, D.C.

BETTY CHEN, MD [28]
Clinical Assistant Instructor, Department of Radiology, SUNY–Downstate Medical Center, Brooklyn, New York

CHARLES J. CHUNG, MD [42, 79]
Assistant Professor of Radiology, Department of Radiology, University of North Carolina, Chapel Hill, North Carolina

HARRIS L. COHEN, MD, FACR [1–5; 8–14; 16–21; 23–31; 66; 82, 83; 93; 95–103; 105–108; 113; 115–117; 120]
Visiting Professor of Radiology; Director, Division of Pediatric Imaging, The Russell H. Morgan Department of Radiology and Radiological Science, Johns Hopkins Medical Institutions, Baltimore, Maryland

Professor of Radiology, SUNY–Downstate Medical Center; Until recently: Director, Division of Ultrasound; Co-Director, Division of Pediatric Radiology, Brooklyn, New York

MICHAEL A. DIPIETRO, MD [35]
Professor of Radiology, University of Michigan; Pediatric Radiologist, C. S. Mott Children's Hospital, Ann Arbor, Michigan

JAMES S. DONALDSON, MD [119]
Professor of Radiology, Northwestern University Medical School; Acting Chairman, Department of Radiology, The Children's Memorial Hospital, Chicago, Illinois

JUDY A. ESTROFF, MD [6]
Associate Clinical Professor of Radiology, Harvard Medical School; Radiologist, Children's Hospital in Boston; Radiologist, Boston Ultrasound Consultants, Boston, Massachusetts

LYNN ANSLEY FORDHAM [55, 56]
Assistant Professor of Radiology, Department of Radiology, University of North Carolina, Chapel Hill, North Carolina

BRIAN GALE, MD [95, 98]
Assistant Professor, Department of Radiology, SUNY–Downstate Medical Center, Brooklyn, New York

ANNA GOLJA, MD [9]
Clinical Assistant Instructor, Chief Resident of Radiology, Department of Radiology, SUNY–Downstate Medical Center, Brooklyn, New York

BETH R. GROSS, MD [7, 15]
Director of Ultrasound, Great Neck Obstetrics and Gynecology, Great Neck, New York

HOWARD T. HARCKE, MD, FACR, FAAP [118]
Professor of Radiology and Pediatrics, Jefferson Medical College; Director of Imaging Research, A. I. Dupont Hospital for Children, Wilmington, Delaware

GORDON HAUGLAND, MD [31]
Assistant Professor of Radiology, Department of Radiology, SUNY–Downstate Medical Center, Brooklyn, New York

*The numbers in brackets following the contributor name refer to chapter(s) authored or co-authored by the contributor.

GEORGE KHORIATY, MD [107]
Clinical Assistant Instructor, Department of Radiology, SUNY–Downstate Medical Center, Brooklyn, New York

MADHURI KIRPEKAR, MD [36, 120]
Assistant Professor of Clinical Radiology, Columbia University School of Medicine; Associate Professor of Radiology, St. Luke's-Roosevelt Hospital Center, New York, New York

KAREN K. MOELLER, MD [102]
Clinical Assistant Professor, SUNY–Downstate Medical Center, Department of Radiology, Brooklyn, New York; Fellow, Children's Hospital of Boston, Boston, Massachusetts

STUART MORRISON, MB, CHB, MRCP [64, 71]
Associate Professor of Radiology, Division of Pediatric Radiology, Rainbow Babies and Children's Hospital, Cleveland Clinic Foundation, Cleveland, Ohio

MELISSA T. MYERS, MD [74, 92]
Assistant Professor of Radiology, Division of Pediatric Radiology, University Hospitals of Cleveland, Cleveland, Ohio

HARRIET J. PALTIEL, MD [94, 104, 114]
Associate Clinical Professor of Radiology, Department of Radiology, Harvard Medical School; Radiologist, Children's Hospital in Boston, Boston, Massachusetts

MARLENA PURSNER, MD [26, 115]
Assistant Clinical Instructor, SUNY–Downstate Medical Center, Brooklyn, New York

DAPHNE ROITBERG-MIZRAHI, MD [117]
Assistant Professor of Radiology, Albert Einstein College of Medicine; Assistant Attending, Beth Israel Medical Center, New York, New York

LYNNE RUESS, MD [69, 72]
Department of Radiology, Tripler Army Medical Center, Honolulu, Hawaii

MARYANNE RUGGIERRO-DELITURRI, MD [93, 97]
Bayridge Radiology, Brooklyn, New York

YAIR SAFRIEL, MD [99, 101]
Clinical Assistant Department of Radiology, SUNY–Downstate Medical Center, Instructor, Brooklyn, New York

JOANNA J. SIEBERT, MD [32, 33]
Professor of Radiology and Pediatrics, University of Arkansas; Director of Radiology, Arkansas Children's Hospital, Department of Radiology, Little Rock, Arkansas

CARLOS J. SIVIT, MD [34; 37; 39–41; 43–46; 48, 49; 51–53; 57–63; 67, 68; 70; 72; 76–78; 80, 81; 84–91; 111, 112]
Director, Division of Pediatric Radiology, Rainbow Babies and Children's Hospital, Professor of Radiology and Pediatrics Case Western Reserve University School of Medicine, Cleveland, Ohio

JEAN TORRISI, MD [108]
Assistant Professor, Department of Radiology, Albert Einstein College of Medicine, Beth Israel Medical Center, New York, New York

DAVID L. WELLS [100]
Clinical Assistant Instructor, Department of Radiology, SUNY–Downstate Medical Center, Brooklyn, New York

ROGER YANG, MD [13, 21]
Clinical Assistant Professor of Radiology, SUNY–Downstate Medical Center, Brooklyn, New York

DANIEL L. ZINN, MD [83, 96, 106]
Assistant Professor of Radiology, SUNY–Downstate Medical Center, Brooklyn, New York

HARRY L. ZINN, MD [103]
Assistant Professor of Radiology, Department of Radiology, SUNY–Downstate Medical Center; Director of CT/MRI, University Hospital of Brooklyn, Brooklyn, New York

Medical illustrations by Elena DuPont, University Imaging, Cleveland, Ohio.

Acknowledgments

The creation of this book requires the acknowledgment of debts owed for the imaging experience necessary to take on the task of authorship. We have to thank and acknowledge many individuals. These include outstanding teachers and colleagues from our fellowship days at Children's National Medical Center and colleagues at Brookdale University Medical Center, SUNY-Downstate. Johns Hopkins Medical Institutions (North Shore University Hospital–Cornell) North Shore University Hospital, and Rainbow Babies and Childrens Hospital, who have helped us develop and hone the skills of our craft. Outstanding pediatricians, pediatric surgeons and obstetrician/gynecologists have provided us with the cases, advice and feedback to keep going in pursuit of clinical answers despite these challenging times in academic medicine. We are grateful to the outstanding sonographers who have assisted us: Jerry Adell, RDMS; Andrew Brown, RDMS; Frank Cervantes, RDMS; Winsome Charles, RDMS; Heather Cross, RDMS; JoAnne Marti-Cartagena, RDMS; Maureen McGeary, RDMS; Dara Muller RDMS, MBA; Deverel Patterson, RDMS; Chakravarth Premkumar, RDMS; Anna Rosenberg, BS; Judy Schwartz, RDMS; Brian Smith, RDMS; and Darnett Williams, RDMS. A large number of residents and fellows have allowed us to improve our work by allowing us to teach sonographic technique review their cases, and question findings and diagnostic conclusions. Our recent and current colleagues, including Kimberly Applegate, M.D., Jane Benson, M.D., Sheila Berlin, M.D., Netta Blittman, M.D., Andrew Campbell, M.D., Thomas Gaston, M.D., Jack Haller, M.D., Stuart Morrison, M.D., Melissa Myers, M.D., Rona Orentlicher, M.D., Melissa Spevale, M.D., Dayna Weinert, M.D., Harry Zinn, and Daniel Zinn, M.D., deserve special mention. One must be surrounded by bright, hard working and enthusiastic people to achieve success.

Special acknowledgements go to Benjamin ("Just call me Ben") Cohen, Lauren Elizabeth Cohen, David (#44) Cohen, and Sandra W. Cohen, M.D., who either filed cases or photographed images or scanned images, Joseph Molter, who photographed images, Valerie Borisa, who helped organize material, and to Elena DuPont, the medical illustrator, who provided art work.

We would also like to acknowledge the efforts of Muza Navrozov, Richard Ruzycka, and the staff of McGraw-Hill who helped to finally bring this book to fruition.

Preface

This book was written with several goals in mind. First, we desired to provide up-to-date information related to the ultrasound analysis of the pediatric patient, from neonatal life through adolescence. Age is an important consideration in differential diagnosis and in determining the normalcy of various imaged structures and imaging findings. We hope that the book will make the reader aware of this fact. Additionally, we desired to provide up-to-date information on the ultrasound analysis of the fetus. Fetal abnormalities may result in clinical problems in the newborn or older child. Early diagnosis of these abnormalities can have significant impact on improved clinical outcomes. Conversely, knowledge of what occurs postnatally to a fetus with an abnormality is important information for sonologists dealing with antenatal diagnosis.

The target audience of any ultrasound text is sonologists and sonographers. We desired to provide the book's information to its typical audience, e.g., fetal and obstetrical ultrasound for the radiologist and obstetrician and pediatric ultrasound for the pediatric radiologist and pediatrician. We also desired to expand the horizons of these groups by providing information that is not typically in their clinical scope but relevant and important to know for those whose clinical concerns are on either side of the life boundary known as birth. Such information has, historically, been used successfully, for example, by obstetricians who adapted neonatal transfontanelle techniques for head ultrasound introduced by pediatric radiologists into their work in the transvaginal analysis of the fetal brain. It is always important to know what physicians in other clinical disciplines are doing for proper education, communication, and improvement of clinical and imaging skills.

The book is meant to be for the education, review, and enjoyment of sonologists, sonographers, and clinicians of various specialties and levels of training. We desired to provide this in a less cut-and-dry manner than the typical textbook by using an unknown case approach. The unknown image cases introduce a variety of topics that are meant to cover the spectrum of work necessary to know in fetal and pediatric ultrasound practice. The unknown images are discussed and reviewed. The case discussions vary, with some geared predominantly to discussing differential diagnosis and some to discussing methods of analysis of various clinical problems by US and, when relevant, other modalities and some cases dealing with clinical aspects of various medical problems. Many of the cases and their discussions are a combination of these three items but with the concept that book space cannot be infinite. The use of different authors, with their own styles, has hopefully kept the book's style from being stilted. Occasional editorial comments underline the fact that there exists much information, but true axioms in medicine and medical imaging analysis are rare. The clinical experience of the senior authors is great, and their comments, on top of what is traditional knowledge, useful. The individual case discussions introduce many other relevant images, which improves the book's scope.

The book can be used as a test-yourself-on-unknown-ultrasound-images exercise. We hope this will help radiology residents studying for their boards and resident clinicians and clinicians studying for other exams. Certainly, we hope it will help those studying for the pediatric radiology certificate of added qualification. Looked at as a whole, the book's images and discussions can be seen, partially, as an atlas of ultrasound findings in the fetus, neonate, child, and adolescent and partially as a text on pediatric and fetal ultrasound. The book can be used as a reference for the topics under discussion. All key areas except pediatric echocardiography are covered. Our desire is that there be something here for everyone. The goal is education and review, with a spoonful of sugar and no bitter aftertaste. We hope that the book will be a fun way to learn and review *Fetal and Pediatric Ultrasound.*

Harris L. Cohen, MD
Carlos J. Sivit, MD

PART 1

THE FETUS

Section A
HEAD AND NECK

1

This is a fetus of 18 weeks gestation. Figures 1-1 and 1-2 are axial views of the brain at slightly different levels. What do you see? Should the parents and physicians be worried?

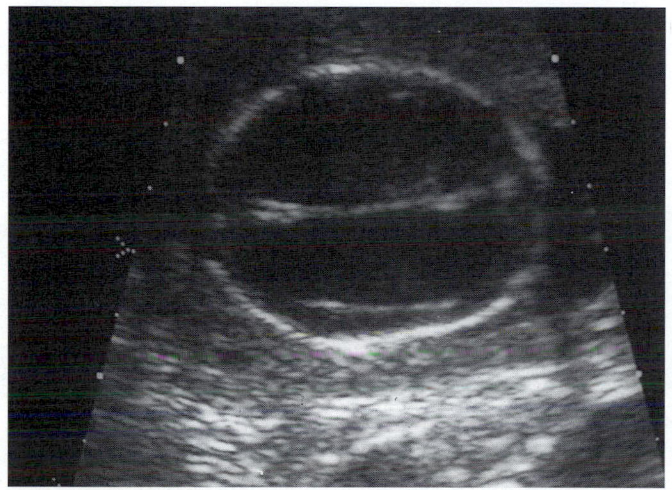

FIGURE 1–1. Fetal head. Axial plane.

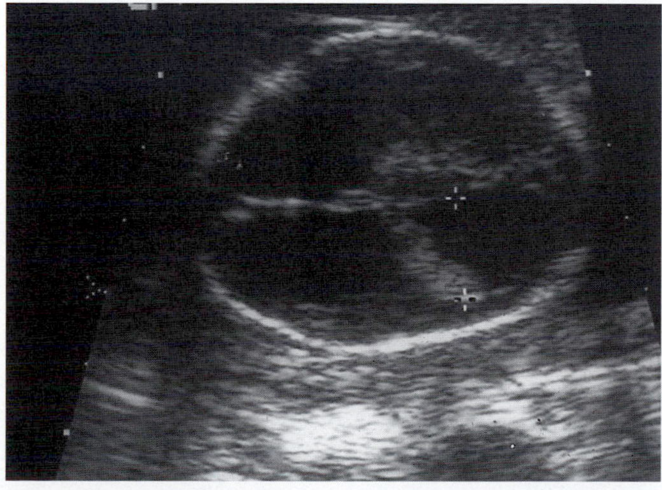

FIGURE 1–2. Fetal head. Axial plane, somewhat inferior to that of Fig. 1-1.

CHAPTER 1

Ventriculomegaly/ Hydrocephalus

HARRIS L. COHEN

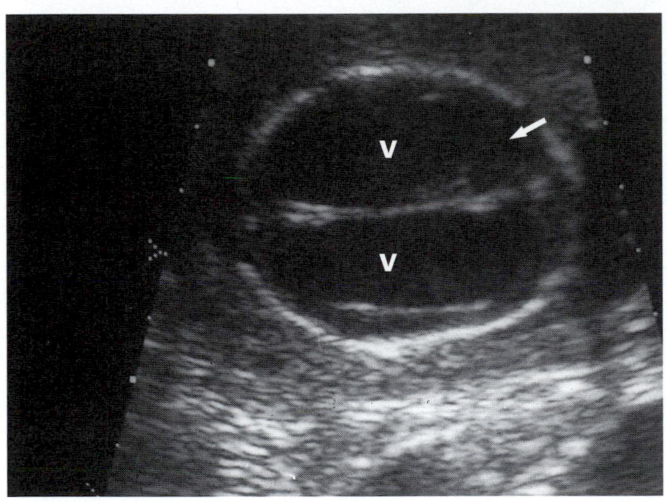

FIGURE 1–3. Annotated version of Fig. 1-1. Hydrocephalus. Axial plane through fetal head. Two cystic areas in the head represent dilated lateral ventricles (V). There is some filling in of the near-field ventricle (*arrow*) with sound due to near-field artifact. This phenomenon, at times, particularly when more echogenic, can hinder the diagnosis and falsely suggest asymmetrical or unilateral ventricular dilatation.

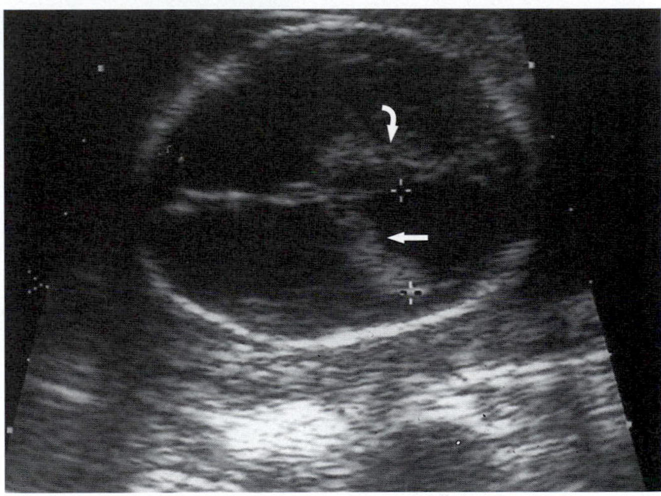

FIGURE 1–4. Annotated version of Fig. 1-2. Hydrocephalus. Axial plane through fetal head. The choroid plexus (*arrow*) of the far-field ventricle dangles within the capacious fluid-filled ventricle. The near-field ventricle's choroid plexus (*curved arrow*) lies horizontally on the medial aspect of its ventricle's surface. It would dangle if its ventricle became the dependent ventricle.

THE UNKNOWN IMAGES

Figures 1-1 (annotated as Fig. 1-3) and 1-2 (annotated as Fig. 1-4) are ultrasound (US) images of a fetus with obvious ventriculomegaly. The fluid-filled spaces represent dilated lateral ventricles. In Fig. 1-4, the choroid plexus in the far field is noted to dangle in the dilated lateral ventricle on the dependent side of the fetal head. This "dangling choroid plexus" phenomenon aids in the diagnosis of hydrocephalus. The next paragraphs will underline reasons to worry about the finding of hydrocephalus.

DEFINITIONS AND CAUSES OF FETAL VENTRICULOMEGALY/HYDROCEPHALUS

Ventriculomegaly is defined as enlargement of the cerebral ventricles, from any cause, nonobstructive or obstructive.

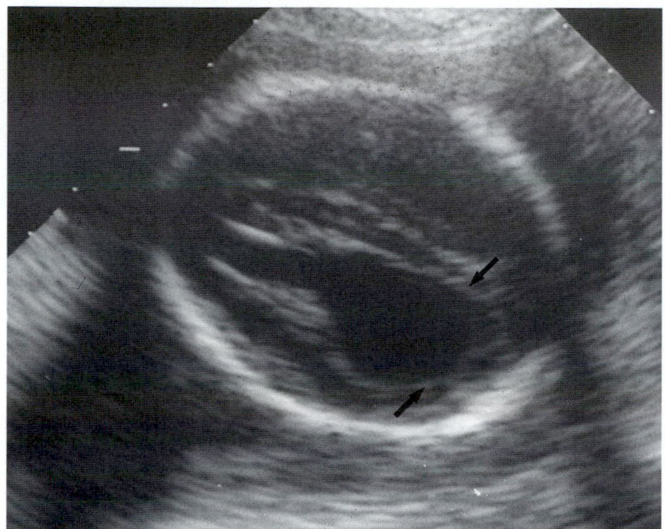

FIGURE 1–5. Colpocephaly. Fetal head. Axial plane. This fetus has ventriculomegaly, but the dilatation is far more prominent in the occipital area (arrows).

Nonobstructive causes of ventriculomegaly include a congenital absence of brain substance, and absence of brain substance secondary to brain destruction. The ventricles become secondarily distended with cerebrospinal fluid (CSF) and fill the intracranial space that has been made excessive by the lack of variable amounts of brain substance. This dilatation is said to be the basis of an ex vacuo phenomenon. Nonobstructive ventriculomegaly may also be due to failure of development of portions of the normal brain. The ventriculomegaly may not be uniform throughout. Colpocephaly (Fig. 1-5) is the nonspecific dilatation of the posterior portion of the lateral ventricles. It can be seen as the "teardrop" posterior ventricles of patients with agenesis of the corpus callosum. In those cases, it is thought to be the result of deficient development of periventricular white matter in the peritrigonal region.

Hydrocephalus is a more specific term for ventricular enlargement that implies that the dilatation is due to pressure from relative or complete obstruction of CSF flow within the pathways from its sites of production, predominantly in the choroid plexus (found within the lateral, third, and fourth ventricles), to its sites of resorption (and eventual entry into the dural and venous sinuses) at the pacchionian or arachnoid granulations within the subarachnoid space at the brain's vertex.

Hydrocephalus may also be divided into communicating and noncommunicating varieties. In noncommunicating hydrocephalus, the obstruction to CSF flow occurs within the ventricular system, perhaps at the foramina of Monro between each lateral ventricle and the third ventricle, at the aqueduct of Sylvius, the CSF pathway between the third and fourth ventricles, or anywhere proximal to CSF egress from the intraventricular system at the median aperture of Magendie or the lateral foramina (apertures) of Luschka.

Communicating hydrocephalus, which is rare in fetuses, is seen with obstructions in the extraventricular CSF pathways between the foramina of Luschka or Magendie and the CSF resorption site at the arachnoid granulations.

A less usual form of ventriculomegaly can occurs with choroid plexus papillomas and the overproduction of CSF within the ventricular system.

Increasing dilatation of the cerebral ventricles over time can confirm an obstructive cause for an imaged hydrocephalus, but a fetus may have obstructive hydrocephalus without evident increasing dilatation. Follow-up US examinations allow determination of the improvement, stabilization, or worsening of a case of ventriculomegaly. This information can be used for decision making with regard to mode of delivery.

THE ANTENATAL DIAGNOSIS OF VENTRICULOMEGALY/HYDROCEPHALUS—WHY IS IT IMPORTANT?

It is most important to make the antenatal diagnosis of hydrocephalus. Hydrocephalus is associated with chromosomal abnormalities, found in as many as 25 percent of affected fetuses, that may or may not be life-threatening. Ventriculomegaly, and more specifically hydrocephalus, is associated with other congenital intracranial and extracranial anomalies that may themselves be associated with significant perinatal and pediatric morbidity and mortality. As many as 80 percent of fetuses with hydrocephalus have associated anomalies.

The antenatal finding of ventriculomegaly is associated with an almost 90 percent sensitivity for the eventual discovery of an associated brain or spinal cord abnormality. Common causes of pediatric ventriculomegaly that can be looked for on antenatal imaging include aqueductal stenosis (reported as the cause of 33 to 43 percent of cases in children), myelomeningocele with the associated Arnold-Chiari II malformation (28 percent), and Dandy-Walker malformation (7 to 13 percent). Another 10% of cases are said to be due to such abnormalities as arachnoid cysts, vein of Galen aneurysms, and agenesis of the corpus callosum. Certainly a major pediatric cause of ventriculomegaly, the intracerebral mass, is a very unusual finding in the fetus. The diagnosis of aqueductal stenosis is made if the the fourth ventricle is normal in size and the third and lateral ventricles are dilated, suggesting obstruction at the aqueduct of Sylvius. Some say that aqueductal stenosis may be overdiagnosed by US as a result of more limited visualization of the fourth ventricle compared to the supratentorial lateral and third ventricles.

Difficult family decisions have to be made with regard to maintenance of the pregnancy as well as the mode (i.e., vaginal delivery vs. cesarean section) and place of delivery (i.e., a tertiary care facility). Only 25 to 30 percent of fetuses with hydrocephalus survive. This reported percentage of survivors is affected, however, by the number of elective terminations of pregnancy performed on those with this antenatal diagnosis. Only about half of survivors are intellectually normal or near normal. Some report an even lesser percentage. Isolated ventriculomegaly is associated with developmental delay in anywhere from 14 to 45 percent of cases. Progressive ventricular dilatation is associated with a poorer intellectual outcome.

THE ANTENATAL DIAGNOSIS OF VENTRICULOMEGALY/HYDROCEPHALUS—HOW IS IT MADE?

Improved Machinery Has Improved Diagnosis

Improvements in US technology over the last two decades have markedly improved our ability to diagnose fetal ventriculomegaly, among other normal and pathologic fetal anatomic findings. Modern machinery with routine transabdominal (TA) scanning using transducers with electronically controlled focal points, cineloop and duplex, and color and power Doppler have aided antenatal diagnosis. Transvaginal (TV) ultrasonography has allowed better imaging of the internal contents of the fetal calvaria (Fig. 1-6), particularly for the fetus in a low cephalic position in the maternal pelvis or for fetuses in whom the mother's TA imaging is limited by body habitus, as a result of, for example, obesity or anterior abdominal wall scarring. TV ultrasonography has markedly improved imaging of the fetal brain in the early second trimester in comparison to routine TA work. In our laboratory we save TV imaging for those few cases in which important clinical questions and decisions remain after routine TA imaging. Certainly we avoid its use when it is clinically interdicted, particularly in the late third trimester and in patients with vaginal bleeding or ruptured membranes.

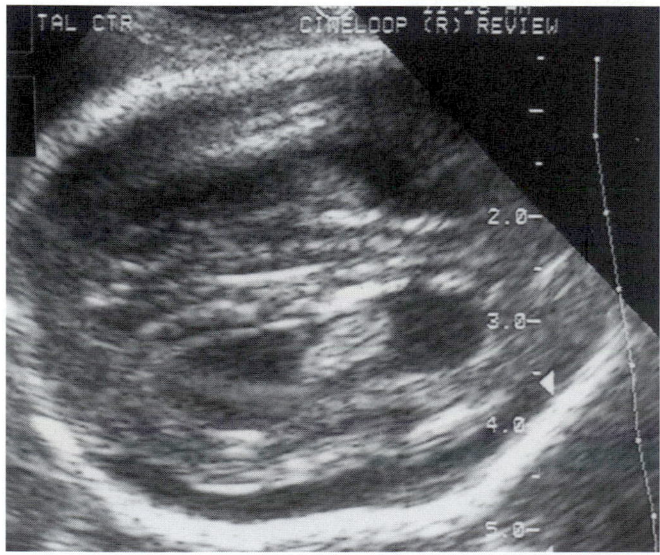

FIGURE 1–6. Hydrocephalus. Fetal head. Transvaginal ultrasound. Axial view. This 20-week fetus's intracranial contents could not be properly imaged through her obese mother's abdominal wall. However, the fetal head was low in the uterus and in good position to be well imaged using a higher-frequency 6.5-MHz transvaginal (TV) transducer with less penetration but better near-field resolution than the 3.5-MHz transabdominal transducer that was used. The choroid plexus (c) dangles somewhat in a 10-mm atrium of the dependent surface's ventricle, suggesting borderline ventriculomegaly and the need to at least follow the fetus.

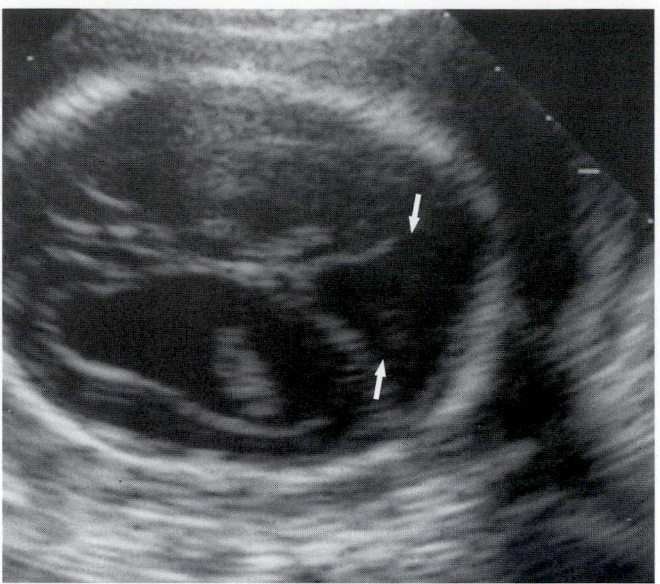

FIGURE 1–7. Dangling choroid plexus in hydrocephalus. Fetal head. Axial view. Another fetus with significant ventriculomegaly and a dangling choroid plexus. The echoless triangle (*arrows*) noted posteriorly is part of the patient's associated subtentorial Dandy-Walker cyst.

An Improved Knowledge Base Has Improved Diagnosis

Anatomic information learned from nearly two decades of neonatal brain analysis by neurosonography [as well as analysis by computed tomography (CT) and magnetic resonance imaging (MRI)] has allowed better fetal intracranial diagnosis.

US Diagnosis of Fetal Hydrocephalus—Diagnosis by Gestalt

Cases with significant ventriculomegaly can be readily identified by noting the prominent echoless ventricles, which take up a significant amount of the intracranial space compared to the brain parenchyma (Fig. 1-7). One has to be wary of overcalling normal findings, particularly the prominent size of the choroid in the mid-second trimester (Fig. 1-8). Less prominent cases of true ventriculomegaly may be diagnosed by noting the presence of intraventricular CSF lateral to the choroid plexus in the axial (Fig. 1-6), coronal, or sagittal plane. The choroid normally fills the lateral ventricular atrium (Fig. 1-9). Because the choroid plexus is heavier than CSF, it will droop into an enlarged ventricle, at least on the dependent side of the calvaria (Figs. 1-2, 1-4, and 1-7)—the so-called dangling choroid sign.

US Diagnosis of Fetal Hydrocephalus—Diagnosis by Measurements

Some sonologists prefer a more "scientific" or mathematical approach to the diagnosis of ventriculomegaly/hydrocephalus. For several years a lateral ventricle/hemisphere (LV/H) ratio (Fig. 1-10) was used to make this determina-

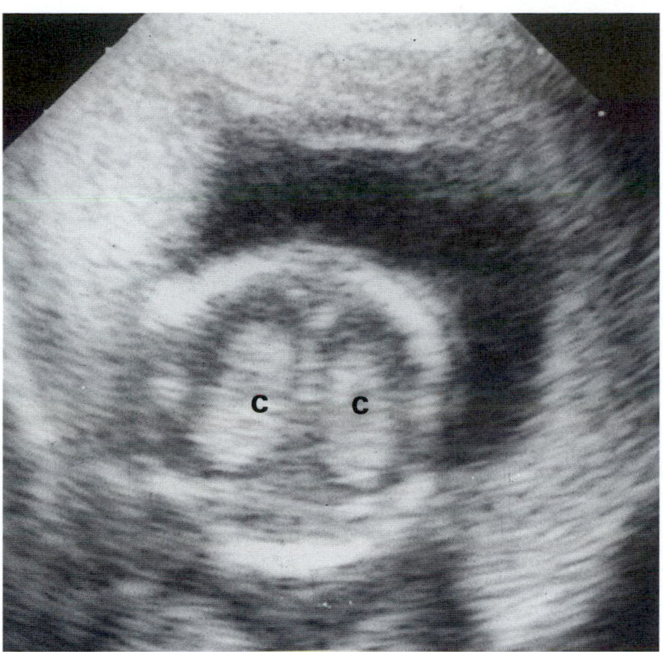

FIGURE 1–8. Normal prominence of the choroid plexus in a younger (16-week) fetus. Fetal head. Coronal plane. The choroid plexus in younger fetuses represents a greater percentage of the intracranial contents. This is a typical example, with choroid (c) representing much of the intracranial contents. While normal biparietal diameter increases by 6 mm from 18 to 20 weeks and by 11 mm from 20 to 23 weeks, choroid plexus thickness grows only 0.8 and 1.2 mm, respectively, proving that the younger fetus has a choroid plexus to cerebral tissue ratio that will decrease as the fetus ages.

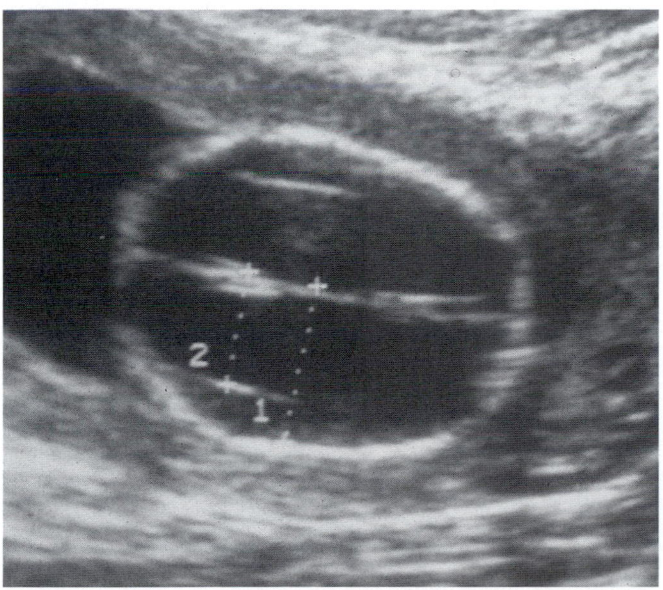

FIGURE 1–10. Measurement of lateral ventricular wall to cerebral hemisphere ratio. Fetal head. Axial plane. Measurement line 1 denotes (a slightly incorrect—not 90°) measurement of the hemisphere width. Measurement line 2 shows the lateral ventricular wall measurement between midline and the most lateral aspect of the lateral ventricle. This ratio, an often unreliable one without definitive last menstrual period date information, was formerly used to diagnose ventriculomegaly.

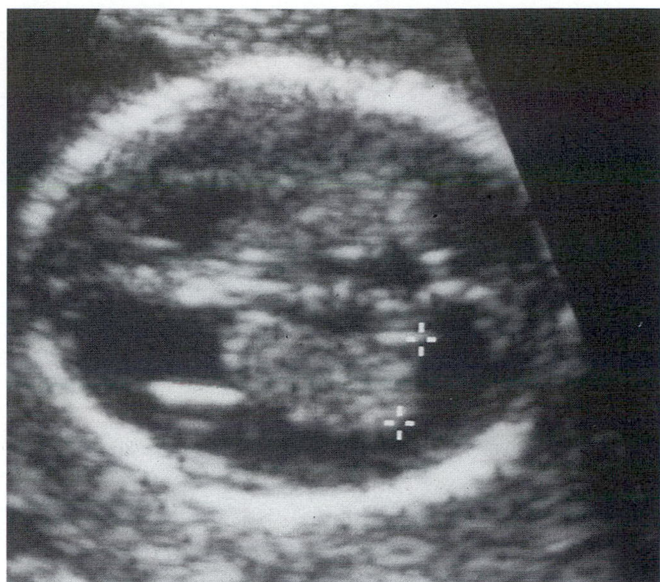

FIGURE 1–9. Measurement of the atrium of the lateral ventricle. Fetal head. Axial plane. Crosshatches mark off the measurement of the atrium of the lateral ventricle. In this case, there is no ventriculomegaly, noted both by the lack of CSF lateral to the choroid and an 8-mm measurement of the atrium of the lateral ventricle.

tion. It consisted of the ratio of a measurement (in the axial plane) from the midline to the lateral aspect of the lateral ventricle (LV) to a measurement from the brain midline to the lateral calvaria (the hemisphere). Unhappily, the LV/H ratio, which was used to make key decisions about the continuation of the pregnancy and the mode and place of delivery, depends on rigorous technique and is hindered by a high standard deviation, which limits the identification of cases with only mild dilatation. The ratio varies for different weeks of gestational age, and since, in cases of hydrocephalus, biparietal diameter (BPD) and head circumference (HC) measurements are unreliable, gestational age determination, in part, requires exact knowledge of the dates of the mother's last menstrual period (LMP) (a phenomenon that is not always straightforward even among the most reliable maternal historians). Without a true LMP, errors in diagnosis can be made.

The ultrasonography group at the University of California at San Francisco helped us deal with our concerns about the LV/H ratio by introducing a better US technique for fetal ventriculomegaly determination. They looked at the measurements of the lateral ventricle itself by measuring the width of the atria of the lateral ventricle (Fig. 1-9). Since the atrium is the first area of the ventricle to dilate in ventriculomegaly, its measurement allows differentiation between a normal and an enlarged ventricle. Cardoza, Goldstein, and Filly noted a normal mean measurement of the ventricular atrium, obtained from the inner medial to the inner lateral wall, of 6 mm. A 10-mm measurement was determined to be four standard deviations (SD) greater than the normal mean. Since the measurement remains the same throughout pregnancy (from 15 to 35 weeks), the need for exact LMP information is precluded. Recent information has indicated that

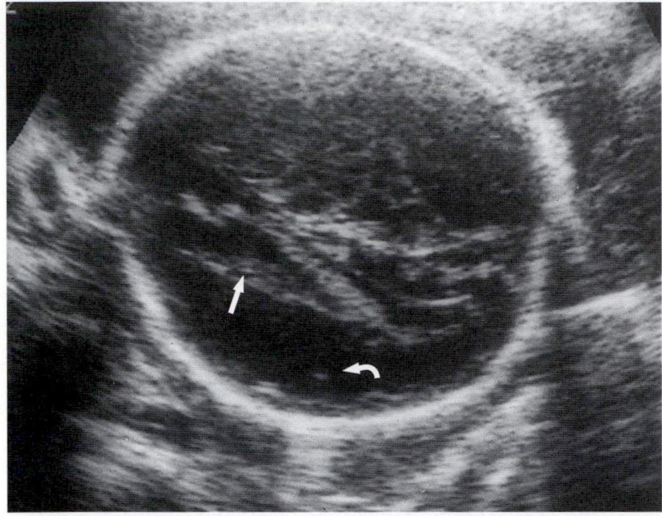

A

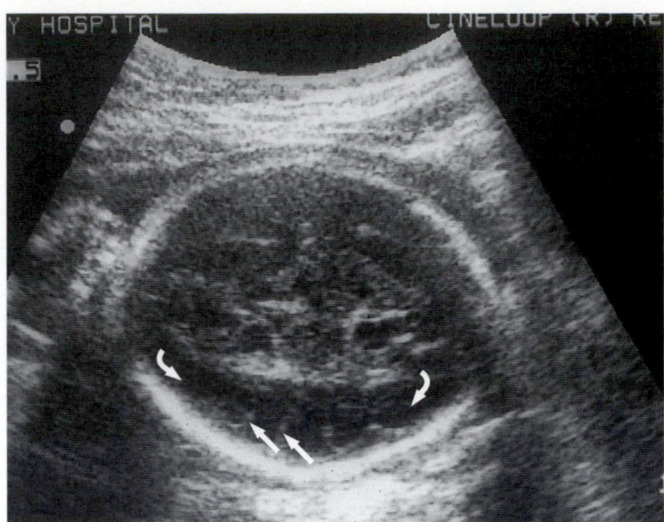

B

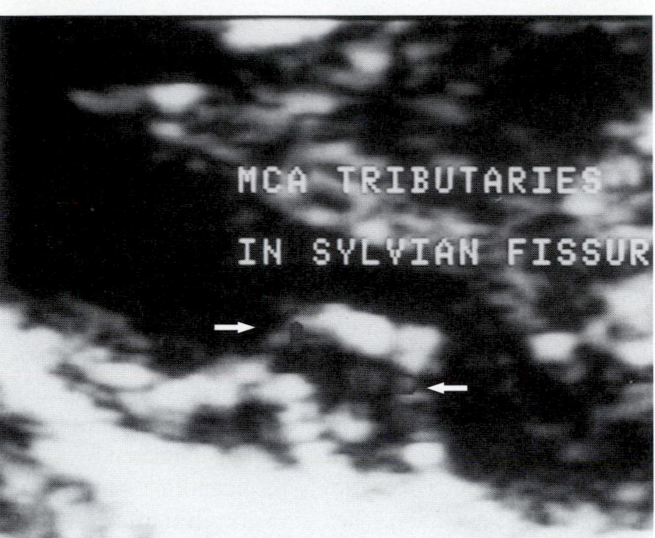

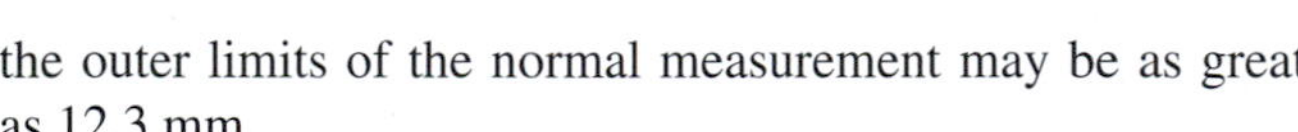

C

FIGURE 1–11. Normal echopenic temporal brain may simulate hydrocephalus. ***A.*** Fetal head, axial view. The choroid plexus (c) is seen to dangle slightly within a normal lateral ventricle. An arrow marks off the lateral ventricular wall, which, if not so readily seen as on this image, would have allowed the choroid plexus to appear to dangle toward the normally echopenic temporal brain (*curved arrows*), simulating hydrocephalus. ***B.*** Fetal head. Axial view. Another patient's echopenic temporal brain (*curved arrows*) is less worrisome because the choroid does not appear to dangle toward it and because small echogenic lines (*straight arrows*) within the brain allow one to identify it as solid brain parenchyma rather than echoless CSF. ***C.*** Close-up of fetal brain periphery at an area similar to the echogenic structures at the periphery of the brain in ***B.*** Color Doppler shows vascular flow (*arrows*) within these structures. This and their spectral patterns confirmed that they were middle cerebral artery tributaries in the Sylvian fissure. (See Color Plate 1.)

the outer limits of the normal measurement may be as great as 12.3 mm.

Of note is the fact that prognosis is best when atrial dilatation is mild (10 to 15 mm) and there is no associated intracranial or extracranial fetal anomaly. Among fetuses that were not terminated electively, 11 percent of those with isolated mild hydrocephalus died, whereas 56 percent of those with mild dilatation but with an associated anomaly died. Therefore, one must remember to search for other anomalies.

OUR MEASUREMENT AND ULTRASOUND POLICY

We use 10 mm as our measurement of concern and consider 10 to 12 mm a grey zone. This information is discussed with the patient during counseling. Follow-up studies can help decide whether there is evidence of increasing ventriculomegaly or evidence of normalcy. We are, however, conservative, in that we try to avoid false-negative results by offering follow-up examinations for fetuses with measurements at 8 mm and beyond, those with prominent amounts of CSF lateral to the choroid plexus (considered by some to be abnormal at 3 mm or greater), and those in whom ventricular fluid appears prominent. We also do this so that a follow-up exam will allow imaging of any interval increase in ventricular size, in case we have picked up the abnormality at an early stage. We try to do the follow-up exam with concern for dates for possible legal termination if that is a parental or clinical consideration. We make a dedicated search of the rest of the fetus, including the heart, to note if there is any other anatomic area of concern or any evidence of chromosomal or syndromic abnormality. Genetic amniocentesis obviously may help as well.

A NOTE OF CAUTION TO THE BEGINNER

An occasional simulator of hydrocephalus is the known phenomenon of the echopenic normal temporal brain (Fig. 1-11). Great care must be taken to avoid overreading ventriculomegaly in these cases. Color Doppler and evidence of flow

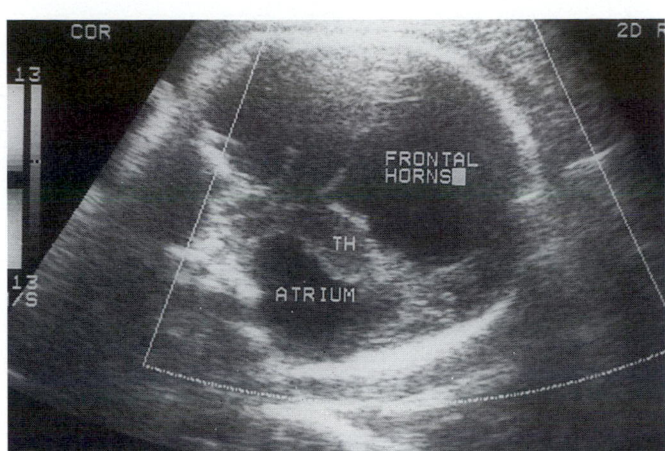

FIGURE 1–12. Fenestration of septi pellucidi simulating their congenital absence. Fetal brain. Coronal view. Vertex to the reader's right. The fetus has hydrocephalus, denoted by dilated frontal horns and dilated ventricular atria. There are no septi pellucidi separating the frontal horns. This simulated absence of the septi pellucidi but was really due to fenestration of the septi pellucidi by long-term hydrocephalus.

in the middle cerebral artery tributaries of the Sylvian fissure (Fig. 1-11*C*; see also Color Plate 1) may help avoid a false-positive diagnosis.

A NOTE OF CAUTION TO ALL OF US

Occasionally we have noted the apparent complete absence (Fig. 1-12) of the septi pellucidi in a fetus with significant hydrocephalus. Although we have to consider the possibility of congenital absence of the septi pellucidi, which is usually associated with other brain abnormalities, we know from neonatal work that the septi can fenestrate over time under the influence of significant intraventricular pressure, and that the apparent absence is the result of multiple fenestrations.

Antenatal US Findings of Ventriculomegaly/Hydrocephalus

1. Dilated ventricles
2. Dangling choroid within ventricle (dependent surface)
3. A 3-mm or greater distance between choroid and lateral atrial/ventricular wall (especially if on dependent surface)
4. A 10-mm (perhaps 12-mm) measure of inner atrial diameter
5. Fenestrated septi pellucidi

References

Cardoza J, Filly R, Podrasky A: The dangling choroid plexus: A sonographic observation of value in excluding ventriculomegaly. *AJR* 151:767–770, 1988.

Cardoza J, Goldstein R, Filly R: Exclusion of fetal ventriculomegaly with a single measurement: The width of the lateral ventricular atrium. *Radiology* 169:711–714, 1988.

Cohen HL, Haller J: Advances in perinatal neurosonography. *AJR* 163:801–810, 1994.

Cohen HL, Haller J, Pollack A: Ultrasound of the septum pellucidum. Recognition of evolving fenestrations in the hydrocephalic infant. *J Ultrasound Med* 9:377–383, 1990.

Filly R: Ultrasound evaluation of the fetal neural axis, in *Ultrasonography in Obstetrics and Gynecology*, 3d ed, Callen PW (ed). Philadelphia, Saunders, 1994:207–215.

Filly R, Goldstein R, Callen P: Fetal ventricle: Importance in routine obstetric sonography. *Radiology* 181:1–7, 1991.

Goldstein R, La Pidus A, Filly R, Cardoza J: Mild lateral cerebral ventricle dilatation in utero: Clinical significance and prognosis. *Radiology* 176:237–242, 1990.

Mahony B, Nyberg D, Hirsch J, et al: Mild idiopathic lateral cerebral ventricular dilatation in utero: Sonographic evaluation. *Radiology* 169:715–721, 1988.

Monteagudo A, Timor-Tritsch I: Fetal neurosonography of congenital brain anomalies, in *Ultrasonography of the Prenatal and Neonatal Brain,* Timor-Tritsch I, Monteagudo A, Cohen HL (eds). Stamford, CT, Appleton & Lange, 1996:178–183.

Sauerbrei E: The fetal brain and skull, in *A Practical Guide to Ultrasound in Obstetrics and Gynecology,* 2d ed, Sauerbrei E, Nguyen K, Nolan R (eds). Philadelphia, Lippincott-Raven, 1998:155–197.

Siegel M: Brain, in *Pediatric Sonography,* Siegel M (ed). New York, Raven, 1995:89–91.

Timor-Tritsch I, Monteagudo A: Normal neurosonography of the prenatal brain, in *Ultrasonography of the Prenatal and Neonatal Brain,* Timor-Tritsch I, Monteagudo A, Cohen HL (eds). Stamford, CT, Appleton & Lange, 1996:11–87.

2

Figures 2-1 and 2-2 are the ultrasound (US) images of the cranium and contents of a 19-week fetus sent for evaluation for fetal age determination. What do you see? What is the diagnosis? What associated anomalies, if any, should be searched for?

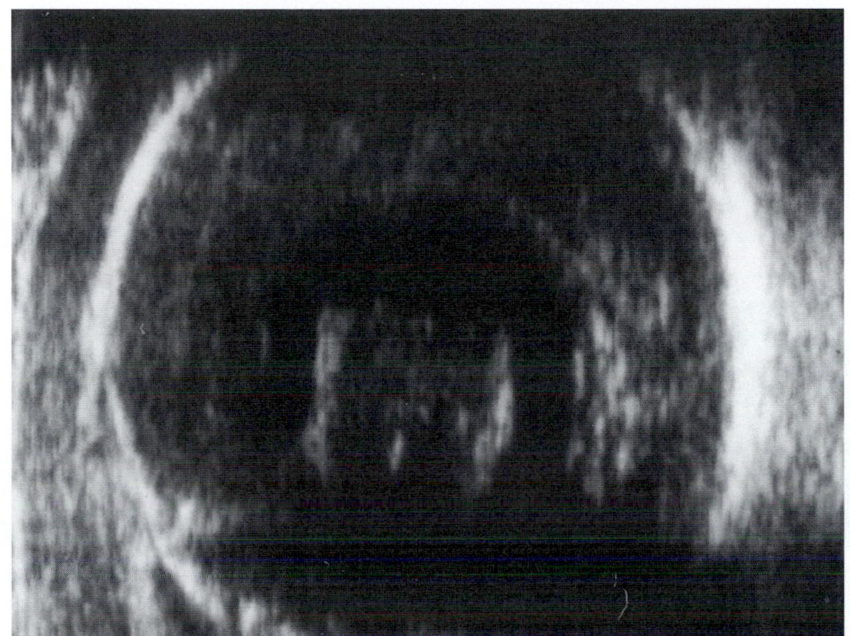

FIGURE 2–1. Ultrasound of the brain. Coronal plane.

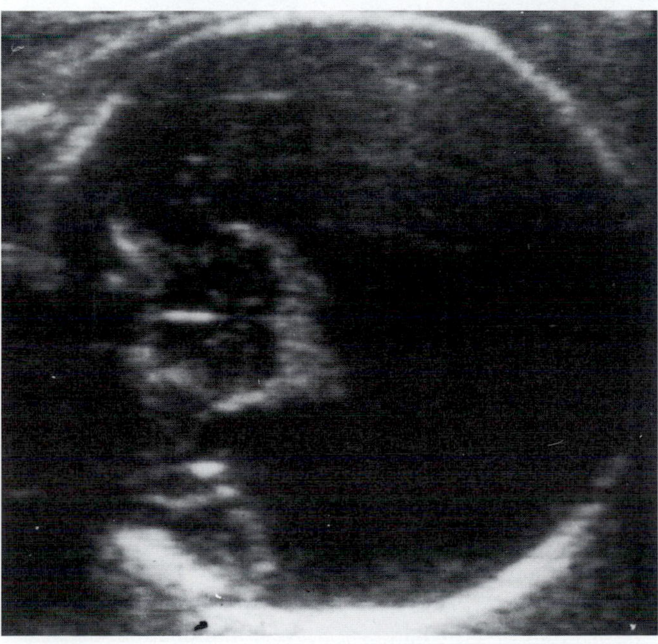

FIGURE 2–2. Ultrasound of the brain. Coronal plane. Fetal head is on its side.

CHAPTER 2

Holoprosencephaly

HARRIS L. COHEN

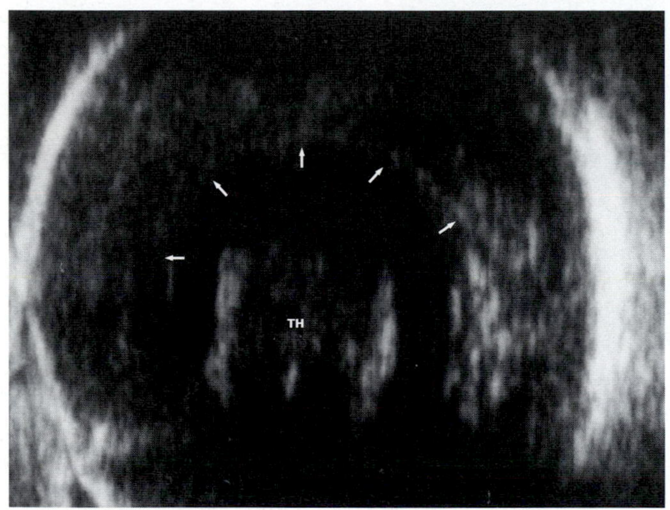

FIGURE 2–3. Annotated version of Fig. 2-1. Alobar holoprosencephaly. Coronal plane. A single ventricle (*arrows*) surrounds fused thalami (th).

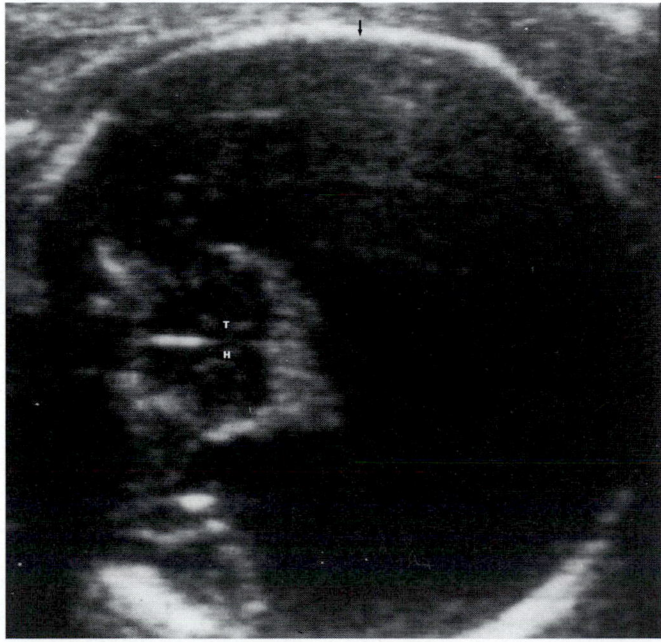

FIGURE 2–4. Alobar holoprosencephaly. Coronal plane. Same patient as in Fig. 2-3. This view was obtained with the fetal head in a dependent position. Asymmetry of the intracranial echogenicity, greater on the nondependent surface (*arrows*), is due to the near-field artifact. The thalami (TH) are fused. There is only a single (uni)ventricle, without any evidence of division of the ventricular system into the normal two lateral ventricles. No dorsal cyst was seen.

Figures 2-3 (an annotated version of Fig. 2-1) and 2-4 (an annotated version of Fig. 2-2) show a single univentricle and fusion of the thalami. These findings are typical of the more severe forms of holoprosencephaly.

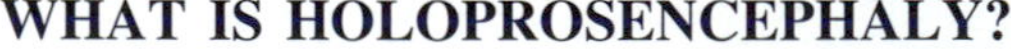

WHAT IS HOLOPROSENCEPHALY?

Holoprosencephaly is a malformation sequence that involves the brain and often the face. This malformation, like many midline brain malformations, occurs early in embryonic life. It is considered one of the disorders of brain diverticulation that involve complete (or partial) failure of cleavage of the cerebral hemispheres. Failure of cleavage results in failure of formation of intracranial midline structures. The beginnings of this cleavage and midline brain development, known as ventral induction, occur between the fourth and eighth weeks of gestation. Errors of development occuring during this time will therefore result in variable degrees of fusion of the olfactory and optic tracts as well as the cerebral hemispheres. Midline brain development is associated with development of the midface, and so are its anomalies. As with many anomalies occuring early in embryologic development, by the time they can be adequately imaged, the examiner can do nothing but see the results.

Holoprosencephaly has been reported in 1 in 16,000 live births but is more common in fetuses and even more so among embryos (as high as 1 in 250), the majority of which do not survive. It can be an isolated finding or part of a syndrome. As many as 34 percent have a cytogenetic abnormality, including cases of trisomies 13–15 and 16–18. As many as 25 percent, particularly those with chromosomal abnormalities, have other associated system abnormalities. Animal work has suggested a possible link to maternal alcohol exposure.

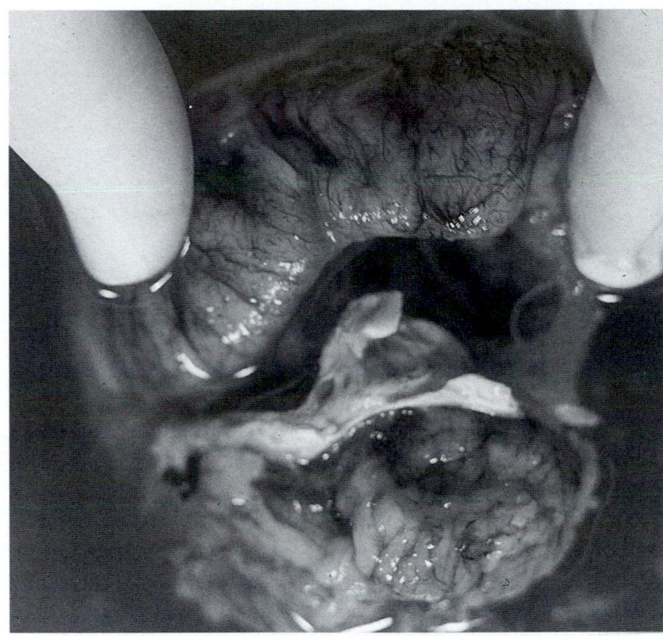

FIGURE 2–5. Monoventricle of holoprosencephaly. Pathology specimen. Coronal plane viewed from the back. The pathologist's fingers are at the boundaries of the brain surrounding the single ventricle, seen as the open space within the brain. The white material is the tentorium, and the cerebellum is seen below it. (See Color Plate 2.)

THE VARIOUS FORMS OF HOLOPROSENCEPHALY

The brain abnormality, as noted, is due to partial or complete failure of the primitive forebrain, the prosencephalon, to cleave in a horizontal plane to allow development of the olfactory and optic bulbs, in a sagittal plane to allow normal development of the telencephalon (which forms the paired cerebral hemispheres), and in a transverse plane to allow proper formation of the telencephalon and diencephalon (the structure that forms the thalamus and hypothalamus).

In the most severe form (i.e., *alobar* holoprosencephaly), there is a unified holosphere (Figs. 2-3 and 2-4). Rather than the normal existence of two communicating lateral ventricles and a third ventricle, there is a single monoventricle (Fig. 2-5; see also Color Plate 2), which most often communicates with a dorsal sac. Often only a thin mantle of anterior brain tissue is seen surrounding the monoventricle. The brain is small. Optic tracts and olfactory bulbs, which would have formed from an evagination of the prosencephalon, are absent. The falx, corpus callosum, fornix, and interhemispheric fissure are not formed. There are no third and fourth ventricles. The midbrain, brainstem, and cerebellum are typically normal unless they are made hypoplastic by mass impression from the large monoventricle and its dorsal sac. The thalami and corpus striatum are usually fused.

In the intermediate form (i.e., *semilobar* holoprosencephaly), there is partial evidence of prosencephalon cleavage. This may include partial separation of the temporal and occipital lobes, the existence of a rudimentary posterior falx or interhemispheric fissure, or the existence of an anterior monoventricle with bilateral rudimentary occipital horns. There is more cerebral tissue and a smaller single ventricle.

In the incomplete and therefore least devastating form (i.e., *lobar* holoprosencephaly), there may be a relatively normal-appearing brain. There may simply be an absent septum pellucidum, yet an evident corpus callosum and perhaps fused or squared frontal horns. Flattening of the roof of the frontal horns is due to the absence of normal midline structures. Rostral fusion may be the only ventricular fusion seen, with the rest of the ventricular system (e.g., the atria and the occipital and temporal horns) apparently separated.

THE ASSOCIATED FACIAL ANOMALIES

When a child is born with a midline facial anomaly, a head ultrasound is always performed to rule out holoprosencephaly. The classic fetal or neonatal axiom "the face predicts the brain" is, like many axioms in medicine, not always true. Facial abnormalities are more variable than would be expected, and the brain does not always predict the face. Facial defects may not be seen at all (Fig. 2-6) or may range from mild facial dysmorphism such as hypotelorism (Fig. 2-7) or unilateral (Fig. 2-8) or bilateral median cleft lip or palate to more severe forms. Facial deformities may be present and yet be missed on US examination, perhaps because of fetal position, maternal body habitus, or happenstance. Cebocephaly is an intermediate facial deformity with hypotelorism and a single-nostrilled nose (Fig. 2-9). In ethmocephaly there is hypotelorism (usually severe), arrhinia, and an interorbital single or double proboscis. Cyclopia consists of a single median orbit with variable pairings of eyes (e.g., anophthalmia, synophthalmia, median monoophthalmia), arrhinia (no nose or median facial bones), and usually a proboscis in a supraorbital location. The more significant facial abnormalities are almost always associated with alobar holoprosencephaly.

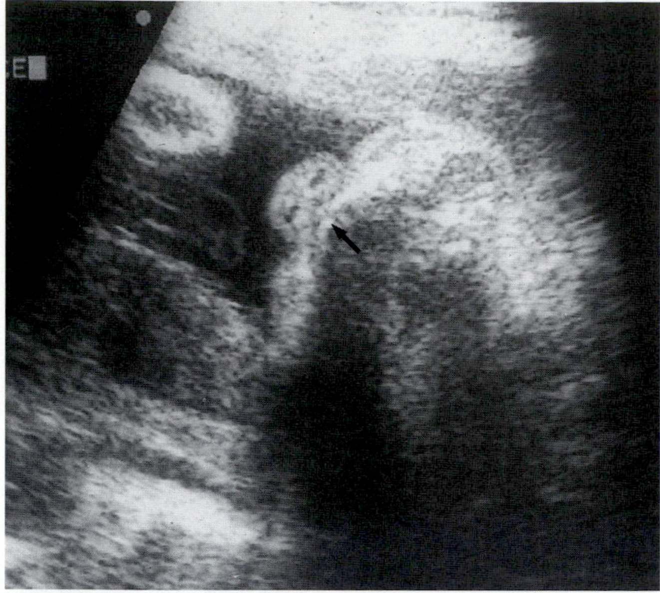

A

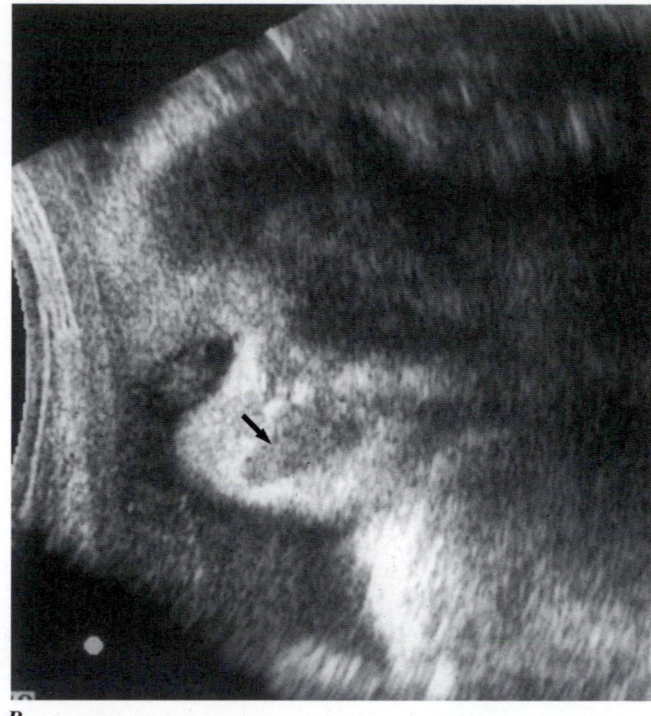

B

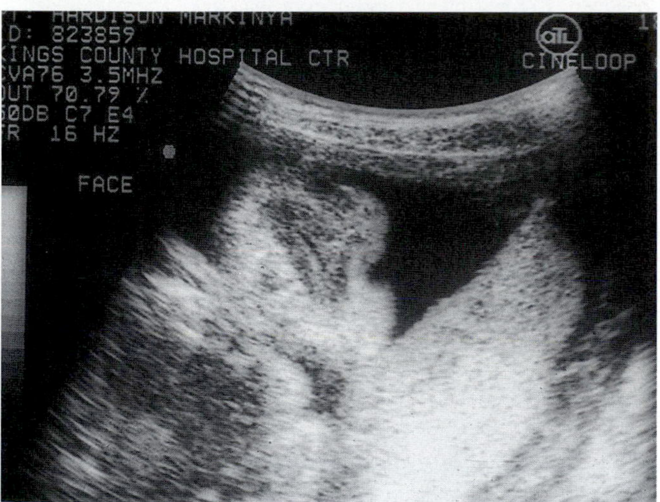

C

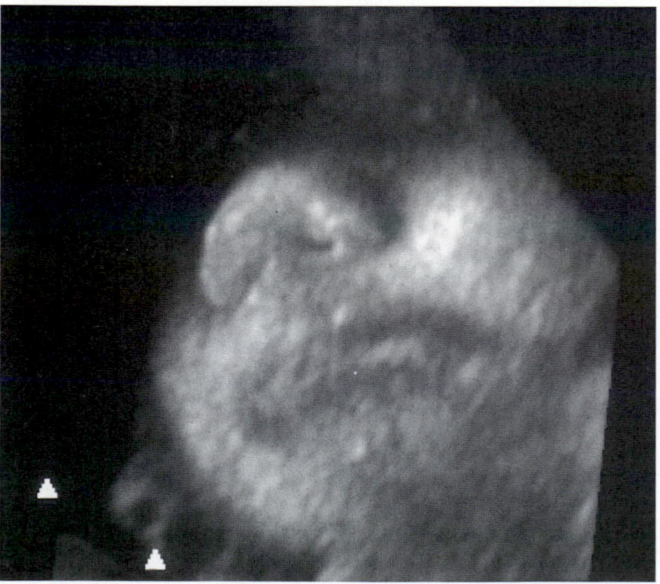

D

FIGURE 2–6. Normal facial ultrasound images. ***A.*** Normal nostrils. Axial view of normal anterior face at level of nostrils. Two nostrils are seen in the nose. C = cheek. An arrow points to the hard palate of this normal fetus. ***B.*** Normal face. Coronal view of face, somewhat obliqued. Complete lips (*arrows*) are noted. One orbit is well seen, the other less so. However, one can get a good concept of the typical rounded orbits and the distance between them. The interorbital distances may vary among fetuses, and charts for their measurement have been created. ***C.*** Normal lips. Coronal view of lips. The thin black line seen between the upper and lower lips is a small amount of amniotic fluid that was being swallowed. Its blackness helped highlight the normalcy (lack of break) of these lips. ***D.*** Normal anterior lower face. Coronal plane. Three-dimensional (3D) ultrasound. The normal lips and nose of this fetus are better imaged using 3D software and hardware. This imaging refinement is available on some high-end US machines as well as with a few units created for 3D imaging alone. *(Image provided courtesy of GE Medical Systems.)*

WHAT ARE THE FETUS'S CHANCES OF SURVIVAL?

For those with severe damage to the brain with associated arhinia or choanal atresia, survival much beyond birth is uncommon. Those with less severe brain and face involvement may live several years but are most commonly hindered by severe neurologic and intellectual impairment. Seizures are common. Even those with lobar holoprosencephaly who may live a normal lifetime are severely retarded. In light of these devastating results, one must remain aware of the risk of recurrence for nonchromosomal cases, which is 12 percent for

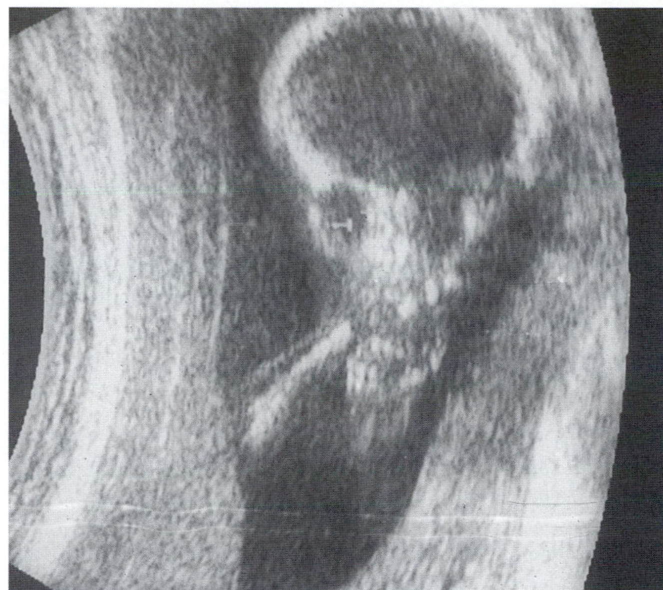

FIGURE 2–7. Hypotelorism in a fetus with holoprosencephaly. The interorbital distance (*arrow*) is abnormally short by gestalt as well as by chart. The orbits are also more elongated than usual. This was an 18-week-old fetus who was aborted.

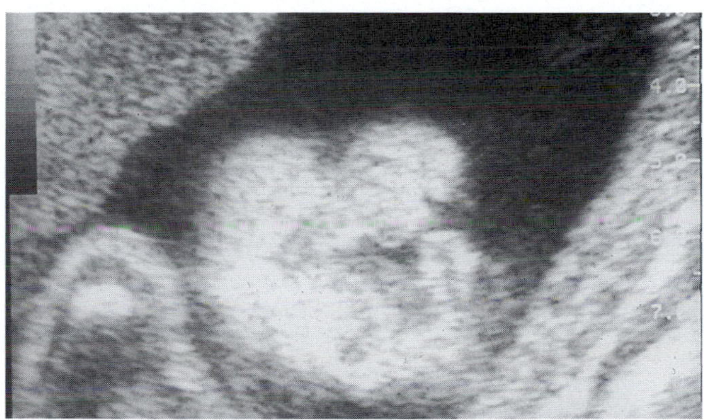

A

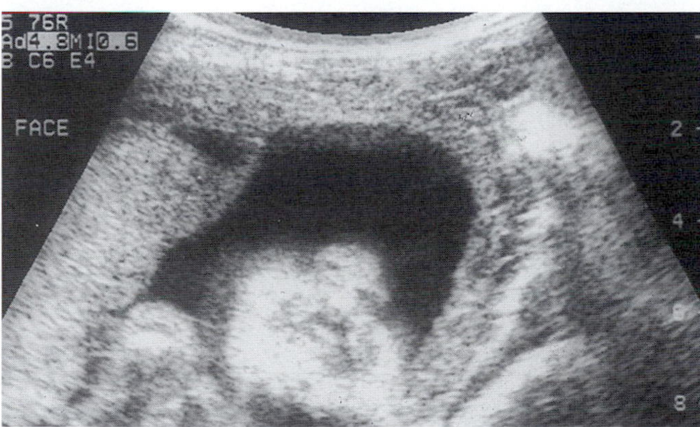

B

FIGURE 2–8. Cleft lip. ***A.*** Median cleft. Coronal plane. Only the lower face is imaged in this plane. The nostrils are normal. Just as the echoless amniotic fluid highlighted the normalcy of Fig. 2-6*C*, echoless fluid highlights a prominent left-sided median cleft (*arrow*) in this fetus. ***B.*** Median cleft not seen. Coronal plane. The diagnosis in Fig. 2-8*A* had almost been missed seconds before when this image only hinted at possible abnormality and the need to devote more time to facial imaging.

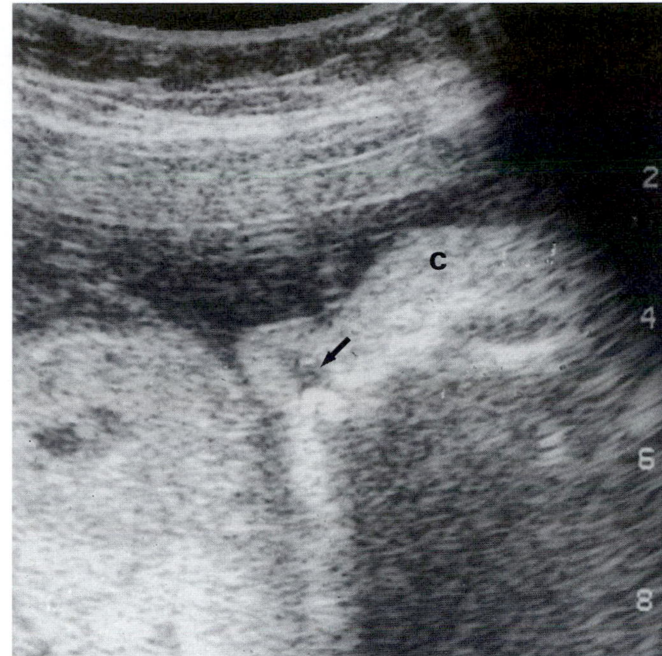

A

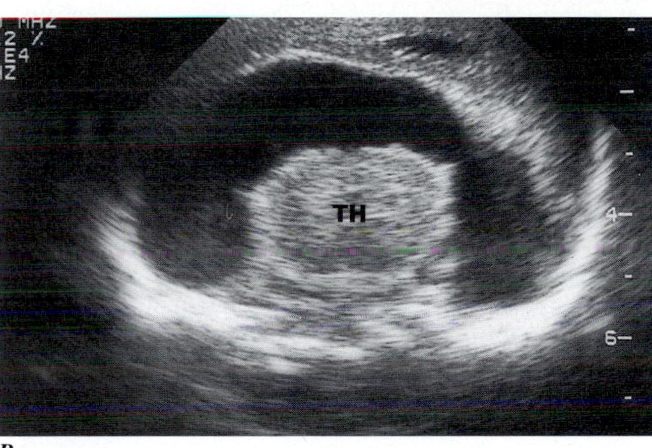

B

FIGURE 2–9. Holoprosencephaly. ***A.*** Abnormal nose in holoprosencephaly. Axial plane. Only a single nostril (*arrow*) was noted in the abnormal nose (proboscis) of this fetus with holoprosencephaly. The fetus's mother was in her forties. C = right cheek. This finding was confirmed at birth. ***B.*** Abnormal brain in holoprosencephaly. Coronal plane. After birth, this patient's fused thalami (th) and monoventricle were confirmed on neonatal neurosonography. The infant died within 48 h. Figure 2-5 is this neonate's pathology specimen.

the next pregnancy. Careful ultrasonography of the next pregnancy is necessary.

ULTRASOUND FINDINGS IN HOLOPROSENCEPHALY AND DIFFERENTIAL DIAGNOSTIC POINTS

Ultrasound findings (Table 2-1) in the more severe alobar holoprosencephaly include: a monoventricle, fused thalami (Fig. 2-3) (which exclude severe hydrocephalus from the dif-

TABLE 2-1
US Findings of Alobar Holoprosencephaly

1. Univentricle
2. Absent falx
3. Absent corpus callosum
4. Fused thalami
5. Facial abnormalities: cyclopia, proboscis, cleft lip/palate.

ferential diagnosis), absent midline structures such as the falx and the septi pellucidi, and a dorsal sac that communicates with the monoventricle. The calvaria appears to be predominantly filled by fluid. Unlike in hydranencephaly, there is a rind of brain even in the most severe cases, although it is displaced cephalically, with none seen around the dorsal cyst. It may be difficult to image the typical dorsal sac that the univentricle communicates with. The two structures may appear as one. A dorsal sac could not be imaged in this unknown case. Despite the smaller brain, the dilated univentricle may add enough size to cause a large biparietal diameter (BPD), although normal and small measurements may also be obtained. Filly points out that the identification of septi pellucidi or their cavum excludes all form of holoprosencephaly.

Septo-optic dysplasia, which some people believe is a related anomaly, can show fusion and squaring of the frontal horns with absence of the septum pellucidum similar to that found in lobar holoprosencephaly. Septo-optic dysplasia's distinctive feature, optic tract hypoplasia, cannot be readily distinguished in fetal life.

Fetuses with hydrocephalus to the point of rupture of the septi pellucidi may seem to have an image simulating that of lobar holoprosencephaly, but their normal midline structures will indent the frontal horn roof. It still may be difficult to differentiate lobar holoprosencephaly from postfenestration hydrocephalus or from agenesis of the corpus callosum.

References

Cohen HL, Haller J: Advances in perinatal neurosonography. *AJR* 163:801–810, 1994.

Filly R: Ultrasound evaluation of the fetal neural axis, in *Ultrasonography in Obstetrics and Gynecology,* 3d ed, Callen PW (ed). Philadelphia, Saunders, 1994:207–215.

Fitz C: Holoprosencephaly and septo-optic dysplasia. *Pediatr Neuroradiol* 4:263–281, 1994.

Herman T, Siegel M: Neurosonographic abnormalities in chromosomal disorders. *Pediatr Radiol* 21:398–401, 1991.

Pilu G, Perolo A, David C: Midline anomalies of the brain, in *Ultrasonography of the Prenatal and Neonatal Brain,* Timor-Tritsch I, Monteagudo A, Cohen HL (eds). Stamford, CT, Appleton & Lange, 1996:241–247.

Pilu G, Sandri F, Perolo A, et al: Prenatal diagnosis of lobar holoprosencephaly. *Ultrasound Obstet Gynecol* 4:65–67, 1994.

Sauerbrei E: The fetal brain and skull, in *A Practical Guide to Ultrasound in Obstetrics and Gynecology,* 2d ed, Sauerbrei E, Nguyen K, Nolan R (eds). Philadelphia, Lippincott-Raven, 1998:155–197.

Siebert J, Lemire R, Cohen M Jr: Aberrant morphogenesis of the central nervous system. *Clin Perinatol* 17:569–595, 1990.

Whiteford M, Tolmie J: Holoprosencephaly in the west of Scotland 1975–1994. *J Med Genet* 33:578–584, 1996.

3

A mother was sent for antenatal evaluation of her 33-week-old fetus because of an abnormal finding (Fig. 3-1) on fetal cardiac ultrasound examination. A fetal head ultrasound (Fig. 3-2) helped make the diagnosis. What is the diagnosis? Would Doppler analysis help?

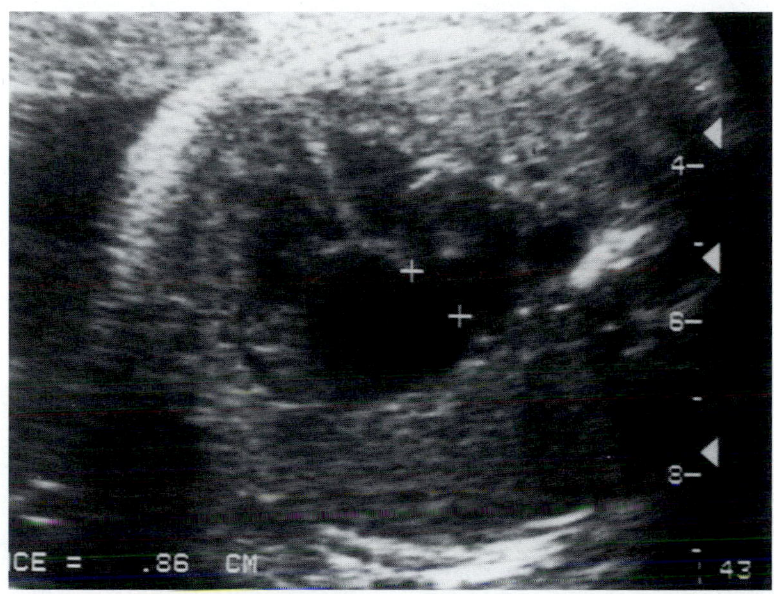

FIGURE 3–1. Fetal heart. Somewhat obliqued axial plane. The two crosshatches are in the area of an intact (although difficult to prove on this image) interatrial septum. *(From Koven et al, with permission.)*

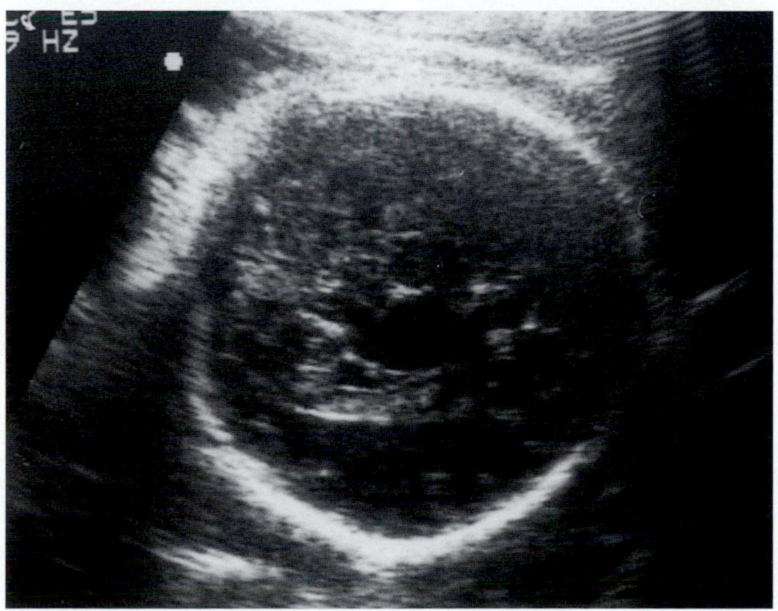

FIGURE 3–2. Fetal head. Axial plane.

CHAPTER 3

Intracranial Arteriovenous Malformation

HARRIS L. COHEN

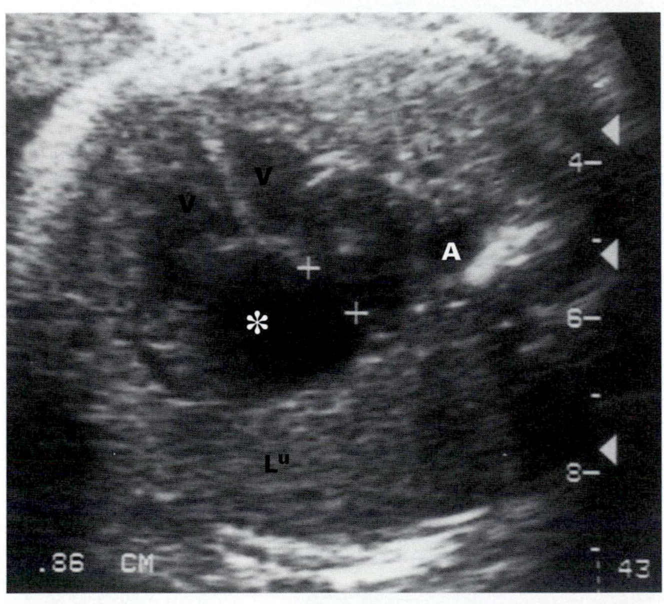

FIGURE 3–3. Annotated version of Fig. 3-1. Fetal heart. Somewhat obliqued axial plane. The right atrium (*) is enlarged. The ventricles (v) are equal in size. The left atrium is anterior to the descending aorta (A). No other cardiac abnormality was noted in the fetus. L = right lung. *(From Koven et al, with permission.)*

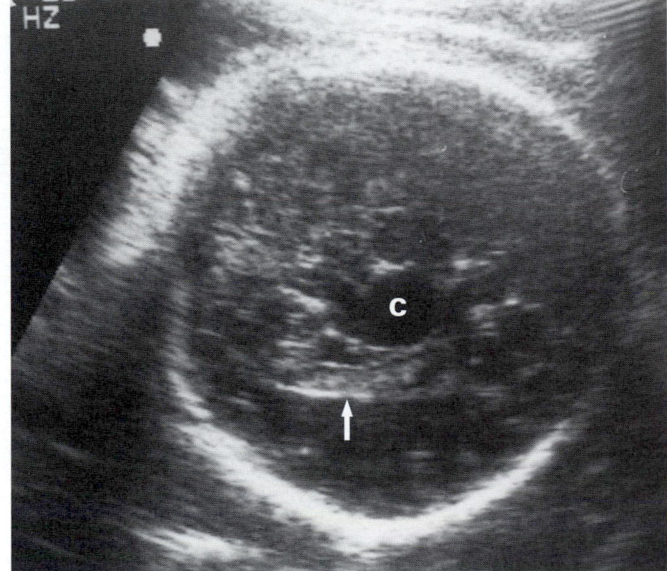

FIGURE 3–4. Annotated version of Fig. 3-2. Fetal head. There is artifactual filling in of the near field, making it more echogenic than the more dependent far-field brain parenchyma. A cystic area (c) is seen in the midline, medial to a normal-sized left lateral ventricle (*arrow*) containing choroid plexus. This fetus, therefore, did not have hydrocephalus. Cystic tubular structures are seen extending into or from the cystic mass. These suggest a vascular mass, particularly in light of the atrial enlargement without associated cardiac disease.

THE ANTENATAL DIAGNOSIS OF AN INTRACRANIAL ARTERIOVENOUS MALFORMATION

Figure 3-3 (the annotated version of Fig. 3-1) shows a dilated right atrium. Right atrial enlargement in the fetal heart may be due to several cardiac abnormalities (see Table 3-1). Lack of fetal hydrops or other evidence of cardiac failure made this an unlikely possibility in this case.

Figure 3-4 (the annotated version of Fig. 3-2) shows a cystic area in the brain with tubular areas extending to it. Seeing the brain's cystic structure alone, one might consider the pos-

TABLE 3-1
Right Atrial Dilatation of the Fetal Heart—Some Differential Diagnostic Considerations

1. Ebstein's anomaly (atrialization of a portion of the right ventricle due to a dysplastic, inferiorly displaced tricuspid valve)
2. Tricuspid valve insufficiency due to any cause
3. Pulmonary atresia with an intact septum
4. Congestive heart failure
5. Extracardiac AVM

sibilities of a congenital subarachnoid cyst or an unusually positioned area of brain destruction. However, when the cystic structure is combined with the finding of an enlarged cardiac chamber (the right atrium), the key diagnostic consideration is a vein of Galen aneurysm (which this proved to be) or some other arteriovenous malformation (AVM) of the brain. The diagnosis can be and in this case was immediately confirmed by duplex and color Doppler evaluation.

USE OF DOPPLER IN CONFIRMING THE DIAGNOSIS OF AVM OF THE FETAL/NEONATAL BRAIN

Doppler imaging allows a rapid differentiation between cystic and vascular areas of the structures, whether they are normal or not. If they are vascular, the Doppler spectral pattern allows one to qualify the type of vascular flow present: arterial, venous, or other.

Color Doppler imaging (CDI) or its enhancement, power Doppler (which provides enhanced motion detection at the sacrifice of directional information), can provide a quick visual answer to questions about vascular flow, whether the vessels are normal (Fig. 3-5) or, as in this case, abnormal and enlarged. CDI (Fig. 3-6; see also Color Plate 3) proved this case to be an AVM.

WHAT IS A VEIN OF GALEN ANEURYSM OR INTRACRANIAL ARTERIOVENOUS MALFORMATION?

Arteriovenous malformations are the most common vascular lesions seen in children. They are congenital lesions formed by the failure of the normal fetal embryonic arteriovenous shunts (communicating between arteries and veins), which normally are replaced by capillaries, to regress. Variable in size, AVMs are of greatest clinical concern when they are large and when they are diagnosed earlier in life.

The most common prenatal venous malformation of the brain is the vein of Galen aneurysm (VGA), which is really a misnomer, since it is not a true aneurysm but an AVM. True aneurysms are very rare in fetuses or neonates. The VGA is more correctly referred to as the galenic arteriovenous malformation. Arterial feeders that are derived from the anterior and posterior cerebral circulations are frequently present. Increased blood flow, essentially "stolen" from the cerebral arterial circulation, results in dilatation of the vein of Galen (VOG). The VOG is a deep cerebral vein that curves under

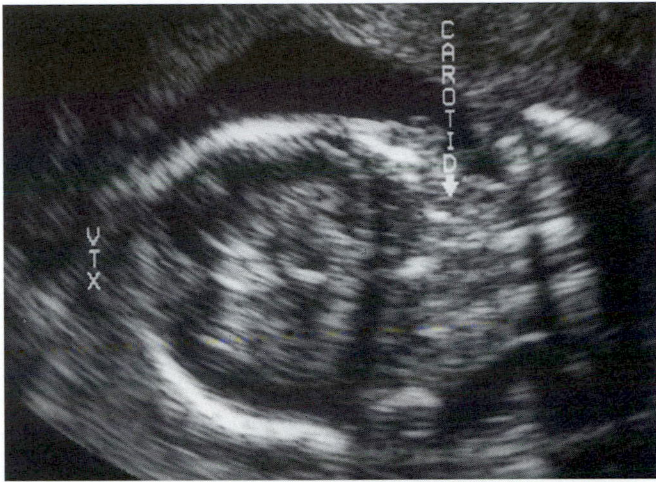

A

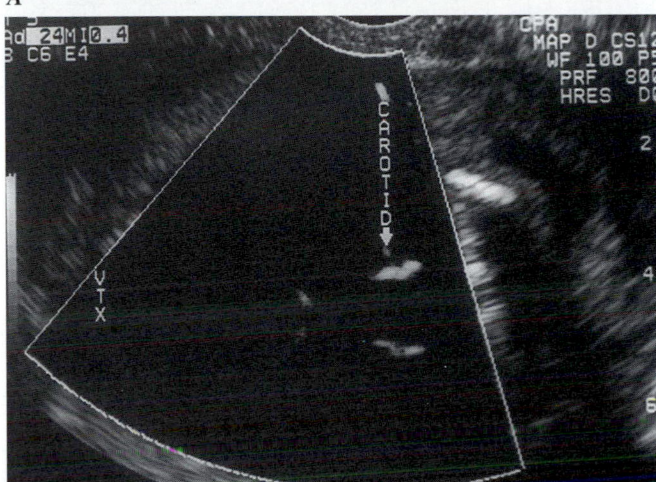

B

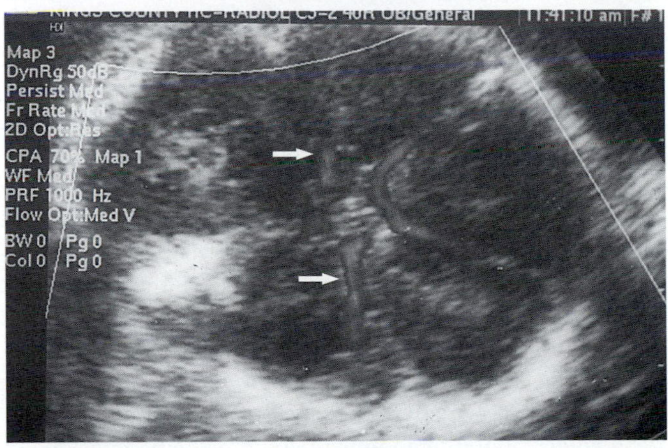

C

FIGURE 3–5. Power Doppler in fetal intracranial vascular analysis. ***A.*** Fetal head and neck. Coronal plane. VTX marks off the vertex of the calvarium. CAROTID marks where left carotid artery pulsations were noted in this fetus. Note that the vessels of the neck are not particularly apparent (compare this to Fig. 3-7, the neck of the fetus used for this unknown case). ***B.*** Fetal head and neck. Power Doppler. Coronal plane. This image is the same as that of ***A*** but with the background blacked out to highlight flow assessment by power Doppler. The word *Carotid* points to flow in the left carotid artery. ***C.*** Fetal head. Power Doppler. Coronal plane, some obliquity and more anterior plane than in ***B.*** Arrows mark off the right and left middle cerebral arteries as they come off an internal carotid artery.

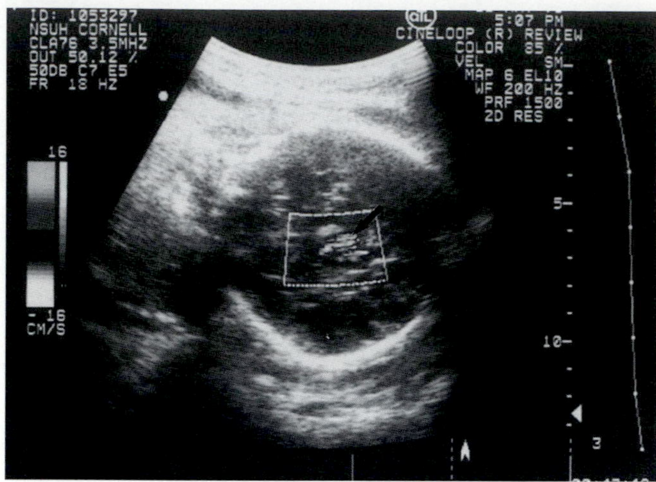

FIGURE 3–6. Fetal head. Color Doppler. Axial plane. The cystic area immediately filled with color (*arrow*), proving it to be vascular. The biphasic and irregular venous spectral pattern obtained showed it to be typical of a vein of Galen "aneurysm" or other arteriovenous malformation. (See Color Plate 3.)

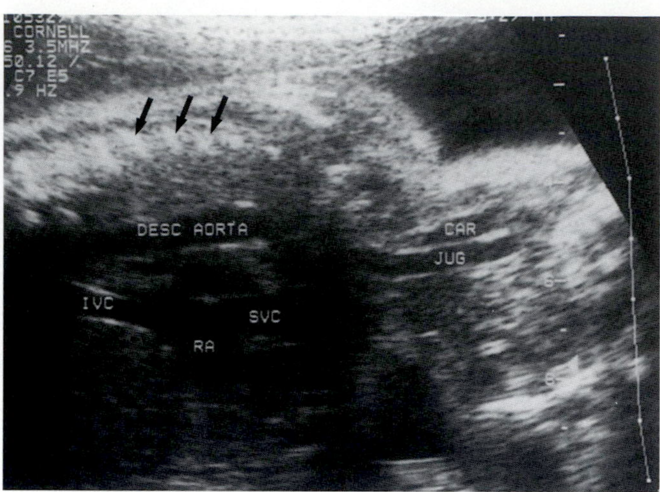

FIGURE 3–7. Fetal neck and thorax in patient with intracranial arteriovenous malformation. Coronal oblique plane. Prominent vascular flow to the large intracranial AVM, which increased in size by birth, was the reason for the inordinately prominent neck vessels (CAR = left carotid artery, JUG = left jugular vein). The superior vena cava (SVC) is wider than the inferior vena cava (IVC) for probably the same reason. RA = right atrium, Desc Aorta = descending aorta. Ribs (*arrows*) can be seen at the left chest periphery.

the splenium of the corpus callosum and unites with the inferior sagittal sinus to form the straight sinus. It is not seen with routine imaging.

CLINICAL INFORMATION REGARDING THE VGA OR GALENIC ARTERIOVENOUS MALFORMATION

When enlarged, a VGA may result in hydrocephalus through its mass effect on the ventricles. Some 40 to 50 percent of postnatally diagnosed cases are discovered early in neonatal life. How many could have been picked up antenatally is unknown. About 95 percent of neonatal presentations are due to cardiac failure as a result of significant arteriovenous shunting. Cardiac catheterization, when performed on such neonates, is typically normal except for rapid filling of the neck venous drainage. The discovery of prominent jugular veins and carotid arteries in a fetus (Fig. 3-7) would suggest a finding similar to that for the catheterized neonate with VGA. Cardiovascular hemodynamic abnormalities may also lead to an antenatal presentation with nonimmune hydrops due to fluid overload and cardiac failure. Brain damage is known to occur in affected neonates as a result of anoxia from the ischemia caused by arterial feeders stealing blood from the posterior choroidal and thalamostriate arteries. This is a cause of significant fetal and neonatal mortality.

US FINDINGS AND DIFFERENTIAL DIAGNOSIS OF FETAL GALENIC AVMs

On ultrasound (US) exam, a cystic structure, whether circular or oval, is typically seen within the brain. Classically, galenic AVMs are found in the midline between the dilated lateral ventricles, posterior to the foramen of Monro and superior to the third ventricle. The AVM is frequently tortuous in shape and seen with its feeding vessels. Doppler spectral flow analysis shows turbulent or biphasic and irregular venous flow, typical of the dilated venous portion of any AVM. Color Doppler imaging rapidly fills the cystic mass, identifying its vascular nature. Vascular dilatation of the posterior cerebral arteries, the arteries of the circle of Willis, the common carotid arteries, and venous structures such as the straight and sigmoid sinuses and the superior vena cava has been noted. The diagnosis of fetal brain AVMs has been limited in the literature to case reports in the third trimester, perhaps because it takes time to develop the enlarged vessels that can be imaged by US.

Lack of flow on Doppler suggests simulation of an AVM by a quadrigeminal plate or other arachnoid cyst that has no vascular flow within it. There are other possible causes of midline or other cystic masses in the fetal or neonatal brain. A cystic area in the midline could also be an enlarged or high-riding third ventricle, as seen in agenesis of the corpus callosum (ACC), or the associated midline interhemispheric cyst seen in this condition, but affected fetuses would have other findings of ACC. Holoprosencephalic patients have a dorsal cyst communicating with the univentricle. Parenchymal cystic neoplasms, as well as porencephalic cysts and clefts as seen in schizencephaly, are typically not midline. The main differential decision for the cause of a midline cystic mass is, again, between a galenic AVM and an arachnoid cyst.

The associated cardiovascular hemodynamic abnormalities in affected fetuses can lead to nonimmune hydrops, which may be suggested by imaging of fetal skin thickening

(>5 mm) as well as pleural effusion, ascites, and pericardial effusion. Classically, there is associated polyhydramnios and placental thickening.

KEY FETAL IMAGING POINT TO THIS CASE

The combination of right atrial enlargement and jugular venous distention in a fetus is highly suggestive of an intracranial arteriovenous malformation. Look in the brain for a cystic mass. Prove its vascular nature by Doppler.

References

Cohen HL: Neurosonography of the infant: Diagnosis of abnormalities, in *Ultrasonography of the Prenatal and Neonatal Brain,* Timor-Tritsch I, Monteagudo A, Cohen HL (eds). Stamford, CT, Appleton & Lange, 1996:259–285.

Cohen HL, Haller J: Review. Advances in perinatal neurosonography. *AJR* 163:801–810, 1994.

Comstock C, Kirk J: Arteriovenous malformations—locations and evolution in the fetal brain. *J Ultrasound Med* 10:361–365, 1991.

Ishimatsu J, Yoshimura O, Tetsuou M, Hamada T: Evaluation of an aneurysm of the vein of Galen in utero by pulsed and color Doppler ultrasonography. *Am J Obstet Gynecol* 164:743–744, 1991.

Koven M, Cohen HL, Goldman M: Fetal intracranial avm presenting as enlarged cardiac chamber. *J Ultrasound Med* 11:177, 1992.

Monteagudo A, Timor-Tritsch I: Fetal neurosonography of congenital brain anomalies, in *Ultrasonography of the Prenatal and Neonatal Brain,* Timor-Tritsch I, Monteagudo A, Cohen HL (eds). Stamford, CT, Appleton & Lange, 1996:178–183.

Rumack C, Johnson M: Intracranial neoplasms, cysts, and vascular malformations, in *Prenatal and Infant Brain Imaging. Role of Ultrasound and Computed Tomography,* Rumack C, Johnson L (eds). Chicago, Year Book, 1984:191–194.

Smythe J: The fetal heart and great vessels, in *A Practical Guide to Ultrasound in Obstetrics and Gynecology,* 2d ed, Sauerbrei E, Nguyen K, Nolan R (eds). Philadelphia, Lippincott-Raven, 1998:255–256.

Volpe J: Brain tumors and vein of Galen malformations, in *Neurology of the Newborn: Neuronal Proliferation, Migration, Organization and Myelination,* 3d ed. Philadelphia, Saunders, 1995:802–806.

Westra S, Curran J, Duckwiler G, et al: Pediatric intracranial vascular malformations: Evaluation of treatment results with color Doppler US. Work in progress. *Radiology* 186:775–783, 1993.

4

This 18-week-old fetus was evaluated on a routine obstetrical exam for determination of gestational age. An axial image (Fig. 4-1) is available for your interpretation. Is this of any concern?

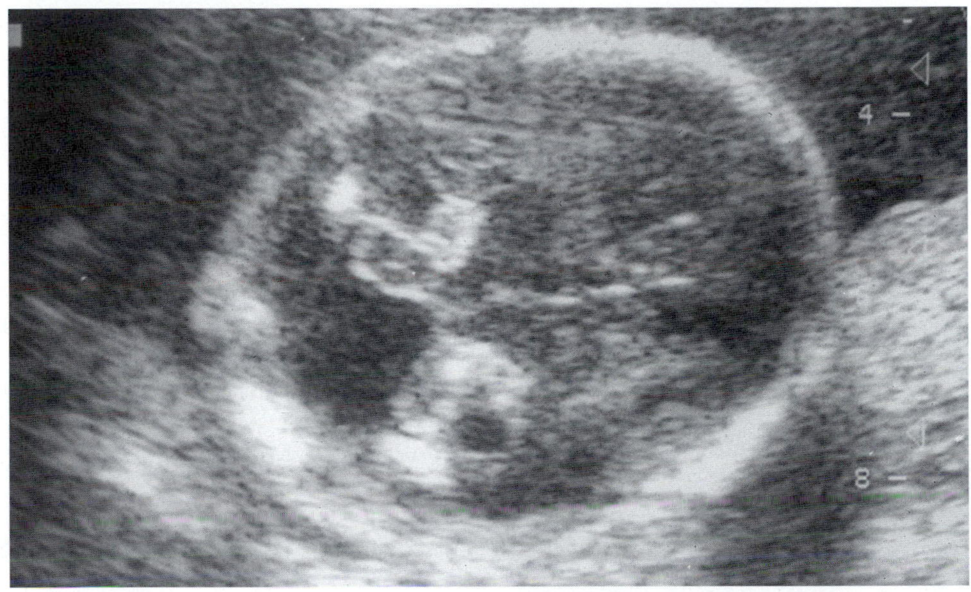

FIGURE 4–1. Fetal brain. Axial view. The anterior calvaria is to the reader's right.

CHAPTER 4

Dandy-Walker Malformation

HARRIS L. COHEN

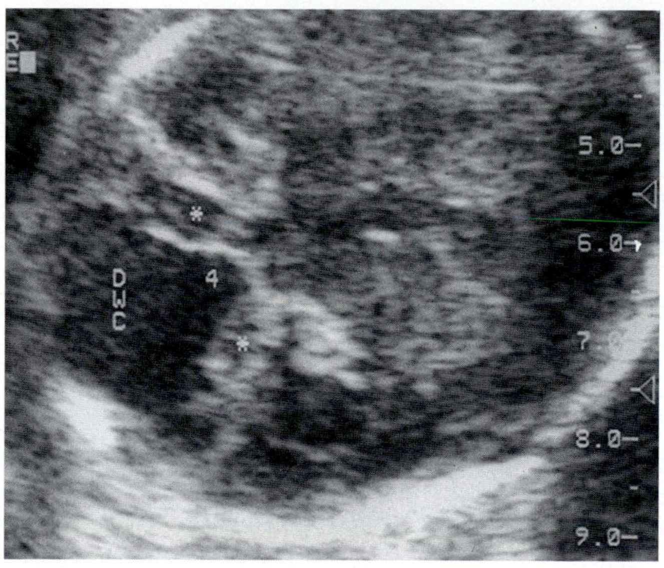

FIGURE 4–2. Fetal brain with Dandy-Walker malformation. Axial view. This figure is a somewhat magnified equivalent of Fig. 4-1. The triangular infratentorial cyst extends from the region of the cisterna magna to the fourth ventricle. This area is too large to be a normal cisterna magna. It is a Dandy-Walker cyst (DWC). The associated vermian dysgenesis allows the distended (due to obstruction) fourth ventricle (4) to extend backward to the most posterior aspect of the calvaria. The starred (*) oval structures on either side of the anterior extent of the fourth ventricle are the dysplastic and displaced cerebellar hemispheres.

There is a large cystic area in the posterior aspect of the fetal brain seen in Fig. 4-2, a slightly magnified view of Fig. 4-1. The cystic area is triangular in shape and extends from its widest point at the posterior calvaria to its narrower apex at the area of the fourth ventricle. Two oval echogenicities seen peripheral to the cyst's apex (at the level of the fourth ventricle) are peripherally displaced cerebellar hemispheres. The cerebellar hemispheres are smaller than normal. A normal central cerebellar vermis (Fig. 4-3), usually situated just posterior to the fourth ventricle, is not seen. What is seen of the supratentorial brain appears unremarkable. This fetus's intracranial findings are classical for the Dandy-Walker malformation (DWM).

WHAT IS THE DANDY-WALKER CYST/COMPLEX/MALFORMATION?

The DWM was first reported as a clinical and pathologic entity by Dandy and Blackfan in 1914. It consists of a spectrum of anatomic abnormalities thought by some to be due to defective development of the posterior medullary velum into what should be the roof of the fourth ventricle at around 7 to 10 weeks of gestation. Others believe that the embryologic abnormality leading to DWM occurs later (and therefore later than most other brain abnormalities), at between the third and fifth months of gestation. There is often, but not always, a lack of patency of one or more of the cerebrospinal fluid (CSF) outlets from the fourth ventricle, i.e., atresia of the foramina of Luschka (the lateral apertures, normally patent by the second trimester) and/or Magendie (the median aperture). This obstruction results in dilatation of the fourth ventricle into a balloon-like membrane filled with ventricular CSF. This thin-walled sac (Fig. 4-4) of obstructed fourth ventricle may vary in size but often fills and expands the posterior fossa, elevating the tentorium (Fig. 4-4*B*), as well as the transverse sinuses and torcular Herophili (confluence of the sinuses). Associated absence of the vermis (33 percent of autopsied cases in one series) or varying degrees of vermian hypoplasia allow the dilated fourth ventricle to extend so far posteriorly that the DWM may simulate a retrocerebellar cyst. The infratentorial cystic mass can displace the cerebel-

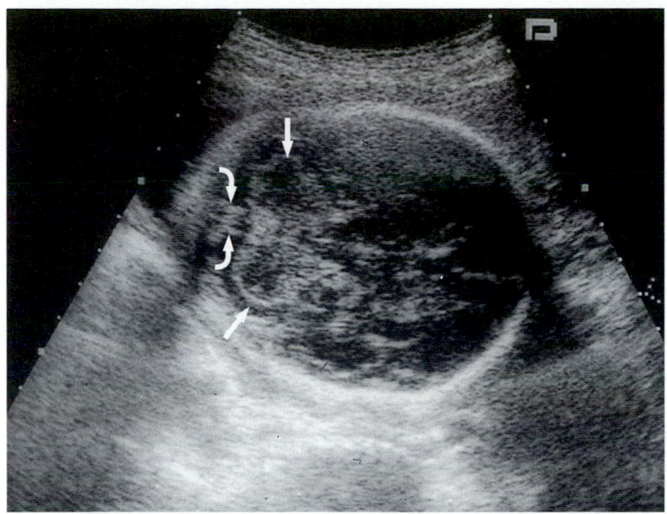

FIGURE 4–3. Fetal brain with normal cerebellum and cisterna magna. Axial view. The infratentorial area of a normal fetal brain on axial view shows a normal peanut-shaped cerebellum. The two rounded structures at the periphery are the cerebellar hemispheres (*arrows*). The brighter central echogenic area is the vermis, which sits behind the fourth ventricle. The fourth ventricle is not well seen on axial view unless it is enlarged. The cystic area behind the cerebellum is the cisterna magna. It is of a normal anteroposterior measurement in this normal fetus. Echogenic lines (*curved arrows*) crossing the cisterna magna from front to back are normal dural folds. Their presence suggests normalcy and the absence of a Dandy-Walker cyst.

lum superiorly and/or displace and compress the cerebellar hemispheres, which are often hypoplastic, laterally. The degree of hemisphere separation is proportional to the size of the cyst. An associated hydrocephalus of variable degrees (Fig. 4-5), involving the lateral ventricles and aqueduct of Sylvius, has been reported in at least 53 to 75 percent of affected infants. The hydrocephalus is most often treated with routine ventriculoperitoneal shunting. The degree of hydrocephalus appears unrelated to the patency of the foramina, the degree of vermian hypoplasia, or the size of the fourth ventricular cyst. Hydrocephalus at birth has been said by some authorities to be unusual. This may be more debatable in these times of excellent antenatal imaging but is consistent with my experience, in which a number of fetuses I have imaged who had DWM did *not* have hydrocephalus at the time of my examination. Hydrocephalus is seen in 75 percent of DWM patients by 3 months of age and in 90 percent of all patients by the time they are clinically diagnosed with DWM (probably because of symptoms of hydrocephalus).

WHAT OTHER ABNORMALITIES ASSOCIATED WITH THE DANDY-WALKER MALFORMATION?

Up to one-third of DWM patients have agenesis or hypogenesis of the corpus callosum. Occipital encephaloceles are seen in 5 to 16 percent. Between 5 and 10 percent of patients have neuronal migration disorders, such as heterotopias and polymicrogyria. While ultrasound (US) can readily diagnose encephaloceles in the fetus and agenesis of the corpus callosum in the fetus and neonate, the diagnosis of hypogenesis of the corpus callosum and certainly the diagnosis of heterotopias and polymicrogyria is more difficult and is markedly improved by magnetic resonance imaging (MRI). Associated aqueductal stenosis and brainstem malformation in DWM patients have been reported.

The most common extracranial abnormality associated with DWM is congenital heart disease, but polysyndactyly, cleft lip and palate, and facial hemangiomata have also been noted. As many as one-third of affected patients are said to have associated chromosomal abnormalities. There is a purported increased incidence of trisomy 21, as well as of the Walker-Warburg, Klippel-Feil, and Ellis-van Creveld syndromes.

VARIANTS—WHAT ARE THEY AND WHY DO WE STILL HAVE TO WORRY ABOUT THEM?

There are two lesser forms of DWM that may be part of one larger spectrum. Both were thought to be of little genetic or clinical concern until recently. The *Dandy-Walker variant* consists of deficiency of only the inferior cerebellar vermis and therefore communication only inferiorly with a cystic and dilated fourth ventricle. There is no enlargement of the posterior fossa. Despite the milder-appearing morphology, we now know that we have to be worried about such fetuses. Two studies have shown 24 percent of Dandy-Walker variant patients with ventriculomegaly, almost half with associated abnormalities beyond the central nervous system, and an incidence of associated chromosomal abnormalities of 29 to 53 percent, perhaps higher than that reported with complete vermian agenesis (i.e., classic DWM).

The *mega cisterna magna* is an isolated enlargement of the cisterna magna. The normal cisterna magna has an anteroposterior (AP) measurement on an (10 to 15° inclined) axial image of 5 ± 3 mm. A measurement greater than 10 mm is considered abnormal. No other morphologic abnormality is noted. But, again, we have to be concerned because of the reported association of mega cisterna magna with trisomy 18. Another group has shown there to be no associated abnormality when this is an isolated finding.

One key technical point: The cisterna magna's normal (2- to 10-mm) AP measurement is obtained in the midline from the posterior aspect of the cerebellar vermis to the inner wall of the occipital bone. One should measure on typical axial images that show the cerebellar hemispheres well in order to avoid the falsely elongated measurements obtained when the plane of insonation is overangulated, resulting in a semicoronal image. This will help one avoid a false-positive diagnosis of Dandy-Walker variant or mega cisterna magna.

Another technical point: Thin echogenic lines within the cisterna magna (Fig. 4-6) extending in an anterior to posterior direction are normal dural folds and indicate that what is imaged is a normal cisterna magna rather than an arachnoid cyst or some other abnormality.

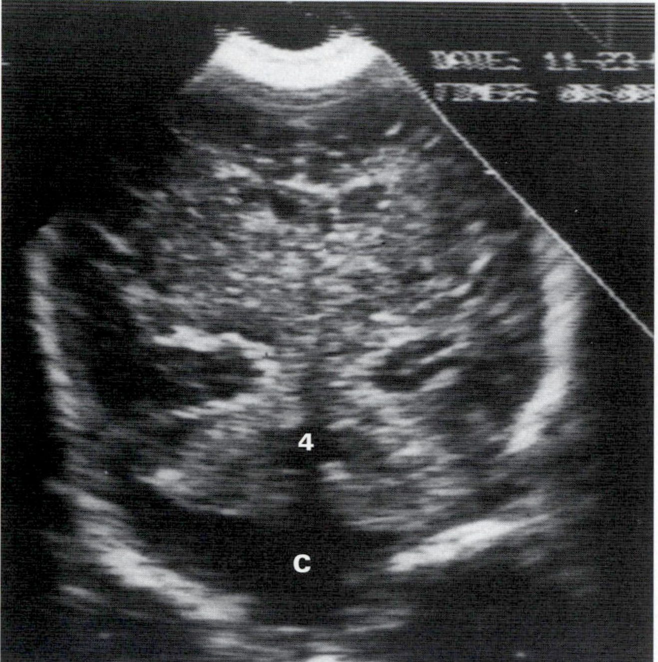

A

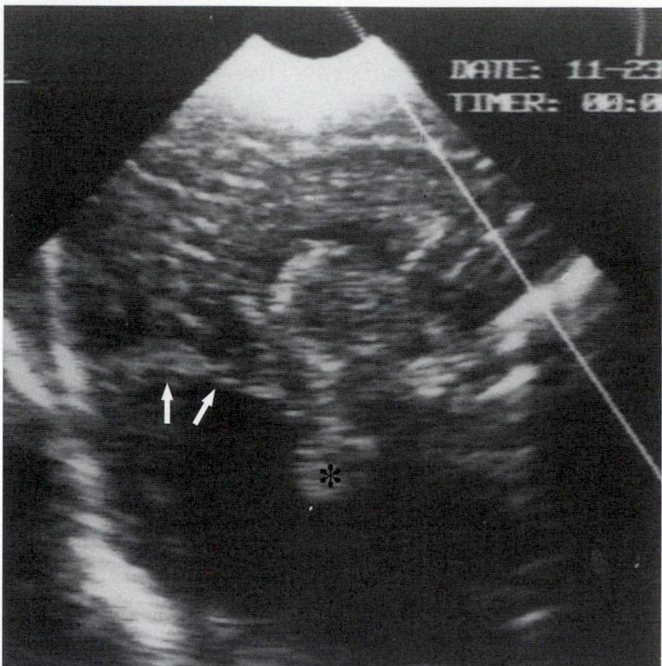

B

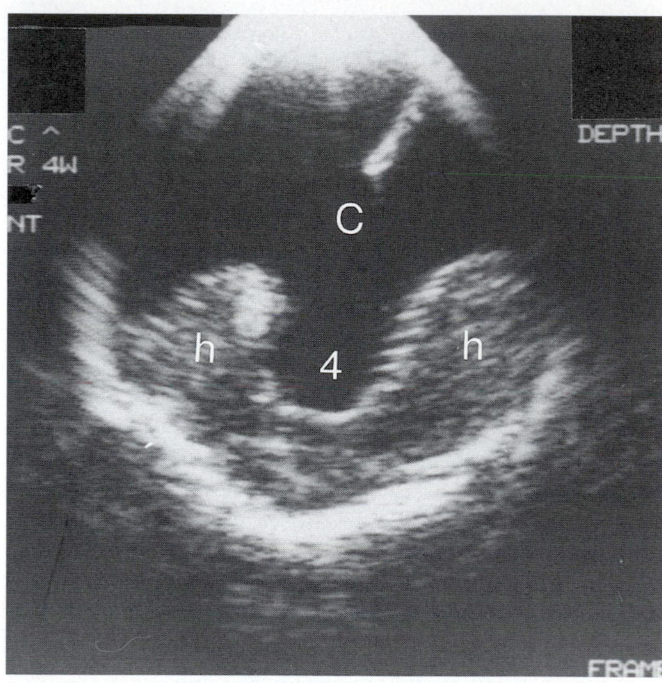

C

FIGURE 4–4. Neonatal brain. Dandy-Walker complex. ***A.*** Coronal plane. Image taken through the anterior fontanelle. A prominent cystic area (c) is seen in the region of this newborn's cisterna magna. It represents fluid in a distended fourth ventricle that can be tracked to its most anterior aspect (4). This can occur only with cerebellar vermian dysgenesis. Hemispheres are seen and are only mildly displaced. There was no hydrocephalus at this time. An arrow points to normal-sized frontal horns. Within weeks, hydrocephalus developed. I have often likened these images to those of a smiling lion or cat, with the smile being the Dandy-Walker cyst. ***B.*** Sagittal (*midline*) plane via the anterior fontanelle. The image is not in standard sagittal image display with anterior structures at the reader's left. Rather, the anterior brain in this image is to the right. A large subtentorial cyst is seen. The tentorium (*arrows*) is lifted superiorly. A star (*) has been placed on what appears to be dysgenetic vermis or another portion of the dysgenetic cerebellum. ***C.*** Coronal plane. Image taken via the posterior fontanelle. Use of the posterior fontanelle view is most helpful in assessing the posterior brain and the subtentorial brain contents. This technique allowed a unique perspective on this Dandy-Walker malformation, showing the cystic mass (c) closest to the transducer (*at the top of the image*) and in a deeper (*or more anterior*) position the laterally displaced hemispheres (H) and extension of the cyst into the anterior aspect of the fourth ventricle (4). This could occur because of the vermian dysgenesis. *(From Cohen, with permission.[4])*

CLINICAL INFORMATION AND PROGNOSIS

Symptoms of DWM are said to be due not to the DWM itself, but to the associated supratentorial abnormalities. The diagnosis has, historically, been made in neonates, children, or even adults with a clinical presentation related to hydrocephalus (e.g., head circumference enlargement, headaches, papilledema). Prognosis is related to the severity of these "other" central nervous system (CNS) abnormalities. There is a 55 percent postnatal death rate. Three-fourths of survivors are mentally retarded. Interference with brainstem function is considered the chief functional complication, which can be associated with worsening of seizure activity in the Lennox-Gastaut syndrome. When DWM is isolated and the brainstem is intact, chance of survival is good and similar to that of patients with treated hydrocephalus.

DANDY-WALKER CYST—WHAT ARE THE DIFFERENTIAL DIAGNOSTIC POSSIBILITIES?

The one key differential possibility is a subtentorial retrocerebellar subarachnoid cyst (Fig. 4-7). These congenital

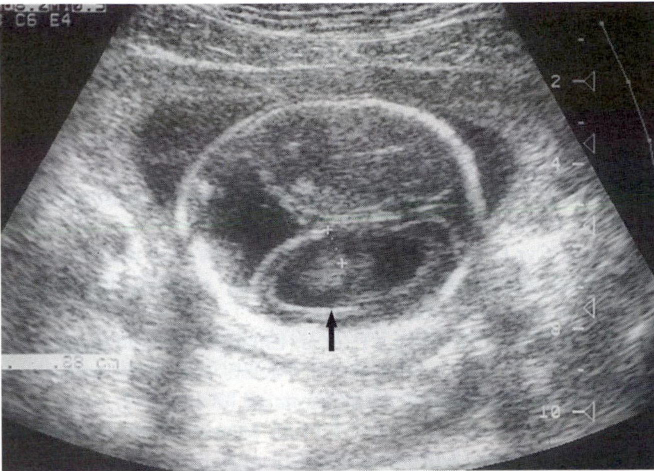

FIGURE 4–5. Fetal brain with Dandy-Walker cyst and hydrocephalus. Axial view. The triangular cyst in the infratentorial region is a Dandy-Walker cyst. It may be simulated by an infratentorial arachnoid cyst. Lateral ventricular dilatation (*arrow*) is due to hydrocephalus, an often accompanying finding.

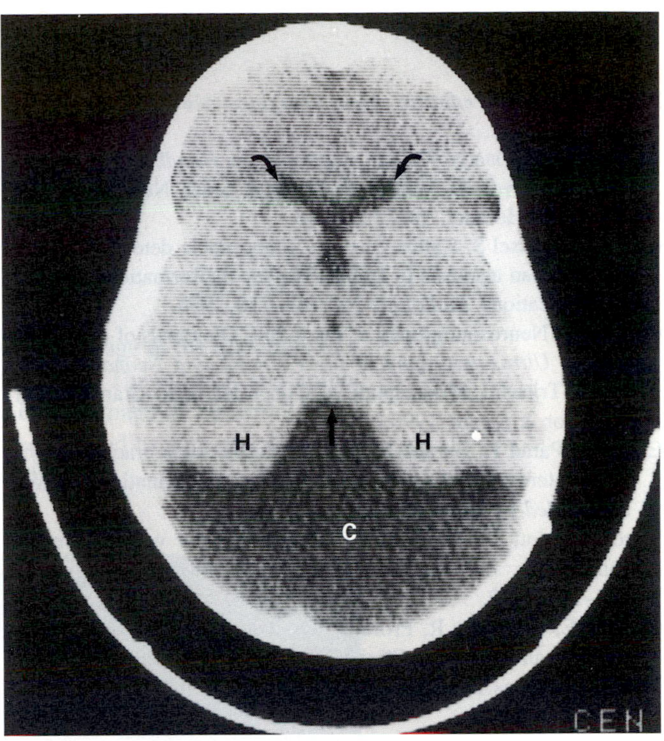

FIGURE 4–6. Dandy-Walker syndrome vs. variant. Computed tomography image. Axial plane. The distended infratentorial cyst (c) is seen taking up most of the imaged infratentorial area. Laterally displaced cerebellar hemispheres (H) with what appears to be at least some vermis (*arrow*) are seen. The frontal horns (*curved arrows*) are mildly distended due to hydrocephalus.

cysts are thought to be the result of maldevelopment of the leptomeninges. Found between the pia-arachnoid layers and communicating with the subarachnoid space, they may grow because of this communication and the accumulation of fluid within them through a ball-valve mechanism. Some are said to have choroid plexus–like tissue in their walls, allowing actual internal CSF secretion and growth. When subtentorial in location, they tend to displace the cerebellum as a unit rather than separating the individual hemispheres as in DWM. Less common and more benign than DWM, subarachnoid cysts may cause a mass impression leading to hydrocephalus but, unlike DWM, are not associated with other CNS anomalies or brain maldevelopment. If symptomatic and treated, they have an excellent outcome.

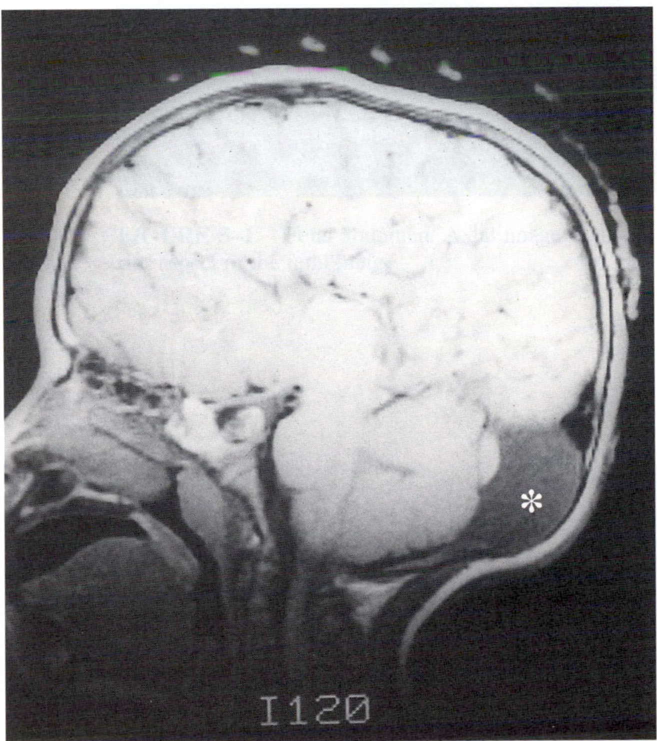

FIGURE 4–7. Retrocerebellar arachnoid cyst. Magnetic resonance (MR) image (T1 weighted). Sagittal plane. A low-intensity cystic mass (*) is seen posterior to normal cerebellar tissue in this 5-year-old's subtentorial region. This proved to be a subarachnoid cyst but can readily simulate the MR image of a Dandy-Walker cyst.

US Findings: Dandy-Walker Syndrome

1. Enlarged posterior fossa cystic space
2. Vermian dysgenesis
3. Displacement of often hypoplastic cerebellar hemispheres
4. Cephalic displacement of tentorium due to enlarged subtentorial space
5. Often, associated hydrocephalus (at least in neonates)

CHAPTER 5

Myelomeningocele

HARRIS L. COHEN

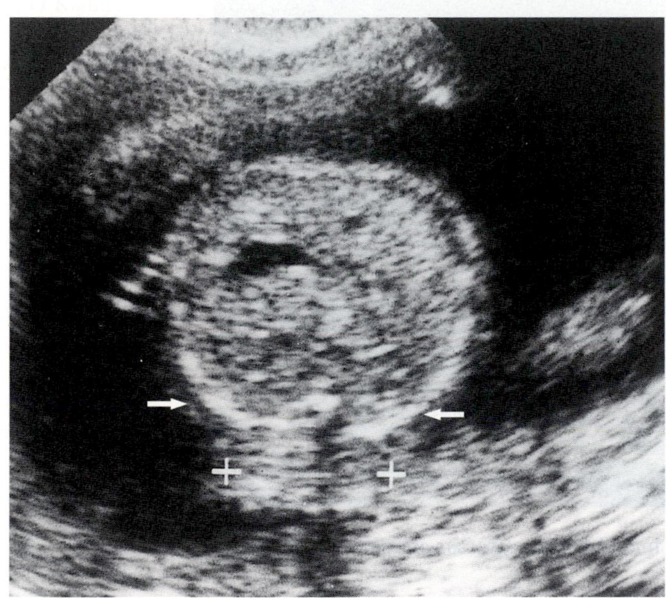

FIGURE 5–2. Annotated version of Fig 5-1. Fetal abdomen. Axial image at mid-abdomen. The solid mass (*crosses*) extends posterior to the lower thoracic ribs (*arrows*).

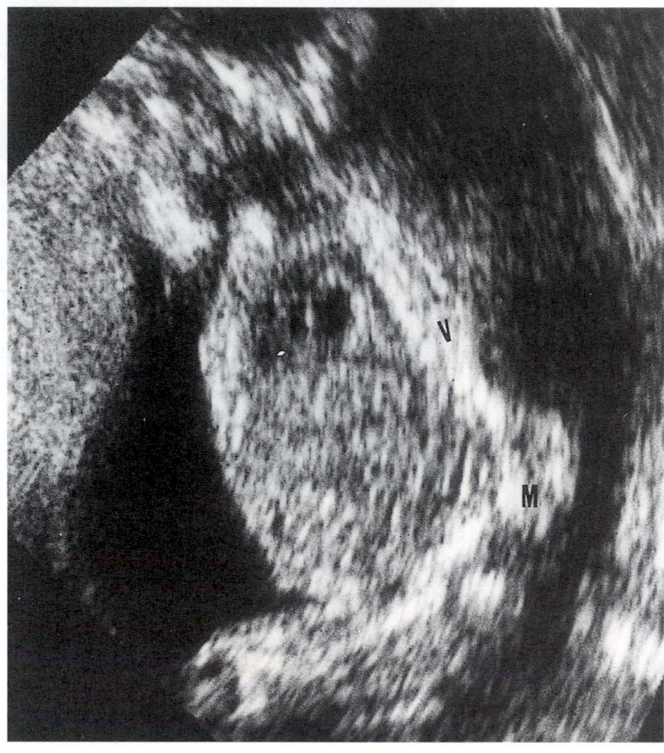

FIGURE 5–3. Fetal chest and abdomen. Sagittal plane, some obliquity. While some obliquity of this view aided the imaging of the mass (M), it limited the imaging of the vertebral bodies (V). The mass is also noted on this view to extend posterior to the vertebral bodies. Its solid nature is consistent with a myelomeningocele. *(From Cohen et al.[3], with permission.)*

In Fig. 5-2 (the annotated version of Fig. 5-1), one can see that the posterior crosses surround a solid mass in the posterior midline of a fetus. The mass is posterior to the vertebral body (V), which is not well seen, and the ribs of the lower thoracic wall. While masses can arise from any of the soft tissue structures in the region, when such a mass involves the fetal midline posteriorly, one must consider the possibility of a myelomeningocele (MMC), which this case proved to be. A 90° turn of the transducer (Fig. 5-3) may allow a better analysis of the mass. In some cases one may more readily identify separated posterior elements of the vertebral column (Fig. 5-4).

WHAT IS A NEURAL TUBE DEFECT? WHAT IS A MYELOMENINGOCELE?

The normal central nervous system begins to form during dorsal induction (also termed primary neuralation), which occurs at 3 weeks after fertilization. A secondary neuralation of the caudal neural tube occurs at 26 to 32 days. Failure of primary neuralation results in cranial (anencephaly),

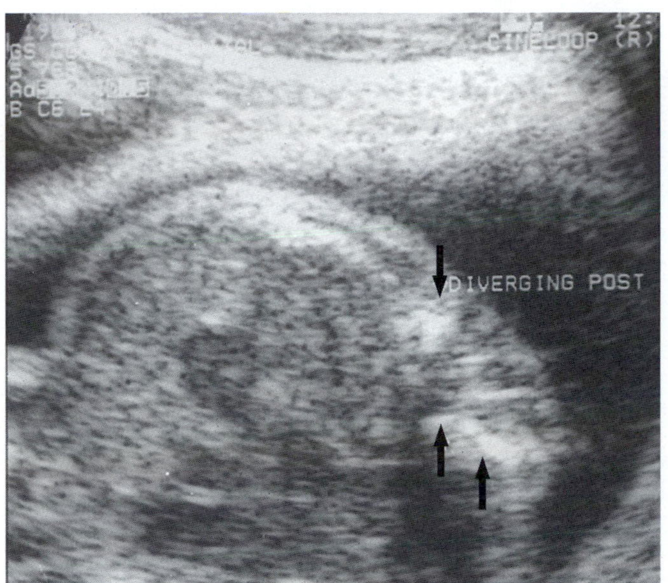

FIGURE 5–4. Myelomeningocele with separation of posterior elements. Axial plane, level of abdomen. A mass (*straight arrow*) consistent with a myelomeningocele is seen posteriorly in this second-trimester fetus. The diverging posterior elements of the vertebral body at that level are marked off.

spinal (myelomeningocele), or craniospinal (craniorachischisis) defects.

HOW ARE NEURAL TUBE DEFECTS DIAGNOSED?

Laboratory Assessment

The diagnosis of neural tube defects (NTDs), with their significant morbidity and mortality, has been aided by the assessment of maternal serum and amniotic fluid for alpha fetoprotein (AFP) and of amniotic fluid for the presence of acetylcholinesterase (ACH). Alphafetoprotein is a glycoprotein synthesized by the fetal liver and gastrointestinal (GI) tract that enters the amniotic fluid by fetal urine or GI secretions. It crosses the placenta and can be found (to a lesser extent than within the fetus or the amniotic fluid) in the maternal serum. When it is found at a 2.5 or greater multiple of the normal median of AFP in a pregnant woman's serum, one may suspect an open defect in the calvarium or spine of the fetus. There are, however, other reasons for these increases that are unrelated to a neural tube defect (Table 5-1). Acetylcholinesterase, an enzyme derived from neural tissue and not normally found in amniotic fluid, is another indicator of an open neural tube defect that may help differentiate the cause of high AFP levels (although nerves involved in an open abdominal wall defect can be the source of high amniotic ACH levels).

These laboratory assessments, particularly the assessment of maternal serum AFP levels as a screening examination, have greatly aided the early diagnosis of NTDs. There are, however, difficulties that make the use of fetal ultrasound (US) a highly desirable modality. Since AFP peaks in the fetus at 12 weeks and continues to rise in the maternal serum during pregnancy, knowledge of true gestational age is most important for accurate AFP analysis. Since only open NTDs are not covered by skin, closed NTDs may be missed by laboratory testing.

Anencephaly and Its Ultrasound Assessment

The most common NTD is anencephaly. Anencephaly is a lethal anomaly that is said to occur in 1 in every 1000 pregnancies. Three-fourths of such births are stillborn, and essentially all such patients die within the first 48 h of life. Anencephaly is now thought to be due to a combination of dysraphia (skull defect) and exencephaly (exposure of a well-developed brain outside the skull), followed by anencephaly (disintegration of the exposed brain during the fetal period). The anencephalic has no cranial vault seen above the orbits. If tissue is seen in the area of what would be the brain, it is angiomatous stroma (Fig. 5-5).

Myelomeningocele and Its Ultrasound Assessment

Myelomeningocele is the second most common open NTD. It occurs in 0.2 to 0.4 case per 1000 births. Masses extending beyond the vertebral bodies may be cystic or solid. The presence of neural tissue as well as meninges distinguishes a myelomeningocele from the less clinically problematic meningocele, which consists only of meninges. Myelomeningoceles occur most often in the lumbar or thoracolumbar area. Sacral and cervical lesions are less common. About 86 percent of MMC patients survive beyond 10 years of age but have morbidity related to the level of their spinal defect. Patients with myelomeningocele have variable neurologic defects related to the size and position of the lesion vis-à-vis the spinal cord and its nerves. The higher lesions are more significant. Paraparesis, minor anesthesia, and problems with micturition and stooling are common. Morbidity is also related

TABLE 5-1
Some of the Many Causes of High Maternal Serum AFP

Key considerations in the fetus:

1. Neural tube defect
2. Myelomeningocele
3. Omphalocele
4. Gastroschisis

Other considerations:

5. Fetal death
6. Multiple pregnancies
7. Renal abnormalities (e.g., agenesis, recessive polycystic kidney disease, congenital nephrosis)
8. Intestinal atresia
9. Congenital fetal skin disorders, i.e., epidermolysis bullosa
10. Sacrococcygeal teratomas
11. Cystic hygroma
12. Congenital cystic adenomatoid malformation
13. Others: Oligohydramnios, placental hemangioma, abdominal pregnancy, maternal infection

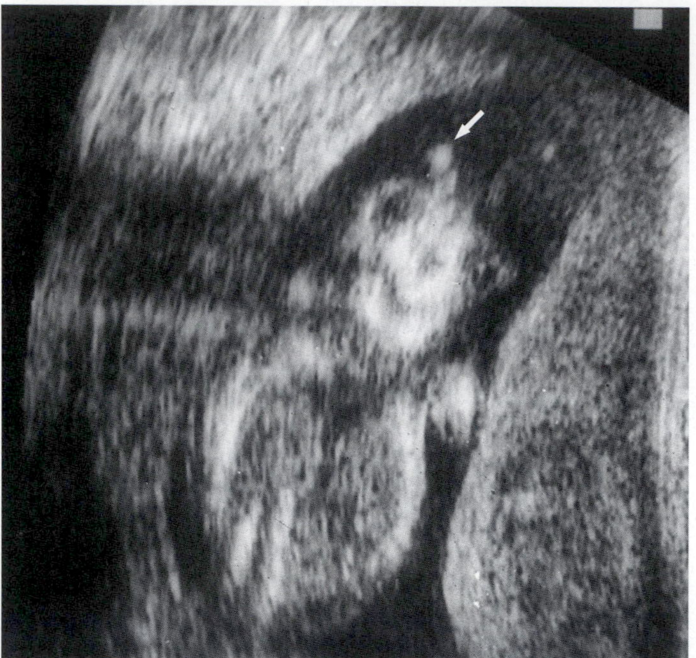

FIGURE 5–5. Anencephaly. Coronal plane through fetal face. The orbits are seen with nothing superior to them except a small echogenicity (*arrow*) that represented angiomatous stroma simulating normal brain tissue.

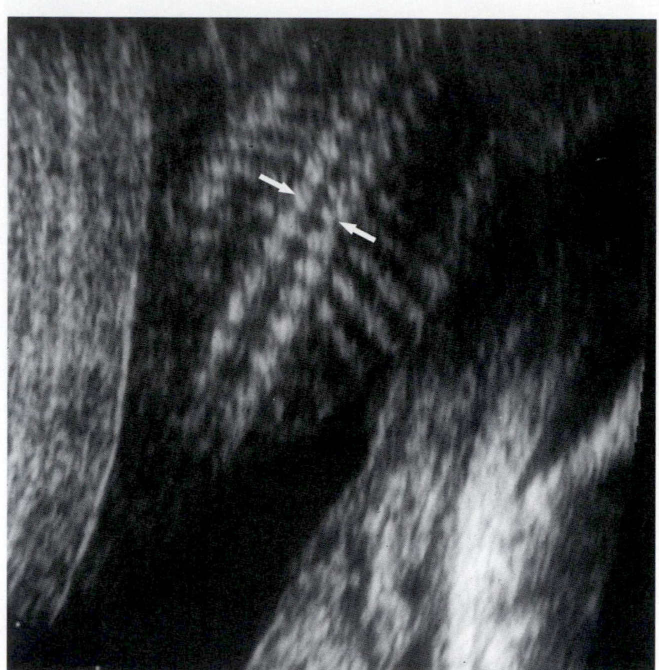

A

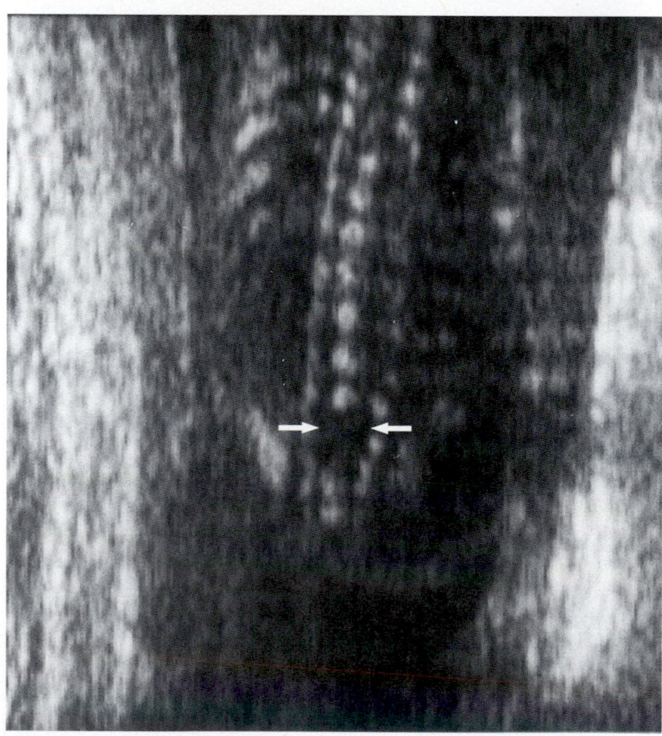

B

FIGURE 5–6. Coronal plane for imaging fetal spine. ***A.*** Normal spine. Coronal plane. Fetal spine and ribs are seen. Pedicles (*arrows*) appear to be separated equally at the different vertebral body levels, with no obvious splaying that might suggest an MMC. ***B.*** MMC. Coronal plane. There is a lack of vertebral ossification centers in an area (*arrow*) of the lumbosacral spine. This proved to be due to spinal dysraphism from an MMC.

to any associated anomalies, which usually are neurologic, often related to the associated Chiari II malformation, and musculoskeletal, associated with foot deformities and hip dislocation. Some 2 percent of those born with MMC die in neonatal life, and 50 percent have some form of learning disability. Those with hindbrain and brainstem symptoms (pain, weakness, arm spasticity) have a 33 percent mortality from respiratory failure. As a general rule, patients with smaller lesions involving fewer vertebral levels, lower lesions, or closed lesions and those without hindbrain and brainstem problems do better.

MYELOMENINGOCELE DIAGNOSIS BY ULTRASOUND

Past Problems Using Spine Images Alone

Despite our unknown image's ready portrayal of the mass of the MMC, an MMC can still be missed antenatally. Classic imaging of the spine in axial or transverse, sagittal or coronal planes (Fig. 5-6) can be limited for the diagnosis of MMC. In the early 1980s I had personal experience with a case that we examined 12 times, knowing that the AFP was increased, without being able to see the actual spinal defect, which proved to be one lamina large. In a proper study, each vertebral body must be imaged in axial and sagittal planes. Not all can be perfectly well seen in every patient. The normal axial image of a vertebra denotes three ossified elements of the fetal spine (Fig. 5-7*A*); the anterior element is the vertebral

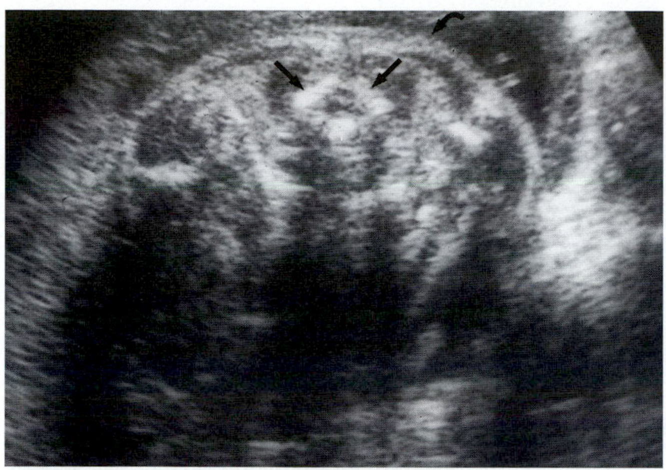

A

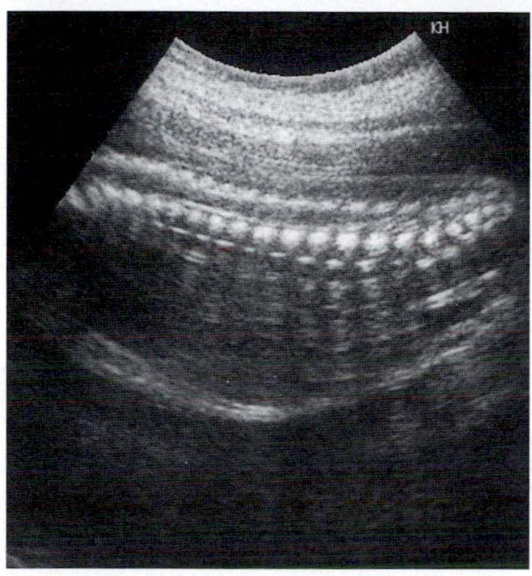

B

FIGURE 5–7. Normal fetal spine. ***A.*** Normal spine. Transverse plane. The fetus is prone. The two posterior elements *(arrows)* of this cervical spine converge posteriorly. The skin line (*curved arrow*) is intact. These findings go against a myelomeningocele at this level. ***B.*** Normal spine. Sagittal plane. The fetal head is to the reader's left. Most of the fetal spine is seen. However, one can see no more than two of the three ossified elements in this or any sagittal plane.

body, and the two posterior elements are the lamina, which will become the rest of the eventually fully ossified vertebral body. At each vertebral level, each of these elements must be seen. Fetal positioning often prevents this. At each level, the posterior elements should converge to the center of the spine rather than diverge laterally. An intact posterior skin line should be seen, but this may be obscured by the fetal spine being next to the uterine wall or placenta and no amniotic fluid being seen between them. Fetal positioning may obscure imaging of the mass itself. The meningocele itself may burst and the typically cystic portion not be seen, creating diagnostic difficulty. The posterior elements may be parallel to each other; this is usually an indicator of normalcy but does not give the examiner 100 percent assurance. While the tedious analysis of each vertebral body in axial view can be accomplished if fetal positioning is fortunate, analysis of the vertebral bodies in the sagittal plane (Fig. 5-7*B*) is limited because only two of the three elements can be imaged in a given plane.

TABLE 5-2
Signs of Myelomeningocele or the Chiari II Malformation

1. Mass extending beyond the skin of the back (sac may not be intact)
2. Mass extending through divergent ecogenic posterior elements of the vertebral body
3. Defect in the skin of the fetal back
4. Chiari II malformation
    - 4a. Banana-shaped cerebellum
    - 4b. Lemon-shaped calvarium
    - 4c. Effaced cisterna magna

How Intracranial and Cranial Findings Help

Recognition over the last several years of the intracranial sonographic findings of the Chiari II malformation (Table 5-2) has proven to be a major breakthrough in the antenatal diagnosis of MMC. Virtually all patients with Chiari II malformations have an associated MMC. Although viewing the spinal column, particularly in the most typical MMC locations (the lumbosacral and, to a lesser extent, thoracolumbar spine areas), is still necessary, the indirect findings of a "lemon-shaped" calvarium, a "banana-shaped" cerebellum, or an effaced cisterna magna coupled with the common associated finding of hydrocephalus (44 to 86 percent of cases) help to identify fetuses with MMC. A recent study has shown that the degree of hydrocephalus is unrelated to the size or spinal level of the MMC.

The fetal cerebellum should be easily imaged anterior to the cisterna magna, which normally measures 2 to 10 mm in an anteroposterior (AP) direction. An inability to image the cerebellum as a bilobed peanut-shaped structure (Fig. 5-8), in combination with a cisterna magna measurement of less than 2 mm, suggests the Chiari II malformation, in which the small posterior fossa and low tentorial attachment allow the cerebellum to be indented and the pons, medulla, and cervical spine to be stretched inferiorly. The downward displacement of these structures effaces the cisterna magna and flattens and elongates the cerebellum into a more tubular shape, referred to as the "banana" configuration (Fig. 5-9).

The "lemon" sign refers to the inward depression of the calvarium's frontal bones, deforming it from the shape of an oval to one of a lemon. The imaging of a lemon-shaped calvarium (Fig. 5-9) does not, however, make the diagnosis of MMC or NTD. Although when it was first reported in 1986, the sign was noted in all of a group of fetuses with spina bifida, Nyberg imaged it in only two-thirds of a group of MMC patients that he studied. It was, however, seen in 89 percent of his MMC patients of less than 24 weeks gestation. One must also note that 1 percent of normal fetuses without spina bifida show the lemon sign. It is also a nonspecific sign, since one group noted it in 5 of 23 fetuses with intracranial or

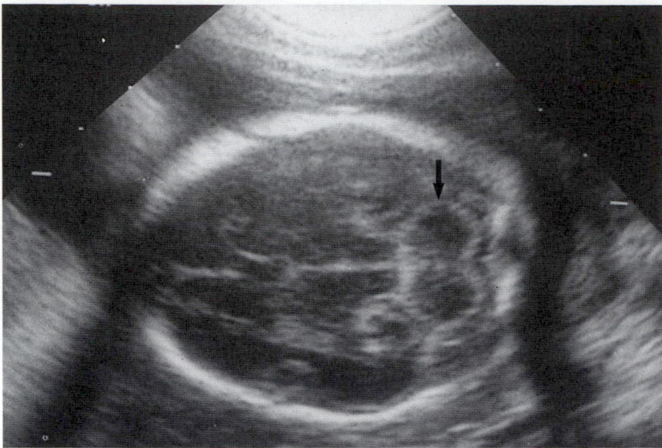

FIGURE 5–8. Normal fetal cerebellum (and calvarial shape). Axial plane. The normal cerebellum (*arrow*) is peanut-shaped or bilobed. There is a fluid-filled cisterna magna posterior to it that is not well seen on this image. The calvarial shape is smooth, with no inward flattening of the frontal bones.

extracranial abnormalities but no MMC or encephalocele. The absence of a lemon sign, however, is a helpful antenatal cue, since it has a negative predictive value for NTD of 99.5 percent. If you don't see a lemon, chances for an MMC are <0.5 percent.

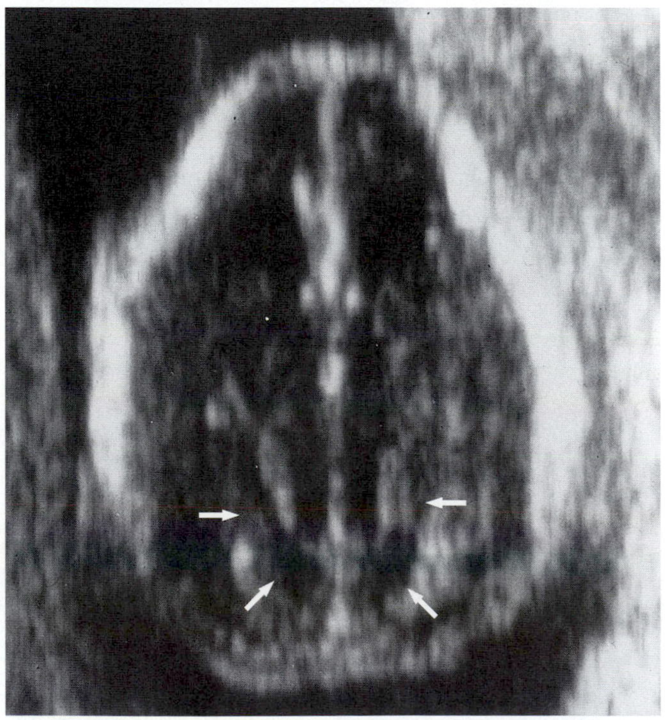

FIGURE 5–9. Abnormal or banana-shaped cerebellum and lemon-shaped calvarium of MMC. Fetal head. Axial plane. The frontal bones are at the superior portion of this print. No cisterna magna is noted. It has been effaced in this fetus with a Chiari II malformation associated with an MMC. The usually rounded cerebellar hemispheres have been flattened into a C-shaped or banana-shaped structure (*arrows*). The calvaria are depressed in the frontal area, allowing the complete skull to look like a lemon on this view.

GENETIC IMPLICATIONS OF THE DIAGNOSIS OF MMC

Slightly over 4 percent of the siblings of children born with closed or occult dysraphia have a disorder of primary neuralation such as meningocele or anencephaly. While in the United States (the risks are greater for people of Wales and less for people in Japan) there is a 1 to 2 per 1000 case risk for MMC, the risk becomes greater with a positive family history. If one parent has an MMC, the likelihood of a child's being born with one is 5 percent. If a single sibling has an MMC, the risk is 2 percent; if two siblings have an MMC, the risk is 2 to 5 percent. It will be interesting to know whether these percentages will decrease with active treatment of mothers with folate supplementation, to correct a deficiency that has been linked to NTDs.

A TAKE HOME MESSAGE

We are lucky that clinical US research has shown us that there are *both* vertebral and cranial signs that allow us to pick up MMCs. That fact obligates us to look at the infratentorial contents of the brain as well as the shape of the calvarium, even if the entire spine can be imaged. Look for the fruit—i.e., the associated cranial lemon and banana signs of MMC. Since 44 to 86 percent of MMC patients have hydrocephalus, the discovery of hydrocephalus should force us to take a second look at the cerebellum and cisterna magna.

References

Babcook C, Drake C, Goldstein R: Spinal level of fetal myelomeningocele: Does it influence ventricular size? *AJR* 169:207–210, 1997.

Benacerraf B, Stryker J, Frigoletto J Jr, et al: Abnormal US appearance of the cerebellum (banana sign): Indirect sign of spina bifida. *Radiology* 171:151–153, 1989.

Cohen HL, Haller JO: Advances in perinatal neurosonography. *AJR* 163:801–810, 1994.

Cohen HL, Muller D, Zinn DL: Abnormal fetal chest, abdomen, pelvis, in *Obstetrics and Gynecology*, 2d ed, Berman MC, Cohen HL (eds). Philadelphia, Lippincott,1997:285–320.

Goldstein R, Podrasky A, Filly R, Callen P: Effacement of the fetal cisterna magna in association with myelomeningocele. *Radiology* 172:409–413, 1989.

Monteagudo A, Timor-Tritsch I: Fetal neurosonography of congenital brain anomalies, in *Ultrasonography of the Prenatal and Neonatal Brain,* Timor-Tritsch I, Monteagudo A, Cohen HL (eds). Stamford, CT, Appleton & Lange, 1996:147–219.

Nicolaides K, Gabbe S, Campbell S, Guidetti R: Ultrasound screening for spina bifida: Cranial and cerebellar signs. *Lancet* 2: 272–274, 1986.

Nyberg D, Mack L, Hirsch J, Mahony B: Abnormalities of fetal cranial contour in sonographic detection of spina bifida: Evaluation of the "lemon" sign. *Radiology* 167:387–392, 1988.

Sauerbrei E, Toi A: The fetal spine, in *Diagnostic Ultrasound,* Rumack C, Wilson S, Charboneau J (eds). St Louis, Mosby–Year Book, 1998:1283–1302.

6

Figure 6-1 is the sagittal view of a 12.1-week fetus (crown–rump length 51 mm). The mother was 41 years old and was referred for ultrasound because of uncertain dates. What is seen? What is the diagnosis? Should you be concerned?

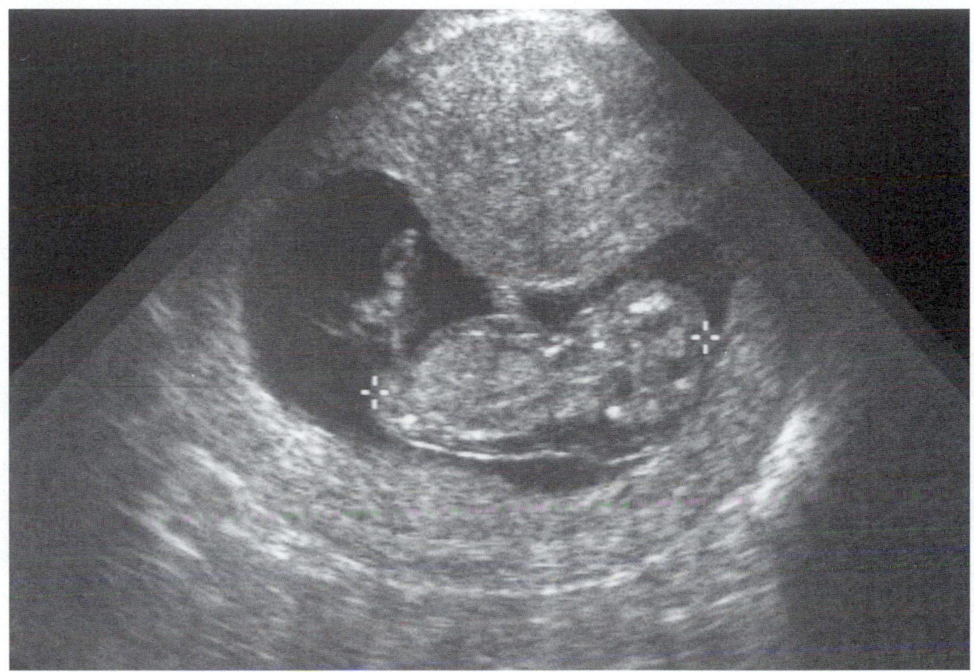

FIGURE 6–1. Intrauterine pregnancy. Sagittal plane through uterus and fetus.

CHAPTER 6

Nuchal Translucency in Turner Syndrome

JUDY A. ESTROFF

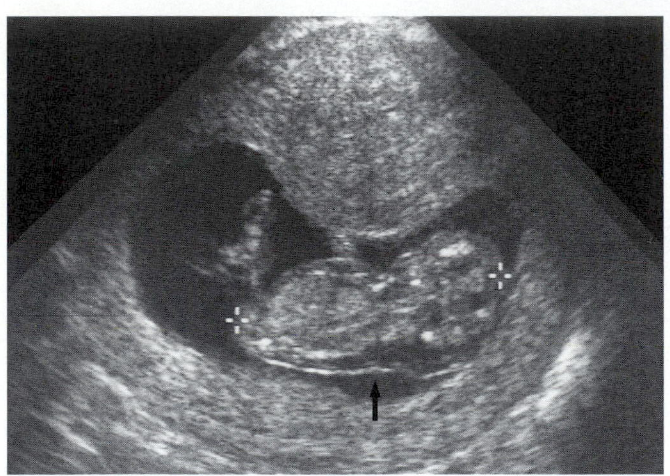

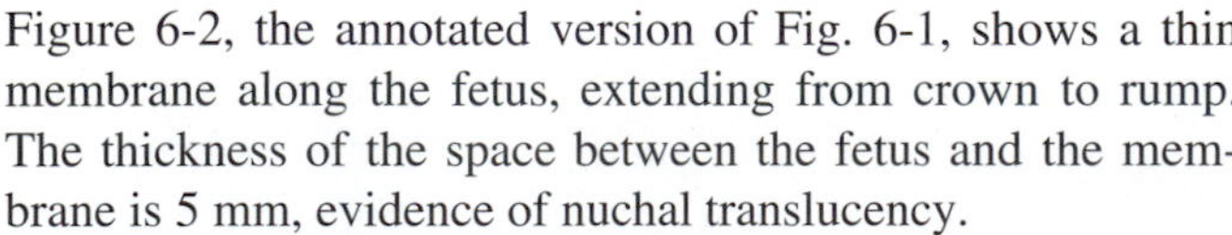

FIGURE 6–2. Annotated version of Fig. 6-1. Intrauterine pregnancy. Sagittal plane through uterus and fetus. The cursor on the reader's left denotes the fetal rump, and the cursor on the reader's right, the fetal cranium. A thin membrane (*arrow*) can be seen extending from the fetal crown to the rump. The thickness of the space between the fetus and the membrane was measured at 5 mm, consistent with nuchal translucency.

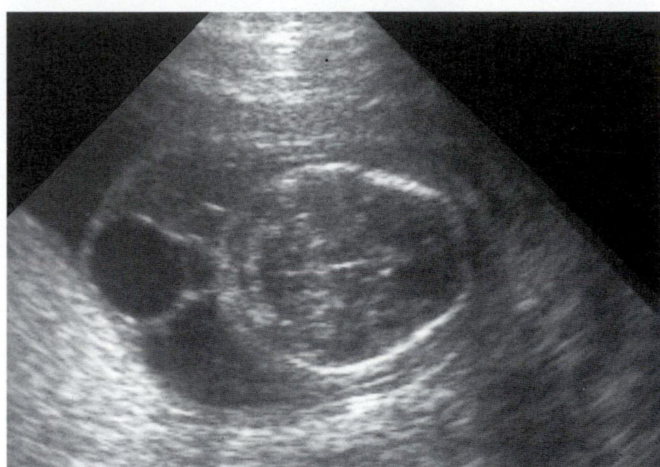

FIGURE 6–3. Cystic hygroma. Fetal head and neck. Axial plane. A septated cystic mass is noted posterior to the calvarium. It proved to be a cystic hygroma in a fetus who on chromosomal analysis proved to have trisomy 18.

Figure 6-2, the annotated version of Fig. 6-1, shows a thin membrane along the fetus, extending from crown to rump. The thickness of the space between the fetus and the membrane is 5 mm, evidence of nuchal translucency.

Nuchal translucency is a commonly used term for abnormal thickness of the skin or tissue at the posterior aspect of the neck and along the back of a first-trimester fetus (i.e., one with a gestational age of less than 13 weeks). When seen in an older fetus, the same finding is often called *cystic hygroma*, *nuchal fold,* or *nuchal thickening* (see Fig. 6-3).

Figures 6-1 and 6-3 can be viewed as a continuum, with the first-trimester nuchal translucency in this case (as in others) progressing to an evident cystic hygroma in the second trimester. Both findings, for the trimester they are discovered in, have similar differential diagnoses. Figure 6-4 is an example of equivalent images for normal fetuses in the first and the second trimester, respectively.

Nuchal translucency and cystic hygroma are associated with the possibility of serious fetal abnormality. This includes karyotype abnormalities such as trisomies 13, 18, and 21; Turner's syndrome (45 XO), and triploidy. It is said that as many as 65 percent of fetuses with cystic hygroma have karyotype abnormalities, with Turner's syndrome being the most common. Some authorities have linked the webbed neck of Turner's syndrome to the residua of the cystic hygroma, which can disappear in later pregnancy.

The presence of nuchal translucency or cystic hygroma is also associated with various congenital anomalies, including

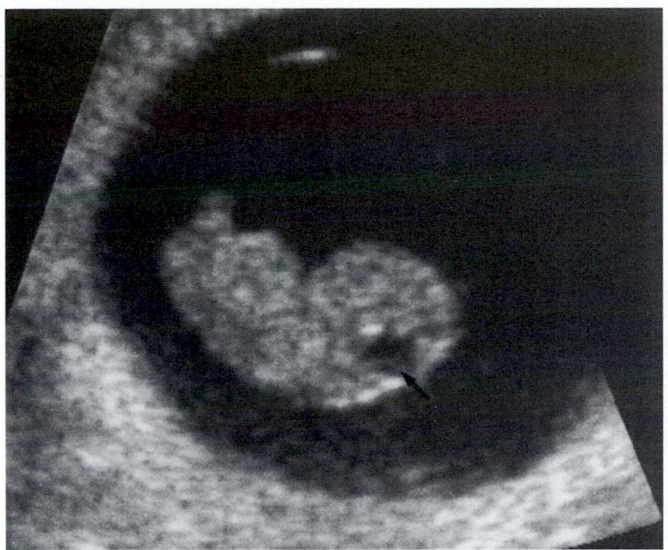

FIGURE 6–4. Normal first-trimester fetus. Sagittal plane through uterus and fetus. The fetal head is on the reader's right. The echopenic area (*arrow*) in the posterior region of this 8.4-week head is the normal rhomboencephalon of the brain, which will eventually become the pons, cerebellum, and medulla oblongata. This area should not be confused with a nuchal translucency because there is no paralleling line separating it from the fetus.

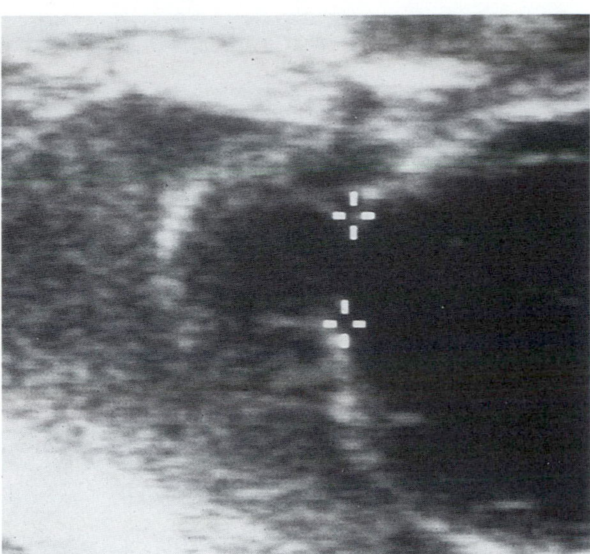

FIGURE 6–5. Encephalocele off posterior calvaria. Axial view. A cystic area is noted posterior to the calvaria of this second-trimester fetus. There is, however, an associated calvarial defect, marked off by crosses. This helped prove the mass to be an encephalocele. Other views that showed brain parenchyma extruding through the defect helped confirm this.

congenital heart disease, renal anomalies, and anterior abdominal wall defects. Cystic hygromas are often present in association with fetal hydrops. Increased alpha fetoprotein levels have been noted in fetuses with cystic hygromas who have Turner's syndrome.

The pathophysiology of nuchal translucency/cystic hygroma is uncertain, but it is generally thought to involve an abnormality in the development of the fetal jugular lymphatic circulatory system.

THE ULTRASONOGRAPHIC DIAGNOSIS

The ultrasonographic diagnosis of nuchal translucency/cystic hygroma depends primarily upon adequate imaging of the fetus, which at times can be improved by the higher-frequency transducers of transvaginal examination, particularly in the first trimester, but usually can be well seen using modern state-of-the-art equipment and routine transvesicle/transabdominal technique. The nuchal region can be visualized and measured in the axial or sagittal plane of section. Overangulation of the plane of measurement, which would produce incorrectly elongated measurements, should be avoided.

MEASUREMENT CRITERIA—WHAT IS ABNORMAL THICKNESS FOR THE NUCHAL AREA?

Controversy exists over what constitutes an abnormal nuchal thickness measurement. What is the threshold measurement that separates normal nuchal area thickness from abnormal? Many ultrasound practitioners consider a measurement of >3 mm in the first trimester to be abnormal and suggest the need for karyotyping. Some will allow thicknesses of up to 4 mm, while others will not accept measurements greater than 2.5 mm. Fetal position and gestational age, as well as the transducer type, the frequency used, and, as mentioned, the ultrasound (US) technique, may lead to difficulties in evaluating the nuchal area and in measuring its thickness. These factors may also affect the reproducibility of measurements obtained by different observers.

Despite the controversies, measurement of the fetal nuchal region has proved to be a significant first-trimester clue to abnormality. Most examiners have found that a septated nuchal translucency (Fig. 6-3) or cystic hygroma carries a poorer prognosis and higher risk of aneuploidy than simple, nonseptated nuchal thickening.

DIFFERENTIAL DIAGNOSIS OF CYSTIC POSTERIOR NECK MASS IN THE SECOND TRIMESTER

When one sees a cystic mass in the posterior neck, one must consider cystic hygroma, but also an occipital encephalocele (Fig. 6-5) and a cervical meningocele. These three possibilities may be readily differentiated if one can see the skull and vertebral body adequately. The encephalocele has an associated calvarial defect, and the meningocele has a vertebral body defect. Only the cystic hygroma has septations within the cystic mass posterior to the neck.

A key point to remember: Whenever nuchal translucency or nuchal thickening is identified, in either the first or the second trimester, chromosomal analysis is warranted. Even if

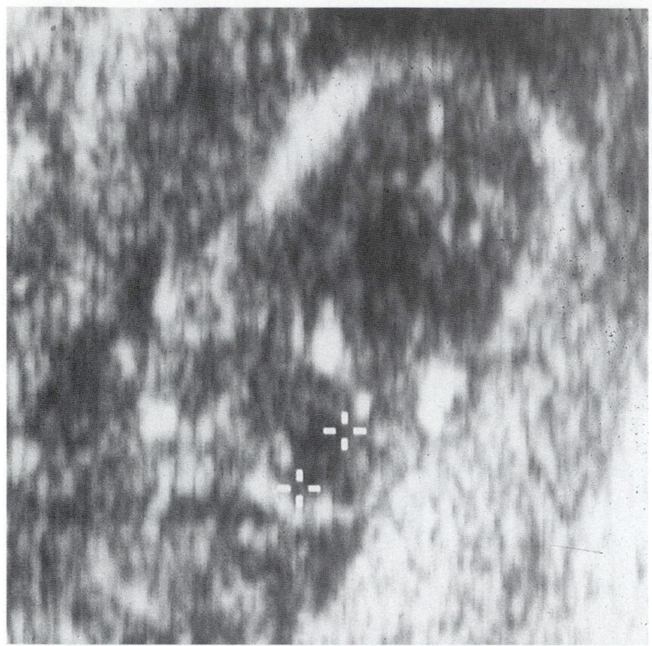

FIGURE 6–6. Small cystic hygroma. Fetal face, neck, and chest. Coronal view. A small cystic hygroma on the left side of this fetus's neck is marked off by arrows.

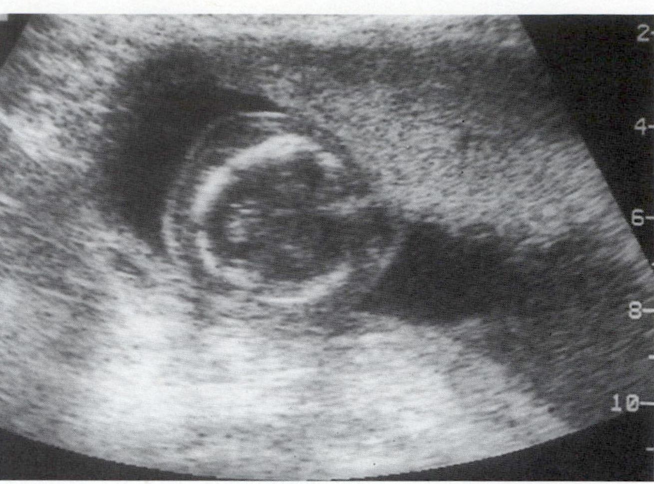

FIGURE 6–7. Fetal hydrops. Fetal head. Axial view. The fetal head is surrounded by a soft tissue density that is not exclusive to the back of the neck. This 16-week-old fetus had hydrops. This represented soft tissue edema. The fetus died soon after this study.

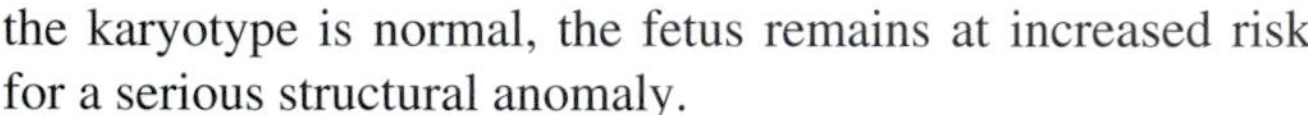

the karyotype is normal, the fetus remains at increased risk for a serious structural anomaly.

Note: Not all cystic hygromas are linked to other abnormalities. Some may be small and difficult to image (Fig. 6-6) and will prove to be only cosmetic problems after birth. Cystic hygromas associated with pleural effusion, ascites, and hydrops fetalis (Fig. 6-7) are to be most worried about.

References

Brambati B, Cislaghi C, Tului L, et al: First-trimester Down's syndrome screening using nuchal translucency: A prospective study in patients undergoing chorionic villus sampling. *Ultrasound Obstet Gynecol* 5:9–14, 1995.

Bronshtein M, Bar-Hava I, Blumenfeld I, et al: The difference between septated and non-septated nuchal cystic hygroma in the early second trimester. *Obstet Gynecol* 81:683–687, 1996.

Bronshtein M, Rottem S, Yoffe N, Blumenfeld Z: First-trimester and early second-trimester diagnosis of nuchal cystic hygroma by transvaginal sonography: Diverse prognosis of the septated from the nonseptated lesion. *Am J Obstet Gynecol* 161:78–82, 1989.

Cha'ban FK, Van Splunder P, Loss FJ, Wladimiroff JW: Fetal outcome in nuchal translucency with emphasis on normal fetal karyotype. *Prenat Diagn* 16:537–541, 1996.

Comas C, Martinez JM, Ojuel J, et al: First-trimester nuchal edema as a marker of aneuploidy. *Ultrasound Obstet Gynecol* 5:26–29, 1995.

Crane JP, Gray DL: Sonographically measured nuchal skinfold thickness as a screening tool for Down syndrome: Results of a prospective clinical trial. *Obstet Gynecol* 77:533–536, 1991.

Hertzberg BS, Bowie JD, Carroll BS, et al: Normal sonographic appearance of the fetal neck late in the first trimester: The pseudomembrane. *Radiology* 171:427–429, 1989.

Hyett JA, Perdu M, Sharland GK, et al: Increased nuchal translucency at 10–14 weeks of gestation as a marker for major cardiac defects. *Ultrasound Obstet Gynecol* 10:242–246, 1997.

Nadel AN, Bromley B, Benacerraf BR: Nuchal thickening or cystic hygromas in first- and early second-trimester fetuses: Prognosis and outcome. *Obstet Gynecol* 82:43–46, 1993.

Nguyen K: The fetal face and neck, in *A Practical Guide to Ultrasound in Obstetrics and Gynecology,* 2d ed, Sauerbei E, Nguyen K, Nolan R (eds). Philadelphia, Lippincott-Raven, 1998: 228–239.

Nicolaides KH, Azar G, Byrne D, et al: Fetal nuchal translucency: Ultrasound screening for chromosomal defects in first trimester of pregnancy. *Br Med J* 304:867–869, 1992.

Pandya PP, Kondylios A, Hilbert L, et al: Chromosomal defects and outcome in 1015 fetuses with increased nuchal translucency. *Ultrasound Obstet Gynecol* 5:15–19, 1995.

Pandya PP, Snijders RJM, Johnson SP, et al: Screening for fetal trisomies by maternal age and fetal nuchal thickness at 10–14 weeks of gestation. *Br J Obstet Gynaecol* 12:957–962, 1995.

Reynders CS, Pauker SP, Benacerraf BR: First trimester isolated fetal nuchal lucency: Significance and outcome. *J Ultrasound Med* 16:101–105, 1997.

Taipale P, Hiilesmaa V, Salonen R, Ylostalo P: Increased nuchal translucency as a marker for fetal chromosomal defects. *N Engl J Med* 337:1654–1658, 1997.

Section B
FETAL CHEST

7

The mother of this fetus was referred to you for a routine fetal anatomic survey. Figures 7-1 and 7-2 represent two images of the fetal chest. What is your diagnosis?

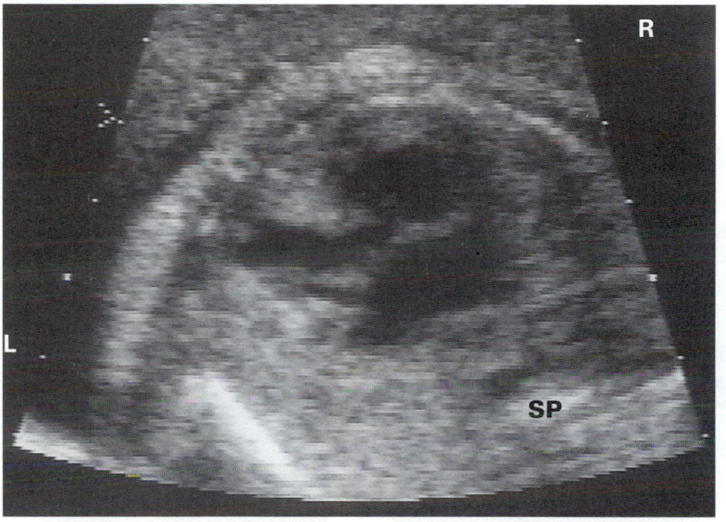

FIGURE 7–1. Fetal chest. Transverse view during systole. L = left, Right = right, SP = spine.

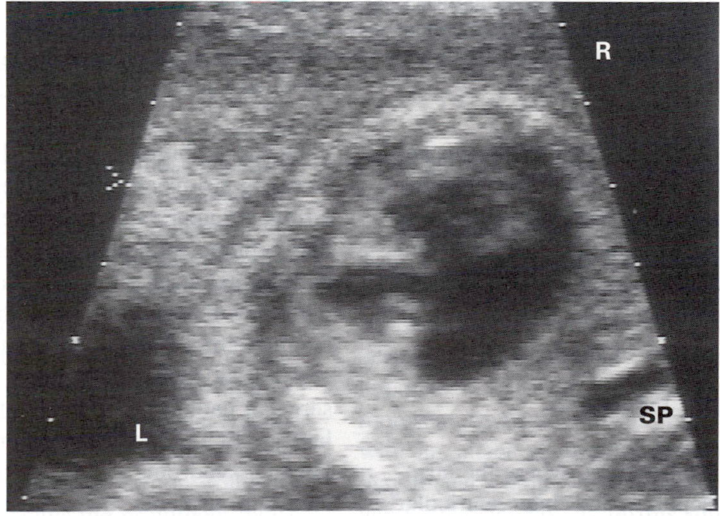

FIGURE 7–2. Fetal chest. Transverse view during diastole. L = left, Right = right, SP = spine.

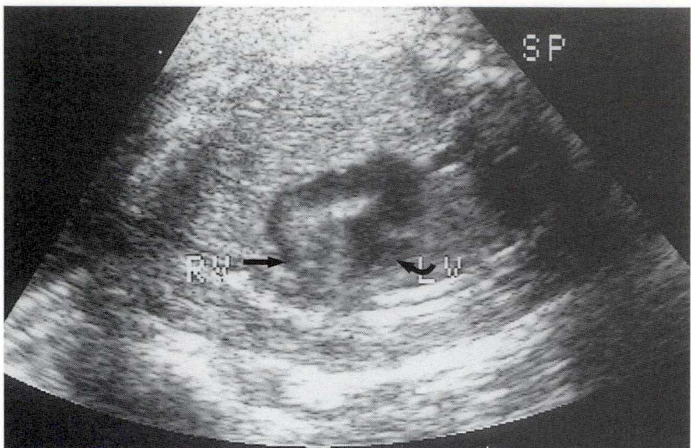

FIGURE 7–8. Abnormal four-chamber heart view—tricuspid atresia. This fetus of 28 weeks gestation has a right ventricular cavity that is significantly smaller than the left ventricular cavity. The fetus proved to have tricuspid atresia.

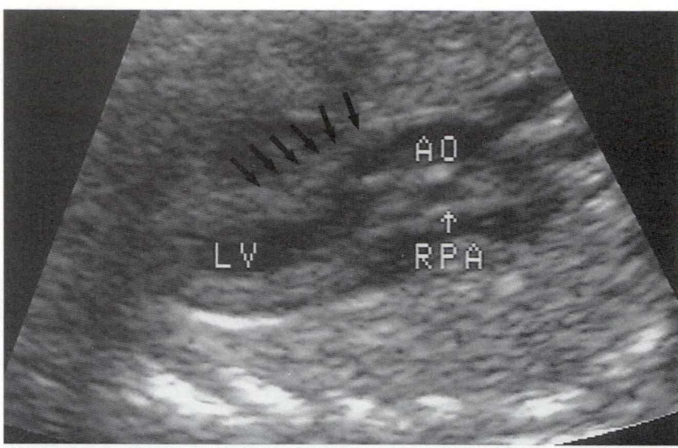

FIGURE 7–9. Normal long-axis view of the left ventricular outflow tract. There is evident continuity between the interventricular septum and the anterior wall of the aorta.

Analysis of Outflow Tracts

Although current standards for fetal ultrasound evaluation indicate the four-chamber heart view as necessary for every comprehensive fetal anatomic ultrasound examination, limiting evaluation of the fetal heart to this standard view will limit diagnosis. Certainly, abnormalities of the great vessels, such as tetralogy of Fallot (TOF), transposition of the great vessels (TOGV), or truncus arteriosus, may by missed if the outflow tracts are not visualized. The identification of the outflow tracts in addition to the four-chamber view may significantly increase the sensitivity for diagnosing heart anomalies. This can be difficult, but one should try. When studying the outflow tracts, one must identify the origins of the great vessels from the ventricles, identify the bifurcation or even trifurcation into right and left pulmonary arteries and ductus arteriosus, and note the aorta and its arch vessels. One should confirm that the aorta and pulmonary artery cross each other and are of comparable size, which is the normal state. Paralleling great vessels on this view suggests abnormality.

To do a complete outflow tract examination, attempt to obtain long- and short-axis views through the right and left ventricular outflow tracts. The long-axis view of the left ventricular outflow can be obtained by angling toward the fetal head from the four-chamber view and rotating the transducer (Fig. 7-9). The aorta originates from the center of the heart, and the ascending aorta extends toward the right. Demonstration of the continuity between the anterior wall of the aorta and the interventricular septum is crucial for excluding an overriding aorta, which is seen in cases of TOF or double-outlet right ventricle (DORV). Further superior angulation of the ultrasound beam will reveal the right ventricular outflow in a plane perpendicular to the aorta (Fig. 7-10). Scanning between the right and left long-axis views enables appreciation of the "crisscross" relationship of the great vessels. The right ventricular outflow tract is more anterior than the left ventricular outflow tract and is directed posteriorly toward the descending aorta. Long-axis views of the outflow tracts will enable visualization of membranous VSDs, as well as the assessment of semilunar (aortic, pulmonic) valve motion.

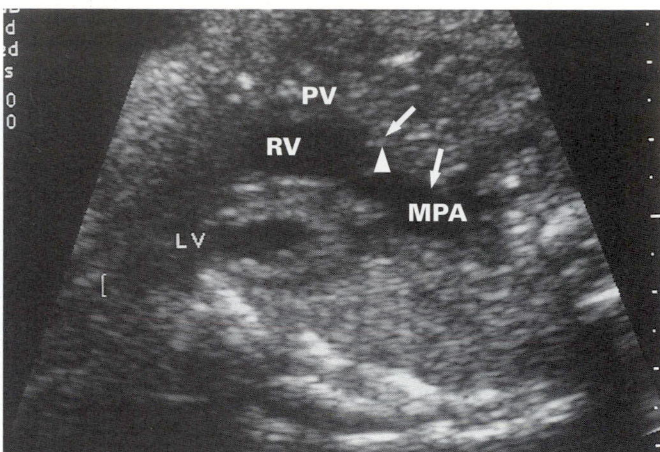

FIGURE 7–10. Normal long-axis view of the right ventricular outflow tract. The right ventricular outflow tract is anterior to the left ventricular outflow tract. An arrow points to the main pulmonary artery and an arrowhead points to the pulmonic valve, which are both normal.

A New Recently Described View (by Yoo)—The Three-Vessel View

If, when angling cephalically from the four-chamber heart view, one increases the angle in an even more cephalic direction through the superior mediastinum of the fetus, one has the "three-vessel view," whereby one can identify the main pulmonary artery, ascending aorta, and superior vena cava (SVC) in a straight line of decreasing size (Fig. 7-11). In this view, one can image the main pulmonary artery running perpendicular to the ascending aorta and see the full length of the ductus arteriosus. This three-vessel view can reveal pathology related to abnormalities of vessel size, alignment,

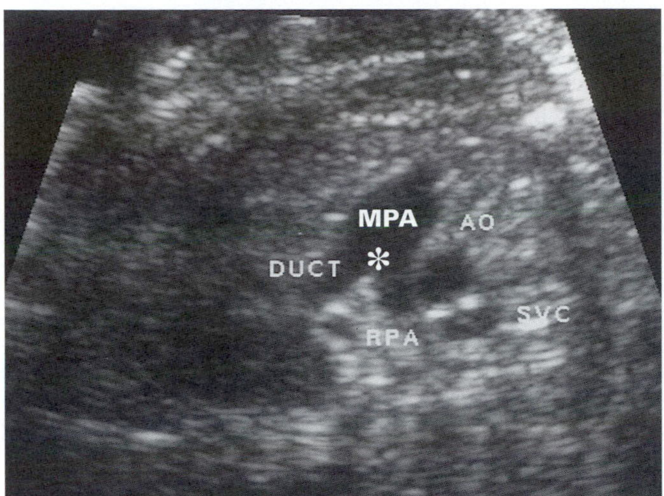

FIGURE 7–11. Normal three-vessel view of the fetal heart. An asterisk denotes the bifurcation of the main pulmonary artery into the ductus arteriosus (DUCT) and right pulmonary artery (RPA), which courses posterior to the ascending aorta (AO).

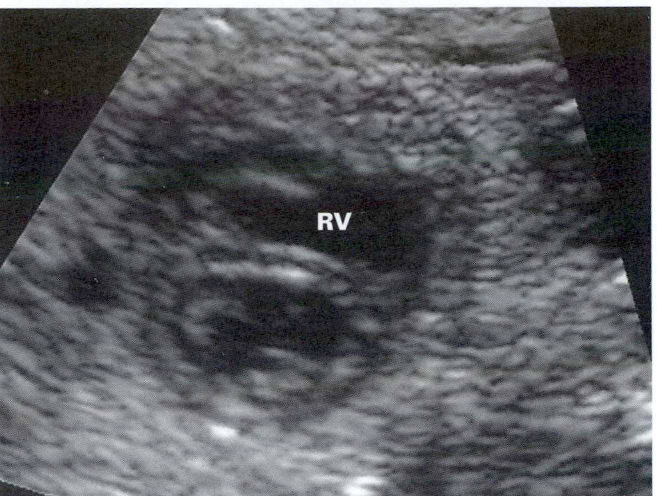

FIGURE 7–12. Normal short-axis view through the cardiac ventricles. The right ventricle is anterior to the more posterior left ventricle.

position, and number. Such abnormalities can be seen in cases of TOF, DORV, and complete and corrected TOGV. In complete TOGV, the aorta and the pulmonary artery are abnormally parallel, with the aorta being the more anterior vessel.

Short-Axis Views

Finally, short-axis views (Fig. 7-12) can be obtained by orienting the transducer parallel to the fetal spine and gently rocking from left to right through the fetal heart. Starting on the left, the short axis through the ventricles offers a view of the papillary muscles that enhances one's ability to assess ventricular contractility and to note VSDs. As one sweeps the transducer's field of view toward the right of the fetus, one can again confirm the normal perpendicular relationship of the great vessels by imaging the pulmonary artery wrapping around the aorta, seen in cross section (Fig. 7-13). The pulmonary valve should be identified to the left of the aortic valve and in a position more anterior to it.

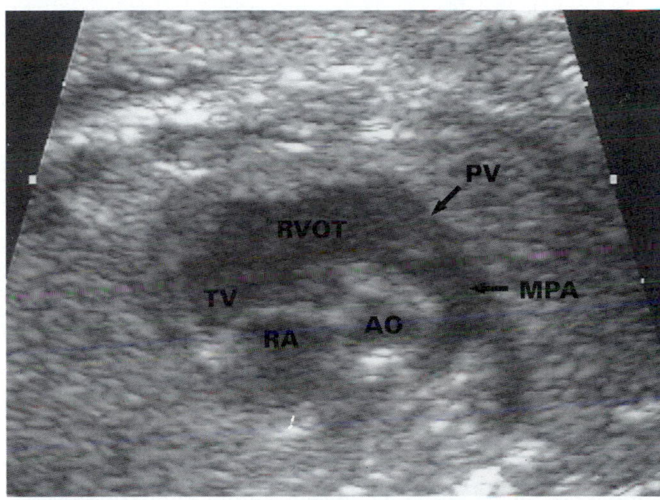

FIGURE 7–13. Normal short-axis view through the cardiac great vessels. This view is obtained in a more cephalic plane of the fetus than Fig. 7-12. The right ventricular outflow tract (RVOT) wraps around the aorta (AO). (RA = right atrium, TV = tricuspid valve, MPA = main pulmonary artery.) An arrowhead points to the pulmonic valve (PV).

FINAL THOUGHTS REGARDING THE DIAGNOSIS OF AV CANAL DEFECTS

The common atrioventricular valve that exists in a fetus's AV canal defect is readily imaged in the four-chamber heart view. The atrioventricular defect is best seen during diastole (Figs. 7-2 and 7-4). During systole (Figs. 7-1 and 7-3), the atrial defect is easily seen, but the ventricular defect may be harder to visualize. This is due to the attachment of the chordae tendineae of the common atrioventricular valve to the crest of the ventricular septum, and the resultant obscuration of the defect. Assessment of chamber size in an AV canal defect is important, since one ventricle may be dominant in these defects. The origin of the aorta can also be difficult to discern, as it has lost its normal origin from the center of the heart. Attempts should be made to follow the course of the ventricular outflow tracts, since TOGV may be an associated abnormality. Other associated defects include TOF, DORV, aortic coarctation, pulmonic stenosis, and pulmonary atresia. Although color Doppler is not necessary for diagnosing an AV canal defect, color and pulsed Doppler can aid in the detection of atrioventricular valve incompetence, as well as help in identifying great vessel abnormalities.

Note: In discussing examination of the fetal heart, which requires rigorous practice to perfect technique and in difficult cases is best accomplished by cardiac ultrasound specialists, one must remember key pieces of information to provide the requesting clinician that are truly within the scope of all ultrasound practitioners. Some of these are summarized in

TABLE 7-1
Fast Facts: The Normal Fetal Heart

RV = LV (the right ventricle is essentially equal in size to the left ventricle)
RA = LA (the right atrium is essentially equal in size to the left atrium)
RV contains an echogenic area (the moderator band)
AO = PA (the aorta and pulmonary artery are essentially equal in size when exiting the heart)
PA is anterior (the pulmonary artery takes off from the anterior heart and bifurcates)
AO is posterior (the aorta arises from the middle of the heart and has branches off its arch)

Key: AO = aorta, LA = left atrium, LV = left ventricle, PA = pulmonary artery, RA = right atrium, RV = right ventricle.

TABLE 7-2
Important Points to Note Even If Intracardiac Anatomy Is Poorly Seen

1. **Cardiac Rate:** be wary when greater than 180 bpm or less than 100 bpm
2. **Cardiac Position:** be wary when cardiac apex is on the opposite side of the stomach
3. **Cardiac Axis:** be wary of angulation of the heart to midline of less than 25 and greater than 65°

Table 7-1. In addition, one should look for a regular heartbeat at a rate, in the second trimester and beyond, of 140 to 160. Heart rate can be assessed through M-mode techniques and a software analysis of time between beats. This method can also be used to note dissociations of atrial and ventricular rates. One should worry about tachycardia when cardiac rates are 180 beats per minute or greater, particularly when there is dissociation of atrial and ventricular rates. Bradycardia is of concern at a rate below 100 beats per minute. Anasarca, pleural effusion, and ascites are obviously of great concern and may signify cardiac failure.

A particularly important point in surveying for possible congenital heart disease (CHD), even if the cardiac anatomy may not be well imaged, is the position of the stomach in relation to the cardiac apex. Chances of CHD are greater than 90 percent when the cardiac apex is on the side opposite to that of the fetal stomach. Chances of CHD are less than 1 percent when the cardiac apex and the stomach are on the left and about 5 percent when the cardiac apex and stomach are on the right (cardiac and abdominal situs inversus). Because of the above, we specifically seek this information on all our exams (Table 7-2).

The heart should also maintain an angle (relative to a line drawn down the midline on axial views of the chest) of 45 ± 20°. Significant deviation from this, even when the apex is on the left, is associated with heart defects. An angle of greater than 75° has been linked to a 75 percent chance of cardiac abnormality.

References

Benacerraf BR: Sonographic detection of fetal anomalies of the aortic and pulmonary arteries: Value of four-chamber view vs. direct images. *AJR* 163:1483–1489, 1994.

Brown DL, DiSalvo DN, Frates MC, et al: Sonography of the fetal heart: Normal variants and pitfalls. *AJR* 160:1251–1255, 1993.

Copel JA, Morotti R, Hobbins JC, Kleinman CS: The antenatal diagnosis of congenital heart disease using fetal echocardiography: Is color flow mapping necessary? *Obstet Gynecol* 78:1–8, 1991.

DeVore GR: The aortic and pulmonary outflow tract screening examination in the human fetus. *J Ultrasound Med* 11:345–348, 1992.

DeVore GR: Color Doppler examination of the outflow tracts of the fetal heart: A technique for identification of cardiovascular malformations. *Ultrasound Obstet Gynecol* 4:463–471, 1994.

Drose J: Scanning: Indications and technique, in *Fetal Echocardiography,* Drose J (ed). Philadelphia, Saunders, 1998:15–58.

Ferencz C, Rubin JD, McCarter RJ, et al: Cardiac and noncardiac malformations: Observations in a population-based study. *Teratology* 35:367–378, 1987.

Kirk JS, Riggs TW, Comstock CH, et al: Prenatal screening for cardiac anomalies: The value of routine addition of the aortic root to the four-chamber view. *Obstet Gynecol* 84:427–431, 1994.

Machado MVL, Crawford DC, Anderson RH, Allan LD: Atrioventricular septal defect in prenatal life. *Br Heart J* 59:352–355, 1988.

McGahan JP: Sonography of the fetal heart: Findings on the four-chamber view. *AJR* 156:547–553, 1991.

Shipp T, Bromley B, Hornberger L: Levorotation of the fetal cardiac axis: A clue for the presence of congenital heart disease. *Obstet Gynecol* 85:97–102, 1995.

Wigton TR, Sabbagha RE, Tamura RK, et al: Sonographic diagnosis of congenital heart disease: Comparison between the four-chamber view and multiple cardiac views. *Obstet Gynecol* 82:219–224, 1993.

Yoo SJ, Lee H, Kim ES, et al: Three-vessel view of the fetal upper mediastinum: An easy means of detecting abnormalities of the ventricular outflow tracts and great arteries during obstetric screening. *Ultrasound Obstet Gynecol* 9:173–182, 1997.

8

Figure 8-1 is an axial view of a second-trimester fetal chest. The sonographer is perturbed by the image. Are you? What, if anything, should be considered or done?

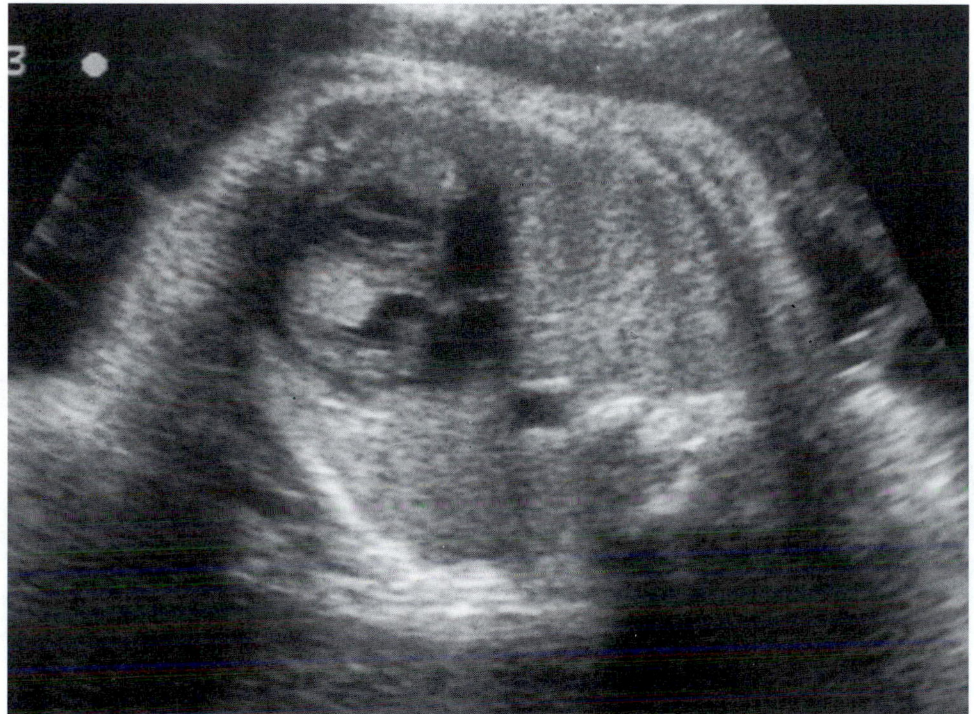

FIGURE 8–1. Fetal chest. Axial view.

CHAPTER 8

Cardiac Rhabdomyoma

HARRIS L. COHEN

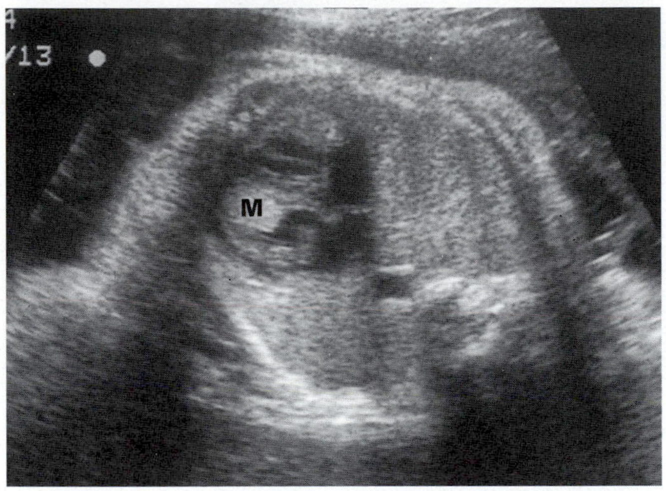

FIGURE 8–2. Annotated version of Fig. 8-1. Fetal chest. Axial view. An echogenic mass is noted in the left cardiac ventricle. This proved to be a cardiac rhabdomyoma.

Figure 8-2, the annotated version of Fig. 8-1, shows two normally and symmetrically echogenic lungs. The heart accounts for only one-third of the intrathoracic contents. Four cardiac chambers and two atrioventricular valves are noted. The two cardiac ventricles and two atria appear to be of equal size. All these findings are normal. However, there is an echogenic mass within the heart's left ventricle. It is too big to be a commonly seen echogenic focus. A tumor must be the diagnosis of concern. This mass proved to be a cardiac rhabdomyoma. Its implications and the differential diagnosis of such a mass will be discussed.

WHAT ARE THE POSSIBLE FETAL CARDIAC MASSES?

In fetal life, the cardiac ventricles are equal in size. Although the right ventricle has somewhat more contained echogenicity as a result of the presence of the normal moderator band, the normal ventricular chambers are essentially symmetrical in their contents, and predominantly echoless (Fig. 8-3) because of the contained circulating blood. These chambers should contain no masses. If a mass is seen, a tumor must be ruled out.

Congenital cardiac tumors or masses are rare in fetal life, with an occurrence rate of 0.027 percent. Rhabdomyomas are the most common pediatric cardiac tumors (Fig. 8-4), representing 60 percent of cases. Another 21 percent are teratomas, which are not truly cardiac but usually pericardial and are imaged as a mass of cystic and calcified areas. If a mass is seen within the pericardium or extending elsewhere in the chest but not within the heart itself, a more specific diagnosis of teratoma can be made. Some 13 percent of pediatric cardiac tumors are fibromas, but these have not, as yet,

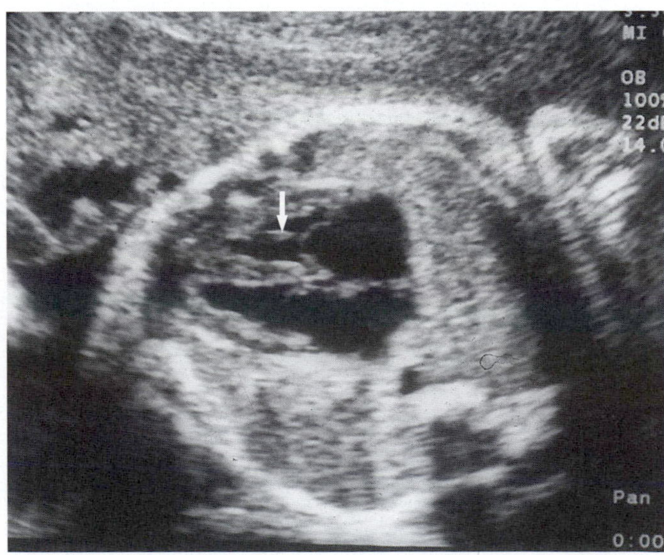

FIGURE 8–3. Normal fetal heart. Axial view of chest. The fetal left side is on the reader's left. No mass is seen in the ventricular chambers. A small echogenicity (*arrow*) in the right chamber is related to a small portion of the normally contained moderator band.

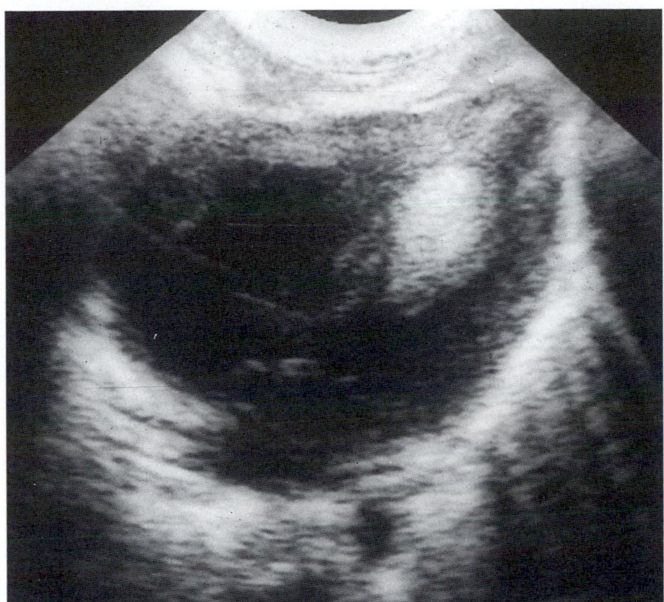

FIGURE 8–4. Neonatal heart. Longitudinal plane. This is an image of our unknown case's heart after birth. The echogenic mass is again noted in the left lateral ventricle attached to the interventricular septum. It proved to be a rhabdomyoma in a patient with tuberous sclerosis.

been identified in a fetus. Atrial myxoma, which is the most common cardiac tumor in adults, is rare in the neonate.

Pediatric cardiac tumors are typically benign, with less than 10 percent becoming malignant. Symptoms may arise from inflow or outflow obstruction or arrhythmia, which can lead to congestive heart failure (CHF). In the fetus, one must therefore be wary of the associated development of pleural effusion, ascites, pericardial effusion, and generalized edema (anasarca). All cardiac tumors can potentially cause arrhythmia. On occasion, cardiac tumors may be simulated by intrathoracic masses that may compress or displace the heart. These may include cystic adenomatoid malformations or pulmonary sequestrations.

WHAT ARE THE CHARACTERISTICS OF THE CARDIAC RHABDOMYOMA?

Cardiac rhabdomyomas can be found as echogenic masses within any and all of the four cardiac chambers. They typically, as in this case, arise from the ventricular septum and can be multiple. If multiple cardiac tumors are noted, the diagnosis is rhabdomyoma until disproven. Unusually, they may infiltrate the myocardium, simulating ventricular hypertrophy.

Fetuses and children with rhabdomyomas may have supraventricular tachycardia. This is thought to be due to accessory conductive pathways in the tumor itself. Intrauterine growth retardation (IUGR) has been reported in some affected fetuses. Spontaneous regression of the tumor has been reported. Between 50 and 86 percent of patients with cardiac rhabdomyomas also have tuberous sclerosis.

WHAT IS TUBEROUS SCLEROSIS?

Tuberous sclerosis is a multisystem disease. It is usually inherited in an autosomal dominant pattern with a variable to high degree of penetrance. It can occur sporadically in the offspring of unaffected families. Its classic triad of symptoms includes mental retardation, seizures, and adenoma sebaceum, a facial hamartomatous condition that can resemble acne but is made up of sebaceous glands and fibrovascular tissue. Only one-fourth of affected patients have mental retardation or seizures. After birth, hypomelanotic skin macules are often seen. Many of these patients have associated cortical tubers and subependymal hamartomas that can result in noncalcified masses as well as calcified intracranial masses, which may be noted on computed tomography (CT) (Fig. 8-5). These patients may also suffer from associated retinal hamartomas, renal hamartomas, and periungual fibromas.

WHAT ABOUT THE COMMONLY SEEN TINY BRIGHT ECHOGENIC FOCUS IN THE FETAL HEART—SHOULD ONE WORRY?

Our unknown case showed an obvious mass, which is different from the often-seen single tiny bright focus in the fetal heart (Fig. 8-6). These foci are seen in the left ventricle 93

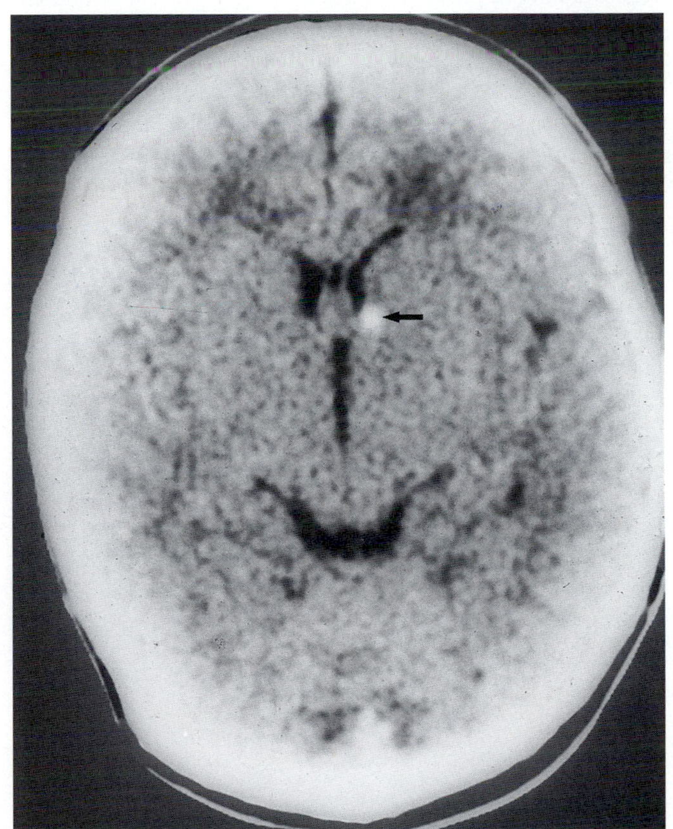

FIGURE 8–5. Tuberous sclerosis. Head CT. A calcified subependymal hamartoma (*arrows*) is seen in the left subependymal area of this neonate. Other calcified masses were seen at different intracranial levels. This is the same patient as in Figs. 8-1, 8-2, and 8-4.

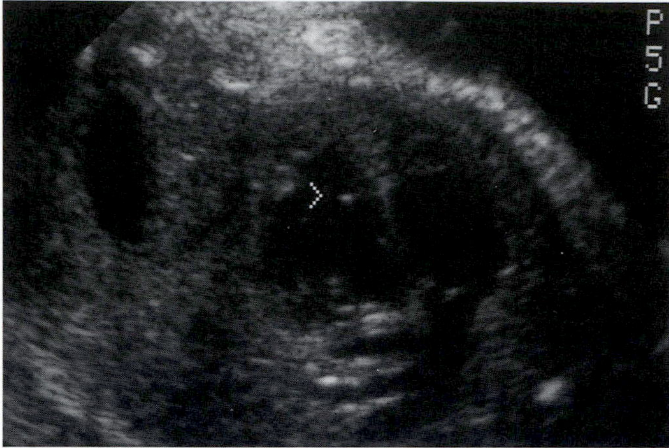

FIGURE 8–6. Bright echogenic focus. Four-chamber heart view. A tiny bright focus (*arrowhead*) is noted in the left ventricle. It is thought to be due to echogenic reflection from a papillary muscle. Some echogenicity in the right ventricle is due to the normal moderator band. The fetus showed no other anatomic abnormality and was normal after birth.

percent of the time and are imaged in 0.46 to 4.8 percent of all normal fetuses. The finding is therefore not uncommon. These foci are thought to be due to a reflection from either papillary muscle or chordae tendineae. For many years their presence was considered completely innocuous. However, over the last 5 years, one group has found an 18 percent incidence among a group of trisomy 21 patients, and another group, a 10 percent incidence among trisomy 13 patients. An autopsy study showed a 2 percent incidence of this calcification, proven pathologically to be due to papillary muscle calcification, in normal fetuses but as high an incidence as 16.5 percent among fetuses with trisomy 21 and 38.9 percent among fetuses with trisomy.

REMEMBER: WHEN SEEING A BRIGHT ECHOGENIC FOCUS IN THE FETAL HEART, CONSIDER A POSSIBLE TRISOMY

Yes, if an echogenic focus is seen, one has to worry. After ruling out the possibility of a rhabdomyoma or teratoma, one must still, at the very least, study the fetal anatomy carefully for any other abnormality or sign suggestive of associated trisomy 13 or 21. However, it is seen in many normal fetuses.

References

Benacerraf B: The second-trimester fetus with Down syndrome: Detection using sonographic features. *Ultrasound Obstet Gynecol* 7:147–155, 1996.

Callen P: Cardiac echogenic focus (bright papillary muscle), in *An Interactive Diagnostic Ultrasound Text and Journal Focusing on Obstetrics and Gynecology,* Callen P (ed). San Francisco, Ultrasound Educational Press, 1998.

Cyr D, Guntheroth W, Smith K, Winter T: Fetal echocardiography, in *Diagnostic Medical Sonography. A Guide to Clinical Practice. Obstetrics and Gynecology,* Berman M, Cohen HL (eds). Philadelphia, Lippincott, 1997:321–343.

Dennis M, Appareti K, Manco-Johnson M, et al: The echocardiographic diagnosis of multiple fetal cardiac tumors. *J Ultrasound Med* 4:327–329, 1985.

Drose J: Scanning: Indications and technique, in *Fetal Echocardiography,* Drose J (ed). Philadelphia, Saunders, 1998:15–58.

Harding C, Pagon R: Incidence of tuberous sclerosis in patients with cardiac rhabdomyoma. *Am J Med Genet* 37:443–446, 1990.

Lehman C, Nyberg D, Winter T, et al: Trisomy 13 syndrome: Prenatal US findings in a review of 33 cases. *Radiology* 194: 217–222, 1995.

Manco-Johnson M, Drose J: Congenital cardiac tumors, in *Fetal Echocardiography,* Drose J (ed). Philadelphia, Saunders, 1998: 241–251.

Platt L, Devore G, Horenstein J, et al: Prenatal diagnosis of tuberous sclerosis: The use of fetal echocardiography. *Prenat Diagn* 7:407–411, 1987.

Roberts D, Genest D: Cardiac histologic pathology characteristics of trisomy 13 and 21. *Hum Pathol* 23:1130–1140, 1992.

Romero R, Pilu G, Jeanty P, et al: *Prenatal Diagnosis of Congenital Anomalies.* Norwalk, CT, Appleton & Lange, 1988:182–183.

Smythe J: Fetal heart and great vessels, in *A Practical Guide to Ultrasound in Obstetrics and Gynecology,* 2d ed, Sauerbrei E, Nguyen K, Nolan R (eds). Philadelphia, Lippincott-Raven, 1998:240–277.

Smythe J, Dyek J, Smallhorn J, et al: Natural history of cardiac rhabdomyomas in infancy and childhood. *Am J Cardiol* 66:1247–1249, 1990.

9

An axial view through this fetal chest (Fig. 9-1) is of concern. What is the diagnosis? Are there any other possible diagnoses?

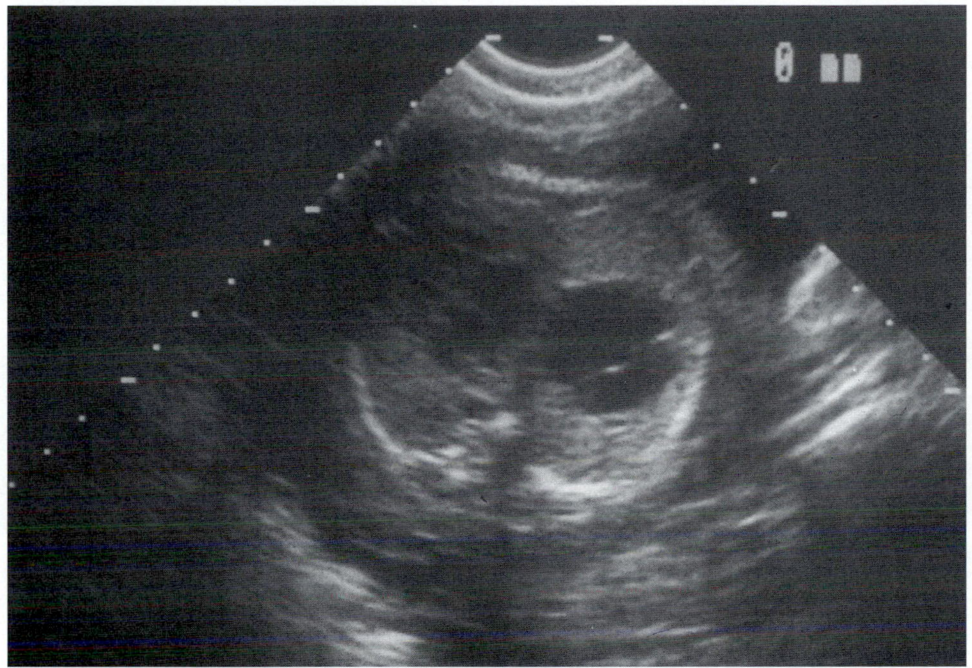

FIGURE 9–1. Fetal chest. Axial plane.

CHAPTER 9

Bronchogenic Cyst

HARRIS L. COHEN AND ANNA GOLJA

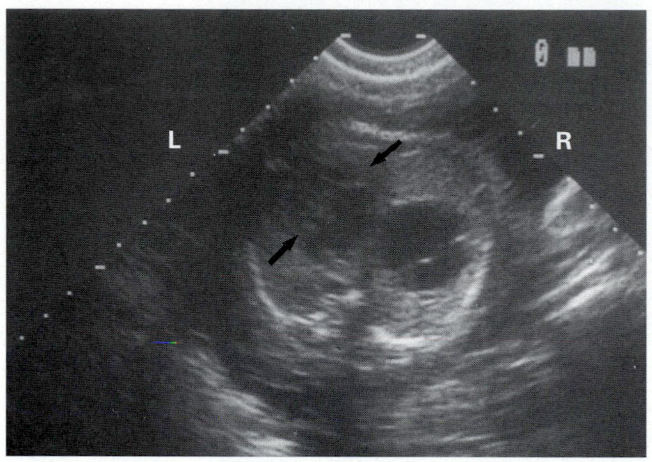

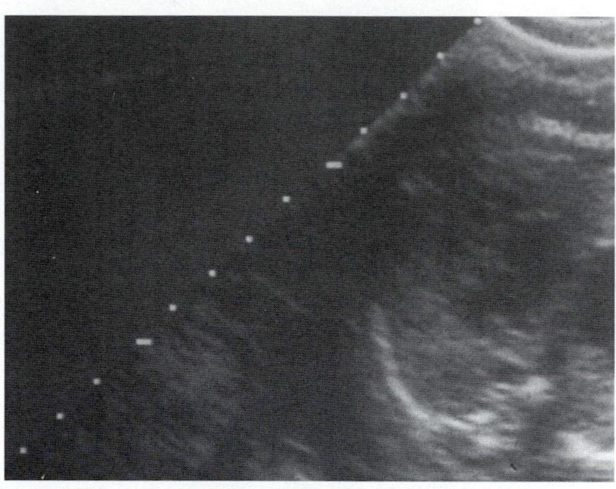

A *B*

FIGURE 9–2. Bronchogenic cyst. ***A.*** Annotated version of Fig. 9-1. Fetal chest. Axial plane. The heart (*arrows*), denoted by its two ventricles, can be seen in the left chest. There is some apparent mass impression from the right lung, which is somewhat enlarged due to a contained cystic mass with an apparent septation. The mass is completely surrounded by more echogenic lung parenchyma. It proved to be a bronchogenic cyst. ***B.*** Fetal chest. Longitudinal plane through right chest. The cystic mass is again seen surrounded by lung parenchyma in this orthogonal plane. R = right, L = left, INF = inferior, SUP = superior.

Figure 9-2*A*, the annotated version of Fig. 9-1, and 9-2*B*, a longitudinal view, shows a cystic mass in the right lung. This is abnormal, since the fetal lungs should be homogeneous in echogenicity, with the only echoless area being the heart chambers that separate them. All cases in which there are deviations in lung echogenicity pattern from homogeneous and solid should be suspect for abnormality. Those lung masses that communicate with the bronchus may fill with amniotic fluid and appear echoless. This fetus was proven as a neonate to have a bronchogenic cyst.

FETAL LUNG MASSES AND LUNG HYPOPLASIA

Fetal lung masses include only a few differential diagnostic possibilities. A bronchogenic cyst is statistically a less likely possibility than the cystic adenomatoid malformation or pulmonary sequestration. The key concern, regardless of the pathology of the mass, is whether there is significant lung compression and whether there is significant compromise to the intrathoracic space necessary for further lung growth and development. This is not a great clinical concern for this fetus. However, such compression of the lung may lead to the development of pulmonary hypoplasia (Fig. 9-3), which is a significant clinical concern, depending on its degree, after birth. The greater the degree of pulmonary hypoplasia, the more difficult is survival when breathing becomes necessary. Lung masses may push the diaphragm inferiorly and the mediastinum and contralateral lung away. This can lead to compromise of these structures as well. Long-term lung compression has been linked to persistent fetal pulmonary circulation in the neonate.

The development of pulmonary hypoplasia is not caused only by pulmonary masses. It also occurs when there is re-

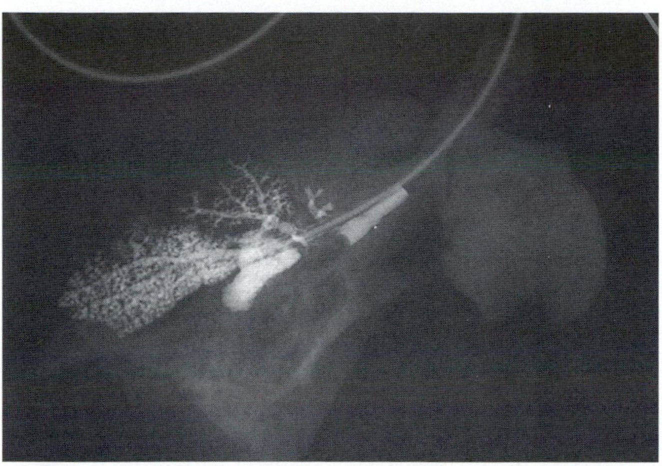

FIGURE 9–3. Lung hypoplasia. Pathology specimen. Contrast is seen in the bronchi and alveoli of the normal lung. Moderate to significant hypoplasia is seen in the contralateral lung. This neonate died shortly after birth. The hypoplasia was secondary to the long-term mass effect of a diaphragmatic hernia.

striction of growth of the thoracic cavity, either because of decreased amniotic fluid, e.g., in patients with bilateral renal agenesis or obstruction, or when there are skeletal deformities that limit thoracic growth. Masses from below the diaphragm, such as the diaphragmatic hernia, can do the same, compromising the lung or lungs and leading to morbidity and mortality on the basis of pulmonary hypoplasia, even with proper surgical repair. Various intrathoracic masses that may occur in the fetus are noted in Table 9-1.

TABLE 9-1
Fetal Intrathoracic Masses

Common
Hydrothorax—pleural effusion—surrounds the lung with echless fluid
Congenital diaphragmatic hernia—bowel, organs in chest, no left upper quadrant stomach
Cystic adenomatoid malformation—cystic (types I and II) and solid (type III—tiny cysts)
Pulmonary sequestration—normal pulmonary tissue, abnormal vascular supply
Less common
Bronchogenic cyst—usually unilocular; can be multilocular
Neurenteric cyst—associated spinal defect
Enteric cyst—rare duplication of the esophagus; may image as cyst in thorax
Bronchial atresia with distended distal lung
Rarer
Rhabdomyoma, fetal goiter, intrathoracic cystic hygroma, pericardial or mediastinal teratoma, neuroblastoma

From Cohen, Torrisi, and Schwartz; and Nolan, with permission.

UNILATERAL FETAL LUNG MASS—WHAT SHOULD I CONSIDER IN THE DIAGNOSIS?

Half of all fetal intrathoracic abnormalities are pleural effusions. They are echoless and surround the lung (Fig. 9-4). Pleural effusion is rarely due to an intrathoracic mass and its associated compression. It is most often part of an extrathoracic process such as fetal hydrops.

The key intrathoracic masses to consider are the bronchogenic cyst and, even more so, cystic adenomatoid malformation and pulmonary sequestration, all of which appear to be part of the lung parenchyma. These masses may be cystic or solid. Solid masses that are isoechoic to the lung parenchyma are the most difficult to image, especially if they are small and not creating a cardiac or mediastinal shift through the mass effect.

The predominant cystic masses of the lung are bronchogenic cysts, which are most often unilocular, and cystic adenomatoid malformations, of which types I and II are seen as multicystic masses. Pulmonary sequestration appears solid.

WHAT IS A BRONCHOGENIC CYST?

A few cases of antenatally detected bronchogenic cysts, including this one (Figs. 9-1 and 9-2), have been reported. They are not common. I have imaged only two such cases. Bronchogenic cysts are thought to occur as the result of abnormal budding or branching of the tracheobronchial tree between the fourth and sixth weeks of fetal life. These cysts may be unilocular or multilocular. They are not associated with other congenital anomalies. They may displace mediastinal structures or cause bronchial obstruction, although this is an uncommon finding in neonatal life. They are lined by epithelium similar to that of a normal bronchus and may contain cartilage, muscle, or mucus glands. They may be found within the lung parenchyma or mediastinum, and they often communicate with the trachea or mainstem bronchi.

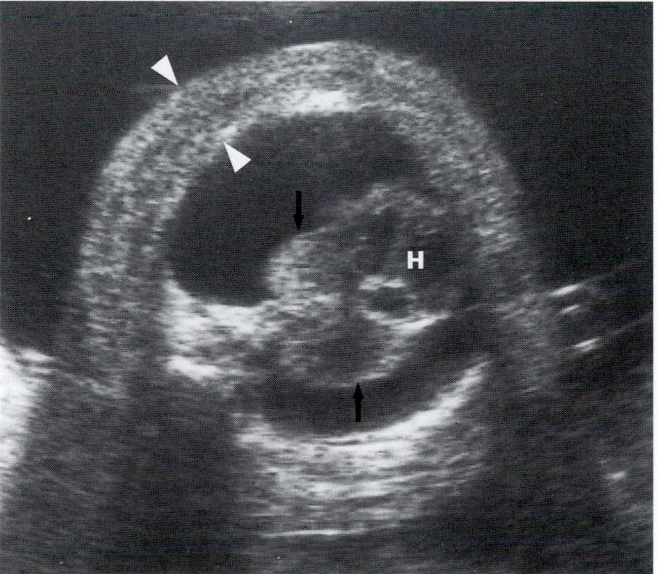

FIGURE 9–4. Pleural effusion. Fetal chest. Axial view. Echoless fluid surrounds the heart (*H*) and atelectatic lungs (*arrows*). The patient who has effusion related to fetal hydrops has very thick (hydropic) skin (*arrowheads*).

WHAT IS A CYSTIC ADENOMATOID MALFORMATION?

Excluding diaphragmatic hernias, a cystic adenomatoid malformation (CAM) is the most frequently identified mass in the fetal chest. Typically unilateral, it accounts for 25 percent of congenital lung malformations. It may involve an entire lobe or only part of one. Only rarely does a CAM involve an entire lung. Bilateral involvement may occur. Mediastinal shift is seen in almost 90 percent of cases. CAM is characterized histologically as an adenomatoid increase of terminal respiratory elements, leading to the development of a pathologic mass consisting of multiple cysts of different sizes. The vascular supply to this lung mass is normal.

Three forms of CAM have been described. Type I consists of a single or multiple large cysts of at least 2 cm (usually 3 to 7 cm) with a trabeculated wall and, often, smaller cystic outpouchings. Broad fibrous septa and mucigenic cells are thought to be responsible for areas of echogenicity noted within the mass. Type II CAM is a mass containing multiple uniform-sized cysts of about 1.5 to 2 cm or less diameter. Types I and II appear cystic on ultrasound examination (Fig. 9-5). Type III CAM consists of multiple very small cysts (0.3 to 0.5 mm) that, like the multiple small cysts of infantile polycystic kidney disease, present numerous reflecting surfaces to the ultrasound beam. Since these small cysts cannot be resolved individually, the CAM appears as a single, solid, homogeneously echogenic mass.

Patients with CAM may have associated renal (particularly agenesis), cardiac, and/or gastrointestinal malformations. Fetuses with CAM, like those with other space-occupying lung masses, may have associated fetal hydrops, ascites, and polyhydramnios, which are poor prognostic signs, as is a larger area of lung involvement. The mass of the CAM may expand and cause an increase in thoracic diameter as well as inversion of the diaphragm. As with other lung masses, there have been reports of significant size decrease or spontaneous resolution of CAMs antenatally. Stillbirth and premature labor are common among fetuses with CAM. Many neonates with CAM who survive will have respiratory distress at birth, but the majority will be asymptomatic. These patients usually do well after surgical excision of these masses.

The differential diagnosis of the type III, solid-appearing, CAM includes pulmonary sequestration, rhabdomyoma, mediastinal teratoma, and herniated solid abdominal contents, which may include liver, spleen, or, rarely, kidney.

There has been some debate as to which of the CAM types is worst. There are those who say that the cystic forms (types I and II) have a better prognosis than do solid-appearing CAMs (type III). Others disagree. Some say that anomalies are more common in type II cases. There is controversy over whether surgery can be avoided in the apparently resolving CAM, since malignancies have been reported in cases that have not been operated. This includes cases of rhabdomyosarcoma in toddlers and bronchoalveolar carcinoma in children and adults.

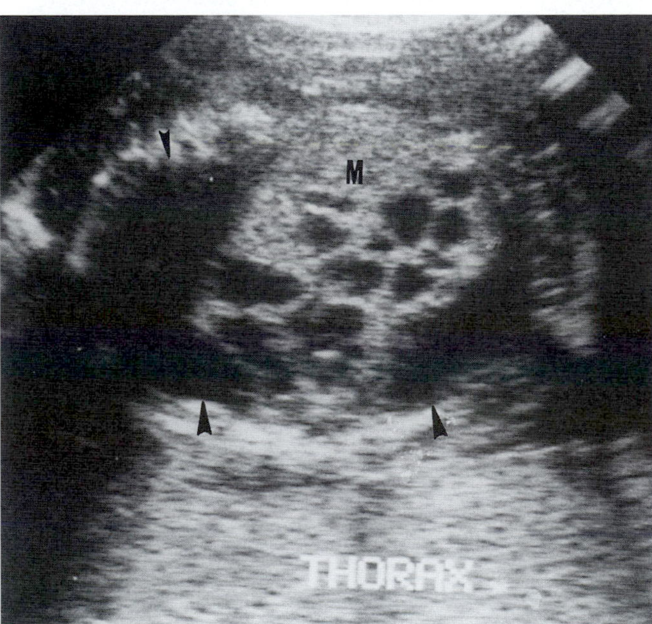

FIGURE 9–5. Cystic adenomatoid malformation, type II, fetal chest. Axial plane. Multiple cysts are noted in the lung parenchyma of this patient with cystic adenomatoid malformation (*M*) and surrounding pleural effusion (*arrowheads*). *(From Cohen, Muller, and Zinn, with permission.)*

PULMONARY SEQUESTRATION

A pulmonary sequestration is a solid (Fig. 9-6), nonfunctioning mass of lung tissue that lacks communication with the tracheobronchial tree and has a systemic arterial blood supply (and in the specific case of the extralobar variety a systemic venous drainage, usually the hemiazygos or portal vein, as well). The intralobar variety, so called because it is contained within the lung's visceral pleura, has venous drainage to the pulmonary veins. There is a 14 percent association of this variety with congenital anomalies. The lung mass is usually spherical on axial view and often wedge-shaped on sagittal view (Fig. 9-6). It is highly echogenic and is often found at the lung base. Bronchiectatic forms have been described that could simulate a type I or II CAM. Color Doppler (Fig. 9-7) has been used to identify this lung mass's abnormal vascular supply and help differentiate it from other diagnostic possibilities.

TECHNICAL TIPS

1. After diagnosing an abnormal fetus in the pregnancy noted in Fig. 9-6, a few of our staff had difficulty proving the presence of the mass in axial views through the chest on follow-up examination. The sagittal views (Fig. 9-6*B* and *C*) performed at that time helped confirm and, in fact, cement our suspicions that the finding was real. My point: Always attempt to look from an orthogonal view—i.e., change the paradigm.

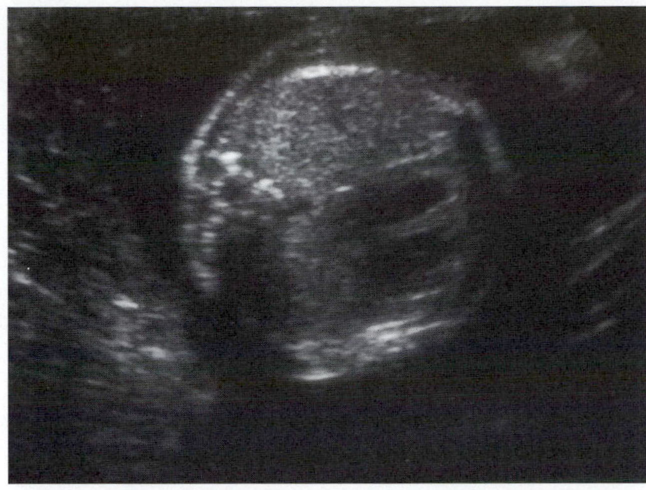

A

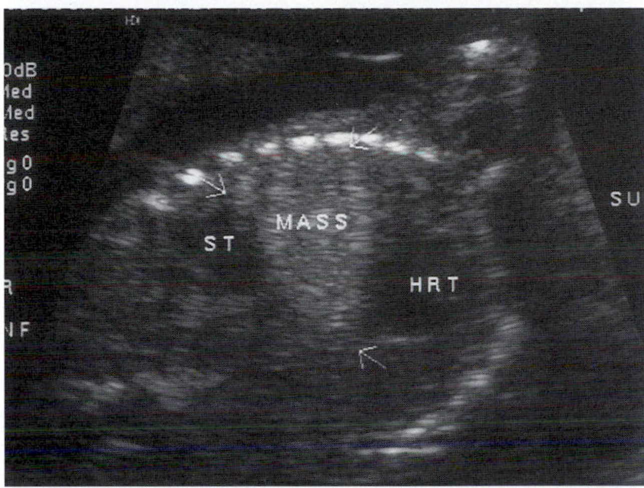

B

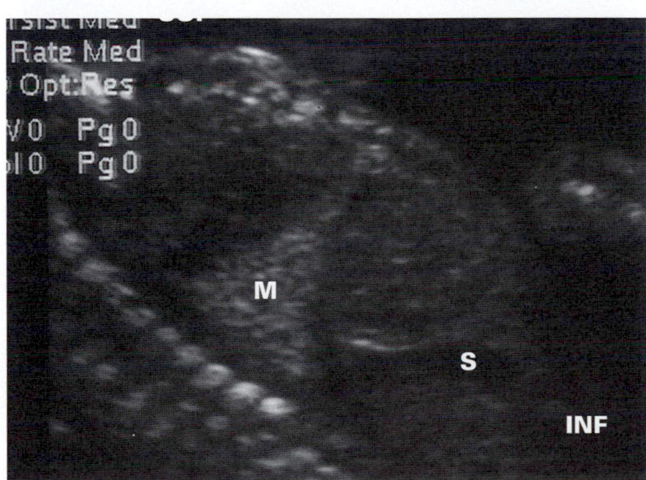

C

FIGURE 9–6. Pulmonary sequestration. ***A.*** Fetal chest. Axial plane. The heart is shifted to the right (the lower half of the image) by a somewhat more-echogenic-than-normal lung mass. ***B.*** Fetal chest. Sagittal oblique plane through left chest. Arrows point to an echogenic wedge-shaped mass (*MASS*) which is superior to the stomach (*ST*) and inferior to the heart. ***C.*** Fetal chest. Sagittal plane through left chest. The echogenic, solid, and wedge-shaped nature of the mass (*arrows*) is confirmed in this view.

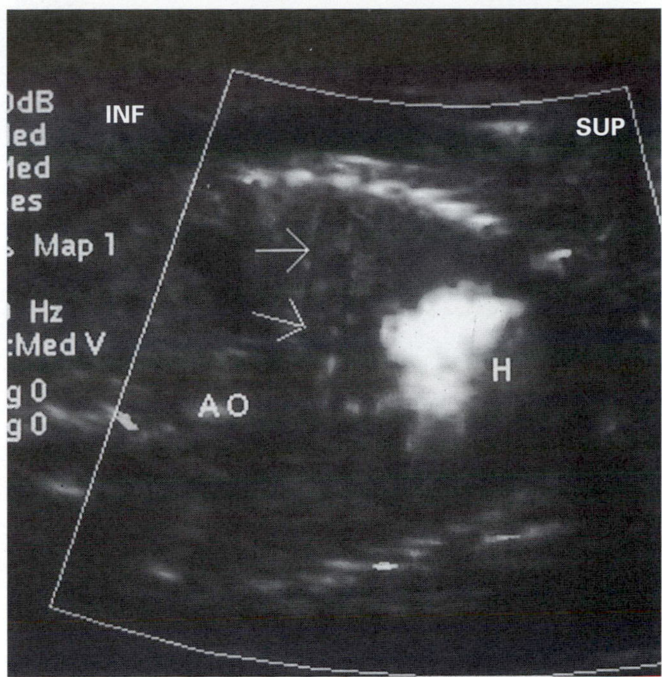

FIGURE 9–7. Fetal chest. Sagittal oblique plane through left chest. Color Doppler used with black-and-white filming. Two arrows point to the arterial supply to the sequestration coming off the aorta. This helped prove that it was a pulmonary sequestration.

2. Try using color or power Doppler to diagnose a sequestration. If you see flow to the intrathoracic sequestration from subdiaphragmatic vessels or from the thoracic or abdominal aorta, you have made the diagnosis and separated the mass from a possible CAM. If you can't differentiate between the two, at least you tried.

References

Adzick N, Harrison M: Management of the fetus with a cystic adenomatoid malformation. *World J Surg* 17:342–349, 1993.

Albright E, Crane J, Shackelford G: Prenatal diagnosis of bronchogenic cyst. *J Ultrasound Med* 7:91–95, 1988.

Avni E, Vanderelst A, Van Gansbeke D, et al: Antenatal diagnosis of pulmonary tumours: Report of two cases. *Pediatr Radiol* 16:190–192, 1986.

Cohen HL, Muller D, Zinn D: Abnormalities of the fetal chest, abdomen and pelvis, in *Diagnostic Medical Sonography. A Guide to Clinical Practice. Obstetrics and Gynecology,* 2d ed, Berman M, Cohen H (eds). Philadelphia, Lippincott, 1997:285–319.

Cohen HL, Torrisi J, Schwartz J: Ultrasound of the normal fetal chest, abdomen and pelvis, in *Diagnostic Medical Sonography. A Guide to Clinical Practice. Obstetrics and Gynecology,* 2d ed, Berman M, Cohen H (eds). Philadelphia, Lippincott, 1997: 269–284.

Comstock C: Fetal masses: Ultrasound diagnosis and evaluation. *Ultrasound Q* 6:229–256, 1988.

D'Agostino S, Bonoldi E, Dante S, et al: Embryonal rhabdomyosarcoma of the lung arising in cystic adenomatoid malformation: Case report and review of the literature. *J Pediatr Surg* 32: 1381–1383, 1997.

Fine C, Adzick N, Doubilet P: Decreasing size of a congenital cystic adenomatoid malformation in utero. *J Ultrasound Med* 7: 405–408, 1988.

Goldstein R: Ultrasound evaluation of the fetal thorax, in *Ultrasonography in Obstetrics and Gynecology*, 3d ed, Callen P (ed). Philadelphia, Saunders, 1994:333–346.

Kaslovsky R, Purdy S, Dangman B, et al: Bronchioalveolar carcinoma and congenital cystic adenomatoid malformation. *Chest* 112:548–551, 1997.

MacGillivray T, Harrison M, Goldstein R, Adzick N: Disappearing fetal lung lesions. *J Pediatr Surg* 28:1321–1324, 1993.

Miller J, Corteville J, Langer J: Congenital cystic adenomatoid malformation in the fetus: Natural history and predictors of outcome. *J Pediatr Surg* 31:805–808, 1996.

Nolan R: The fetal thorax, in *Practical Guide to Ultrasound in Obstetrics and Gynecology,* 2d ed, Sauerbrei E, Nguyen K, Nolan R (eds). Philadelphia, Lippincott-Raven, 1998:288–290.

Pezzuti R, Isler R: Antenatal ultrasound detection of cystic adenomatoid malformation of lung: Report of case and review of the recent literature. *J Clin Ultrasound* 11:342–346, 1983.

Stocker T, Madewell J, Drake RT: Congenital cystic adenomatoid malformation of the lung: Classification and morphologic spectrum. *Hum Pathol* 8:155–171, 1977.

Weiss J, Cohen H, Haller J: Cystic abnormalities of the fetal thorax. Sonographic evaluation. *J Diagn Med Sonogr* 3:172–176, 1987.

10

A radiology resident had difficulty getting an abdominal circumference measurement on this fetus. The fetal stomach was not definitively seen. You are presented with this axial view of the fetal chest (Fig. 10-1). Are you worried?

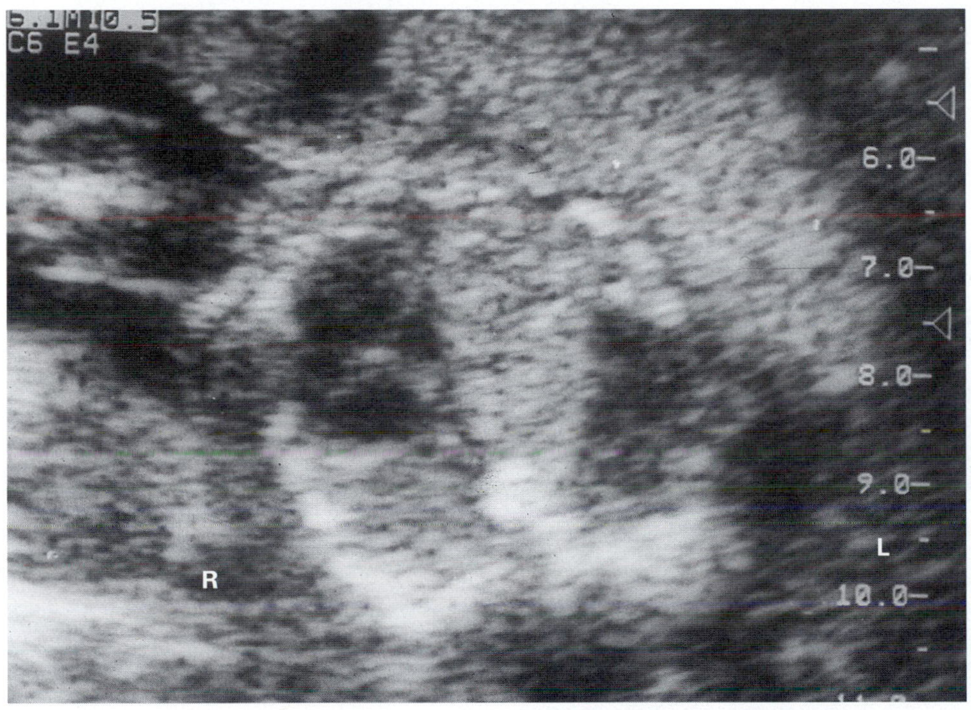

FIGURE 10–1. Fetal chest. Axial view. R = right side of chest, L = left side of chest.

CHAPTER 10

Congenital Diaphragmatic Hernia

HARRIS L. COHEN

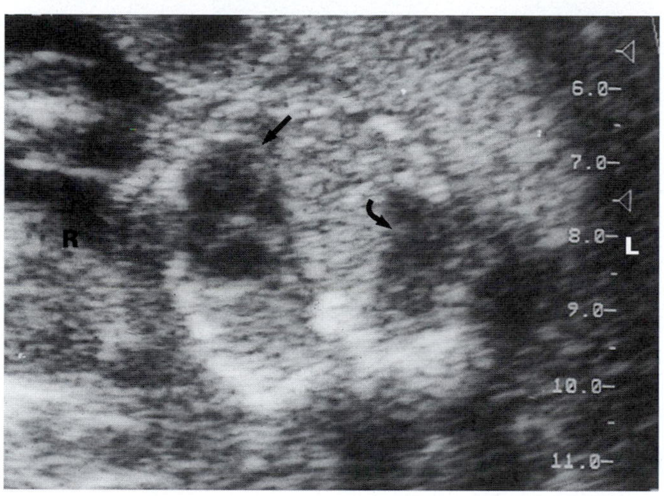

FIGURE 10–2. Fetal chest. Axial view. The fetal heart (*arrow*) has been pushed to the right (*R*) side of the chest by a large left-sided intrathoracic mass. The mass is echogenic anteriorly and echopenic posteriorly. The echopenic area, probably fluid-filled bowel (*curved arrow*), is seen posterolaterally on the left. The entire mass is part of the herniated bowel contents of a congenital diaphragmatic hernia.

Figure 10-2, the annotated version of Fig. 10-1, shows two echoless/echopenic areas in the chest. The anterior one contained the echogenic lines of the atrioventricular valves of the fetal heart. The contralateral and posterior echopenic area appears to be part of a larger mass, including a more echogenic component than normal lung, that has deviated the heart to the right. Since this is not a true cyst or cysts, the possibility of a bronchogenic cyst or the cystic adenomatoid malformation, types II and III, is unlikely. Since no intraabdominal stomach was seen on abdominal circumference views, you must worry about a congenital diaphragmatic hernia (CDH), which this case proved to be.

WHAT IS A CONGENITAL DIAPHRAGMATIC HERNIA? SHOULD YOU WORRY ABOUT IT?

Congenital diaphragmatic hernia has an incidence of 1 in every 2000 to 5000 live births. The diaphragm develops between the fourth and twelfth weeks of fetal life (usually at 8 weeks gestational age) as a result of fusion of the septum transversum centrally, the posterolateral pleuroperitoneal membranes, the dorsal mesentery of the esophagus, which will become the diaphragmatic crura, and the body wall, which contributes the last and most posterior portion of the diaphragm. Failure of these structures to fuse into a complete diaphragm will result in a diaphragmatic defect and a CDH. Abdominal viscera may then protrude into the thoracic cavity (Fig. 10-3), resulting in a CDH. The mass of abdominal viscera, whether echogenic solid organs or cystic or echopenic fluid-filled bowel, and depending on its size can compress the lungs and push the heart and mediastinum out of its path. Compressed lungs are at great risk for pulmonary hypoplasia in general and poor acinar development in particular, as well as persistent fetal circulation. Pulmonary hypoplasia is a major cause of neonatal morbidity and mortality.

The vast majority of diaphragmatic defects (92 percent) are posterolateral, Bochdalek hernias. I remember this because they are in the "bock." The remaining congenital diaphragmatic problems include other retrosternal hernias, anteromedial (Morgagni—incidence of 1 in 100,000 births) hernia, diaphragmatic eventration (congenitally defective muscle leading to focal aponeurotic bulging), hiatal hernia (a congenitally large esophageal hiatus) (Fig. 10-4), and, uncommonly, the complete absence of a diaphragm. Congential diaphragmatic hernia occurs five times more often on the left than on the right. The liver may perhaps be a protective barrier to herniation on the right (decreasing symptoms and improving prognosis) unless the defect is very large and the

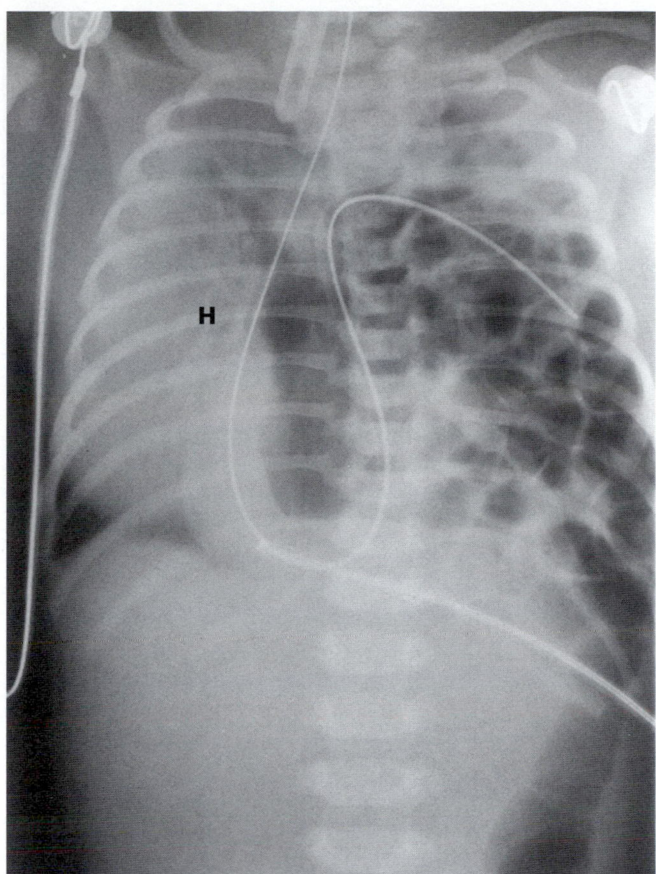

FIGURE 10–3. Diaphragmatic hernia. Anteroposterior chest film. The heart (*H*) of this neonate has been pushed to the right by the radiolucent mass of bowel that has herniated from below the diaphragm via a diaphragmatic defect. The baby soon died of respiratory failure due to significant bilateral pulmonary hypoplasia.

liver itself herniates. Sporadic cases of CDH are unilateral 96 percent of the time. There is a slight male predominance. A familial form of CDH is more often bilateral (20 percent) and has a 2:1 male predominance. Pulmonary hypoplasia may be bilateral despite a unilateral diaphragmatic lesion. Overall mortality from CDH is 50 to 86 percent, which includes 35 percent stillbirths. It is associated with several syndromes (e.g., Beckwith-Wiedemann, Marfan, and Cornelia de Lange) as well as with karyotype abnormalities, including trisomies 13, 18, and 21. Associated anomalies of several body systems are noted. Cardiovascular and central nervous system anomalies are the most lethal. Amniocentesis and careful ultrasound (US) evaluation for other anomalies help in parental counseling. There is a 2 percent risk of recurrence of CDH among subsequent siblings.

DIAGNOSTIC ULTRASOUND FINDINGS

Ultrasound findings in CDH are reviewed in Table 10-1. Those associated with a poorer prognosis are found in Table 10-2. Fluid-filled herniated structures, usually in the posterior thorax (Fig. 10-1), are readily differentiated from normal ho-

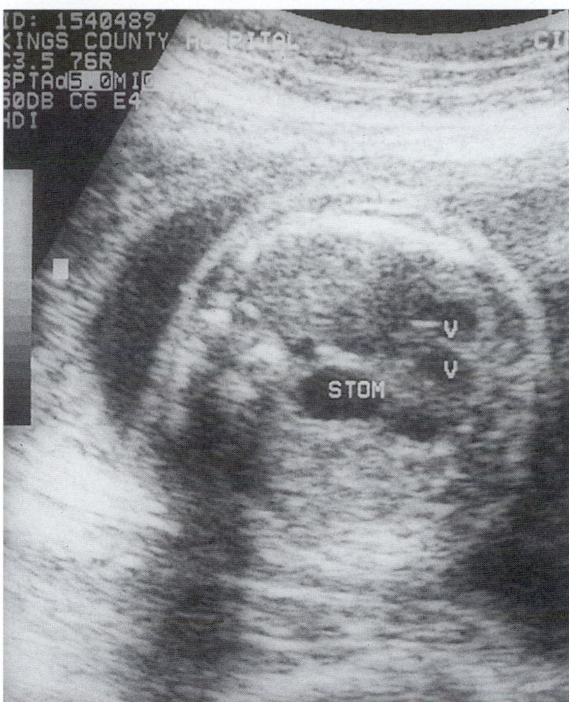

A

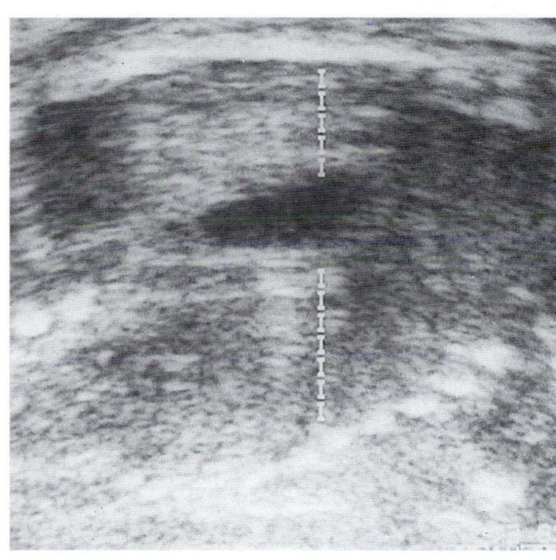

B

FIGURE 10–4. Hiatal hernia. ***A.*** Fetal chest. Axial plane. The cardiac ventricles (v) are seen in the anterior chest. The fluid-filled stomach (STOM) is seen in a midthoracic position. On this view alone, one must consider the possibility of congenital diaphragmatic herniation. ***B.*** Fetal chest/abdomen. Longitudinal plane. Only a small portion of the stomach, however, was in the chest. A string of I's is placed at the level of the diaphragm to illustrate this point. This case proved to be a hiatal hernia. SUP = superior.

TABLE 10-1
Ultrasound Findings in CDH

1. Intrathoracic mass deviating heart and mediastinum to the contralateral side
2. Intrathoracic fluid-filled bowel (occasional peristalsis) or stomach
3. Absent intraabdominal stomach
4. Smaller than normal abdominal circumference

TABLE 10-2
US Findings in CDH Suggesting Poorer Prognosis

1. Large defect/large intrathoracic mass/severe mediastinal shift
2. Little visible lung in thorax
3. Significant amount of intrathoracic liver—poor in utero surgery results
4. Concurrent cardiovascular, central nervous system, and other anomalies
5. Intrauterine growth retardation
6. Polyhydramnios
7. Hydrops fetalis
8. Early detection (<25 weeks)
9. Dilated intrathoracic stomach

mogeneously echogenic lung. Visualization of the contents of the thorax is aided by views in several planes, including the axial, sagittal, and coronal (Fig. 10-5). Multiple imaging planes, and avoiding an overangulated view through part of the fetal chest and fetal abdomen, help prevent a false-positive diagnosis of intrathoracic bowel. Imaging an intraabdominal stomach and, if possible on sagittal views, an intact diaphragm (Fig. 10-6) makes the diagnosis of CDH unlikely.

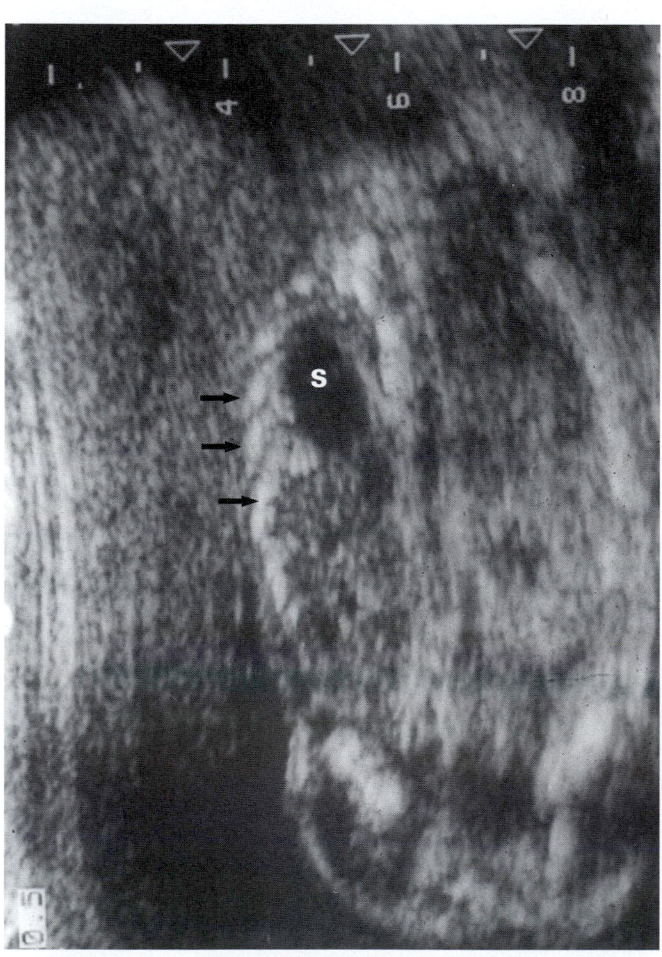

FIGURE 10–5. Congenital diaphragmatic hernia. Fetal stomach/abdomen. Coronal plane. The cystic stomach (*S*) is seen high in the thorax, near the ribs (*arrows*).

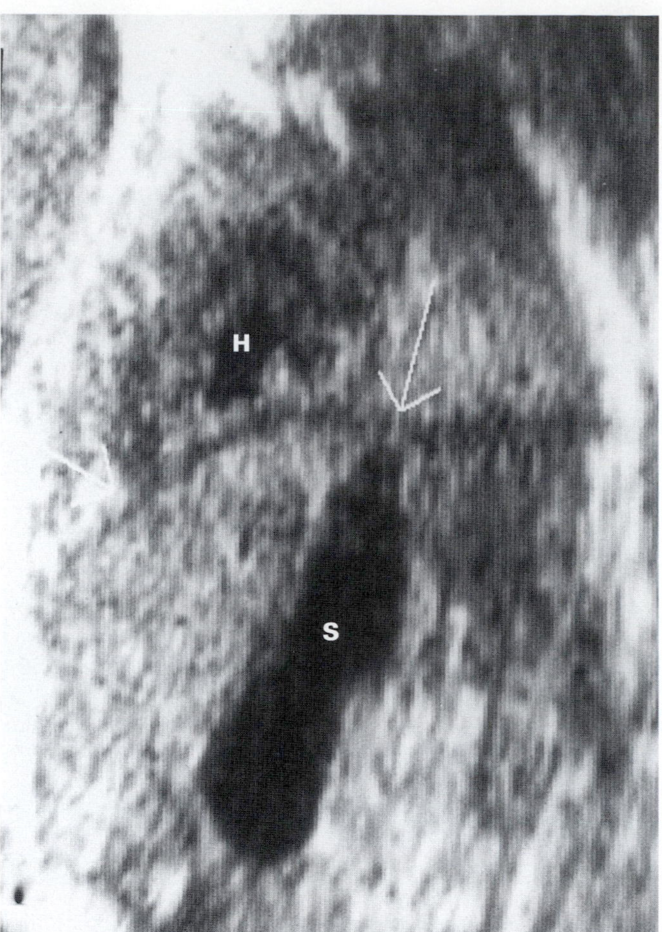

FIGURE 10–6. Normal diaphragm. Fetal chest/abdomen. Left parasagittal plane. Arrows point to the diaphragm, which appears as an echopenic line between the echogenic lung and the abdominal contents. The fluid-filled stomach (*S*) is seen below the diaphragm. Its intraabdominal presence is helpful in ruling out CDH. H = heart.

The fetal stomach should be seen by 15 weeks gestational age. Polyhydramnios and pleural effusions may be noted. The presence of polyhydramnios, thought to be due to impression of the CDH mass on the esophagus, is associated with poorer prognosis. One series noted only an 11 percent survival when CDH was associated with polyhydramnios but a 55 percent survival when amniotic fluid levels were normal. Those with smaller diaphragmatic defects or herniations that represent an isolated anomaly and occur later in gestation have a better prognosis.

SOME POINTS ON MANAGEMENT OF PATIENTS WITH CDH

After discovery of CDH, patients are karyotyped, undergo echocardiography, and are scheduled for delivery at a tertiary center. Early delivery does not improve prognosis. At the University of California at San Francisco (UCSF), in utero surgery has been performed if the fetus cannot wait for a later delivery, the CDH (diagnosed before 24 weeks) is the only anomaly, the fetus has a normal karyotype, and the mother is in good health. Previously, the surgical goal was to remove the compressing mass to allow the lung to grow and, it was hoped, avoid the development of significant pulmonary hypoplasia. The pioneering fetal surgery group at UCSF reported poor results when the CDH included large portions of herniated liver because of difficulties with kinking of the liver vessels when the liver is herniated and therefore with vascularization of the liver after its repositioning into the abdomen. The US diagnosis of liver herniation, however, can be confusing, since fetal liver may be isoechoic to fetal lung. Color Doppler can help predict herniation by revealing bowing of the umbilical segment of the portal vein to the left of midline or coursing of the lateral segment of the left lobe's portal veins at a level at or above the diaphragm. Imaging of the intrathoracic stomach in the middle or posterior third of the thorax in the axial plane is an excellent predictor of liver herniation. All this information may be moot in that the newest surgical technique involves artificially clipping the fetal trachea to force the lung to remain in a more distended state, helping to push the abdominal mass back into the abdomen and avoiding some of the lung hypoplasia.

References

Adzick N, Harrison M, Glick P, et al: Diaphragmatic hernia in the fetus: Prenatal diagnosis and outcome in 94 cases. *J Pediatr Surg* 20:357–361, 1985.

Bootstaylor B, Filly R, Harrison M, Adzick N: Prenatal sonographic predictors of liver herniation in congenital diaphragmatic hernia. *J Ultrasound Med* 14:515–522, 1995.

Cohen HL, Muller D, Zinn D: Abnormalities of the fetal chest, abdomen and pelvis, in *Diagnostic Medical Sonography. A Guide to Clinical Practice. Obstetrics and Gynecology,* 2d ed, Berman M, Cohen H (eds). Philadelphia, Lippincott, 1997:285–319.

Geary M, Chitty L, Morrison J, et al: Perinatal outcome and prognostic factors in perinatally diagnosed congenital diaphragmatic hernia. *Ultrasound Obstet Gynecol* 12:107–111, 1998.

Goldstein R: Ultrasound evaluation of the fetal thorax, in *Ultrasonography in Obstetrics and Gynecology*, 3d ed, Callen P (ed). Philadelphia, Saunders, 1994:333–346.

Goldstein R: The fetal thorax, in *Diagnostic Obstetrical Ultrasound,* McGahan J, Proto M (eds). Philadelphia, Lippincott, 1994:239–256.

Guibaud L, Filiatrault D, Garel L, et al: Fetal congenital diaphragmatic hernia: Accuracy of sonography in the diagnosis and prediction of the outcome after birth. *AJR* 166:1195–1202, 1996.

Harrison M, Adzick N, Flake A: Prenatal management of the fetus with a correctable defect, in *Ultrasonography in Obstetrics and Gynecology*, 3d ed, Callen P (ed). Philadelphia, Saunders, 1994:536–547.

Hirata G, Medearis A, Platt L: Fetal abdominal abnormalities associated with genetic syndromes. *Clin Perinatol* 17:675–702, 1990.

McNamara J, Eraklis A, Gross R: Congenital posterolateral diaphragmatic hernia in the newborn. *J Thorac Cardiovasc Surg* 55:55–59, 1968.

Moore KL: Body cavities, primitive mesenteries and the diaphragm, in *Before We Are Born. Basic Embryology and Birth Defects,* 3d ed. Philadelphia, Saunders, 1989:126–132.

Nolan R: The fetal thorax, in *A Practical Guide to Ultrasound in Obstetrics and Gynecology,* Sauerbrei E, Nguyen K, Nolan R (eds). Philadelphia, Lippincott-Raven, 1998:288–292.

Norio R, Kaarininen H, Rapola J, et al: Familial congenital diaphragmatic defects. Aspects of etiology, prenatal diagnosis and treatment. *Am J Med Genet* 17:471–483, 1984.

Section C
ABDOMEN

11

The abdomen (Figs. 11-1 and 11-2) of this 16-week-5-day-old fetus looks unusual. What is the problem? Could this be a normal finding? Is this an abnormal finding? What is your diagnosis?

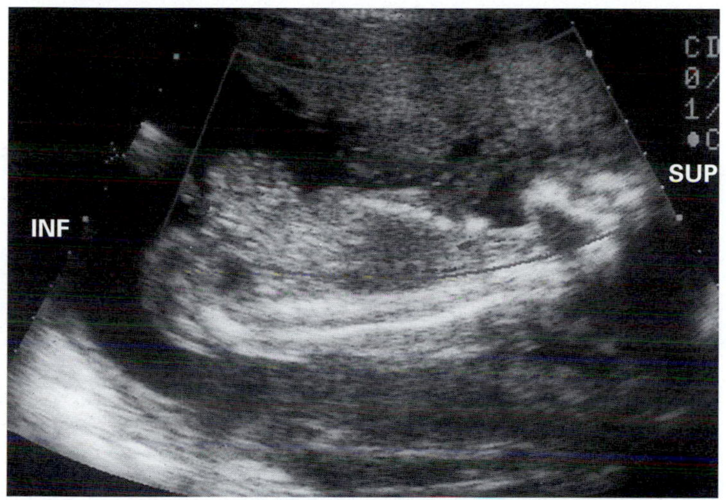

FIGURE 11–1. Fetal chest/abdomen. Sagittal plane, mild obliquity. Color flow imaged in black and white.

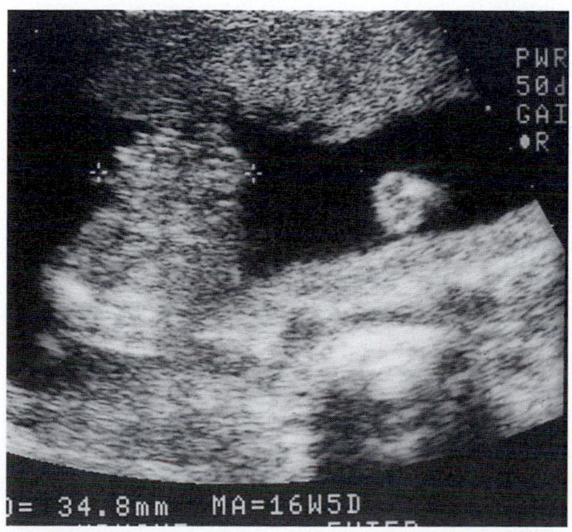

FIGURE 11–2. Fetal abdomen. Axial plane.

CHAPTER 11

Abdominal Wall Defect: Gastroschisis

HARRIS L. COHEN

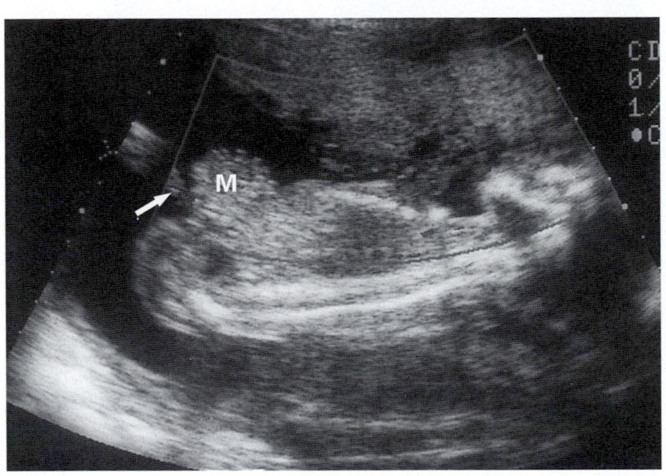

FIGURE 11–3. Annotated version of Fig. 11-1. Gastroschisis. Fetal chest/abdomen. Sagittal plane, mild obliquity. Color flow imaged in black and white. The fetal head is to the reader's right. A mass (M) is noted protruding from the anterior abdominal wall. It is not surrounded by a membrane. Its borders are irregular, suggesting individual loops of bowel. A blood vessel (*arrow*) inferior to the mass is part of the umbilical cord. The findings are consistent with gastroschisis.

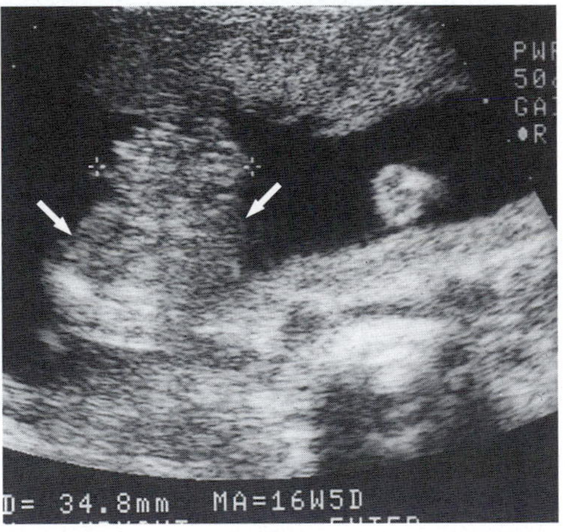

FIGURE 11–4. Annotated version of Fig. 11-2. Gastroschisis. Fetal abdomen. Axial plane. Crosses mark off the borders of a mass extending from the abdomen (*arrows*). Its irregular borders suggest that it is bowel without a covering membrane, suggesting gastroschisis.

Figures 11-3 and 11-4, the annotated versions of Figs. 11-1 and 11-2, respectively, show a mass extending above the anterior abdomen, suggesting an anterior abdominal wall defect. The mass is irregular in contour, suggesting individual loops of bowel and no covering membrane. On Fig. 11-3, an umbilical cord vessel is seen below the mass. These findings help make the diagnosis of gastroschisis. Fetal gross pathology views (Fig. 11-5) confirmed this. One might have considered the possibility that this was an omphalocele, but certainly the unknown image is not part of a normal physiologic process—e.g., the normal extracoelomic bowel herniation, which should not be seen beyond 12 weeks gestational age—nor is there an artifactual simulator of abnormality—e.g., a pseudoomphalocele (Fig. 11-6).

APPROACH TO ABDOMINAL WALL CONTOUR ANALYSIS BY ULTRASOUND—WHAT SHOULD YOU LOOK FOR?

All fetal anatomy surveys should include a general fetal abdominal survey. At that time, one should denote the contours of the abdominal walls, particularly the anterior abdominal wall, and ensure that they are intact (Fig. 11-7). This is most important at the site of umbilical cord entry (Fig. 11-8). Protrusions from the abdominal side walls should also be searched for, but they are unusual.

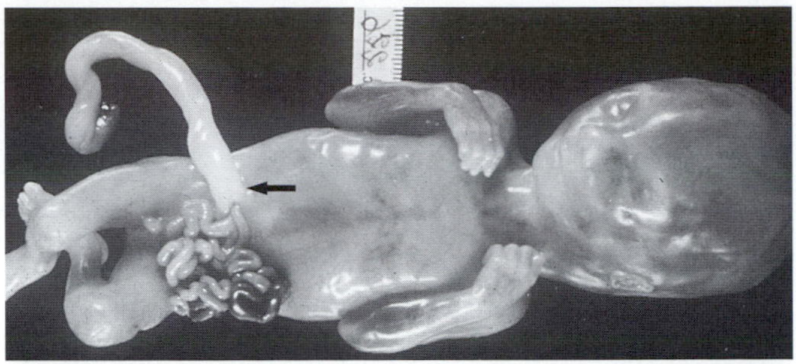

A

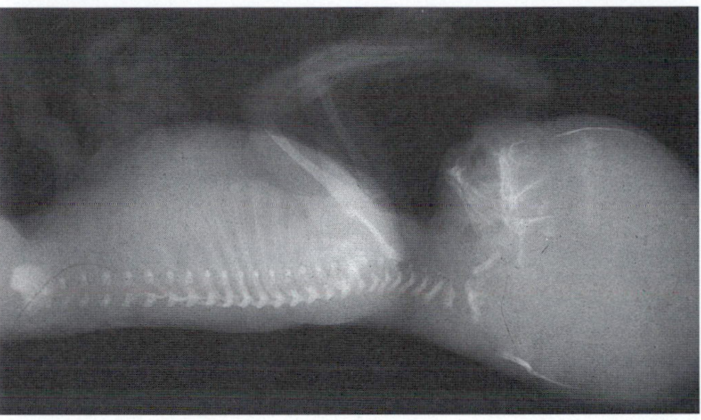

B

FIGURE 11–5. Gastroschisis. Pathology specimen. ***A.*** Fetus with gastroschisis. Autopsy specimen. Frontal projection. The umbilical cord (*arrow*) is in its normal midline position. The mass extending from the left of the midline abdominal wall defect is small bowel (see Color Plate 4). ***B.*** Fetus with gastroschisis. Plain film of autopsy specimen. Lateral view. The mass (*curved arrow*) is superior and is unrelated to the normal cord (*arrow*) imaged below it.

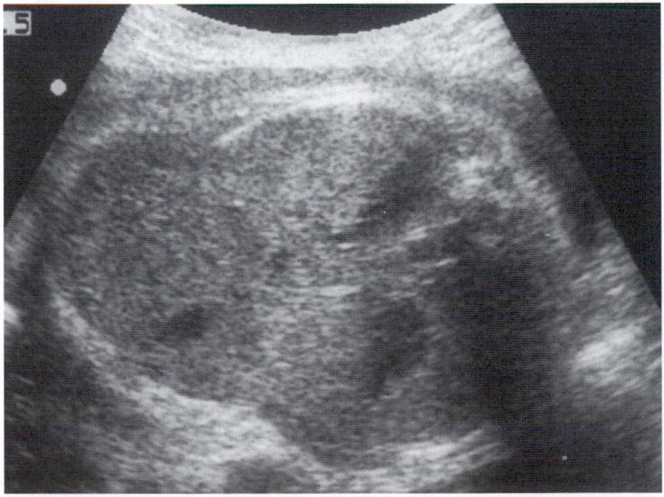

FIGURE 11–6. Pseudoomphalocele. Fetal abdomen. Transverse plane. The anterior abdominal wall (to the reader's left) is somewhat pinched in, simulating a wide anterior wall defect. This pseudoomphalocele image may be simulated for brief periods of time by nearby uterine contractions. This is even more likely when the fetus is surrounded by lesser amounts of amniotic fluid.

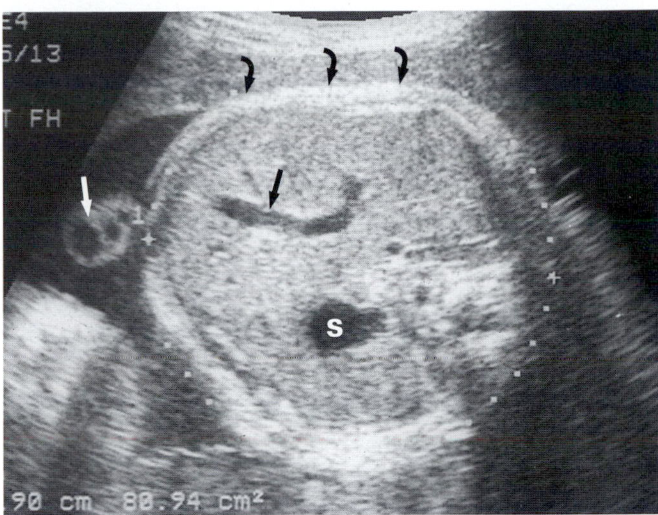

FIGURE 11–7. Normal abdomen. Axial view. This is an axial view through the upper abdomen that could be used for determination of abdominal circumference. One can see the fluid-filled stomach (S), the vertebral body (v), and the intrahepatic portion of the umbilical vein (*arrow*), although we perhaps see too much of the portal vein. The right anterior abdominal wall, seen highlighted by amniotic fluid, is obviously intact. A portion of the umbilical cord (*white arrow*) is anterior to the wall. The left side of the anterior abdominal wall was also intact, but on this view that analysis is limited by the fetus's position up against the uterine wall (*curved arrow*). This analysis would also be difficult when there is oligohydramnios.

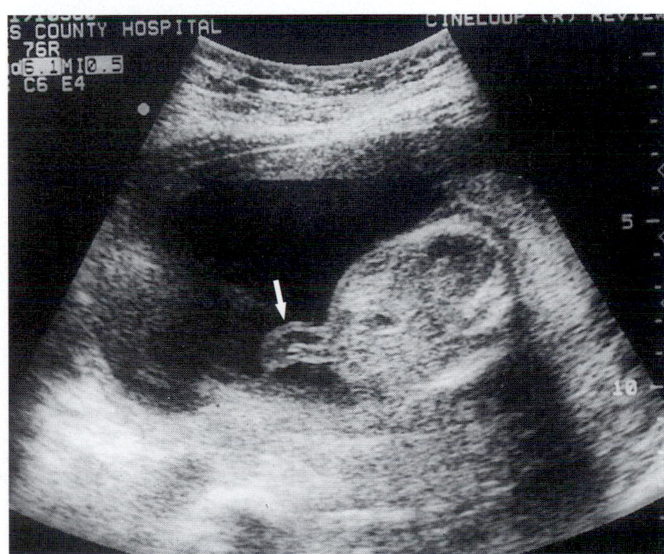

FIGURE 11–8. Intact low abdominal wall. Axial/oblique view. The umbilical cord is seen exiting the low anterior abdominal wall of this fetus. No mass is seen involving the cord. Such a view helps rule out an omphalocele.

TABLE 11-1
Differences between Omphalocele and Gastroschisis

ITEM	GASTROSCHISIS	OMPHALOCELE
Position of defect	Off-midline, usually on right	Midline
Membrane covering hernia	No	Yes
Contents of hernia	Bowel > other >> liver	Liver > other
Associated anomalies	Essential malrotation or or other gastrointestinal	Many, from many systems

FETAL ANTERIOR ABDOMINAL WALL DEFECTS

Abdominal wall defects vary in type and complexity. The two most common types (Table 11-1), omphalocele and gastroschisis, will be discussed here. Other defects that occur range from the mundane umbilical hernia (linea alba defect and protruding bowel covered by skin and subcutaneous tissue) to complicated defects resulting from amniotic band syndrome or resulting in limb–body wall complex.

The anterior abdominal wall develops from the fusion of four ectomesodermal folds: a cephalic, a caudal, and a pair of lateral folds. Abdominal wall defects are one of the causes of high alpha fetoprotein (AFP) levels in amniotic fluid or maternal serum. Knowledge of the particular wall defect and its associated abnormalities is necessary for proper decision making with regard to continuation of pregnancy, method of delivery, and surgical treatment.

Omphalocele

An omphalocele (Figs. 11-9 and 11-10) is a midline defect that occurs in 1 in 4000 births. It may be due to failure of fusion of the lateral ectomesodermal folds or to persistence of the body stalk in an area normally occupied by abdominal wall. Abdominal muscle, fascia, and skin fail to develop at the area of the defect. On ultrasound (US), abdominal viscera, covered by an amnion/peritoneal sac, protrude through the midline defect into the base of the umbilical cord. The defect is usually 2 to 10 cm wide. Most often, liver is contained in the omphalocele, but any of the abdominal/pelvic contents, usually large or small bowel, can be present, with or without liver. There is often associated fetal ascites. Besides the typical omphalocele—which is limited to the anterior abdominal wall at the level of the umbilical cord—less typical varieties, associated with failure of closure of the caudal or cephalic fold at the umbilical ring, can occur. These include the low omphalocele of cloacal or bladder extrophy and the high omphaloceles associated with ectopia cordis (externalization of the heart), which may be part of the pentalogy of Cantrell.

The majority (50 to 70 percent) of fetuses with omphalocele have associated anomalies whose presence affects the prognosis for the worse. Some 30 to 50 percent of these anomalies are gastrointestinal; the most common is bowel malrotation, but there can also be atresia or stenosis of the small bowel, bowel duplication, biliary atresia, tracheoesophageal fistula, or imperforate anus. Half of the anomalies are cardiovascular, including ventricular and atrial septal defects, tetralogy of Fallot, pulmonary artery stenosis, and great vessel abnormalities.

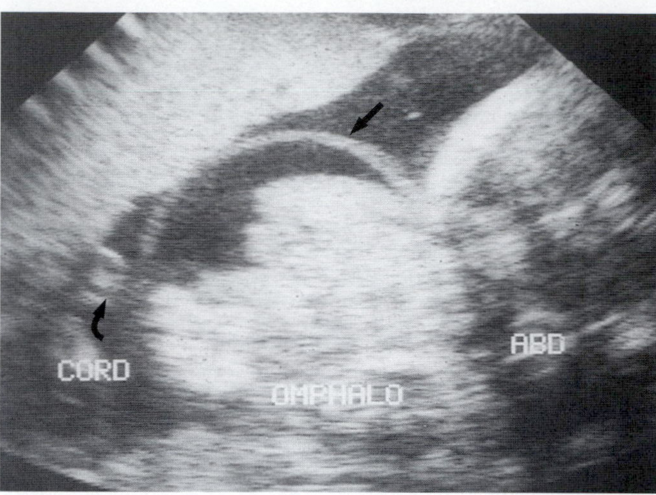

FIGURE 11–9. Omphalocele. Axial plane. The abdomen (ABD) is seen to the reader's right. It is smaller than a large mass (OMPHALO) that has a membrane (*arrow*) surrounding contained fluid and solid mass that consists of bowel and liver. This large omphalocele extends into the base of the umbilical cord (CORD) (*curved arrow*).

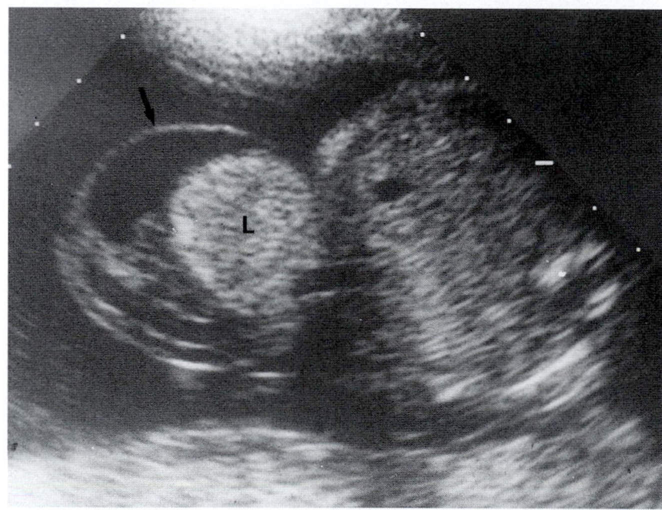

FIGURE 11–10. Omphalocele. Axial plane. Another example of a large omphalocele. The mass contains liver (*L*). The peritoneal membrane (*arrow*) is readily seen. There are times at delivery when the peritoneal covering ruptures and an exact differentiation of omphalocele from gastroschisis cannot be made.

A large number (40 to 60 percent) of patients with omphaloceles have chromosomal disorders, such as trisomy 13, 18, or 21; Turner's or Klinefelter's syndrome; or triploidy. Chromosomal abnormalities seem to be more common in cases without contained liver in the omphalocele. Omphaloceles are part of several fetal malformation syndromes. One in every seven cases of omphalocele is associated with Beckwith-Wiedemann syndrome and its associated organomegaly, macroglossia, hypoglycemia, hemihypertrophy, and increased risk for Wilms' tumor.

The smaller the abdominal wall defect and the fewer the associated anomalies, the better the prognosis. Defects greater than 5 cm tend to a more adverse outcome. The presence of spleen or heart in the sac has also been associated with a poor outcome. Poor outcome is usually related to the associated anomalies or karyotype abnormalities rather than to the omphalocele itself, since there is a 25 to 75 percent overall mortality reported but only a 10 percent mortality among those whose problem is only an omphalocele.

Gastroschisis

In gastroschisis, there is a smaller abdominal wall defect than in omphalocele. It occurs 1 to 2 times per 10,000 births, but has a greater incidence among teenage mothers. It is more common in males. The abdominal wall defect tends to be no greater than 4 cm and is paraumbilical, unrelated to the umbilical cord, and typically just to the right of midline. The viscera that herniate into a gastroschisis are usually the small or large bowel. Obviously, other structures may be included, but the presence of liver is rare. Lack of a covering membrane may lead to the development of a thickened, fibrinous coating on the herniated bowel, probably as the result of chemical peritonitis produced by its contact with fetal urine in the amniotic fluid. Free-floating bowel (without a surrounding membrane) is the typical US image of gastroschisis (Figs. 11-1 to 11-4).

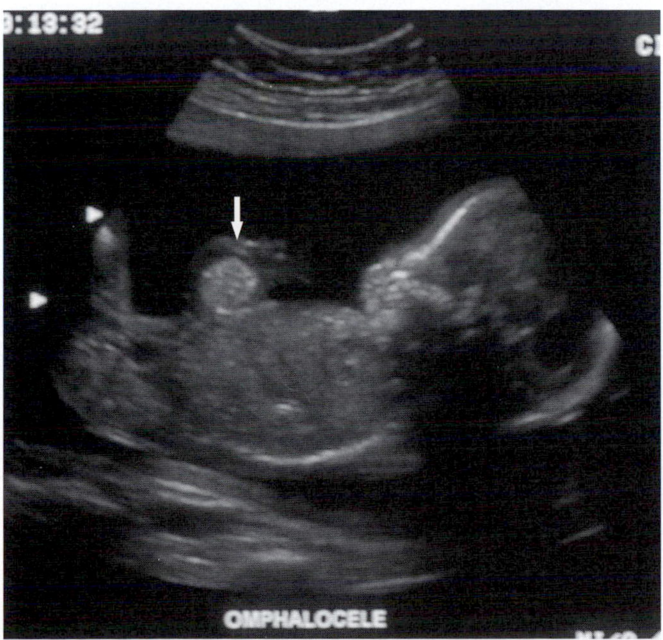

FIGURE 11–11. Omphalocele. Fetal chest/abdomen. Sagittal plane. A small omphalocele extends from the anterior abdominal wall of this first-trimester fetus. Despite the difficulties in making an early diagnosis, its size (greater than 7 mm) helped assure the examiner of the diagnosis. *(Image provided courtesy of GE Medical Systems.)*

Theoretical causes for this anomaly include abnormal involution of the right umbilical vein (with resultant poor development of vascular flow to the periumbilical region) and disruption of the omphalomesenteric artery.

Except for bowel malrotation and jejunal or ileal atresia, probably related to vascular compromise of malrotated bowel, associated anomalies are far less common than with omphalocele. There is only an 11 percent antenatal mortality rate. Only about 24 percent of neonates born with gastroschisis have intrauterine growth retardation (IUGR), despite reports of IUGR rates as great as 50 percent among fetuses. This is probably due to the overestimation of IUGR based on smaller abdominal circumference measurements because of the herniations.

Although there is active debate over the method of delivery, many clinicians favor cesarean section to avoid further contamination of the uncovered eviscerated bowel. Surgical closure is done primarily or in stages; a Silastic covering is placed over the bowel and abdominal wall defect between operations.

A WARNING: DO NOT ATTEMPT TO MAKE BOLD DIAGNOSES BEFORE 12 WEEKS, UNLESS…

Normal bowel rotates 270° in fetal life to achieve its normal postnatal course, and 90° of this rotation occurs extracoelomically within the base of the cord. Since this actual physiologic herniation of bowel into the umbilical cord occurs between weeks 6 and 10 of life, one must be cautious about the diagnosis of omphalocele prior to this time. We use a 12 weeks gestational age cutoff (by which time physiologic bowel rotation has finished) before we are definitive about a subtle or small omphalocele (Fig. 11-11). A definitive first-trimester diagnosis is made by some imagers only if the omphalocele is larger than the abdomen itself. Bowerman reported that an omphalocele may be suggested early in pregnancy if the cord containing midgut has a maximal dimension of 7 mm or greater or the mass is seen after a crown-to-rump length of 44 mm (the equivalent of 11.2 weeks).

AN INTERESTING WARNING REGARDING AFP RELIABILITY IN OMPHALOCELE DIAGNOSIS

Anterior abdominal wall defects are associated with high AFP levels as a result of the diffusion of this fetal liver product into the amniotic fluid, but trisomies are often associated with low AFP levels. The AFP levels in fetuses with a combination of an omphalocele (which involves lower AFP levels than gastroschisis because of its surrounding membrane) and an associated trisomy may, therefore, not be as high as expected.

References

Bowerman R: Sonography of fetal midgut herniation: Normal size criteria and correlation with crown-rump length. *J Ultrasound Med* 5:251–254, 1993.

Callen P: Gastroschisis, in *An Interactive Diagnostic Ultrasound Text and Journal Focusing on Obstetrics and Gynecology,* Callen P (ed). San Francisco, Ultrasound Educational Press, 1998.

Cohen HL, Muller D, Zinn D: Abnormal fetal chest, abdomen, pelvis, in *Diagnostic Medical Sonography. A Guide to Clinical Practice. Obstetrics and Gynecology,* 2d ed, Berman M, Cohen H (eds). Philadelphia, Lippincott, 1997:285–320.

DeVries P: The pathogenesis of gastroschisis and omphalocele. *J Pediatr Surg* 15:245–251, 1980.

Fries M, Filly R, Callen P, et al: Growth retardation in prenatally diagnosed cases of gastroschisis. *J Ultrasound Med* 12:583–588, 1992.

Goncalves LF, Jeanty P: Ultrasound evaluation of abdominal wall defects, in *Ultrasonography in Obstetrics and Gynecology,* 3d ed, Callen P (ed). Philadelphia, Saunders, 1994:370–388.

Hill L: Sonographic detection of fetal gastrointestinal anomalies. *Ultrasound Q* 6:35–68, 1988.

Kim S: Omphalocele. *Surg Clin North Am* 56:361–371, 1976.

Moore T: Gastroschisis and omphalocele: Clinical differences. *Surgery* 82:561–568, 1977.

Nicolaides K, Snijders R, Cheng H, Gosden C: Fetal gastrointestinal and abdominal wall defects: Associated malformations and chromosomal abnormalities. *Fetal Diagn Ther* 7:102–115, 1992.

Raynor B, Richards D: Growth retardation in fetuses with gastroschisis. *J Ultrasound Med* 16:13–16, 1997.

Romero R, Pilu G, Jeanty P, et al (eds). The abdominal wall, in *Prenatal Diagnosis of Congenital Anomalies.* East Norwalk, CT, Appleton & Lange, 1988:209–232.

Sauerbrei E: The fetal abdominal wall, in *A Practical Guide to Ultrasound in Obstetrics and Gynecology,* Sauerbrei E, Nguyen K, Nolan R (eds). Philadelphia, Lippincott-Raven, 1998:297–305.

12

This sagittal image of a fetal kidney (Fig. 12-1) of a 32-week-old fetus measures 4.7 cm in length. The level of amniotic fluid surrounding the fetus was normal. You know that fetal renal lengths are thought by some to be equivalent to 1 mm for each week of gestation. Fetal renal lengths may be increased in several conditions, including recessive polycystic kidney disease (a/k/a infantile polycystic kidney disease), hydronephrosis, and renal duplication. What is happening in this case?

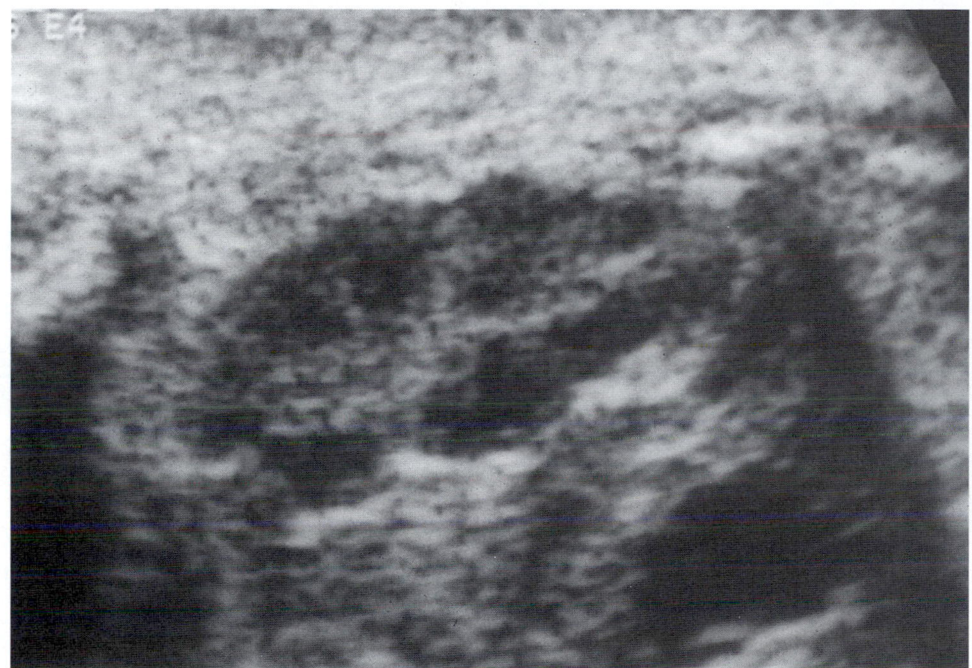

FIGURE 12–1. Fetal kidney. Sagittal plane.

CHAPTER 12

Normal Fetal Kidney

HARRIS L. COHEN

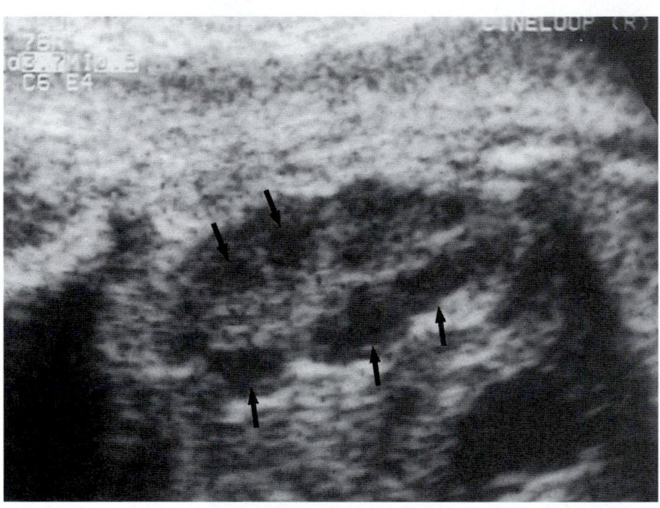

FIGURE 12–2. Annotated version of Fig. 12-1. Normal fetal kidney. Sagittal plane. The central echogenicity is central renal fat. The echopenic areas (*arrows*) noted in a regular pattern within the renal parenchyma are the normal renal pyramids.

The unknown image in Fig. 12-2 (the annotated version of Fig. 12-1) shows the sagittal view of a kidney that is 4.7 cm long. It appears normal in shape. There is no obstructed upper pole to suggest a duplicated system. There is no increased echogenicity to suggest recessive polycystic kidney disease (RPK) (see Fig. 12-3), which should not be considered in light of a normal amniotic fluid level at 32 weeks. Recessive polycystic kidney disease can show renal enlargement prior to evident increases in echogenicity. Hence, it is important to know what the normal fetal renal length is. The kidney contains regularly spaced echopenic areas that are normal pyramids. An obstructed or distended pyelocaliceal system would have a larger central echoless area representing the renal pelvis and smaller surrounding echoless areas consistent with dilated calices (Fig. 12-4).

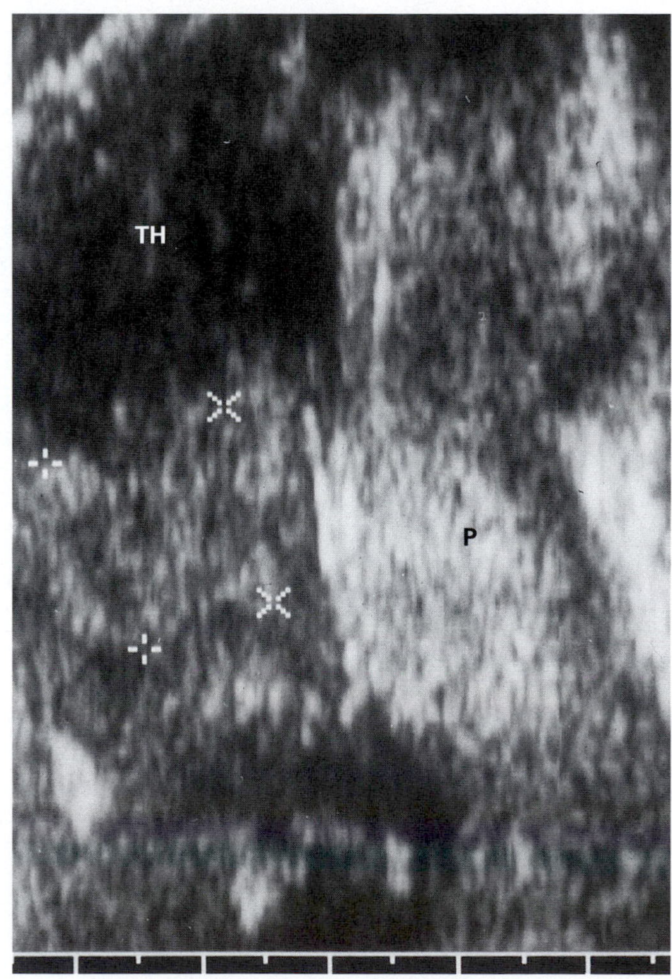

FIGURE 12–3. Recessive polycystic kidney disease (RPK). Chest/abdomen. Coronal plane. Two echogenic kidneys (*marked off by crosses*) were imaged as much longer than expected in this 18-week fetus. On axial views, the kidneys took up most of the abdominal space. Enlarged echogenic kidneys are typical for RPK. No cysts are seen because they are too small to be imaged, and the kidneys appear echogenic because the small cysts present multiple interstices for the ultrasound beam. Eventually this fetus stopped producing urine, leading to oligohydramnios. P = adjacent placenta, TH = fetal thorax.

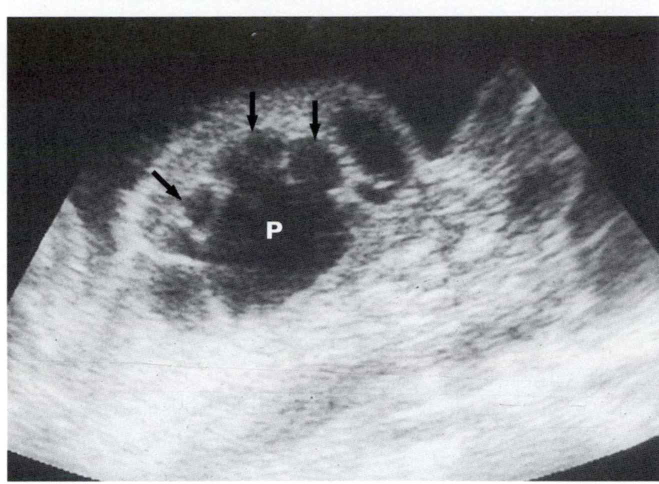

FIGURE 12–4. Pyelocaliceal system dilatation. Kidney. Sagittal plane. The central renal pelvis is more dilated than surrounding and communicating calices (*arrows*). Findings are typical of obstruction or significant reflux. P = pelvis.

The key message of this unknown case, however, is that the axiom that normal fetal kidney measurements should not vary much from approximately 1 mm per week of gestation is wrong. Our table of normal mean measurements and normal confidence limits (Table 12-1) was the result of research that was done after dealing with the very anxious parents of several second-trimester fetuses that were sent to us as "enlarged kidneys—r/o recessive polycystic kidneys." Since amniotic fluid levels may be normal or low normal in the early course of RPK and decisions had to be made with regard to genetic counseling and possible termination before 24 weeks, we wanted to confirm our anecdotal opinion that fetal kidneys were greater in size than was commonly thought—i.e., "Bigger than you think."

FETAL KIDNEYS—WHAT SIZE IS NORMAL?

Table 12-1 confirms the larger than 1 mm/week sizes of fetal kidneys. This case's 4.7-cm-long kidney fits into the normal 95 percent confidence interval for a 32-week fetus. Our measurements showed a larger mean and a wider confidence interval than those previously accepted. Yet our measurements fit well with those of premature neonates (Fig. 12-5). The knowledge of the actual normal mean measurement for fetal kidney length is not as important as a knowledge of the true wider range of normal lengths. The normal newborn's kidney ranges between 3.5 and 5.5 cm in length.

TABLE 12-1
Normal Fetal Kidney Lengths

Gestational Age, weeks	Mean Kidney Length, cm	95% Confidence Interval, cm
18	2.2	1.6–2.8
19	2.3	1.5–3.1
20	2.6	1.8–3.4
21	2.7	2.1–3.2
22	2.7	2.0–3.4
23	3.0	2.2–3.7
24	3.1	1.9–4.4
25	3.3	2.5–4.2
26	3.4	2.4–4.4
27	3.5	2.7–4.4
28	3.4	2.6–4.2
29	3.6	2.3–4.8
30	3.8	2.9–4.6
31	3.7	2.8–4.6
32	4.1	3.1–5.1
33	4.0	3.3–4.7
34	4.2	3.3–5.0
35	4.2	3.2–5.2
36	4.2	3.3–5.0
37	4.2	3.3–5.1
38	4.4	3.2–5.6
39	4.2	3.5–4.8
40	4.3	3.2–5.3
41	4.5	3.9–5.1

SOURCE: *From Cohen, Cooper, Eisenberg, et al. With permission.*

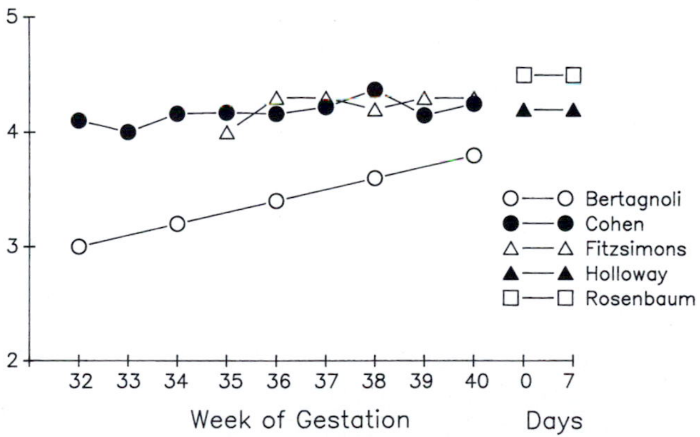

FIGURE 12–5. Plot of kidney length with age. Our measurements (Cohen) in late pregnancy are larger than the fetal kidney measurements of Bertagnoli et al but similar to the premature neonatal kidney measurements of Fitzsimons. Measurements by Holloway et al and Rosenbaum et al in the first week after birth are used for reference. *(Reprinted from Cohen, Cooper, Eisenberg, et al, with permission.)*

ULTRASOUND IMAGING OF THE FETAL KIDNEY

The fetal kidneys can be seen as early as the 15th week after last menstrual period (LMP) by transabdominal imaging and perhaps earlier by transvaginal scanning. Essentially all should be imaged on exams performed between weeks 17 and 22. On transverse images (Fig. 12-6), the kidneys are hypoechoic ovoid masses on either side of the spine. The ratio

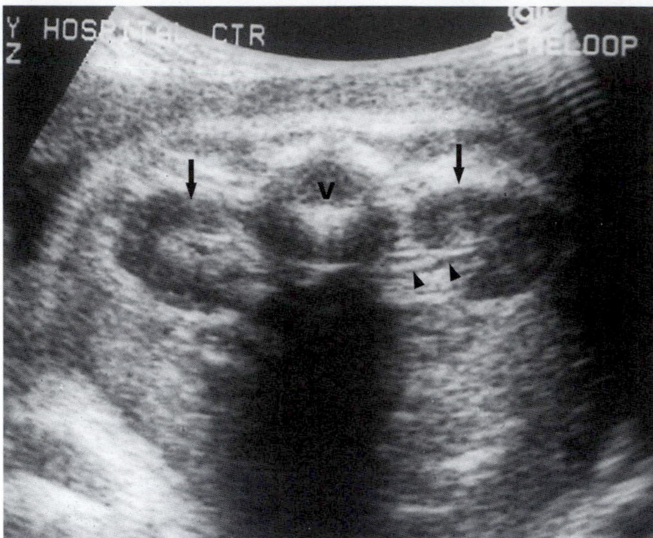

FIGURE 12–6. Normal fetal kidneys. Midabdomen. Axial plane. The fetus is prone. Two oval masses (*arrows*) are seen, each to the side of the vertebral body (v). Thin echoless lines (*arrowheads*) extending medially from these kidneys are normal vessels.

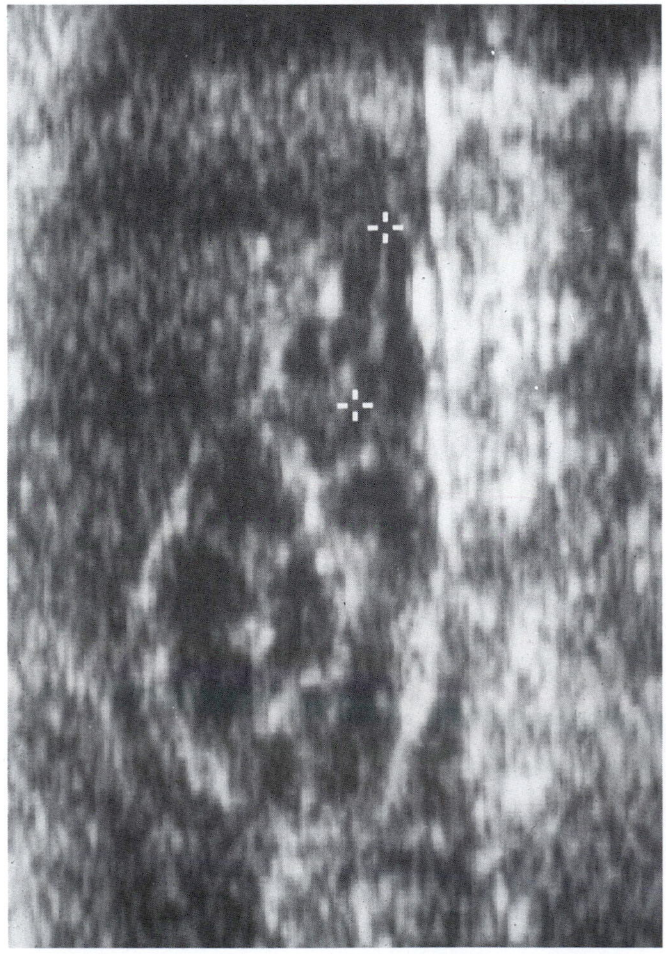

FIGURE 12–7. Normal fetal adrenal gland. Sagittal plane through the fetal kidney. A triangular adrenal gland, marked off by crosses, is seen above a normal fetal kidney. Echopenic pyramids are seen in the kidney.

of kidney circumference to abdominal circumference remains approximately 0.3 throughout pregnancy. Parasagittal views of each kidney show the kidneys to be paraspinous and bean-shaped. As in neonates, and as already stated, the normal hypoechoic renal pyramids may be seen arranged in anterior and posterior rows around the renal pelvis and should not be mistaken for renal cysts.

The contralateral kidneys of fetuses with nonfunctioning multicystic dysplastic kidneys are noted to undergo the phenomenon of compensatory hypertrophy. This is a well-known growth phenomenon seen among children and at least younger adults, in which when one kidney is damaged or surgically removed, the remaining kidney grows to a greater degree to compensate for the absence of the contralateral kidney. The fetal ureters are not normally visualized unless there is significant genitourinary system reflux or obstruction.

SOME INFORMATION ON IMAGING THE FETAL ADRENAL GLAND

The adrenals are ovoid, triangular (Fig. 12-7), or heart-shaped masses that are often imaged in the suprarenal area of the fetus. On transverse view, the adrenals may appear oval and therefore reniform, particularly in association with ipsilateral renal agenesis (Fig. 12-8). The high retroperitoneal position of the adrenals and their position often near and not on top of the kidney can limit their imaging.

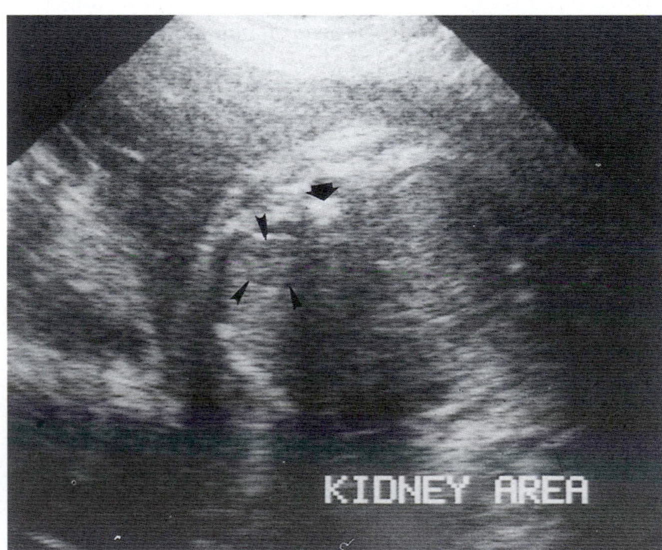

FIGURE 12–8. Rounded adrenal gland in a case of renal agenesis. Midabdomen. Axial plane. A thick arrow points to the vertebral body in this prone fetus. Arrowheads point to a round structure in the "kidney area." Orthogonal views proved that there were no kidneys. When there is no kidney, adrenal glands can appear rounder and simulate a kidney. This fetus died as a newborn of pulmonary hypoplasia associated with bilateral renal agenesis. *(Reprinted from Cohen, Torrisi, and Schwartz, with permission.)*

References

Bertagnoli L, Lalatta F, Gallicchio R, et al: Quantitative characterization of the growth of the fetal kidney. *JCU* 11:349–356, 1983.

Cohen HL, Cooper J, Eisenberg P, et al: Normal length of fetal kidneys: Sonographic study in 397 obstetric patients. *AJR* 157: 545–548, 1991.

Cohen HL, Haller JO: Diagnostic sonography of the fetal genitourinary tract. *Urol Radiol* 9:88–98, 1987.

Cohen HL, Torrisi J, Schwartz J: Normal fetal chest, abdomen, pelvis, in *Diagnostic Medical Sonography. A Guide to Clinical Practice. Obstetrics and Gynecology,* 2d ed, Berman MC, Cohen HL (eds). Philadelphia, Lippincott, 1997:269–284.

Corteville J, Gray D, Crane J: Congenital hydronephrosis: Correlation of fetal ultrasonographic findings with infant outcome. *Am J Obstet Gynecol* 165:384–388, 1991.

Fitzsimons R: Kidney length in the newborn measured by ultrasound. *Acta Paediatr Scand* 72:885–887, 1983.

Glazebrook K, McGrath F, Steele B: Prenatal compensatory renal growth: Documentation with US. *Radiology* 189:733–735, 1993.

Grignon A, Filion R, Filiatrault D, et al: Urinary tract dilatation in utero: Classification and clinical applications. *Radiology* 160: 645–647, 1986.

Holloway H, Jones T, Robinson A, et al: Sonographic determination of renal volumes in normal neonates. *Pediatr Radiol* 13: 212–214, 1983.

Konje J, Okaro C, Bell S, et al: A cross-sectional study of changes in fetal renal size with gestation in appropriate and small-for-gestational-age fetuses. *Ultrasound Obstet Gynecol* 10:22–26, 1997.

Lawson T, Foley W, Berland L, et al: Ultrasonic evaluation of fetal kidneys: Analysis of normal size and frequency of visualization as related to stage of pregnancy. *Radiology* 138:153–156, 1981.

Rosenbaum D, Korngold E, Teele R: Sonographic assessment of fetal renal lengths in normal children. *AJR* 142:467–469, 1984.

Rosenberg E, Bowie J, Andreotti R, et al: Sonographic evaluation of fetal adrenal glands. *AJR* 139:145–147, 1982.

Schoenecker S, Cyr D, Mack L: Sonographic diagnosis of bilateral fetal renal duplication with ectopic ureteroceles. *J Ultrasound Med* 4:617–618, 1985.

TABLE 13-2
Causes of Fetal Pyelectasis and Hydronephrosis

Obstruction
UPJ construction
UVJ obstruction
Posterior urethral values
Reflux
Vesicoureteral reflux
Mesodermal defect
Prune-belly syndome
Physiological causes
Filled bladder

Key: UPJ = ureteropelvic junction; UVJ = ureterovesical junction.

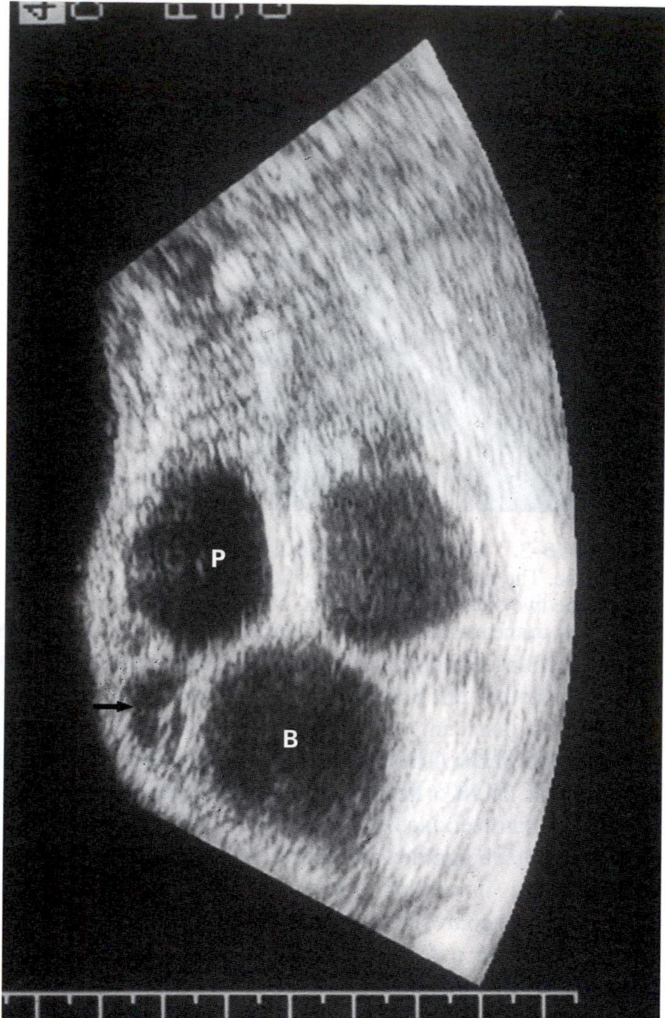

FIGURE 13–5. Significant pelvic dilatation due to prune-belly syndrome in a fetus with trisomy 21. Fetal chest/abdomen/pelvis. Coronal plane. This fetus was aborted at 20 weeks for many abnormalities. The renal pelves (*p* = left renal pelvis) are very dilated, as was the bladder (B). Autopsy data suggested the diagnosis of prune-belly syndrome. This mesodermal defect often involves tortuous dilated ureters. The amount of renal pelvic dilatation is far more than I have previously seen. Whether the dilatation is in part related to the trisomy 21 karyotype or not is unknown. An arrow points to a portion of the left ureter.

CAUSES OF FETAL PYELECTASIS AND HYDRONEPHROSIS

The etiologies of fetal pyelectasis are similar to those of neonatal and pediatric hydronephrosis. The renal pelvis may be dilated because of a distal obstruction, which could be at the UPJ, at the ureterovesical junction (UVJ), or at the bladder outlet and urethra, e.g., posterior urethral valves (PUV).

Nonobstructive Causes of Renal Pelvic Dilatation

Vesicoureteral reflux is the most common cause of pathologic renal pelvic dilatation without obstruction. There may also be apparent ureteral and possible renal pelvic dilatation (Fig. 13-5) that is not obstructive but associated with the mesodermal defect of prune-belly syndrome. Benacerraf et al have linked mild fetal renal pelvis dilatation to an increased risk for Down's syndrome. However, amniocentesis has not been recommended (because of the potential fetal loss from the procedure itself) if the only abnormality seen is renal pelvis dilatation and there are no other imaging findings associated with trisomy 21.

Obstructive Causes of Renal Pelvic Dilatation

Ureteropelvic junction obstruction is the most common obstructive cause of renal pelvic dilatation. One-third of cases have bilateral but asymmetric involvement. Patients with bilateral completely obstructive UPJs cannot survive. The early neonatal death, if the fetus survives fetal life, would usually be due to pulmonary hypoplasia. In following fetuses with UPJ obstruction, one can see progressive hydronephrosis antenatally, especially with higher grades of obstruction.

Ureterovesicular junction obstruction is far less common. A hydroureter should be imaged on the affected side to the level of the bladder. Fetuses with renal duplication anomalies (Fig. 13-6) have partial obstructions, usually of the upper pole moiety. The upper pole moiety may appear cystlike secondary to a distal obstruction associated with the ectopic placement of the distal ureter into the bladder, often in association with a ureterocele. There is usually VUR into the lower pole moiety. Both moieties can therefore appear dilated on ultrasound (US) examination.

Bladder outlet obstructions will be discussed elsewhere in Chap. 17.

WHICH FETUSES SHOULD BE FOLLOWED BY ULTRASOUND AND HOW?

In an attempt to capture as many true positive cases as possible, we adhere to Corteville's suggestions and follow fetuses with dilated renal pelves as small as 4 mm every 4 to 6 weeks. We do this when the 4-mm measurement is noted in the second trimester. We usually follow fetuses greater than

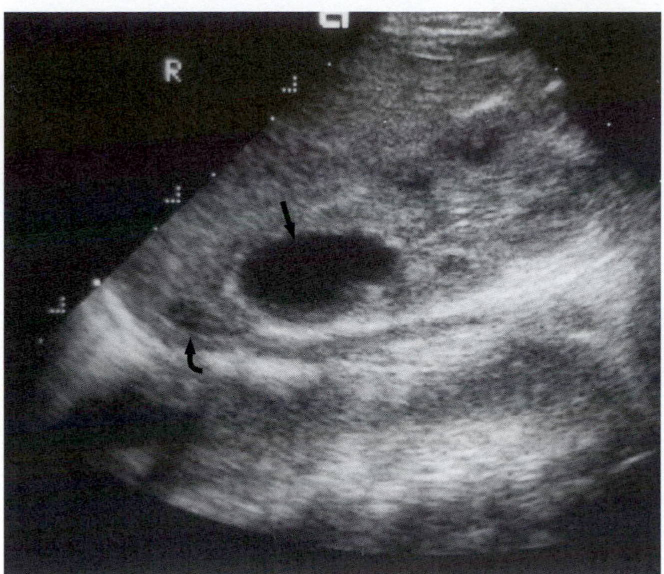

FIGURE 13–6. Obstructed upper moiety. Neonatal kidney. Longitudinal plane. There is dilatation of the pelvis (*arrow*) of the upper one-third of the kidney. This was an obstructed upper pole moiety of a duplication anomaly. This obstructed area was associated with a ureterocele. The remainder of the kidney's pyelocaliceal system is not distended, since there was no vesicoureteral reflux into the lower pole moiety of the duplication. Note the triangular adrenal (*curved arrow*) seen superior to (to the reader's left of) the kidney.

30 weeks only if the measurement is 7 mm or greater. This close follow-up, however, is only for those with possible bilateral involvement, since these fetuses are at risk for the development of oligohydramnios, and frequent clinical and sonographic assessment of the genitourinary system and the amniotic fluid volume can help in clinical decision making. In the presence of a contralateral functional and nondilated kidney, one may be less stringent about follow-up obstetric ultrasound until after birth. We tend to do at least one third-trimester follow-up if unilateral abnormality is noted in the second trimester. After birth, there is a relative hypovolemia among infants because of relative dehydration and relatively low glomerular filtration rates. This may result in a falsely normal appearance of the newborn renal pelvis if it is evaluated on the first day of life. Antenatal confirmation of hydronephrosis should, therefore, be performed on day 2 or 3 of life. With all this "scientific" planning and follow-up, one must emphasize that the majority of kidneys with prenatal pyelectasis prove to be normal at birth and that fetuses without any abnormality on antenatal examination may still develop obstruction or reflux that can be imaged after birth. In fact, according to one group, prenatal US is less sensitive than postnatal US in detecting obstructive uropathies.

AN IMPORTANT CLINICAL CONSIDERATION

Avoid immediate postbirth analysis of the neonatal kidney to rule out hydronephrosis or to evaluate antenatally detected pyelectasis. This postnatal analysis for hydronephrosis is one of several instances in clinical US where one does the patient a disservice by doing an immediate "emergency" examination. Day 2 or 3 of life is the best time to look.

AN IMAGING POINT TO REMEMBER

Fetal renal dilatations of 10 mm or greater warrant assessment for pathologic causes of hydronephrosis. Extending the grey zone of concern to as low as 4 mm in the very young fetus and 7 mm in the third-trimester fetus will help avoid missing some cases. Infants can develop obstructive hydronephrosis despite normal fetal exams.

IS THERE A GENETIC PREDISPOSITION TO PYELECTASIS?

There may be a genetic predisposition to fetal renal pyelectasis. Among a group of mothers whose normal fetuses had mild pyelectasis on antenatal US, 67 percent of their next pregnancies had a fetus with pyelectasis.

References

Benacerraf B, Mandell J, Estroff J, et al: Fetal pyelectasis: A possible association with Down syndrome. *Obstet Gynecol* 76:58–60, 1990.

Cohen H, Haller J: Diagnostic sonography of the fetal genitourinary tract. *Urol Radiol* 9:88–98, 1987.

Cohen HL, Muller D, Zinn DL: Abnormal fetal chest, abdomen, pelvis, in *Diagnostic Medical Sonography. A Guide to Clinical Practice, Obstetrics and Gynecology,* 2d ed, Berman MC, Cohen HL (eds). Philadelphia, Lippincott, 1997:285–320.

Cohen HL, Torrisi J, Schwartz J: Normal fetal chest, abdomen, pelvis, in *Diagnostic Medical Sonography. A Guide to Clinical Practice. Obstetrics and Gynecology,* 2d ed, Berman MC, Cohen HL (eds). Philadelphia, Lippincott, 1997:269–284.

Corteville J, Gray D, Crane J: Congenital hydronephrosis: Correlation of fetal ultrasonographic findings with infant outcome. *Am J Obstet Gynecol* 165:384–388, 1991.

Degani S, Leibovitz Z, Shapiro I, et al: Fetal pyelectasis in consecutive pregnancies: A possible genetic predisposition. *Ultrasound Obstet Gynecol* 10:19–21, 1997.

Dremsek P, Gindl K, Voitl P, et al: Renal pyelectasis in fetuses and neonates—diagnostic value of renal pelvic diameter in pre- and postnatal sonographic screening. *AJR* 168:1017–1019, 1997.

Grignon A, Filiatrault D, Homsy Y, et al: Ureteropelvic junction stenosis: Antenatal ultrasonographic diagnosis, postnatal investigation and follow-up. *Radiology* 160:649–651, 1986.

Grignon A, Filion R, Filiatrault D, et al: Urinary tract dilatation in utero. Classification and clinical applications. *Radiology* 160:645–647, 1986.

Hoddick W, Filly R, Mahony B, et al: Minimal renal pyelectasis. *J Ultrasound Med* 4:85–89, 1985.

Laing F, Burke V, Wing V, et al: Postpartum evaluation of fetal hydronephrosis: Optimal timing for follow-up sonography. *Radiology* 152:423–424, 1984.

Mayor G, Genton N, Torado A, et al: Renal function in obstructive nephropathy: Long-term effects of reconstructive surgery. *Pediatrics* 56:740–743, 1975.

Petrikovsky B, Cohen HL, Cuomo M, et al: Degree of fetal hydronephrosis depends on the fetal bladder size [abstr]. *Am J Obstet Gynecol* 170:363, 1994.

Seeds J: Antenatal sonographic assessment of the genitourinary tract, in *Ultrasound Annual 1986,* Sanders R, Hill M (eds). New York, Raven, 1986:67–97.

Wilson R, Lynch S, Lessoway V: Fetal pyelectasis—comparison of postnatal renal pathology with unilateral and bilateral pyelectasis. *Prenat Diagn* 17:451–455, 1997.

14

Figure 14-1 is a view of a second-trimester fetus that is not doing well. Three abnormalities should be noted. What does the patient have?

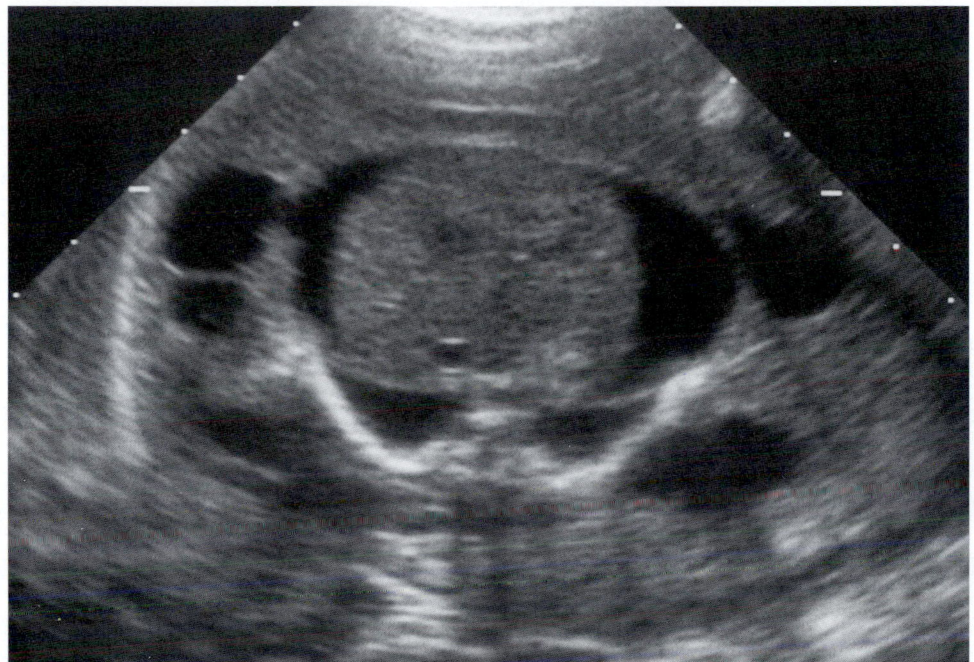

FIGURE 14–1. Fetal abdomen. Axial plane.

CHAPTER 14

Ascites and Pleural Effusion in Hydrops

HARRIS L. COHEN

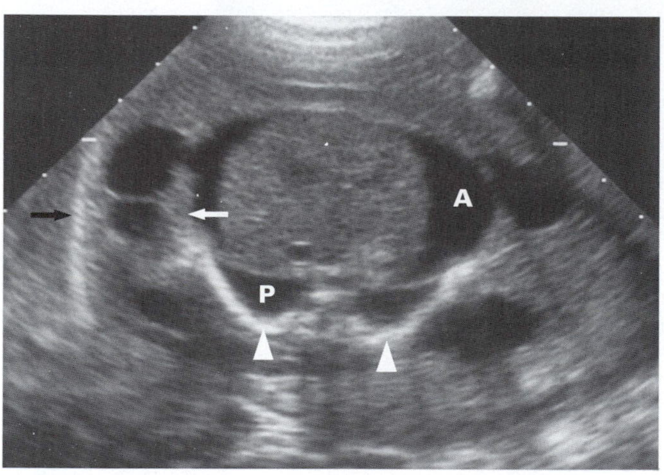

FIGURE 14–2. Annotated version of Fig. 14-2. Fetal hydrops. Abdomen. Axial plane. The fetus is supine; the spine and ribs (*arrowheads*) are seen posteriorly. Fluid surrounds the fetal liver, consistent with ascites (*A*). Pleural fluid (*P*) is seen posterior to the liver and behind the diaphragm. The fetus has severely thickened skin (*arrows*) with contained cystic areas that may be related to the patient's cystic hygroma. The fetus has fetal hydrops and died in utero.

Figure 14-2, the annotated version of Fig. 14-1, shows fluid in the abdomen conforming to the abdominal contours and consistent with ascites. There is pleural fluid, noted as the triangular echoless areas conforming to the pleural space posterior to the diaphragms. One must remember that the posterior costophrenic angles of the lungs descend inferior to the level of the more anterior portions of the diaphragms. The fetus is surrounded by solid and cystic structures that represent severely thickened skin. The cysts may be part of the patient's cystic hygroma. Figure 14-3 provides a coronal view of the pleural effusion, ascites, and cystic masses in thickened skin. The fetus had nonimmune hydrops and died in utero.

FETAL ASCITES, PLEURAL EFFUSION AND FETAL HYDROPS

Any fluid in the peritoneal cavity or pleural space of a fetus of any gestational age is abnormal. Overall mortality for the discovery of a pleural effusion is at least 50 percent; it is highest when the pleural effusion is discovered earlier in the pregnancy, is bilateral in distribution, or is associated with

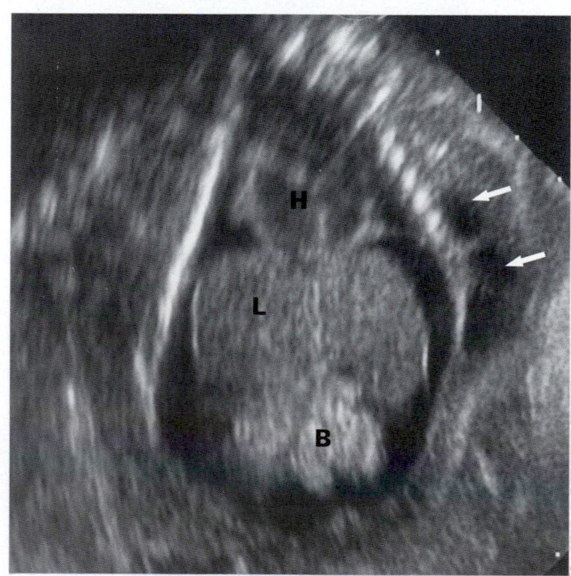

FIGURE 14–3. Fetal chest/abdomen. Coronal plane. This is the same fetus as in the previous figures. Triangular pleural fluid is seen lateral to the heart (H). Ascites is seen lateral to the liver (L) and spleen and lateral and inferior to the more echogenic collapsed small bowel (B). Arrows point to some cystic areas within the thickened skin. This fetus had an abnormal karyotype and an associated cystic hygroma. Ascites and pleural effusion in association with cystic hygroma predicts a poor outcome. *(Reprinted from Cohen et al, with permission.)*

fetal hydrops. Fetal hydrops is a condition in which excessive fluid accumulates within the fetal soft tissues and body cavities. It can be immune or nonimmune in type.

Immune hydrops occurs in a fetus whose mother has been sensitized, usually in previous pregnancies, by a blood factor histoincompatibility, usually Rhesus (Rh) factor but possibly due to any fetal red blood cell antigens. An immune reaction between maternal immunoglobulin G and the fetal blood factor leads to the significant fetal morbidity and mortality. Early warning signs may be a small amount of ascites or pericardial effusion. Obviously the massive signs in this case are consistent with significant fetal decompensation. Polyhydramnios is a sensitive indicator of severe fetal anemia and a harbinger of fetal decompensation and frank immune hydrops. In full-blown immune hydrops, there is sonographic evidence of thick (greater than 5 mm) skin, large pleural and pericardial effusions, ascites, and hepatosplenomegaly. Current obstetric treatment has markedly improved mortality in immune hydrops.

The prognosis for nonimmune hydrops (NIH) remains poor. Mortality is reported at 50 to 98 percent. This may be because NIH is not a disease but the late result of several different fetal diseases or circumstances. The ultrasound (US) findings are similar to those in immune hydrops.

The causes of NIH are quite varied. Lymphatic obstruction associated with Turner's syndrome may be a cause, as may the hypoproteinemia resulting from congenital liver or renal disease (e.g., nephrotic syndrome). Many "idiopathic" cases are thought to really be due to cardiac arrhythmias or anomalies (e.g., hypoplastic left heart and supraventricular tachycardia), which are well-known causes of cardiac failure leading to NIH. Intrauterine TORCH (*t*oxoplasmosis, *o*ther, *r*ubella, *c*ytomegalovirus, *h*erpes) infections may also lead to cardiac failure. Causes of high-output cardiac failure that lead to NIH include severe anemias (e.g., congenital α thalassemia, an extremely common cause in Asia), twin-to-twin transfusion syndrome, or a Galenic arteriovenous malformation. Chromosomal abnormalities (Turner's syndrome, trisomy 18 or 21) are associated with NIH. Fetal masses within the chest [e.g., CCAM (congenital cystic adenomatoid malformation)] or abdomen (e.g., neuroblastoma) can lead to obstruction of venous return and NIH. Maternal causes may include diabetes and toxemia. The increased flow of an occasional placental chorioangioma has also been implicated as a cause.

FETAL ASCITES

Ascites represents fluid in the peritoneum. True fetal ascites is always abnormal. Depending on the amount, the fluid may be seen only in dependent portions of the fetus (e.g., the pelvis in a fetus in breech position). In large amounts, it may be seen surrounding intraperitoneal structures and shifting them superiorly, inferiorly, or laterally. It should be searched for in the subhepatic space, the flanks, and the lower abdominal/pelvic cavity (Fig. 14-4). The retroperitoneal structures such as the kidneys lie posterior to the free fluid (Fig. 14-5).

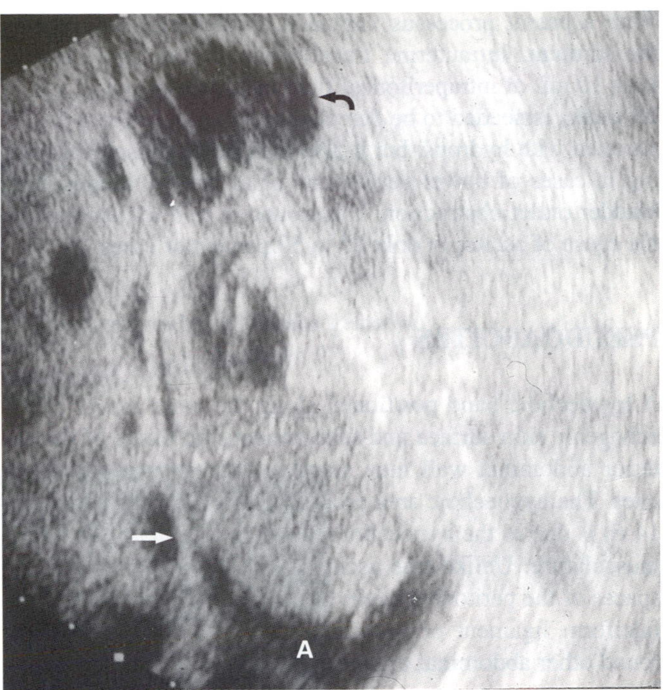

FIGURE 14–4. Early nonimmune hydrops. Fetal neck, chest, and abdomen. Sagittal plane. The fetus is facing the reader's left. Ascites (A) is seen as an echoless area below the bowel. The amount was too small to be imaged to the sides of the liver or spleen on views through the upper abdomen. There is no pericardial effusion at this time. This fetus also has a cystic hygroma in the area of the neck (*curved arrow*). Notice that there is no skin thickening (*arrow*) at this time. This fetus eventually developed full-blown hydrops associated with Turner's syndrome. The baby died in utero.

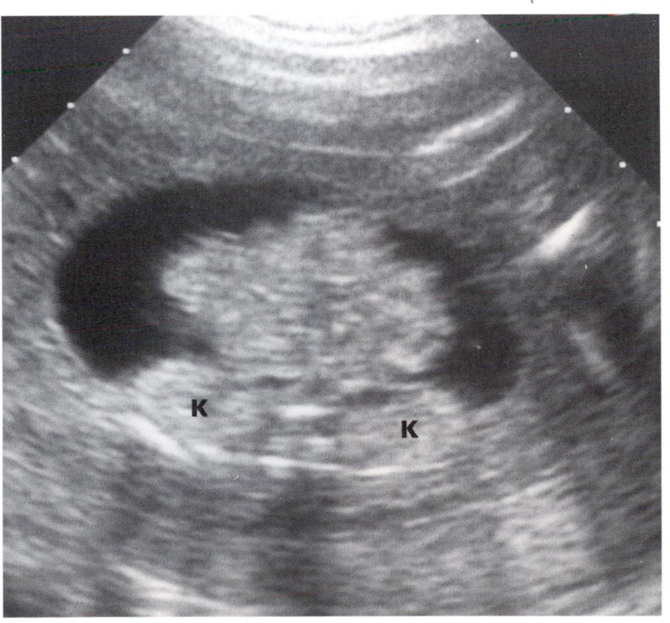

FIGURE 14–5. Fetal ascites. Fetal midabdomen at level of kidneys. Axial plane. Ascites is noted in the peritoneal cavity. It does not surround the retroperitoneal kidneys (Ks).

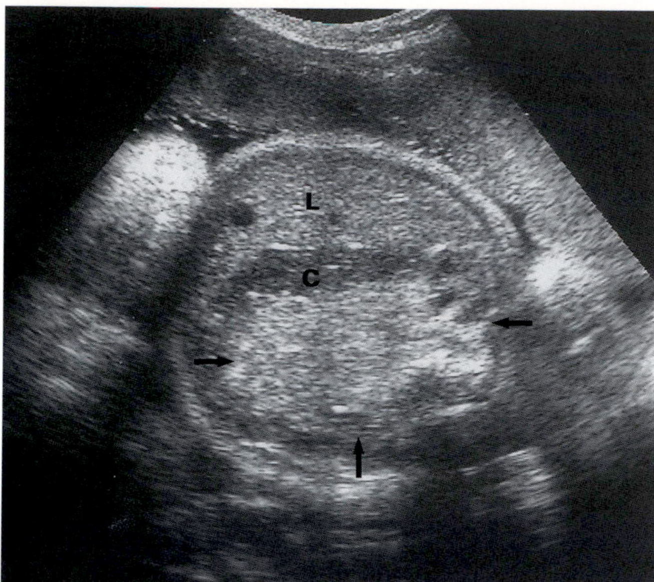

FIGURE 15–8. Normal collapsed echogenic small bowel. Axial section through the midabdomen of a third-trimester fetus. Liver (*L*) is noted in the fetus's right upper quadrant. There is a hypoechoic loop of normal colon (*C*), near which is a large, minimally echogenic (not equal to or greater than the echogenicity of bone) area (*arrows*) that represents normal collapsed small bowel. Large bowel, as in this case, lies peripheral to the more central small bowel.

The ascending and descending colon are found at the periphery of the fetal abdomen (Fig. 15-8). The colon does not normally demonstrate peristalsis, and although the colonic diameter increases linearly with advancing gestation, it should not be greater than 23 mm.

ANTENATAL BOWEL LUMEN DILATATION: SMALL-BOWEL ATRESIA

Fetal bowel dilatation is uncommon. When prenatal sonography reveals multiple interconnecting loops of dilated bowel, this is usually due to a mechanical obstruction. An actual level of obstruction is difficult to localize prior to birth. When small-bowel dilatation is observed, one must consider the diagnoses listed in Table 15-1. Small-bowel atresia is thought to be secondary to an in utero vascular insult and occurs in 1 in 3000 to 5000 live births. Atresias (Fig. 15-9) are more common than stenoses and are often multiple. Although there is a low rate of associated extraintestinal anomalies in cases of bowel atresia, other gastrointestinal (GI) anomalies are found in 45 percent of cases and include bowel malrotation, volvulus, duplication, meconium ileus, esophageal atresia, and microcolon. Since fetal swallowing begins at 16 to 17 weeks, bowel dilatation and the polyhydramnios that is associated with it in cases of proximal GI tract obstruction are observed only later in pregnancy, in the the late second and third trimesters. Polyhydramnios is far less likely to be noted in association with more distal obstructions. Progressive small-bowel dilatation during the third trimester and hyperperistalsis are strong predictors of an underlying small-bowel obstruction.

TABLE 15-1
Differential Diagnostic Consideration—Fetal Small-Bowel Dilatation

Common possibilities
1. Jejunal, ileal, or jejunoileal atresia
2. Midgut volvulus
3. Meconium ileus
4. Intestinal duplication
5. Internal hernias
6. Colonic obstruction
Rarer possibilities
7. Megacystis-microcolon–intestinal hypoperistalsis syndrome
8. Syphilis
9. Congenital chloride diarrhea

MECONIUM PERITONITIS, CYSTIC FIBROSIS, ECHOGENIC BOWEL

Fetal ascites, observed in combination with other signs of bowel obstruction, suggests the possibility of a spontaneous bowel perforation with subsequent meconium peritonitis. Intraabdominal calcifications, specifically peritoneal calcifications, are highly suggestive of meconium peritonitis and are frequently observed after fetal bowel rupture. Foreign body

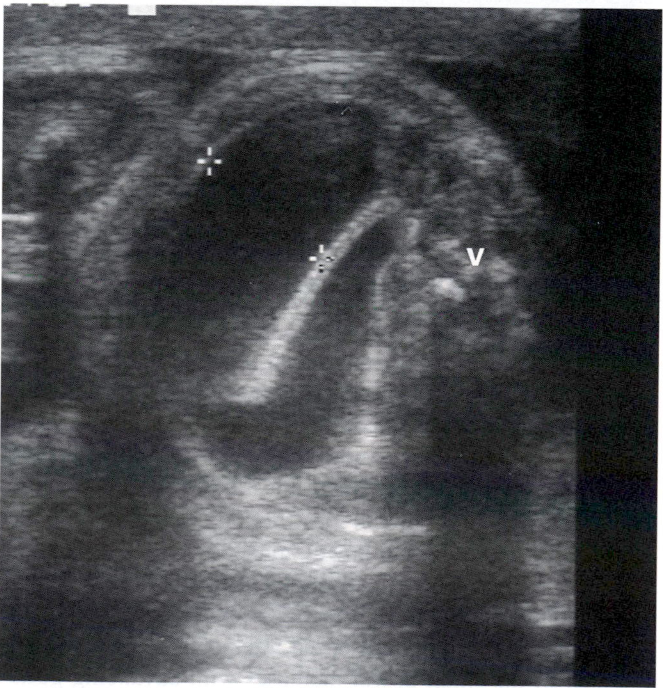

FIGURE 15–9. Jejunal atresia. Transverse plane through low abdomen/pelvis. There is a moderately dilated bowel loop, which was the only antenatal evidence of what proved to be an isolated area of jejunal atresia. The vertebral body (v) is to the reader's left.

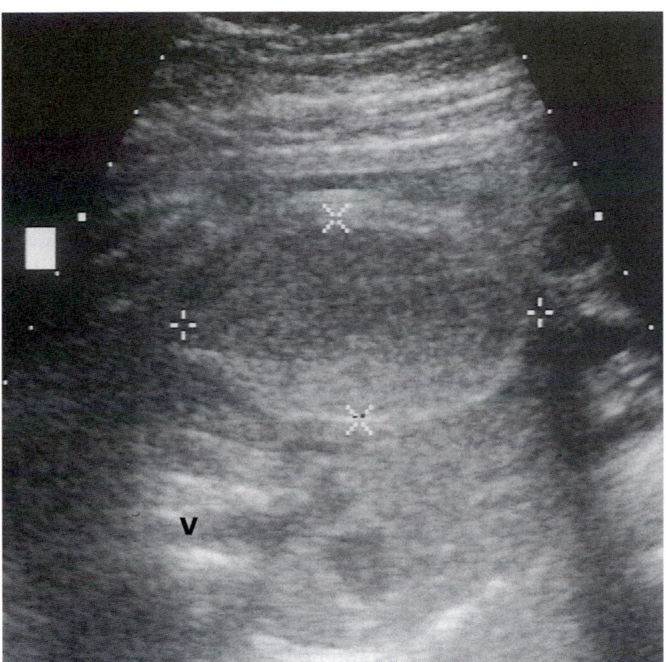

FIGURE 15–10. Meconium pseudocyst. Transverse plane through lower fetal abdomen. A complicated cystic mass (*marked off by crosses*) containing a debris-debris level consistent with meconium pseudocyst is seen. It developed as a complication of the jejunal atresia associated with gastroschisis that this fetus proved to have. V = vertebral body.

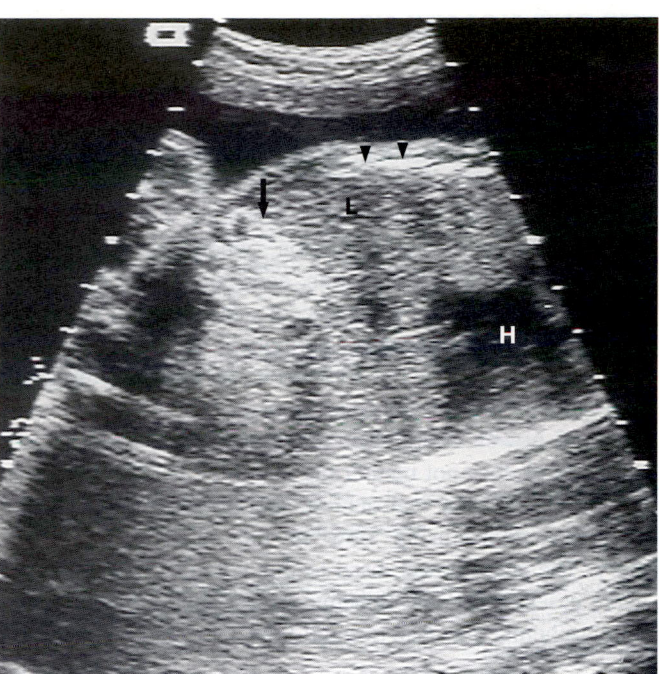

FIGURE 15–11. Cystic fibrosis. Fetal abdomen. Coronal plane. Echogenic fetal bowel (*arrow*) was noted to have an echogenicity equal to or greater than nearby fetal bone (*arrowheads*). This suggested that the echogenic bowel was of greater concern than normal. The fetus proved to have cystic fibrosis. L = liver, H = heart.

giant cells' inflammatory reaction with calcium deposition is responsible for the ultrasound (US) image of linear or punctate echogenicities, which are often best imaged in such cases at the periphery of the liver .

A meconium pseudocyst (Fig. 15-10) may be observed after bowel rupture if the meconium is localized to a particular area of the peritoneum. It appears as a thick-walled intraabdominal cystic mass that may contain debris, septations, or calcifications. Although among many fetuses, bowel perforations may close and the associated meconium peritonitis resolve without sequelae, there are others who may need surgery to correct the bowel obstruction or other cause of perforation soon after birth. Fetuses with peritoneal calcification or meconium pseudocysts should therefore be followed antenatally to note any development of associated bowel obstruction.

The development of meconium peritonitis is most commonly caused by small-bowel atresia, volvulus, intussusception, or viral infections such as cytomegalovirus (CMV). Internal hernias are said to be the cause in as many as 50 percent of cases. At least 15 percent of cases of meconium peritonitis, and perhaps as many as 40 percent, are found in fetuses with cystic fibrosis (CF) and underlying meconium ileus. In one reported series, one-third of fetuses with dilated bowel had CF.

Meconium ileus represents an obstruction secondary to inspissated meconium in the distal ileum and almost always implies underlying CF. The observation of echogenic bowel (Fig. 15-11) in fetuses with CF is related to these inspissated intestinal contents. Other antenatal sonographic features of CF are secondary to the complications of perforation and associated meconium peritonitis. The discovery of echogenic bowel in association with dilated bowel is more predictive of CF than the identification of dilated bowel alone. At times the US image of a fetus with meconium ileus is indistinguishable from that of a fetus with small-bowel atresia. The two conditions may also coexist. The detection of fetal bowel dilatation warrants testing for CF.

Again, echogenic bowel may be a normal variant. A review of the other differential diagnostic possibilities can be found in Table 15-2. Isolated second-trimester echogenic bowel has been associated with increased risk of adverse perinatal outcome and third-trimester growth restriction.

TABLE 15-2
Differential Diagnosis of Echogenic Bowel

1. Normal variant
2. Cystic fibrosis
3. Congenital infections (cytomegalovirus, toxoplasmosis)
4. Fetal trisomies
5. Severe fetal growth restriction
6. Intraamniotic bleeding with secondary swallowing of blood by the fetus

16

Figure 16-1 is a coronal view of a fetus. Is any abnormality seen? What problems should we consider?

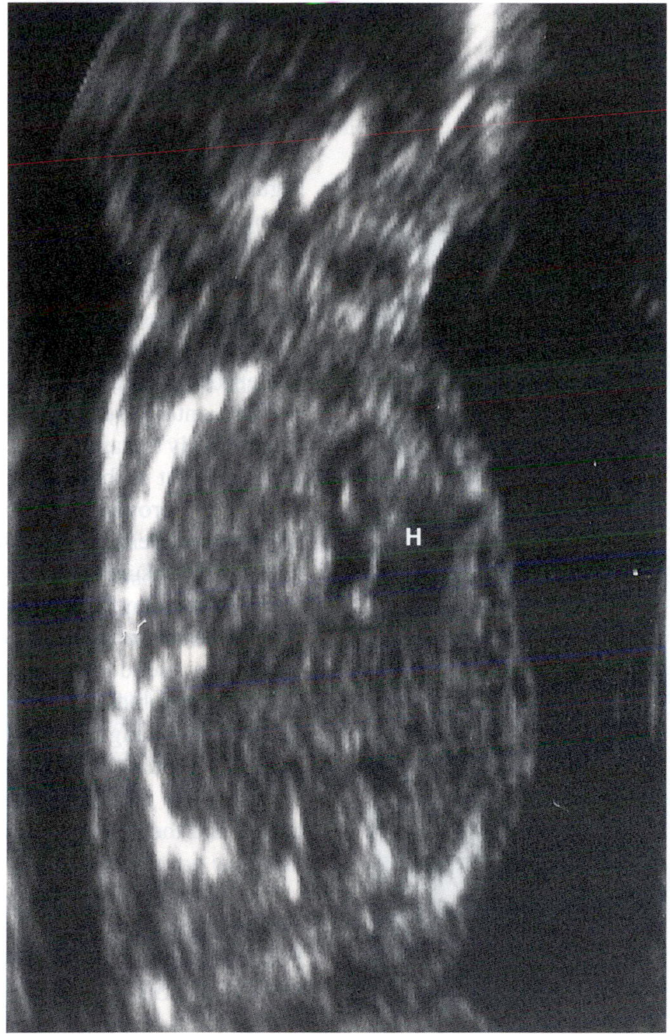

FIGURE 16–1. Fetal head, neck, thorax, and abdomen. Coronal plane, some obliquity. H = heart.

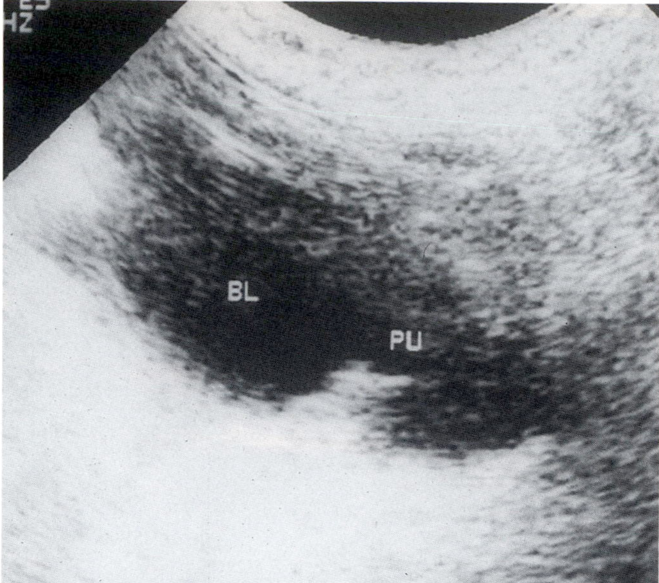

FIGURE 17–6. Keyhole sign. Bladder/urethra. Coronal plane. There is significant distention of the bladder (BL) and lesser distention of the posterior urethra (PU). They appear as a keyhole, with the larger portion of the key fitting through the bladder and the smaller portion through the urethra. Seeing both distended suggests PUV, although there are other differential diagnostic considerations (Table 17-1).

The imaging of hydronephrosis is most helpful in diagnosing PUV, since it is seen in 90 percent of children with PUV. The imaging of a dilated bladder and dilated posterior urethra (Fig. 17-6, Table 17-1) has been called the keyhole sign and suggests PUV.

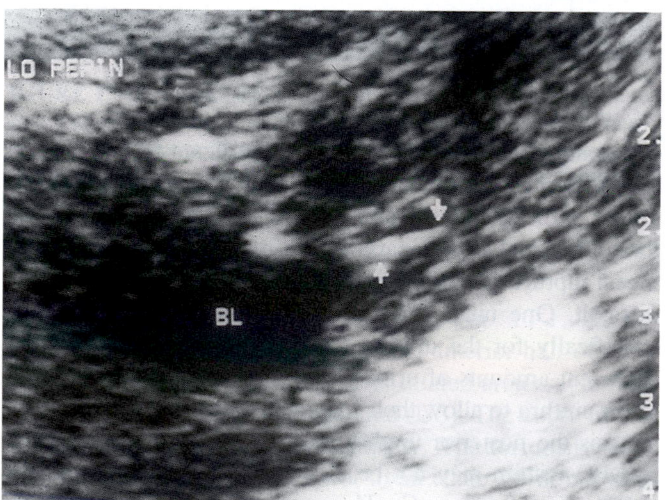

FIGURE 17–7. Valve seen in fetal posterior urethra. Bladder/urethra. Transperineal view. Coronal plane. An echogenic linear structure (*arrows*) is seen in the distended posterior urethra of this fetus with PUV. BL = bladder.

TABLE 17-1
Differential Diagnosis Considerations in Ultrasound Assessment for PUV

Dilated Posterior Urethra
1. Posterior urethral valve due to obstruction
2. Urethral atresia due to obstruction
3. Prune-belly (Eagle-Barrett) syndrome due to mesodermal defect

Bladder Outlet Obstruction
1. Posterior urethral valve (PUV)
2. Urethral atresia
3. Caudal regression syndrome

Dilated Ureters
1. Vesicoureteral reflux
2. Ureterovesicle junction obstruction
3. Posterior urethral valve
4. Primary megaureter—does not have associated pyelocaliceal system dilatation

A RECENT ULTRASOUND FINDING FOR DIAGNOSING PUV

In recent years, we have been able to image a linear echogenicity (Fig. 17-7) within the dilated posterior urethra of three fetuses that has proved to be the posterior valve itself. Certainly, if this is seen, a more definitive diagnosis of PUV can be made.

IMAGING TIP

Consider PUV in all cases of hydronephrosis. If the fetus is a male, try to find the posterior urethra and try to note if the bladder is distended or its wall thickened.

References

Aaronson I: Posterior urethral valve: A review of 120 cases. *S Afr Med J* 65:418–422, 1984.

Blumhagen J: Echographic findings in posterior urethral valves. Presented at the 26th annual meeting of the Society for Pediatric Radiology, Atlanta, GA, 1983.

Cohen HL, Haller JO: Diagnostic sonography of the fetal genitourinary tract. *Urol Radiol* 9:88–98, 1987.

Cohen HL, Susman M, Haller JO, et al: Posterior urethral valve: Transperineal US for imaging and diagnosis in male infants. *Radiology* 192:261–264, 1994.

Cohen HL, Zinn H, Patel A, et al: Prenatal sonographic diagnosis of posterior urethral valves: Identification of valves and thickening of the posterior urethral wall. *JCU* 26:366–370, 1998.

Cremin B, Aaronson I: Ultrasonic diagnosis of posterior urethral valves in neonates. *Br J Radiol* 56:435–438, 1983.

Currarino G, Wood B, Majd M: Abnormalities of the pelvocaliceal system, ureter, bladder, and urethra, in *Caffey's Pediatric X-Ray Diagnosis: An Integrated Imaging Approach*, 9th ed, Silverman F, Kuhn J (eds). St. Louis, Mosby, 1993:1284–1303.

Freedman AL, Bukowski TP, Smith CA, et al: Fetal therapy for obstructive uropathy: Specific outcomes diagnosis. *J Urol* 156: 720–723, 1996.

Kaplan GW, Scherz HC: Posterior urethra, in *Clinical Pediatric Urology*, 3d ed, Kelalis P, King L, Belman AB (eds). Philadelphia, Saunders, 1992:835–849.

Macpherson R, Leithiser R, Gordon L, Turner W: Posterior urethral valves: An update and review. *Radiographics* 6:753–791, 1986.

Mahoney BS: Ultrasound evaluation of the fetal genitourinary system, in *Ultrasonography in Obstetrics and Gynecology*, 3d ed, Callen PW (ed). Philadelphia, Saunders, 1994:389–419.

Young HH, Frontz WA, Baldwin JC: Congenital obstruction of the posterior urethra. *J Urol* 3:289–354, 1919.

CHAPTER 18

Multicystic Dysplastic Kidney

HARRIS L. COHEN

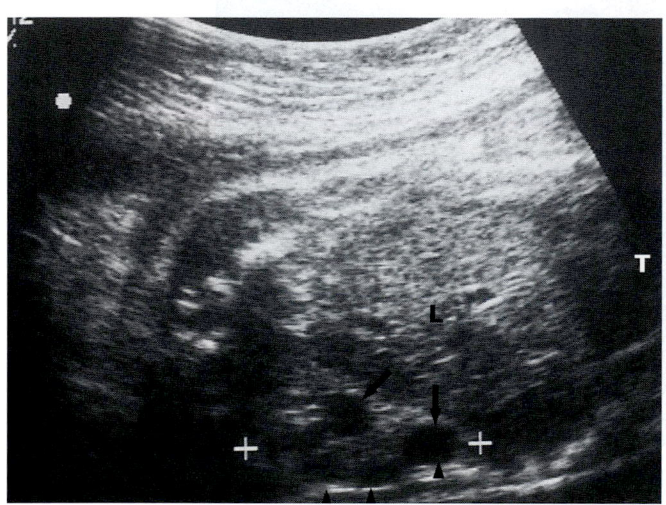

FIGURE 18–2. Annotated version of Fig. 18-1. Multicystic dysplastic kidney (MDK). Fetal abdomen. Sagittal plane. The fetal chest is to the reader's right. The kidney (*marked off by crosses*) contains at least two cysts (*arrows*). Three smaller cysts that may simulate echopenic pyramids are also seen (*arrowheads*). None of the cysts are central, suggesting that cystic disease rather than obstruction with a dilated central renal pelvis is the cause. This was a multicystic dysplastic kidney. L = liver, T = thorax.

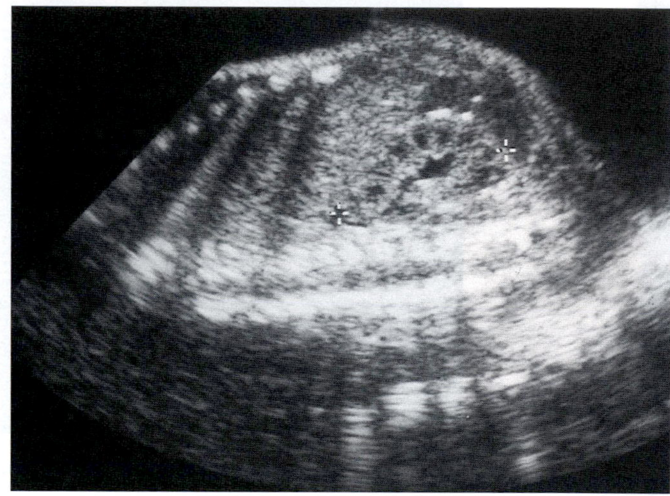

FIGURE 18–3. Mild pyelectasis. Fetal chest/abdomen. Sagittal plane through the kidney. The fetal chest is to the reader's left. The kidney (*marked off by crosses*) has a mildly fluid-filled pelvis consistent with pyelectasis. The more superficial anterior of the anterior and posterior rows of normal echopenic pyramids surrounding the pelvis is seen. V = vertebal bodies.

Figure 18-2 (the annotated version of Fig. 18-1) shows a right kidney with two larger and three smaller cysts (confirmed on other views). There is no central cyst which might have suggested hydronephrosis with surrounding dilated calices or even pyelectasis with surrounding echopenic pyramids (Fig. 18-3). This was a unilateral multicystic dysplastic kidney (MDK). When this is discovered in fetal life, one must search the contralateral kidney for abnormality, as will be discussed. If the contralateral kidney is normal, the prognosis is excellent. The MDK is one of several renal dysplasias.

WHAT ARE THE RENAL DYSPLASIAS?

Renal dysplasias are said to occur at the rate of 2 to 4 cases for every 1000 births. Multicystic dysplastic kidney, as well as the other cystic renal dysplasias, is thought to be the result

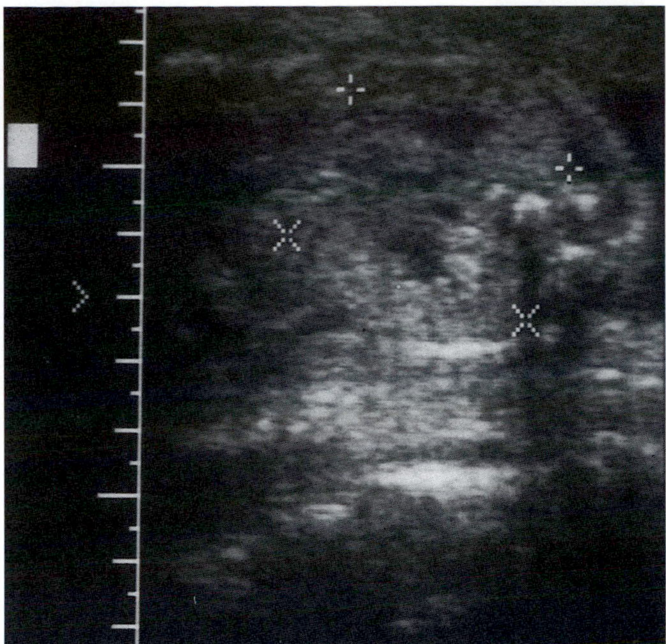

FIGURE 18–4. Autosomal recessive polycystic kidney disease (ARPKD). Fetal abdomen. Coronal plane. This fetus was 17 weeks old, yet had enlarged and echogenic kidneys (*marked by crosses*) of 3.6 to 3.9 cm. This suggested recessive polycystic kidney disease. The fetus had two deceased siblings with ARPKD. A central echoless area noted in each kidney represented urine in the renal pelvis from still-functioning glomeruli and gave hope to some observers that the fetus would survive. However, during the late second trimester, nonvisualization of the bladder and significant oligohydramnios suggested that urine production had ceased. The fetus died soon after birth and proved to have classic APRKD.

of abnormal metanephric tissue differentiation early in gestation. Early obstructions or atresias are thought to be the cause of abnormal metanephric bud and metanephric blastema interactions that lead to abnormal induction and maturation of glomeruli as well as abnormal development of the collecting system, including the collecting tubules, calices, and ureters. Disorganized epithelial structures and fibrous tissue are found in place of normally functioning glomeruli and tubules. Dysplastic areas remain abnormal throughout life. It is the cysts of these dysplasias that often permit their early antenatal diagnosis. Bilateral renal dysplasias are not compatible with long life, predominantly because poor antenatal renal production results in oligohydramnios, which, when severe, leads to lung hypoplasia. Early death is due to pulmonary hypoplasia and renal failure.

Osthanondh and Potter classified cystic dysplasias of the kidneys into four types: type I, autosomal recessive polycystic kidney disease (ARPKD), also known as infantile polycystic kidney disease; type II, multicystic dysplastic kidney, or MDK (now divided into IIa, the classic pelvoinfundibular atresia type of our unknown case, and IIb, a form that simulates a hydronephrotic kidney); type III, autosomal dominant polycystic kidney disease (ADPKD), once known as adult polycystic kidney disease; and type IV, cystic renal dysplasia (due to urethral obstruction).

FACTS ABOUT THE OTHER RENAL DYSPLASIAS

Autosomal recessive polycystic kidney disease affects both kidneys. It occurs in 1 in 16,000 to 55,000 births. There is a 25 percent recurrence rate in affected families. The 1- to 2-mm saccular dilatations of the collecting tubules seen on gross pathology examination are too small to be resolved as individual cysts on ultrasound (US). This is said to occur because the multiple collecting tubule walls present multiple interstices to the ultrasound beam, resulting in a prominent area of increased echogenicity, similar to what happens with multiple small fat cells, which also are imaged as a coalescent area of increased echogenicity. In ARPKD, therefore, kidneys classically appear on US as enlarged, homogeneously echogenic kidneys, often taking up most of the abdomen's space and having a circumference that goes beyond the classic normal kidney circumference–to–abdominal circumference ratio of 0.3. Some renal function may persist early in gestation, and central echoless renal pelves may be seen (Fig. 18-4). Ultrasound imaging of ARPKD in the second trimester (a time when possible abortion decisions have to be made) can look normal, and these abnormal kidneys and their decreased amniotic fluid production may first be noted only in the late second or third trimester.

Autosomal dominant polycystic kidney disease or adult polycystic kidney disease is a very common cause of renal failure in middle-aged to older adults but is rarely seen in antenatal life. Case reports note cysts interspersed in the cortex and medulla of bilaterally enlarged kidneys. Small cysts may not be resolved, and the kidneys may appear similar to those of autosomal recessive disease (ARPKD). Asymmetry of involvement with only decreased or normal amniotic fluid levels has been reported.

Type IV cystic renal dysplasia and MDK are the most common renal dysplasias. Type IV cystic renal dysplasia is thought to be secondary to an early obstruction of the lower genitourinary tract. It may be noted in severe cases of posterior urethral valves but is more commonly seen in association with urethral atresia (Fig. 18-5) and caudal regression syndrome. Sonographically, involvement is bilateral, with the kidneys enlarged, echogenic, and containing small peripheral capsular and/or parenchymal cysts that can be individually imaged.

THE MULTICYSTIC DYSPLASTIC KIDNEY

The MDK is the most common of the cystic renal dysplasias. When, as is typical, it is a unilateral finding, the intrauterine amniotic fluid level is normal and fetal lung development is unhindered. Contralateral abnormalities, however, often occur. When they do occur and there is no urine production or whatever urine is produced does not enter first the bladder and then the amniotic cavity, the fetus/neonate will not survive. There is a 19 percent incidence of bilateral MDKs.

Section D
GENITAL CYST

19

Figure 19-1 is an image of a fetus's pelvis. Two cystic structures are noted. One is the bladder. What could the other be? What key antenatal finding could help in differential diagnosis?

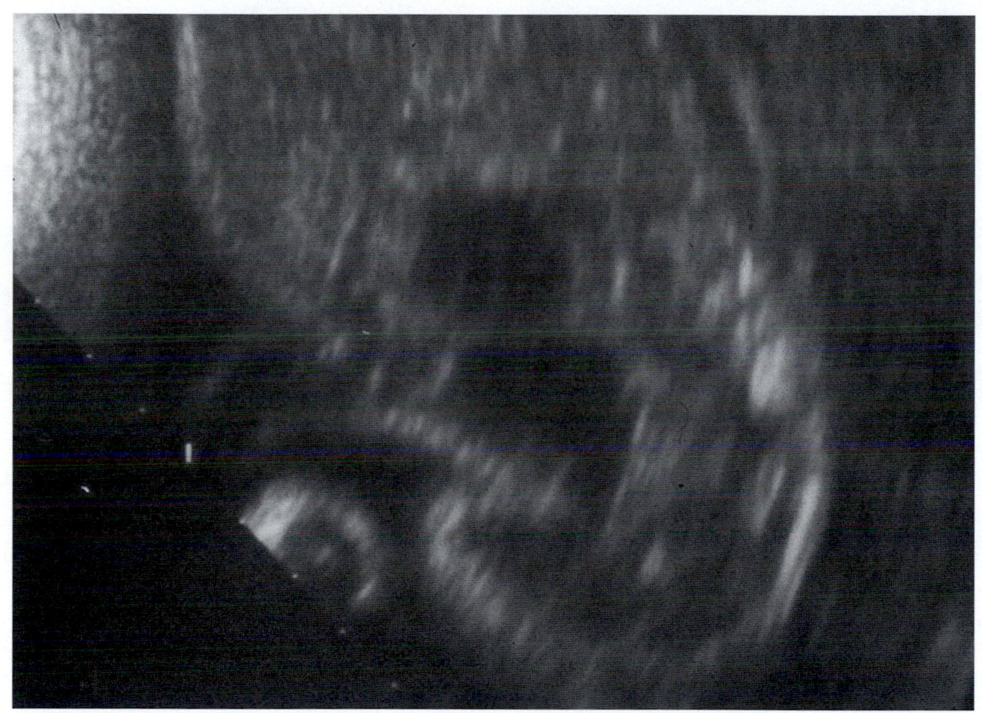

FIGURE 19–1. Fetal pelvis/lower abdomen. Sagittal plane. The fetus is facing the reader's left.

CHAPTER 19

Fetal Ovarian Cyst

HARRIS L. COHEN

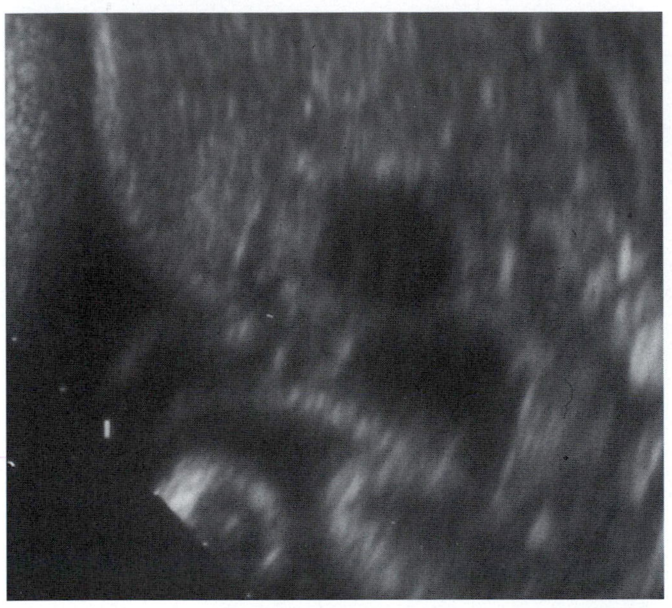

IGURE 19–2. Annotated version of Fig. 19-1. Fetal pelvis/lower abdomen. Sagittal plane. Two cystic areas are noted in the fetal pelvis. The more inferior one is the bladder. The cystic area (*arrow*) superior to it contains septations or the walls of smaller cysts. In a female fetus, the first consideration is an ovary. If several follicles/cysts can be seen, an endocrinologically stimulated ovary must be considered. Only normal adnexa with a few contained smaller follicles were noted in this child after birth.

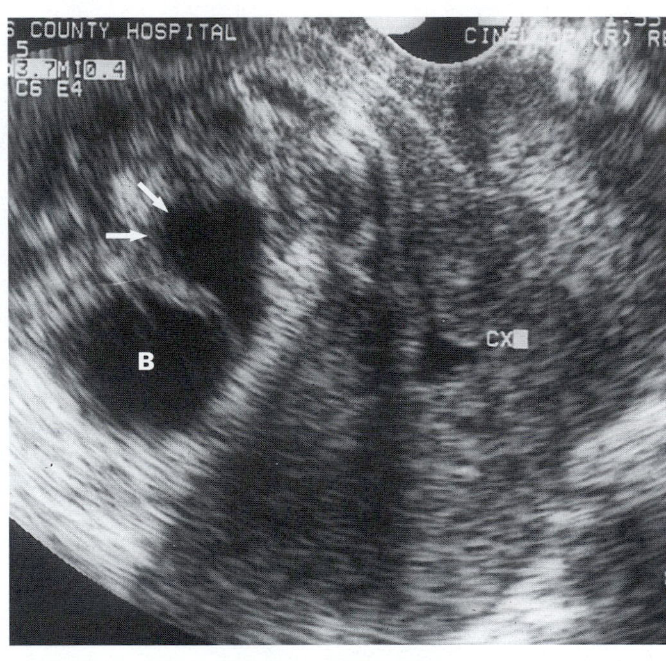

FIGURE 19–3. Unilocular fetal ovarian cyst. *A*. Sagittal plane through maternal cervix. Transvaginal technique. Two cystic pelvic masses were noted. Arrows point to the ovary.

Figure 19-2, the annotated version of Fig. 19-1, is a midline view of the fetal lower abdomen and pelvis. A multiseptated cystic structure is noted superior to the bladder. Differential diagnosis includes mesenteric cyst or lymphangioma, both of which are usually larger and have more irregularly interspersed septations; a urachal cyst, which should be in a more anterior position communicating with the bladder; and a bowel duplication, which is usually not septated. Fetal genital identification allowed correct gender determination, forcing consideration of a stimulated ovary with contained follicles, which is what this case proved to be.

THE FETAL OVARY

Despite maternal hormone stimulation, the normal fetal ovary is not typically seen. When ovaries are prominent because of contained cysts, they are seen on occasion. The follicles/cysts develop in response to normal but prominent maternal hormonal stimulation. Small follicular cysts that were not visualized on fetal examination are found in many autopsy specimens and are certainly a common finding in the ovaries of normal neonates.

Ovarian follicles/cysts are the predominant and usual cause of enlarged ovaries, which appear as unilocular (Fig. 19-3) or multiseptate (Fig. 19-2) cystic masses in the fetus. When enlarged, these ovaries may rise out of the pelvis and into the abdomen. If the fetal adnexa contain hemorrhage or a fluid debris level, one would have to consider the possibility of a torsed ovary, and postnatal surgery would be considered. Follow-up fetal, but more so neonatal, exams can help prove that what was noted was an ovary with prominent follicles.

A POINT TO REMEMBER

Some fetuses, like some adolescents, under normal but prominent hormone stimulation may develop more follicles/cysts than others.

References

Cohen HL: The female pelvis, in *Syllabus: Current Concepts: A Categorical Course in Pediatric Radiology*, Siebert J (ed). Chicago, RSNA Publications, 1994.

Cohen HL, Muller D, Zinn DL: Abnormal fetal chest, abdomen, pelvis, in *Diagnostic Medical Sonography. A Guide to Clinical Practice. Obstetrics and Gynecology,* 2d ed, Berman MC, Cohen HL (eds). Philadelphia, Lippincott, 1997:285–320.

Cohen HL, Shapiro M, Mandel F, Shapiro M: Normal ovaries in neonates and infants: A sonographic study of 77 patients 1 day to 24 months old. *AJR* 160:583–586, 1993.

Comstock C: Fetal masses: Ultrasound diagnosis and evaluation. *Ultrasound Q* 6:229–256, 1988.

Polhemus D: Ovarian maturation and cyst formation in children. *Pediatrics* 11:588–594, 1953.

Preziosi P, Fariello G, Moiorana A, et al: Antenatal sonographic diagnosis of complicated ovarian cysts. *JCU* 14:196–198, 1986.

20

You have a large number of obstetric cases on your schedule. You are running from room to room confirming findings and looking at fetal anatomy. Two sets of parents are besieging you and your staff for information regarding their child's gender. Figure 20-1 is handed to you; is the patient a boy or a girl? Figure 20-2 is handed to you; it looks like a boy; is the scrotum normal or not? When is gender identification most useful?

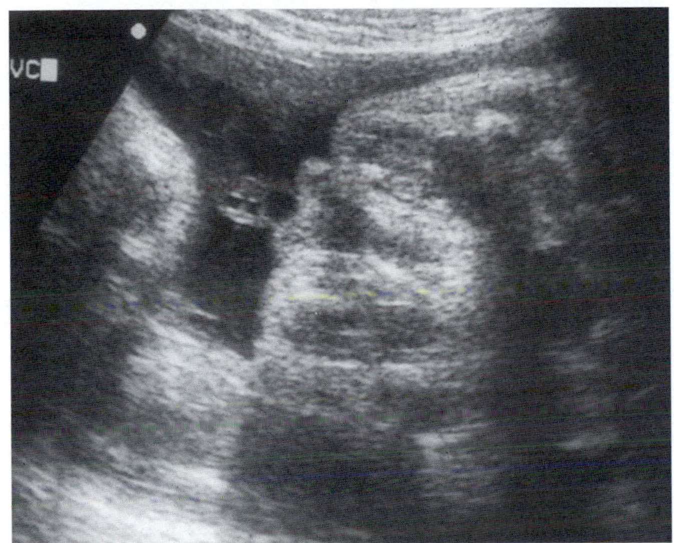

FIGURE 20–1. Fetal groin. Coronal plane.

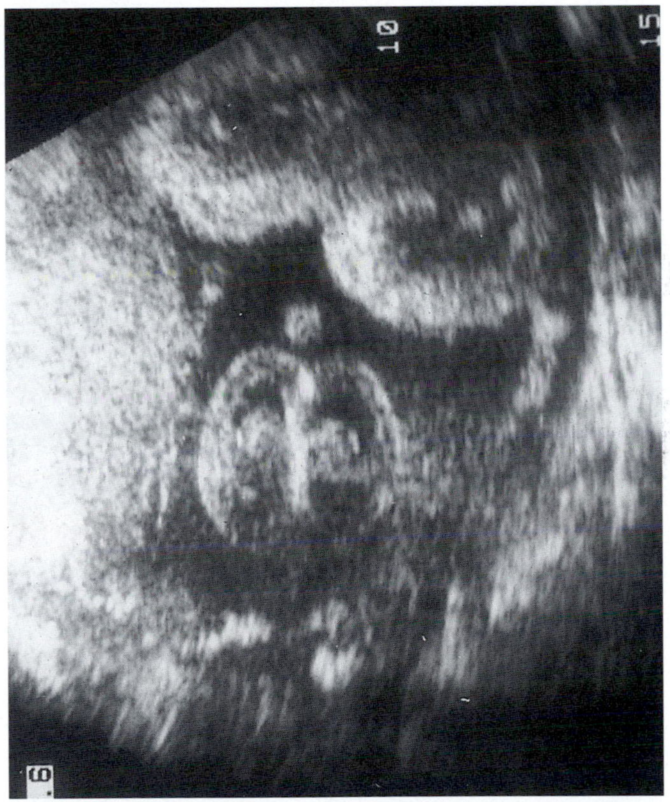

FIGURE 20–2. Fetal scrotum. Coronal plane.

CHAPTER 20

Fetal Genital Identification and Hydrocele

HARRIS L. COHEN

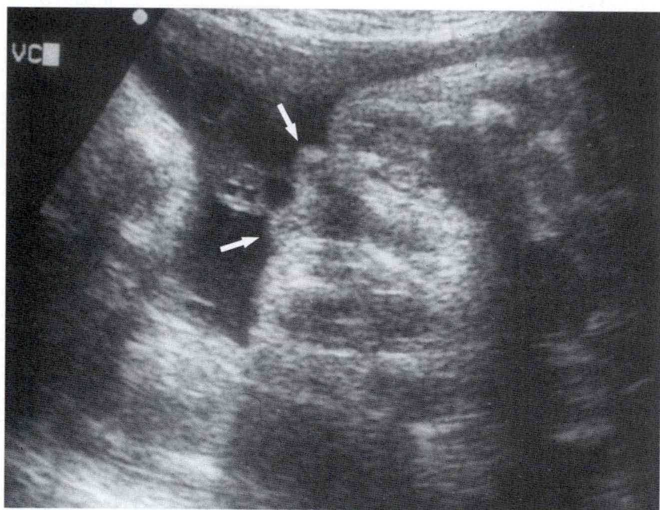

A

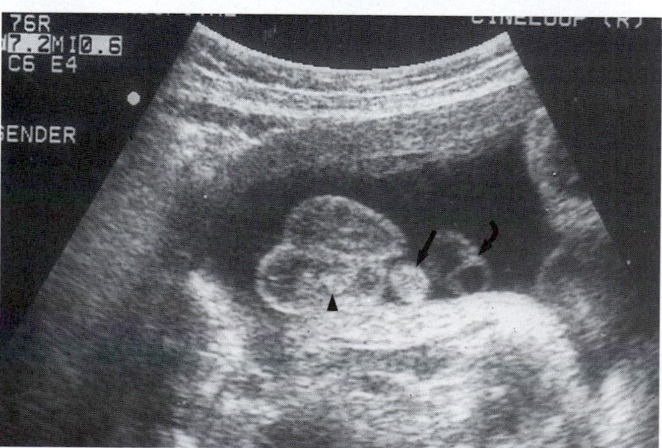

B

FIGURE 20–3. Annotated version of Fig. 20-1. Difficult determination of gender without other views. ***A.*** Fetal groin. Coronal plane. A V-shaped soft tissue structure (*arrows*) is seen. This appears to be widely separated labia but without a central echogenic line for the labia minora. ***B.*** Fetal scrotum. Coronal plane. A penis (*arrow*) is seen in cross section. A scrotum is seen, with perhaps the dependent testicle (*arrowhead*) seen well within it. This was a normal male. The image in *A* was probably caused by steep angulation through the very top of the scrotum. Without the use of orthogonal views, gender identification may prove to be incorrect.

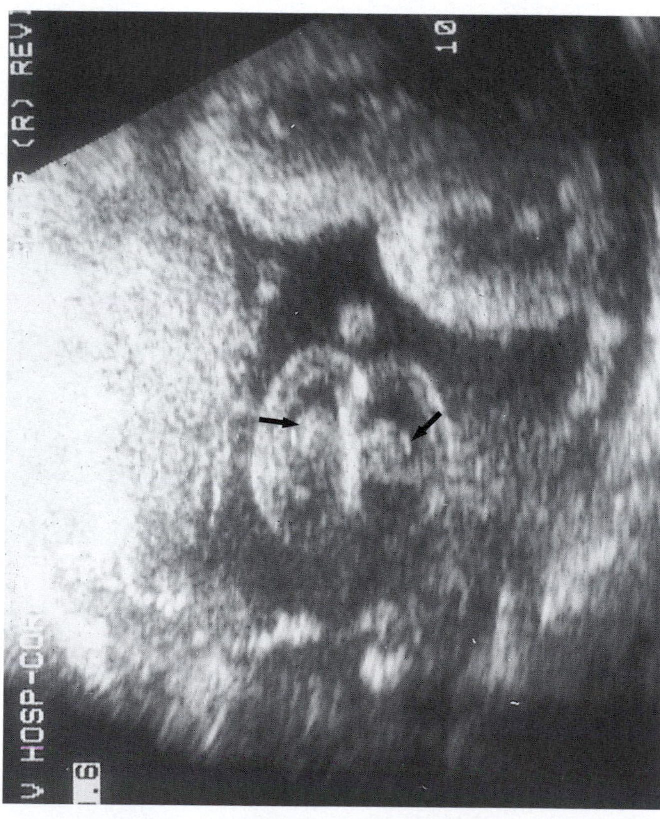

FIGURE 20–4. Annotated version of Fig. 20-2. Hydroceles. Fetal scrotum. Coronal plane. Two testes (*arrows*) are seen in the scrotum. Echoless fluid is seen between the testicle and the scrotal wall on each side. The fetus has hydroceles bilaterally.

Figure 20-3*A*, the annotated version of Fig. 20-1, shows a confusing V-shaped soft tissue structure at the perineum of this fetus. Other views (Fig. 20-3*B*), obtained after having the mother turn and after the fetus was in another position, helped show this to be a normal scrotum. The fetus is a boy. The V-shaped structure is probably the most cephalad portion of the scrotum as it hangs off the perineum. (This could have been a male with a bifid scrotum, a form of ambiguous genitalia that because of limited masculinization and associated hypospadias has testes within soft tissue structures on each side of the penis that I think look visually like scrotum.) The point is: Gender identification is not always straightforward.

Figure 20-4 is an obvious scrotum in a male. The penis size cannot be determined on this view, in which it is imaged in cross section. Fluid surrounds both testes, consistent with bilateral hydrocele. This is a not uncommon finding in a fetus.

ULTRASOUND IN FETAL GENDER IDENTIFICATION

It is well known that errors can be made in the identification of fetal genitalia. Proper evaluation requires a good image of the perineal area, which can be obtained only with sufficient surrounding fluid and a fetus positioned in such a way that one can actually image the genitalia. A flexed thigh can hide a scrotum. Legs held side to side can obscure any genital identification. Inadequate visualization of genitalia has been reported in up to 30 percent of cases. The actual physical differences in genitalia are not very prominent before 16 weeks. Even with fetuses that are adequately imaged, two groups have reported error rates of 3 to 3.3 percent in gender identification among fetuses younger than 24 weeks. Birnholz reported an overall error rate of 1.7 percent.

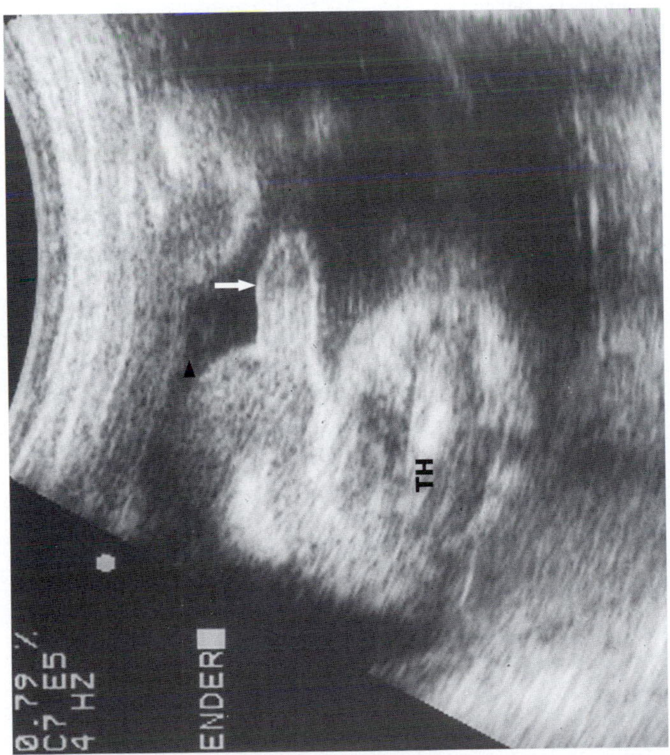

FIGURE 20–5. Normal male genitalia. Just superficial to fetal pelvis. Sagittal/oblique plane through genitalia. The scrotum (*arrowhead*) and penis (*arrow*) are noted. The penis is erect. This is not an unusual finding. The echogenic line within the center of the penis is the normal nondistended urethra. TH = thigh.

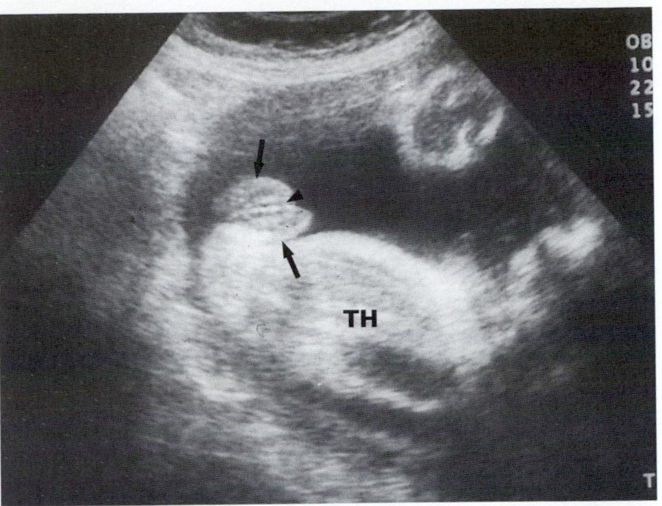

FIGURE 20–6. Normal female genitalia. Axial plane through labia. Superficial to the medial aspect of the fetal thigh (*TH*) are the two convex C-shaped labia majora (*arrows*). Anteriorly, there is a small space between the two labia. Between them is an echogenic line (*arrowhead*) representing the coapted labia minora.

WHAT DO NORMAL FETAL GENITALIA LOOK LIKE?

In the male, the penis and scrotum are readily visualized between the thighs. The penis, when viewed in a longitudinal plane, often has a central echogenic line, which represents the urethra (Fig. 20-5). Occasionally an overzealous tyro sonologist may mistake the umbilical cord for the penis. Color Doppler or a true sagittal view of the fetus can dispel this possibility. One may, on occasion, see actual voiding into the amniotic fluid. This is seen as echogenicity as the turbulent voided urine enters the relatively static fluid of the amniotic cavity. Erections are not unusual in fetal life.

The scrotum, when well imaged, will be oval to round. Testes are not always easily seen within the scrotum. At times, this is because they are not present. After 32 weeks, however, in more than 90 percent of cases, testicles should have descended into the scrotum, where they can be noted as echogenic masses.

In females, genitalia are noted as an oval consisting of C-shaped labia majora (Fig. 20-6) on axial view with a central linear echogenicity representing the labia minora. The normal ovaries, uterus, and vagina typically are not visualized in a normal fetus, and their visualization cannot be used to help gender identification.

WHEN CAN GENDER IDENTIFICATION BE IMPORTANT CLINICALLY?

Gender identification can be important clinically in families that carry severe X-linked inherited disorders, such as hemophilia or Duchenne's muscular dystrophy. In these situations, the female fetus would carry the trait, but the male fetus would have the disease. Monozygotic twins have several clinical problems that dizygotic twins do not, e.g., twin-to-twin transfusion syndrome. Noting separate sexes in the twins helps confirm dizygosity. As noted in Chap. 19, the differential diagnosis of cystic masses in the pelvis is affected by knowledege of the sex of the fetus.

Certainly, if it is clinically necessary to know the gender of the fetus, karyotype information may also be obtained from chorionic villus sampling or amniocentesis for chromosomal gender determination. If a karyotype is known and the external genitalia appear different from what is expected, particularly if the karyotype is 46XY and the fetus appears to be a female, this suggests the possibility of a rare intersex problem, particularly testicular feminization syndrome, in which the affected individual has a male karyotype but, because of end-organ insensitivity to androgen stimulation, female genitalia.

WHAT ARE HYDROCELES? HOW COMMON ARE THEY?

Fetal hydroceles (Fig. 20-4) are common. Pretorius et al noted an incidence of 15 percent among 123 male fetuses between 17 and 41 weeks gestational age. Others have reported an incidence as high as 58 percent. They tend to be first seen in the late second to third trimester. In the hydrocele, there is a variable amount of echoless fluid (which remains from normal testicular descent) imaged in the scrotum, surrounding the testes. This type of hydrocele does not increase in size and is resorbed within the first 9 months of life. If an imaged hydrocele increases in size, one must consider the possibility that there is a patent processus vaginalis that allows peritoneal contents into the scrotum. This may be seen in a case of inguinal hernia, although I have not identified one antenatally. More commonly, the scrotum may fill with fetal ascites as well as perforated meconium, which can calcify and actually be noted on ultrasound (US) as one or more small echogenic masses and can be palpated on physical examination of the newborn. The normal fetal testicle is homogeneous in echogenicity. Heterogeneity suggests the possibility of testicular torsion.

References

Birnholz J: Determination of fetal sex. *N Engl J Med* 309:942–944, 1983.

Cohen H, Haller J: Diagnostic sonography of the fetal genitourinary tract. *Urol Radiol* 9:88–98, 1987.

Cohen HL, Muller D, Zinn DL: Abnormal fetal chest, abdomen, pelvis, in *Diagnostic Medical Sonography. A Guide to Clinical Practice. Obstetrics and Gynecology,* 2d ed, Berman MC, Cohen HL (eds). Philadelphia, Lippincott, 1997:285–320.

Elejalde B, de Elejalde M, Heitman T: Visualization of the fetal genitalia by ultrasonography: A review of the literature and analysis of its accuracy and ethical implications. *J Ultrasound Med* 4:633–639, 1985.

Gross B, Cohen HL, Schlessel J: Perinatal diagnosis of bilateral testicular torsions: Beware of torsions simulating hydroceles. *J Ultrasound Med* 12:479–482, 1993.

Kenney P, Spirt B, Ellis D, Patil U: Scrotal masses caused by meconium peritonitis: Prenatal sonographic diagnosis. *Radiology* 154: 362, 1985.

Mahony B: The genitourinary system, in *Ultrasonography in Obstetrics and Gynecology*, 2d ed, Callen P (ed). Philadelphia, Saunders, 1988:254–276.

Meizner I, Katz M, Zamora E, et al: In utero diagnosis of congenital hydrocele. *JCU* 11:449–451, 1983.

Pretorius D, Halsted M, Abels W, et al: Hydroceles identified prenatally: Common physiologic phenomenon? J *Ultrasound Med* 17:49–52, 1998.

Seeds J: Antenatal sonographic assessment of the genitourinary tract, in *Ultrasound Annual,* Sanders R, Hill M (eds). New York, Raven, 1986:67–97.

Stephens J: Prenatal diagnosis of testicular feminization. *Lancet* 2:1038, 1984.

Section E
MUSCULOSKELETAL SYSTEM

21

Figures 21-1 and 21-2 were obtained on a routine obstetric ultrasound. These are images of the fetal thoracic and lumbar spine area. No vertebral body anomaly was noted. What is seen? What is the diagnosis? What is the clinical concern?

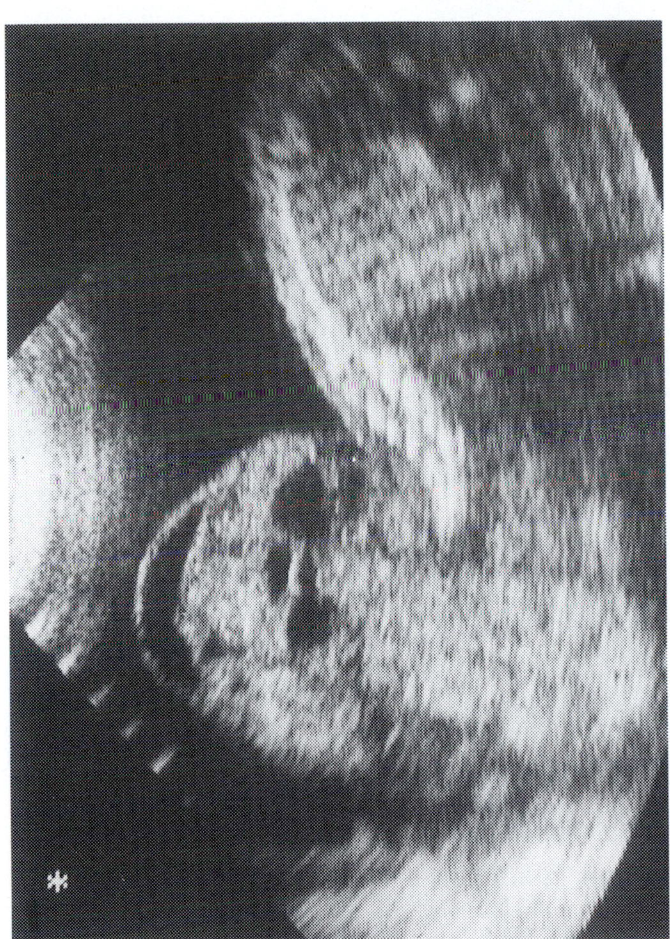

FIGURE 21–1. Fetal thorax/abdomen/pelvis area. Sagittal plane. Fetus facing reader's right. *(From Cohen et al, with permission.)*

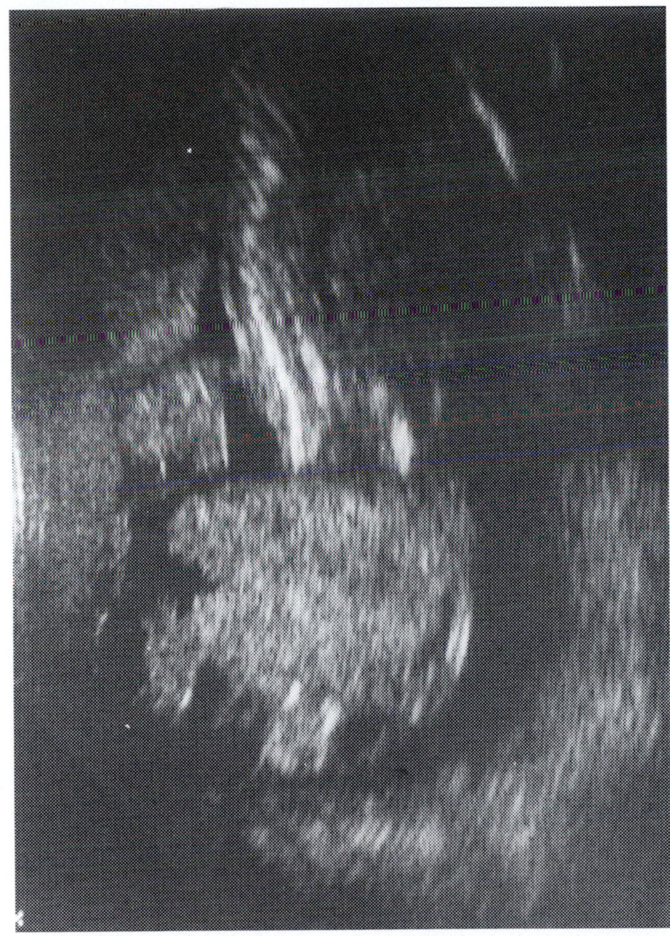

FIGURE 21–2. Fetal thorax/abdomen/pelvis area. Coronal plane.

CHAPTER 21

Sacrococcygeal Teratoma

HARRIS L. COHEN AND ROGER YANG

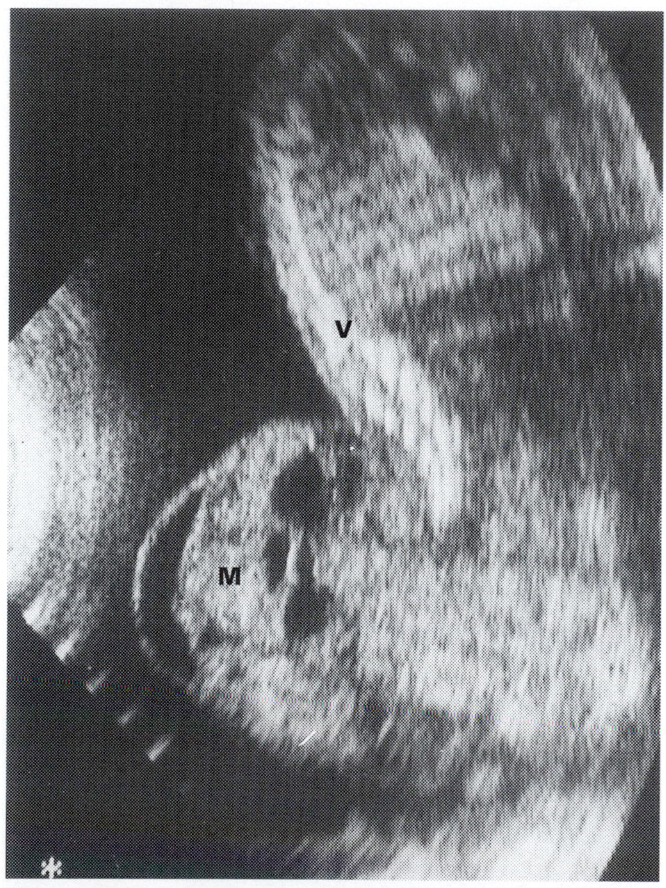

FIGURE 21–3. Annotated version of Fig. 21-1. Sacrococcygeal teratoma. Fetal thorax/abdomen/pelvis area. Sagittal plane. Fetus facing reader's right. A large mass (*M*) is seen posterior to the sacral area. It contains cystic and solid elements. It is a sacrococcygeal teratoma. No vertebral column (*V*) abnormality was noted. *(From Cohen et al, with permission.)*

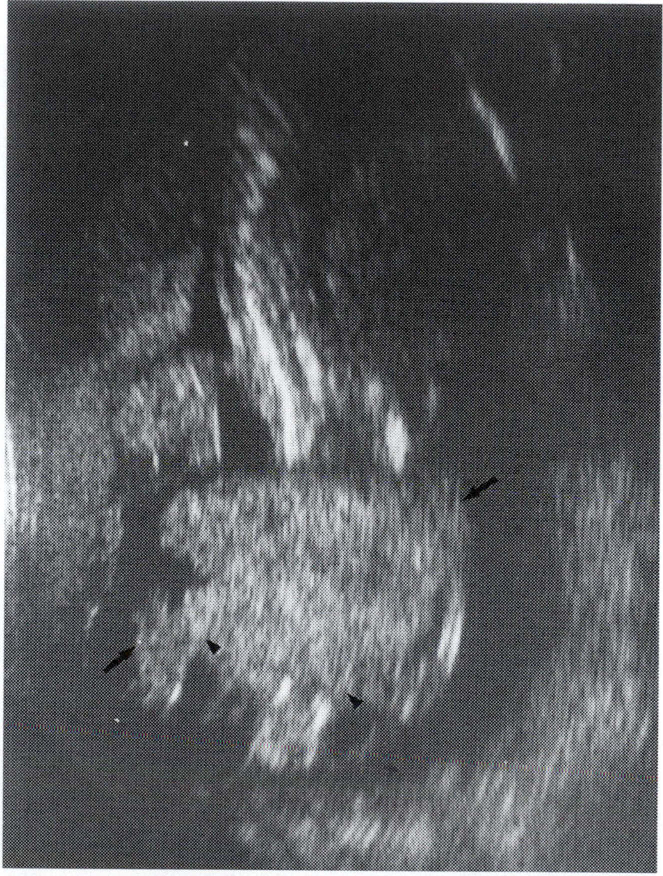

FIGURE 21–4. Annotated version of Fig. 21-2. Sacrococcygeal teratoma. Fetal thorax/abdomen/pelvis area. Coronal plane. Fetus facing reader's right. The complex mass (*arrows*) is seen inferior to lumbar vertebrae. It is predominantly solid with cystic elements (*arrowheads*).

Figure 21-3, the annotated version of Fig. 21-1, shows a complex mass extending posteriorly off the area of the caudal vertebral column. Figure 21-4, the annotated version of Fig. 21-2, shows this mass with solid and cystic components on coronal view. Little if any intrapelvic extension of this mass was seen. The vertebral ossification centers that were seen on these and other views of this fetus showed no obvious abnormality. The posterior elements of the vertebral bodies were intact. This appearance is consistent with a sacrococcygeal teratoma (SCT). The most important differential diagnostic consideration with the predominantly external SCT is a meningomyelocele (MMC), but that is when the SCT is cystic. A solid MMC of this size is unlikely and would be found in association with a defect of the vertebral body's posterior elements, which this patient did not have.

WHAT IS A SACROCOCCYGEAL TERATOMA?

The SCT is the most common tumor discovered in newborns. Its incidence is 1 in 35,000 births. There is a 3 or 4 to 1 female predominance. It occurs more commonly in twins. These tumors, like all fetal teratomas, arise from pluripotential cells. The sacrococcygeal area and the gonads are the most likely areas of occurrence, but teratomas can occur anywhere from the fetal crown to the rump, most typically in the midline. The area of origin of the SCT, in particular, is a region, known as Hensen's node or the primitive knot, that is anterior to the coccyx. The pluripotentiality of the cells that make up teratomas allow these tumors to be made up histologically of cells differentiated along many different germ lines. Sacrococcygeal teratomas most often include cells of respiratory, gastrointestinal, and neurologic origin.

Most cases of SCT are asymptomatic and are discovered after birth if no antenatal imaging is performed. There are, however, several causes for increased morbidity and mortality among fetuses with SCT. These can be related to preterm labor and associated premature birth, thought often to be due to an associated polyhydramnios. Obstetric complications of preeclampsia, dystocia, and traumatic delivery can occur with these fetuses and their large sacrococcygeal-area masses. Intratumoral hemorrhage can occur and account for mass enlargement. Antenatal diagnosis is therefore important. Elective vaginal deliveries are attempted when there is an SCT mass of less than 4.5 cm and no associated fetal anomaly or problem. An even more important reason for early antenatal diagnosis of SCT is that some fetuses develop placentomegaly and fetal hydrops, which are often associated with fetal demise. These findings are due to high-output cardiac failure, which probably occurs because of the prominent arteriovenous shunting that occurs in SCTs, particularly the solid ones and the larger ones. If hydrops is discovered in a fetus that is too young to deliver (less than 28 weeks) and "amenable to easy resection," Harrison et al have suggested consideration of intrauterine resection, obviously in specialized centers. Because of the possibility of hydrops development, fetuses with SCTs should be followed via interval ultrasound (US) exams during the pregnancy.

Sacrococcygeal teratoma growth tends to parallel the growth of the fetus during antenatal life. The pregnancy is often large for gestational age. Sacrococcygeal teratomas may have significant intrapelvic extensions and have been classified in accordance with the degree of their exterior and/or intrapelvic component. Fetuses with SCT have no associated sacral vertebral anomalies. There is, however, an increased incidence of associated vertebral anomalies in other locations.

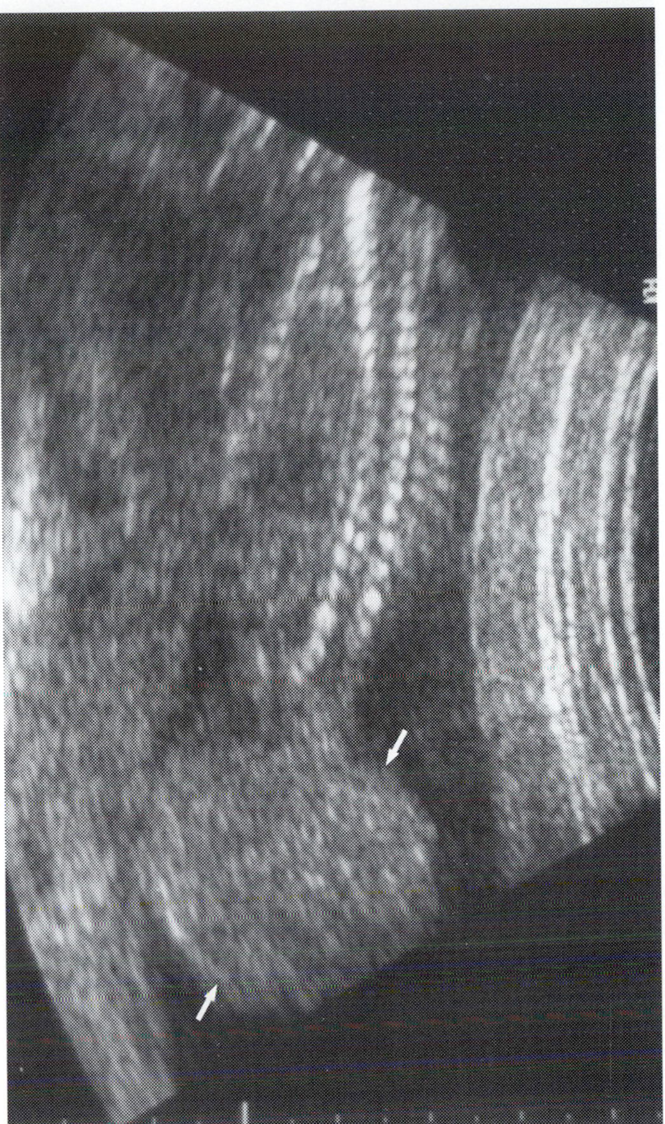

FIGURE 21–5. Solid fetal sacrococcygeal teratoma. Lumbosacral area. Coronal plane. A solid mass (*arrows*) is seen inferior to the lumbar vertebral bodies. The mass is actually posterior to unremarkable sacral vertebrae. *(Courtesy of Madhuri Kirpekar, MD.)*

THE ANTENATAL AND POSTNATAL IMAGING OF SACROCOCCYGEAL TERATOMA

An SCT is typically noted as a large mass off the fetal buttock region (Fig. 21-3). Those fetuses with external masses are the easiest to diagnose. The masses are usually posterior or inferior to the buttock region. They are usually solid (Fig. 21-5) or of mixed echogenicity (Fig. 21-3) with interspersed or peripheral cystic components. About 15 percent of SCTs are purely cystic. These are the key masses to be differentiated from myelomeningoceles. There is little correlation between size and consistency of the SCTs and ultimate prognosis, as long as there is no significant arteriovenous shunting. Many of the solid masses (36 percent) have contained calcifications (Fig. 21-6) that may be noted as shadow-

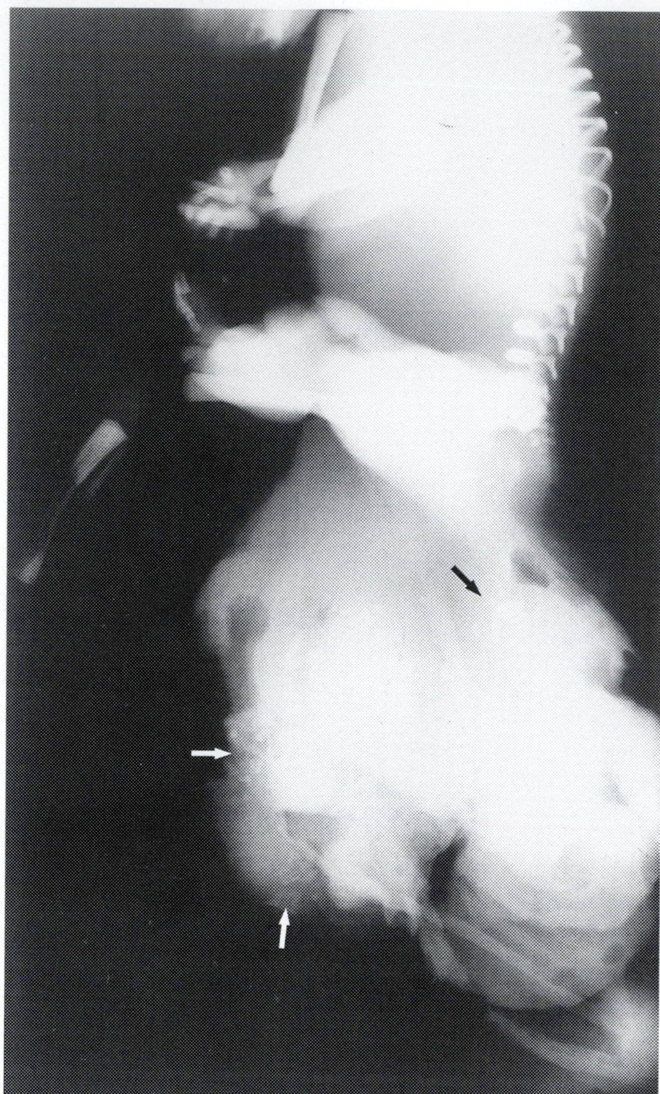

FIGURE 21–6. Sacrococcygeal teratoma with contained calcification. Radiograph of pathology specimen. Fetus on its side. A predominantly solid mass extends off the sacrococcygeal area inferiorly. Scattered areas of significant radiodensity (*arrows*) within the mass are consistent with contained calcifications. This is not an uncommon finding in sacrococcygeal teratoma, which this stillbirth had. *(Courtesy of William J. McSweeney, MD.)*

ing from the echogenic mass. The intrapelvic component of the SCT is less easily imaged. It must be considered, even if not imaged, if mass effect causes bowel or ureteral dilatation or if there is compression of the bladder. Cystic intrapelvic SCTs, which are predominantly benign, may be unilocular or multilocular. They may simulate anterior meningoceles, neurenteric cysts, ovarian cysts, bowel duplications, or the normal bladder. They may, on occasion, be simulated by the normal near-term meconium-filled rectosigmoid. An abscess may be considered in the child. One must be more concerned about malignancy with predominantly solid SCTs. When imaging a solid internal presacral mass, one must consider SCT as well as other solid masses, including neuroblastomas, neurogenic tumors, soft tissue sarcomas, chordomas, and sacral bone tumors.

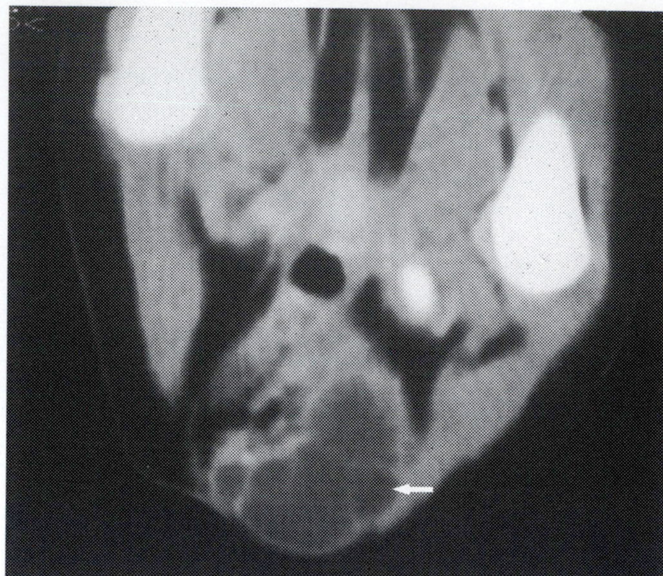

FIGURE 21–7. Sacrococcygeal teratoma. CT image. Axial plane. Level of low pelvis. A low-density mass (*arrow*) that is multilocular is seen posterior to the rectum. It is predominantly internal (Type III SCT).

Sacrococcygeal teratomas may be classified by US in antenatal life according to the positioning of the components of the mass. The type 1 SCT, the most common (47 percent of all) variety, consists essentially of an external component with a small presacral component. Type 2 tumors (34 percent) are external masses with a significant internal component. Type 3 tumors (9 percent) are predominantly internal masses that may be pelvic or extend into the abdomen and have a smaller external component. Type 4 tumors (10 percent) are entirely internal and presacral. They have no external or abdominal component. This evaluation, however, is more easily made postnatally by computed tomography (CT) (Fig. 21-7) or magnetic resonance imaging (MRI). These modalities help provide a surgical map of the lesion. The tumors are usually removed with the coccyx.

WHAT SHOULD WE WORRY ABOUT IF AN SCT IS IMAGED?

We have already discussed the possibility of fetal demise and the need to analyze the fetus for any evidence of hydrops. We have already noted that the mass may create difficulties with delivery. However, the SCT itself is of concern because of its malignant potential. There is an incidence of malignancy in SCTs operated on before 2 months of age of 2 to 10 percent. The incidence of malignancy in SCTs is increased to about 60 percent (67 percent for boys and 50 percent for girls) among those undergoing surgery after the second month of life. This increase in malignant components discovered in SCTs, as time goes on, suggests the need for early diagnosis and excision in neonatal life to prevent malignant degeneration. Malignant tumors as noted are somewhat more common in males.

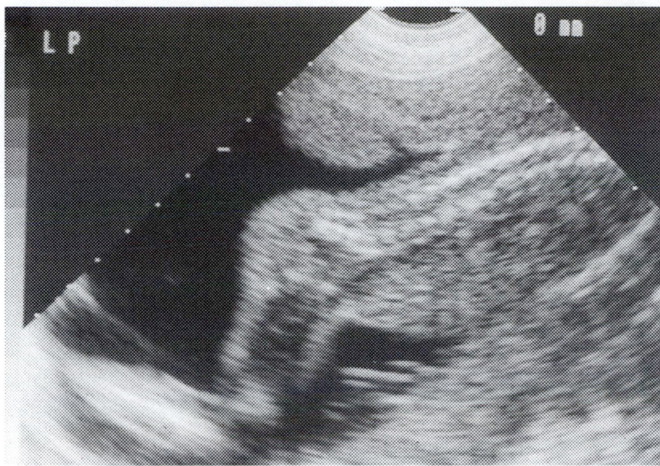

FIGURE 21–8. Normal fetal buttock area. Sagittal image. The fetus is prone and facing the reader's right. Sufficient surrounding amniotic fluid allows a clear image of the buttock area, showing no external mass and therefore no evidence of a sacrococcygeal teratoma, particularly one with any external component.

TECHNICAL POINT IN SCT DIAGNOSIS

One should try to analyze other areas of the fetal pelvis on images obtained of the bladder to rule out intrapelvic masses. This is easiest when the masses are cystic. Views of the fetal buttock area (Fig. 21-8) should be obtained to rule out masses extending off the sacrococcygeal area. As with all masses beyond the fetal body confines, e.g., myelomeningocele, one must hope that there are sufficient amounts of amniotic fluid between the mass and the uterine and/or body wall to enable imaging of the abnormality.

References

Altman RP, Randolph JG, Lilly JR: Sacrococcygeal teratoma: American Academy of Pediatrics surgical section survey. *J Pediatr Surg* 9:389–398, 1974.

Bloechle M, Ballman R, Zienert A, et al: Fetal teratoma: Diagnosis and management. *Zentralbl Gynakol* 114:175–180, 1992.

Burgess I, Hines B, Stevenson P: Cystic type IV sacrococcygeal teratoma detected at 18-week prenatal ultrasound. *Ultrasound Obstet Gynecol* 11:305, 1998.

Cohen HL, Muller D, Zinn DL: Abnormal fetal chest, abdomen, pelvis, in *Diagnostic Medical Sonography. A Guide to Clinical Practice. Obstetrics and Gynecology,* 2nd ed, Berman MC, Cohen HL (eds). Philadelphia, Lippincott, 1997:285–320.

Ein SH, Adeyemi SD, Manur K: Benign sacrococcygeal teratoma in infants and children: A 25 year review. *Ann Surg* 191:382–384, 1980.

Flake AW, Harrison MR, Adzick NS, et al: Fetal sacrococcygeal teratoma. *J Pediatr Surg* 21:563–566, 1986.

Harrison M, Adzick N, Flake A: Prenatal management of the fetus with a correctable defect, in *Ultrasonography in Obstetrics and Gynecology*, 3d ed, Callen P (ed). Philadelphia, Saunders, 1994:536–547.

Hogge W, Thiagarajah S, Barber V, et al: Cystic sacrococcygeal teratoma. Ultrasound diagnosis and management. *J Ultrasound Med* 6:707–710, 1987.

Karcnik T, Rubenstein J, Swayne L: The fetal presacral pseudomass: A normal sonographic variant. *J Ultrasound Med* 10: 579–581, 1991.

Sauerbrei E: The fetal spine, in *A Practical Guide to Ultrasound in Obstetrics and Gynecology,* 2d ed, Sauerbrei E, Nguyen K, Nolan R (eds). Philadelphia, Lippincott-Raven, 1998:198–227.

Shackelford G: Adrenal glands, pancreas, and other retroperitoneal structures, in *Pediatric Sonography,* 2d ed, Siegel M (ed). New York, Raven, 1995:301–355.

Sherer DM, Fromberg RA, Rindfusz DW: Color doppler aided prenatal diagnosis of type I cystic sacrococcygeal teratoma simulating a myelomeningocele. *Am J Perinatol* 14:13–15, 1997.

Sheth S, Nussbaum AR, Sanders RC, et al: Prenatal diagnosis of sacrococcygeal teratoma: Sonographic-pathologic correlation. *Radiology* 169:131–136, 1988.

Werner J, Taybi H: Presacral masses in childhood. *AJR* 109: 403–410, 1970.

Winderl L, Silverman R: Prenatal identification of a completely cystic internal sacrococcygeal teratoma (Type IV). *Ultrasound Obstet Gynecol* 9:425–428, 1997.

22

Figure 22-1 is a longitudinal view of the right femur of a 19-week fetus. The femur is short and measured at the fifth percentile for length for 19 weeks. What else do you see? Figure 22-2 is the fetal clavicle. Other images showed that the vertebral bodies were of normal echogenicity, and the calvaria had ultrasonographic evidence of poor mineralization. What is the diagnosis?

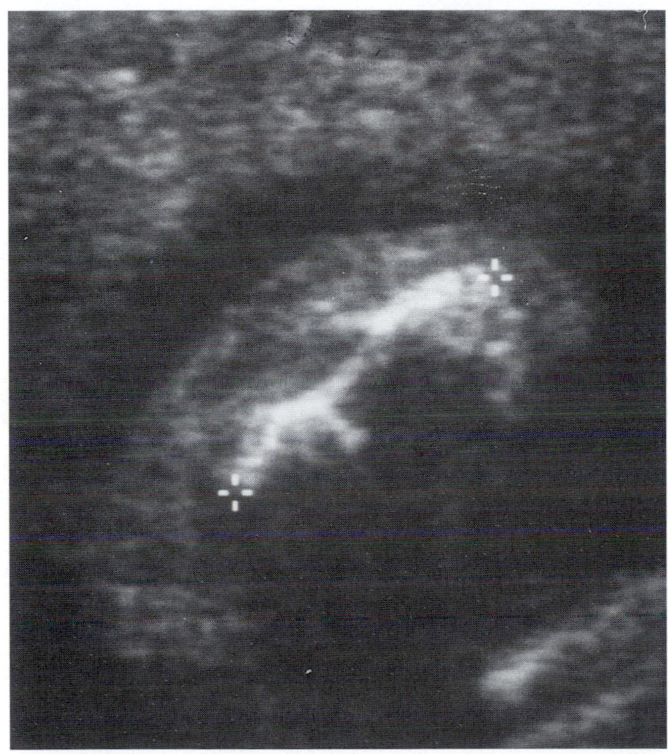

FIGURE 22–1. Fetal thigh. Longitudinal plane.

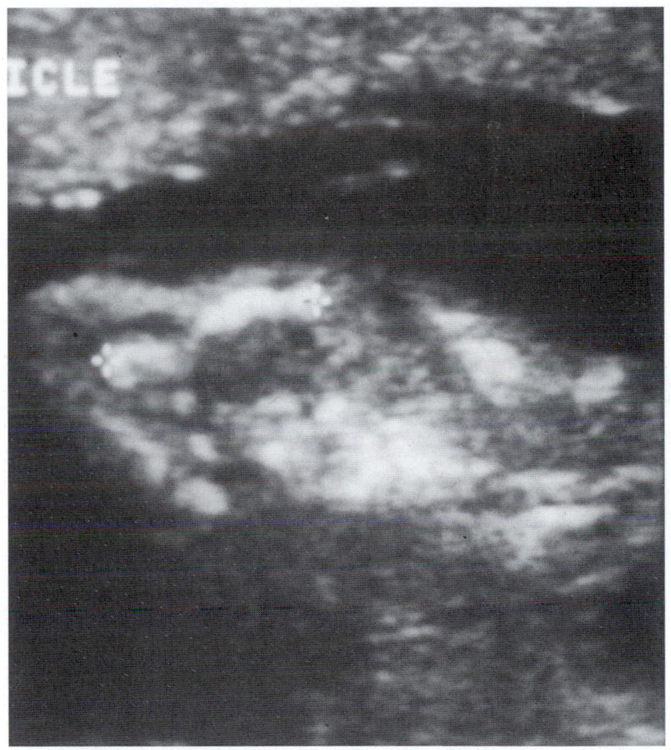

FIGURE 22–2. Fetal left clavicle. Coronal plane.

CHAPTER 22

Osteogenesis Imperfecta in a Fetus

DOROTHY I. BULAS

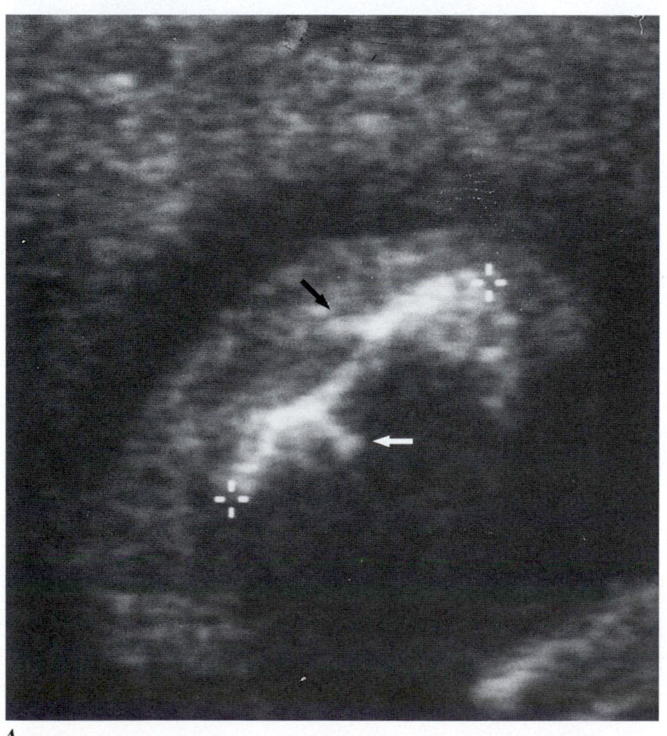

A

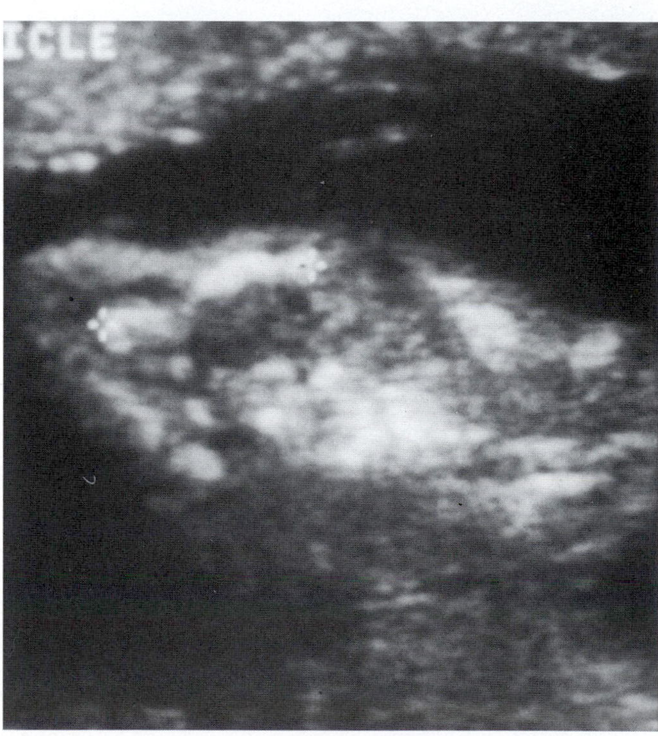

B

FIGURE 22–3. Osteogenesis imperfecta—19-week fetus. ***A.*** Annotated version of Fig. 22-1. Fractured femur. Fetal thigh. Longitudinal plane. The femur is irregular in shape, with bony spicules (*arrows*) extending horizontally from its middle thirds. These suggest fractures of a short (less than fifth percentile) femur. ***B.*** Annotated version of Fig. 22-2. Fractured clavicle. Fetal left clavicle. Coronal plane. The clavicle (*marked off by crosses*) is irregular, suggesting fracture. ***C.*** Fetal body radiograph. Anteroposterior. The family electively terminated the pregnancy at 20 weeks gestation. The radiograph confirmed the presence of osteopenia (note how thin the calvaria are) and fractures of the femora and left clavicle. Other fractures were seen. Skin biopsy revealed that the fetus had osteogenesis imperfecta.

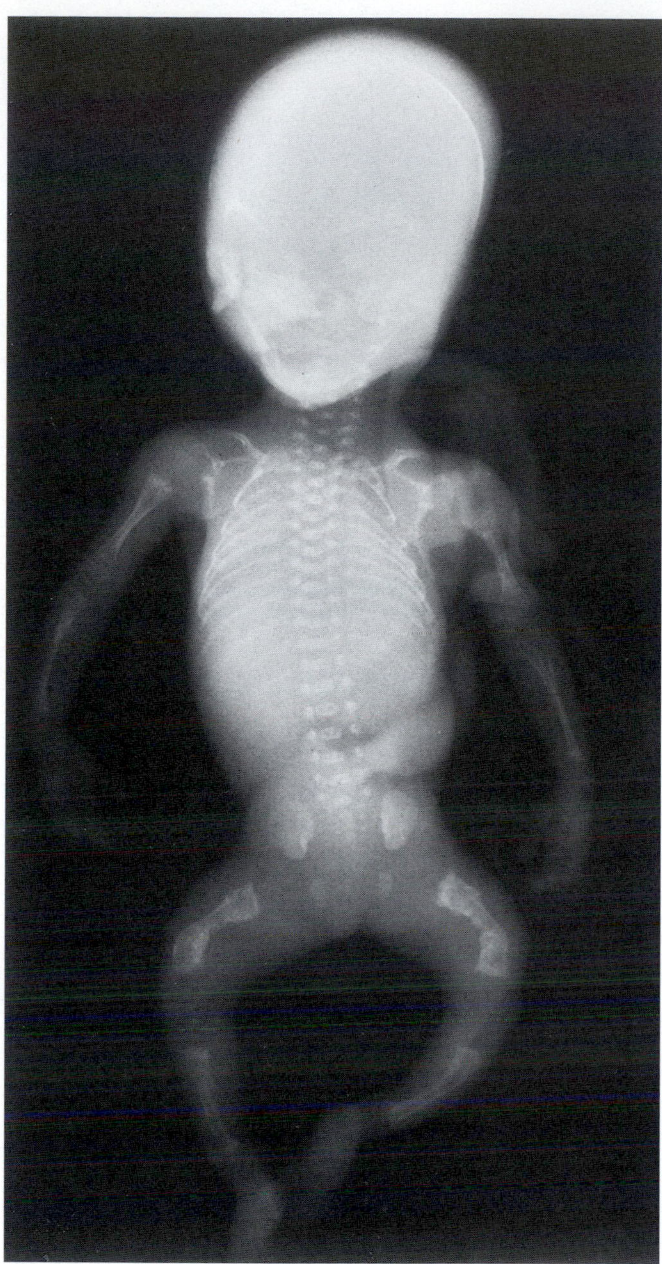

C

FIGURE 22–3 (*continued*).

Figure 22-3*A* and *B,* the annotated version of Figs. 22-1 and 22-2, respectively, shows an irregular femur that has been measured as short and an irregular clavicle. Bowing of bone may be caused by various bone dysplasias. Bony irregularity or a lack of a smooth cortical contour in a fetal bone suggests fracture. Fractures or bowing may be seen in several conditions (Table 22-1). Skull or other bony demineralization can also be seen in several conditions (Table 22-2). The combination of skull demineralization with bone fractures certainly suggests the diagnosis of osteogenesis imperfecta (OI). The fact that vertebral body mineralization appears relatively normal makes the alternative possibility of achondrogenesis based on fractures and demineralization far less likely. The complex information necessary to evaluate bone dysplasias is well beyond the scope of this unknown case. Certain key findings to look for, however, in analyzing fetuses for possible dysplasia will be discussed in the following section.

TABLE 22-1
Bowed or Fractured Bones in a Fetus

1. Osteogenesis imperfecta type II
2. Camptomelic dysplasia
3. Achondrogenesis
4. Hypophosphatasia
5. Thanatophoric dysplasia

SOURCE: From Nolan.

TABLE 22-2
Fetal Bone Hypomineralization

1. Osteogenesis imperfecta—predominantly calvarial
2. Hypophosphatasia—almost a complete lack of mineralization
3. Achondrogenesis—particularly the spine

SOURCE: From Nolan.

WHAT IS OSTEOGENESIS IMPERFECTA?

Osteogenesis imperfecta is a heterogeneous group of disorders of type I collagen, the principal collagen found in bone. Decreased collagen synthesis leads to osteopenia and, clinically, osteoporosis. The group of disorders making up OI includes both lethal and nonlethal types. Common clinical features in life include fractures, short limbs, progressive deafness, defective dentition, and blue sclera. Clinical expression ranges from the severe (stillbirth) to the mild (mild osteoporosis).

OSTEOGENESIS IMPERFECTA: CLASSIFICATION

Sillence et al attempted to classify these disorders into four types based on clinical, radiographic, and genetic criteria. Type I OI has autosomal dominant inheritance, and its sufferers have only mild bone fragility. Their prognosis is good, with deafness, noted in 35 percent, their most significant clinical problem. Type II OI (Fig. 22-4), on the other hand, is lethal during the perinatal period. Type II OI may have autosomal dominant inheritance, although many cases are due to spontaneous mutation. The classic type II OI has severe bone shortening and innumerable fractures. It is seen in 1 in every 60,000 births. Cases of autosomal recessive type II have been reported. Type III has autosomal recessive inheritance, moderate femur shortening, and many fractures. Survivors have severe handicaps. Type IV (Fig. 22-5) OI patients usually live and have only occasional fractures or none, normal bony mineralization (which in a fetus would be noted as normal echogenicity), and a good clinical outcome. However, these patients may be born with significant bowing. Inheritance is usually autosomal dominant. While the

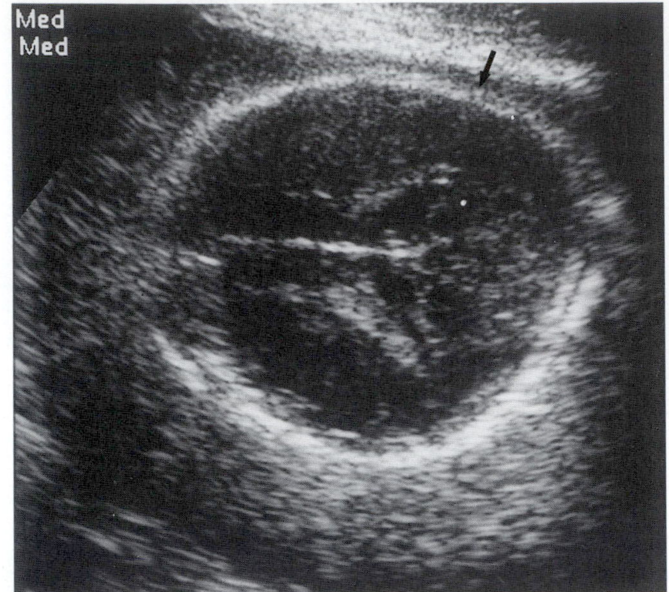

A

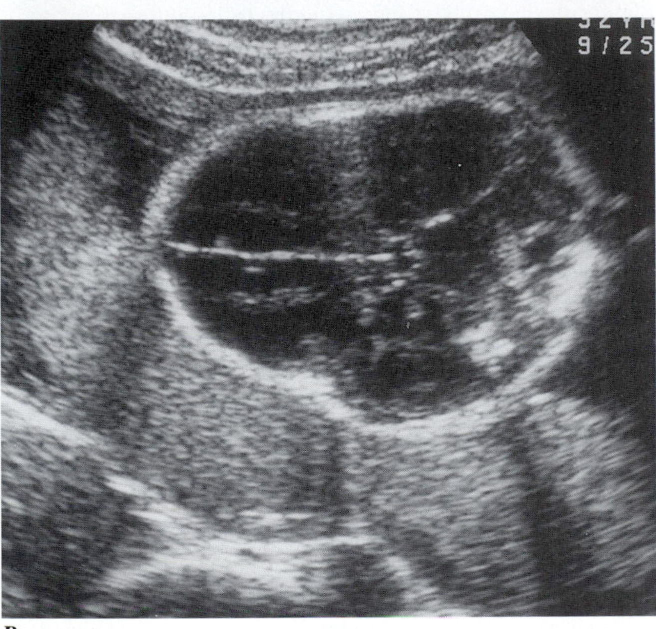

B

FIGURE 22–4. Fetus with osteogenesis imperfecta type II. ***A.*** Fetal skull. Axial plane. This 24-week fetus has decreased skull ossification. This can be noted by the lack of near-field artifact and the thinner near-field calvaria (*arrow*). This image was obtained routinely and without significant compression by the transducer on the fetal skull (NON COMP). ***B.*** Fetal skull. Axial plane. When compression was applied to the fetal skull, it proved to be deformable, confirming poor ossification.

FIGURE 22–5. Fetus with osteogenesis imperfecta type IV. ▶ ***A.*** Fetal tibia and fibula. Coronal longitudinal plane with some obliquity. This fetus is at 26 weeks gestation and has bowing of the tibia and fibula. Both were short, as were the tibia and fibula on the contralateral side. ***B.*** Neonatal left leg. The femur is bowed anteriorly at its midshaft (*arrow*). Subtle anterior bowing is also seen in the fibula. The femur is bowed (*arrowhead*). Bony sclerosis is noted posteriorly at the apex of the convexity. An asterisk of the femur and tibia (*).

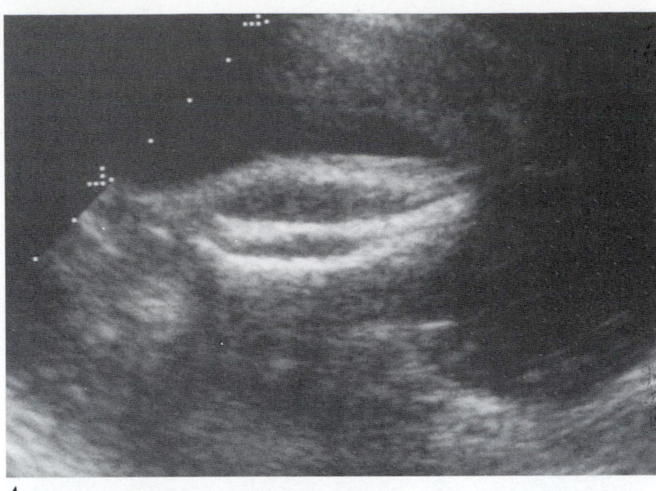

A

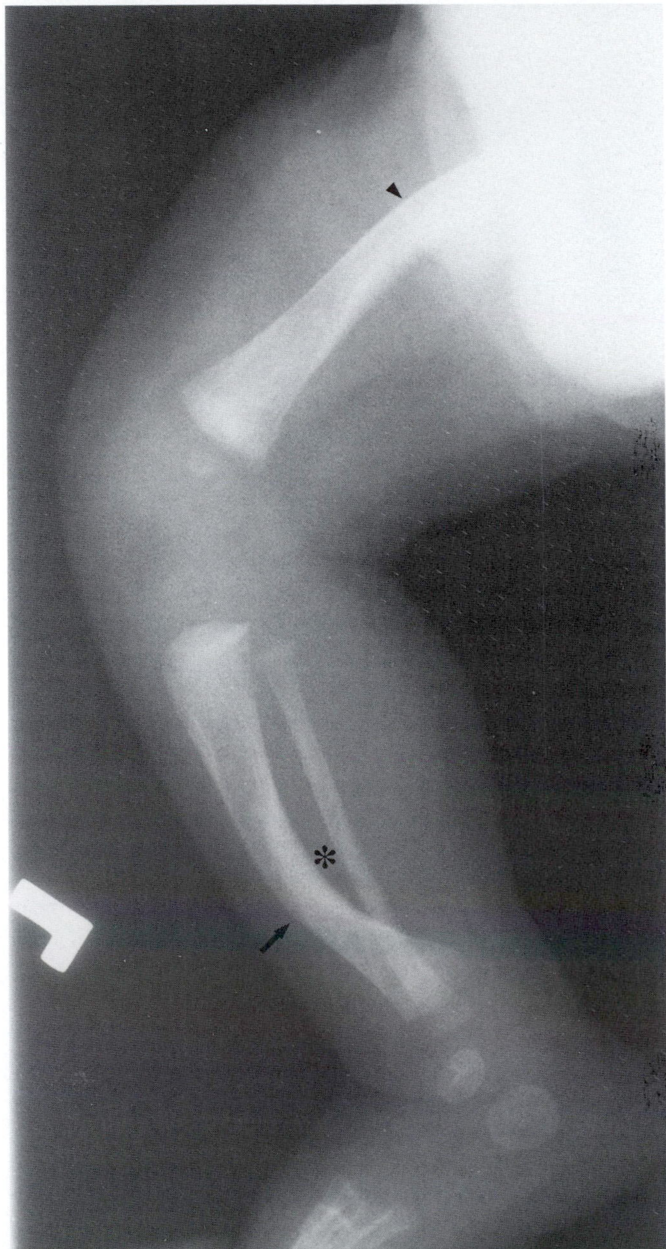

B

Sillence classification is widely used, a sizable number of OI patients do not fit any of the types. Maroteaux et al suggested using prognosis as an extension of the Sillence classification. They noted three forms of prognosis: lethal, severe, and regressive.

OI IN THE FETUS

Just as there is wide variation in clinical presentation, the findings necessary for prenatal sonographic identification are variable as well. The prenatal appearance of the more severe forms of OI, specifically the lethal type II, includes multiple fractures and bowing (Table 22-1), extremity shortening with femur length more than 3 standard deviations below the mean for gestational age, and evidence of calvarial and/or other bony demineralization, seen as skeletal hypoechogenicity and diminished acoustical shadowing from the fetal bones (Fig. 22-3*C*), which in the case of the calvaria allows greater penetration of the skull (Fig. 22-4*A*) and a more ready image of its contents, particularly in the near field. Fetuses with the less severe (nonlethal) types of OI have variable ultrasound (US) exams, which can range from those with abnormal skeletal findings to those that appear completely normal.

The classic finding of short, irregular, angled, or bowed long bones (Fig. 22-3) in the early second trimester is most suggestive of lethal OI type II. Additional features such as polyhydramnios, rib fractures, platyspondyly, soft skull (Fig. 22-4), and hypoechogenic skeleton may aid in confirming the diagnosis. In utero radiographs may be useful to confirm the presence of severe osteoporosis (Fig. 22-3C), if deemed necessary for diagnosis. The differential diagnosis includes congenital hypophosphatasia and achondrogenesis type I, which also are lethal (Table 22-2). The sonographic findings in OI type II are often striking and have been noted as early as 15 weeks gestation.

Severe progressively deforming OI type III has been identified prenatally as early as 15 weeks gestation, although abnormalities may not develop until the late second trimester.

The later clinical onset of the regressive and nonlethal forms of OI, types I and IV, is also why the early (or even later) prenatal diagnosis of OI in such fetuses is limited and difficult. Extremity shortening and bowing may be mild (Fig. 22-5) and progressive. Ultrasonographic findings may be limited to an isolated fracture or limb bowing late in the third trimester. Thus, normal prenatal sonograms do not exclude milder forms of OI, which can take years of life before clinical symptoms actually develop.

SOME MORE DIFFERENTIAL DIAGNOSTIC CONSIDERATIONS AND POINTS

The diagnosis of nonlethal OI should be considered when congenital bowing with normal mineralization is identified prenatally. The differential diagnosis includes camptomelic dysplasia (CD), an autosomal recessive skeletal dysplasia. Early neonatal death may occur in CD because of respiratory complications from maldeveloped tracheal cartilage. In CD, bowing is more marked in the tibia, with hypoplastic fibula and scapula. The presence of hydrocephalus, a flat nasal bridge, and talipes equinovarus can help differentiate this entity from OI, but this is usually done after birth.

Hypophosphatasia, a disease with alkaline phosphatase deficiency and hence poor mineralization, may show significant demineralization and shortened long bones as in severe cases of OI, but does not have the long bone fractures or their subsequent thickening due to healing that are seen in OI.

Key Points

Osteogenesis imperfecta is a progressive disorder with a variable prenatal appearance. If short, demineralized, fractured bones are identified in the early second trimester, severe forms of OI must be considered. When isolated skeletal bowing is identified, milder forms of OI should be excluded.

EDITOR'S COMMENTS

Differentiating among skeletal dysplasias can be confusing antenatally and postnatally. The goal of the sonographer and sonologist is to note several things during antenatal evaluation:

- *Are the bones normal or abnormal in appearance?*
- *Does mineralization appear normal?* Or is there a compressible skull or too easily penetrated brain parenchyma? Note the mineralization of the skull as compared to that of vertebral bodies and extremities.
- *Are the bones markedly shortened?* This includes the question as to whether vertebral bodies are of normal height or flattened. Remember that the nonlethal forms of OI may have normal bone length.
- *Are the bone contours smooth, or is there bowing or irregularity suggesting fracture?* Bowing certainly does not always mean fracture. However, shortening or irregularity of bone contour may be due to fracture, and the fractured bone may subsequently appear bowed or shortened, particularly if fractured portions are pulled inward like an accordion, a typical finding in the classic OI films of neonates. Consider very thick bones as possible evidence of callus formation. Consider discontinuity of bony cortex or sharp angulation as evidence of possible fracture.
- *Are there particular body areas of abnormality?* The thorax is unusually small in asphyxiating thoracic dysplasia, but this finding may also suggest lethal OI with its typical thoracic circumference of <2.5th percentile. Certainly if there are rib fractures, OI is the diagnosis. Look at the spine, skull, and pelvis as well for findings typical of the various individual dysplasias.
- *Is the bony shortening diffuse* (micromelia), as in OI, or does it involve just the middle or distal portions of the skeleton, suggesting rhizomelic or mesomelic types of dwarfism?

References

Brons JTJ, van der Harten HJ, Wladimiroff JW, et al: Prenatal ultrasonographic diagnosis of osteogenesis imperfecta. *Am J Obstet Gynecol* 159:176–181, 1988.

Bulas DI, Stern HJ, Rosenbaum KN, et al: Variable prenatal appearance of osteogenesis imperfecta. *J Ultrasound Med* 13:419–427, 1994.

Constantine G, McCormack J, McHugo J, Fowlie A: Prenatal diagnosis of severe osteogenesis imperfecta. *Prenat Diagn* 11: 103–110, 1991.

Cordone M, Lituania M, Zampatti C, et al: In utero ultrasonographic features of camptomelic dysplasia. *Prenat Diagn* 9:745–750, 1989.

Mahony B: Ultrasound evaluation of the fetal musculoskeletal system, in *Ultrasonography in Obstetrics and Gynecology*, 3d ed, Callen P (ed). Philadelphia, Saunders, 1994:254–290.

Marini JC: Osteogenesis imperfecta: Comprehensive management. *Adv Pediatr* 35:391–426, 1988.

Maroteaux P, Frezal J, Cohen-Solail, Bonaventure J: Les formes antenatales de l'osteogenese imparfaite. *Arch Fr Pediatr* 43: 235–241, 1986.

Munoz C, Filly RA, Golbus MS: Osteogenesis imperfecta type II: Prenatal sonographic diagnosis. *Radiology* 174:181–185, 1990.

Nolan R: The fetal musculoskeletal system, in *A Practical Guide to Ultrasound in Obstetrics and Gynecology,* 2d ed, Sauerbrei E, Nguyen K, Nolan R (eds). Philadelphia, Lippincott-Raven, 1998:348–376.

Phillips OP, Shulman LP, Altieri LA, et al: Prenatal counselling and diagnosis in progressively deforming osteogenesis imperfecta: A case of autosomal dominant transmission. *Prenat Diagn* 11: 705–710, 1991.

Robinson LP, Worthen NJ, Lachman RS, et al: Prenatal diagnosis of osteogenesis imperfecta type III. *Prenat Diagn* 7:7–15, 1987.

Sanders RC, Greyson-Fleg RT, Hogge WA, et al: OI and camptomelic dysplasia: Difficulties in prenatal diagnosis. *J Ultrasound Med* 13:691–700, 1994.

Sillence DO, Senn A, Danks DM: Genetic heterogeneity in osteogenesis imperfecta. *J Med Genet* 16:101–116, 1979.

Thompson EM: Non-invasive prenatal diagnosis of osteogenesis imperfecta. *Am J Med Genet* 45:201–206, 1993.

Section F
GENERAL OBSTETRICS AND MISCELLANEOUS

23

Figure 23-1 is one of the images from an ultrasound (US) exam performed on a mother without prior prenatal care who appeared "too large for dates" to the examining physician. What is the diagnostic finding? What are the possible causes?

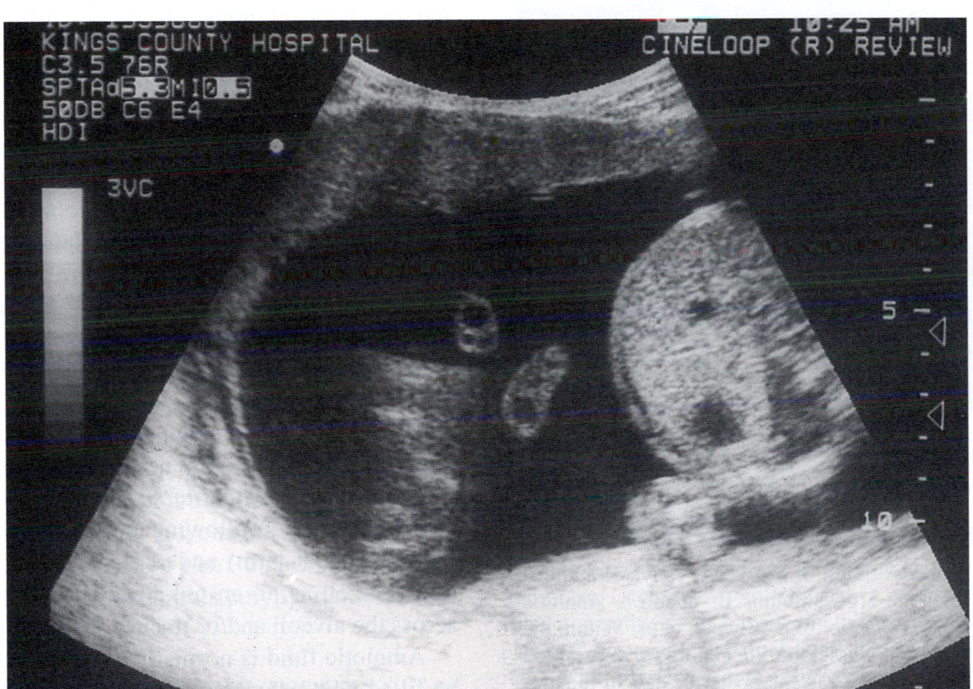

FIGURE 23–1. Uterus. Longitudinal plane.

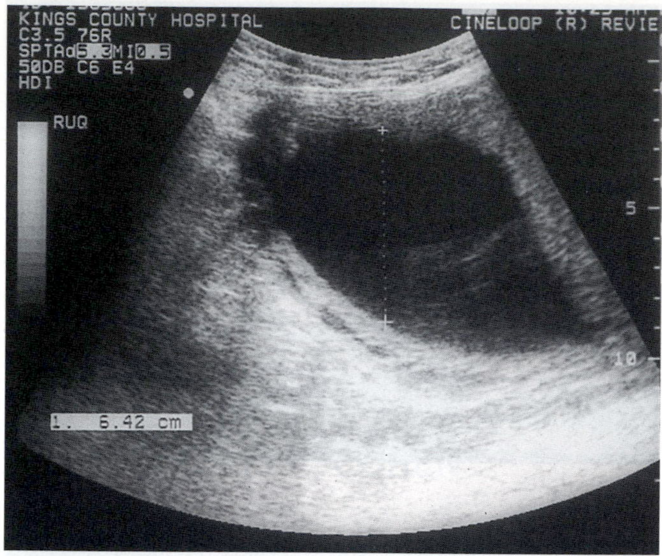

FIGURE 23–5. Vertical amniotic fluid depth determination. Superior portion of uterus, to the right of midline. Longitudinal plane. The markers show a 6.4-cm depth, which would be somewhat greater if measured more medially. This patient had an AFI of 28 cm, consistent with polyhydramnios.

OLIGOHYDRAMNIOS

Normal amniotic fluid volume may be maintained by one functioning kidney and a nonobstructed genitourinary (GU) tract. Oligohydramnios of fetal origin is due to abnormality of the GU tract. This may include bilateral renal agenesis; bilateral nonfunctional renal dysplasias, such as infantile (recessive) polycystic kidney disease or multicystic renal dysplasia; bilateral obstructions proximal to the bladder, such as bilateral ureteropelvic junction obstructions; or obstructions beyond the bladder, such as posterior urethral valves or urethral atresia. The analysis of fetal anatomy is hindered, sometimes significantly, by oligohydramnios, which limits the imaging window about the fetus. Imaging the fetal bladder goes against the possibility of bilateral renal obstruction or dysplasia.

Oligohydramnios may also be idiopathic or be associated with chromosomal abnormalities, postterm pregnancy (as a result of decreased urine production), and treatment of polyhydramnios with indomethacin (which also decreases urine production). The two key and usual abnormalities, besides GU anomalies, that we see in a busy daily practice are asymmetric intrauterine growth retardation (IUGR) [associated also with decreased abdominal circumference (AC) measurements, normally maintained femur length (FL) measurements, and, at times, prematurely aged placenta] and premature rupture of membranes, which will on occasion not be clearly known by the patient, especially the young adolescent. Polyhydramnios in association with symmetric IUGR (both AC and FL measurements are abnormally small) is often associated with chromosomal abnormalities and has a poor prognosis.

WHAT ARE CAUSES OF POLYHYDRAMNIOS?

Most cases of mild to moderate polyhydramnios (also known as hydramnios) have an idiopathic cause. These represent 60 percent of all cases of polyhydramnios. One-fifth of cases have a maternal cause, including poorly controlled diabetes and Rh or other histoincompatibility.

Only 20 percent of polyhydramnios cases are due to a fetal abnormality, but 75 percent of the severe cases have a fetal cause. These causes include gastrointestinal anomalies, particularly proximal bowel obstructions with resultant decreases in gastrointestinal tract absorption of swallowed amniotic fluid; central nervous system anomalies such as neural tube defects, hydranencephaly, and holoprosencephaly, which may allow increased amniotic fluid from transudation across the meninges; neurologically impaired fetal swallowing; or a lack of antidiuretic hormone, leading to polyuria. Thoracic abnormalities such as thanatophoric dwarfism, diaphragmatic hernia, or cystic adenomatoid malformation may allow compression of the esophagus or poor absorption of fluid via the trachea or alveoli and result in polyhydramnios.

KEY THINGS TO REMEMBER

Be wary of AFIs less than 9 cm and greater than 20 cm. Most mild to moderate cases of polyhydramnios are idiopathic and prove not to be of true clinical concern. In cases of severe polyhydramnios, look for a fetal anomaly. If none is seen, look again!

References

Brown D, Polger M, Clark P, et al: Very echogenic amniotic fluid: Ultrasonography-amniocentesis correlation. *J Ultrasound Med* 13:95–97, 1994.

Cohen H, Haller J: Diagnostic sonography of the fetal genitourinary tract. *Urol Radiol* 9:88–98, 1987.

Cohen HL, Muller D, Zinn DL: Abnormal fetal chest, abdomen, pelvis, in *Diagnostic Medical Sonography. A Guide to Clinical Practice. Obstetrics and Gynecology,* 2d ed, Berman MC, Cohen HL (eds). Philadelphia, Lippincott, 1997:285–320.

Doubilet P, Benson C: Ultrasound evaluation of amniotic fluid, in *Ultrasonography in Obstetrics and Gynecology*, 3d ed, Callen P (ed). Philadelphia, Saunders, 1994:475–486.

Dubbins P, Kurt A, Wapner R, et al: Renal agenesis: Spectrum of in utero findings. *J Clin Ultrasound* 9:189–193, 1981.

Goldstein R, Filly R: Sonographic estimation of amniotic fluid volume: Subjective assessment versus pocket measurements. *J Ultrasound Med* 7:363–369, 1988.

Hashimoto B, Kramer D, Brennan L: Amniotic fluid volume: Fluid dynamics and measurement technique. *Semin Ultrasound CT MR* 14:40–55, 1993.

Moore T, Cayle J: The amniotic fluid index in normal human pregnancy. *Am J Obstet Gynecol* 162:1168–1173, 1990.

Nolan R: The placenta, membranes, umbilical cord and amniotic fluid, in *A Practical Guide to Ultrasound in Obstetrics and Gynecology,* 2d ed, Sauerbrei E, Nguyen K, Nolan R (eds). Philadelphia, Lippincott-Raven, 1998:435–486.

Sohaey R: Amniotic fluid and the umbilical cord: The fetal milieu and lifeline. *Semin Ultrasound CT MR* 19:355–369, 1998.

Wladimiroff J: Effect of furosemide on fetal urine production. *Br J Obstet Gynaecol* 82:221–224, 1975.

24

A cross-sectional view of the umbilical cord (Fig. 24-1) in a second-trimester pregnancy is seen. The examination of another mother with a similar pregnancy showed a peculiar-looking fetal chest area (Fig. 24-2). What is the problem, if any, with these pregnancies?

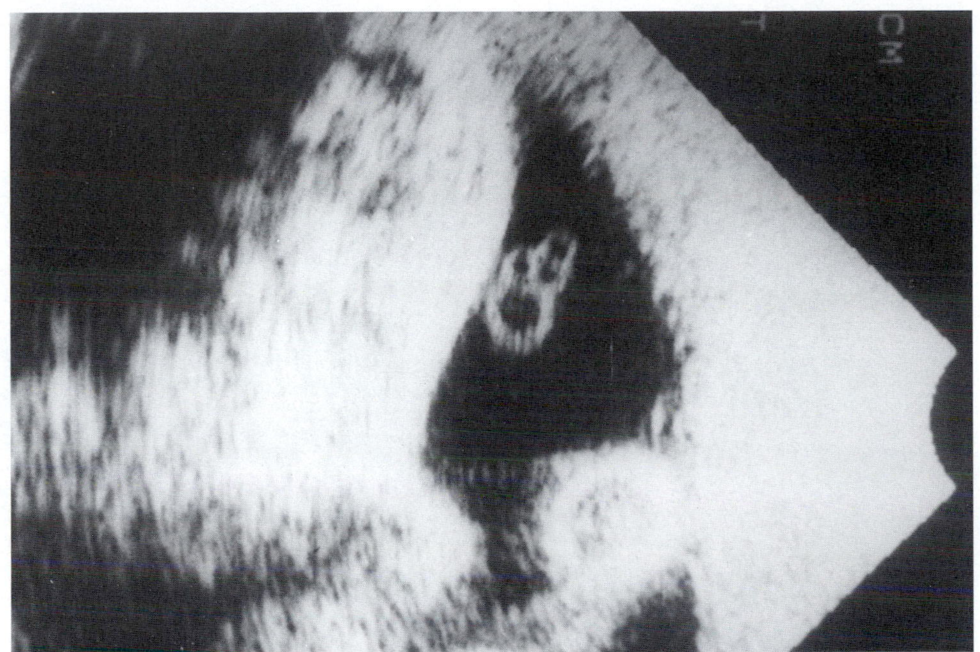

FIGURE 24–1. Umbilical cord. Axial plane.

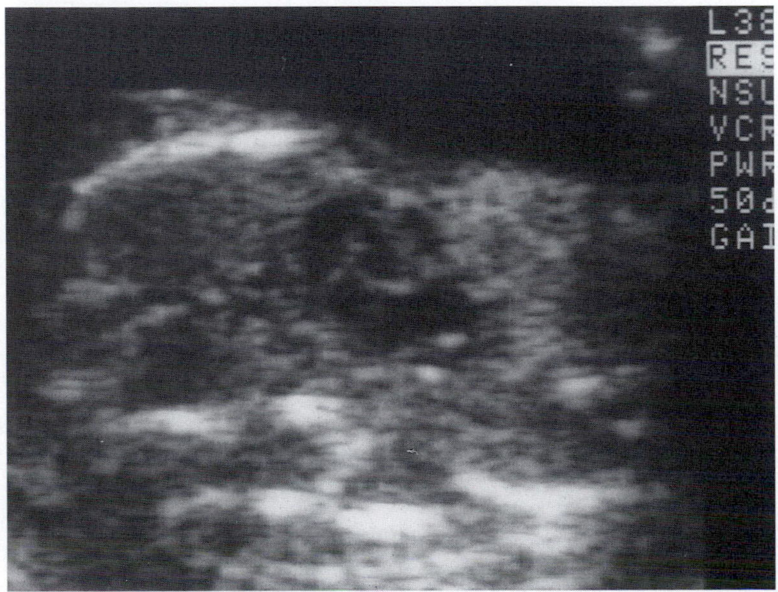

FIGURE 24–2. Fetal chest area. Axial plane.

CHAPTER 24

Multivessel Umbilical Cord in Conjoined Twinning

HARRIS L. COHEN

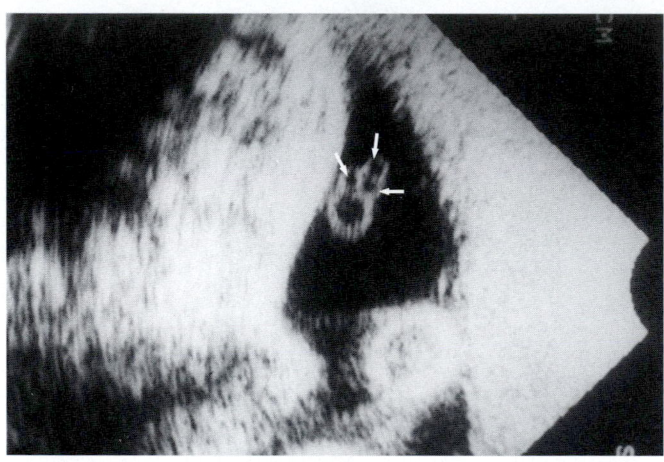

FIGURE 24–3. Annotated version of Fig. 24-1. Umbilical cord. Axial plane. The umbilical cord has four vessels. The three smaller echoless circular areas (*arrows*) are three umbilical arteries. The larger circle is an umbilical vein. The presence of more than two umbilical arteries can be seen in cases of conjoined twins, which this was. These twins did not survive an operation to separate them that would have sacrificed at least one of them. *(Image reprinted from Cohen et al, with permission.)*

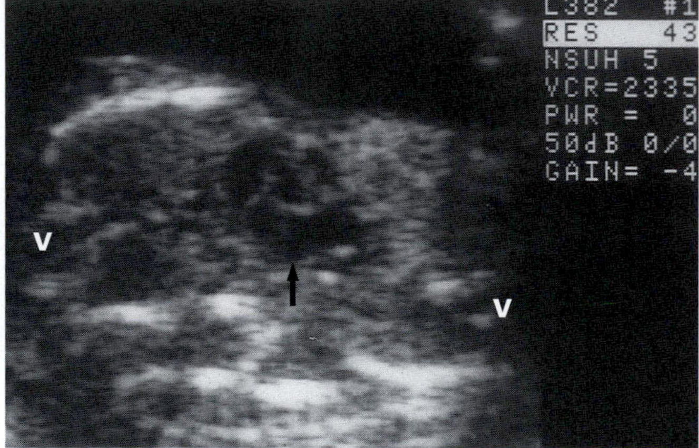

FIGURE 24–4. Annotated version of Fig. 24-2. Conjoined twins. Fetal chest area. Axial plane. A single heart (*arrow*) with an unknown number of chambers is seen between two conjoined thoraces. V = vertebrae. This fetal pair proved to have five chambers between them. They were aborted.

Figure 24-3, the annotated version of Fig. 24-1, shows a multivessel umbilical cord consisting of three umbilical arteries and a single umbilical vein. Figure 24-4, the annotated version of Fig. 24-2, shows a fetal heart in the center of two fetal thoraces that are joined anteriorly. The diagnosis is conjoined twinning. Multivessel umbilical cords have been reported in conjoined twins.

THE UMBILICAL CORD AND ITS BLOOD VESSELS

The normal umbilical cord consists of two umbilical arteries and a single umbilical vein (Fig. 24-5). Color Doppler (Fig. 24-6) may be used to confirm this. These vessels are derived from the stalk of the yolk sac and the allantois. The arteries have a mean width of 2.4 mm. The vein, at 8 mm, is three to four times greater in width.

The Single Umbilical Artery

In 1 of every 100 pregnancies, the right umbilical artery either regresses or does not form at all, and the patient has just a single umbilical artery (SUA). The finding is more common in twin pregnancies. The finding of an SUA has usually been considered of no clinical significance for the majority of patients but has been seen to a greater than normal extent among fetuses with trisomy, fetuses that have intrauterine

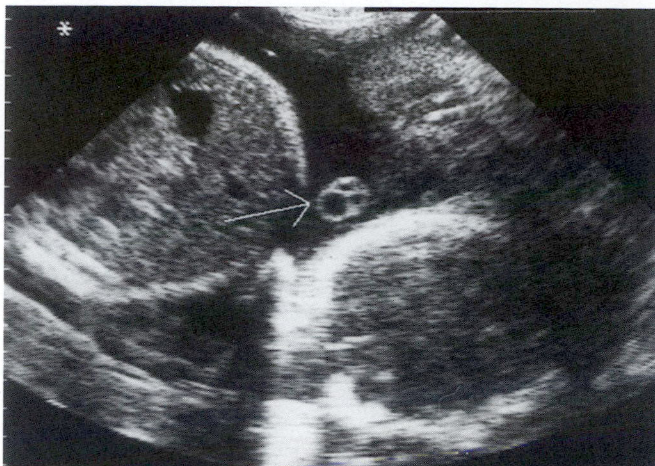

FIGURE 24–5. Normal umbilical cord. Axial plane through the cord. An arrow points to the normal umbilical blood vessels of a fetus. The arrow's point is closer to the larger umbilical vein. The two umbilical arteries are smaller and resemble the eyes, if the vein can be considered the mouth of a "Mr. Bill"–like image.

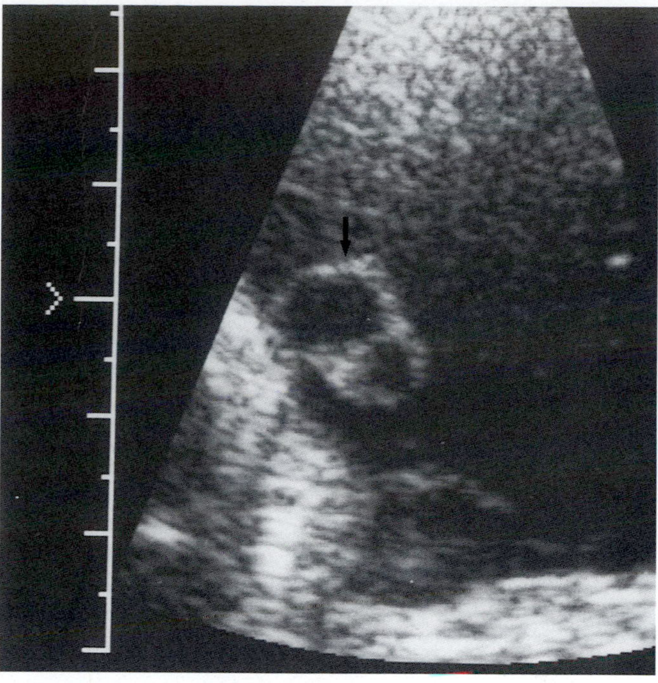

FIGURE 24–7. Single umbilical artery. Umbilical cord. Axial view. This two-vessel cord was seen in an otherwise normal fetus. There is one umbilical vein, the larger vessel (*arrow*), and one umbilical artery. The single umbilical artery is larger than normal.

growth retardation or are born with low birth weights (<2500 g), twins, the children of diabetic mothers, stillborn infants, and infants with major congenital abnormalities of the cardiovascular, genitourinary, and central nervous systems. A recent study reported a tremendous association of SUA with fetal structural abnormality, noting it in 31 percent of 167 studied fetuses. The same group also noted a 7 percent incidence of structural anomalies in neonates born with SUA despite an apparently normal fetal ultrasound (US) exam.

Often a *single* umbilical artery (Fig. 24-7) has a greater width (4 mm) than would be normal (2.4 mm) for either of a typical pair of umbilical arteries. This fact should help the examiner make the correct diagnosis and avoid considering a technical cause for an apparent SUA on a limited US examination if the imaged artery is wider than normal. Many umbilical cords with an SUA, especially when examined near the fetal end, have lost the classic braided appearance of the normal umbilical vessels (Fig. 24-8). In one study, fetuses with noncoiled umbilical cords had an almost five times

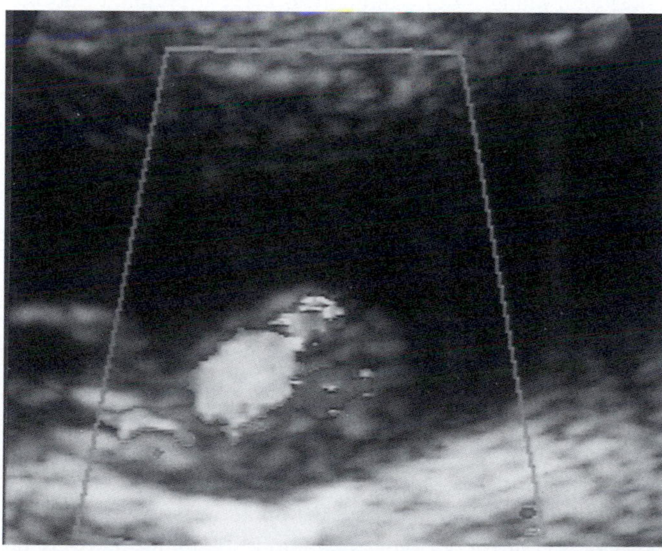

FIGURE 24–6. Normal umbilical cord. Axial plane through the cord. Using color Doppler, one can note that the direction of flow in the larger vessel, the vein, is pink/red, indicating flow in a direction opposite to the flow (blue) in the arteries. The spectral patterns of these vessels confirmed these facts. (See Color Plate 5.)

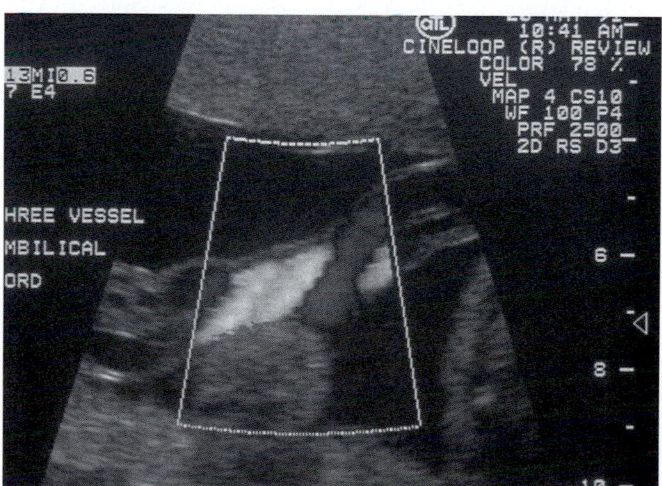

FIGURE 24–8. Normal umbilical braiding or coiling. Color Doppler image. Longitudinal oblique plane through umbilical cord. There is a normal three-vessel cord, with the two arteries (in red) coiled about the single umbilical vein (blue). This coiling or braiding of vessels about one another is not found in cases of SUA. (See Color Plate 6.) *[Image used with permission of Advanced Technology Laboratories (ATL).]*

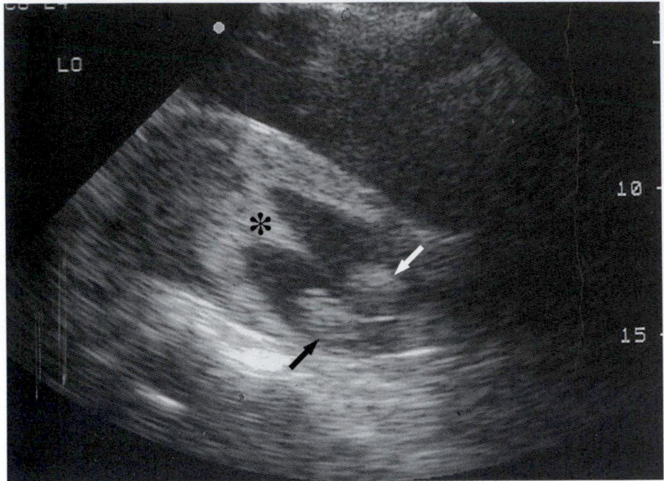

FIGURE 24–9. Dichorionic, diamniotic twins—"twin peak" sign. Uterus. Longitudinal plane. Two amniotic cavities each contain a fetal pole (*arrows*). The amniotic cavities are separated by a membrane, suggesting that this is a dichorionic rather than a monochorionic twinning. The triangle of thickening at the upper end of the membrane (*arrow*) is the "twin peak" sign that may help confirm this. Dichorionic, diamniotic twins have better perinatal survival statistics than other types of twins.

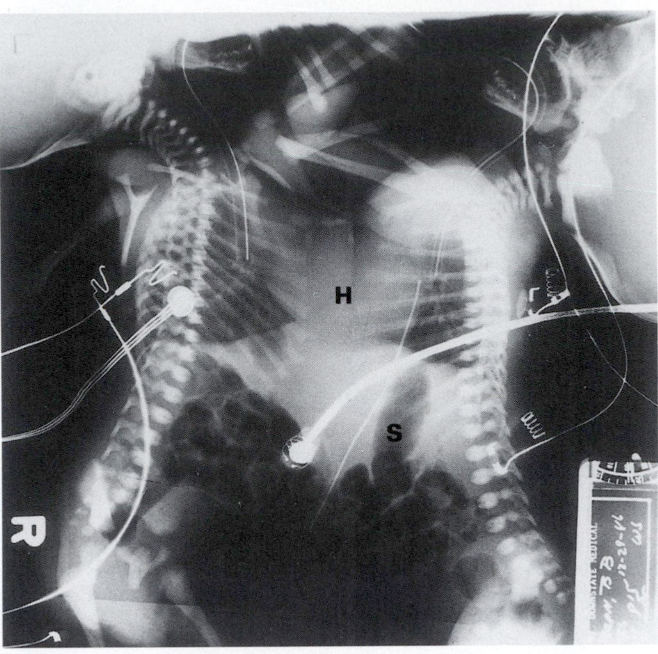

FIGURE 24–10. Thoracoomphalopagus conjoined twins. *A.* Skull/chest/abdomen/pelvis. Lateral film. This film confirmed the neonatal physical exam finding of a conjoined chest and upper abdomen. An H has been placed over the conjoined heart, which ultrasound and cardiac catheterization proved to be of five chambers. *(Images reprinted from Cohen et al, with permission.)*

greater incidence (16 percent) of fetal anomalies or death compared to a group with normal umbilical coiling (3.5 percent).

The Multivessel Umbilical Cord

Reports of an umbilical cord with more than three vessels, i.e., a multivessel cord, are uncommon. Multivessel cords have been seen in normal infants as well as those with congenital anomalies. They have, however, been reported in at least five cases of conjoined twins. It has been theorized that the multivessel cord may be a result (as is conjoined twinning) of incomplete separation of the embryonic disc. Gore et al's classic review of the x-ray and US findings of conjoined twinning introduced the concept that an umbilical cord with more than three vessels may be an indicator, among other findings, of conjoined twinning.

WHAT ARE THE VARIOUS TYPES OF TWINS?

Twins occur once every 80 to 90 births. Their perinatal mortality (14 percent) is almost 5 times that of singleton pregnancies (3.3 percent). Twins may be dizygotic, the result of two separately fertilized oocytes. All dizygotic twins have separate chorions and separate amnions—i.e., they are dichorionic and diamniotic. This group has the fewest of the complications of twinning and represents 70 percent of all twin pregnancies.

Twins may be monozygotic, the result of the division into two of a single fertilized oocyte (zygote) or the products of the oocyte's early mitotic divisions, the morula or the blastocyst. The result is a set of twins of the same genetic makeup. Division of the zygote within 4 days of fertilization results in the least serious of the types of monozygotic twinnings, i.e., the dichorionic (two placentas, which can appear fused), diamniotic (separate amniotic cavities) twin pregnancy. Dichorionic twins have a 9 percent perinatal mortality rate. Blastocyst division at between 4 and 8 days results in monochorionic, diamniotic twinning (26 percent perinatal mortality), and that at between 8 and 13 days, in monochorionic, monoamniotic twinning. Monochorionic, monoamniotic twins are at risk for several clinical problems, including twin-to-twin transfusion syndrome and cord entanglement. Monochorionic, monoamniotic twins have a 50 percent perinatal mortality rate. There is a significant ultrasound literature that discusses differentiating dichorionic, diamniotic twins from monochorionic, diamniotic twins (with their greater perinatal risk) based on intertwin dividing membrane thickness. The greater thickness (2 mm or greater) is due to, and found in the twin type with, the greater number of membranes, i.e., the dichorionic group. However, finding the intertwin membrane is not always easy. In addition, these membranes can stretch in pregnancy and appear overly thin or even rupture, confusing this US differentiation. Finberg has shown that triangular thickening (Fig. 24-9) at one edge of the intertwin membrane is evidence of dichorionic, diamniotic twinning and has labeled this the "twin peak" sign. Certainly if the genitalia of the twins show evidence that they are of opposite sexes, there is a 100 percent likelihood of a dichorionic, diamniotic dizygotic twin pregnancy.

WHAT IS CONJOINED TWINNING?

Conjoined twinning is a rare abnormality noted in 1 in 50,000 to 100,000 pregnancies and in only 1 in 600 twin pregnancies. It is a sporadic event resulting from an arrest in the division of the inner cell mass or embryonic disk after the 13th day of fertilization. These same-sex twins are monochorionic, monoamniotic, and incompletely separated from each other. Most are born premature, and the majority are stillborn. Whether they survive or not depends upon where they are joined, what organs are shared, and what organs remain separate and individual. The most common site of fusion (28 percent) is thoracoabdominal (with the resultant conjoined twins labeled thoracoomphalopagus) (Figs. 24-4, 24-10). Solitary fusion of the thorax (thoracopagus) (18 percent) and solitary fusion of the abdomen (omphalopagus) (10 percent) are less common. Other forms of fusion include those of buttocks (pyopagus) and lower spine (20 percent), the head (craniopagus) (6 percent), and the pelvis (ischipagus) (5 percent).

The antepartum diagnosis of conjoined twins is important for maximizing fetal viability and reducing maternal morbidity. Prior to the development of ultrasound, the diagnosis could be suggested at labor if (1) there were three or more presenting limbs, (2) if two right or two left extremities were felt on vaginal exam after the membranes had ruptured, or (3) if it was impossible to move one fetus up or down in relation to the other.

Ultrasound has made evaluation easier. This is particularly true when there is obvious fusion of the head, thorax, or abdomen. In conjoined twins with chest fusion, 90 percent share pericardium and 75 percent have some form of cardiac fusion. Be wary of a single Doppler waveform or a single heart rate when examining the fetal heart, since this is suggestive of cardiac fusion. Associated abdominal fusions include the liver in 100 percent of cases and the gastrointestinal tract in 50 percent. There are usually two umbilical cords leading to the monochorionic placenta. However, with wide anterior thoracic, abdominal, or thoracoabdominal fusions, the cords may become fused, resulting in a *single* multivessel umbilical cord. Reports of such multivessel cords include those with combinations of two to four arteries and one to four veins.

IN SUMMARY

Multivessel umbilical cords may suggest conjoined twins. Be wary of possible conjoined twins if you find monochorionic twins and there is/are

1. A single umbilical cord
2. Too many body parts in one area
3. Decreased independence of movement for any of the twins or twin parts

Breathe a sigh of relief if there are

1. Two separate placentas
2. A membrane between the two fetuses

because then you are dealing with dichorionic, diamniotic twinning, and fusion may be excluded.

References

Barth R, Filly R, Goldberg J, et al: Conjoined twins: Prenatal diagnosis and assessment of associated malformations. *Radiology* 177:201–207, 1990.

Benirschke K, Sullivan M, Marin-Padilla M: Size and number of umbilical vessels. A study of multiple pregnancy in man and the armadillo. *Obstet Gynecol* 24:819–834, 1964.

Chase L: The placenta and umbilical cord, in *Diagnostic Medical Sonography. A Guide to Clinical Practice. Obstetrics and Gynecology,* 2d ed, Berman MC, Cohen HL (eds). Philadelphia, Lippincott, 1997:415–447.

Chow J, Benson C, Doubilet P: Frequency and nature of structural anomalies in fetuses with single umbilical arteries. *J Ultrasound Med* 17:765–768, 1998.

Cohen HL, Shapiro M, Haller J, Schwartz D: The multivessel umbilical cord: An antenatal indicator of possible conjoined twinning. *JCU* 20:278–282, 1992.

Eddmonds L, Layde P: Conjoined twins in the United States, 1970–77. *Teratology* 25:301–308, 1982.

Finberg H: The "twin peak" sign: Reliable evidence of dichorionic twinning. *J Ultrasound Med* 11:571–577, 1992.

Finberg HJ: Ultrasound evaluation in multiple gestation, in *Ultrasonography in Obstetrics and Gynecology*, 3d ed, Callen P (ed). Philadelphia, Saunders, 1994:102–128.

Gore R, Filly R, Parker J: Sonographic antepartum diagnosis of conjoined twins: Its impact on obstetric management. *JAMA* 247:3351–3353, 1982.

Kalchbrenner M, Weiner S, Tempelton J, Losure T: Prenatal ultrasound diagnosis of thoracopagus conjoined twins. *JCU* 15: 59–63,1987.

Lam Y, Sin Y, Lee C, et al: Prenatal sonographic diagnosis of conjoined twins in the first trimester: Two case reports. *Ultrasound Obstet Gynecol* 11:289–291, 1998.

Nolan R: Multiple gestation, in *A Practical Guide to Ultrasound in Obstetrics and Gynecology,* 2d ed, Sauerbrei E, Nguyen K, Nolan R (eds). Philadelphia, Lippincott-Raven, 1998:417–434.

Nolan R: The placenta, membranes, umbilical cord and amniotic fluid, in *A Practical Guide to Ultrasound in Obstetrics and Gynecology,* 2d ed, Sauerbrei E, Nguyen K, Nolan R (eds). Philadelphia, Lippincott-Raven, 1998:435–486.

Strong T, Finberg H, Mattox J: Antepartum diagnosis of noncoiled umbilical cords. *Am J Obstet Gynecol* 170:1729–1731, 1994.

Wu M, Chang F, Shen M, et al: Prenatal sonographic diagnosis of single umbilical artery. *JCU* 25:425–430, 1997.

25

Images of the fetal abdomen (Fig. 25-1) and the fetal cranium (Fig. 25-2) of a 24-week fetus are worrisome. What do you see? What do you think the fetus has?

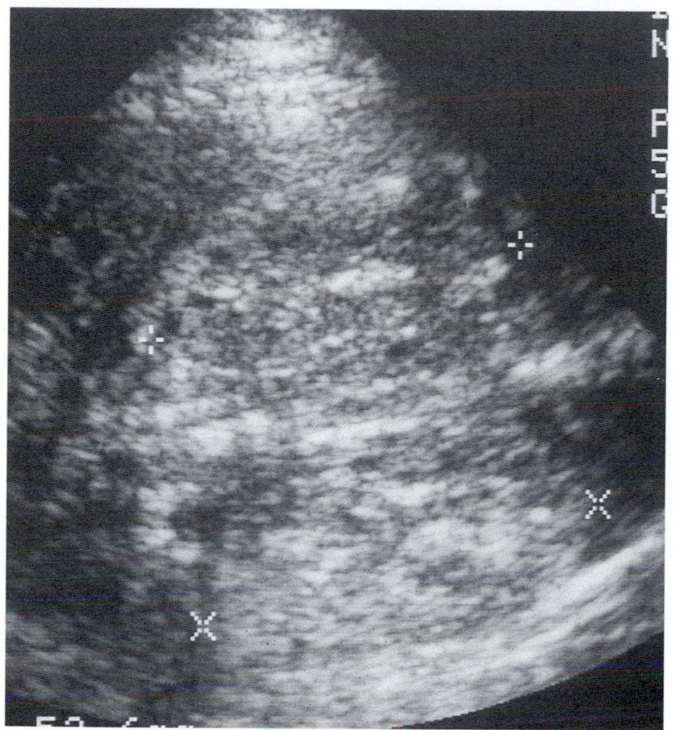

FIGURE 25–1. Fetal kidneys. Coronal view. The kidneys measure 5.3 cm in length.

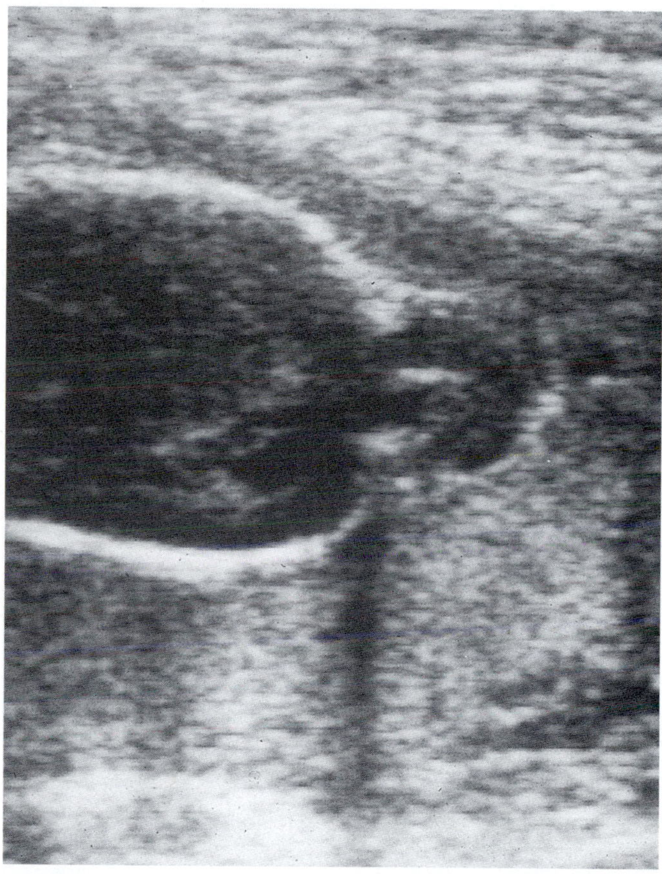

FIGURE 25–2. Fetal calvaria. Axial view. Posterior is to reader's right.

CHAPTER 25

Meckel-Gruber Syndrome

HARRIS L. COHEN

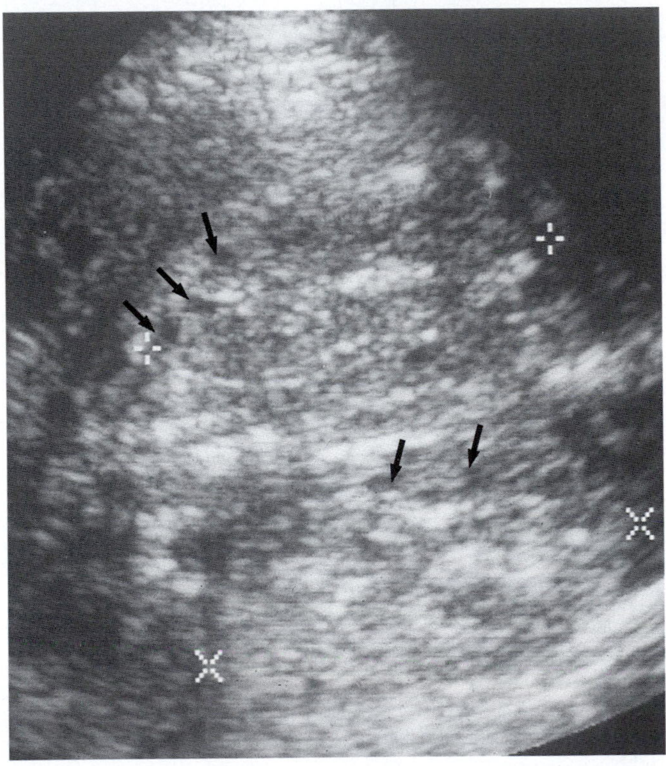

FIGURE 25–3. Annotated version of Fig. 25-1. Cystic renal dysplasia. Fetal kidneys. Coronal view. The kidneys are echogenic and enlarged, with measurements around 5.3 cm. The kidneys also contain tiny scattered cysts (*arrows*), best seen in the near-field kidney.

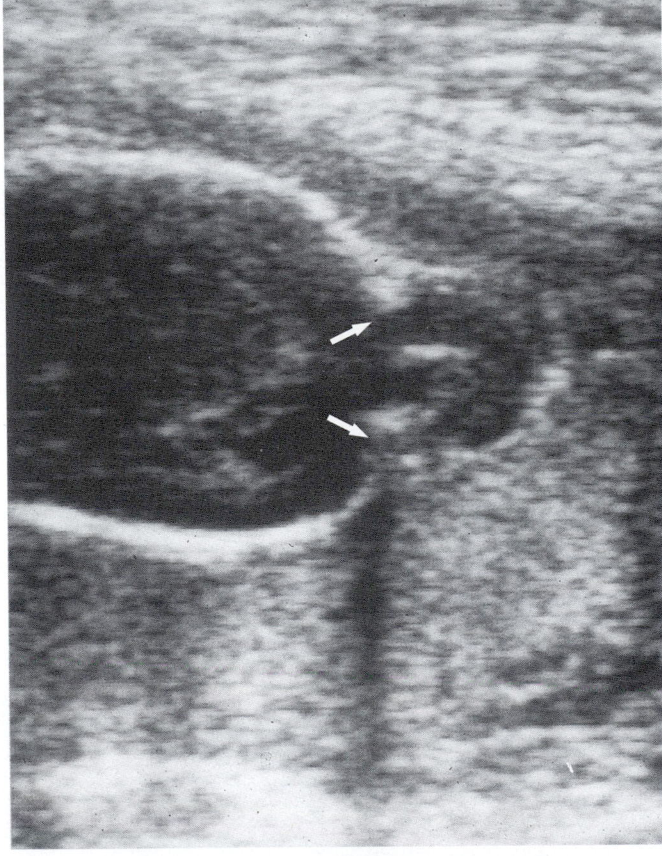

FIGURE 25–4. Annotated version of Fig. 25-2. Encephalocele. Fetal cranium. Axial view. There is a defect (*arrow*) in the posterior cranium of this patient. Brain parenchyma extends through it, consistent with the diagnosis of encephalocele.

Figure 25-3, the annotated version of Fig. 25-1, shows echogenic fetal kidneys, each containing scattered cysts. The 5.3-cm length for each kidney is far greater than normal. If the only abnormal finding were that of the kidneys themselves, then their increased echogenicity and enlargement would suggest cystic renal dysplasia. Potter type I cystic renal dysplasia—i.e., recessive polycystic kidney disease (RPKD)—would be a consideration. However, in the typical case of RPKD, where, pathologically, tiny scattered renal cysts result from 1- to 2-mm saccular dilatation of collecting tubules, the cysts are usually too small to be individually resolved by ultrasound (US) and so are not seen as cysts by US.

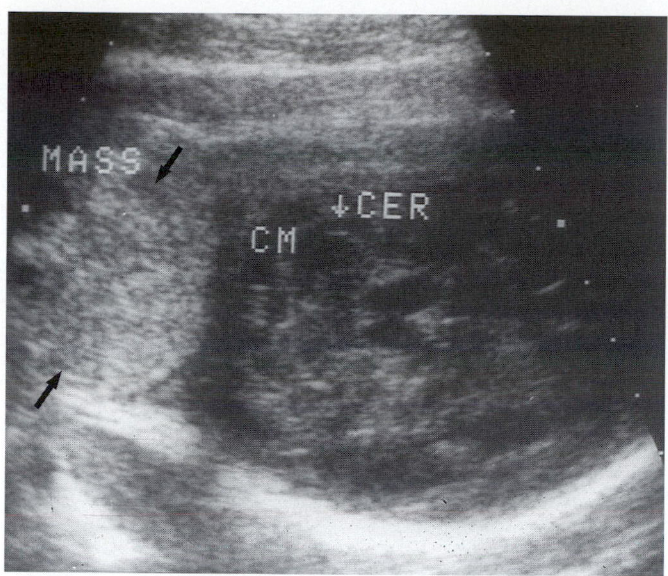

FIGURE 25–5. Occipital teratoma. Fetal brain. Axial plane. A highly echogenic mass (*MASS*) is seen posterior to the cisterna magna (*CM*) and cerebellum (*CER*) of a fetus. This and other views showed no skull defect. The mass is also more echogenic than normal brain. It proved to be an occipital teratoma. Masses beyond the cranium can simulate encephaloceles. The diagnosis of encephalocele should not be made unless a definitive defect in the calvaria can be imaged.

Rather, the multiple cyst walls create multiple interstices for the US beam, resulting in the kidneys appearing solid and highly echogenic. The image seen in Fig. 25-3 is more typical of Potter type IV cystic renal dysplasia, often considered the result of early genitourinary tract obstruction. (However, genitourinary tract obstruction is sometimes thought to be the cause of all cystic renal dysplasias, particularly by those who believe that all types are part of a broad spectrum of abnormality and that their differences are not as clearly defined as may have once been believed.)

In addition to the cystic renal dysplasia that this fetus has, Fig. 25-4, the annotated version of Fig. 25-2, shows a fetal calvaria in which the smooth contour is interrupted by an "outpouching" that contains brain parenchyma. The brain has extended through a calvarial defect as an encephalocele.

The combination of cystic renal disease and encephalocele in a fetus suggests Meckel-Gruber syndrome, which was what this fetus proved to have.

WHAT IS AN ENCEPHALOCELE?

An encephalocele is a neural tube defect involving the cranium that allows brain parenchyma to extend beyond its confines. (In the case of a meningocele, meninges extend beyond the confines of the skull.)

Although an encephalocele may be seen in the parietal area (13 percent) or the frontal area (12 percent) of the cranium, in the Western world, 75 percent of these lesions are occipital and usually midline. Encephaloceles are usually due to a neural tube defect, but they can be seen as part of an amniotic band syndrome (if an amniotic band crosses over and destroys part of the cranial vault) or as part of various malformation syndromes, including Meckel-Gruber syndrome. An encephalocele may be simulated by any mass beyond the confines of the cranium (Fig. 25-5), particularly one that appears similar on US examination to either brain (e.g., occipital hemangioma) or fluid-filled meninges (e.g., cystic hygroma). Therefore, to be assured of a correct diagnosis, one must be able to image a definitive skull defect and continuity of the mass to intracranial contents. Encephaloceles are, logically, associated with microcephaly and are often associated with hydrocephalus.

WHAT IS THE MECKEL-GRUBER SYNDROME?

Meckel-Gruber syndrome, also known as dysencephalia splanchnocystica and as Gruber's syndrome, is an autosomal recessive syndrome (an aggregate of signs, symptoms, and/or findings) that has several associated fetal abnormalities. These include a posterior encephalocele, seen in 80 percent of affected fetuses; postaxial polydactyly (usually six fingers and toes, or hexadactyly), seen in 75 percent; and cystic dysplasia of the kidneys, seen in 95 percent. It has also been associated with other central nervous system abnormalities, some of which we have described as associated with encephaloceles. These include microcephaly, ventriculomegaly, cerebellar hypoplasia, Dandy-Walker syndrome, the Arnold-Chiari malformation, and agenesis of the corpus callosum. Facial defects such as microphthalmia, micrognathia, and cleft palate have been noted. These fetuses may have cardiac defects, genital anomalies, and perhaps omphalocele. They often have fibrotic or cystic changes of the liver. Hepatic fibrosis is a common finding in RPKD patients, often to a degree inversely proportional to the degree of significance of their renal disease. Affected fetuses often have oligohydramnios because of the associated fetal renal dysfunction. They may have associated absence of the renal pelvis or aplasia or hypoplasia of the ureters. The enlarged echogenic kidneys containing cysts often, as with solitary cases of RPKD or cystic renal dysplasia type IV, take up essentially all the fetal abdominal space at the fetal renal level (Fig. 25-6).

The fetal diagnosis has been made as early as 10 to 11 weeks gestation because of polydactyly and encephalocele. It takes longer, sonographically, to note cystic renal dysplasia or to denote oligohydramnios based on poor renal function, since fetal urine production starts having a dominant effect on amniotic fluid levels at 18 to 20 weeks. The fetal bladder will not be imaged in these fetuses. The encephalocele may be diagnosed by laboratory findings of high alpha fetoprotein levels.

Meckel-Gruber syndrome is lethal. It has been noted in 1 in 140,000 British births, 1 in 50,000 Ashkenazi Jewish births, 1 in 13,250 Massachusetts births, 1 in 3000 Belgian births, and 1 in 1300 Gujarati Indian births. One-third of affected fetuses are stillborn. The vast majority, if they survive

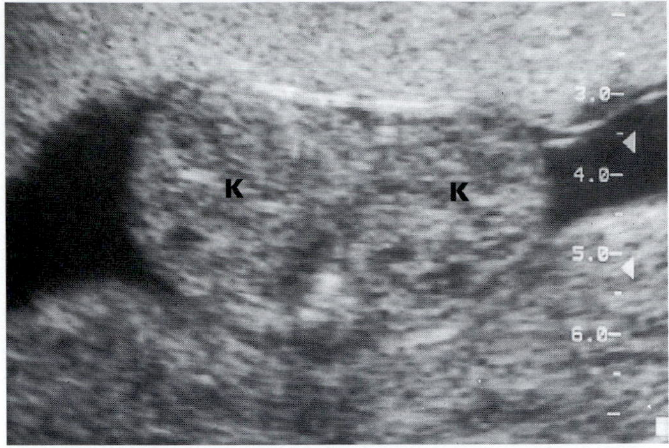

A

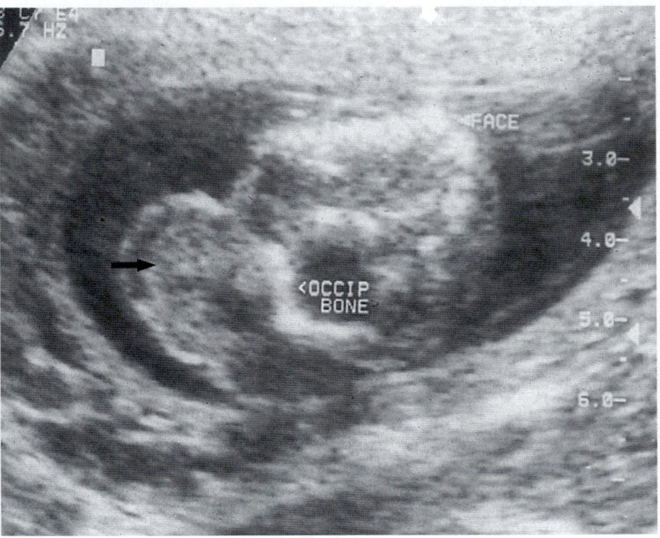

B

FIGURE 25–6. Meckel-Gruber syndrome. 16-week-old fetus. ***A.*** Fetal abdomen, level of kidneys. Axial plane. The abdominal contents at this level are made up solely of two enlarged kidneys (*arrows*). Subtle cysts are hard to see. ***B.*** Fetal posterior cranium. Sagittal oblique plane. Brain parenchyma (*arrow*) is seen beyond the confines of the cranium. The occipital bone (*Occip Bone*) appears oddly angulated on this view. This helped point toward a cranial defect and allow an early diagnosis of Meckel-Gruber syndrome.

intrauterine life, will live for only hours. Scattered reports of individuals surviving for months or even several years exist.

POINTS TO REMEMBER

As with all syndromes, to make a diagnosis, you have to know the syndrome's components and put two and two together. A wise pediatric radiologist once told me that you don't have to know them all by heart. You just have to know where the information is and arm yourself with those books. I do.

In the case of Meckel-Gruber syndrome, think of it when there is a combination of cystic renal disease and encephalocele. If you are fortunate, you may also image the polydactyly. I have not.

References

Benacerraf B: *Ultrasound of Fetal Syndromes.* New York, Churchill Livingstone, 1998:51–53, 125–127.

Cohen HL, Haller JO: Diagnostic sonography of the fetal genitourinary tract. *Urol Radiol* 9:88–98, 1987.

Cohen HL, Muller D, Zinn DL: Abnormal fetal chest, abdomen, pelvis, in *Diagnostic Medical Sonography. A Guide to Clinical Practice. Obstetrics and Gynecology,* 2d ed, Berman MC, Cohen HL (eds). Philadelphia, Lippincott, 1997:285–320.

Salonen R: The Meckel syndrome: Clinicopathological findings in 67 patients. *Am J Med Genet* 18:671–689, 1984.

Sauerbrei E: Fetal brain and skull, in *A Practical Guide to Ultrasound in Obstetrics and Gynecology,* 2d ed, Sauerbrei E, Nguyen K, Nolan R (eds). Philadelphia, Lippincott-Raven, 1998: 155–197.

Sepulveda W, Sebire N, Souka A, et al: Diagnosis of the Meckel-Gruber syndrome at eleven to fourteen weeks gestation. *Am J Obstet Gynecol* 176:316–319, 1997.

Streltzoff J, Gurewitsch E, Chervenak F: Sonographic assessment of the fetal head, neck and spine, in *Diagnostic Medical Sonography. A Guide to Clinical Practice. Obstetrics and Gynecology,* 2d ed, Berman MC, Cohen HL (eds). Philadelphia, Lippincott, 1997:243–268.

Taybi H, Lachman R: *Radiology of Syndromes, Metabolic Disorders and Skeletal Dysplasias,* 3d ed. Chicago, Year Book, 1990:294–295.

Wiedenmann H, Kunze J: *Clinical Syndromes,* 3d ed. New York, Year Book, 1997:92–93.

26

An axial view of the head of a fetus (Fig. 26-1) of 21 weeks gestational age is handed to you. What do you see? Do you have any concerns?

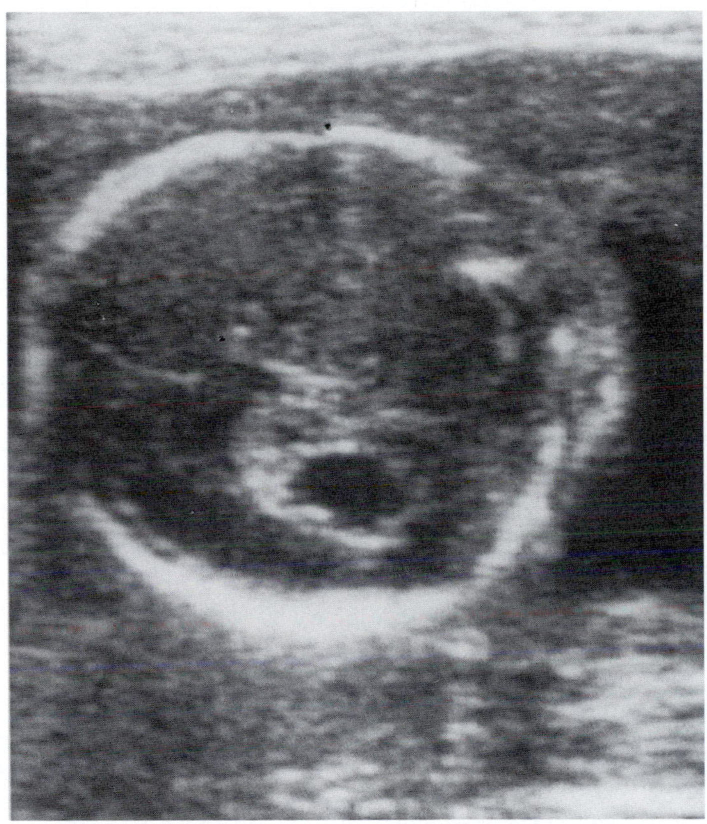

FIGURE 26–1. Fetal head. Axial plane.

CHAPTER 26

Choroid Plexus Cyst

HARRIS L. COHEN AND MARLENA PURSNER

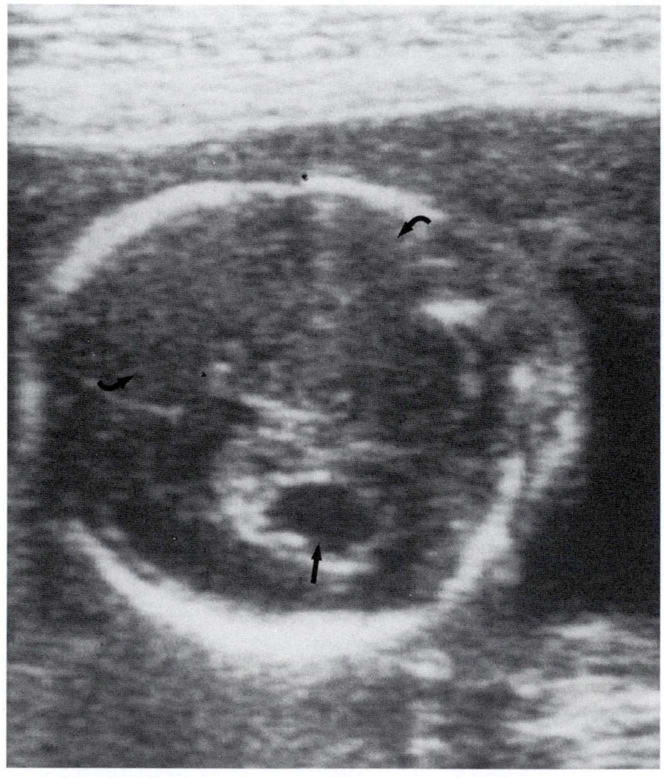

FIGURE 26–2. Annotated version of Fig. 26-1. Choroid plexus cyst. Fetal head. Axial plane. A large (10-mm) cyst (*arrow*) is seen in an echogenic area consistent with the choroid plexus in the atrium of the far field's lateral ventricle. Near-field artifact (*curved arrows*) obscures the intracranial contents of the near field's ventricular system. The fetus had a normal karyotype.

Figure 26-2, the annotated version of Fig. 26-1, shows a 1-cm cyst in the choroid plexus in the atrium of the left (far-field) lateral ventricle. It is not difficult to image or diagnose a choroid plexus cyst (CPC). Most fetuses with CPCs are normal, as this one was. Some have karyotype abnormalities. The difficulty with the CPC, as with other findings that are associated with normal fetuses as well as with those with chromosomal abnormality (e.g., the echogenic focus in the fetal heart or echogenic small bowel), is what to do about this possible indicator of aneuploidy (any karyotype abnormality) once it is discovered.

WHAT IS THE CHOROID PLEXUS CYST AND WHY ARE WE WORRIED ABOUT IT?

The choroid plexus is the normal cerebrospinal fluid–producing tissue of the cerebral ventricular system. It is found in the lateral ventricles as well as the roof of the third ventricle. It is readily imaged in the lateral ventricles. Choroid plexus cysts are most often thin-walled cysts that develop in the choroid plexus. They are a common finding in the second-trimester fetus and are imaged in 0.67 to 3.6 percent of routine obstetric ultrasound (US) studies. Although they are said to disappear in the late second and early third trimester, particularly beyond 22 to 26 weeks gestation, an incidence of 3 percent has been reported in routine head ultrasonography of neonates. Perhaps they do not all disappear.

The problem, and therefore the controversy, with regard to CPCs is that they are associated with fetal karyotype abnormalities. The exact percentage of fetuses with CPCs that also have a karyotype abnormality varies among clinical reports, ranging from 0 to 7.2 percent. Some 5 percent of CPC cases have trisomy 18 (Edwards' syndrome). Trisomy 18 represents 76 percent of the aneuploidies associated with CPCs. About 1 percent of fetuses with CPCs have another karyotype abnormality, often trisomy 21 (Down's syndrome). One group, however, believes that the prevalence of CPCs in fetuses with trisomy 21 is no different from their prevalence in fetuses without trisomy 21. They suggest that the presence of a CPC does not increase the calculated risk of a fetus's having Down's syndrome. There is at least one report that claims a 0 percent incidence of karyotype abnormality with CPCs.

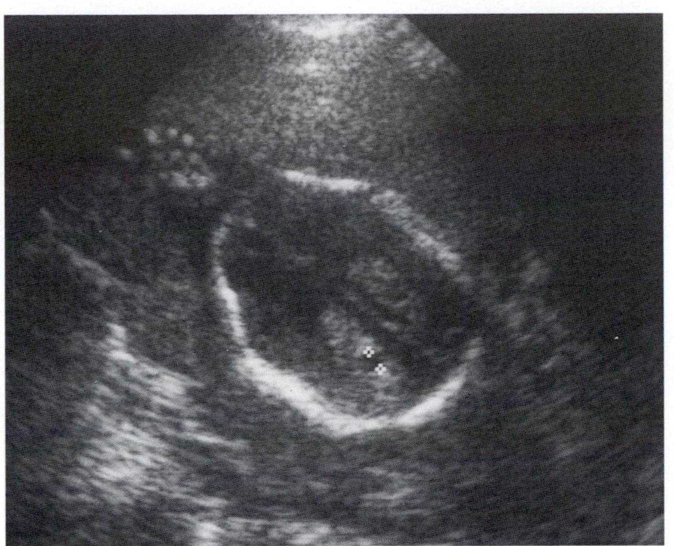

FIGURE 26–3. Trisomy 18. Fetal head. Axial plane. This fetus had an abnormal karyotype (trisomy 18) but only a unilateral 3.5-mm choroid plexus cyst (*marked off by crosses*). The calvaria appears lemon-shaped on this image. No other structural abnormality was found in this fetus.

Initially, amniocentesis was recommended only if large (10 mm or greater) and bilateral CPCs were discovered. However, cases of karyotype abnormality in fetuses whose CPCs are small and/or unilateral (Fig. 26-3) have been reported. Some authorities have suggested that amniocentesis be performed only when an associated structural abnormality was imaged as well as a CPC. While the risk of aneuploidy in the presence of a solitary CPC can be as great as 7.2 percent, the risk is much higher (1 in 3), when the CPC is found in combination with a structural abnormality. However, associated structural abnormalities are found in only 84 percent of affected fetuses. The classic clenched fist and overlapping fingers typical of trisomy 18 neonates are not found in as many as 20 percent of cases.

The controversy—to recommend amniocentesis or not—arises from the fact that amniocentesis itself is not without danger. The reported 1 in 200 to 250 incidence of miscarriage after amniocentesis must be weighed against the risk of occurrence of a case of trisomy 18 or other karyotype abnormality in a particular mother. In the case of trisomy 21, this is often linked to maternal age. The occurrence of trisomy 18 has also been linked to increased maternal age.

This same type of thinking vis-à-vis amniocentesis in the fetus with a CPC has been applied in deciding whether amniocentesis should be performed because of other discovered associations between relatively inconsequential structural findings and an abnormal karyotype. This includes the link between pyelocaliceal system dilatation, seen relatively often and not considered of significance in the third-trimester fetus when less than 10 mm, and trisomy 21, which has been linked to lesser degrees of pyelocaliceal system dilatation.

WHAT ARE THE CURRENT THOUGHTS ON WHAT TO DO WITH CASES OF CPC?

The controversy rages. Information from various groups is divergent (see Table 26-1). A 1997 study of 13,690 pregnant women with 84 (0.6 percent) fetuses with CPCs found 6 cases of aneuploidy, all with structural abnormalities. That group recommended US evaluation and no amniocentesis when a CPC is discovered. Their recommendation (which other groups are in agreement with) is that meticulous anatomic survey by US should be performed for fetuses with CPCs. They believe that the low incidence of karyotype abnormalities among fetuses with isolated CPCs may not justify the risk of amniocentesis. A 1994 study of 15,565 pregnancies with 152 (0.98 percent) CPCs, however, found 2.6 percent of the CPC group to have aneuploidy, with none of the 4 cases having a positive US image for associated structural abnormality. *That* group recommends (as do others) amniocentesis for isolated CPCs after 19 weeks gestation. Still another group found that the risk of trisomy 18 is only 12 times greater if there is one structural abnormality rather than an isolated CPC, but almost 600 times greater if there are two structural abnormalities. They believe that ma-

TABLE 26-1
Sample of Divergent Clinical Findings in Cases of CPC and Aneuploidy

GROUP	PREGNANT POPULATION (n =)	% WITH CPC	% OF CPC WITH ANEUPLOIDY	POINT MADE
Geary et al (1997)	13,690	0.6 (n = 84)	7	All cases of isolated cysts were chromosomally normal—do US, not amniocentesis
Walkinshaw et al (1994)	15,565	0.98 (n = 152)	2.6	4 aneuploidy cases (3 trisomy 18), none with structural defect—do amniocentesis

ternal age should be the deciding factor for amniocentesis unless there are two structural abnormalities.

Most groups seem to agree that bilaterality is not helpful in predicting aneuploidy. Some authorities say the same about the size of the cysts, while others still regard the large or septated cyst as more indicative of possible abnormality. Cyst disappearance is considered common beyond 22 weeks and should not infer normalcy.

BEWARE THE PSEUDOCYST!

Oblique or coronal views through the atrium of the lateral ventricle may allow the normal corpus striatum to project into the corpus callosum and appear as an ovoid hypoechoic mass or choroid pseudocyst. Ultrasound imaging from other angles and an attempt to obtain a true transaxial plane can help to avoid this problem.

WHAT DO *WE* DO?

As one of the clinical research groups that found aneuploidy, particularly trisomy 18, in fetuses without significant structural abnormality, we remain confused, knowing that there are variations in reported clinical experience. We are more concerned about larger cysts, but we know that small cysts can be linked to aneuploidy as well. We offer the option of amniocentesis to the family after they have been informed of both the risks for aneuploidy and the risks of amniocentesis. We attempt to make as meticulous an exam of the fetus as the amniotic fluid levels, fetal lie, maternal body habitus, and other factors in the performance of fetal examination allow us. If necessary, we will reexamine the fetus on another day.

WHAT IS TRISOMY 18? WHAT ARE THE FINDINGS?

Trisomy 18 or Edwards' syndrome infants either have three rather than two 18th chromosomes or have a chromosome 18 with three times the normal genetic material. The affected fetus is usually female, and the incidence of this trisomy is 1 in 8000 births. These infants die young. By age 5, all affected males have died and only 15 percent of affected females are living.

These infants have many abnormalities. Trisomy 18 patients have low birth weight, are mentally retarded in most cases, and are hypotonic at birth. They later develop hypertonia. They have characteristic facial features, including upward-slanting palpebral fissures, a short philtrum, micrognathia, and other facial deformities involving the lip, jaw, palate, and ears that may not be readily picked up on fetal examination. They have a classic so-called clenched fist based on the position of the fingers. The first digit is adducted; the first, second, and fifth fingers at least partially extended; and the third and fourth fingers flexed and sometimes overlapping (Fig. 26-4). Foot deformities such as rocker bottom feet are common. Anomalies of the cardiovascular (ventricular septal defect, patent ductus arteriosus, ectopia cordis), central nervous system (myelomeningocele, microcephaly), genitourinary (hypospadius, cryptorchidism, hydronephrosis), and gastrointestinal (omphalocele, diaphragmatic hernias) systems are common, as are hernias (umbilical and inguinal). There is an increased incidence among these patients for the development of central nervous system and liver neoplasms and of Wilms' tumors.

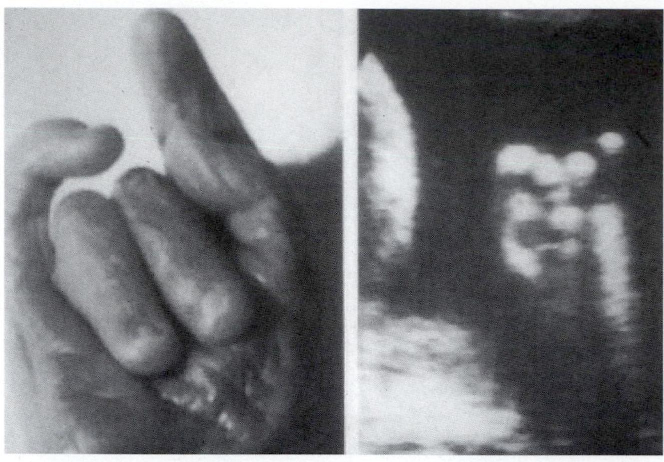

FIGURE 26–4. Trisomy 18 hand. The left side of the image shows a clinical view of a trisomy 18 hand with classically flexed third and fourth fingers and extended first, second, and fifth fingers. The right side of the image shows this in a fetus. *(Reprinted from Nguyen, with permission.)*

Affected fetuses have an increased incidence of single umbilical arteries, intrauterine growth retardation, and polyhydramnios. Microcephaly is common.

Making an antenatal diagnosis could spare parents much grief. The controversy and difficulty in knowing what to do after discovering a CPC is heavily affected by the above. Imaging an open fetal hand (Fig. 26-5) goes against trisomy 18, but is not a guarantee.

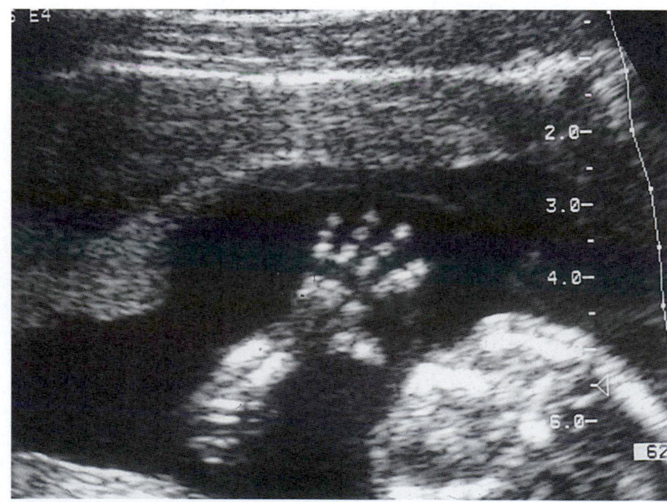

FIGURE 26–5. Open hand. Fetal hand. Coronal plane. The fingers are extended. This image goes against the possibility of trisomy 18 and its classic "clenched fist."

As a last point: Exact answers are not easy to come by. Ultrasound is still an art as well as a science. Hopefully, we can all continue to be open to new information and data.

References

Benacerraf B, Harlow B, Frigoletto I: Are choroid plexus cysts an indication for second-trimester amniocentesis? *Am J Obstet Gynecol* 162:1001–1006, 1990.

Bromley B, Lieberman E, Benacerraf B: Choroid plexus cysts: Not associated with Down syndrome. *Ultrasound Obstet Gynecol* 8:232–235, 1996.

Burrows A, Ramsden GH, Frazer MI: Choroid plexus cysts in the fetal brain. *Aust N Z J Obstet Gynaecol* 33:262–264, 1993.

Cohen HL, Haller JO: Review. Advances in perinatal neurosonography. *AJR* 163:801–810, 1994.

Geary M, Patel S, Lamont R: Isolated choroid plexus cysts and association with fetal aneuploidy in an unselected population. *Ultrasound Obstet Gynecol* 10:171–173, 1997.

Gupta J, Cave M, Lilford R, et al: Clinical significance of fetal choroid plexus cysts (see comments). *Lancet* 346:724–729, 1995.

Kurtz A, Middleton W: *Ultrasound: The Requisites.* St Louis, Mosby–Year Book, 1996:221–225.

McGahan JP: The fetal head: Borderlines. *Semin Ultrasound CT MR* 19:318–328, 1998.

Nadel AS, Bromley BS, Frigoletto FD Jr, et al: Isolated choroid plexus cysts in the second-trimester fetus: Is amniocentesis really indicated? *Radiology* 185:545–548, 1992.

Nguyen K: Chromosomal abnormalities, in *A Practical Guide to Ultrasound in Obstetrics and Gynecology,* Sauerbrei E, Nguyen K, Nolan R (eds). Philadelphia, Lippincott-Raven, 1998:394–395.

Ostlere S, Irving H, Lilford R: Fetal choroid plexus cysts: A report of 100 cases. *Radiology* 175:753–755, 1990.

Perpignano M, Cohen HL, Klein V, et al: Fetal choroid plexus cysts: Beware the smaller cyst. *Radiology* 182:715–717, 1992.

Snijders RJ: Isolated choroid plexus cysts: Should we offer karyotyping? *Ultrasound Obstet Gynecol* 8:223–224, 1996.

Snijders RJ, Shawa L, Nicolaides KH: Fetal choroid plexus cysts and trisomy 18: Assessment of risk based on ultrasound findings and maternal age. *Prenat Diagn* 14:1119–1127, 1994.

Walkinshaw S, Pilling D, Spriggs A: Isolated choroid plexus cysts—the need for routine offer of karyotyping. *Prenat Diagn* 14:663–667, 1994.

Wiedenmann H, Kunze J: *Clinical Syndromes,* 3d ed. New York, Year Book, 1997:98–99.

PART 2

THE PEDIATRIC PATIENT

Section A
CENTRAL NERVOUS SYSTEM

27

Two coronal ultrasound (US) images of a neonate of 26 weeks gestation are handed to you. The first, Fig. 27-1, was obtained in the first week of life. The second, Fig. 27-2, was obtained when the neonate was 11 weeks old. What do you see? What is the diagnosis?

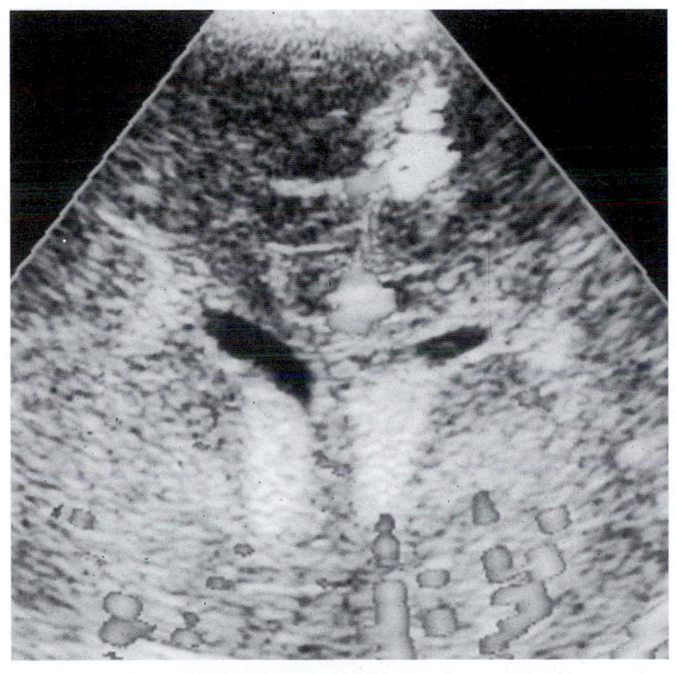

FIGURE 27–1. Head Ultrasound. Coronal plane. Ignore imaged vascular flow.

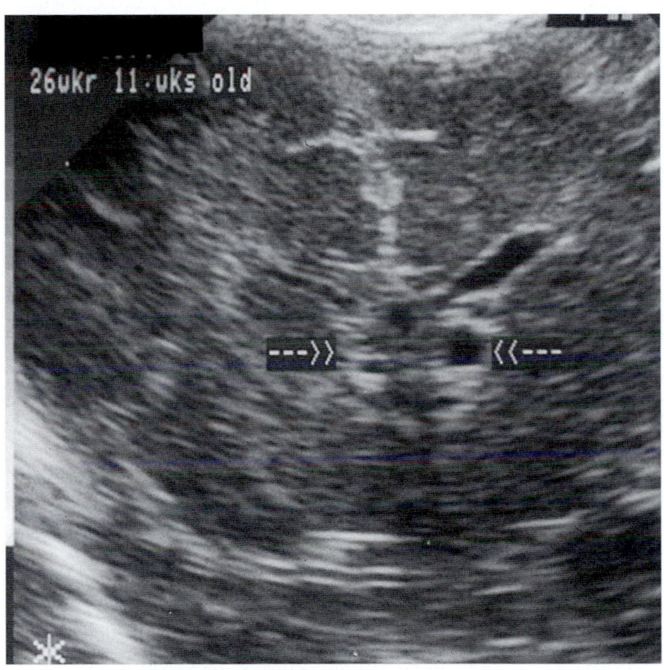

FIGURE 27–2. Head Ultrasound. Coronal plane.

CHAPTER 27

Subependymal Hemorrhage and Cysts

HARRIS L. COHEN

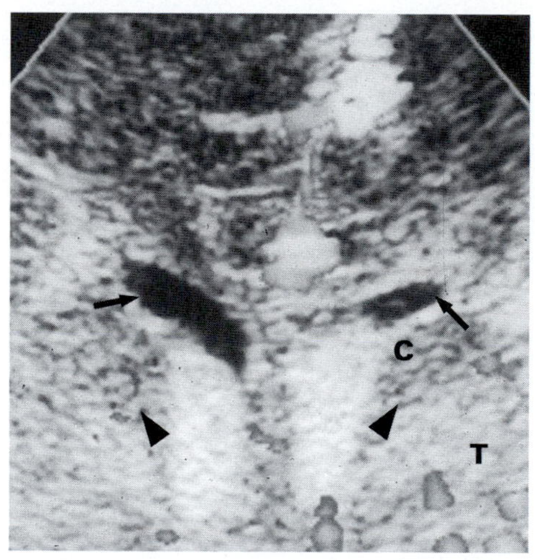

FIGURE 27–3. Annotated version of Fig. 27-1. Bilateral subependymal hemorrhage. Head ultrasound. Coronal plane. This image is a relative close-up of the frontal horn region of the lateral ventricles. It is, incidentally, a color Doppler image that was photographed in black and white. The frontal horns (*arrows*) are black because of their contained echoless cerebrospinal fluid. They are normal in size, with the one on the right slightly full. Inferior to the frontal horns, on this image, are two highly echogenic areas (*arrowheads*) that (at least on the right) appear definitively outside the ventricular system. Other views proved this. The image is consistent with bilateral grade I hemorrhage in a premature infant. The head of the caudate nucleus (C) is just lateral to the hemorrhage. The thalami (T) are slightly more echogenic than the caudate heads and, incidentally, show normal thalamostriate vessel flow, best seen on the left.

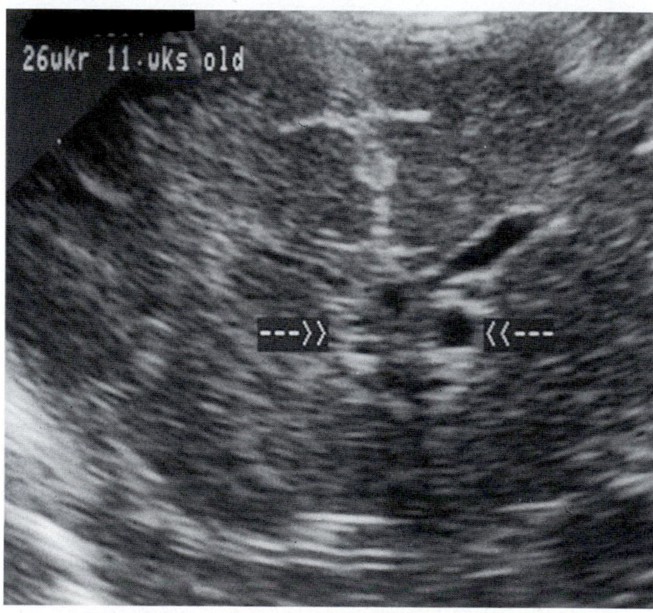

FIGURE 27–4. Annotated version of Fig. 27-2. Subependymal cysts that developed in bilateral subependymal hemorrhage (SEH). Head ultrasound. Coronal plane. On a follow-up exam at the tenth week of life, several cysts are noted in the formerly homogeneously echogenic subependymal area (*arrows*). This is a commonly seen finding in resolving SEH. If the prior hemorrhage had not been seen, other clinical considerations for their etiology (see text) would have to be considered.

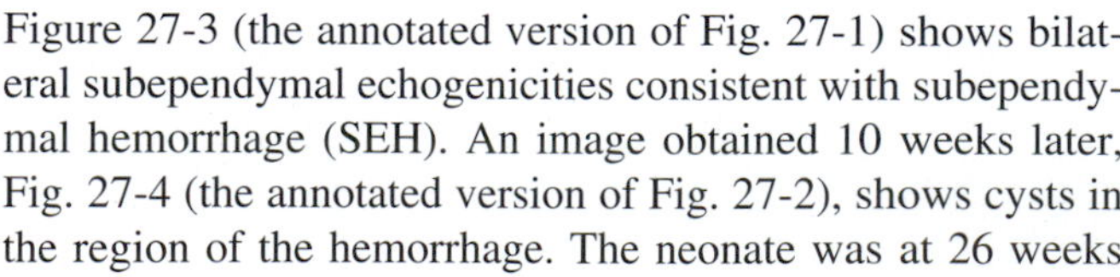

Figure 27-3 (the annotated version of Fig. 27-1) shows bilateral subependymal echogenicities consistent with subependymal hemorrhage (SEH). An image obtained 10 weeks later, Fig. 27-4 (the annotated version of Fig. 27-2), shows cysts in the region of the hemorrhage. The neonate was at 26 weeks gestation at birth. Premature infants of less than 32 weeks gestational age at birth and/or less than 1500 g birth weight are at particularly great risk for SEH and intraventricular hemorrhage (IVH). The imaging of residual cysts in the subependymal areas as SEH hemorrhages resorb is not uncommon.

NEONATAL NEUROSONOGRAPHY

History/Technical Factors

Previous chapters in this book have discussed the analysis of the *fetal* brain with US. A great deal of the information used to analyze US images of the fetal brain has come from work performed in the neonatal head. Although the concept that US could help evaluate the neonatal brain was clear for many years, the practical and wide-scale implementation of this concept awaited the development of satisfactory real-time US equipment and the discovery of a satisfactory ultrasound window to bypass the difficulty in imaging brain deep to the bony calvaria. In 1980, the anterior fontanelle was discovered to be a satisfactory US window. Since then, many other calvarial openings (posterior fontanelle, metopic suture) have been used as well. Whereas in 1980 premature neonates waited days to weeks until they were able to be safely transported to computed tomography (CT), by 1981 neonates were analyzed by US in the comfort and clinical security of a monitored isolette in the neonatal intensive care unit (NICU).

The infant brain is typically imaged with high-frequency transducers, usually 7.5 MHz for premature neonates, 5 to 7.5 MHz for full-term infants. The brain can also be imaged, in a less satisfactory manner, after fontanelle closure by using the better-penetrating low-frequency transducers (e.g., 3.5 MHz) at the sacrifice of near-field resolution. Duplex and color and power Doppler have allowed us to obtain additional anatomic and physiologic information.

Why Look?

Neonatal neurosonography allows analysis of anomalies, e.g., hydranencephaly, hydrocephalus, or holoprosencephaly (particularly in a neonate presenting with a midline facial anomaly). Anomaly detection has helped clinicians and parents make important clinical and social decisions. Fetal intracranial US has helped clinicians make some of these diagnoses earlier. However, intracerebral abnormalities may first show up only *after* the usual 18- to 21-week gestational age view of fetal anatomy. What is most important to note in the premature neonate is IVH and its sequelae, which, although occasionally imaged in a fetus (Fig. 27-5), are primarily a problem of the premature neonate.

THE NEONATAL HEAD ULTRASOUND EXAM—HOW IS IT DONE?

The typical exam (see the American Institute of Ultrasound in Medicine's guidelines) requires a review of the infant brain in the coronal and sagittal planes. In the coronal plane, the brain is examined from front to back (Fig. 27-6). Representative coronal views are obtained anterior to the frontal horns (Fig. 27-7), in the plane of the frontal horns (Fig. 27-8), in the plane of the body of the lateral ventricles (Fig. 27-9), and more posteriorly, if possible. These images are obtained by holding the transducer steadily but lightly in the anterior fontanelle and using subtle wrist angulation to obtain the desired plane of insonation.

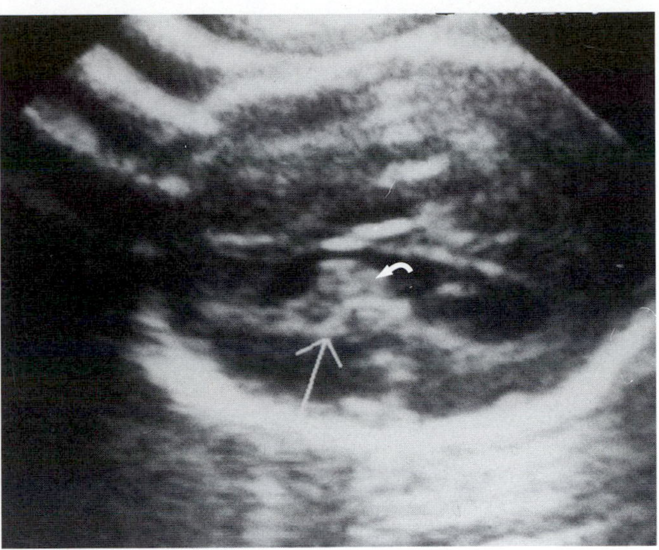

FIGURE 27–5. Intraventricular hemorrhage in fetus. Fetal head. Axial oblique plane. The near field is filled in by artifact. An arrow points to a dilated lateral ventricle in the far field. Within it is an echogenic mass (*curved arrow*) that was a hemorrhage. Ventricular dilatation and intraventricular hemorrhage are consistent with grade III IVH. This fetus was distressed at this time, about 36 weeks gestation. After birth, the hemorrhage resolved, and she did well. *(Reprinted from Cohen HL, Haller J, Gross B. Diagnostic sonography of the fetus: A guide to evaluation of the neonate.* Pediatr Ann *21:87–98, 1992, with permission.)*

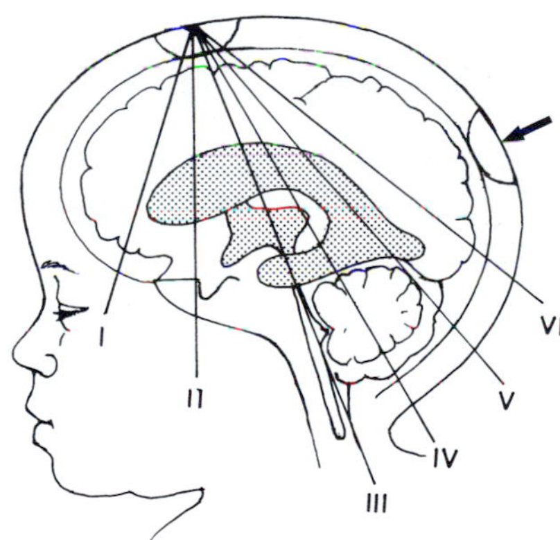

FIGURE 27–6. Neonatal neurosonography technique. Schematic drawing of various coronal planes. Lines extend from the area of the anterior fontanelle. The drawing reflects the different planes of section that can be obtained with different angling of the transducer. Just as these lines can be drawn from the anterior fontanelle, others could be drawn from the posterior fontanelle (*arrow*). Posterior fontanelle views have been used in the identification of subtle intraventricular hemorrhage and in the analysis of subtentorial anomalies such as the Dandy-Walker cyst. *(Reprinted from Cohen and Sanchez, with permission.)*

The images in the sagittal plane are obtained from the brain's periphery, the sylvian fissure (Fig. 27-10) on one side to that on the other side (Fig. 27-11). Key and necessary are a midline image—to note the corpus callosum (Fig. 27-12) and whether there is abnormality to the midline third or fourth ventricles—and both left (Fig. 27-13) and right parasagittal images through the body of the lateral ventricles and the caudothalamic area

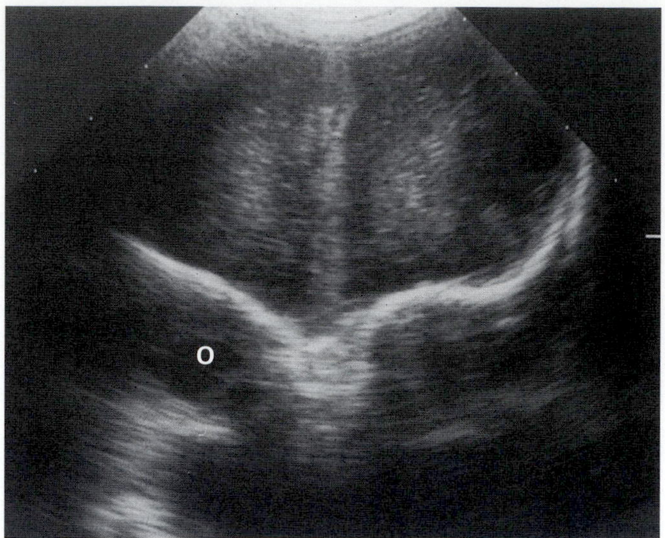

FIGURE 27–7. Neonatal head ultrasound. Coronal plane. Significant anterior angulation. This image was obtained far anterior to the frontal horns. It shows normal brain of the frontal lobe superior to the orbits. O = right orbit.

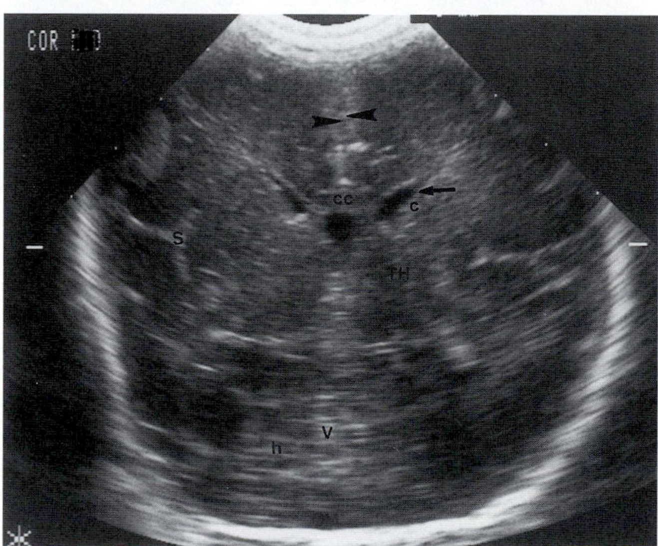

FIGURE 27–8. Neonatal head ultrasound. Coronal plane. Some anterior angulation. This image passed through the frontal horns. Many structures can be imaged. Normal frontal horns and lateral ventricles can be slitlike. The frontal horns in this normal patient are slightly fuller. An arrow points to the left frontal horn, which is somewhat more evident than the right frontal horn on this image. Arrowheads point to the interhemispheric fissure where the two frontal lobes meet. If there was volume loss, fluid in the interhemispheric space would be between the lobes, and the single thin echogenic line seen here would disappear. At the inferior aspect of the interhemispheric fissure on this image can be noted the corpus callosum (cc). Th = left thalamus; T = right temporal brain; S = the Y-shaped sylvian fissure; V = vermis of the cerebellum; h = right cerebellar hemisphere; CM = cisterna magna.

(Fig. 27-14). The parasagittal images allow one to diagnose hydrocephalus as well as SEH or IVH. Certainly all the brain parenchyma that can be imaged should be reviewed for the less common intraparenchymal hemorrhage (Fig. 27-15), possible extraaxial collections (which allow the brain borders to be too easily seen when separated from the calvaria), and anomalies. Doppler, in all its forms, may be used to analyze normal (Fig. 27-16; see also Color Plate 7*A* and *B*) and abnormal vessels (see Chap. 3) and the flow within them.

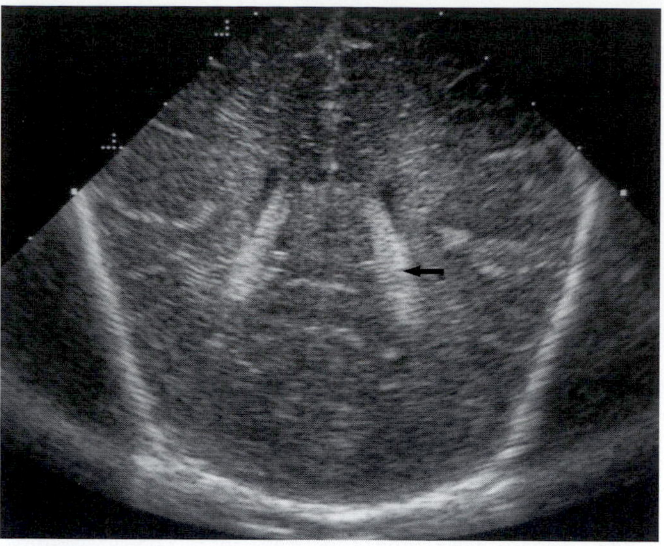

FIGURE 27–9. Neonatal head ultrasound. Coronal plane. Mid to posterior angulation. This imaging plane cuts through the bodies of the lateral ventricles. The echogenic choroid plexus (an arrow points to the left choroid) is hugged by the lateral ventricular wall. This argues against hydrocephalus. As we shall note, relatively acute hemorrhage is as echogenic as the normal choroid.

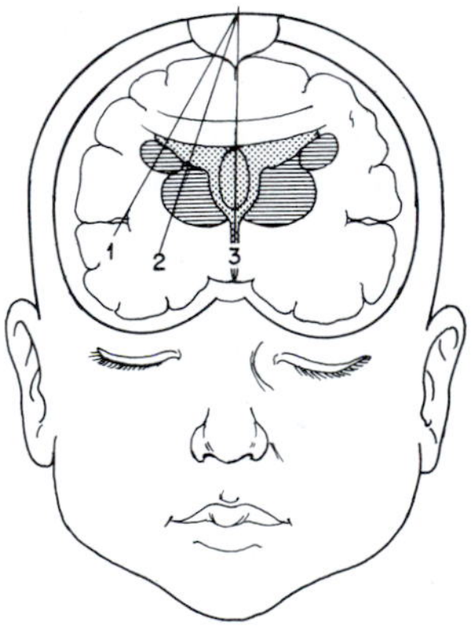

FIGURE 27–10. Neonatal neurosonography technique. Schematic drawing of sagittal and parasagittal planes. Line 1 cuts through the sylvian fissure area at the brain periphery. Line 2 cuts through the caudothalamic groove, a key area to evaluate for subependymal hemorrhage. Line 3 cuts through the midline.

WHAT ARE SUBEPENDYMAL AND INTRAVENTRICULAR HEMORRHAGES?

WHY DO THEY OCCUR? HOW ARE THEY CLASSIFIED?

The germinal matrix (GM) is an area of spongioblasts and neuroblasts that eventually develop into neurons and glial cells that will migrate into the cerebral cortex and basal gan-

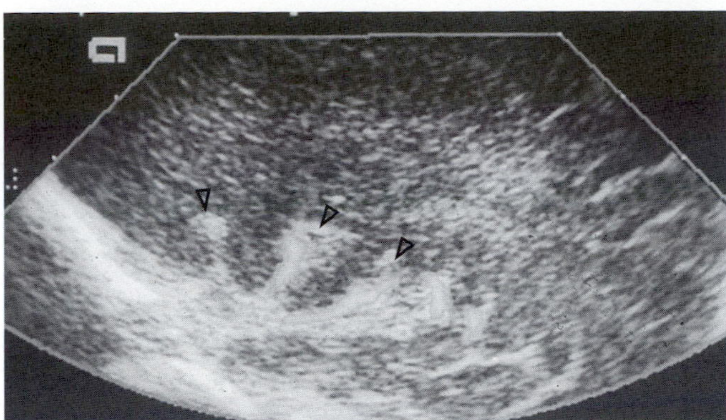

FIGURE 27–11. Neonatal head ultrasound. Parasagittal plane. This image is obtained at the far left periphery of the brain. An arrow points to the calvaria. The echogenic lines (*arrowheads*) represent the sylvian fissure and its contained middle cerebral artery tributaries.

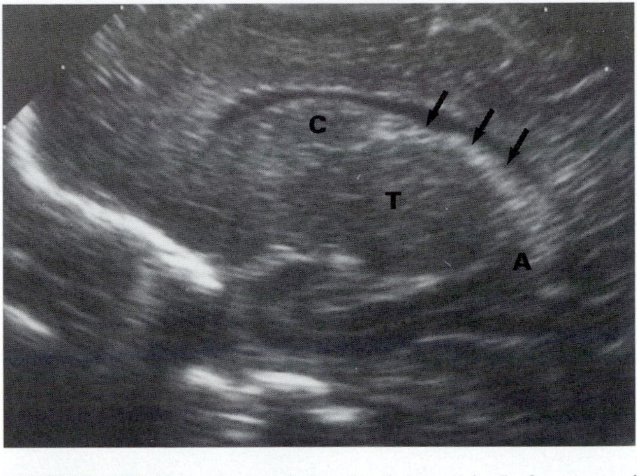

FIGURE 27–13. Neonatal head ultrasound. Left parasagittal plane. This plane cuts through the body and atrium of the left lateral ventricle of a 26-week, 1800-g neonate. C = head of the caudate; T = thalamus. The choroid is the echogenic mass (*arrows*), seen best at the widest point of the lateral ventricle and the first area to dilate in hydrocephalus, the atrium (A). The ventricle is not dilated. The neonate was normal.

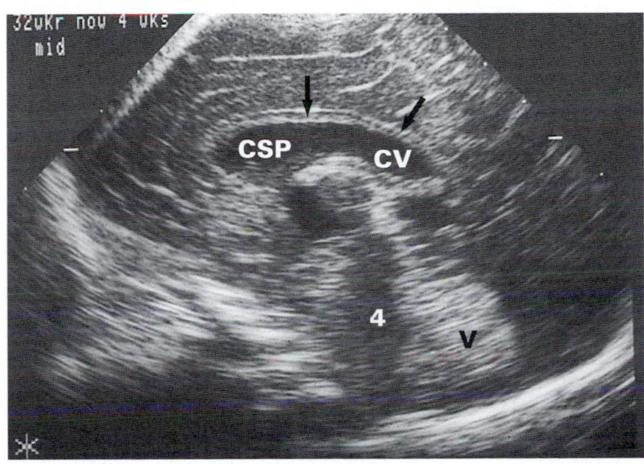

FIGURE 27–12. Neonatal head ultrasound. Midline sagittal plane. The corpus callosum (*arrows*) is seen superior to and surrounding the cavum septum pellucidum (CSP) and its cavum vergae (CV) posterior extension. This is a more common finding in premature infants than in full-term infants. The fourth ventricle (4) is just anterior to the very echogenic vermis of the cerebellum (*small arrows*). Few gyri and sulci are noted because of the neonate's young gestational age. The gyri/sulci can be seen to relatively parallel the corpus callosum.

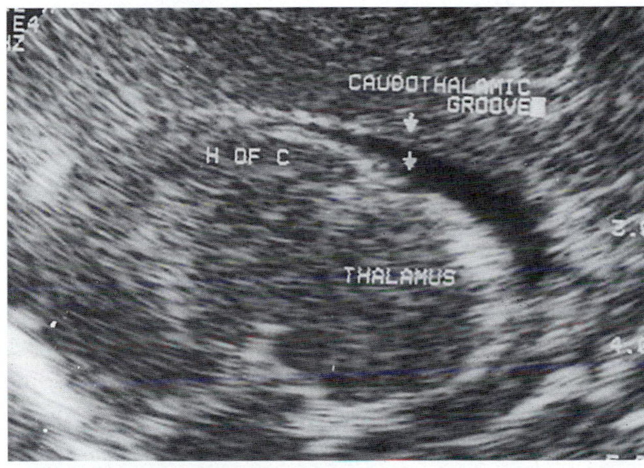

FIGURE 27–14. Caudothalamic groove. Neonatal head ultrasound. Right parasagittal plane. This is a close-up of the caudothalamic groove area of a neonate. No hemorrhage (i.e., echogenic material) is seen at the groove (*arrows*) between the head of the caudate (H of C) and the thalamus (thalamus).

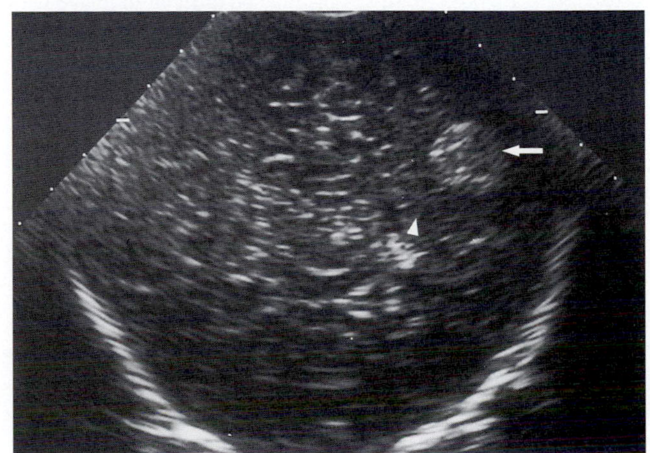

FIGURE 27–15. Intraparenchymal hemorrhage. Coronal plane. ▶ This neonate had no ventriculomegaly and no obvious intraventricular hemorrhage. However, an echogenic circular mass (*arrow*) in the posterior aspect of the right frontal lobe proved to be one of several hemorrhages due to a bleeding disorder. An arrowhead points to a nondilated left lateral ventricle.

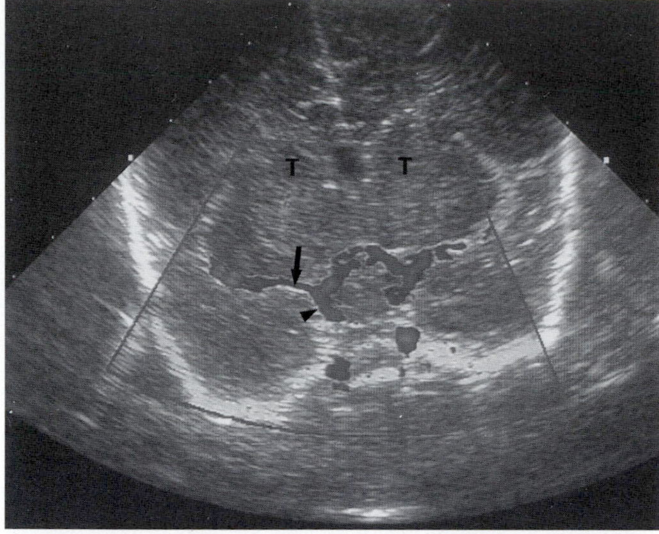

A

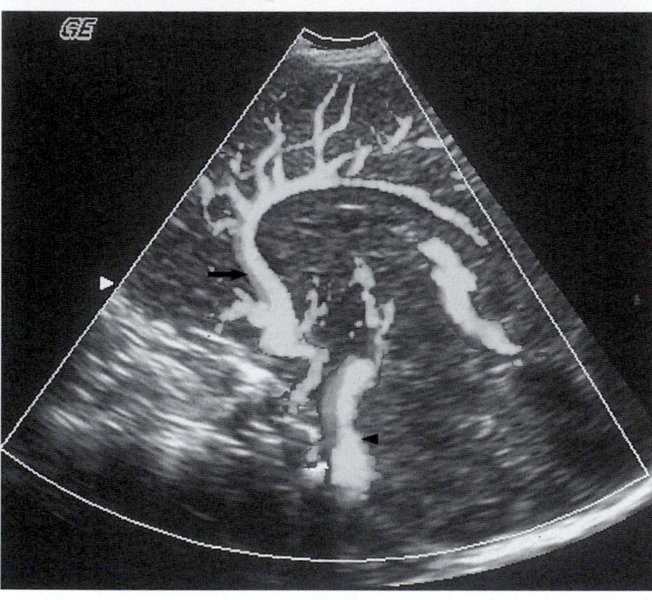

B

FIGURE 27–16. Power Doppler used in neonatal neurosonography. ***A.*** Neonatal head. Coronal plane. Several of the vessels of the circle of Willis are noted. An arrow points to the right middle cerebral artery. An arrowhead points to the right posterior communicating artery. Tiny vessels in the area of the thalami (T) are thalamostriate arteries. These vessels may be difficult to image with routine color Doppler, which relies on Doppler frequency shift data. Power Doppler, which relies on the overall amplitude of the Doppler signal and has improved decibel sensitivity at the loss of directional information, readily shows these vessels. ***B.*** Neonatal head. Sagittal plane. Power Doppler readily shows the anterior cerebral artery and its branches. Arrowhead points to ICA (internal carotid artery). *(Image provided by GE Medical Systems.)* (See Color Plate 7*A* and *B*.)

glia. In the first trimester, this area is large and is found along the caudate nucleus and all along the floor of each lateral ventricle from frontal to temporal horn. With time, the area becomes smaller. At 32 weeks gestational age, it is found only along the ventricular surface of the caudate nucleus and at the border of this nucleus with the thalamus, the caudothalamic groove (Fig. 27-14). The GM area contains many fragile, thin-walled vessels with little connective tissue support. Increased blood flow into this area in the pressure passive brains of premature infants may lead to hemorrhage and destruction of potentially important neural cells.

Subependymal hemorrhage and IVH of GM origin are the most common intracranial abnormalities in premature infants, particularly those who weigh less than 1500 g at birth or are born at 32 weeks gestation or younger. The incidence in premature infants has been going down over the last decade, perhaps because of better medical care. Occurrence rates for SEH and IVH are still quoted at 25 to 40 percent in prematures less than 1500 g, compared to 2 to 4 percent for full-term infants. These hemorrhages are graded, with some minor modification, according to the Papile et al grading system. Grade I hemorrhage is subependymal, remaining in the GM area and not extending into the ventricle. The typical SEH is imaged as an echogenic area (Fig. 27-17) at the caudothalamic groove, although it may involve the entire head of the caudate nucleus.

Grade I hemorrhages are of little immediate clinical significance. Like all hemorrhages, they are echoless at first but very quickly become echogenic with fibrin deposition and clot formation. New clot is homogeneously echogenic. With time, however, clots break down. The SEH clot often liquefies centrally and may be imaged for several months as a cyst, before disappearing. These residual cysts are said to resolve without clinical consequence or pathologic change to the brain. Subependymal hemorrhage cysts (Fig. 27-18), except when seen within an echogenic area of hemorrhage, appear no different from subependymal cysts of other etiologies, including ischemia (Fig. 27-19), the probable cause for occasional cysts, and periventricular leukomalacia (PVL), seen in the offspring of cocaine abusers. Subependymal GM cysts have also been seen in infants with congenital viral infections (most notably cytomegalovirus and rubella) and as a consequence of neonatal ventriculitis or as part of Zellweger (cerebrohepatorenal) syndrome. Subependymal cysts have been reported in patients with no evidence of hemorrhagic or viral disease. There have, in fact, been several studies noting subependymal cysts of unknown etiology, including hemorrhage, in as many as 4 percent of full-term infants. This is a far greater percentage than I have seen.

Hemorrhage within but not distending the lateral ventricle (Fig. 27-20; see also Color Plate 8) is labeled as grade II IVH. Unlike grade I and grade II hemorrhages, intraventricular hemorrhage with significant ventricular dilatation (grade III) or with significant ventricular dilatation and an associated intraparenchymal hemorrhage (grade IV) do have significant morbidity and mortality.

SOME NEWER INFORMATION—GERMINAL MATRIX HEMORRHAGE IS A *VENOUS* EVENT

A recent pathology report assessed the microvasculature of GM and perihemorrhagic autopsy tissues of a small number of full-term infants, very low birth weight prematures, and

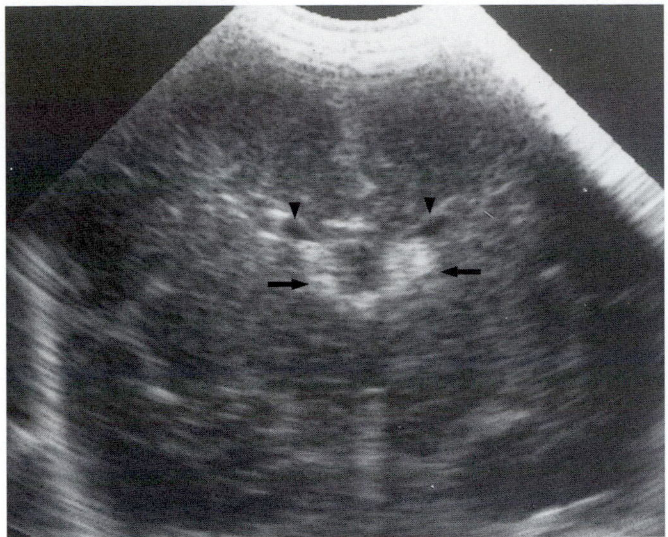

A

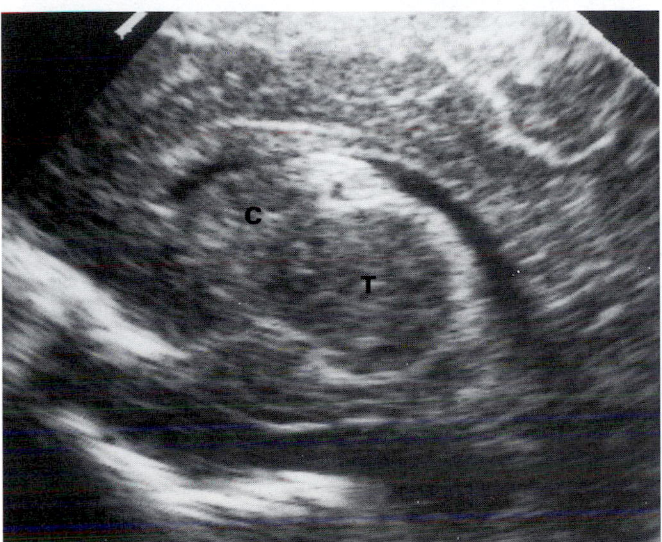

B

FIGURE 27–17. Subependymal (grade I) hemorrhage. ***A.*** Bilateral grade I SEH. Coronal plane. Bright echogenicity (arrows) is seen below the frontal horns *(arrowheads)*. Sagittal views showed the echogenic masses to be outside the ventricle and in the caudothalamic groove, consistent with grade I SEH. ***B.*** Grade I SEH with minimal cyst development. Left parasagittal plane. Between the head of the caudate (C) and the thalamus (T), within the area of the caudothalamic groove, is significant echogenicity, consistent with grade I hemorrhage.

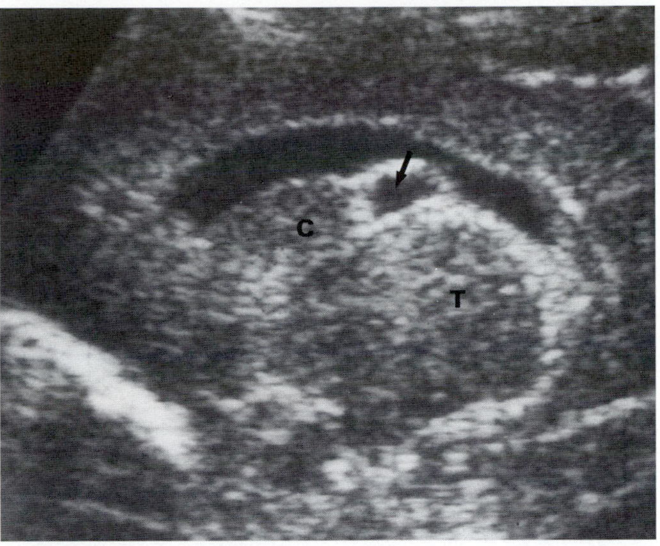

FIGURE 27–18. Subependymal cyst due to hemorrhage. Right parasagittal plane. A cystic area *(arrow)* is seen in the caudothalamic groove. It was the residua of hemorrhage in a 30-week gestation who was 3 months old at the time of this image.

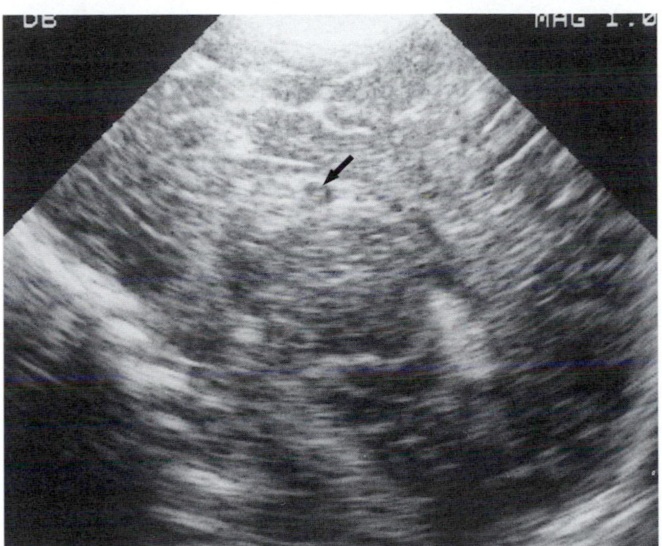

FIGURE 27–19. Subependymal cyst due to cocaine use by mother. Left parasagittal plane. A small echopenic area *(arrow)*, proven on other images to be real, was the only abnormal finding on the head ultrasound of a full-term infant with significant maternal exposure to cocaine. Whether this was residua from brain ischemia as a direct effect of cocaine on the cerebral arteries or related to placental vasoconstriction is unknown. There was no evidence of hemorrhage, although this possibility cannot be ruled out entirely.

full-term beagles. A stain for alkaline phosphatase ectoenzyme, taken up by the plasma membrane of afferent arteries but not by veins, was used. The authors noted that by 31 weeks gestation, subependymal veins are the largest intracranial vessels without any wall reinforcing tissue such as collagen or smooth muscle. Germinal matrix hemorrhages lay near veins and not arterioles. They concluded that rupture of periventricular veins is the prominent feature in premature GM bleeding.

According to a commentary by Taylor, hypoxemia, systemic hypotension, and decreased hemoglobin concentrations lead to decreases in oxygen delivery to the premature brain. Much of the brain injury from hypoxemia is due to large accumulations of glutamic acid, among other excitatory amino acids, at neural synapses. This accumulation leads to cell membrane depolarization and autolysis of neurons. Glutamic acid also stimulates nitric oxide production by inducing nitric oxide synthase. Nitric oxide is a potent vasodilator (as per SUNY–Downstate's Dr. Robert Furchgott's work, which

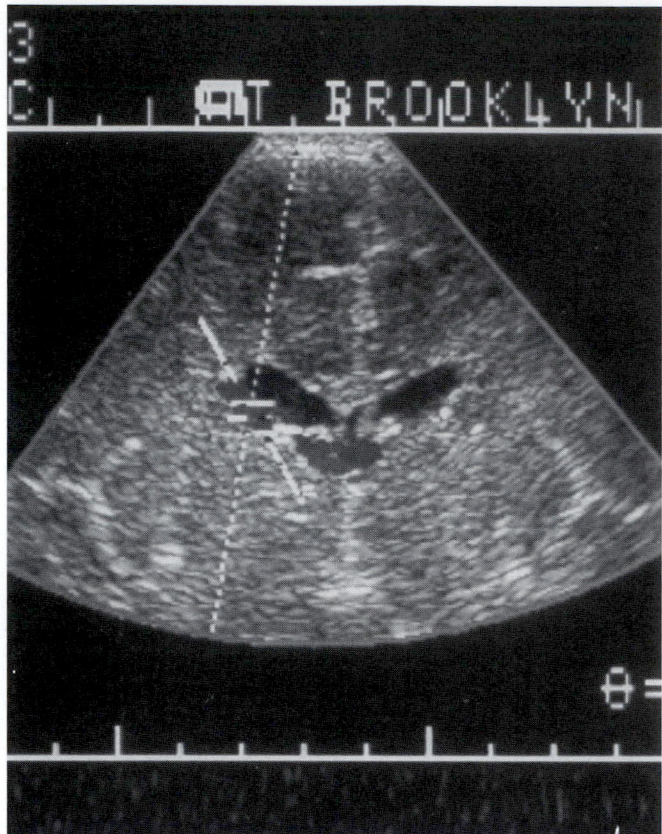

FIGURE 27–20. Normal terminal vein. Coronal plane. Color Doppler. This triplex (gray-scale image, color Doppler, and spectral pattern) image of the frontal horn area of a premature infant with known grade I SEH shows flow *(insonated blue line)* in the right terminal vein. A normal venous spectral pattern *(arrow)* showing a typical continuous sinusoid pattern (slight change in peak flow with respiratory motion) is seen. With slight angulation, a normal left terminal vein was noted on another image. This helped prove the terminal veins to be normal and unaffected by the grade I SEH (not seen on this image). (See Color Plate 8.)

earned him part of the 1998 Nobel Prize in Medicine), responsible for a hyperemia of three to four times normal blood flow in the area of injured brain. This increased flow increases the risk of hemorrhage. In addition, endotracheal tube suctioning, mechanical ventilation, and high ventilator peak inspiratory pressures, very common NICU actions, have been implicated in increasing intracranial venous flow, leading to increased risk of venous hemorrhage. Venous bleeding leads to perivenous blood leakage and mass impression on larger veins. Intraparenchymal hemorrhage is now thought to be due in part to venous infarction caused by obstruction of terminal veins that typically course just inferior and then lateral to the frontal horns on coronal view. Taylor has used color Doppler to show that these veins may be obstructed by large GM hemorrhages.

References

American Institute of Ultrasound in Medicine (AIUM) Education Committee: Guidelines for performance of the pediatric neurosonology ultrasound examination. Rockville, MD, AIUM Publications, 1999.

Babcock D, Han B: The accuracy of high resolution real-time ultrasonography of the head in infancy. *Radiology* 139:665–676, 1981.

Ben-Ora A, Eddy L, Hatch G, Solida B: The anterior fontanelle as an acoustic window to the neonatal ventricular system. *JCU* 8:65–67, 1980.

Cohen HL: Neurosonography of the infant: Diagnosis of abnormalities, in *Ultrasonography of the Prenatal and Neonatal Brain*, Timor-Tritsch I, Monteagudo A, Cohen HL (eds). Stamford, CT, Appleton & Lange, 1996:259–286.

Cohen HL, Haller J: Review. Advances in perinatal neurosonography. *AJR* 63:801–810, 1994.

Cohen HL, Sanchez J: Neurosonography of the infant: The normal examination, in *Ultrasonography of the Prenatal and Neonatal Brain*, Timor-Tritsch I, Monteagudo A, Cohen HL (eds). Stamford, CT, Appleton & Lange, 1996:221–240.

Cohen HL, Sloves J, Laungani S, et al: Neurosonographic findings in full-term infants born to maternal cocaine abusers: Visualization of subependymal cysts and periventricular cysts. *JCU* 22:327–333, 1994.

Ghazi-Birry H, Brown W, Moody D, et al: Human germinal matrix: Venous origin of hemorrhage and vascular characteristics. *AJNR* 18:219–229, 1997.

Grant E: Neurosonography: Germinal matrix-related hemorrhage, in *Neurosonography of the Pre-term Neonate,* Grant E (ed). New York, Springer-Verlag, 1986:33–68.

Grant E, Borts F, Schellinger D, et al: Real-time ultrasonography of neonatal intraventricular hemorrhage and comparison with computed tomography. *Radiology* 139:687–691, 1981.

London D, Carroll B, Enzmann D: Sonography of ventricular size and germinal matrix hemorrhage in premature infants. *AJR* 135:559–564, 1980.

Mito T, Ando Y, Takeshita K, et al: Ultrasonography and morphologic examination of subependymal cystic lesions in maturely born infants. *Neuropediatrics* 20:211–214, 1989.

Papile L, Burstein J, Burstein R, Koffler H: Incidence and evolution of subependymal and intraventricular hemorrhage: A study of infants with birth weights less than 1500 gm. *J Pediatr* 92: 529–534, 1978.

Sudakoff G, Mitchell D, Stanley C, Graziani L: Frontal periventricular cysts on the first day of life. A one year clinical follow-up and its significance. *J Ultrasound Med* 10:25–30, 1991.

Taylor G: New concepts in the pathogenesis of germinal matrix intraparenchymal hemorrhage in premature infants. *AJNR* 18: 231–232, 1997.

Volpe JJ: Intraventricular hemorrhage in the premature infant—current concepts: Part I. *Ann Neurol* 25:3–11, 1989.

28

Figure 28-1 was obtained in a neonate of 26 weeks gestation who was 7 days old at the time of this examination. The neonate was intubated in the neonatal intensive care unit, and his hematocrit had dropped. What do you see? What is the diagnosis?

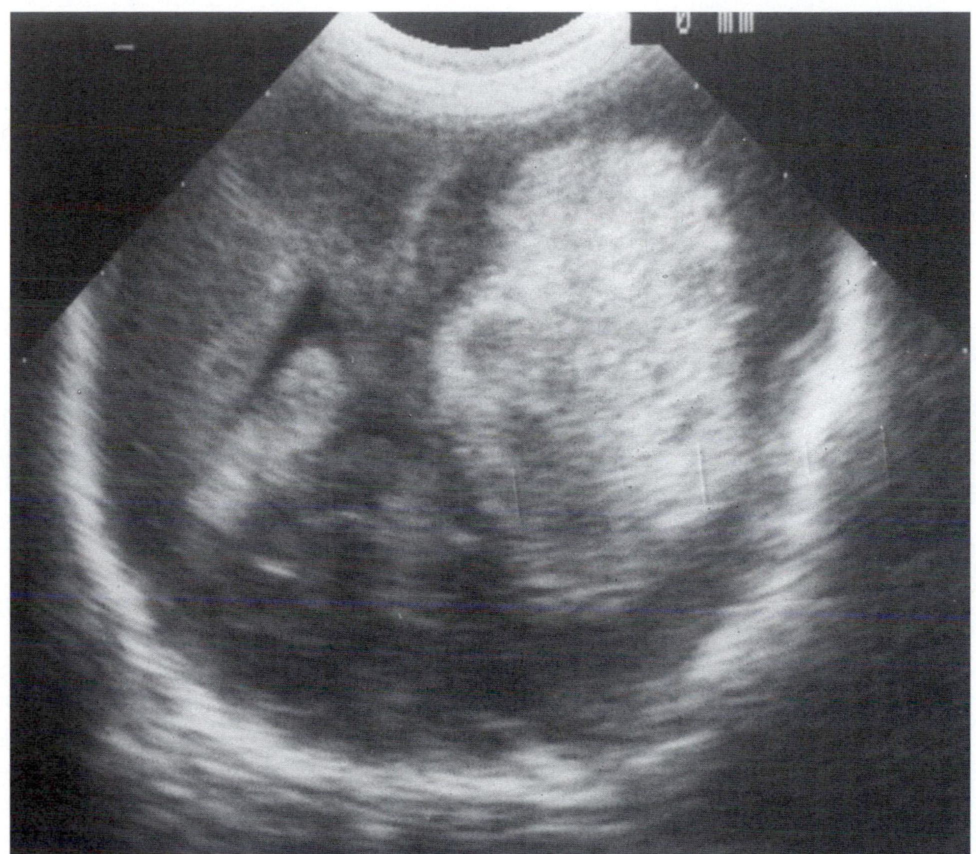

FIGURE 28–1. Head ultrasound. Coronal plane.

CHAPTER 28

Grade IV Hemorrhage

HARRIS L. COHEN AND BETTY CHEN

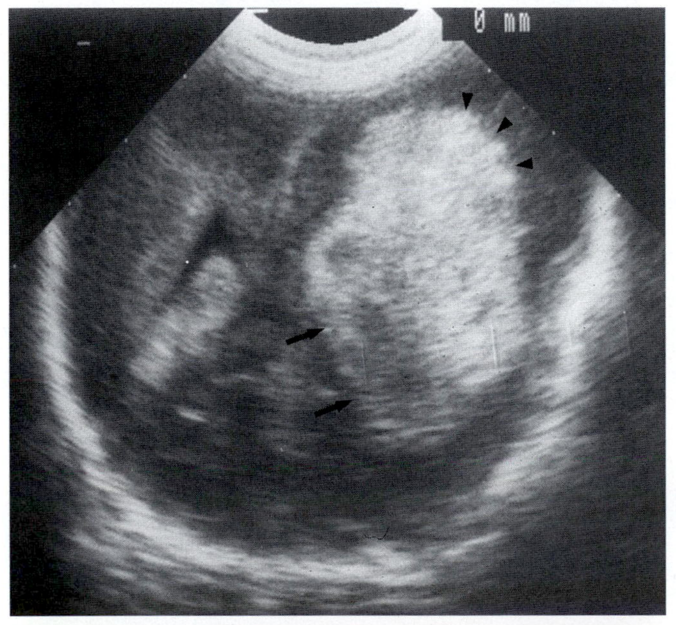

FIGURE 28–2. Annotated version of Fig. 28-1. Left grade IV germinal matrix hemorrhage. Head ultrasound. Coronal plane. The right lateral ventricle appears normal in size and contains the homogeneously echogenic choroid plexus. The left lateral ventricle is dilated and filled with echogenic material. Somewhat more echogenic material extends beyond the confines of the left ventricle if we use the frontal area of the right lateral ventricle as a guide. These findings are consistent with a grade IV germinal matrix hemorrhage/hemorrhagic infarction that includes clot in a dilated lateral ventricle and hemorrhage in the adjacent frontal lobe. The lesser echogenicity of the ventricular clot and the greater echogenicity of the extraventricular hemorrhage go along with Volpe's explanation of grade IV hemorrhage as an intraparenchymal hemorrhage that occurs in a temporally delayed manner compared to the usually associated intraventricular hemorrhage (IVH).

Figure 28-2, the annotated version of Fig. 28-1, shows a large echogenic mass expanding the left lateral ventricle and apparently extending frontally and laterally within the left frontal lobe. This is a classic grade IV germinal matrix hemorrhage. However, the classic explanation for the image has changed over the years.

GRADING OF INTRAVENTRICULAR HEMORRHAGE

As discussed in Chap. 27, there is a grading system for germinal matrix (GM) hemorrhages (see Table 28-1). Subependymal or grade I hemorrhages are usually confined to the GM region at the caudothalamic groove. Hemorrhage within but not distending the lateral ventricle(s) is labeled as grade II intraventricular hemorrhage (IVH). Patients with grade I and II hemorrhages usually do well clinically. The

TABLE 28-1
Germinal Matrix Hemorrhage Classification

Grade I hemorrhage
Hemorrrhage is confined to the subependymal area.
Grade II hemorrhage
Hemorrhage extends into lateral ventricle with little, if any, ventricular dilatation.
Grade III hemorrhage
Hemorrhage is noted in a distended lateral ventricle.
Grade IV hemorrhage
There is intraparenchymal hemorrhage, usually associated with a clot-filled and distended lateral ventricle.

hemorrhages associated with significant neonatal morbidity and mortality are the grade III and grade IV hemorrhages.

Grade III hemorrhage is defined as IVH with ventricular dilatation. Grade IV hemorrhage, in which, classically, there is a dilated ventricle with hemorrhage as well as adjacent intraparenchymal hemorrhage (IPH), was once thought to be caused by direct extension of the IVH into the brain parenchyma.

NEW CONCEPTS ABOUT GRADE IV HEMORRHAGE

Pathology studies and clinical ultrasound (US) examinations, however, showed that the IPH component of the grade IV hemorrhage was typically found on US examination 2 days (usually at day 4 of life) after the IVH (which usually occurred at day 1 or 2 of life). Volpe therefore suggested that the IPH did not occur by direct extension of the IVH into the brain parenchyma, but rather by venous infarction resulting from mechanical obstruction of the medullary veins of the periventricular white matter that drain the terminal veins of the subependymal area. Obstruction of these veins leads to venous congestion and ischemia, with hemorrhagic infarction or reperfusion injury developing as a result of the hypoperfusion.

EPIDEMIOLOGIC INFORMATION REGARDING GM HEMORRHAGE—WORK IN PROGRESS

Over the last several years, a lot of epidemiologic work has been done in an attempt to find linkages between IVH and IPH development and a variety of prenatal, perinatal, and neonatal conditions and treatments. The information can be confusing. Here are some facts/opinions.

1. *The incidence of IVH increases progressively with decreasing gestational age.* In one study of 5286 German infants reviewed in 1997 (but carried out between 1984 and 1988), 1.6 percent of infants born at 38 to 43 weeks gestational age had peri/intraventricular hemorrhage, whereas 50 percent of those born at 24 to 30 weeks did. Intraventricular and periventricular hemorrhage is also increased, according to some, in growth-retarded neonates, those with cord blood pH less than 7.29, the offspring of mothers with preeclampsia or premature rupture of membranes, and neonates with low Apgar scores. In the German study, among premature infants with hemorrhage, there was an inverse relationship between Apgar score and the degree of hemorrhage, while among more mature newborns, the incidence of hemorrhage was linked only to those with poor Apgar scores (0 to 4).

2. *The relationship between IVH/IPH and mode of delivery is not simply vaginal vs. cesarian section.* According to one group, there is no difference in IVH/IPH incidence when modes of delivery are compared as simply vaginal vs. cesarian section. Others suggest an increase in hemorrhage related to vaginal delivery and suggest greater consideration of cesarian section. Another report suggests that early IVH (within the first hour of life—which may not be the best time to evaluate such infants and obtain the most sensitive determination of IVH) among fetuses of less than 1750 g is related to mode of delivery in a more sophisticated way, with the incidence increasing from cesarian without labor (11 percent) to cesarian with latent labor to vaginal delivery with forceps to cesarian with active labor to its most significant percentage (28 percent) in vaginal delivery without forceps. On the other hand, this group noted that the development of IVH at a later point in neonatal life was more common among cesarian deliveries, particularly those performed with active-phase labor. They concluded that the active phase of labor may predispose to early periventricular and intraventricular hemorrhage and that early use of forceps or cesarian section may prevent this, but that cesarian section does not protect the infant from later-onset IVH. Their work and that of others show why there are confusing reports linking increased hemorrhage to vaginal delivery, cesarian delivery, or forceps delivery. Obstetrics is obviously an art as well as a science, and a clear-cut answer on the issue of mode of delivery does not seem to be currently available.

3. *It is known that the incidence of higher-grade hemorrhage is decreasing.* Is this because of the use of surfactant therapy in the newborn? One Turkish study noted that surfactant therapy decreased IVH incidence by 23 percent and bronchopulmonary dysplasia (BPD) incidence by 32 percent. The increased use of perinatal steroids, the better use of respirator technology, or a combination of these and improved clinical knowledge may be the reason. It is known that neonates who need ventilator therapy have an increased incidence of IVH, IPH, and white matter disease. Then again, some believe that genetics and/or environmental factors may also play a role, as one group suggested after noting higher PVL and lower IVH among African prematures compared to other groups from temperate climates.

ULTRASOUND IMAGING OF GRADE III AND GRADE IV HEMORRHAGE

From a US imaging point of view, the diagnosis of grade III and IV IVH is relatively easy—or is it? With experience, it is.

In grade III hemorrhage, one has to look for echogenicity in a dilated lateral ventricle. How much dilatation is needed to separate grade II from grade III? I call a hemorrhage with any dilatation beyond that consistent with the presence of the actual mass of a small imaged intraventricular clot a grade III. Any large hemorrhage, any moderate or greater dilatation of the lateral ventricle is a grade III IVH. I would rather be more conservative and diagnose the higher grade of hemorrhage, than undergrade the hemorrhage, so as to warn my clinician of the need for greater vigilance in the clinical and US follow-up analysis of the neonate. Difficulties in US diagnosis will occur if one does not evaluate orthogonal views to confirm findings

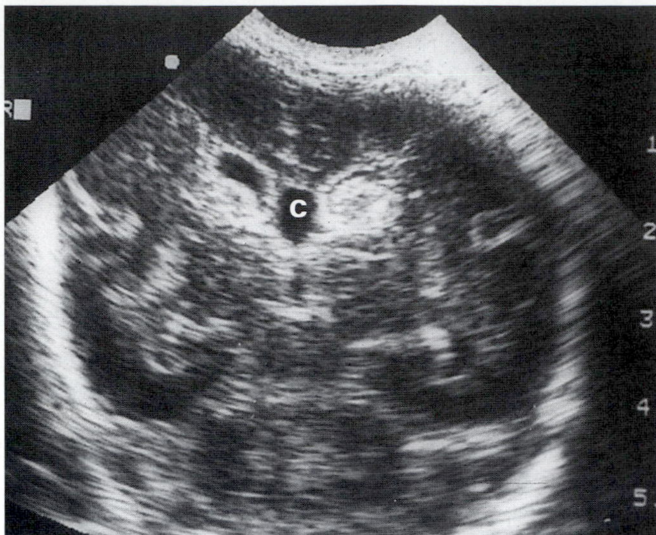

FIGURE 28–3*A*. Grade I intraventricular hemorrhage (IVH) may be difficult to separate from grade III IVH. Grade I IVH simulating grade III IVH. Head ultrasound. Coronal plane. There is echogenicity in the caudate head/subependymal region on the right, typical of grade I subependymal hemorrhage (SEH). However, on the left, the germinal matrix echogenicity is large and appeared to be within the frontal horn. It wasn't. An orthogonal, left parasagittal view proved that this was a large SEH and not an IVH. The left frontal horn, with its thin rim of fluid, was impressed upon by the hemorrhage but not dilated by the presence of hemorrhage within it. This can be a confusing image if it is noted in only one plane. The cavum septum pellucidum (C), often seen in premature infants, is seen between the two frontal horns. An arrow points to the third ventricle, in its normal and more posterior position.

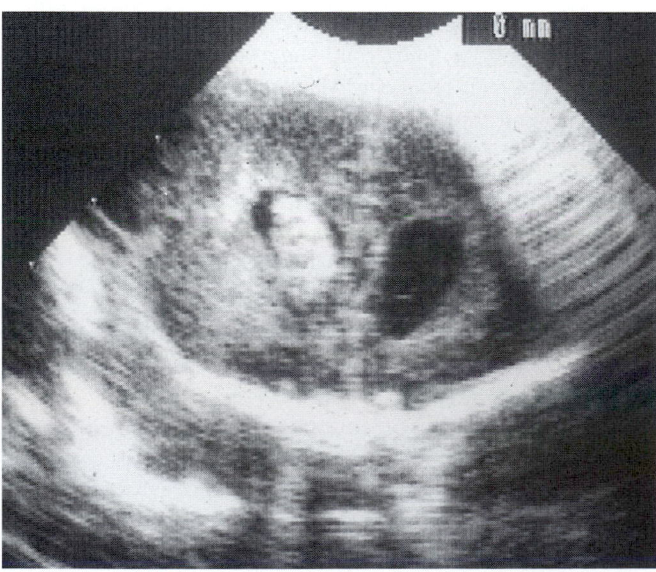

FIGURE 28–3*B*. Grade III–IV IVH. Head ultrasound. Coronal plane. Cerebrospinal fluid (CSF) surrounds clot in the right frontal horn, confirming that this is at least a grade III IVH and not a grade I SEH. A parasagittal image should still be obtained to confirm this. Increased echogenicity surrounding the right frontal horn that is asymmetric from that around the left frontal horn suggests that this is, perhaps, a grade IV hemorrhage. Later images proved this to be a right grade IV IVH.

imaged in only one plane. Large grade I subependymal hemorrhages may appear as if they are within the frontal horns and simulate grade III hemorrhage (Fig. 28-3).

The normal choroid plexus is as echogenic as acute clot. However, the two can be separated. Clot has no vascular flow within it. Color Doppler can, however, show vascular flow within normal choroid plexus (Fig. 28-4; see also Color Plate 9). The choroid plexus is normally smooth. Irregularity of its border (Fig. 28-5) requires consideration of hemorrhage hanging off the choroid. If in doubt, one may look through

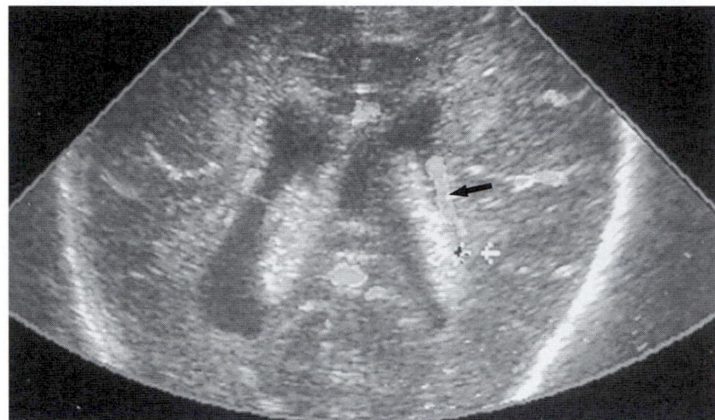

FIGURE 28–4. Color Doppler flow in choroid plexus. Head ultrasound. Coronal view. Power Doppler. Occasionally one may need to prove that an echogenic structure is the normal choroid rather than an acute clot. Only choroid has vascular flow within it. This is an image of flow (*arrow*) in a normal left choroid plexus. (See Color Plate 9.)

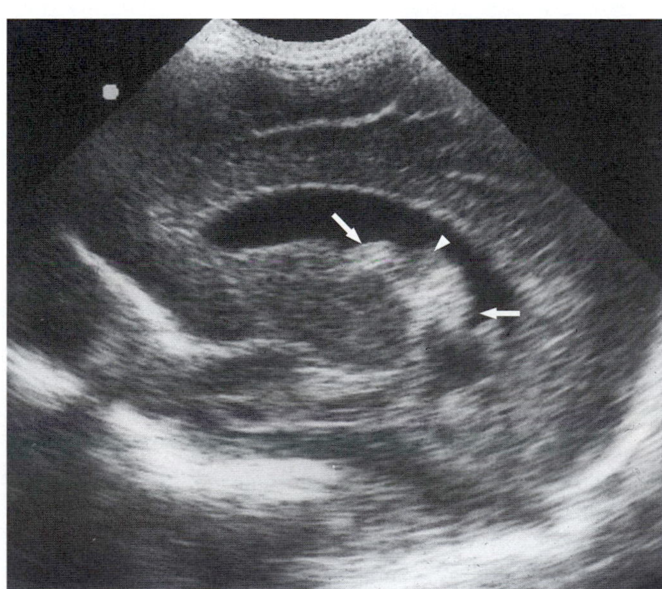

FIGURE 28–5. Subtle grade III intraventricular hemorrhage (IVH)—look for irregular choroid plexus contour. Head ultrasound. Right parasagittal plane. There is moderate dilatation of the right lateral ventricle in this neonate of 30 weeks gestation (at 22 days old). We were suspicious for hemorrhage because what appeared to be choroid was slightly irregular in contour (*arrow*). One can also note a slightly more echopenic area (*arrowhead*) within this region. Both findings suggested IVH rather than normalcy. This was proven on orthogonal projections.

the posterior fontanelle, a method that allowed one group to note 14 otherwise unseen hemorrhages, or wait to see evidence of clot aging as opposed to the unchanging image of normal choroid. As it ages, clot usually becomes more echopenic centrally (Fig. 28-6), often maintaining its bright echogenicity peripherally, before dissolving.

Grade IV hemorrhages have clot in the dilated ventricle as well as hemorrhage beyond the ventricle (Fig 28-7). Because of different days of occurrence, the older intraventricular clot may be more echopenic than the more acute intraparenchymal

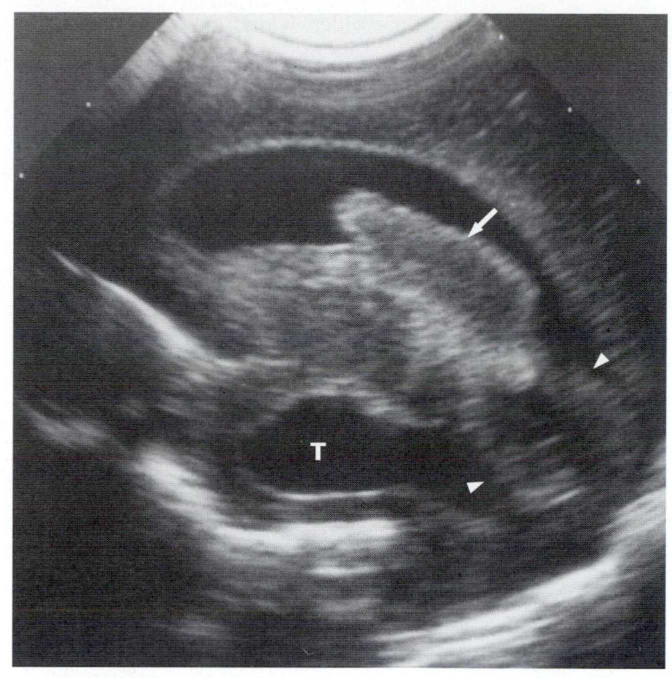

FIGURE 28–6. Subacute grade III intraventricular hemorrhage (IVH). Head ultrasound. Right parasagittal plane. Echopenic clot (*arrow*) with brighter echogenicity peripherally is seen within a moderately dilated lateral ventricle. This allowed ready identification of this as somewhat older-than-acute clot. It is sitting on top of homogeneously bright choroid plexus. Clot (*arrowheads*) is also seen in the atrium and occipital horn of the lateral ventricle. T = temporal horn of lateral ventricle.

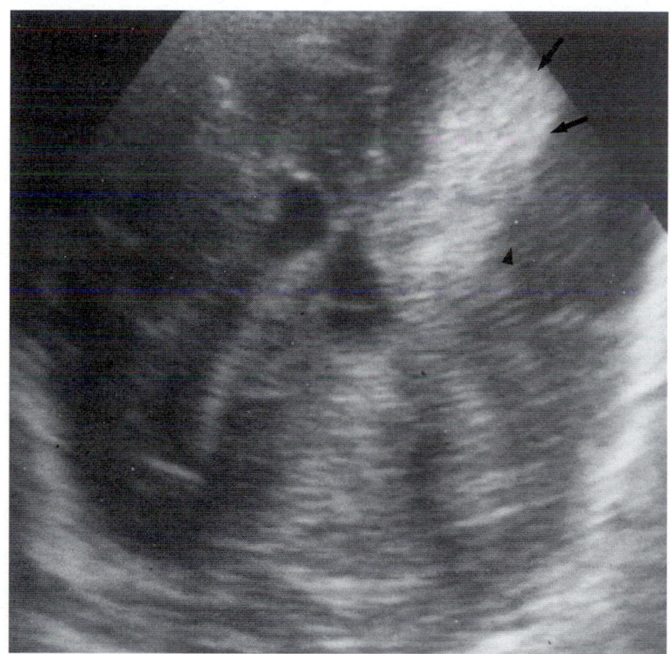

A

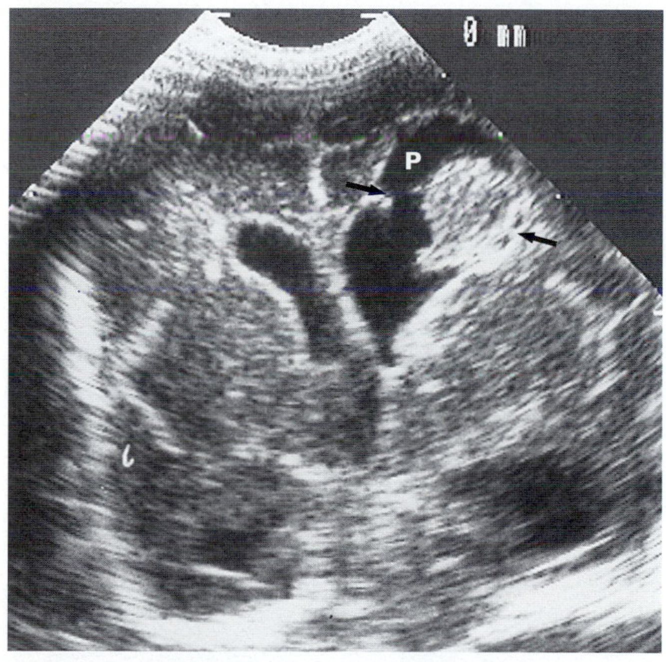

B

FIGURE 28–7*A*. Grade IV germinal matrix hemorrhage (IVH/IPH). ***A.*** Acute grade IV hemorrhage. Coronal plane. The right lateral ventricle is mildly dilated. Significant abnormality is noted on the left. Homogeneously echogenic (i.e., relatively acute) clot is seen distending the left frontal horn (*arrowhead*) and is noted within a large portion of the frontal lobe (*arrows*).

FIGURE 28–7*B*. Older grade IV hemorrhage. Coronal plane. The left frontal horn of a different patient is more dilated than the mildly dilated right frontal horn. Crossing between the expected border (*arrows*) of the left lateral ventricle and a porencephalic cyst (P) is a clot. The clot is less echogenic centrally, suggesting that it is not a new clot. This makes sense, since time has to have passed since the original hemorrhage/infarction to account for the presence of a porencephalic cyst.

clot. Obviously, if both are older, it may be more difficult to know the difference in the age of occurrence of each. When the hemorrhage of both areas (parenchymal and intraventricular) resolves/lyses, all that may remain is a dilated ventricle communicating with a porencephalic cyst.

TABLE 28-2
Tips for Making the Diagnosis of Germinal Matrix Hemorrhage

1. *Use the orthogonal view* to confirm your findings and be more exacting about the grade of hemorrhage.
2. *Consider other US windows.* If you are unsure about the presence of hemorrhage using the anterior fontanelle, consider use of the posterior fontanelle or other calvarial openings.
3. *Separate the choroid plexus from clot.* This can be accomplished by noting blood flow on Doppler evaluation of normal choroid, using tincture of time to see aging of the clot, and looking for nonsmoothness (Figs. 28-5 and 28-8) of the choroid plexus or "choroid" that extends anterior to the foramen of Monro (Fig. 28-9).
4. *Look for fluid debris levels* (Fig. 28-10).
5. *Be aware of normal structures.* Know that there is normal peritrigonal echogenicity on parasagittal views and often mild normal periventricular echogenicity on coronal views. Symmetry with the other side of the brain may help.

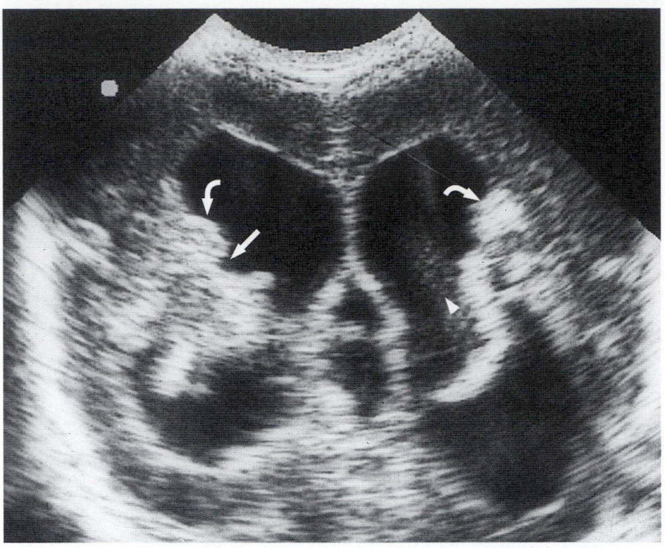

FIGURE 28–8. Grade III intraventricular hemorrhage (IVH). Head ultrasound. Coronal plane. This patient has posthemorrhagic hydrocephalus, which makes imaging of the ventricular contents easier. The left lateral ventricle contains a thin echogenic choroid plexus (*arrowhead*). It appears thinner than usual because of the surrounding hydrocephalus. On the right side, what might be considered choroid rather than clot is too large (*arrow*) and also too irregular to be only choroid and is therefore clot and choroid plexus. On both sides, there is also clot (*curved arrows*) at the far periphery of the lateral ventricles.

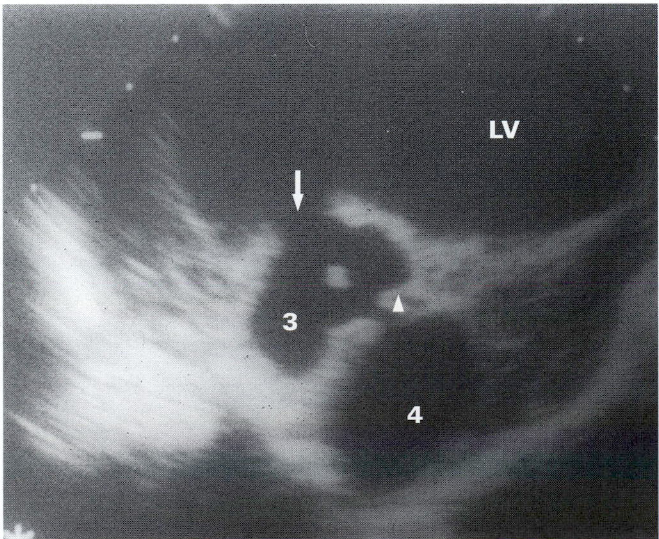

FIGURE 28–9. Foramen of Monro. Head ultrasound. Obliqued sagittal midline plane. This neonate has significant posthemorrhagic hydrocephalus. This image shows no hemorrhage, but its subtle obliquity from midline allows an excellent image of the foramen of Monro (*arrow*), the entry point of lateral ventricular cerebrospinal fluid into the third ventricle. The aqueduct of Sylvius (*arrowhead*) can be seen extending inferiorly from the third ventricle. LV = dilated lateral ventricle, 3 = third ventricle with contained echogenic massa intermedia, 4 = dilated fourth ventricle.

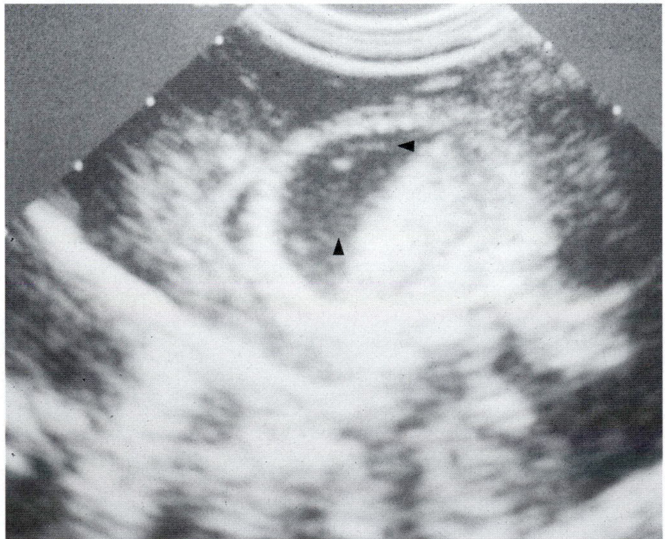

FIGURE 28–10. Hemorrhage/cerebrospinal fluid (CSF) level. Head ultrasound. Parasagittal image. This is an image of a newborn with a sudden drop in hematocrit. This exam was done almost immediately after the acute clinical event. The developing clot in the lateral ventricle layered out (the way a hematocrit tube would), with the lighter CSF remaining superior to the heavier blood (*arrowheads*). The level was parallel to the neonate's head as it lay propped—at an angle in the isolette.

WHY IS NEONATAL NEUROSONOGRAPHY AN IMPORTANT ISSUE?

Simply put, there are key clinical consequences to the presence of GM hemorrhage. Mortality rates in neonatal life are directly proportional to the severity of IVH. Major spastic motor defects and intellectual or developmental deficits (cerebral palsy and mental retardation) can be seen in later pediatric life as a result of IVH and IPH. However, IVH is only a moderate risk factor for disabling cerebral palsy. The most powerful predictors of disabling cerebral palsy are its sequelae. Which are … (keep reading).

References

Allan W, Riviello J Jr: Perinatal cerebrovascular disease in the neonate. Parenchymal ischemic lesions in term and preterm infants. *Pediatr Clin North Am* 39:621–650, 1992.

Anderson N, Allan R, Darlow B, Malpas T: Diagnosis of intraventricular hemorrhage in the newborn: Value of sonography via the posterior fontanelle. *AJR* 163:893–896, 1994.

Berger R, Bender S, Sefkow S, et al: Peri/intraventricular haemorrhage: A cranial ultrasound study on 5286 neonates. *Eur J Obstet Gynecol Reprod Biol* 75:191–203, 1997.

Cohen HL: Neurosonography of the infant: Diagnosis of abnormalities, in *Ultrasonography of the Prenatal and Neonatal Brain*, Timor-Tritsch I, Monteagudo A, Cohen HL (eds). Stamford, CT, Appleton & Lange, 1996:259–286.

Cohen HL, Haller J: Review. Advances in perinatal neurosonography. *AJR* 63:801–810, 1994.

DiPietro M, Brody B, Teele R: Peritrigonal echogenic "blush" on cranial sonography: Pathologic correlates. *AJR* 146:467–471, 1986.

Hesser U, Katz-Salamon M, Mortensson W, et al: Diagnosis of intracranial lesions in very-low-birthweight infants by ultrasound: Incidence and association with potential risk factors. *Acta Paediatr* 419(Suppl):16–26, 1997.

Kaske T, Rumack C, Harlow C: Neonatal and infant brain imaging, in *Diagnostic Ultrasound,* 2d ed, Rumack C, Wilson S, Charboneau J (eds). St Louis, Mosby–Year Book, 1998:1443–1501.

Milner A: Surfactant and respiratory distress syndrome. *Turk J Pediatr* 38:37–43, 1996.

Papile L, Burstein J, Burstein R, Koffler H: Incidence and evolution of subependymal and intraventricular hemorrhage: A study of infants with birth weights less than 1500 gm. *J Pediatr* 92:529–534, 1978.

Perlman J, Rollins N, Burns D, Risser R: Relationship between periventricular intraparenchymal echodensities and germinal matrix–intraventricular hemorrhage in the very low birth weight neonate. *Pediatrics* 91:474–480, 1993.

Shaver D, Bada H, Korones S, et al: Early and late intraventricular hemorrhage: The role of obstetric factors. *Obstet Gynecol* 80:831–837, 1992.

Takashima S, Mito T, Ando Y: Pathogenesis of periventricular white matter hemorrhages in preterm infants. *Brain Dev* 8:25–30, 1986.

Volpe JJ: Intraventricular hemorrhage in the premature infant—current concepts: Part I. *Ann Neurol* 25:3–11, 1989.

Yang R, Cohen H: Sonography in periventricular leukomalacia and intraventricular hemorrhage, in *Textbook of Neonatal Ultrasound*, Haller J (ed). New York, Parthenon, 1998:53–64.

29

Figures 29-1 and 29-2 are single images from two premature neonates who had known germinal matrix hemorrhages within the first week of life. Figure 29-1 was obtained from patient A in the third week of life. Figure 29-2 was obtained from patient B in the fourth week of life. What are the findings? What is patient A's diagnosis? What is patient B's diagnosis? The findings in both cases are significant. Why?

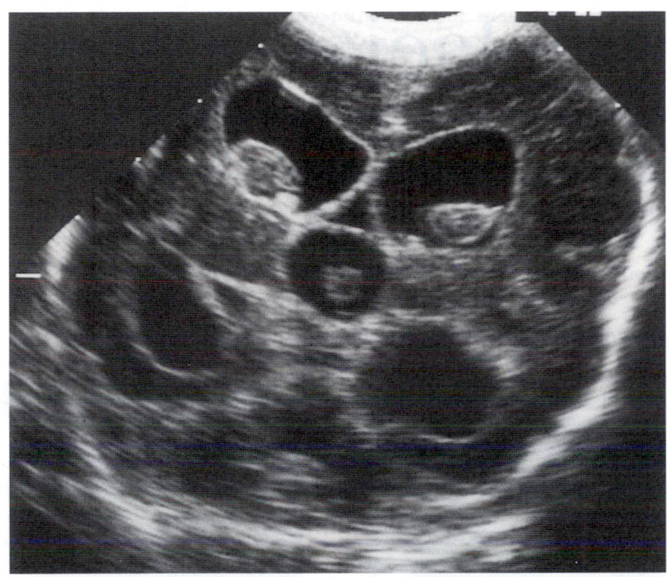

FIGURE 29–1. Head ultrasound. Coronal plane.

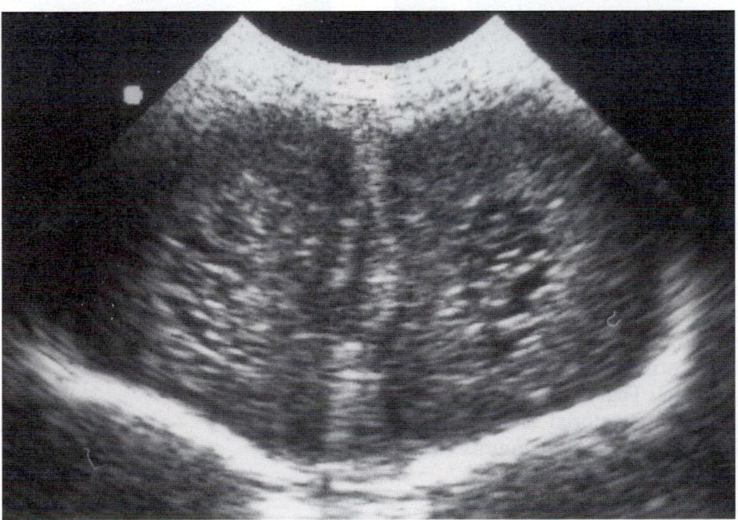

FIGURE 29–2. Head ultrasound. Coronal plane anterior to frontal horns.

TABLE 29-2
Suggested Timing for Neonatal Neurosonography in the Asymptomatic, Apparently Normal Premature Neonate

First exam: at day 4–7. Facts: median dates of observation, day 2 to 3; 36–50% of IVH picked up day 1, 90% by day 6.
Follow-up exam: at 2–3 weeks. Facts: median onset of ventricular dilatation, days 15–20; cystic PVL develops in 2–3 weeks; good time to rule out posthemorrhagic hydrocephalus and to note presence of cystic PVL.
Follow-up (if necessary): at 3 months. Concern for head growth charts readings, delay in milestones to pick up late hydrocephalus.

SOURCES: From Siegel; and Cohen.

week after a hemorrhage, most cases of posthemorrhagic hydrocephalus will have developed. This is why many sonologists recommend a 2-week follow-up head US (Table 29-2).

Even when the patient is beyond the initial month(s) of close neonatal intensive care unit (NICU) examination and US analysis, clinical suspicion of hydrocephalus may be aroused by the neonate's head circumference growing beyond what is expected from the growth charts. This, however, may simply be due to the normal "catch-up" growth in the premature or to an unusual family head shape. Sonography can make a quick and easy diagnosis.

THE ULTRASOUND DIAGNOSIS OF POSTHEMORRHAGIC HYDROCEPHALUS

As with any form of obstructive hydrocephalus, the US examiner should examine the ventricles for their size. In the case of posthemorrhagic hydrocephalus, the presence of contained clot (Fig. 29-3) helps make the diagnosis. Dilatation of the individual lateral ventricles may best be determined by parasagittal views (Fig. 29-5). The atrium is usually the first area of the lateral ventricle to dilate (which is why the measurement of the fetal atrium is an important issue in diagnosing fetal hydrocephalus). The sagittal midline view allows evaluation of dilatation of the third or fourth ventricle. It is the coronal views (Fig. 29-6), using anterior-to-posterior angulation, however, that allow comparison of the lateral ventricles to each other. Coronal views also allow evaluation of the temporal horn tips, as well as the third and fourth ventricles, for size.

One must remember that ventriculomegaly (ventricular enlargement, a term usually used when there is no obstruction or continuous dilatation) may occur on an ex vacuo basis as a result of brain atrophy or dysgenesis and particularly as a result of PVL (to be discussed). In cases of ex vacuo hydrocephalus, the interhemispheric fissure (IHF) is distended, as are the extraaxial spaces. When the extraaxial spaces are fluid-filled and distended, one can image the brain's borders, which are normally obscured on US examination by the adjacent calvaria.

When the IHF (Fig. 29-7) becomes prominent, the normally thin echogenic lines between the frontal brain's two hemispheres (the anchor sign) are separated by the fluid in

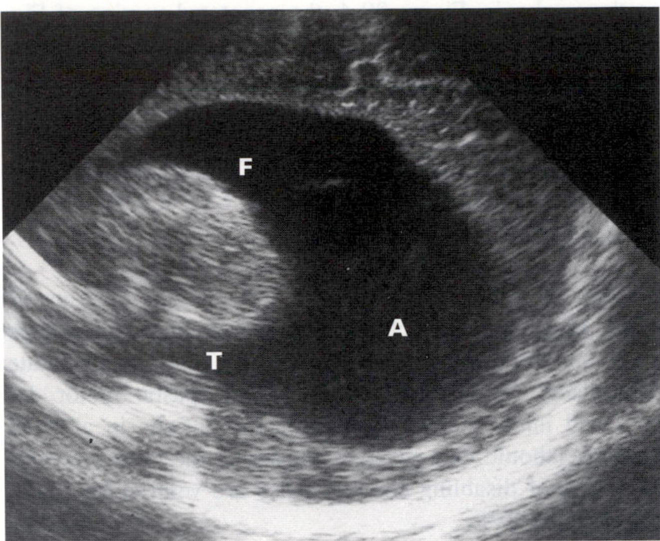

FIGURE 29–5. Hydrocephalus. Head ultrasound. Left parasagittal plane. There is significant dilatation of the lateral ventricle by echoless cerebrospinal fluid. The atrium (A) is the area with the most significant dilatation. F = frontal horn, T = temporal horn tip of the lateral ventricle.

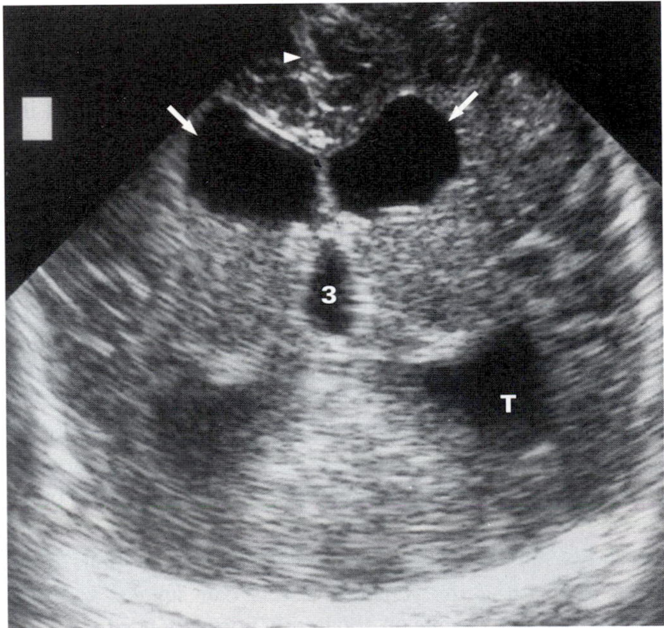

FIGURE 29–6. Hydrocephalus. Head ultrasound. Coronal plane. The frontal horns (*arrows*) are dilated, as is the third ventricle (3), which usually shows little, if any, fluid on coronal view. An arrowhead points to the interhemispheric fissure, which is, in this case, a potential space that is not filled with fluid. Without intervening fluid, the two lobes of the frontal horn touch and the medial walls of each make up one of the two echogenic lines of the "anchor." T = left temporal horn tip.

the IHF. Some patients may have evidence of hydrocephalus and brain atrophy at the same time, which makes an exact diagnosis difficult. Most sonologists read neonatal ventriculomegaly by a gestalt developed over time, rather than by using actual measurements. Visual clues to neonatal ven-

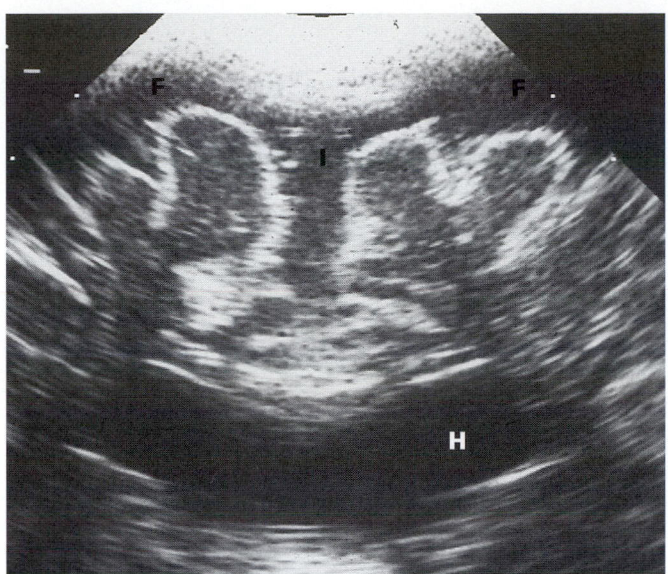

FIGURE 29–7. Ex vacuo hydrocephalus. Head ultrasound. Coronal plane at the level of the frontal horns with magnification of the interhemispheric fissure region. Volume loss of brain substance is responsible for the fluid (F) separating the two frontal lobes and contained in the interhemispheric fissure (I). The anterior brain border is also too readily seen, consistent with fluid in the extraaxial space. Physiologic subdural "effusions" of infancy may show a similar pattern. Note the dilated frontal horns. H = left frontal horn.

triculomegaly include imaging CSF lateral to the choroid plexus (the lateral ventricular wall typically hugs the choroid plexus, with little, if any, CSF seen between the two) and noting the choroid droop into the fluid-filled dependent ventricular surface, if the patient is examined on his/her side.

SEPTAL FENESTRATION MAY DEVELOP DUE TO OBSTRUCTIVE HYDROCEPHALUS

Neurosonography may demonstrate fenestrations (Fig. 29-8) of one or both leaves of the septi pellucidi in cases of untreated hydrocephalus. These fenestrations may increase in size and number over time. Their recognition prevents confu-

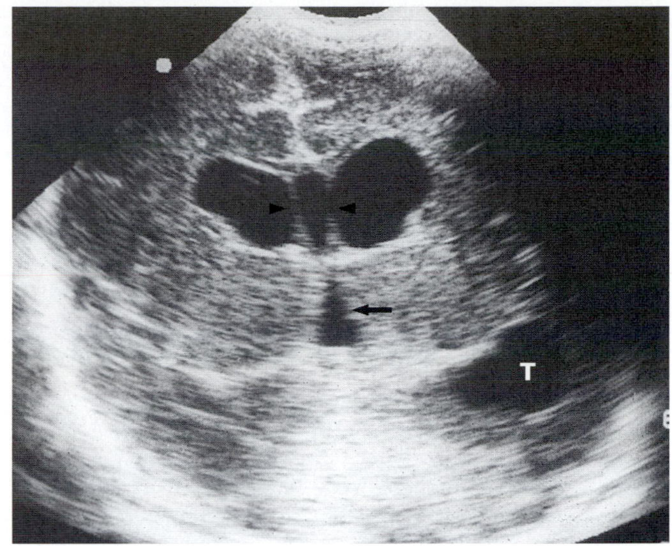

A

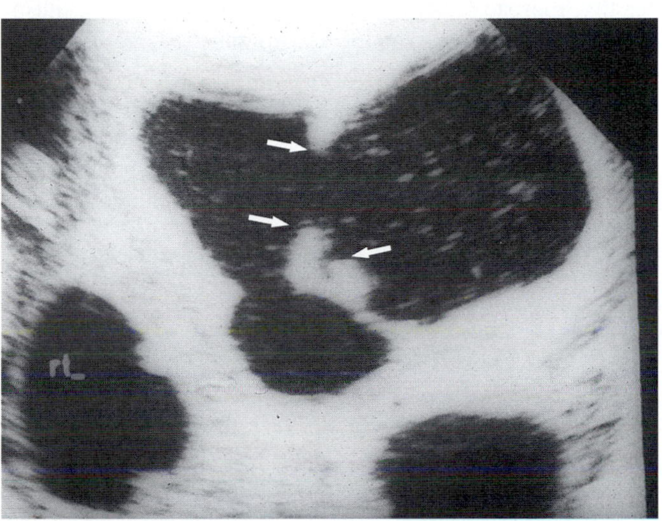

B

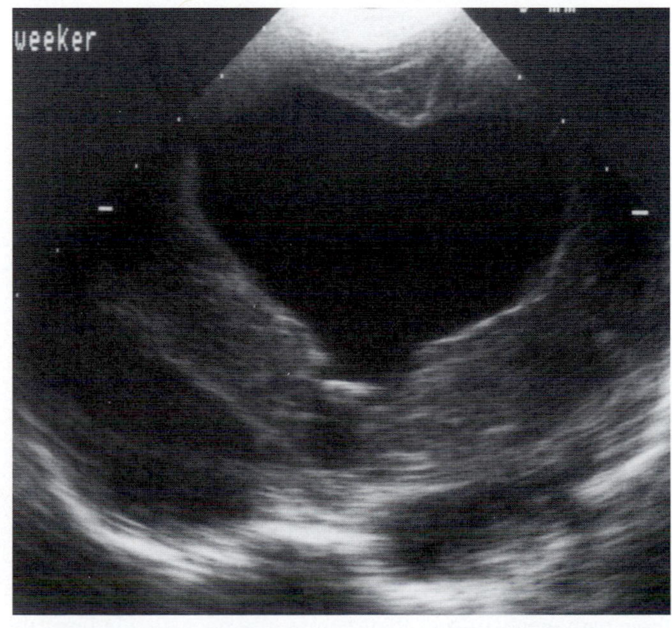

C

FIGURE 29–8. Fenestration of the septi pellucidi in hydrocephalus. ***A.*** Normal septi pellucidi. Coronal plane. A small amount of fluid is seen between the septi pellucidi (*arrowheads*). This is the cavum septi pellucidi. A normal finding, it is more common in premature than in full-term infants. This neonate has mild to moderate ventriculomegaly. Arrow points to third ventricle. T = temporal horn tip. ***B.*** Evolving fenestration of the septi pellucidi. Coronal plane. This neonate has hemorrhage, seen as echogenic material in his ventricles. It was responsible for posthemorrhagic hydrocephalus, which over a few weeks was noted to create bigger and bigger holes in the septi (arrows point to remains of septi). This can be seen on sagittal planes as well but requires the examiner to create an en face view of the individual septum. ***C.*** Ruptured septi pellucidi simulating congenital absence of the septi pellucidi. Coronal plane. Two months after a diagnosis of grade IV intraventricular hemorrhage, this neonate, who had evolving fenestration over time, finally appears to have had no septi pellucidi at all. If this was the neonate's first ultrasound, it might be wrongly assumed that he has absence of the septi pellucidi.

sion with congenital absence of the septum pellucidum, which is often associated with other neuroanatomic abnormalities.

TECHNICAL NOTE: TRANSCRANIAL US MAY BE USED BEFORE OR AFTER FONTANELLE CLOSURE

After closure of the anterior fontanelle, usually at around 10 to 12 months, transcranial US, using the thin squamous portion of the temporal bone (Fig. 29-9) and a low-frequency (e.g., 3 MHz) transducer to penetrate the bone of the skull, may allow continued analysis of ventricular size by US. We do this occasionally in older infants/children (e.g., 12 to 14 months) whose parents are very interested in avoiding any exposure of their child to radiation. Evaluation of the brain periphery is more limited than for neonates, but the size of the central ventricular system can be gauged. We sometimes use this approach (albeit with a higher-frequency transducer, at times as high as our routine transfontanelle 7.5-MHz transducer) in evaluating neonates because it provides a good position to insonate the middle cerebral artery on the near-field side of the transducer. When necessary information can no longer be obtained by ultrasound, the clinician should obtain it by another imaging modality, most often computed tomography.

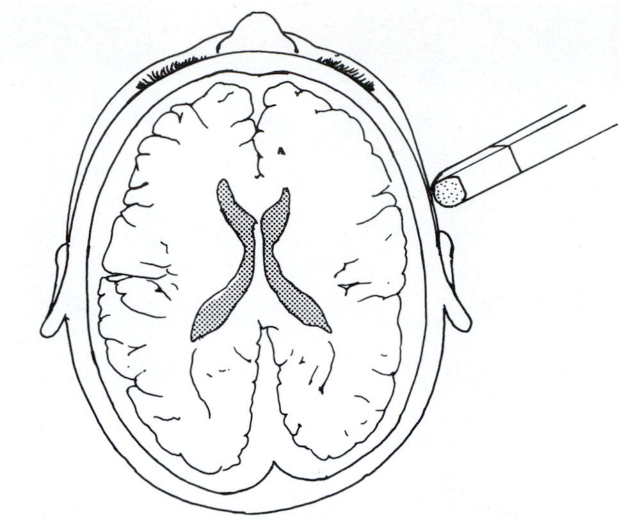

A

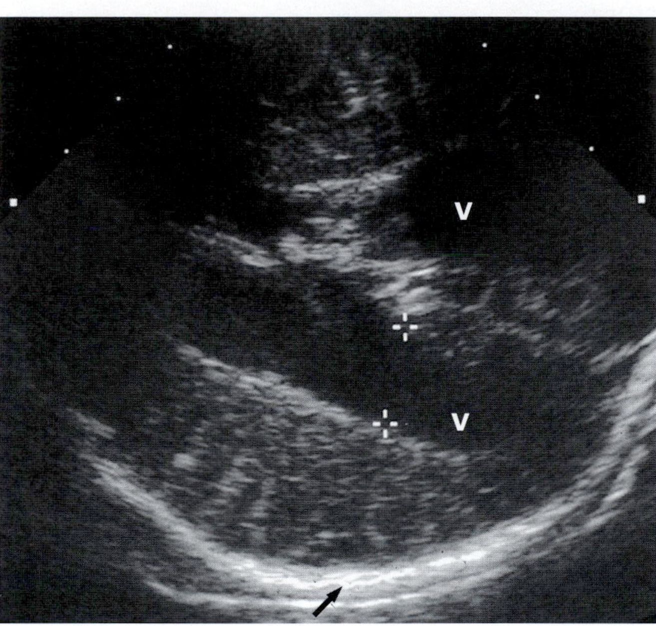

B

FIGURE 29–9. Transcranial ultrasound. ***A.*** Diagram. The transducer, usually of a lower frequency to help penetrate the calvaria, is placed anterior to the mid-ear. One can see how the ventricles, if properly penetrated, would be imaged. This is a particularly good approach if one wants to image or insonate the near-field middle cerebral artery. ***B.*** Head ultrasound. Axial plane. Using a transcranial approach, the cerebral ventricles are noted to be enlarged. Crosses mark off the far-field lateral ventricle's atrium, which is dilated. The patient was a premature infant with a thin calvaria that allowed excellent penetration to the far-field parietal bone (*arrow*) despite the use of a high-frequency transducer (7 MHz). This patient was imaged transcranially, not because the fontanelles were closed, but to improve the imaging of his hydrocephalus.

WHAT IS PERIVENTRICULAR LEUKOMALACIA?

Periventricular leukomalacia describes infarcted periventricular white matter. Areas of PVL occur in the frontal and parieto-occipital lobes. Poor autoregulation of the premature brain's vascular system coupled with systemic stress has been thought to lead to ischemia in arterial watershed areas. Obviously other theories exist, particularly with the newer information regarding venous infarction associated with compression of terminal and perhaps other veins as a cause of brain injury. Immature and actively differentiating glial cells are more prone to injury and cell death. The incidence of PVL in low birth weight infants is reported to be between 12 and 40 percent. Screening for PVL in premature infants is recommended because of its high incidence. A US exam 2 to 3 weeks after birth is thought to pick up the majority of cases. The ischemic abnormality leading to PVL is thought to be responsible for the later development of spastic diplegia and prominent intellectual deficits, which are also seen in survivors of posthemorrhagic ventricular dilatation. Periventricular leukomalacia is associated with a low mortality rate. However, morbidity rates are high, with the degree of neurologic deficit directly related to the size and severity of the PVL lesions. The spastic diplegia may be due to the fact that the lesions in PVL typically affect the corticospinal tracts innervating the lower extremities.

Periventricular leukomalacia and IVH share similarities in their pathogenesis, and they commonly coexist. Findings of PVL are seen in 36 percent of IVH cases, and IVH is seen in 59 percent of PVL cases. In autopsies of PVL patients, 25 percent of the brains may demonstrate intrinsic hemorrhage that may not have been seen on imaging studies.

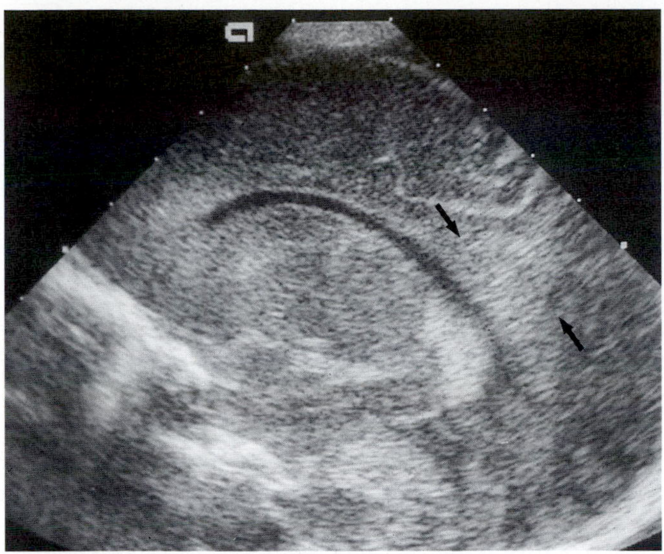

FIGURE 29–10. Normal increased peritrigonal echogenicity. Head ultrasound. Sagittal plane. DiPietro et al showed on pathology studies that an area equivalent to the echogenic triangular area (*arrows*) posterior to the atrium of this normal-sized lateral ventricle is a normal finding. This neonate was normal.

WHAT DOES PVL LOOK LIKE SONOGRAPHICALLY? HOW DO I MAKE THE DIAGNOSIS?

In the acute phase, PVL can be seen as well-defined areas of hyperechogenicity lateral to the frontal horns and trigones of the lateral ventricles. The problem for the diagnosis of this acute echogenic phase of PVL is that the normal neonate has somewhat prominent echogenicity at these periventricular sites as well. This includes the classic areas of involvement: the optic radiation at the trigone (Fig. 29-10) of the lateral ventricle and the cerebral white matter, just anterior and lateral to the frontal horns (Fig. 29-11). Although the early images of periventricular echogenicity may resemble the images of normal brain, these echogenic areas will become cystic within 2 to 3 weeks, and readily diagnosed periventricular cysts can be seen (Fig. 29-12) in true areas of PVL. The cysts and cavities are seen as encephalomalacia develops. Gliosis, however, may fill in the affected areas within months. After gliosis fills the cysts in, the US images of the affected brain will look normal.

TIMING OF NEUROSONOGRAPHY TO PICK UP GERMINAL MATRIX HEMORRHAGE SEQUELAE

Table 29-2 shows one approach to following asymptomatic premature infants using US. In a cost-conscious world but with a concern for correct diagnosis, the goal is to obtain correct and maximal amounts of information using the least number of examinations. This imaging plan is based on several facts. Only 33 to 50 percent of IVHs can be diagnosed on the first day of life. Nine out of ten hemorrhages will have occurred by the sixth day of life. Hemorrhages that first occur after day 6 often are limited to the subependymal area and are not intraventricular. Unless there is an urgent clinical concern, i.e., a sudden drop in hematocrit requiring immediate neurosonography, a first scan should be performed between days 4 and 7 of life. Obviously, a request for a stat examination on an asymptomatic neonate in the first day of life may prove a disservice to the patient. *Stat is not always right!*

POINTS TO REMEMBER

1. Be wary of periventricular areas of increased echogenicity—they may prove to be PVL. Look in 2 to 3 weeks.
2. Look carefully posterior to the atrium and anterolateral to the frontal horns for cystic encephalomalacia.
3. Both PVL and posthemorrhagic hydrocephalus are worrisome findings for the child's future health and educability.
4. Not all cases that appear to be agenesis of the septum pellucidum are—they may be evidence of complete fenestration due to significant hydrocephalus.

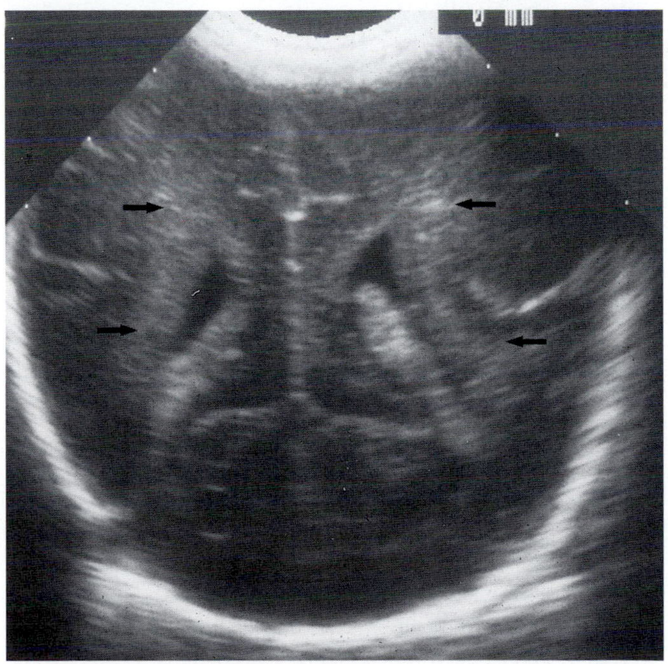

FIGURE 29–11. Normal periventricular echogenicity. Head ultrasound. Coronal plane. A subtle prominent echogenicity (*arrows*) surrounds the mildly prominent lateral ventricles of this neonate. This may be seen in normal patients. Symmetry and subtlety force one to diagnose the patient as normal. However, clinical correlation may help to confirm this. If there was true PVL, a 2-week follow-up exam should show cysts within the area of concern. This infant was normal.

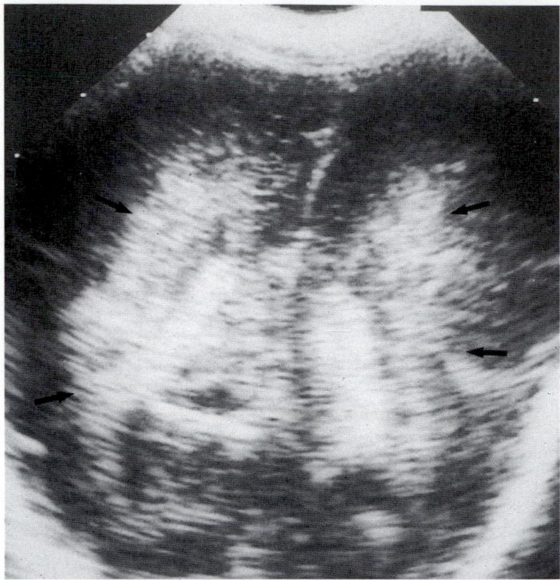

A

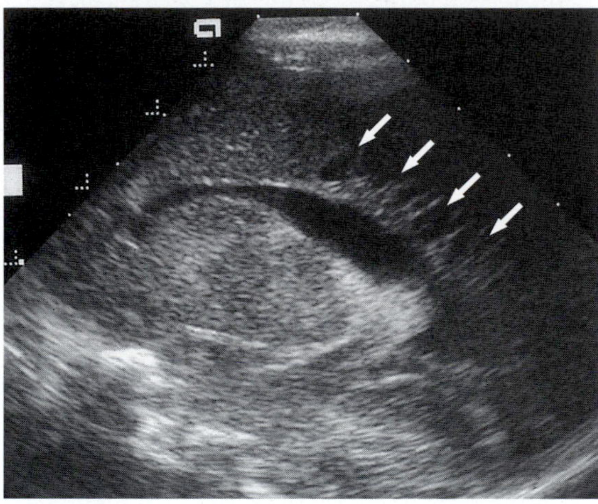

B

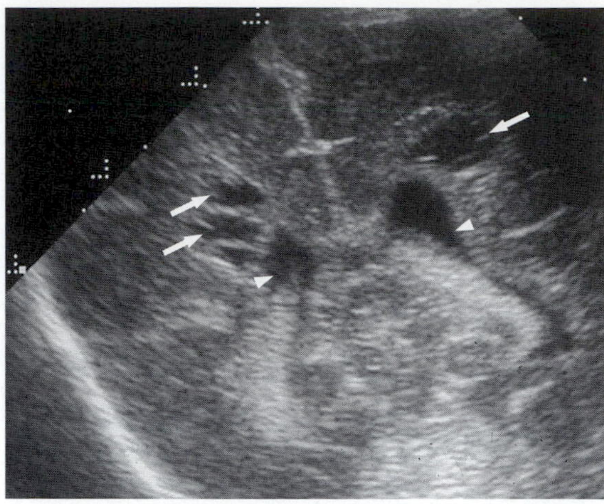

C

FIGURE 29–12. Periventricular leukomalacia. ***A.*** Echogenic PVL. Head ultrasound. Coronal plane. The periventricular echogenicity is more prominent than in Fig. 29-11. We worried because of this and because the patient's clinical course was stormy. We would have worried more if there had been any asymmetry of the periventricular echogenicity. In 2 weeks these echogenic areas were cystic. ***B.*** Cystic PVL. Head ultrasound. Left parasagittal plane. A few cysts (*arrows*) are seen just posterior to the body and atrium of the lateral ventricle. This is cystic encephalomalacia in what has been described as the posterior watershed area. ***C.*** Cystic PVL. Head ultrasound. Coronal plane. Cysts are noted anterior and lateral to the frontal horns of the lateral ventricles (*arrows*). This is the classic anterior watershed area of involvement. Certainly cystic areas of PVL can surround any of the areas of the lateral ventricle. Arrowheads point to the frontal horns of the lateral ventricles.

References

Armstrong D, Norman MG: Periventricular leukomalacia in neonates: Complications and sequelae. *Arch Dis Child* 49: 367–375, 1974.

Cohen HL: Neurosonography of the infant: Diagnosis of abnormalities, in *Ultrasonography of the Prenatal and Neonatal Brain*, Timor-Tritsch I, Monteagudo A, Cohen HL (eds). Stamford, CT, Appleton & Lange, 1996:259–286.

Cohen HL, Haller J: Review. Advances in perinatal neurosonography. *AJR* 63:801–810, 1994.

Cohen HL, Haller J, Pollack A: Ultrasound of the septum pellucidum: Recognition of evolving fenestrations in the hydrocephalic infant. *J Ultrasound Med* 9:377–383, 1990.

DiPietro MA, Brody AB, Teale RL: Peritrigonal echogenic "blush" on cranial sonography: Pathologic correlates. *AJR* 146: 1067–1072, 1986.

Jacobi P, Weissman A, Zimmer E, Blazer S: Survival and long-term morbidity in preterm infants with and without a clinical diagnosis of periventricular, intraventricular hemorrhage. *Eur J Obstet Gynecol Reprod Biol* 46:73–77, 1992.

Larroche JC: Hypoxic brain damage in fetus and newborn. Morphologic characters. Pathogenesis. Prevention. *J Perinat Med* 10: 29–31, 1982.

Levene MI, Wigglesworth JS, Dubowitz V: Hemorrhagic periventricular leukomalacia in the neonate: A real-time ultrasound study. *Pediatrics* 71:794–797, 1983.

Monset-Couchard M, Szwalkiewicz-Warowicka E, de Bethmann O: Chronology of ultrasonographic course of neonatal intraventricular hemorrhage stage III [French]. *Pediatrie* 48:69–75, 1993.

Schellinger D, Grant EG, Richardson JD: Cystic periventricular leukomalacia: Sonographic and CT findings. *AJNR* 5:439–445, 1984.

Siegel MJ: Brain, in *Pediatric Sonography,* 2d ed, Siegel MJ (ed). New York, Raven, 1991:18–25.

Volpe JJ: Intracranial hemorrhage: Subdural, primary subarachnoid, intracerebellar, intraventricular (term infant) and miscellaneous, in *Neurology of the Newborn,* 2d ed, Volpe JJ (ed). Philadelphia, Saunders, 1987:282–310.

Volpe JJ: Current concepts of brain injury in the premature infant. *AJR* 153:243–251, 1989.

Volpe JJ: Brain injury in the premature infant—from pathogenesis to prevention. *Brain Dev* 19:519–534, 1997.

Whitaker A, Feldman J, Van Rossem R, et al: Neonatal cranial ultrasound abnormalities in low birth weight infants: Relation to cognitive outcomes at six years of age. *Pediatrics* 98:719–729, 1996.

Yang R, Cohen H: Sonography in periventricular leukomalacia and intraventricular hemorrhage, in *Textbook of Neonatal Ultrasound*, Haller J (ed). New York, Parthenon, 1998:53–64.

30

Single images from the exams of two different newborns are presented to you. Figure 30-1 is from a 7-week-old with a history of seizures. Figure 30-2 is from a newborn who was examined to "rule out intraventricular hemorrhage." What do you see? What do the children have?

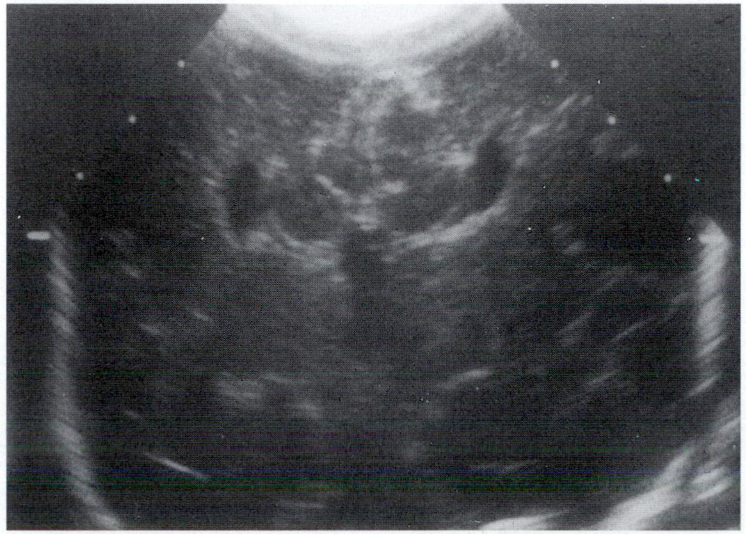

FIGURE 30–1. Head ultrasound. Coronal plane. Level of frontal horns.

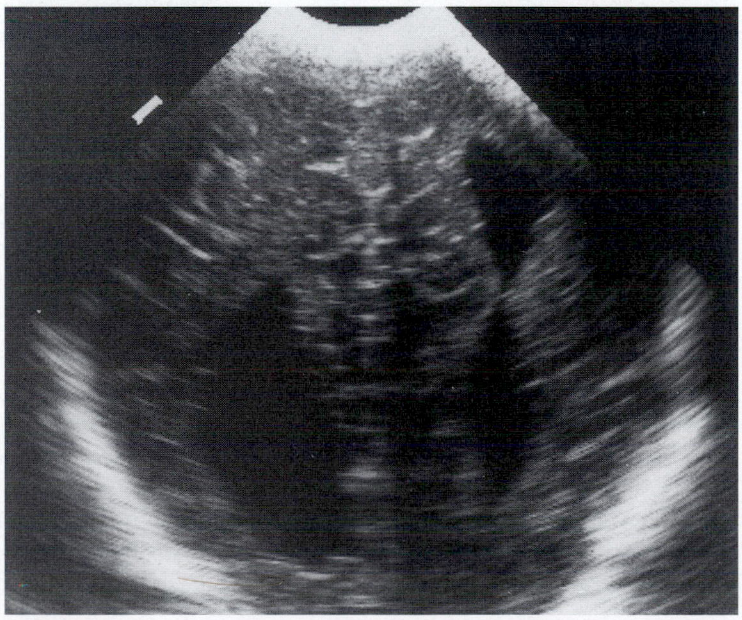

FIGURE 30–2. Head ultrasound. Coronal plane. Level of bodies of lateral ventricles.

CHAPTER 30

Agenesis of the Corpus Callosum

HARRIS L. COHEN

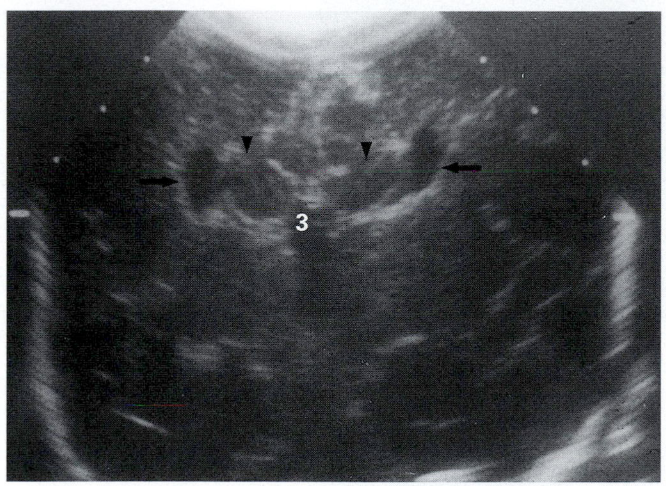

FIGURE 30–3. Annotated version of Fig. 30-1. Agenesis of the corpus callosum. Head ultrasound. Coronal plane. Level of frontal horns. The frontal horns (*arrows*) are widely separated. The third ventricle (3) is somewhat higher than typical, with its most superior aspect seen at the level of the frontal horns. Probst bundles (*arrowheads*) run as two separate white matter bundles parallel to the interhemispheric fissure and medial to the frontal horns. This image is classic for ACC.

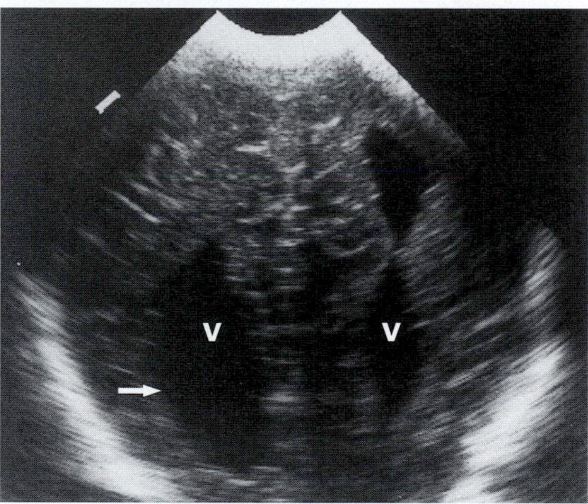

FIGURE 30–4. Annotated version of Fig. 30-2. Agenesis of the corpus callosum (ACC). Head ultrasound. Coronal plane. Level of bodies of lateral ventricles. The bodies of the lateral ventricles (V) are widely separated. They appear to parallel each other rather than extend toward each other anteriorly. The anterior portion of the right lateral ventricle is not imaged (it was not dilated), but its posterior aspect (*arrow*) is dilated, consistent with nonspecific colpocephaly, which can be seen with ACC.

Figure 30-3, the annotated version of Fig. 30-1, shows widely separated frontal horns and perhaps a high-riding third ventricle. Figure 30-4, the annotated version of Fig. 30-2, shows parallel lateral ventricles and perhaps colpocephaly on the right.

WHAT IS AGENESIS OF THE CORPUS CALLOSUM?

The corpus callosum (Fig. 30-5) is the largest of the medial interhemispheric commissures that allow communication between the two halves of the brain. It develops upwardly and from front to back between the 8th and 20th weeks of gestation. The genu is the first area to develop. When complete, the corpus callosum consists of the rostrum, the most anteroinferior portion; the genu, which curves anteriorly and superiorly; the body, which parallels the cavum septum pellucidum; and finally the splenium, which turns posteriorly and behind the cavum.

Partial Agenesis of the Corpus Callosum

The normal development sequence is anterior to posterior (despite the fact that a portion of the anterior genu and rostrum actually develop at the same date or just after the development of the most posterior splenium), which allows one to distinguish between a partial primary callosal dysgenesis and secondary dysgenesis of the corpus callosum. In primary dysgenesis, the callosal development sequence is normal until an insult, usually thought to be inflammatory or vascular in nature, occurs before 12 weeks gestational age. At that time, callosal development posteriorly ends. In other words, if there is an injury to the brain before callosal development is complete, the anterior portion will be formed, but not the posterior portion. In cases of secondary dysgenesis, caused by partial or complete destruction after callosal development, there is no evidence of normal sequential growth, and posterior structures may be imaged without anterior structures being present.

In partial agenesis of the corpus callosum, there will usually be a normal genu, but often the body will be absent and the splenium and rostrum will almost certainly be small or absent. This is not true in cases of holoprosencephaly, however, where callosal anomalies are atypical, with the rostrum often present and the genu absent. The diagnosis of partial agenesis can be more difficult with ultrasound (US) than with magnetic resonance imaging (MRI).

Complete Agenesis (Absence) of the Corpus Callosum—Clinical Information

There are times when there is complete absence of the corpus callosum. When this occurs as a solitary abnormality, the patient is usually asymptomatic. However, callosal development occurs at the same time as cerebral and cerebellar development, and therefore agenesis of the corpus callosum (ACC) is associated with other brain anomalies in 80 percent of cases. These anomalies include polymicrogyria and cortical heterotopias, which are best evaluated by MRI, but they also include septo-optic dysplasia, encephalocele, aqueductal stenosis, midline intracerebral lipoma, interhemispheric arachnoid cyst, hydrocephalus, Dandy-Walker cyst, and Chiari II malformation, all of which may be diagnosed by US.

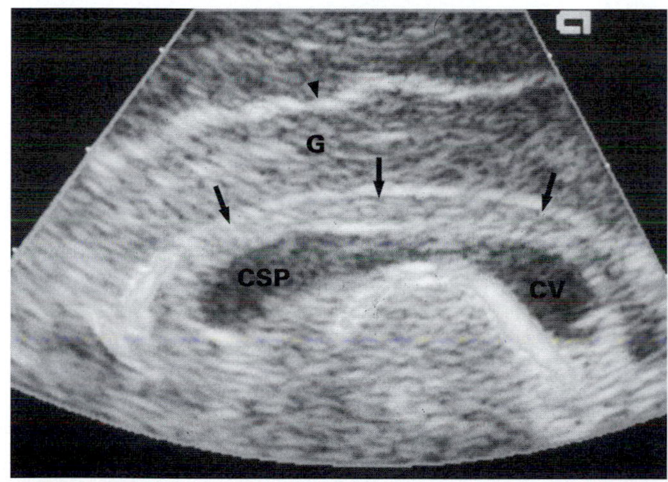

A

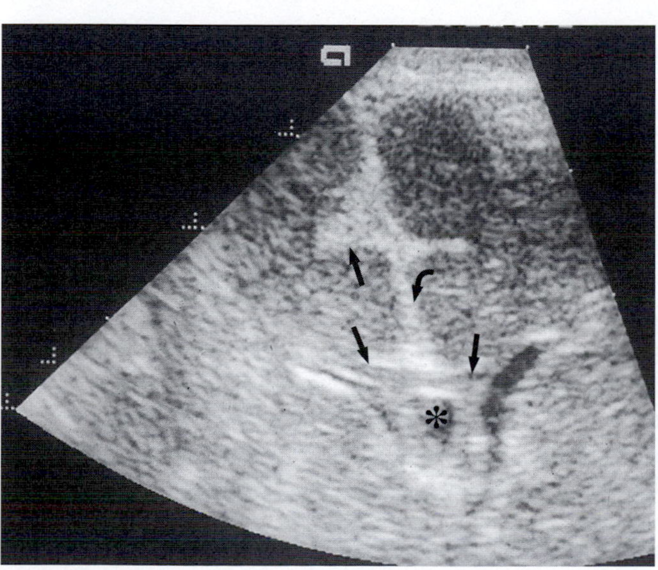

B

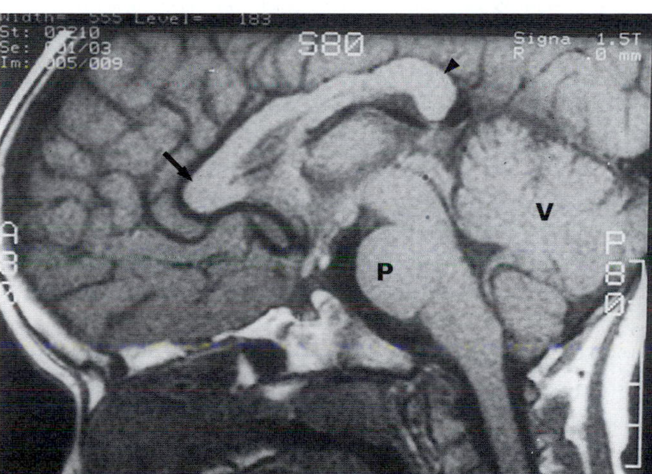

C

FIGURE 30–5. Normal corpus callosum. ***A.*** Head ultrasound. Sagittal plane. This is a magnified image obtained to highlight the presence of the "gray" echogenic corpus callosum (*arrows*). An arrowhead points at its rostrum. CSP = cavum septum pellucidum, CV = cavum vergae, G = cingulate gyrus, which normally parallels the corpus callosum. Arrowhead = cingulate sulcus. ***B.*** Head ultrasound. Coronal plane. This is a magnified image to highlight the presence of the normal corpus callosum (*arrows*) inferior to the interhemispheric fissure (*curved arrow*), above the cavum septum pellucidum (*), and between the frontal horns. ***C.*** Magnetic resonance imaging. Sagittal plane. T1 weighting. The normal corpus callosum is seen in an adult. An arrow points to the genu. An arrowhead points to the rostrum. P = pons, V = vermis of cerebellum. *(Image contributed by Emil Shih, MD.)*

TABLE 30-1
US Findings Suggesting Agenesis of the Corpus Callosum

1. Widely separated (normal-sized) frontal horns
2. Paralleling of lateral ventricular bodies
3. High-riding third ventricle—at or above the level of the frontal horns (possible midline interhemispheric cyst)
4. Gyri that appear to head toward the third ventricle—"sunburst sign"
5. Colpocephaly, greater dilatation of the posterior portion of the lateral ventricle (the least specific of these findings)

Callosal anomalies are found in several syndromes, including the X-linked Aicardi syndrome with its infantile spasms, chorioretinitis, and abnormal electroencephalography. The abnormality is usually sporadic in its occurrence and of unknown etiology. There have, however, been reported cases associated with trisomies 8, 13 to 15, and 18. It is the associated anomalies of the brain that lead to the symptoms of patients with ACC, including mental retardation, seizures, macrocephaly, and hypothalamic dysfunction.

AGENESIS OF THE CORPUS CALLOSUM: ULTRASOUND DIAGNOSIS

The ultrasound diagnosis of ACC (Table 30-1) is consistent with the anatomic findings. An absent corpus callosum allows the frontal horns to be markedly separated (Figs. 30-3 and 30-6) in position. Probst bundles (Fig. 30-3), which represent the axons that would have crossed through the corpus callosum, but now run as two separate white matter bundles that parallel the interhemispheric fissure (IHF), can be imaged as soft tissue structures medial to the frontal horns. Mass impression on the frontal horns may give them a crescentic shape (Fig. 30-6), especially frontally. The presence of the caudate head and lentiform nuclei lateral to the frontal horns keeps them from dilating in their normally nonobstructed state. The bodies of the lateral ventricles, no longer held medially by the corpus callosum, run parallel (Figs. 30-4 and 30-7) to each other. The posterior portion of the lateral ventricles is usually more dilated than the anterior portion. This sign, known as colpocephaly, is not specific to ACC. Patients with ACC have a large foramen of Monro. In addition, the development of a normal corpus callosum inverts the cingulate gyrus. Without a corpus callosum present, the cingulate gyrus remains everted, and the sulci of the medial cerebral hemisphere appear to radiate toward the third ventricle (Fig. 30-8) rather than paralleling the corpus callosum. This has been called the "sunburst sign." In the absence of a corpus callosum superior to it, the third ventricle is higher than normal, extending superiorly in the IHF as an "interhemispheric cyst" (which is not seen in this case). If this cyst grows or is loculated, it may compress and obstruct the ventricular system. With adequate shunting, prognosis for such ACC patients is good.

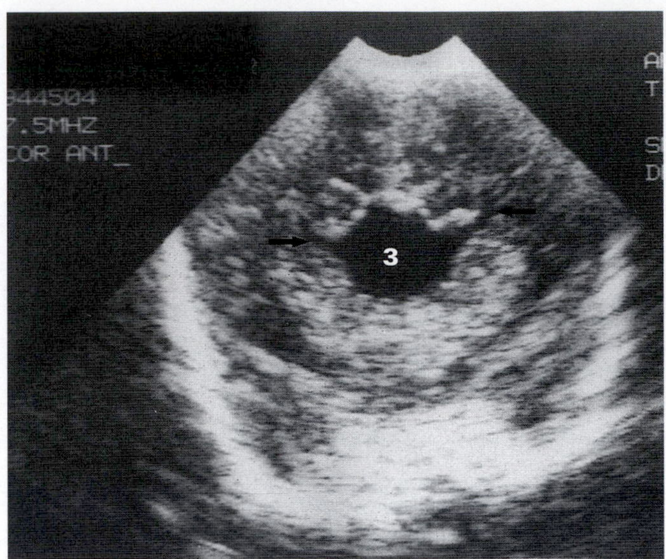

A

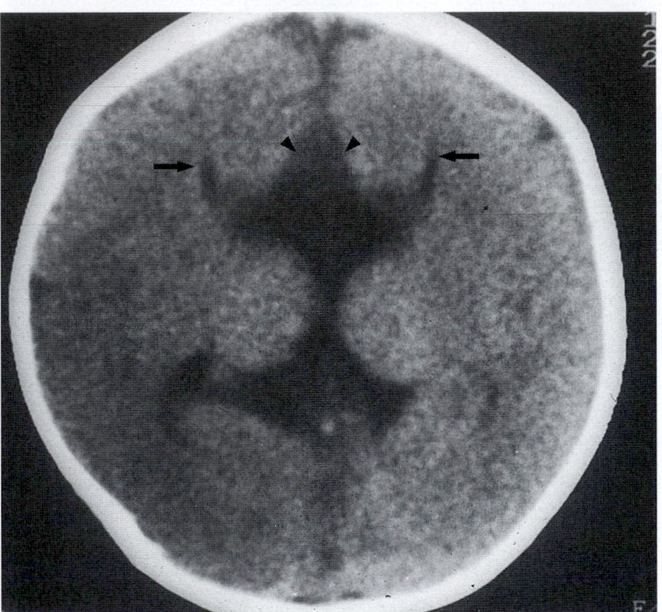

B

FIGURE 30–6. Agenesis of the corpus callosum—marked separation of frontal horns. ***A.*** Ultrasound. Coronal plane. Small nondilated frontal horns (*arrows*) are separated by a large, high-riding third ventricle (3). This image has been likened to a Viking's helmet or bull's horns. ***B.*** Computed tomography. Axial plane. The small frontal horns (*arrows*) are widely separated. The high-riding third ventricle (*arrowheads*) actually extends superior to the frontal horns. *(Reprinted from Rosenthal and Cohen, with permission.)*

IMAGING THE CORPUS CALLOSUM—ULTRASOUND TECHNIQUE

On midline sagittal views, the normal corpus callosum should be readily imaged superior to the cavum septum pellucidum. On coronal views, its anterior portion can be seen at the inferior extent of the IHF "anchor" (Fig. 30-5*C*). An exact identification of the corpus callosum on antenatal studies is somewhat more difficult. Certainly, a good sagittal

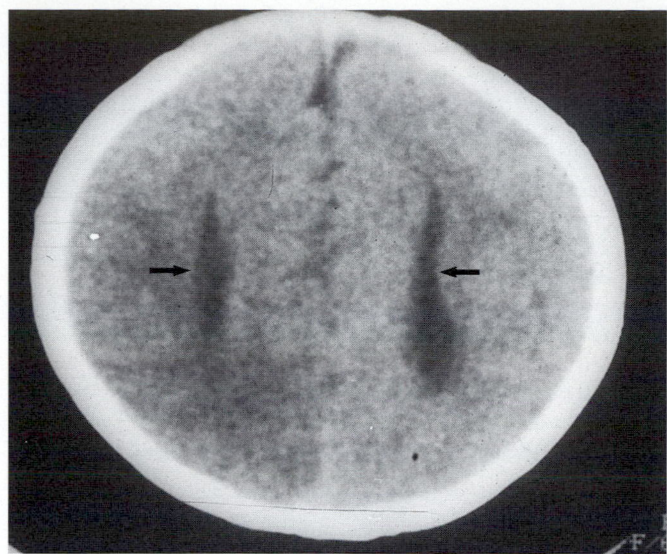

A

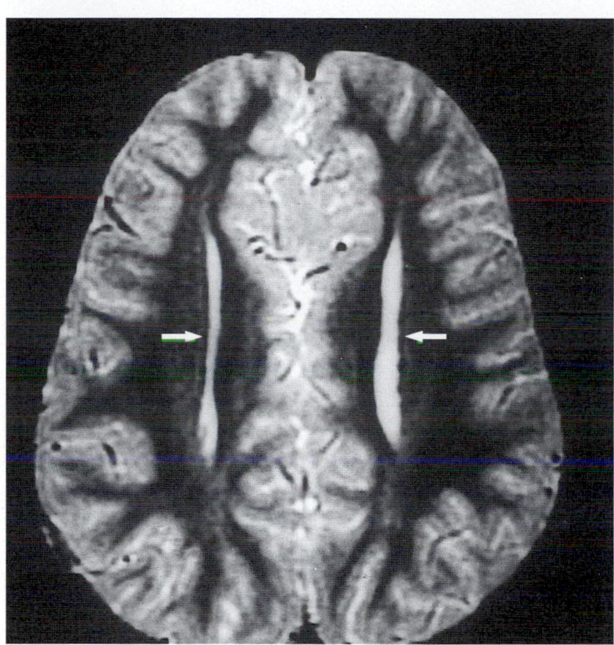

B

FIGURE 30–7. Agenesis of the corpus callosum—parallel lateral ventricles. ***A.*** Computed tomography. Axial plane. The lateral ventricular bodies (*arrows*) are separated from each other and run parallel to each other in agenesis of the corpus callosum. ***B.*** Magnetic resonance imaging (MRI). Axial plane. T2 weighting. The parallel lateral ventricles (*arrows*) can be seen on MRI as well. They are normal in size. *(Image contributed by John Loh, MD.)*

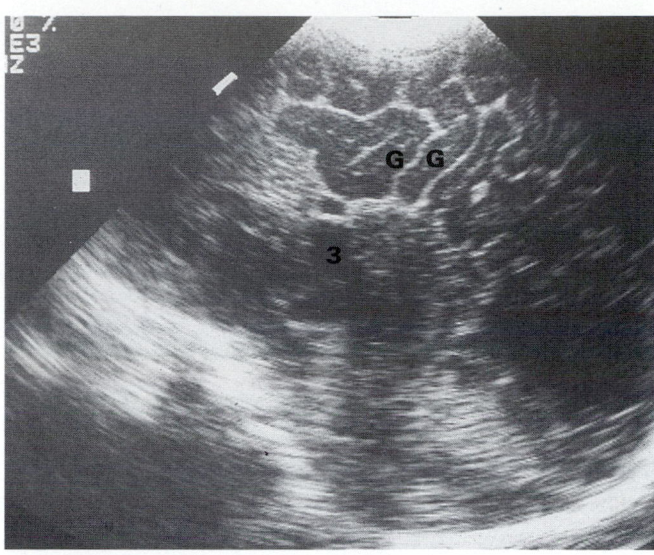

FIGURE 30–8. Agenesis of the corpus callosum—sunburst sign. Ultrasound midline sagittal image. The gyri (g) of the mesial brain seem to point toward the third ventricle (3) rather than appearing, as they normally do, in a curve similar to that of the corpus callosum or cavum septum pellucidum. The cingulate gyrus is absent.

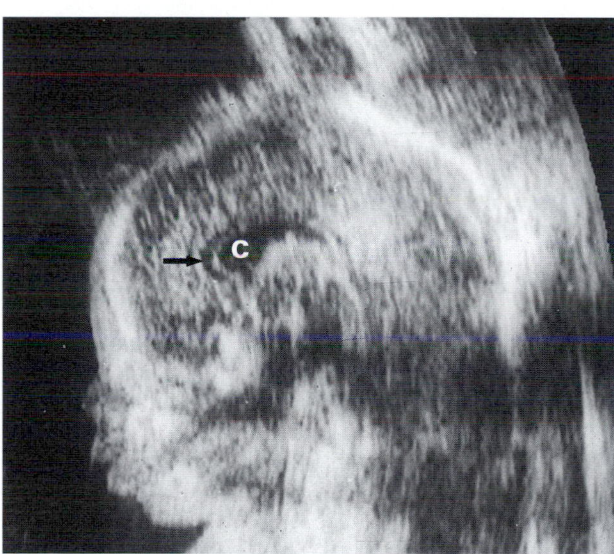

FIGURE 30–9. Corpus callosum in a fetus. Fetal head. Sagittal plane. An arrow points to the genu of the corpus callosum, the first area to develop, in a second-trimester fetus who proved to be normal. The corpus callosum is superior and parallels the cavum septum pellucidum (c).

view may show the corpus callosum (Fig. 30-9) in a fetus. One must be wary of making an early diagnosis of ACC, however, since the corpus callosum is not a complete structure until about 20 weeks. One must also know that even if one sees a normal brain, the fetus may be born with ACC. One group noted that 10 of 15 fetuses with a later diagnosis of ACC had normal US examinations at between 16 and 22 weeks gestational age.

FINAL COMMENTS

This was a case of ACC. The neonatal head US exam can be used to diagnose many congenital anomalies. Antenatal neurosonography has made some of this diagnosis less necessary. However, many patients slip through the cracks, and the neonatal neurosonologist must be aware of the array of diagnoses that can be made. This is particularly true with ACC, whose symptomatology and prognosis are based on what *other* anomalies are found in the affected patient.

References

Atlas S, Shkolnik A, Naidich T: Sonographic recognition of agenesis of the corpus callosum. *AJR* 145:167–173, 1985.

Babcock D: The normal, absent and abnormal corpus callosum: Sonographic findings. *Radiology* 151:449–453, 1984.

Barkovich AJ: *Pediatric Neuroimaging,* 2d ed. New York, Raven, 1995:181–188.

Bennett G, Bromley B, Benacerraf B: Agenesis of the corpus callosum: Prenatal detection usually is not possible before 22 weeks gestation. *Radiology* 199:447–450, 1996.

Cohen HL: Neurosonography of the infant: Diagnosis of abnormalities, in *Ultrasonography of the Prenatal and Neonatal Brain*, Timor-Tritsch I, Monteagudo A, Cohen HL (eds). Stamford, CT, Appleton & Lange, 1996:259–286.

Cohen HL, Haller J: Review. Advances in perinatal neurosonography. *AJR* 63:801–810, 1994.

Comstock C, Culp D, Gonzalez J, Boal D: Agenesis of the corpus callosum in the fetus: Its evolution and significance. *J Ultrasound Med* 4:613–616, 1985.

Davidoff L, Dyke C: Agenesis of the corpus callosum: Its diagnosis by encephalography. *AJR* 32:1–10, 1934.

Fisher R, Cremin B: Lipoma of the corpus callosum: Diagnosis by ultrasound and magnetic resonance. *Pediatr Radiol* 18:409–410, 1988.

Funk K, Siegel M: Sonography of congenital midline brain malformations. *Radiographics* 8:11–25, 1988.

Lockwood C, Ghidini A, Aggarwal R, Hobbins J: Antenatal diagnosis of partial agenesis of the corpus callosum: A benign cause of ventriculomegaly. *Am J Obstet Gynecol* 159:184–186, 1988.

Rosenthal C, Cohen HL: Diagnostic challenge: Agenesis of the corpus callosum. *J Diagn Med Sonog* 3:98–102, 1987.

Siegel MJ, Herman T: Congenital brain anomalies. *Ultrasound Quart* 13:153–176, 1996.

31

A newborn was sent to the ultrasound laboratory for evaluation of increasing head circumference. No obvious intracranial bruit was heard. Neurosonographic images in the coronal (Fig. 31-1) and sagittal planes (Fig. 31-2) are presented. What does the patient have? Should the neuroangiographer get ready to do a study?

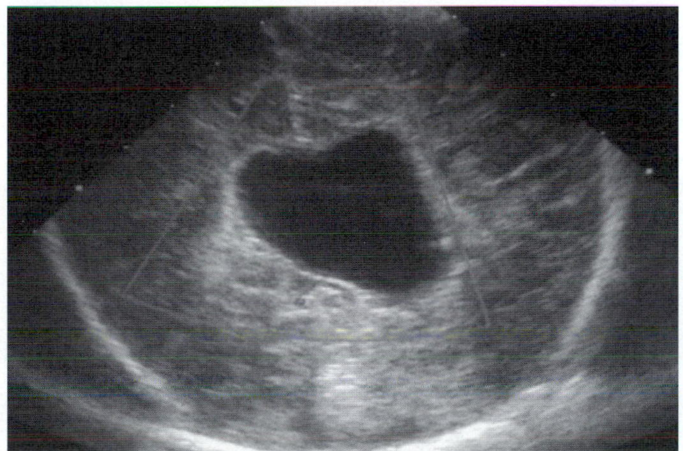

FIGURE 31–1. Neonatal head ultrasound. Coronal plane.

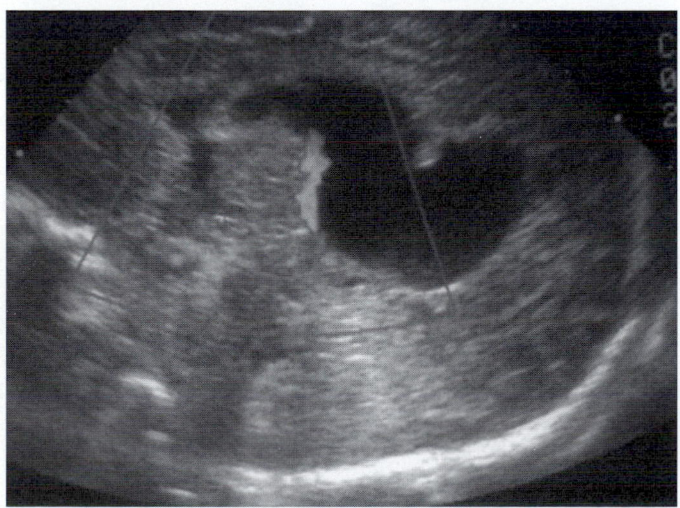

FIGURE 31–2. Neonatal head ultrasound. Sagittal plane. Color Doppler was used.

CHAPTER 31

Arachnoid Cyst Simulating Galenic AVM

GORDON HAUGLAND AND HARRIS L. COHEN

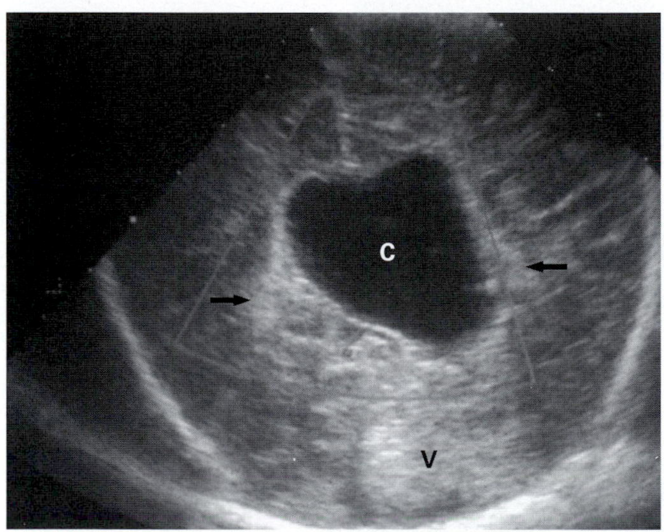

FIGURE 31–3. Arachnoid cyst. Neonatal head ultrasound. Coronal plane. A cystic mass (c) is seen in the middle of the brain parenchyma. Arrows point to nondilated lateral ventricles. V = vermis of the cerebellum.

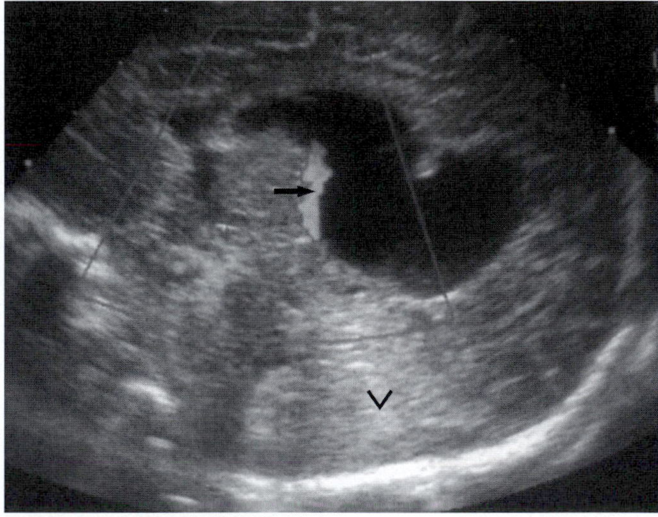

FIGURE 31–4. Arachnoid cyst. Neonatal head ultrasound. Sagittal plane. Color Doppler was used. The cystic mass is tubular but not vascular. The vein of Galen (*arrow*) is the bright linear area within the quadrilateral-shaped area that has been insonated with color Doppler. V = vermis of the cerebellum. By tradition, head ultrasound sagittal images are viewed with the front of the head on the reader's left side.

Figure 31-3, the annotated version of Fig. 31-1, shows a cystic area in the brain on a coronal view. The two lateral ventricles appear somewhat laterally displaced. There is, however, no hydrocephalus. An arteriovenous malformation (AVM) (see Chap. 3) must still be considered.

Figure 31-4, the annotated version of Fig. 31-2, a slightly obliqued midline image, shows the cystic area of the coronal view to be a dilated tubular structure extending posteriorly and inferiorly from the anterior one-third of the brain. Its tubular nature makes the possibility of an AVM, particularly a vein of Galen aneurysm (or, more correctly, a galenic AVM), even more likely. However, the color Doppler proved that the tortuous cystic mass was not a vessel. The true vein of Galen is seen anterior to this cystic structure, which is an arachnoid cyst.

WHAT IS AN ARACHNOID CYST?

Arachnoid cysts represent 1 percent of all intracranial masses. They may be congenital or acquired after hemorrhage or infection. Congenital cysts are thought to be the re-

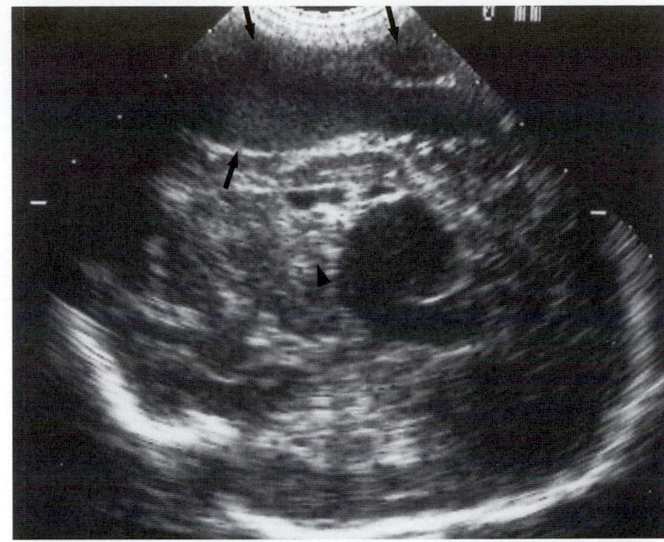

A

B

FIGURE 31–5. Large arteriovenous malformation of the brain. ***A.*** Neonatal head ultrasound. Sagittal plane similar to Figs. 31-2 and 31-4, but in another patient. A tubular cystic structure (*arrowhead*) is seen in the center of the brain. The image has some similarities to the arachnoid cyst in Figs. 31-1 to 31-4. However, although this is not typical, at the top of the calvarium is a much bigger tubular echopenic structure (*arrows*) that proved the central cystic structure to be part of a larger AVM, far greater in size than what was seen at antenatal diagnosis. This neonate died early in life of congestive heart failure. ***B.*** Neonatal head ultrasound. Sagittal plane. Color Doppler. This image concentrated on the echoless tubular structure at the rostrum of this neonate's head. Significant color Doppler flow is now seen in this vessel. Turbulent and biphasic venous Doppler signal proved it to be part of a very large AVM. Similar findings were seen for the central cystic structure as well. (See Color Plate 10.)

sult of maldevelopment of the leptomeninges and are found between the pia-arachnoid layers, communicating with the subarachnoid space. They may grow because of this communication, and fluid is thought to accumulate on a ball-valve basis. Some may have choroid plexus–like tissue in their wall, allowing secretion of cerebrospinal fluid (CSF), which will allow them to enlarge. Often seen in a retrocerebellar location simulating the Dandy-Walker cyst, they are more variable in size and shape when in the larger confines of the supratentorial brain. The accumulated fluid may cause mass effect and hydrocephalus. Arachnoid cysts are not associated with brain maldevelopment and, if treated, have an excellent outcome. Typically a cyst in the quadrigeminal plate area may simulate a galenic AVM (vein of Galen aneurysm) (Fig. 31-5; see also Color Plate 10). Doppler helps make the differentiation (Fig. 31-6).

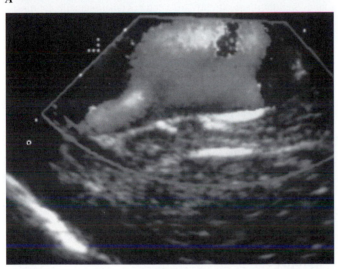

SOME MORE INFORMATION ON AVMS

As discussed in Chap. 3, large lesions may lead to fetal and neonatal mortality as a result of cardiac failure and brain infarction due to a "steal phenomenon" of intracranial arterial flow. Cardiac failure due to the large arteriovenous shunt is the most common presenting symptom in children. Congestive failure with an enlarged aorta on chest radiograph can be the first imaging abnormality, particularly in a child who does not present with associated cranial bruit or enlarged

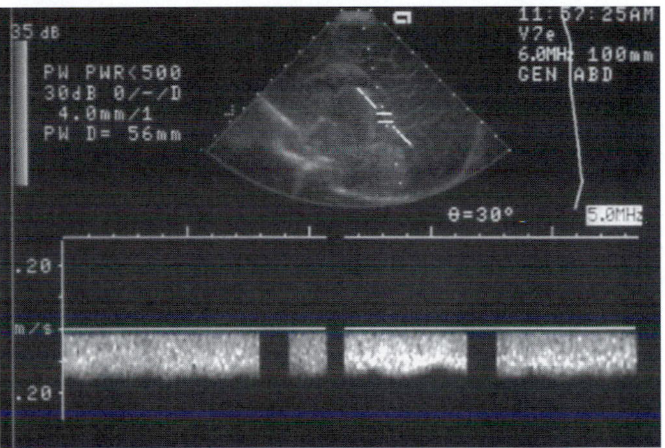

A

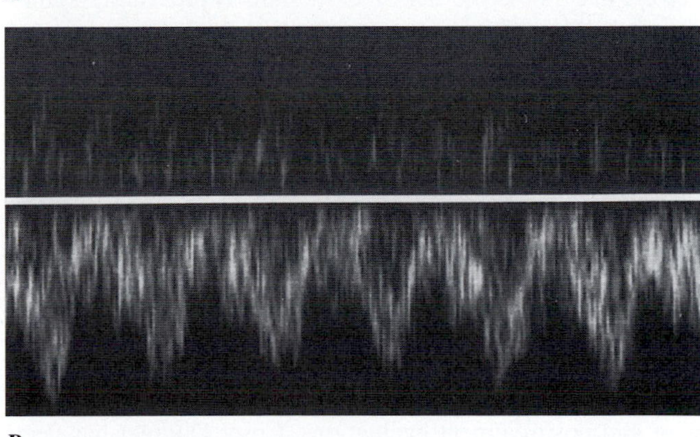

B

FIGURE 31–6. Spectral patterns in normal vein of Galen and in a galenic AVM. ***A.*** Spectral pattern of brain vein. Transfontanelle head ultrasound. Sagittal plane. The Doppler gate is placed in the region of the normal vein of Galen. It was not recognized as an individual structure until color Doppler was performed. A bandlike normal venous pattern with only minimal changes in height based upon respiration is noted. ***B.*** Spectral pattern of galenic AVM. This signal obtained from the venous side of the AVM is abnormal compared to the pattern in ***A.*** This pattern is typical for an intracranial AVM and is described as turbulent or biphasic and irregular.

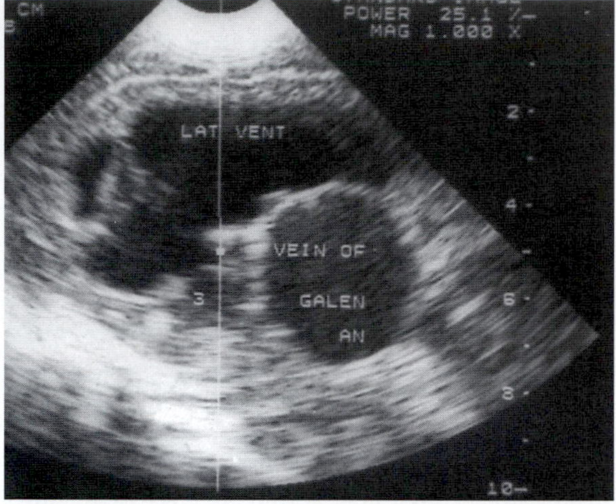

A

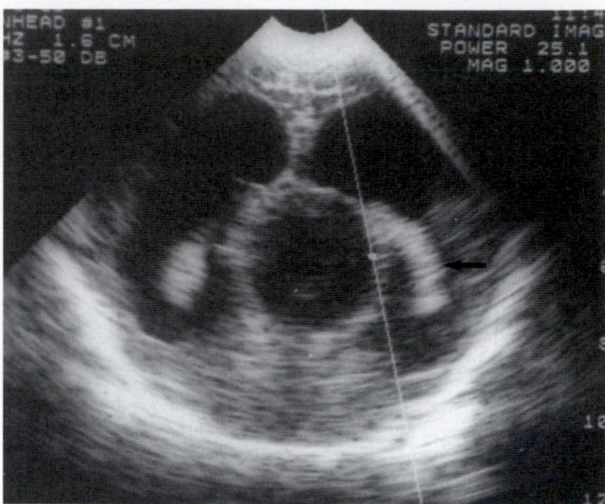

B

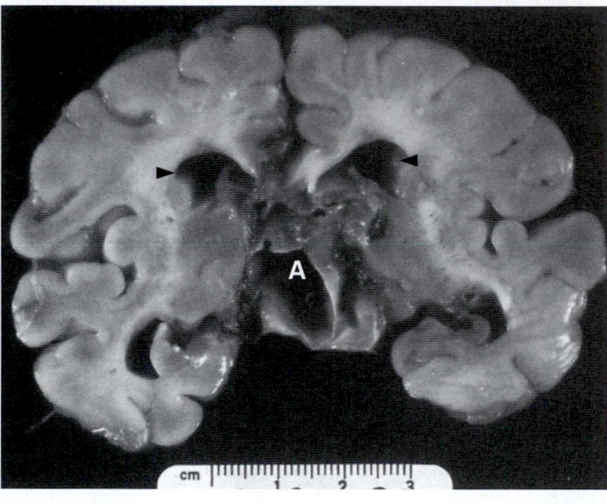

C

FIGURE 31–7. Galenic AVM with hydrocephalus. ***A.*** Head ultrasound. Sagittal plane, slightly off center. Transfontanelle approach. A vein of Galen aneurysm or galenic malformation is seen to be somewhat more echogenic, probably because of swirling or slow-flowing blood, than the dilated lateral ventricle, which is seen only because of slight off-center obliquity of this sagittal image. ***B.*** Head ultrasound. Coronal plane. Transfontanelle approach. The midline cystic structure is the galenic AVM. Its mass effect caused the moderate hydrocephalus. Arrow points to left choroid plexus in the dilated left lateral ventricle. ***C.*** Postmortem brain specimen. Coronal plane. This patient died soon after birth. Arrows point to the frontal horns of the lateral ventricles of the specimen. They are more dilated than normal. They sit lateral to the dilated galenic AVM (A). The AVM was the midline cystic mass noted on ultrasound, and its mass impression was responsible for the hydrocephalus. (See Color Plate 11.)

head circumference. Hydrocephalus (Fig. 31-7; see also Color Plate 11) is the next most common presenting symptom. Dilatation of the vein of Galen can cause obstruction of the ventricular system at the level of the third ventricle and aqueduct of Sylvius. Symptoms and prognosis depend on shunt size, with larger shunts presenting earlier and having a poorer prognosis.

TREATMENT OF THE AVM

Endovascular embolization of the feeding vessels is a current treatment option. Doppler has been used as an adjunct to angiography or magnetic resonance angiography in pretreatment and posttreatment evaluations. Color Doppler has been used to note hemodynamic changes after embolization, including improvements of blood flow to uninvolved portions of the brain as well as changes in the caliber and flow of feeder vessels that have not been embolized.

TAKE HOME POINT

Use caution: An arachnoid cyst may simulate an intracranial AVM.

References

Cohen HL, Haller J: Review. Advances in perinatal neurosonography. *AJR* 163:801–810, 1994.

Diakoumakis E, Weinberg B, Mollin J: Prenatal sonographic diagnosis of a suprasellar arachnoid cyst. *J Ultrasound Med* 5: 529–530, 1986.

Filly R: Ultrasound evaluation of the fetal neural axis, in *Ultrasonography in Obstetrics and Gynecology,* 3d ed, Callen PW (ed). Philadelphia, Saunders, 1994:216–217.

Ishimatsu J, Yoshimura O, Tetsuou M, Hamada T: Evaluation of an aneurysm of the vein of Galen in utero by pulsed and color Doppler ultrasonography. *Am J Obstet Gynecol* 164:743–744, 1991.

Rumack C, Johnson M: Intracranial neoplasms, cysts, and vascular malformations, in *Prenatal and Infant Brain Imaging. Role of Ultrasound and Computed Tomography,* Rumack C, Johnson L (eds). Chicago, Year Book, 1984:191–194.

Volpe J: Brain tumors and vein of Galen malformations, in *Neurology of the Newborn: Neuronal Proliferation, Migration, Organization and Myelination,* 3d ed. Philadelphia: Saunders, 1995: 802–806.

32

A term infant with low Apgar scores was examined by head ultrasound (US) (Fig. 32-1). Figure 32-2 shows the spectral pattern of the right anterior cerebral artery. Is the head US normal or abnormal? Is there anything to worry about?

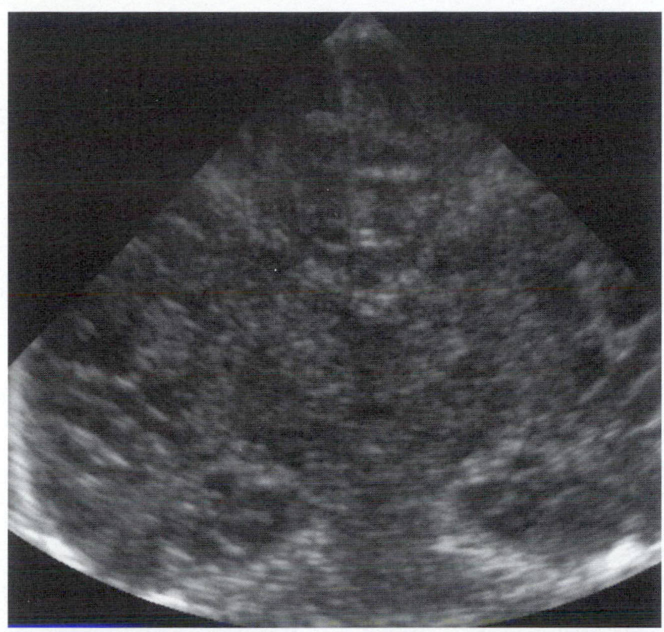

FIGURE 32–1. Neonatal head. Coronal plane. Level of frontal horns.

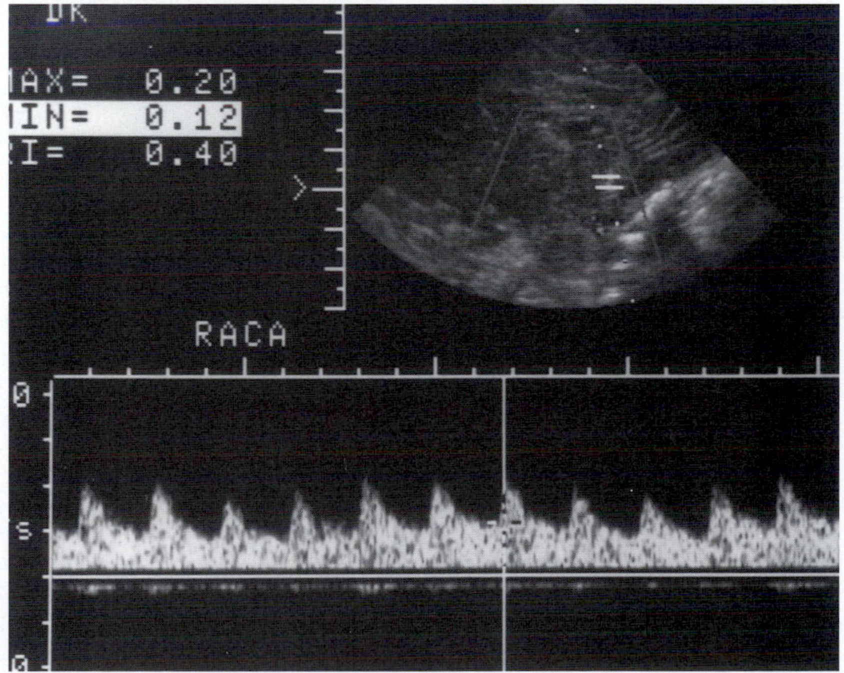

FIGURE 32–2. Neonatal head. Sagittal plane and Doppler with spectral pattern of the right anterior cerebral artery. (The image is not in classic position in that the front of the head is on the reader's right.)

CHAPTER 32

Ischemic Brain Injury in the Newborn

JOANNA J. SEIBERT AND JANICE ALLISON

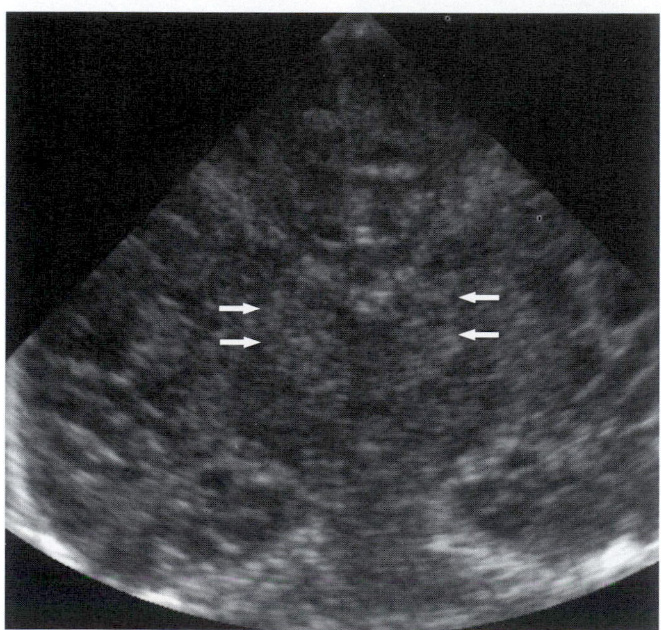

FIGURE 32–3. Annotated version of Fig. 32-1. Increased echogenicity of basal ganglia and thalami. Neonatal head. Coronal plane. Level of frontal horns. The frontal horns are not imaged. Normal patients have no significant ventricular dilatation. At times their frontal horns may be difficult to image, appearing, at most, slitlike. This may also occur with cerebral edema. Of note is the fact that the basal ganglia and thalami (*arrows*) of this term infant with low Apgar scores are of somewhat greater echogenicity than the surrounding brain parenchyma.

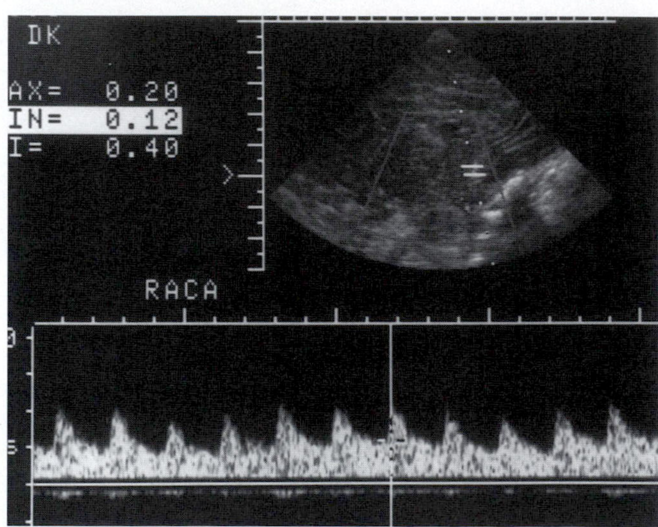

FIGURE 32–4. Annotated version of Fig. 32-2. Lower than normal resistance index. Neonatal head. Sagittal plane and Doppler with spectral pattern of the right anterior cerebral artery. (The image is not in classic position in that the front of the head is on the reader's left.) For this arterial spectral pattern there is a resistive index of 40, which is lower than normal.

Figure 32-3 (the annotated version of Fig. 32-1) shows the gray-scale head US of a term infant with low Apgar scores. Except for a slight increase in echogenicity of the brain in the basal ganglia and thalamus, the image may have appeared normal. Figure 32-4 (the annotated version of Fig. 32-2), on the other hand, shows a resistive index of 40 for the right anterior cerebral artery, which is considered lower than normal. The normal measurements have been determined to be 75 ± 10. Something was amiss. Figure 32-5 is an inversion recovery magnetic resonance image (MRI) that was performed 3 days after the US and proved that there was abnormality. The MRI showed diffuse edema of the brain, evidenced by poor gray-white differentiation. There was increased signal in the basal ganglia and thalamus. The infant expired 1 month later. The US, and particularly the Doppler, had allowed the early recognition of hypoxic-ischemic injury (HII) in this term neonate.

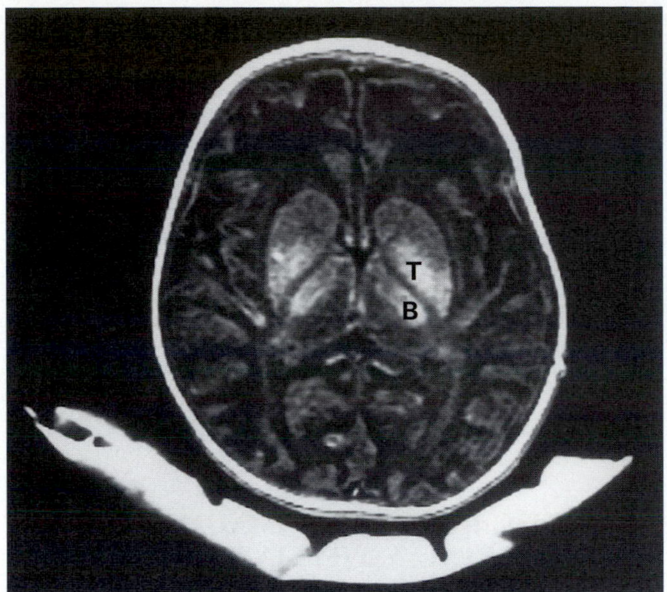

FIGURE 32–5. Diffuse brain edema. Magnetic resonance imaging. Inversion recovery image. Axial plane. This image, obtained 3 days after Figs. 32-3 and 32-4, shows diffuse edema of the brain with poor differentiation of gray and white matter. There is increased signal in the basal ganglia (B) and thalami (T). This is consistent with the subtle increased echogenicity noted in these areas on the ultrasound image of Fig. 32-3.

HYPOXIC-ISCHEMIC INJURY

Clinical Information

Clinical signs of HII in the very young may be nonspecific and may take days to evolve. Knowledge of its presence is important in guiding management and in parental counseling. Gray-scale US has traditionally had a low sensitivity in detecting acute HII, but Doppler resistive indices (RI), reviewed over the last decade, have proved helpful in denoting alterations in cerebral perfusion. A lower than normal Doppler RI of cerebral arteries is thought to reveal post-asphyxia hyperemia and may be the earliest neuroimaging finding of HII in term neonates.

TABLE 32-1
When to Suspect Asphyxia Clinically

Asphyxia should be suspected when two or more of the following criteria are present:

1. Cord blood pH or initial arterial pH of <7.1
2. 5-min Apgar of 5 or less
3. History of abnormal fetal heart rate monitoring
4. Base deficit >10 mEq/L
5. Significant apnea or need for positive-pressure ventilation
6. Clinical seizures and/or abnormal EEG
7. Abnormal neurologic exam indicative of HIE
8. Evidence of asphyxia-associated organ dysfunction, e.g., cardiomyopathy, shock, acute renal failure, hepatic necrosis, necrotizing enterocolitis, DIC

DIC = disseminated intravascular coagulation, EEG = electroencephalogram, HIE = hypoxic-ischemic encephalopathy.

In the brain of a term neonate, HII is the result of a deficit in cerebral oxygen delivery, commonly due to perinatal asphyxia. Table 32-1 shows criteria for the clinical suspicion and diagnosis of asphyxia in the newborn. Asphyxia, an impairment in the exchange of oxygen and carbon dioxide, results in hypoxia and hypercapnia. It occurs in 1 in every 100 to 500 live births.

Asphyxia followed by abnormal neonatal neurologic behavior is known as hypoxic-ischemic encephalopathy (HIE). This disorder is graded as mild, moderate, or severe based on clinical and laboratory indicators. Severe HIE carries a poor prognosis (50 percent mortality), moderate HIE carries a variable prognosis, and mild HIE usually is benign and transient, with a good outcome. The assessment of the severity of HIE, especially in the first 2 or 3 days of life, may be difficult. Long-term deficits of HIE include motor problems (spasticity, choreoathetosis, and ataxia, collectively known as cerebral palsy) as well as seizures and mental retardation.

Pathophysiology and Need for Earlier Ultrasound Diagnosis

Reliable techniques for early assessment of the severity of HII are needed. By the time the neonate is sufficiently stable to undergo MR scanning, many management and treatment decisions have already been made, including continuation of vital support and the use of advanced treatment techniques such as extracorporeal membrane oxygenation (ECMO) and nitric oxide. Ultrasound and Doppler allow examinations early in the neonate's life and at the bedside. Although transfontanelle US images of the brain can be technically excellent, the sensitivity of gray-scale US in the early detection of HIE is low (<50 percent). (The US signs of asphyxia are noted in Table 32-2.)

Doppler, on the other hand, shows promise for the early diagnosis of hypoxic cerebral injury by detecting physiologic changes, i.e., the defective autoregulation of cerebral blood flow that occurs during and after asphyxia, from both hypoxia and, independently, hypercapnia. These may include the maintenance or augmentation of cerebral blood flow, decrease in cerebral metabolic rate, and decrease in intracellular pH. Hypercapnia and hypoxia prevent cerebral autoregulation, the ability to maintain constant cerebral blood flow over a broad range of blood pressures. During the initial phase of asphyxia, an alteration in peripheral vascular resistance results in a larger proportion than normal of the cardiac output being distributed to the brain, heart, and adrenal glands. This redistribution increases total and regional cerebral blood flow, with concomitant loss of vascular autoregulation.

TABLE 32-2
Ultrasonographic Signs of Asphyxia

1. Diffuse increased echogenicity
2. Focal areas of increased echogenicity, especially in the thalamus and basal ganglia (Fig. 32-3)
3. Small ventricles (Fig. 32-3)
4. Indistinct gyri and sulci (Fig. 32-3)

Following asphyxia, there is initial cerebral hyperemia. Possible etiologic factors include increased neuronal excitability, accumulation of vasoactive compounds, and vascular injury. Hyperemia following asphyxia can be detected by transcranial Doppler US because it is frequently associated with a decrease in the resistive index to below 60.

The hyperemic period has been shown to last between 6 and 130 h postnatally. In our experience, this decrease is present for only 24 to 48 h. This initial hyperemic response is followed by a period of decreased cerebral blood flow and diminished cerebral oxygen consumption. Later, there is a decrease in cardiac output with systemic hypotension, which results in decreased cerebral blood flow.

WHAT IS THE RESISTIVE INDEX?

The RI is a reflection of cerebral blood flow. It is defined as the peak systolic velocity (PSV) minus the end-diastolic velocity (EDV) divided by the PSV (Table 32-3). As a ratio, the index is independent of the angle of insonation and absolute flow velocity. As diastolic flow increases relative to systolic flow, the index decreases. The normal values for neonates have been established to be 75 ± 10, based on a published series of 75. The high diastolic flow of early postasphyxial hyperemia decreases the RI to below 60. Although there are numerous systemic causes for an elevated RI, *a low RI is strongly suggestive of the hyperemia of asphyxia.* Other causes of low RIs are ECMO therapy, an arteriovenous malformation, and other intracranial arteriovenous shunts that are usually clinically obvious and/or readily detected by imaging. There is some speculation that hypercapnia itself causes a decrease in the RI. However, a key published study showed that even with Pa_{CO_2} maintained below a certain level, asphyxiated infants still have decreased RIs.

RESULTS OF OTHER DOPPLER STUDIES OF ASPHYXIATED NEWBORNS

Stark and Seibert found that a low RI combined with a history of asphyxia is associated with an adverse outcome and may be among the earliest markers for a poor neurodevelopmental outcome. Half of the patients with asphyxia who had low RIs had a *normal* gray-scale US exam; 10 of 13 (77 percent) of these patients were neurologically abnormal when assessed at 8 months to 1 year. Archer, Levine, and Evans, in a retrospective control study, have shown that low RI in asphyxiated infants correlates strongly with poor outcome. Gray et al also reported a significant association between abnormal anterior cerebral artery flow velocity, low resistive index, and an adverse outcome in infants with perinatal asphyxia examined by Doppler between days 2 and 7 of life.

TABLE 32-3
Definition of Resistive Index

$$\text{Resistive Index} = \frac{\text{Peak Systolic Velocity} - \text{End-Diastolic Velocity}}{\text{Peak Systolic Velocity}}$$

$$\text{or RI} = (\text{PSV} - \text{EDV})/\text{PSV}$$

A technique that may prove promising in evaluating asphyxia in term neonates and that has been performed with premature neonates is the use of power and pulsed-wave Doppler to study regional cerebral blood flow. Blankenberg et al showed that low birth weight infants with periventricular leukomalacia (PVL) and germinal matrix hemorrhage (GMH) have significantly greater mean values and more variable values of vascular cross-sectional area and the product of peak velocity and cross-sectional area than neonates without PVL or GMH. Blankenberg et al also observed significantly lower mean RIs in neonates with PVL and GMH.

MAGNETIC RESONANCE IMAGING FOR NEONATAL ASPHYXIA EVALUATION

Magnetic resonance imaging has been widely accepted as the definitive neuroimaging method for the accurate diagnosis of the changes of HIE, but transporting the sick and unstable newborn for the exam can prove difficult and even hazardous. We perform T1-weighted inversion recovery images, which may be a more sensitive sequence than conventional T1-weighted images for the changes of HIE. Bright signal is typically noted in the basal ganglia, thalami, and brainstem. A similar US finding, echogenic thalami (Fig. 32-3), in neonates with hypoxic ischemia suggests a poor outcome, with 31 percent mortality and 56 percent long-term morbidity.

EDITOR'S NOTES

It is important to diagnose ischemic injury, typically PVL in premature infants and hypoxia in term infants, because of its implications for future morbidity. In the case of both PVL and HIE, the development of cystic areas in the brain helps make the diagnosis, but somewhat later in time (i.e., during the cystic phase of PVL, which usually occurs 2 weeks after the echogenic phase). Increased echogenicity, permitting earlier diagnosis, may not be easily noted using gray-scale imaging alone. It may not be easy, even with a machine that has Doppler capability. Seibert's group, among others, has, however, produced some important work on making this early diagnosis. Further clinical experience will help prove its applicability.

The resistive index is one of several methods of evaluating, mathematically, the spectral pattern obtained by Doppler of an arterial vessel and its systolic and diastolic flow. With the formula (PSV – EDV)/PSV, if there is no diastolic flow, the RI is 1 or, in the method used by Seibert et al, 100. Most of us are quite aware that increased resistance of blood flow into the brain is indicative of abnormality. The brain, like other low-resistance organs such as the testicle, transplanted kidney, and placenta, requires constant blood flow in systole and diastole to maintain its integrity. A high RI in a feed-

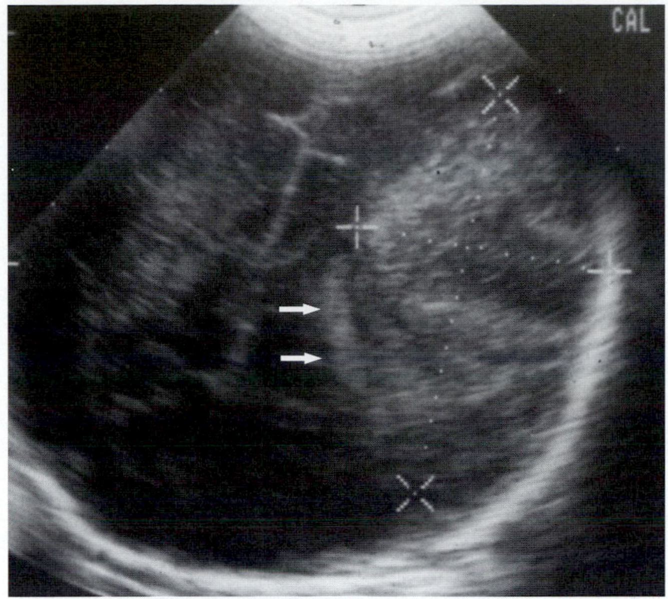

FIGURE 32–6. Brain infarct. Head ultrasound. Coronal plane, angled somewhat to highlight the abnormal area. Crosses mark off the highly echogenic brain parenchyma in the distribution area of the left middle cerebral artery (MCA). This is a relatively easy to diagnose gray-scale image of a left MCA cerebral infarction. Arrows point to normal left choroid plexus.

ing blood vessel suggests decreasing diastolic flow, higher resistance to entering flow, and an organ at risk for ischemia/necrosis. Cerebral edema may so decrease entering blood flow as to cause reversal of diastolic flow. It is Seibert's group and others who have shown that in the term neonate's brain, we must also worry about low-resistance flow—i.e., high diastolic flow in relation to systolic flow, evidence of the poor autoregulation of cerebral vascular blood flow that occurs after hypoxia. Poor autoregulation, if we remember, is a physiologic problem in all low birth weight premature infants.

References

Archer LN, Evans DH, Paton JY, et al: Controlled hypercapnia and neonatal cerebral artery Doppler ultrasound waveforms. *Pediatr Res* 20:218–221, 1986.

Archer LN, Levene MI, Evans DH: Cerebral artery Doppler ultrasonography for prediction of outcome after perinatal asphyxia. *Lancet* 2:1116–1118, 1986.

Babcock DS, Ball W: Postasphyxial encephalopathy in full-term infants: Ultrasound diagnosis. *Radiology* 148:417–423, 1983.

Bada HS, Hajjar W, Chua C: Noninvasive diagnosis of neonatal asphyxia and intraventricular hemorrhage by Doppler ultrasound. *J Pediatr* 95:775–779, 1979.

Barkovich AJ: MR and CT evaluation of profound neonatal and infantile asphyxia. *AJNR* 13:959–972, 1992.

Blankenberg FG, Loh N, Norbash A, et al: Impaired cerebrovascular autoregulation after hypoxic-ischemic injury in extremely low-birth-weight neonates: Detection with power and pulsed wave Doppler US. *Radiology* 205:563–568, 1997.

Connolly B, Kelehan P, O'Brien N, et al: The echogenic thalamus in hypoxic ischaemic encephalopathy. *Pediatr Radiol* 24: 268–271, 1994.

Gray PH, Tudehope DI, Masel JP, et al: Perinatal hypoxic-ischaemic brain injury: Prediction of outcome. *Dev Med Child Neurol* 35:965–973, 1993.

Seibert JJ, McCowan TC, Chadduck WM, et al: Duplex pulsed Doppler US versus intracranial pressure in the neonate: Clinical and experimental studies. *Radiology* 171:155–159, 1989.

Siegel MJ, Shackelford GD, Perlman JM, et al: Hypoxic-ischemic encephalopathy in term infants: Diagnosis and prognosis evaluated by ultrasound. *Radiology* 152:395–399, 1984.

Stark JE, Seibert JJ: Cerebral artery Doppler ultrasonography for prediction of outcome after perinatal asphyxia. *J Ultrasound Med* 13:595–600, 1994.

van Bel F, Hirasing RA, Grimberg MT: Can perinatal asphyxia cause cerebral edema and affect cerebral blood flow velocity? *Eur J Pediatr* 142:29–32, 1984.

Vannucci RC, Perlman JM: Interventions for perinatal hypoxic-ischemic encephalopathy. *Pediatrics* 100:1004–1014, 1997.

Volpe JJ: Hypoxic-ischemic encephalopathy, in *Neurology of the Newborn,* 3d ed, Volpe JJ (ed). Philadelphia, Saunders, 1995:211–369.

33

Two images of a patient with sickle cell disease are shown to you. Figure 33-1 is an image and spectral pattern obtained via a transcranial approach. The patient is 5 years old and without neurologic symptomatology. Figure 33-2 is a similar study performed in the same patient at 9 years of age. Are any of the images/spectra worrisome?

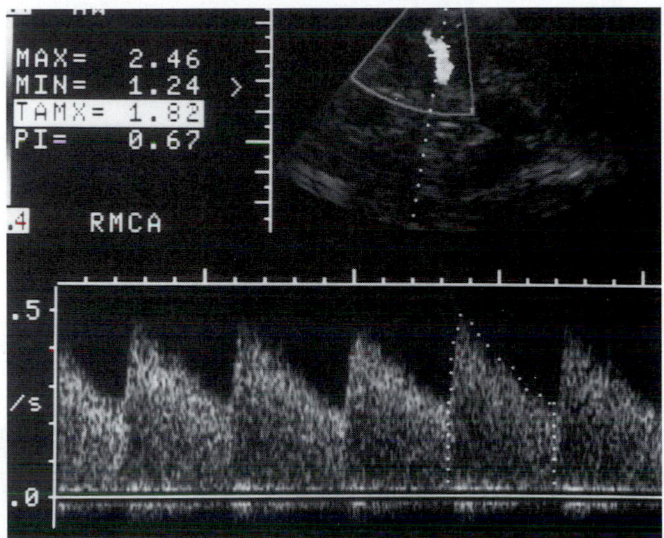

FIGURE 33–1. Transcranial Doppler. Axial plane. Flow in the right middle cerebral artery of a 5-year-old with sickle cell disease is insonated.

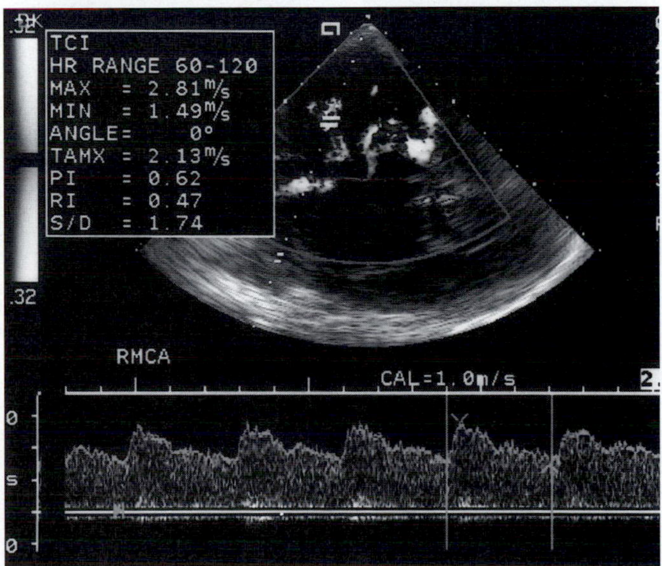

FIGURE 33–2. Transcranial Doppler. Axial plane. Flow in the right middle cerebral artery is again insonated. The patient is now 9 years old.

CHAPTER 33

Abnormal Transcranial Doppler Spectra in Sickle Cell Disease—Predicting Stroke

JOANNA J. SEIBERT AND JANICE W. ALLISON

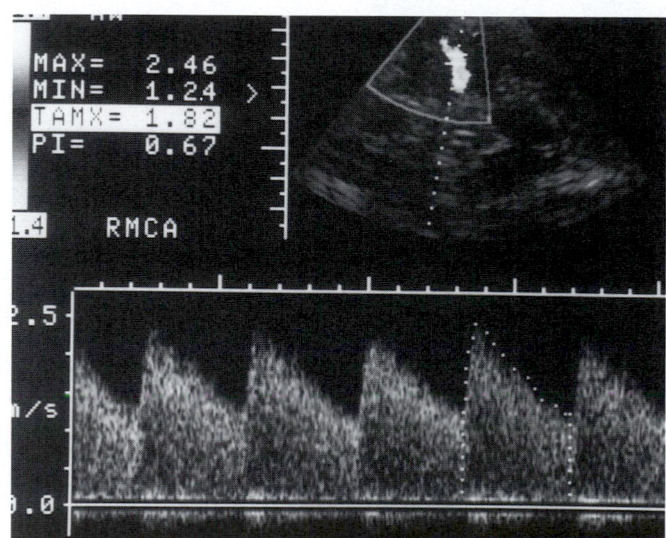

FIGURE 33–3. Annotated version of Fig. 33-1. Abnormal vascular flow. Transcranial Doppler (TCD). Axial plane. Patient is 5 years old. The mean velocity obtained for one spectral waveform (*surrounded by a dotted line*) from the right middle cerebral artery was 1.82 m/s or 182 cm/s. The peak systolic velocity at that point was 246 cm/s. Patients are considered at risk for stroke on the basis of various criteria, including a mean middle cerebral artery (MCA) velocity of 170 to 190 cm/s or greater and a maximum MCA flow of > 200 cm/s. These measurements obtained by TCD indicate that this boy is at risk for a stroke.

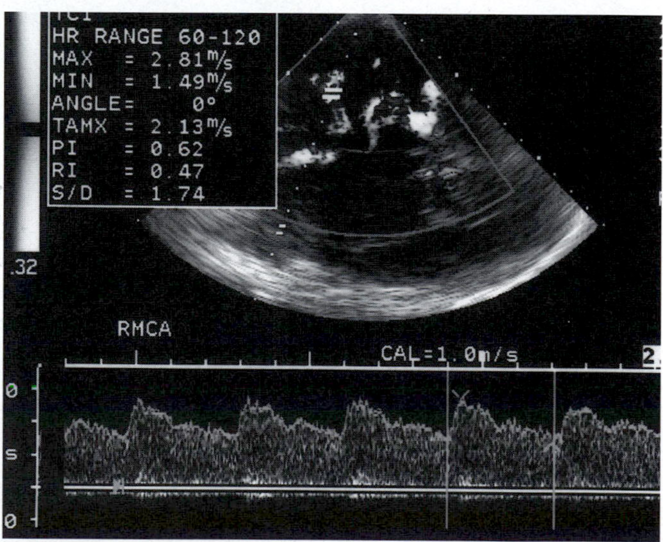

FIGURE 33–4. Annotated version of Fig. 33-2. Abnormal vascular flow in patient with sickle cell disease. Transcranial Doppler (TCD). Axial plane. Patient is now 9 years old. The mean velocity obtained for one spectral waveform (*marked off by vertical lines*) from the right middle cerebral artery was 2.13 m/s or 213 cm/s. The peak systolic velocity at that point was 281 cm/s. These measurements obtained by TCD indicate that this boy is at risk for a stroke.

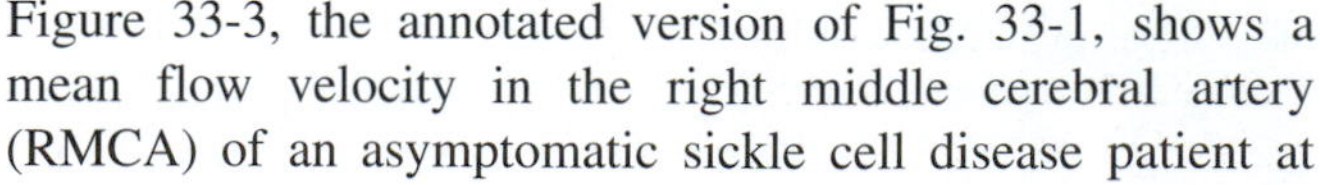
Figure 33-3, the annotated version of Fig. 33-1, shows a mean flow velocity in the right middle cerebral artery (RMCA) of an asymptomatic sickle cell disease patient at age 5 of 182 cm/s. Magnetic resonance angiography (MRA) (Fig. 33-5) performed at the time was normal. Figure 33-4, the annotated version of Fig. 33-2, shows a mean flow veloc-

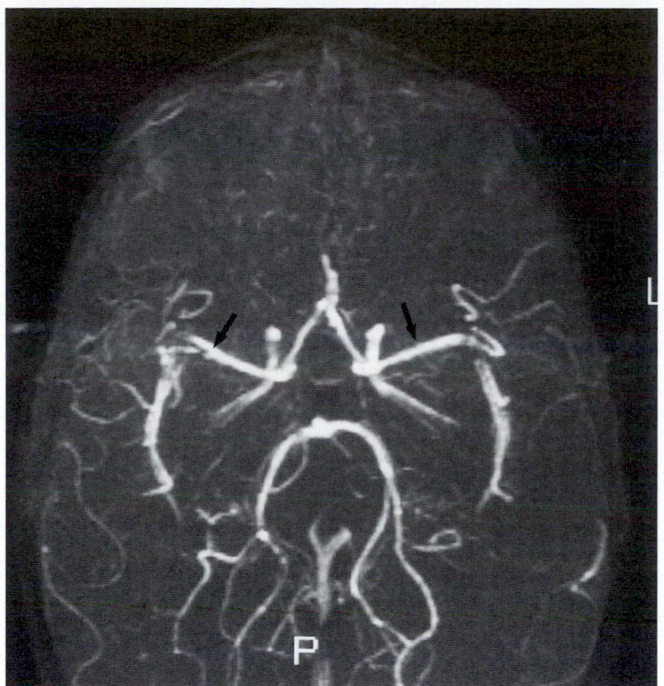

FIGURE 33–5. Normal magnetic resonance angiography (MRA) image. Axial plane. Arrows point to normal middle cerebral arteries within the circle of Willis. This was the MRA of the patient at age 5.

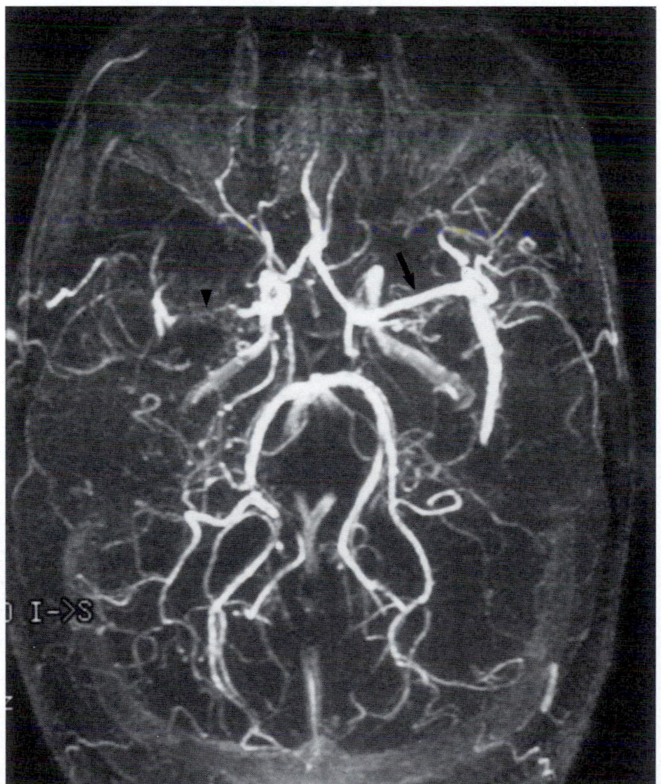

FIGURE 33–6. Abnormal right middle cerebral artery. Magnetic resonance angiography (MRA). Axial plane. An arrow points to the normal left middle cerebral artery. An arrowhead points to an area without flow in the right middle cerebral artery. This proved to be an area of significant stenosis. This was the MRA of the patient at age 9, when his abnormal transcranial Doppler results matched up with abnormal MRA results. He was still asymptomatic at this time.

ity of 213 cm/s in the same patient with sickle cell disease at age 9. The patient still had no neurologic symptoms, but the flow velocities were of concern. An MRA (Fig. 33-6) performed at that time is abnormal. The patient has developed a high-grade stenosis of the right middle cerebral artery.

THE PROBLEM OF STROKES IN PATIENTS WITH SICKLE CELL DISEASE

Cerebral infarction secondary to occlusive vasculopathy is a major complication of patients with sickle cell disease (hemoglobin SS). The reported prevalence of stroke in these patients is 5.5 to 17 percent. These infarctions originate from stenotic lesions involving large vessels in the intracranial internal carotid, middle cerebral, and anterior cerebral artery circulation. These lesions develop and progress for months or years before symptoms develop. Prevention of stroke symptoms by hypertransfusion therapy is theoretically possible in patients at risk. Bone marrow transplantation has also proved curative in young patients with symptomatic sickle cell disease and has led to stabilization of nervous system vasculopathy, as documented by magnetic resonance imaging. Transcranial Doppler (TCD) is the most cost-effective method to screen for children at risk.

USE OF DOPPLER IN PREDICTING SICKLE CELL PATIENTS AT RISK FOR STROKE

Adams first showed the effectiveness of nonduplex (spectra without image) Doppler in screening for cerebrovascular disease in children with sickle cell disease. Using a transtemporal and suboccipital approach, Adams screened 190 asymptomatic sickle cell patients and found in clinical follow-up that a mean flow velocity in the MCA of 170 cm/s or greater was an indicator of a patient at risk for development of stroke. Adams then compared TCD to cerebral angiography in 33 neurologically symptomatic patients and found five criteria for cerebrovascular disease: (1) mean velocity of 190 cm/s, (2) low velocity in the MCA (<70 cm/s), (3) MCA ratio (lower or higher) of 0.5 or less, (4) anterior cerebral artery (ACA)/MCA ratio > 1.2 on the same side, and (5) inability to detect an MCA in the presence of a demonstrated ultrasound window. Using duplex Doppler, MRA, and magnetic resonance imaging (MRI), Seibert et al described their five indicators of cerebrovascular disease in sickle cell patients as (1) a maximum velocity in the ophthalmic artery (OA) > 35 cm/s, (2) mean velocity in the MCA > 170 cm/s, (3) resistive index (RI) in the OA < 50 (0.5), (4) velocity in the OA > that in the ipsilateral MCA, and (5) maximum velocity in the posterior cerebral (PCA), vertebral, or basilar arteries > maximum velocity in the MCA. An 8-year follow-up of 27 neurologically symptomatic and 90 asymptomatic sickle cell patients showed all five original TCD indicators of disease to be still significant. Four additional factors were also significant: (6) evidence of blood flow turbulence, (7) a PCA or ACA visualized without the MCA, (8) any RI < 30 (0.3), and

TABLE 33-1
Some Doppler Criteria for Sickle Cell Patients at Risk for Stroke

1. High velocity in the MCA [TAMX (mean) MCA velocity > 170–200 cm/s]
2. High velocity in the MCA [PSV > 200 cm/s; RI < 30 (or 0.3)]
3. Low velocity in the MCA (PSV < 70–100 cm/s; OA velocity > ipsilateral MCA velocity; or inability to detect MCA flow while noting it in other circle of Willis vessels)
4. High velocity in the OA [PSV – OA > 35 cm/s; RI in OA < 60 (or 0.6); velocity in the OA > that in the ipsilateral MCA]

MCA = middle cerebral artery, OA = ophthalmic artery, PSV = peak systolic velocity, RI = resistive index, TAMX = time averaged mean velocity.

(9) a maximum MCA velocity > 200 cm/s (Table 33-1). Siegel compared transtemporal TCD using duplex equipment to neurologic examination and also found a maximum flow in the MCA of >200 cm/s or <100 cm/s (including no flow) as significant for disease.

Verlhac et al studied sickle cell patients with duplex Doppler with a 3-MHz transducer transtemporally and suboccipitally, as well as with MRA and MRI. Arteriography was performed in cases where a stenosis was suspected on TCD. This group found that patients with a mean velocity of >190 cm/s had stenoses by arteriography. Kogutt et al also evaluated symptomatic sickle cell patients with duplex Doppler, MRI, and MRA and found TCD to have 91 percent sensitivity and 22 percent specificity, using MRA as the standard. Abnormal TCD values included (1) V_{max} and V_{mean} > 2 standard deviations from normal values reported by Adams in sickle cell patients: MCA V_{max} > 168 ± 38 cm/s and V_{mean} 115 ± 31 cm/s, (2) RI < 40, and (3) V_{max} MCA < V_{max} ACA.

TREATMENT POSSIBILITIES FOR THOSE AT RISK FOR STROKE

Adams reported the results of a clinical trial involving 130 sickle cell children between the ages of 2 and 16. In this multicenter controlled study, over 2000 sickle cell children had been screened by TCD for signs of cerebrovascular disease. Children with a mean velocity of the MCA of 200 cm/s or greater on two separate readings were randomized into two groups. One group of 67 children received standard supportive care. The other group of 63 children received periodic blood transfusions to maintain their hemoglobin S levels at or less than 30 percent. After one year, 10 children in the group receiving standard care had had a stroke, while only one child in the transfusion group had suffered a stroke. The results represent a 90 percent relative decline in stroke rate. On the basis of this, the National Institute of Health (NIH) now recommends that all children with sickle cell disease between the ages of 2 and 16 have TCD screening for cerebrovascular disease every 6 months.

ULTRASONOGRAPHIC TCD TECHNIQUE FOR ASSESSING VASCULAR FLOW IN SICKLERS

Our method for screening sickle cell patients with duplex Doppler involves scanning the patient transtemporally to evaluate the MCA, ACA, and PCA with a 2-MHz transducer. The OA should also be evaluated through the eye with a 7-MHz transducer on its lowest power setting. The OA was more sensitive than the MCA for detecting cerebrovascular abnormality in our series. The basilar and vertebral arteries can be evaluated from the occipital approach. This third area for insonation is probably not necessary in routine screening and may be necessary only when a good transtemporal window cannot be obtained. The maximum and mean velocities, as well as the RI, in each of these vessels should be measured at least twice. The highest velocity obtained can be taken as the truest velocity obtained at the best insonating angle. We use the nine described factors as indicators of cerebrovascular disease and recommend that if one of these factors is present, the patient should be evaluated by MRA for stenosis. The sensitivity of Doppler as a predictor of stroke from our investigation was 94 percent with a specificity of 51 percent.

EDITOR'S SOAPBOX

The work of Adams et al, Seibert et al, and others should be lauded. Use of the scientific method and an actual potential improvement in patient morbidity and mortality statistics as a result is an ideal that one often only strives for. They seem to have accomplished it. The time and effort involved in research, including imaging research, can be a most beneficial thing to spend one's tax dollars on.

EDITOR'S PRACTICAL IMAGING POINT

Information can be obtained by ultrasound (US) after closure of the fontanelles. This is obviously true with intraoperative work, where a transducer is placed on the operative site in the brain or spine. I have on occasion needed US to image a known abnormality seen by preoperative imaging examinations but difficult to see at operation. A high-frequency transducer and color Doppler helped. This is also true with transcranial work, discussed in this chapter. Many criteria were discussed. Detecting mean MCA velocities > 170 cm/s can be easy to note with modern machinery, particularly with the position and angle of the near-field MCA almost parallel to the insonating US beam when the transducer is placed in transtemporal position anterior to the ear. Seibert's results with ophthalmic artery insonation (abnormal flow at a maximal velocity of 35 cm/s or greater) even with the warning of limiting eye exposure to ultrasound energy, sounds encouraging.

References

Adams RJ, Aaslid R, Gammal TE, et al: Detection of cerebral vasculopathy in sickle cell disease using transcranial Doppler ultrasonography and magnetic resonance imaging: Case report. *Stroke* 19:518–520, 1988.

Adams R, McKie V, Nichols F, et al: The use of transcranial ultrasonography to predict stroke in sickle cell disease. *N Engl J Med* 326:605–610, 1992.

Adams RJ, Nichols FT III, Aaslid R, et al: Cerebral vessel stenosis in sickle cell disease: Criteria for detection by transcranial Doppler. *Am J Pediatr Hematol Oncol* 12:277–282, 1990.

Adams RJ, Nichols FT, Figueroa R, et al: Transcranial Doppler correlation with cerebral angiography in sickle cell disease. *Stroke* 23:1073–1077, 1992.

Adams RJ, Nichols FT, McKie VC, et al: Transcranial Doppler: Influence of hematocrit in children with sickle cell anemia without stroke. *J Cardiovasc Tech* 8:97–101, 1989.

Huttenlocher PR, Moohr JW, Johns I, Brown FD: Cerebral blood flow in sickle cell cerebrovascular disease. *Pediatrics* 73: 615–621, 1984.

Kogutt MS, Goldwag SS, Gupta KL, et al: Correlation of transcranial Doppler ultrasonography with MRI and MRA in the evaluation of sickle cell disease patients with prior stroke. *Pediatr Radiol* 24:204–206, 1994.

NIH: Clinical alert: Periodic Transfusion Lower Stroke Risk in Children with Sickle Cell Anemia, National Heart Lung Blood Institute (NHLBI), Sept. 18, 1997.

Powars D, Wilson B, Imbus C, et al: The natural history of stroke in sickle cell disease. *Am J Med* 65:461–471, 1978.

Seibert JJ, Glasier CM, Allison JW, et al: Transcranial Doppler (TCD), MRA, and MRI as a screening examination for cerebral vascular disease in patients with sickle cell anemia: A four-year follow-up. Presented at Third Conjoint Meeting, International Pediatric Radiology, Boston, MA, May 1996.

Seibert JJ, Miller SF, Kirby RS, et al: Cerebrovascular disease in symptomatic and asymptomatic patients with sickle cell anemia: Screening with duplex transcranial Doppler US—correlation with MR imaging and MR angiography. *Radiology* 189: 457–466, 1993.

Siegel MJ, Luker GD, Glauser TA, DeBaum MR: Cerebral infarction in sickle cell disease: Transcranial Doppler US versus neurologic examination. *Radiology* 197:191–194, 1995.

Verlhac S, Bernaudin F, Tortrat D, et al: Detection of cerebrovascular disease in patients with sickle cell disease using transcranial Doppler sonography: Correlation with MRI, MRA, and conventional angiography. *Pediatr Radiol* 25:S14–S19.

Waters MC, Patience M, Leisenring W, et al: Bone marrow transplantation for sickle cell disease. *N Engl J Med* 335:369–376, 1996.

34

Figure 34-1 shows a 2-day-old infant with congenital cytomegalovirus infection. What do you see? What are your diagnostic considerations?

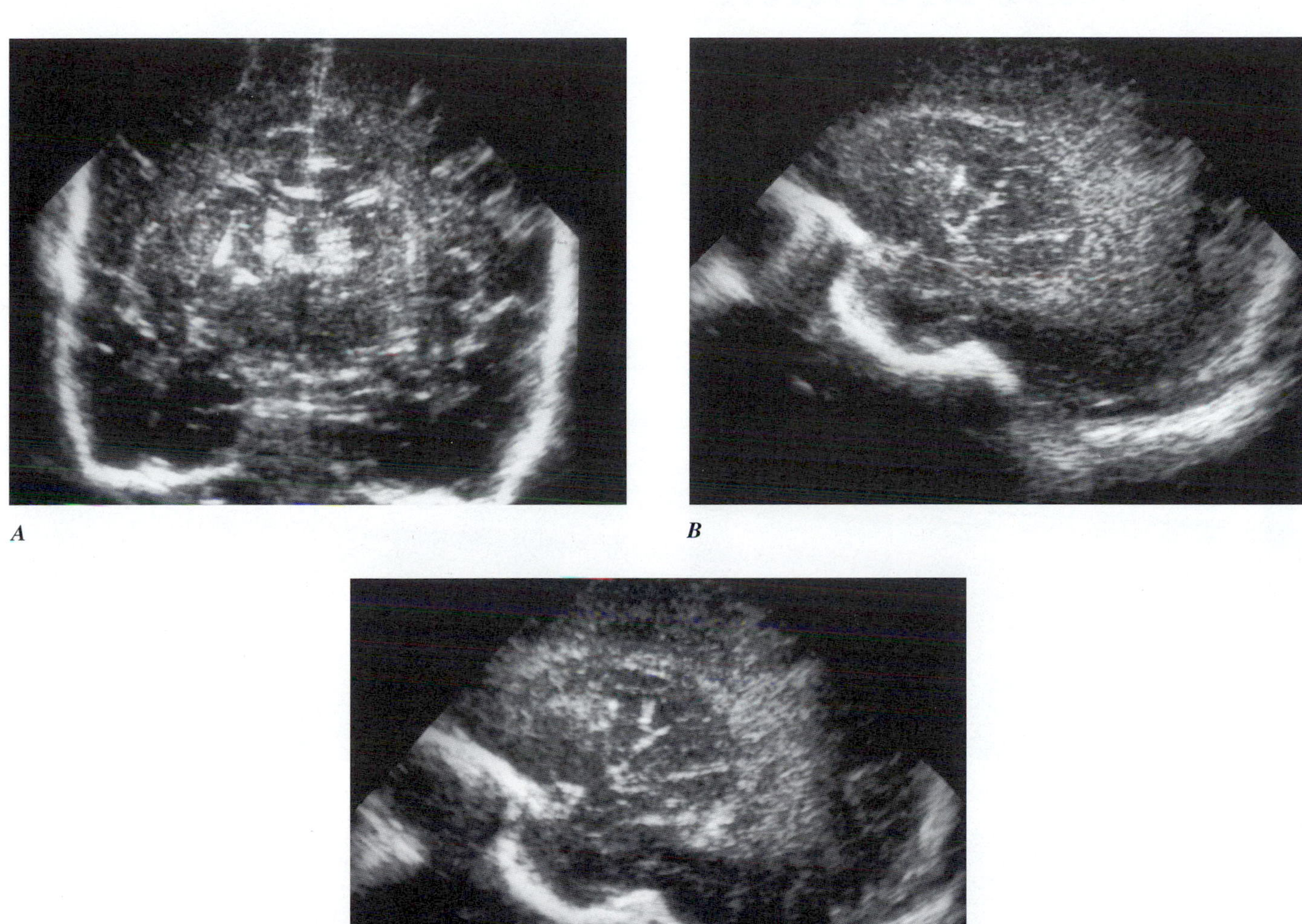

A *B* *C*

FIGURE 34–1. Coronal *(A)*, right longitudinal *(B)*, and left longitudinal *(C)* views through the head.

CHAPTER 34

Lenticulostriate Vasculopathy

CARLOS J. SIVIT

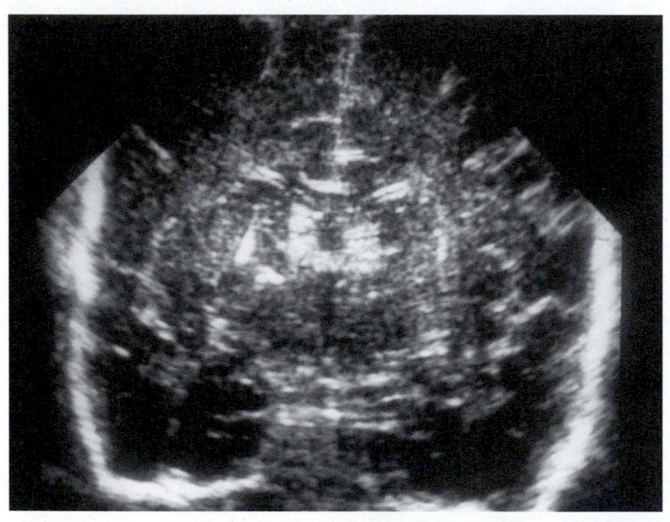

A

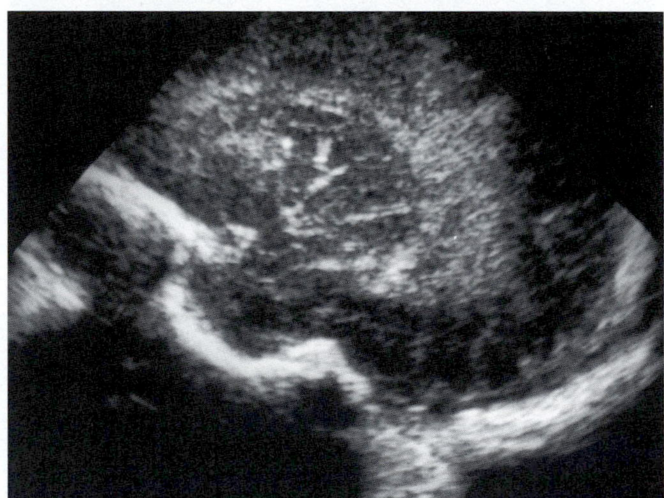

B

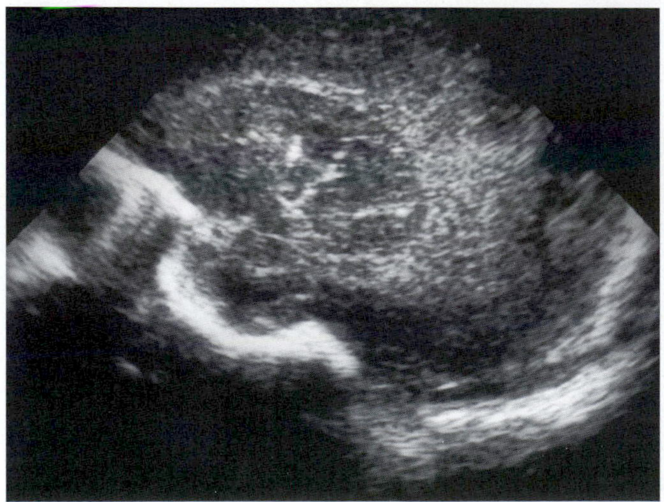

C

FIGURE 34–2. Lenticulostriate vasculopathy. Coronal views at the level of the frontal horns of the lateral ventricles ***(A)*** and longitudinal views through the right ***(B)*** and left ***(C)*** cerebral hemispheres demonstrate linear, branching echogenic areas in the thalamus and basal ganglia bilaterally, consistent with lenticulostriate vasculopathy. Note that there is no posterior acoustic shadowing associated with the echogenic areas.

Linear or branching areas of echogenicity may be demonstrated in the thalami and basal ganglia of some infants (Fig. 34-2). These areas have been shown at histopathology to represent mineralized deposits in arterial walls and perivascular infiltration of mononuclear cells secondary to inflammatory or necrotizing vasculitis. They are predominantly seen surrounding the lenticulostriate branches of the middle cerebral arteries, the medium-sized arteries within the thalamus and basal ganglia. This is a region with active cellular proliferation and high blood flow. The sonographic finding has been termed lenticulostriate vasculopathy. It has been associated

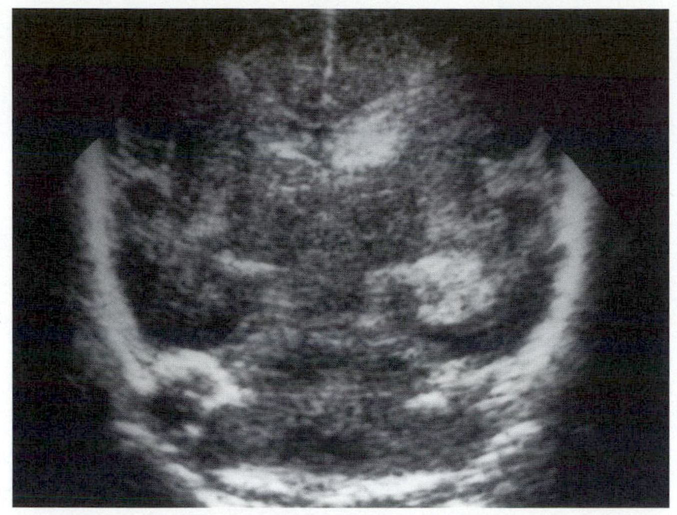

A

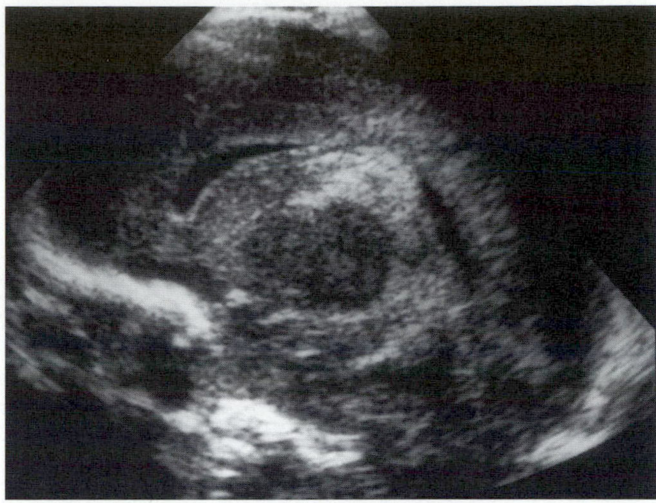

B

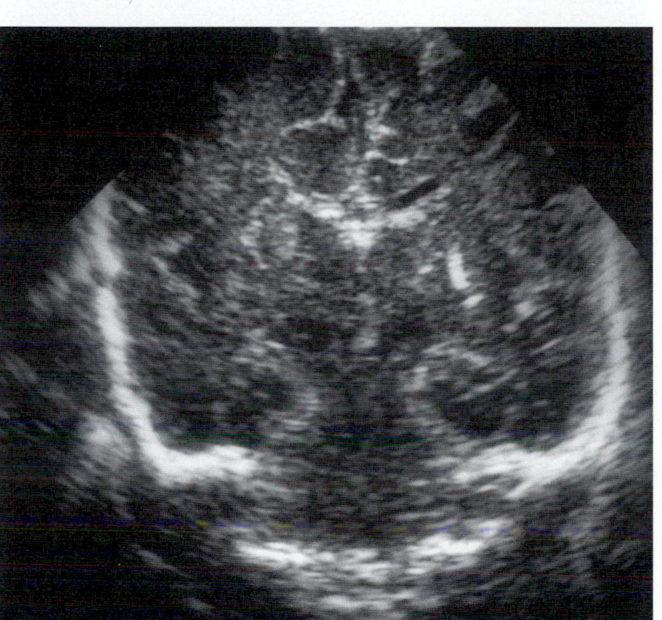

C

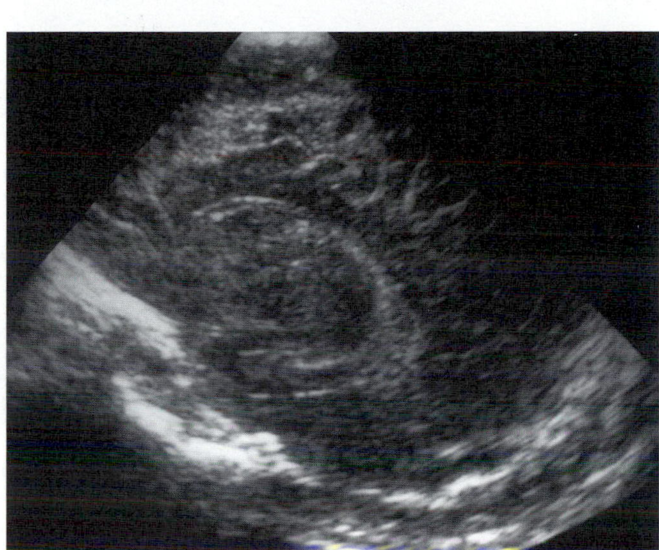

D

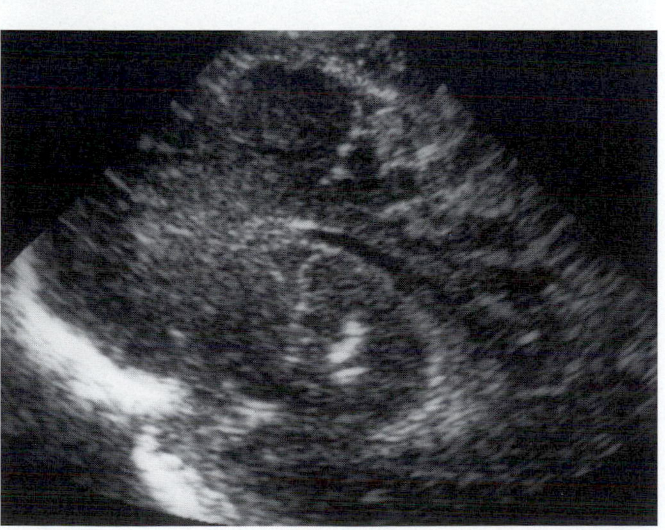

E

FIGURE 34–3. Unilateral lenticulostriate vasculopathy associated with prior intraventricular hemorrhage. Coronal view through the lateral ventricles ***(A)*** and longitudinal view through the left lateral ventricle ***(B)*** in a 5-day-old premature infant demonstrate unilateral, left-sided subependymal and intraventricular hemorrhage. At follow-up examination 3 months later, coronal view through the lateral ventricles ***(C)*** and longitudinal views through the right ***(D)*** and left ***(E)*** lateral ventricles demonstrate resolution of the left-sided intraventricular hemorrhage and the development of unilateral left-sided lenticulostriate vasculopathy.

with various congenital infections, including syphilis, rubella, toxoplasmosis, and cytomegalovirus. The finding has also been associated with chromosomal abnormalities (trisomies 13 and 21), fetal alcohol syndrome, twin-to-twin transfusion syndrome, bacterial meningitis, and perinatal asphyxia. Additionally, in some cases there is no known etiology for this condition. Therefore, lenticulostriate vasculopathy probably represents a nonspecific response to vascular injury.

The sonographic findings of lenticulostriate vasculopathy may be unilateral (Figs. 34-3 and 34-4) or bilateral (Fig. 34-2).

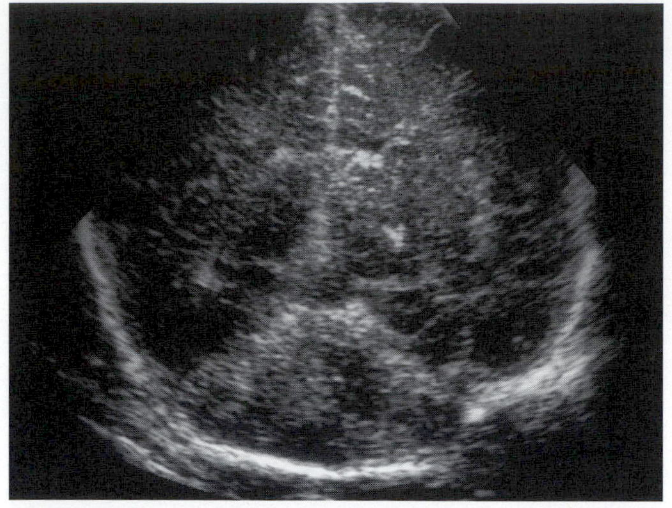

A

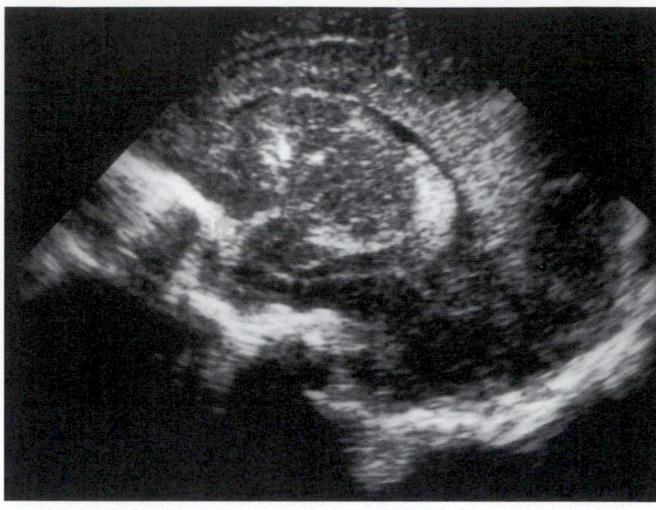

B

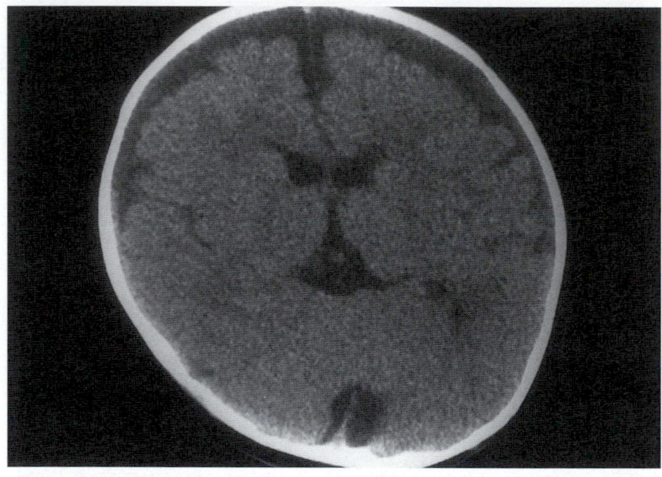

C

FIGURE 34–4. Unilateral lenticulostriate vasculopathy with normal brain parenchyma on computed tomography (CT). Coronal ***(A)*** and left longitudinal ***(B)*** views through the neonatal head demonstrate a linear area of echogenicity consistent with unilateral left-sided lenticulostriate vasculopathy. A CT scan through the level of the basal ganglia and thalamus ***(C)*** in the same infant does not demonstrate any parenchymal abnormalities. Note that there is increased extraaxial fluid in the frontal region.

Unilateral disease is noted in approximately 20 percent of cases. Lenticulostriate vasculopathy may be observed in the first week of life. It also may be initially observed at several months of life in infants who have had prior normal sonograms. The echogenic linear or branching bands typically are not associated with posterior acoustic shadowing. These bands are observed to be in a perivascular distribution when imaged with color Doppler (Fig. 34-5).

Lenticulostriate vasculopathy may be observed as an isolated finding or associated with other abnormalities at neurosonography, including subependymal cysts (Fig. 34-6), periventricular calcifications, and ventriculomegaly. It may also be noted in infants with prior intraventricular hemorrhage (Fig. 34-3). Computed tomography (CT) scanning in infants with lenticulostriate vasculopathy may demonstrate parenchymal calcifications or infarction in the basal ganglia or thalamus. However, the calcifications noted at CT are discrete and punctate. They do not follow a linear "perivascular" pattern, as is seen in sonography. The cranial CT scan may also be normal (Fig. 34-4). Follow-up sonographic assessment in infants with lenticulostriate vasculopathy typically demonstrates persistence of the echogenic regions.

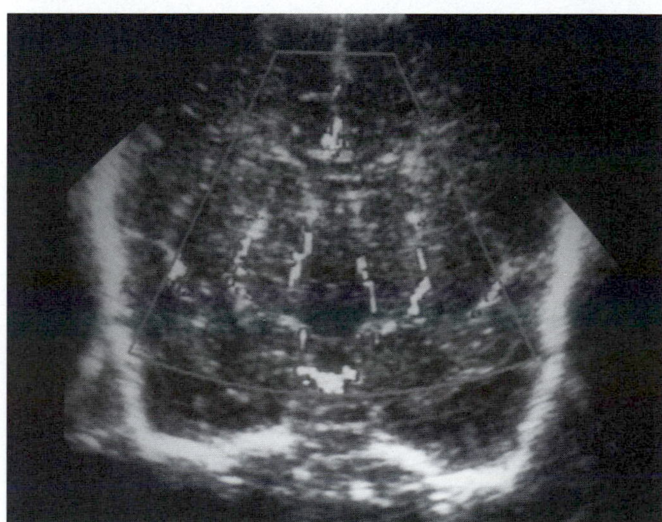

FIGURE 34–5. Color Doppler sonography demonstrating perivascular distribution of lenticulostriate vasculopathy. Coronal view utilizing color Doppler imaging in the same infant as in Fig. 34-1 demonstrates flow in the thalamostriate arteries parallel to the branching echogenic areas seen bilaterally in the thalamus and basal ganglia in Fig. 34-1.

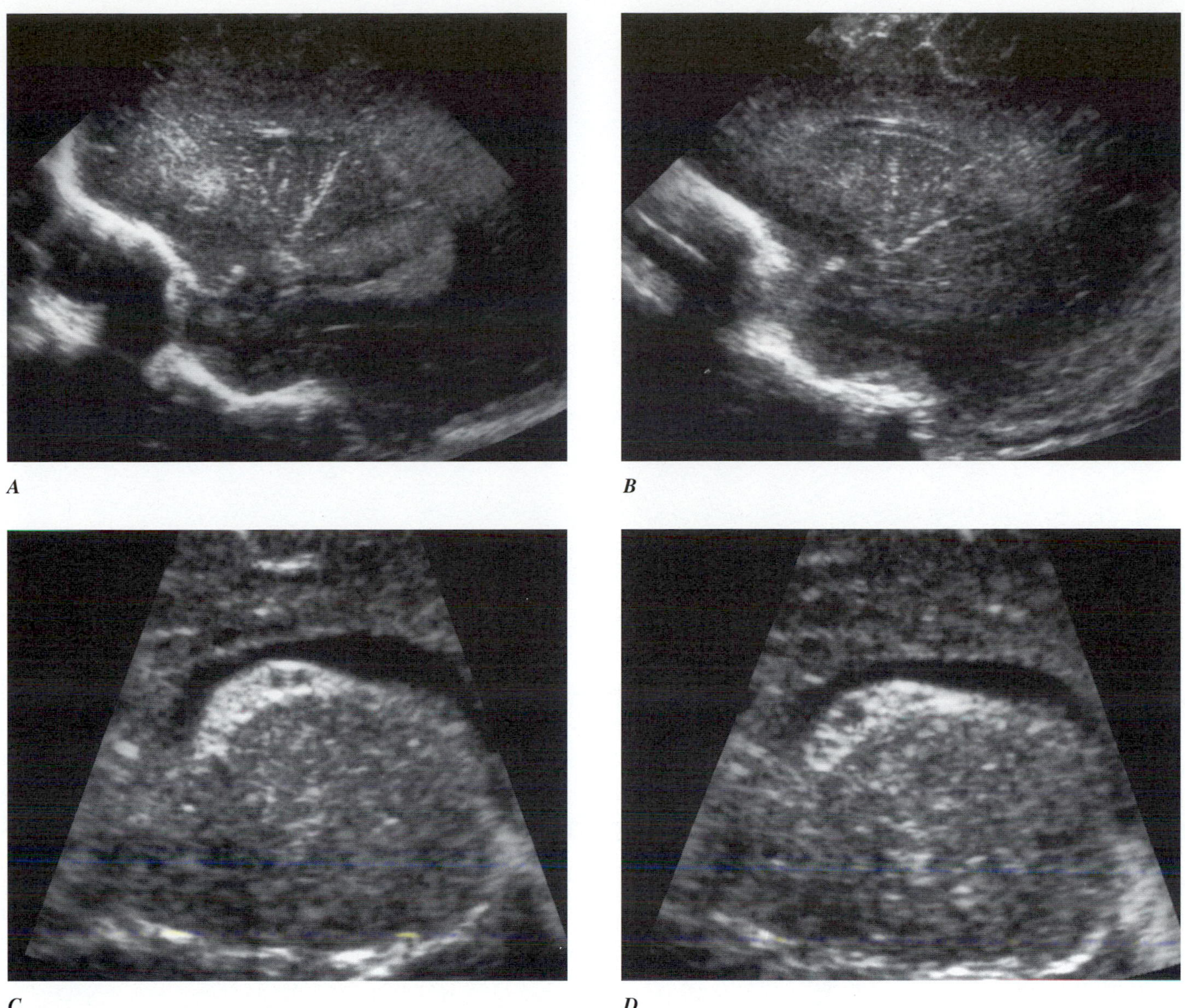

FIGURE 34–6. Lenticulostriate vasculopathy associated with periventricular cysts. Longitudinal views through the right *(A)* and left *(B)* cerebral hemispheres demonstrate branching echogenic areas bilaterally, consistent with lenticulostriate vasculopathy. Longitudinal views at the level of the right *(C)* and left *(D)* lateral ventricles in the same infant demonstrate bilateral subependymal cysts.

The sonographic finding of lenticulostriate vasculopathy should prompt close neurologic and imaging follow-up. The finding is a strong predictor of later neurologic sequelae. This is not surprising, since the lenticulostriate vasculopathy probably represents a nonspecific response to perinatal anoxia or ischemia. Developmental and gross motor delay have been frequently reported on follow-up neurologic assessment in these infants. Deafness may also be seen.

References

Babcock DS, Ball W: Postasphyxial encephalopathy in full-term infants: Ultrasound diagnosis. *Radiology* 148:417–423, 1983.

Ben-Ami T, Yousefzadeh D, Backus M, et al: Lenticulostriate vasculopathy in infants with infections of the central nervous system: Sonographic and doppler findings. *Pediatr Radiol* 20: 575–579, 1990.

DeVries LS, Beek FJA, Stoutenbeck P: Lenticulostriate vasculopathy in twin-to-twin transfusion syndrome: Sonographic and CT findings. *Pediatr Radiol* 25:41–42, 1995.

Grant EG, Williams AL, Schellinger D, et al: Intracranial calcification in the infant and neonate: Evaluation by sonography and CT. *Radiology* 157:63–68, 1985.

Hughes P, Weinberger E, Shaw DWW: Linear areas of echogenicity in the thalami and basal ganglia of neonates: An expanded association. *Radiology* 179:103–105, 1991.

Ries M, Deeg KH, Heininger U: Demonstration of perivascular echogenicities in congenital cytomegalovirus infection by colour doppler imaging. *Eur J Pediatr* 150:34–36, 1990.

Teele RL, Hernanz-Schulman M, Sotrel A: Echogenic vasculature in the basal ganglia of neonates: A sonographic sign of vasculopathy. *Radiology* 169:423–427, 1988.

Wang H, Kuo M, Chang T: Sonographic lenticulostriate vasculopathy in infants: Some associations and a hypothesis. *AJNR* 16:97–102, 1995.

35

A 5-month-old girl with a deep cutaneous dimple in her sacrococcygeal region was examined by ultrasound (US). Figures 35-1, 35-2, and 35-3 are brought to you for interpretation. What do you see? Is there anything to worry about?

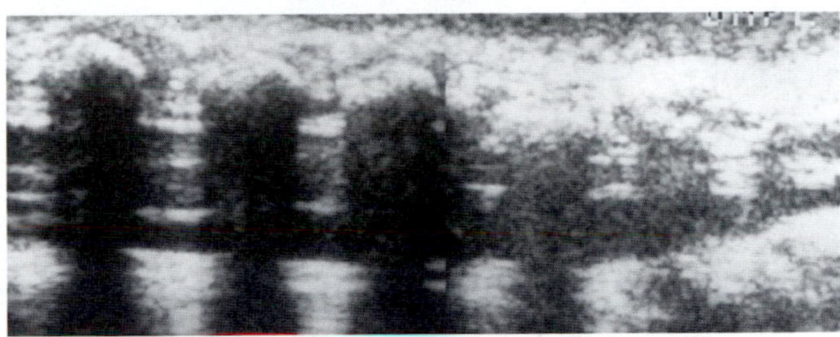

FIGURE 35–1. Ultrasound of spine. Longitudinal midline plane composite sonogram of the lumbosacral region (caudad is toward the reader's right).

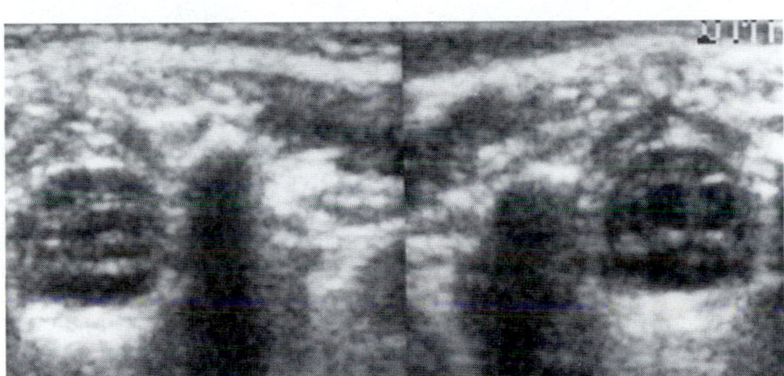

FIGURE 35–2. Ultrasound of spine. Transverse plane at two levels: high lumbar (*on left*) and mid to low lumbar (*on right*).

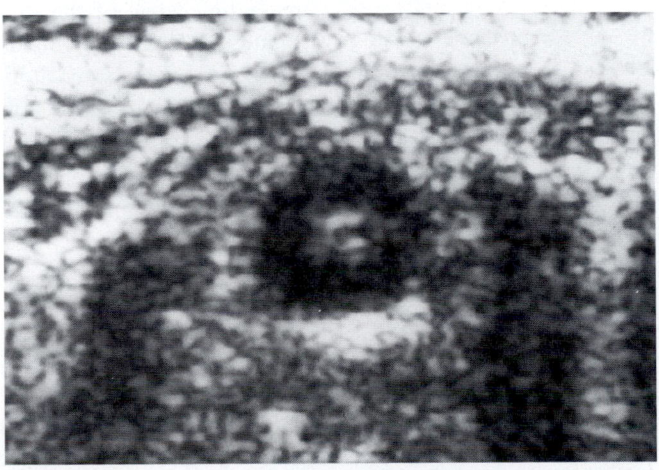

FIGURE 35–3. Ultrasound of spine. Transverse plane at a third level: the sacrum.

CHAPTER 35

Tethered Spinal Cord

MICHAEL A. DIPIETRO

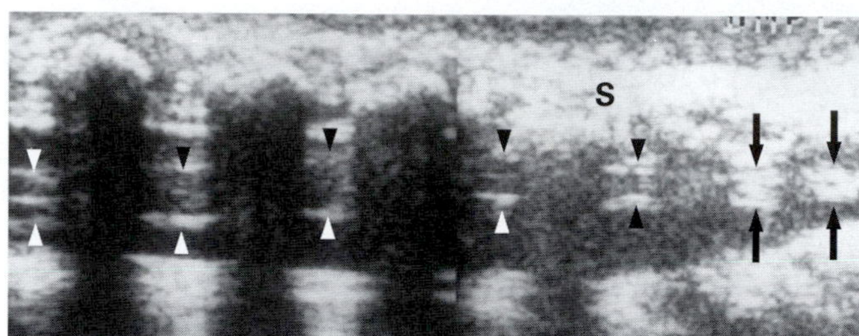

FIGURE 35–4. Annotated version of Fig. 35-1. Tethered cord with thick filum terminale. Ultrasound of spine. Longitudinal midline plane composite sonogram of the lumbosacral region (caudad is toward the reader's right). This composite panoramic view was obtained by carefully aligning views of two adjacent sections of the lumbosacral spine. The spinal cord (*arrowheads*) extends caudally and dorsally into the sacral (S) portion of the spinal canal, far below its normal caudal extent and indicative of being tethered. The cord's most caudal portion, the filum terminale (*arrow*), is abnormally thick and echogenic from infiltrated fat.

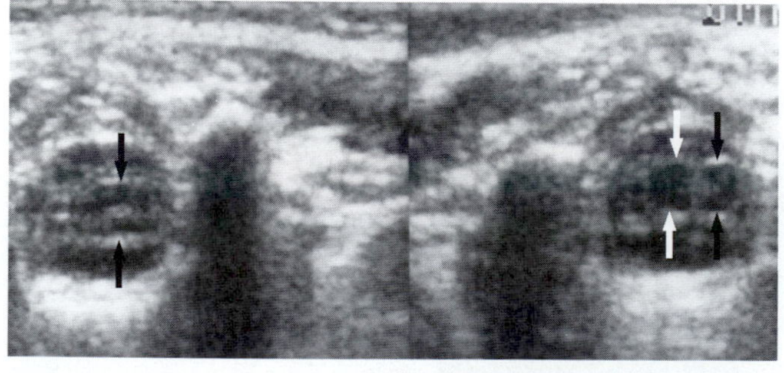

FIGURE 35–5. Annotated version of Fig. 35-2. Tethered cord with caudal diastematomyelia. Ultrasound of spine. Transverse plane at two levels: high lumbar (*on left*) and mid to low lumbar (*on right*). The high lumbar image shows a normal cord (*arrows*) within the vertebral column. The mid to low lumbar image shows the cord to be split into two parts. Arrows point to each hemicord. The splitting of the cord in a lower than normal position suggests a tethered cord with diastematomyelia.

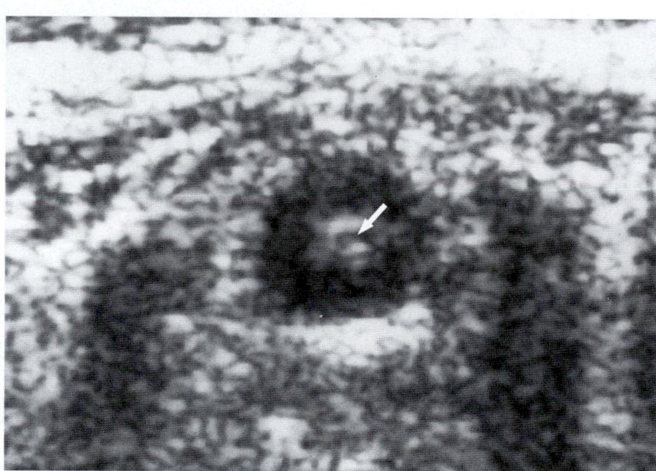

FIGURE 35–6. Annotated version of Fig. 35-3. Ultrasound of spine. Transverse plane at a third level: the sacrum. The cord is far too caudad in the spinal canal. Its most caudal portion, the filum terminale (*arrow*), is thick and echogenic from infiltrated fat.

Figure 35-4, the annotated version of Fig. 35-1, is a panoramic view of the infant's spine in longitudinal plane. Figure 35-5, the annotated version of Fig. 35-2, is a transverse view of the same at high lumbar and mid to low lumbar levels. Figure 35-6 is a transverse view of the cord at sacral level. The cord extends too low in the spinal canal, it is thickened, and it is split caudally. These findings are consistent with a tethered spinal cord with a thick filum terminale and diastematomyelia.

WHAT SHOULD BE SEEN NORMALLY IN A SPINAL CORD ULTRASOUND

The unknown figures can be compared to those of a normal infant (Fig. 35-7), whose cord termination, the tip of the conus medullaris, is usually at vertebral body L2 level. Only the echogenic cauda equina extends into the lower lumbar and sacral canal.

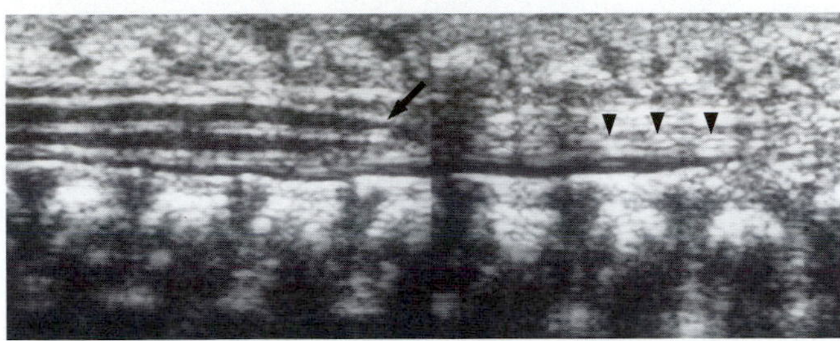

FIGURE 35–7. Normal spinal cord. Longitudinal midline plane composite sonogram of the lumbosacral region (caudad is toward the reader's right). Note that unlike in Fig. 35-4, the cord ends in the high lumbar region (*arrow*). This proved to be the level of the second lumbar vertebral body (L2). Only the cauda equina (*arrowheads*) extends into the lower lumbar and sacral canal.

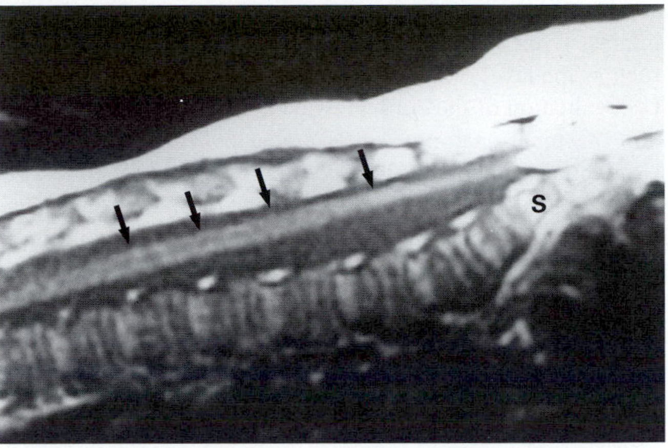

FIGURE 35–8. Tethered cord. Magnetic resonance imaging. Longitudinal plane. T1-weighted images. The cord is the medium-signal tubular structure (*arrows*) that extends caudally into the sacral area (S). This is far below the acceptable inferior extent of the conus just above the L2–L3 disc space.

MORE IMAGING INFORMATION ABOUT THE TETHERED CORD—MAGNETIC RESONANCE IMAGING AND OSCILLATIONS ON REAL-TIME ULTRASOUND

Corresponding longitudinal (Fig. 35-8) and transverse (Fig. 35-9) magnetic resonance (MR) images of the tethered cord corroborate the US findings. During real-time sonography, oscillations of the caudal portion of the tethered spinal cord were noted to be dampened, i.e., less apparent than usual. Normal brisk oscillations of the cord at the heart's rate were noted at the upper lumbar and thoracic levels. A focal dampening of oscillation would suggest that the cord is not as free as usual and therefore suggests tethering. This tethered cord, evaluated by US and MR, shows the classic "low down, stuck up" location of a tethered cord within the spinal canal.

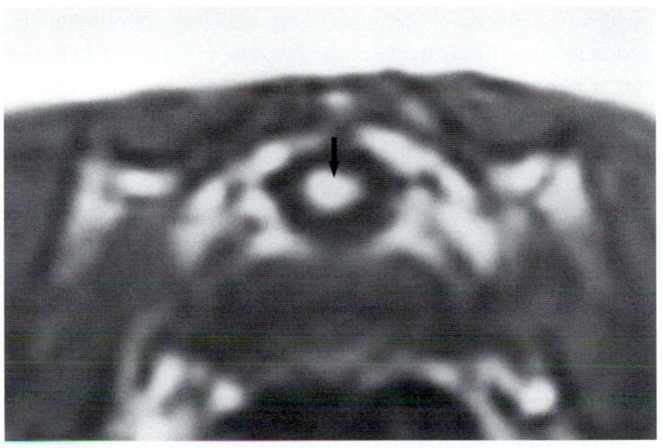

FIGURE 35–9. Tethered cord. Magnetic resonance imaging. Transverse plane. Low lumbar/sacral area. T1-weighted image. The image is positioned as if the baby were prone. Fat is of great signal intensity on T1-weighted images. The white material (*arrow*) within the spinal canal is consistent with the fat that has infiltrated the filum terminale.

SURGICAL FINDINGS AND THERAPY

No osseous, cartilaginous, or fibrous band separating the hemicords was evident on either sonography or MRI. However, a midline fibrous band was revealed at surgery. It extended dorsally from between the arachnoid coverings of each hemicord to a common dura, to which it was tethered at several points. A thick, fat-infiltrated filum terminale arose from the caudal aspect of the reunited cord. The cord was untethered by releasing the fibrous bands of the diastematomyelia and by cutting the thick filum terminale caudal to any functional neural elements.

WHAT IS SPINAL CORD TETHERING AND WHY IS THE DIAGNOSIS IMPORTANT?

Spinal cord tethering refers to abnormal fixation of the cord. There are multiple pathologic causes, including a mass such as an intraspinal lipoma; an osseous, fibrous, or cartilaginous septum in cases of diastematomyelia; or fibrous or fatty infiltration of the cord's distal filum terminale. Early diagnosis and treatment can prevent the cord ischemia that develops secondary to traction as the child grows in height. Progressive neurologic, urologic, and orthopedic deformity may occur if the tethered cord is not diagnosed and treated.

This case is somewhat unusual because it had abnormal fixation from both fatty infiltration of the filum terminale and a diastematomyelia. The case is also clinically unusual because the vast majority of dorsal midline cutaneous dimples found in the *low* sacrococcygeal region are not associated with an occult tethered cord. The usual tethered cord is seen in conjunction with a higher sacral or lumbar dimple or with other midline dorsal cutaneous and subcutaneous stigmata, such as lipomas, hemangiomas, sinuses, hairy tufts, and aplasia cutis.

Many infants with cutaneous dimples undergo a screening sonogram of their spinal cord, which in this case demonstrated all the pathology. Subsequent MRI showed the fatty filum more dramatically, but was otherwise merely confirmatory and revealed no new finding. Carefully performed sonography can reveal much or all of the pathology in such infants. Even in older children, at least limited information, such as the level of the conus medullaris, may be obtained by US evaluation of the cord. However, the difference in resolution of spinal anatomy demonstrated by MRI, compared to US, increases markedly beyond infancy and early childhood. As the spinal column becomes larger and more bony, penetration by a high-frequency transducer for fine resolution of the cord becomes more and more difficult. That is not to say that fine resolution of the cord cannot be obtained using such transducers intraoperatively.

TECHNIQUE OF SPINAL SONOGRAPHY

Ultrasound of the spine is performed over the back. Neonates and infants are most easily scanned, but limited views can be obtained in older children. The patient is usually prone, but a decubitus or sitting posture can also be used. It is most important that the patient be flexed adequately to separate the posterior vertebral elements and thereby maximize the acoustic window. However, one must be careful not to hyperflex a neonate or infant and compromise respiration. I prefer to use a linear array transducer at the highest frequency (usually between 7 and 12 MHz) that allows adequate penetration to the anterior border of the spinal canal. The superficial tissues should be studied at the higher frequencies.

The tip of the conus medullaris is normally at or above the superior aspect of L3. In contrast, the tethered cord usually extends too far caudally. It is also usually eccentric (often dorsal) within the low lumbar and sacral spinal canal. A cause for the tethering, such as a lipoma or a thick filum terminale, is often identified. After the first postnatal month, the spinal cord and cauda equina usually oscillate briskly at the cardiac rate. (The normal neonatal cord might *not* oscillate.) This oscillation can be documented on M mode, but I have not found that to be useful. Oscillation is usually more apparent when the persistence or frame averaging is minimized or eliminated. In cases of tethered spinal cord, the oscillations are often progressively damped as one scans closer to the point of tethering. However, the cord often oscillates normally at points distant (sometimes only a few vertebral levels) from the area of tethering. In the young infant, oscillations may be brisk and not be damped at the point of tethering. If the cord is not untethered, damping will develop as the child grows and presumably the cord is stretched. This dynamic property of the spinal cord is more easily demonstrated on sonography than on MRI. I have been asked to look for cord oscillations in cases with equivocal MRI findings.

EDITOR'S NOTE

For those who do not perform spine US, it is fun, it is easy, and the information is useful. The last paragraphs of this chapter provide some key technical tips from an expert on this examination.

References

Brühl K, Schwarz M, Schumacher R, et al: Congenital diastematomyelia in the upper thoracic spine. Diagnostic comparison of CT, CT-myelography, MRI and US. *Neurosurg Rev* 13:77–82, 1990.

DiPietro MA: The conus medullaris: Normal US findings throughout childhood. *Radiology* 188:149–153, 1993.

DiPietro MA: The pediatric spinal canal, in *Diagnostic Ultrasound,* 2d ed, Rumack CM, Wilson SR, Charboneau JW (eds). Chicago, Mosby–Year Book,1998:1589–1615.

Gusnard DA, Naidich TP, Yousefzadeh DK, et al: Ultrasonic anatomy of the normal neonatal and infant spine: Correlation with cryomicrotome sections and CT. *Neuroradiology* 28: 493–511, 1986.

Kirpekar M, Cohen HL: Ultrasonography of the neonatal spine, in *Ultrasonography of the Prenatal and Neonatal Brain,* Timor-Tritsch I, Monteagudo A, Cohen HL (eds). Stamford, CT, Appleton & Lange, 1996:287–298.

Korsvik HE, Keller MS: Sonography of occult dysraphism in neonates and infants with MR imaging correlation. *Radiographics* 12:297–306, 1992.

Nelson MD Jr, Segall HD, Gwinn JL: Sonography in newborns with cutaneous manifestations of spinal abnormalities. *Am Fam Physician* 40:198–203, 1989.

Raghavendra BN, Epstein FJ, Pinto RS, et al: Sonographic diagnosis of diastematomyelia. *J Ultrasound Med* 7:111–113, 1988.

Rohrschneider WK, Forsting M, Darge K, Troger J: Diagnostic value of spinal US: Comparative study with MR in pediatric patients. *Radiology* 200:383–388, 1996.

Wolf S, Schneble F, Troger J: The conus medullaris: Time of ascendance to normal level. *Pediatr Radiol* 22:590–592, 1992.

Zieger M, Dörr U: Pediatric spinal sonography. Part I: Anatomy and examination technique. *Pediatr Radiol* 18:9–13, 1988.

Zieger M, Dörr U, Schulz RD: Pediatric spinal sonography. Part II: Malformations and mass lesions. *Pediatr Radiol* 18:105–111, 1988.

36

This is a newborn with a hairy tuft in the skin at the lumbar area of the spine. Figure 36-1 is a transverse section through the thoracic spine. What do you see? What is the diagnosis?

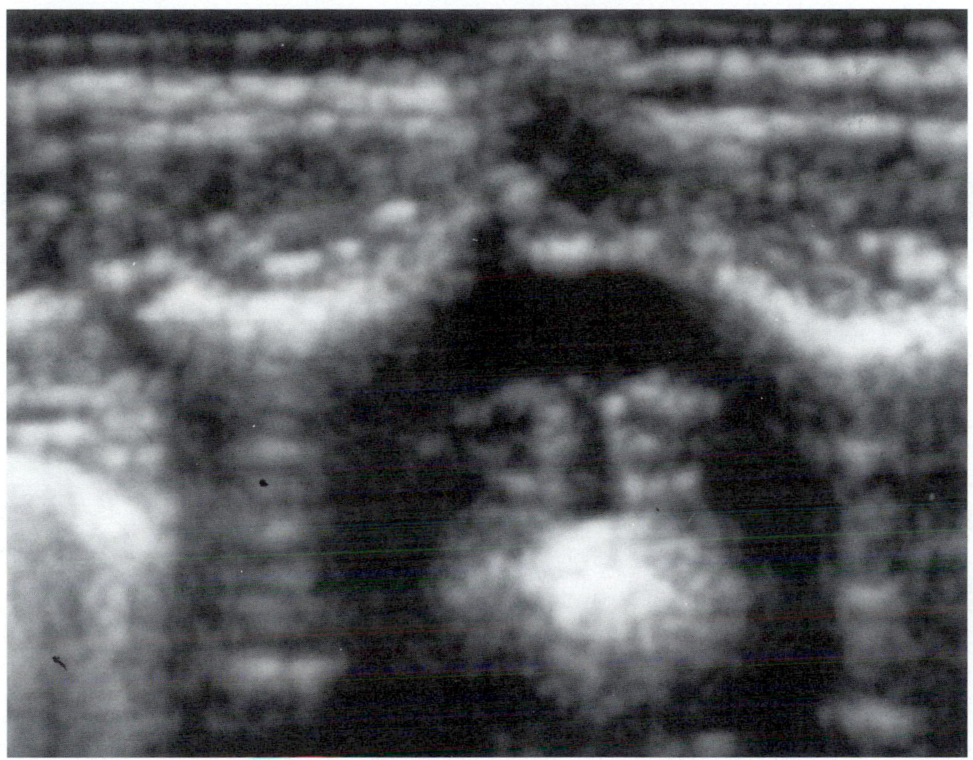

FIGURE 36–1. Spinal ultrasound. Axial view.

CHAPTER 36

Diastematomyelia

MADHURI KIRPEKAR

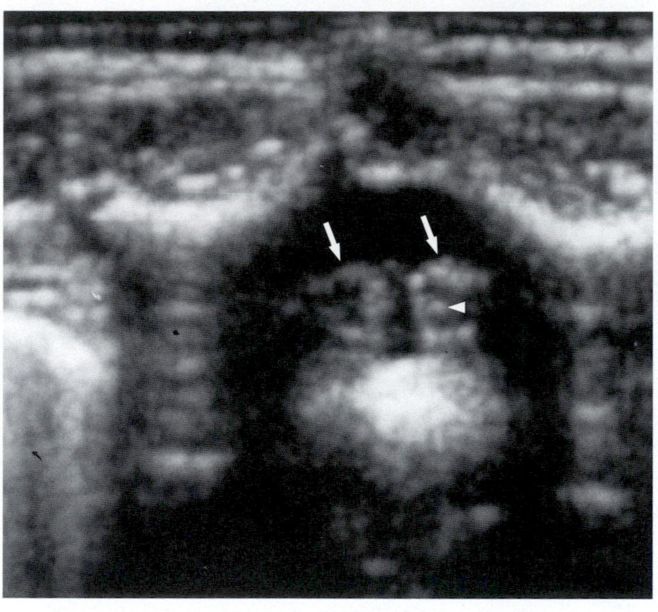

FIGURE 36–2. Annotated version of Fig. 36-1. Diastematomyelia. Spine ultrasound. Transverse plane. The examined child is in prone position. Two hemicords (*arrows*) are noted within the vertebral canal. The small white dot (*arrowhead*) in the hemicord on the reader's right is what has been labeled by some as the spinal canal and by others as its simulator caused by decussating neural fibers near the spinal canal.

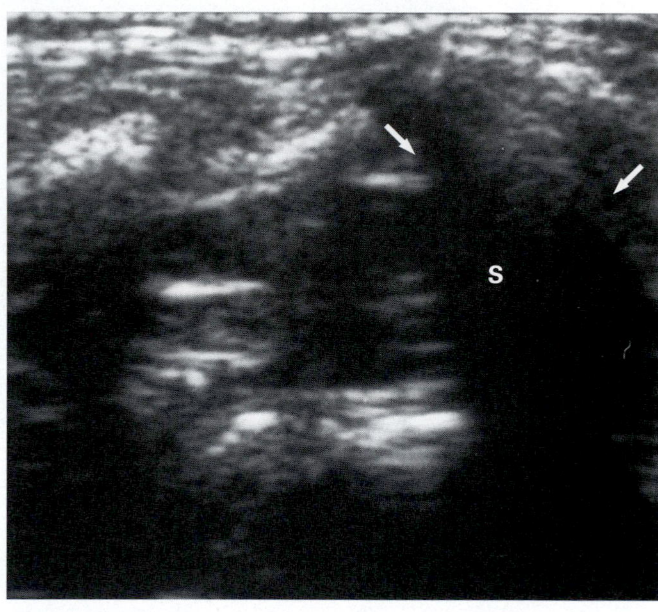

FIGURE 36–3. Diastematomyelia with associated bone spur. Spine ultrasound. Longitudinal plane. Arrows define an area with posterior shadowing (s) deep to it. This is due to a bony spur that split the cord. The hemicords could not be well imaged at this site.

Figure 36-2, the annotated version of Fig. 36-1, is the ultrasound (US) image of a newborn with two hemicords rather than a single spinal cord found within his vertebral canal. Each hemicord contains its own central canal. On a longitudinal view of the spine (Fig. 36-3), there is a linear echogenic density that crosses the spinal canal and causes posterior shadowing of the US image. This is due to a bony spur. When present in the spinal column, bony spurs can cause abnormal fixation of the spinal cord and symptomatology. The diagnosis in this case is two hemicords, or diastematomyelia.

WHAT IS DIASTEMATOMYELIA?

The term *diastematomyelia* is derived from the Greek *diastema*, meaning "cleft." It is a form of spinal dysraphism involving a sagittal cleft in the spinal cord with splaying of the posterior spinal elements. The cleft may be caused by a bony, fibrous, or cartilaginous spur and results in a segmental duplication of the cord with the formation of two hemicords (Fig. 36-4). Each hemicord contains a central canal and one set of ventral and dorsal nerve roots, as would be seen in the

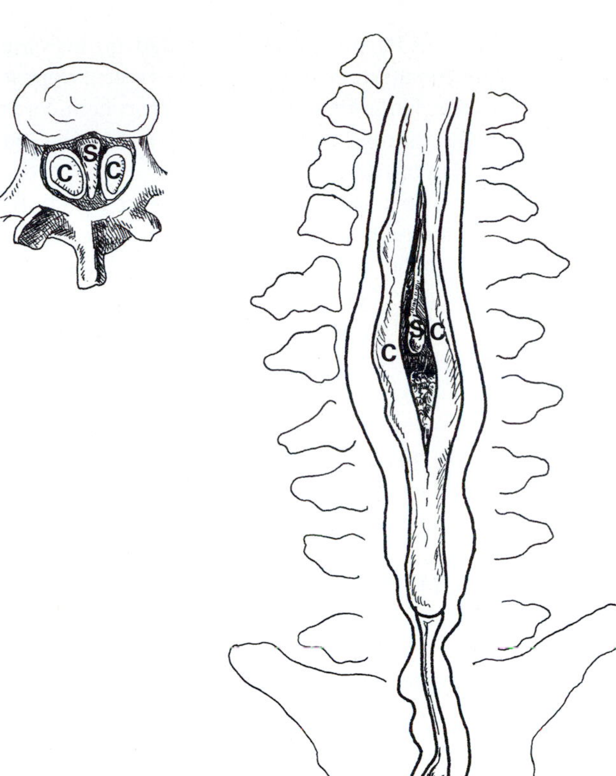

FIGURE 36–4. Drawings of diastematomyelia. The drawing on the reader's left shows two hemicords (C) within a vertebral body. A bony spur (S) is seen between them. V = anterior vertebral body. The drawing on the reader's right is a coronal view of the spinal column with the anterior and posterior vertebral body elements removed. The two hemicords (C) are seen to connect both superiorly and inferiorly. The bony spur (S) is seen between them.

single normal cord. In 50 percent of cases, the two hemicords share a single dural tube. In the remaining 50 percent, the two hemicords are enveloped by separate dural sacs. The two hemicords of diastematomyelia may be asymmetric. They may rejoin as a single cord at a point caudal to the cleft. They are typically side by side in position but can also acquire some degree of ventral-dorsal relationship, especially if the patient has an associated scoliosis.

ASSOCIATED SPINE AND CORD ABNORMALITIES

As might be expected, diastematomyelia is frequently associated with vertebral malformations. A large percentage of these patients have congenital scoliosis. The most frequent concomitant cord abnormality is hydromyelia, in which there is a dilated fluid-filled central spinal canal or other cystic fluid-containing area within the cord substance. Typically, patients with diastematomyelia have a low-lying conus medullaris, as discussed in Chap. 35. In over 90 percent of

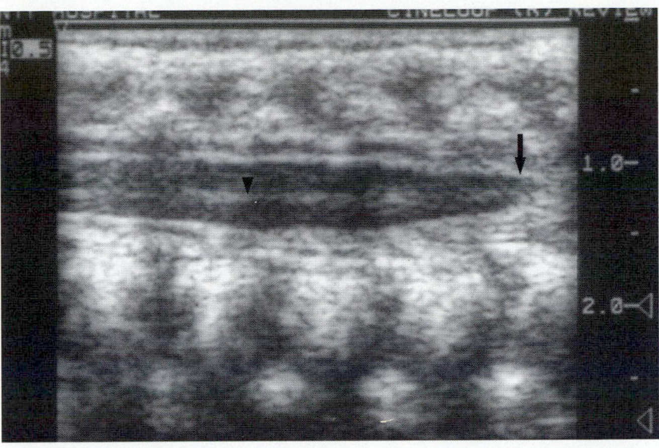

A

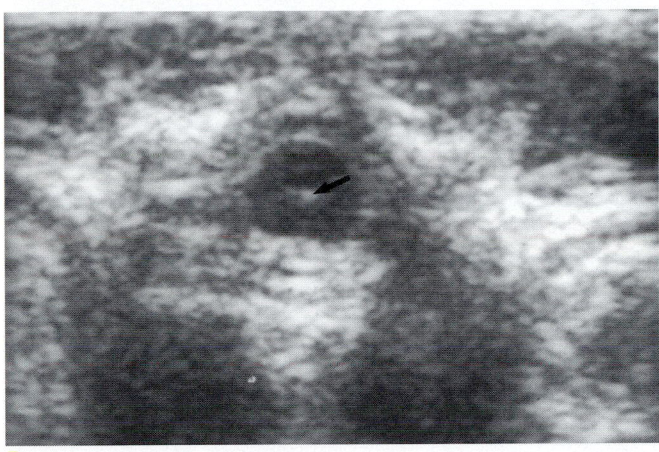

B

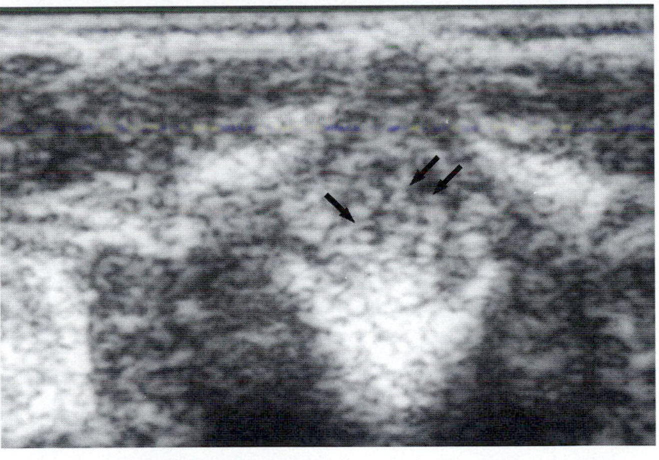

C

FIGURE 36–5. Normal spine ultrasound. ***A.*** Normal cord. Longitudinal plane. The tubular cord ends in a normal tapered point (*arrow*). The central canal (*arrowhead*) or simulating anterior decussating fibers are seen centrally and are echogenic. V = vertebral body. ***B.*** Normal cord. Transverse plane. Thoracic level. Prone patient. The normal cord is echopenic and round, with an echogenic "central canal." ***C.*** Normal canal below end of cord. Transverse plane. Low lumbar level. The round echopenic cord is not seen. It typically ends at L2. What is seen here, however, are the echogenic lines (*arrows*) of nerves extending from below the actual spinal cord, in the fashion of a horse's tail or cauda equina.

affected patients, the area of diastematomyelia is confined to the low thoracolumbar region. Diastematomyelia is more common in girls.

THE ASSOCIATED SKIN FINDINGS

A variety of skin lesions may mark the site of the defect. Associated cutaneous manifestations may include tufts of hair (hypertrichosis), cutaneous dimples, subcutaneous lipomas, vascular malformations, hemangiomatous skin discoloration, and the presence of a congenital dorsal dermal sinus. As many as 50 percent of patients have hypertrichosis, i.e., a hairy tuft of skin.

WHAT ARE THE CLINICAL SYNDROMES AFFECTING PATIENTS WITH DIASTEMATOMYELIA?

Two distinct clinical syndromes have been reported to occur in patients with diastematomyelia. The first is unilateral, in which one hypoplastic lower extremity is enervated by a hypoplastic segment of the cord and there is hypotonia and weakness of that extremity. In the second syndrome, there is bilateral involvement, with weakness and spasticity of both lower extremities and a resultant awkward gait. There are often atrophy of the leg muscles, skeletal deformities of the feet, and bladder and rectal incontinence. The clinical findings are often slowly progressive over a period of months to years. There are two theories concerning the pathogenesis of these clinical syndromes. The first is that the cord becomes impaled by the bony spur and that differential growth of the vertebral column and the spinal cord, particularly with the child's longitudinal growth, results in stretching of the cord above its point of fixation, with resultant neurologic abnormality. An alternative theory is that progressive neurologic damage results from trauma and traction at the spur when the child flexes his or her head or neck. The acquired neurologic deficits may be reversible. Prophylactic surgery to remove the bony spur from an affected infant is indicated to prevent the development of neurologic sequelae. The goal is to free the cord from the effects of traction injury.

IMAGING TECHNIQUES FOR DIAGNOSING DIASTEMATOMYELIA

Several imaging techniques can be used for the diagnosis of diastematomyelia. Plain films of the spine may show widening of the interpedicular distance, vertebral body anomalies, calcified midline bony spur, and scoliosis. Common vertebral body anomalies are hemivertebrae, vertebral body fusion, and small vertebrae.

High-resolution spinal sonography, as noted in this case, can be diagnostic for diastematomyelia. The typical appearance, as in this case, is the demonstration of two hemicords, each with its own central canal. The bony or fibrous spur may sometimes be imaged.

Magnetic resonance imaging (MRI) is useful for confirmation of the sonographic abnormalities and allows the demonstration of concomitant abnormalities, particularly hydromyelia and spinal cord tethering. It may also better demonstrate the bony, but particularly the nonosseous (i.e., fibrous), septum.

Diastematomyelia has been diagnosed prenatally. Boulot et al described a 33-week fetus in whom the diagnosis of diastematomyelia was made based on the visualization of a bony spur and spinal canal enlargement.

EDITOR'S TECHNICAL NOTE ON DETERMINING CORD LEVEL

It was not our original intention to have two similar cases side by side. However, we have them, and the discussions are from different perspectives. Here's a third perspective: In analyzing cord position to determine the level of the conus, we image the cord in longitudinal and transverse planes using a linear array transducer. We confirm in two planes where the cord ends and then mark this position with a clip taped to the child's back. A plain film is taken to confirm the vertebral body level of the clip. The film is taken in prone position so as to not disturb the taped clip. One can avoid the film if the caudal end of the spine is normal (tapered) (Fig. 36-5) and it is in a line cranial to one drawn to the posterior midline from the last palpated ribs. This is usually at L2 or above. Figure 36-5 shows some normal US images of the neonatal spine.

References

Boulot P, Ferran JL, Charlier C, et al: Prenatal diagnosis of diastematomyelia. *Pediatr Radiol* 23:67–68, 1993.

Fitz CR: Diagnostic imaging in children with spinal disorders. *Pediatr Clin North Am* 32:1537–1558, 1985.

Kirpekar M, Cohen HL: Ultrasonography of the neonatal spine, in *Ultrasonography of the Prenatal and Neonatal Brain,* Timor-Tritsch I, Monteagudo A, Cohen HL (eds). Stamford, CT, Appleton & Lange, 1996:287–298.

Korsvik HE, Keller MS: Sonography of occult dysraphism in neonates and infants with MR imaging correlation. *Radiographics* 12:297–306, 1992.

Linn RM, Ford LT: Adult diastematomyelia. *Spine* 19:852–854, 1994.

Raghavendra BN, Epstein FJ, Pinto RS, et al: Sonographic diagnosis of diastematomyelia. *J Ultrasound Med* 7:111–113, 1988.

Walker HS, Dietrich RB, Flannigan BD, et al: Magnetic resonance imaging of the pediatric spine. *Radiographics* 7:1129–1152, 1987.

Section B
HEPATOBILIARY SYSTEM

37

Figure 37-1 shows an 18-month-old boy with a palpable abdominal mass. What do you see? What are your diagnostic considerations?

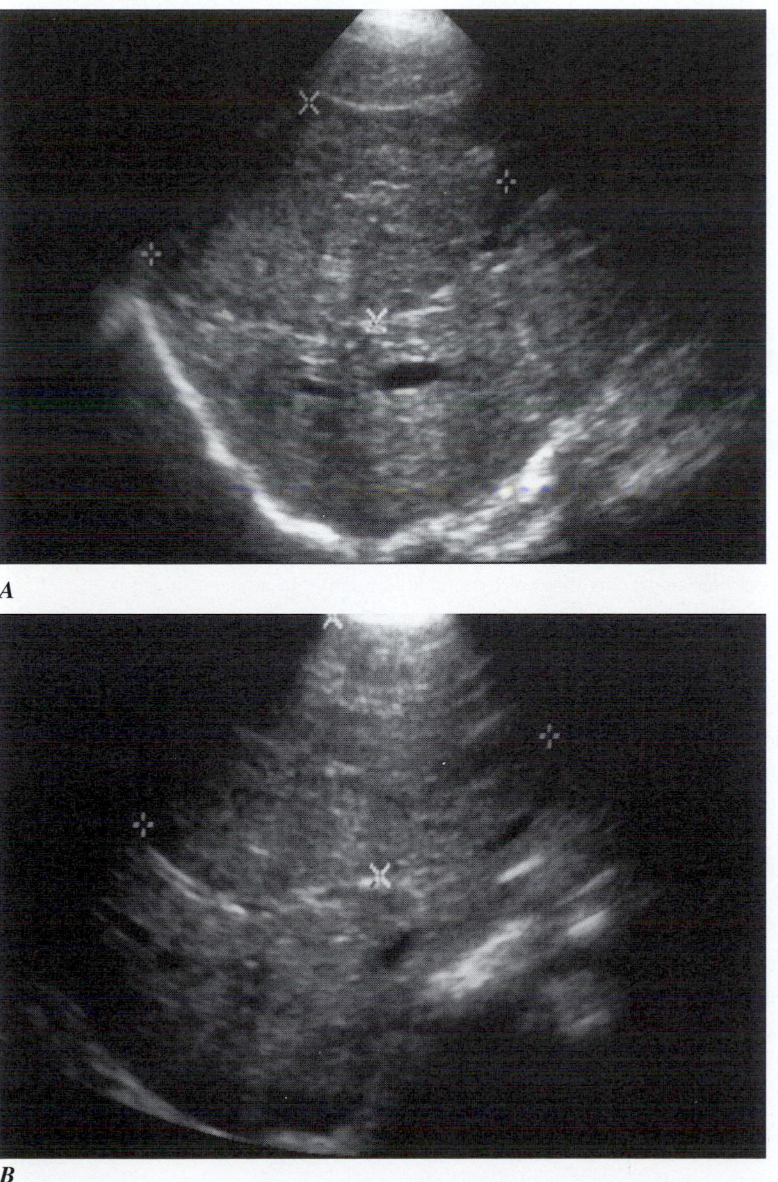

FIGURE 37–1. Transverse *(A)* and longitudinal *(B)* views through the liver.

CHAPTER 37

Hepatoblastoma

CARLOS J. SIVIT

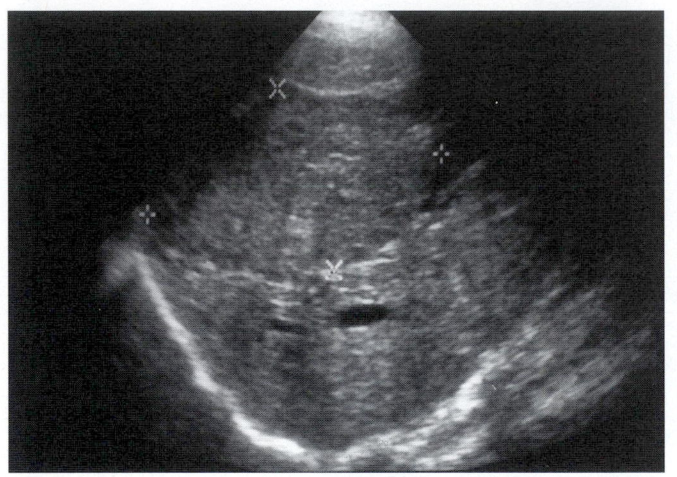

A

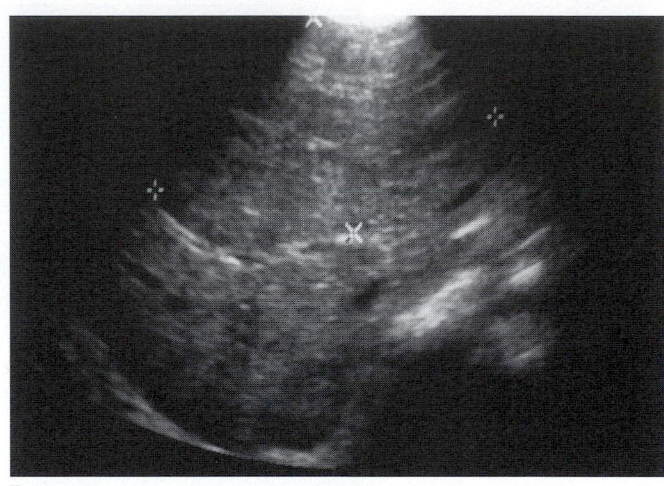

B

FIGURE 37–2. Hepatoblastoma. Transverse *(A)* and longitudinal *(B)* views through the liver demonstrate a well-circumscribed, solid mass (*between electronic calipers*). Note the variable echotexture, with areas that are hypoechoic and areas that are hyperechoic relative to adjacent normal hepatic parenchyma.

Hepatoblastoma is the most common malignant hepatic tumor in children. The tumor is seen exclusively in children under the age of 5 years, with approximately one-half of children presenting in the first year of life. The neoplasm arises within a previously normal liver, in contrast to hepatocellular carcinoma, which is usually associated with chronic liver disease when presenting in children. Hepatoblastoma is more common in boys than in girls by a nearly 2:1 ratio. There is an association of hepatoblastoma with Beckwith-Wiedemann syndrome, familial adenomatous polyposis, and trisomy 18.

Hepatoblastoma is more commonly observed in the right lobe of the liver than in the left. However, it is not unusual for both lobes of the liver to be affected as a result of either direct extension or multifocal involvement. The mass is usually quite large at the time of initial diagnosis, with one-half of these neoplasms exceeding 10 cm. Microscopically, the neoplasm is characterized by epithelial cells and mesenchymal elements such as osteoid, cartilage, and muscle. Calcification is present in approximately one-half of cases. The tumor is classified on the basis of the epithelial cell type as fetal, embryonal, or small cell undifferentiated (anaplastic).

Most children with hepatoblastoma are asymptomatic until the mass is quite large. The most common presenting sign is a palpable right upper quadrant abdominal mass. Other clinical features include abdominal pain, vomiting, anorexia, and weight loss. Jaundice is unusual. The serum alpha fetoprotein is elevated in over 90 percent of children with hepatoblastoma. This marker is also utilized to monitor disease recurrence after initial therapy.

Long-term survival of children with hepatoblastoma depends on complete surgical resection of the tumor. Approximately one-half of tumors are unresectable at presentation.

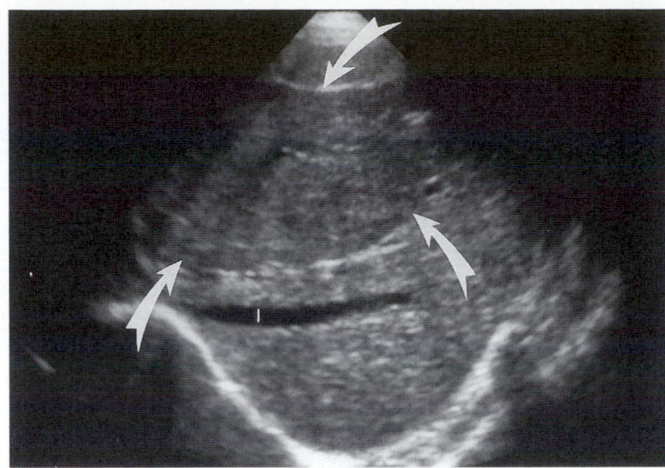

FIGURE 37–3. Hepatoblastoma with a hypoechoic appearance relative to adjacent hepatic parenchyma. Longitudinal view through the liver demonstrates a large solid mass (*arrows*) that is hypoechoic relative to surrounding hepatic parenchyma. I = inferior vena cava.

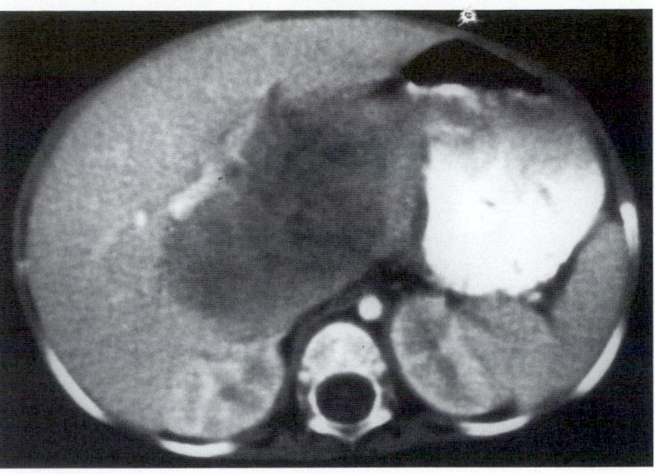

FIGURE 37–5. Hepatoblastoma. Contrast-enhanced computed tomography scan through the liver demonstrates a single large, well-circumscribed hepatic mass of mixed attenuation, displacing the portal vein anteriorly.

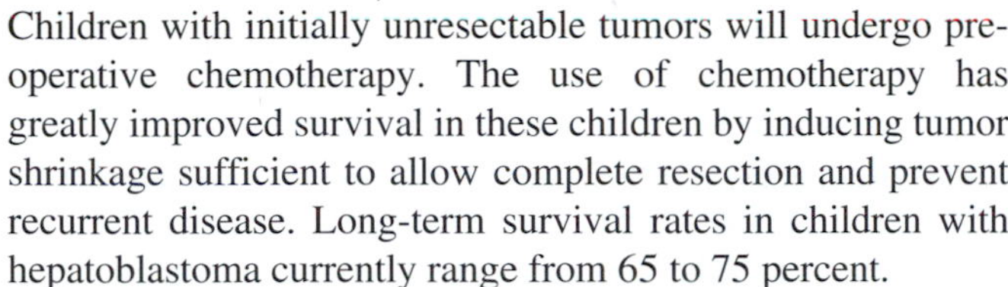

Children with initially unresectable tumors will undergo preoperative chemotherapy. The use of chemotherapy has greatly improved survival in these children by inducing tumor shrinkage sufficient to allow complete resection and prevent recurrent disease. Long-term survival rates in children with hepatoblastoma currently range from 65 to 75 percent.

Sonography is often the initial imaging examination performed in children with a hepatoblastoma. A normal examination is useful in excluding a hepatic mass lesion. Most tumors will be entirely or primarily solid, and heterogeneous in appearance (Fig. 37-2). The neoplasm has a variable echotexture at sonography; it may be anechoic, hypoechoic (Fig. 37-3), or hyperechoic in appearance (Fig. 37-4). Anechoic or cystic areas are usually small and represent tumor necrosis. Calcification may be noted within the mass. Sonography is also useful for evaluation of vascular structures, including hepatic veins, portal veins, and inferior vena cava, for the presence of tumor thrombus. An additional finding associated with hepatoblastoma at duplex Doppler is the presence of high-frequency shifts (exceeding 4 kHz), probably associated with tumor neovascularity. Sonography is limited in the definitive evaluation of hepatoblastoma, as it cannot accurately determine the size and extent of the lesions. The tumor margins are often not well identified at sonography. As a result, sonography is not very accurate in determining surgical resectability.

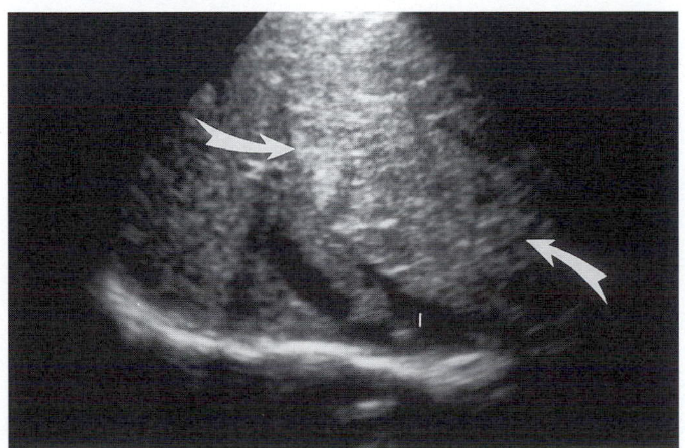

FIGURE 37–4. Hepatoblastoma with a hyperechoic appearance relative to adjacent hepatic parenchyma. Transverse view through the upper liver demonstrates a large solid mass (*arrows*) that is hyperechoic relative to surrounding hepatic parenchyma. I = inferior vena cava.

Cross-sectional imaging with computed tomography (CT) or magnetic resonance imaging (MRI) is the primary means of evaluating and staging a hepatoblastoma and determining surgical resectability. The CT appearance of hepatoblastoma is variable. Most neoplasms will have heterogeneous attenuation on contrast-enhanced CT. The enhancement pattern is nonspecific. The majority of the lesion will demonstrate lower attenuation than the adjacent normal contrast-enhanced hepatic parenchyma. The attenuation will be much lower if areas of necrosis are noted. The pattern of hepatic involvement varies and includes a large single lesion (Fig. 37-5), multiple lesions (Fig. 37-6), or diffuse parenchymal involvement. Calcification is noted at CT in approximately 40 percent of cases. Magnetic resonance imaging has several important advantages in the evaluation of hepatoblastoma, including its multiplanar imaging potential and its ability to clearly visualize the vascular anatomy. However, as with CT, the MRI appearance of hepatoblastoma is variable and nonspecific.

The differential diagnosis of a large solid hepatic mass or multifocal masses at sonography in a young child includes primary hepatic masses such as hemangioendothelioma, hepatocellular carcinoma, and rhabdomyosarcoma of the biliary tree. Additionally, metastatic disease from neuroblastoma, lymphoma, or leukemia may have a similar appearance. He-

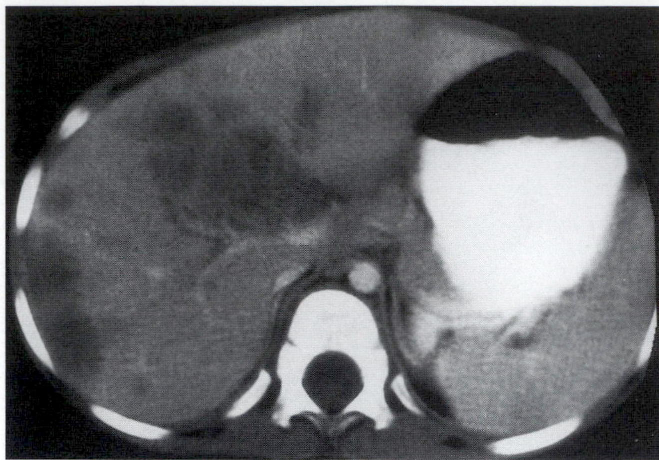

FIGURE 37–6. Hepatoblastoma. Contrast-enhanced computed tomography scan through the liver demonstrates multifocal masses of varying size and mixed attenuation. Note that all of the lesions have lower attenuation than normal adjacent contrast-enhanced hepatic parenchyma.

mangioendothelioma is a highly vascular neoplasm and can usually be differentiated on the basis of its pronounced vascularity. Hepatocellular carcinoma is typically seen in an older age group. In children, it arises only in individuals with preexisting liver disease. Biliary rhabdomyosarcoma is a very rare tumor in children that arises from the porta hepatis. Children with neuroblastoma and hepatic involvement can be differentiated by identification of the primary tumor, most commonly in the adrenal, although it may be in an extra-adrenal location in approximately one-third of cases. Lymphoma and leukemia with hepatic involvement will usually demonstrate involvement of other organs, particularly the spleen, pancreas, and kidneys. Additionally, there is often associated abdominal lymphadenopathy.

References

Abramson SJ, Lack EE, Teele RL: Benign vascular tumor of the liver in infants: Sonographic appearance. *AJR* 138:629–632, 1982.

Bates SM, Keller MS, Ramos IM, et al: Hepatoblastoma: Detection of tumor vascularity with duplex doppler US. *Radiology* 176:505–507, 1990.

Boechat MI, Kangarloo H, Ortega J, et al: Primary liver tumors in children: Comparison of CT and MR imaging. *Radiology* 169:727–732, 1988.

Dachman AH, Pakter RL, Ros PR, et al: Hepatoblastoma: Radiologic-pathologic correlation in 50 cases. *Radiology* 164:15–19, 1987.

Jabra AA, Fishman EK, Taylor GA: Hepatic masses in infants and children: CT evaluation. *AJR* 158:143–149, 1992.

King SJ, Babyn PS, Greenberg ML, et al: Value of CT in determining the resectability of hepatoblastoma before and after chemotherapy. *AJR* 160:793–798, 1993.

Miller JH, Greenspan BS: Integrated imaging of hepatic tumors in childhood. I. Malignant lesions (primary and metastatic). *Radiology* 154:83–90, 1985.

Ohtsuka Y, Takahashi H, Ohnuma N, et al: Detection of tumor thrombus in children using color Doppler ultrasonography. *J Pediatr Surg* 32:1507–1510, 1997.

38

Figure 38-1 shows a 2-day-old infant with congestive heart failure. What are the sonographic findings? What is the differential diagnosis?

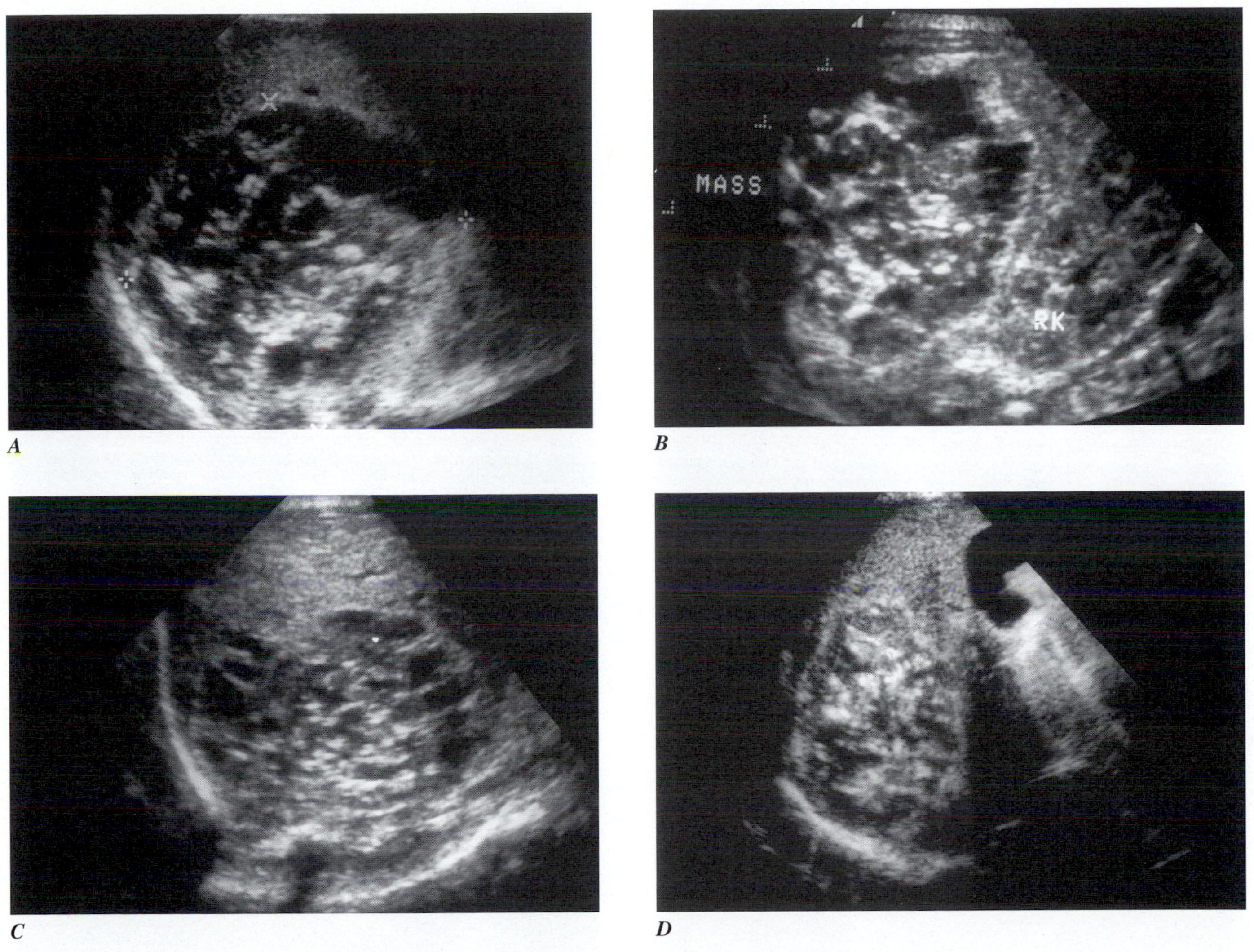

FIGURE 38–1. Transverse views through the upper *(A)* and lower *(B)* aspects of the right lobe of the liver and longitudinal views through the upper *(C)* and lower *(D)* aspects of the right lobe of the liver.

CHAPTER 38

Hemangioendothelioma

SHEILA BERLIN

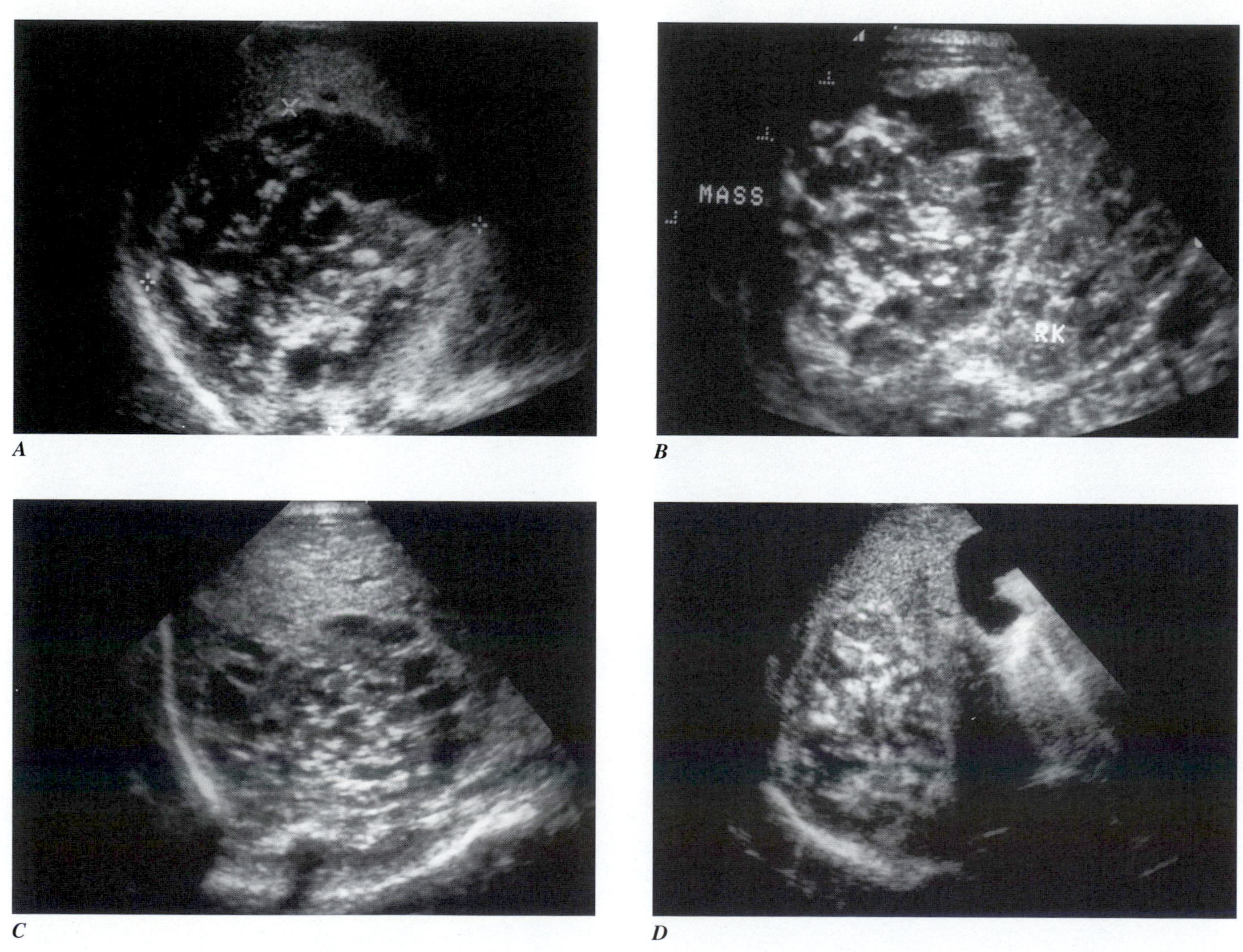

A B C D

FIGURE 38–2. Hemangioendothelioma. Transverse *(A, B)* and longitudinal *(C, D)* views through the right lobe of the liver show a well-circumscribed, solid, heterogeneous intrahepatic mass. Note the variable echotexture within the mass, including peripheral anechoic areas that represent dilated vascular channels. RK = right kidney.

Hemangioendothelioma is an uncommon, histologically benign tumor seen primarily in infants and young children. Some 95 percent of hemangioendotheliomas present in the first year of life. These tumors account for approximately 20 percent of hepatic neoplasms seen in this age group. A female predilection has been reported, with a female-to-male ratio ranging from 1.5:1 to 2:1. Hemangioendotheliomas appear grossly as multiple or single nodules ranging from a few millimeters to 20 centimeters in size. They are variably cystic or solid and usually exhibit hemorrhagic, highly vascular areas alternating with fibrous foci of less vascularity. The lesions are well circumscribed by a pseudocapsule of compressed normal hepatic tissue. Microscopically, internal vascular channels show lining with a single layer of plump endothelial cells. Tumors with pleomorphism and multilayer hyperplasia of the endothelial lining are designated type II hemangioendothelioma. It is felt that these lesions may represent a low-grade form of angiosarcoma.

Most infants with hemangioendothelioma present with a palpable abdominal mass or hepatomegaly. Congestive heart failure secondary to systemic arteriovenous shunting may be a presenting sign or may develop during the course of treatment. Arteriovenous shunting may contribute to fetal hydrops in some patients. A bleeding diathesis due to tumor platelet sequestration or disseminated intravascular coagulopathy may develop in up to 50 percent of affected infants. This condition, known as the Kasabach-Merritt syndrome, is often associated with vascular tumors of the trunk or extremities. Jaundice, anemia, and hemoperitoneum related to hepatic rupture occur less commonly. On physical examination, a loud systolic bruit may be heard over the site of the tumor. There may be associated cutaneous hemangiomas. The serum alpha fetoprotein is typically mildly to moderately elevated.

Sonographic findings are typically diagnostic of hemangioendothelioma, making biopsy of the tumor unnecessary. The typical sonographic appearance is that of a well-circumscribed solid hepatic mass (Fig. 38-2). The echotexture of the lesion is typically quite heterogeneous. This contrasts with the homogeneous, hyperechoic appearance of a cavernous hemangioma of the liver. Calcifications may occasionally be noted within the mass (Fig. 38-3). Internal anechoic areas within the tumor are commonly noted (Fig. 38-2). These areas represent dilated vascular channels on color Doppler imaging. Evaluation with color Doppler demonstrates increased vascularity within the tumor (Fig. 38-4; see also Color Plate 12). Additionally, enlargement of the hepatic artery (Fig. 38-5) and the proximal abdominal aorta (Fig. 38-6) is noted. There is usually also decreased diameter of the abdominal aorta below the celiac axis (Fig. 38-6). High flow volumes through the lesion may also cause secondary enlargement of the hepatic veins.

Cross-sectional imaging with computed tomography (CT) or magnetic resonance imaging (MRI) is often performed to determine the extent of the lesion. The characteristic CT appearance of hemangioendothelioma is that of a large, well-circumscribed solid mass with early peripheral enhancement following intravenous contrast administration and delayed central filling (Fig. 38-7). However, there is some variability in the enhancement pattern seen on CT. Larger lesions with hemorrhage or infarct may not enhance centrally at any time, whereas smaller multifocal lesions may enhance uniformly. If there is replacement of most of the liver with tumor, a heterogeneous pattern of hepatic enhancement may be noted, characterized by areas of increased attenuation mixed with areas of normal attenuation (Fig. 38-8). On MRI, hemangioendotheliomas typically show high signal intensity on T2-weighted images (Fig. 38-9) and diminished signal on T1-weighted images relative to normal hepatic parenchyma (Fig. 38-10), except at sites of flow, hemorrhage, or calcification. Flow voids appear at sites of high blood flow, and various signals of blood by-products at sites of prior hemorrhage.

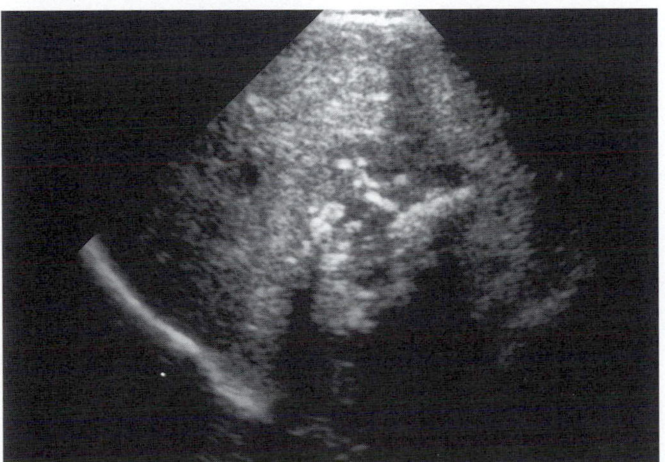

FIGURE 38–3. Hemangioendothelioma with internal calcifications. Transverse view through the right lobe of the liver in an infant with hemangioendothelioma demonstrates a solid mass with multiple echogenic foci, with acoustic shadowing representing calcifications.

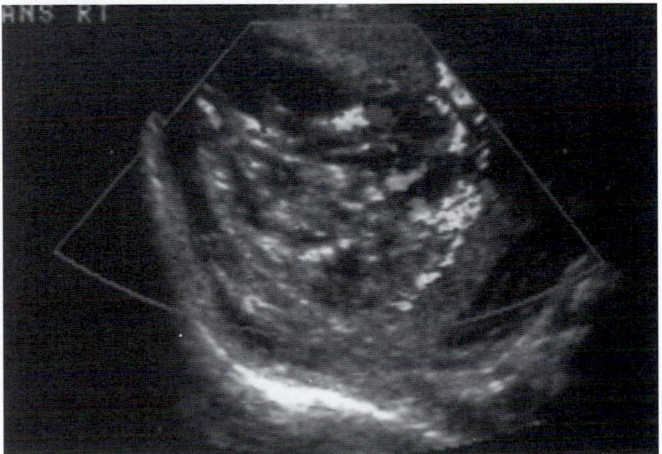

FIGURE 38–4. Hemangioendothelioma on color Doppler sonography. Transverse view through the liver in the same child as in Fig. 38-1 demonstrates increased blood flow within the hemangioendothelioma. (See Color Plate 12.)

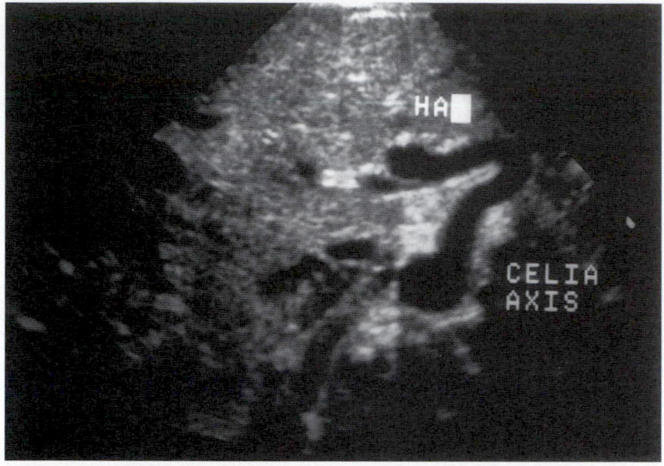

A

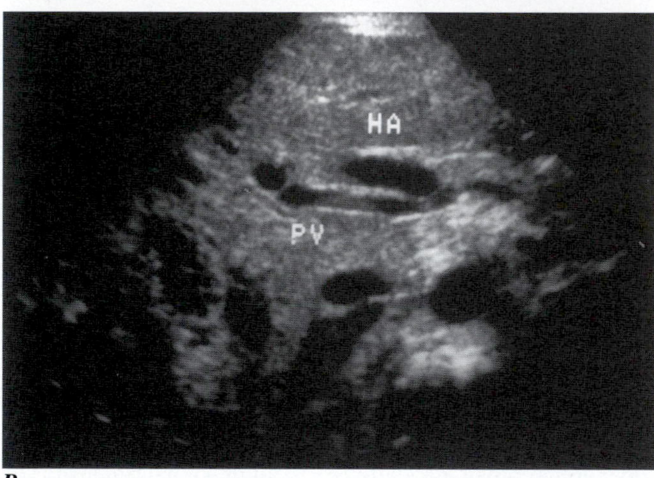

B

FIGURE 38–5. Dilated celiac axis and hepatic artery associated with hemangioendothelioma. ***A.*** Transverse view at the level of the celiac axis in an infant with hemangioendothelioma demonstrates dilatation of the celiac artery and hepatic artery. ***B.*** Longitudinal view through the porta hepatis in the same infant demonstrates a dilated hepatic artery (HA). PV = portal vein.

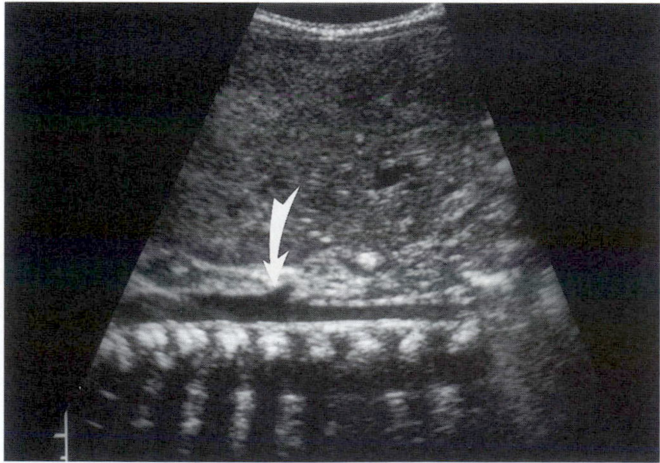

FIGURE 38–6. Dilated proximal abdominal aorta and proximal celiac artery associated with hemangioendothelioma. Longitudinal view through the upper abdomen in an infant with a hemangioendothelioma demonstrates a caliber difference in the abdominal aorta above and below the celiac artery (*arrow*). The aorta demonstrates an increased diameter above the celiac artery compared to below the celiac artery.

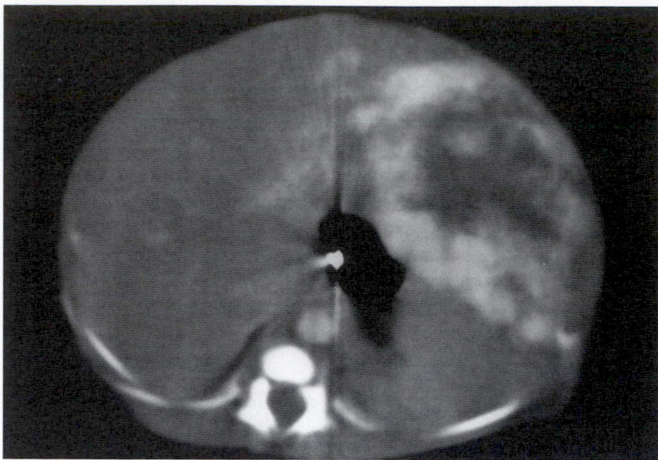

FIGURE 38–7. Hemangioendothelioma. Contrast-enhanced computed tomography through the liver in an infant with hemangioendothelioma demonstrates a large, well-circumscribed, lobulated lesion within the left hepatic lobe. Note the intense contrast enhancement around the periphery of the lesion, associated with a low-attenuation center.

The differential diagnosis of a large solid hepatic mass or multifocal masses in an infant or young child includes hepatoblastoma, rhabdomyosarcoma of the biliary tree, and metastatic neuroblastoma. Hepatoblastoma is rare in infancy and typically presents beyond 1 year of age. The alpha fetoprotein is usually markedly elevated. In contrast to a hemangioendothelioma, hepatoblastoma is not a highly vascular mass. Rhabdomyosarcoma of the biliary tree is also rare in infancy and not highly vascular. Hepatic masses related to metastatic neuroblastoma are typically associated with an adrenal mass. Additionally, these are also relatively avascular lesions, and therefore they typically demonstrate decreased attenuation relative to normal hepatic parenchyma (Fig. 38-11).

The prognosis in children with hemangioendothelioma is variable. The natural history of a hemangioendothelioma is to

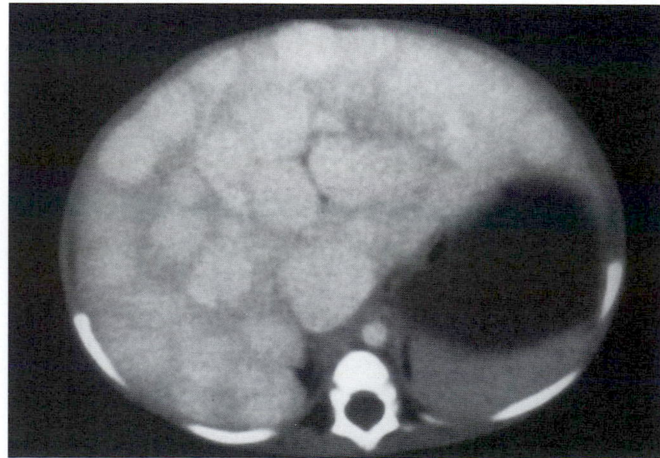

FIGURE 38–8. Hemangioendothelioma diffusely involving the liver. Contrast-enhanced computed tomography through the liver in a child with hemangioendothelioma demonstrates diffuse, multifocal areas of increased enhancement throughout the liver.

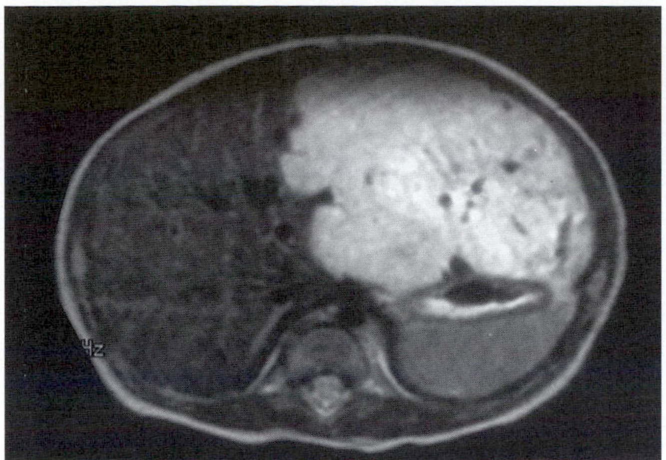

FIGURE 38–9. Hemangioendothelioma. T2-weighted axial image through the liver shows a large, well-circumscribed, lobulated mass in the left hepatic lobe that demonstrates high signal intensity relative to normal hepatic parenchyma in the right lobe of the liver. This appearance is characteristic for hemangioendothelioma.

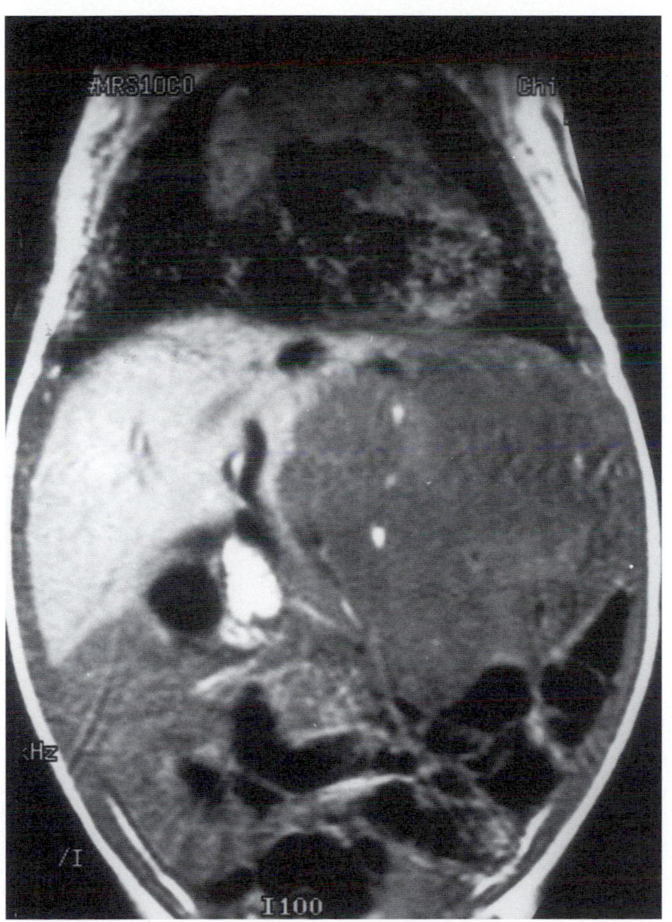

FIGURE 38–10. Hemangioendothelioma. T1-weighted coronal image through the liver in the same child as in Fig. 38-7 demonstrates low signal intensity within the mass relative to the normal right lobe of the liver.

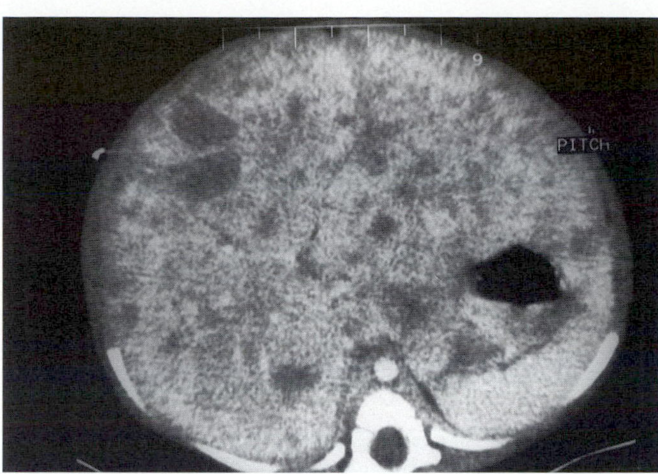

FIGURE 38–11. Hepatic metastases from neuroblastoma. Contrast-enhanced computed tomography scan through the liver in a child with metastatic neuroblastoma demonstrates multiple metastatic lesions throughout the liver. Note that the metastatic lesions demonstrate low attenuation relative to normal hepatic parenchyma.

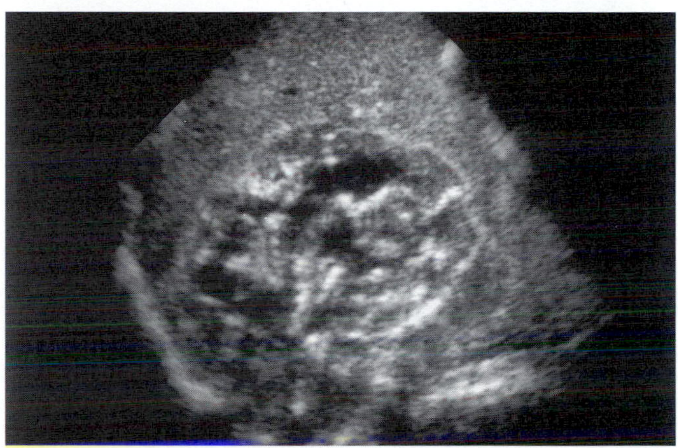

A

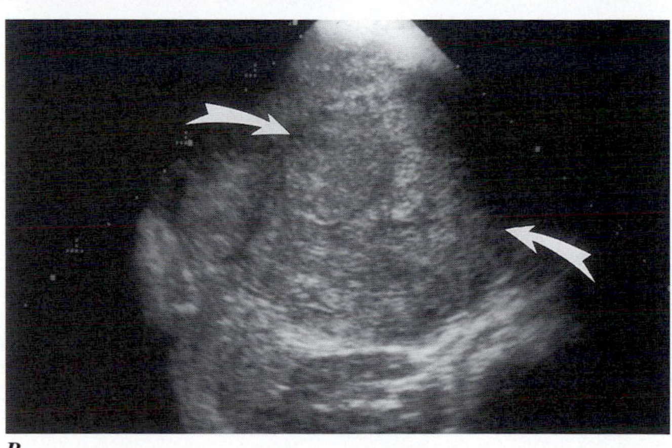

B

FIGURE 38–12. Involution of hemangioendothelioma. ***A.*** Transverse view through the liver in the same child as in Fig. 38-1 at age 6 months shows a decrease in the size of the hepatic mass. Note that there has also been a marked diminution in the size of the peripheral anechoic areas that represent dilated vascular channels. Transverse ***(B)*** view through the liver in the same child at age 9 months show a further decrease in the size of the intrahepatic mass (*arrows*). Also note that the mass no longer contains the anechoic vascular spaces along the periphery.

undergo spontaneous involution over a period of 8 to 12 months following a proliferative phase in the first 6 months of life. In the absence of symptoms, no therapy may be necessary, and serial follow-up sonograms can document tumor regression (Fig. 38-12). Infants presenting with heart failure have a mortality of 75 percent if untreated. Heart failure is initially treated medically. If such a regimen fails, arterial embolization or surgical resection may be necessary. Liver transplantation may be the only option in children with diffuse hepatic involvement.

References

Boechat MI, Kangarloo H, Ortega J, et al: Primary liver tumors in children: Comparison of CT and MR imaging. *Radiology* 169:727–732, 1988.

Burrows PE: Variations in the vascular supply to infantile hepatic hemangioendotheliomas. *Radiology* 181:631–632, 1991.

DeCampo M, deCampo JF: Ultrasound of primary hepatic tumours in childhood. *Pediatr Radiol* 19:19–24, 1988.

Fok TF, Chan MSY, Metreweli C, et al: Hepatic haemangioendothelioma presenting with early heart failure in a newborn: Treatment with hepatic artery embolization and interferon. *Acta Paediatr* 85:1373–1375, 1996.

Keslar PJ, Buck JL, Selby DM: Infantile hemangioendothelioma of the liver revisited. *Radiographics* 13:657–670, 1993.

Orthodoxos OA, Buist LJ, Kelly DA, et al: Unresectable hepatic tumors in childhood and the role of liver transplantation. *J Pediatr Surg* 31:1563–1567, 1996.

Paley MR, Farrant P, Kane P, et al: Developmental intrahepatic shunts of childhood: Radiological features and management. *Eur Radiol* 7:1377–1382, 1997.

Park CH, Hwang HS, Hong J, et al: Giant infantile hemangioendothelioma of the liver: Scintigraphic diagnosis. *Clin Nucl Med* 21:293–295, 1996.

Williams RA, Ferrell LD: Pediatric liver tumors. *Pathology* 2:23–43, 1993.

Woltering MC, Robben S, Egeler RM: Hepatic hemangioendothelioma of infancy: Treatment with interferon. *J Pediatr Gastroenterol Nutr* 24:348–351, 1997.

39

Figure 39-1 shows a 2-year-old boy with a palpable right upper quadrant mass. What do you see? What are the diagnostic considerations?

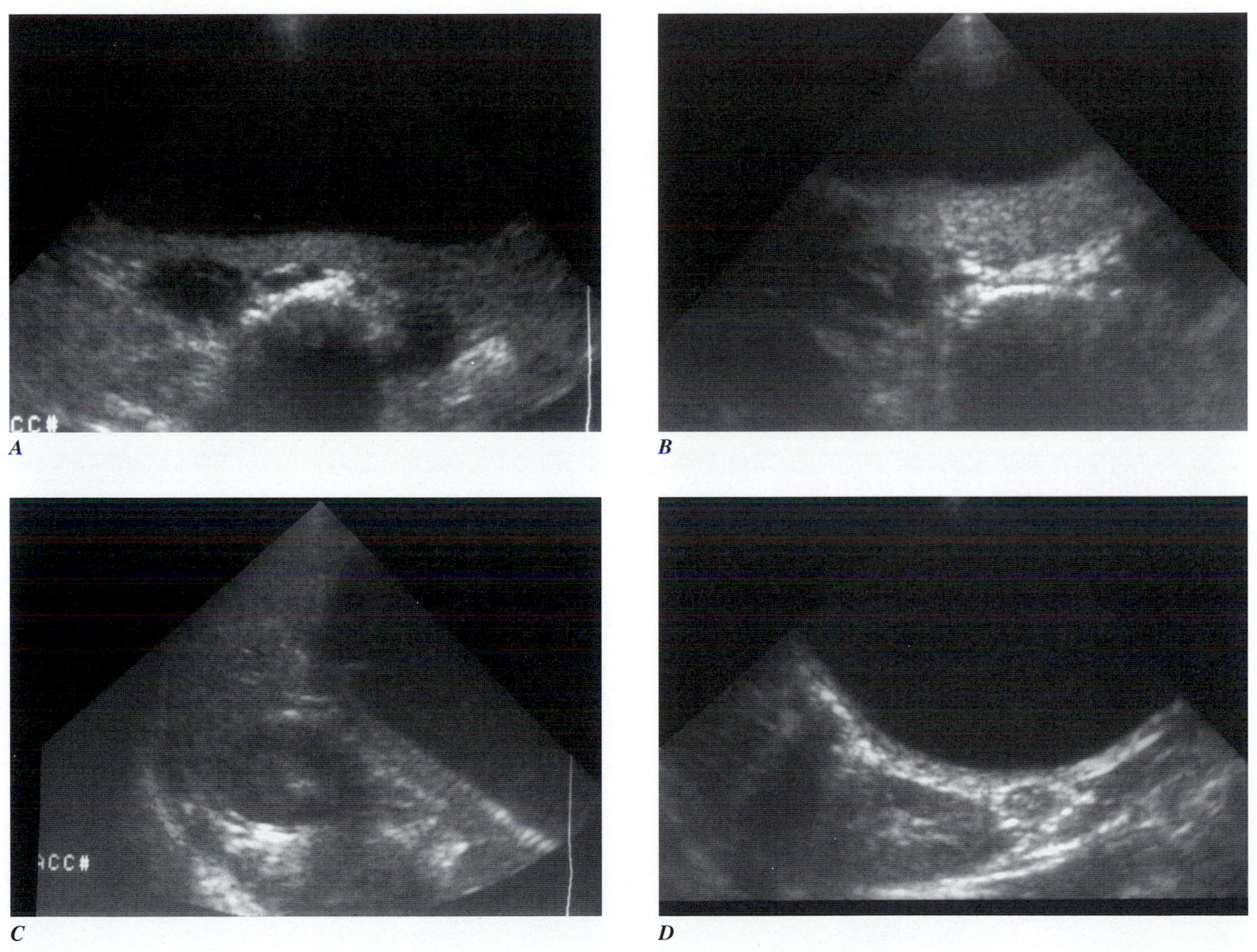

FIGURE 39–1. Transverse *(A–C)* and longitudinal *(D)* views through the liver.

CHAPTER 39

Mesenchymal Hamartoma of the Liver

CARLOS J. SIVIT

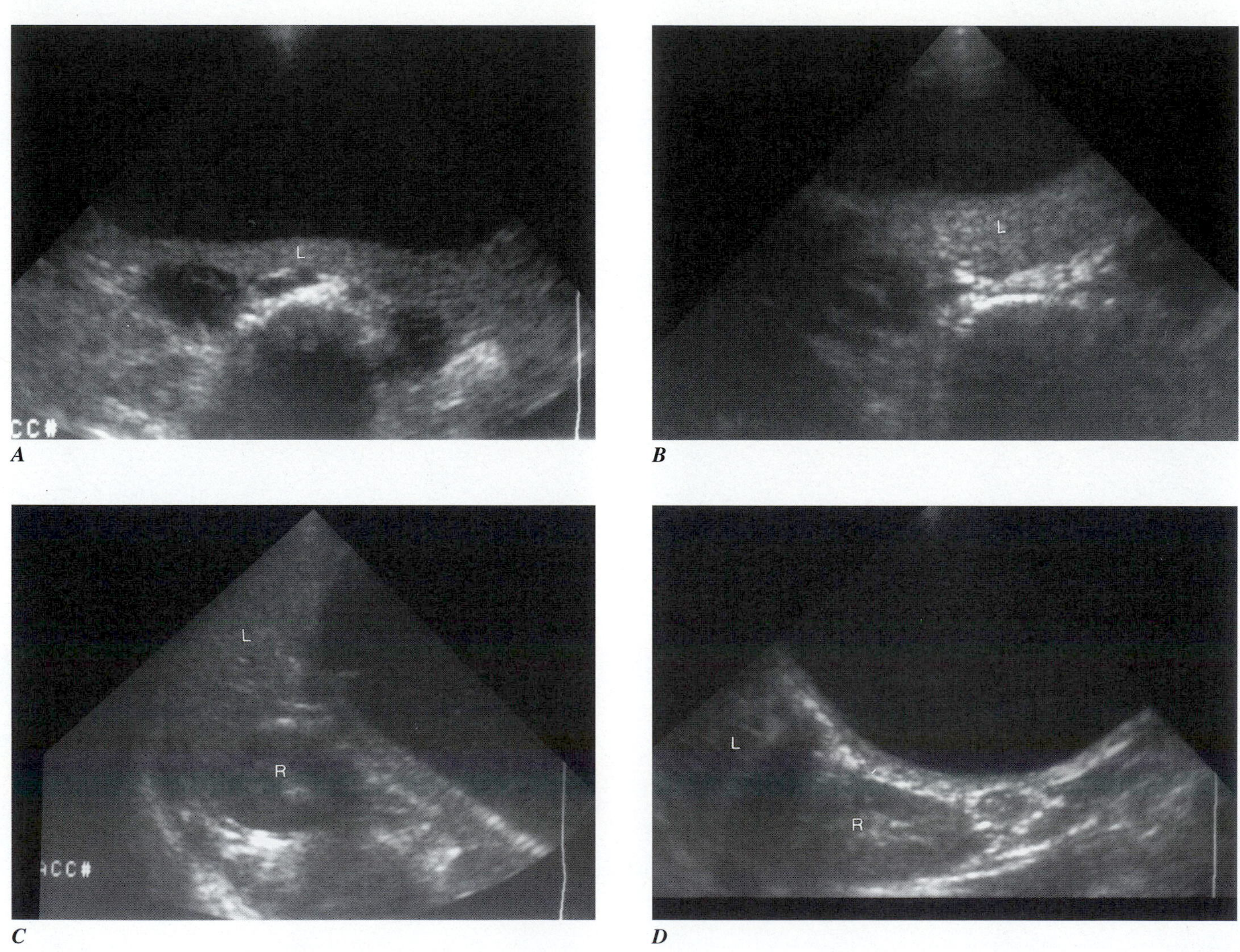

FIGURE 39–2. Mesenchymal hamartoma of the liver. Transverse *(A–C)* and longitudinal *(D)* views through the liver demonstrate a large, well-circumscribed, oval-shaped, cystic intrahepatic mass. At surgery, this was noted to be a mesenchymal hamartoma of the liver. R = right kidney, L = liver.

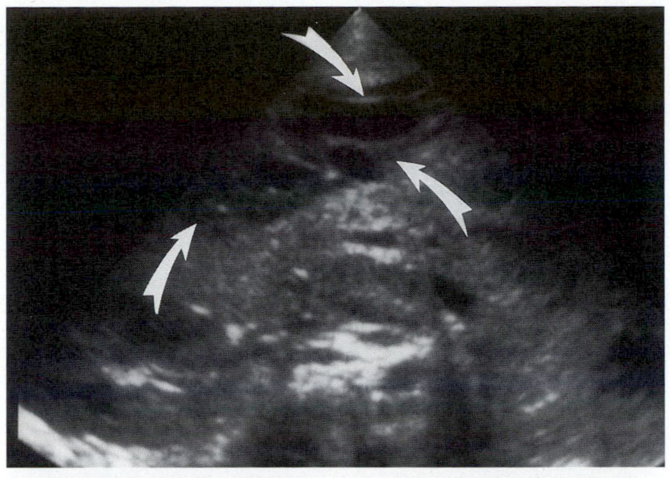

A

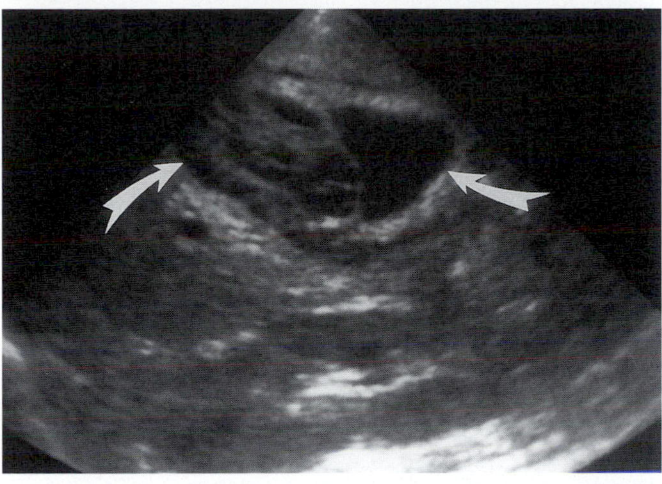

B

FIGURE 39–3. Mesenchymal hamartoma of the liver containing solid and cystic areas and septations. Transverse *(A)* and longitudinal *(B)* views through the liver in a child with a mesenchymal hamartoma demonstrate a complex mass (*arrows*) with solid and cystic areas. Note the presence of several septa within the cystic areas. R = right kidney.

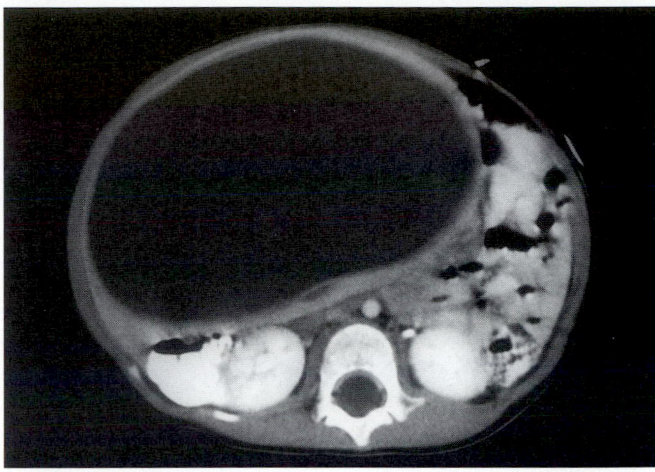

FIGURE 39–4. Mesenchymal hamartoma of the liver. Contrast-enhanced computed tomography (CT) scan through the upper abdomen in the same patient as in Fig. 39-1 shows a large, well-circumscribed, oval-shaped, low-attenuation mass within the liver. There is absence of contrast enhancement within the mass. Note the thin rim of hepatic parenchyma surrounding the mass, allowing characterization of its intrahepatic origin.

Mesenchymal hamartoma is a rare primary hepatic tumor of mesenchymal origin. It is a benign lesion resulting from excessive focal overgrowth of mature normal cells and stroma that are native to the liver but abnormal in quantity, proportion, and arrangement. Thus, it is not a true neoplasm. Grossly, mesenchymal hamartoma is characterized by multiple cysts of varying size. The cysts are filled with either gelatinous material or fluid. They are sharply demarcated but not encapsulated. Microscopically, the tumor is characterized by cystic areas, biliary epithelium, hepatocytes, and mesenchymal elements. Mesenchymal hamartoma is typically noted in younger children. The usual age of presentation is between 4 months and 2 years. It is more common in males than in females. The most common clinical presentation of a mesenchymal hamartoma is that of a palpable right upper quadrant mass. Most patients are asymptomatic. The presence of jaundice or elevated liver enzymes is rare in this condition. Mesenchymal hamartoma is usually surgically resected, although there are case reports of lesions that have undergone spontaneous involution. There are no reports of malignant degeneration of this lesion.

The sonographic appearance of a mesenchymal hamartoma is that of a cystic intrahepatic mass (Fig. 39-2). It may contain solid areas representing fibrous stroma or smaller cysts (Fig. 39-3), but it is usually predominantly or entirely cystic. The cystic areas may be anechoic or may contain low-level internal echoes representing mucoid or gelatinous material. They commonly contain septations (Fig. 39-3). Calcifications in the cyst wall have been described but are rare. The lesions may be quite large, often in excess of 8 cm in diameter. There may be pronounced arterial flow to these lesions with arteriovenous shunting, resulting in enlargement of the aorta proximal to the celiac axis, enlargement of hepatic veins, and increased vascularity surrounding the lesion on Doppler sonography. These findings may overlap with those for vascular hepatic lesions such as hemangioendothelioma and cavernous hemangioma. Localizing the liver as the organ of origin in large mesenchymal hamartomas may be difficult, and computed tomography (CT) is useful in this regard. The typical CT appearance of a mesenchymal hamartoma is that of a large, multilocular, cystic mass (Fig. 39-4). A variable pattern of enhancement is noted on CT, ranging from absence of enhancement to peripheral and septal enhancement with partial centripetal fill-in of enhancement on delayed imaging.

The differential diagnosis of a mesenchymal hamartoma includes hepatic abscess, simple hepatic cyst, and choledochal cyst if the lesion is primarily cystic, and hemangioma and hemangioendothelioma if the lesion is primarily solid with increased vascularity. Hepatic abscess can usually be excluded on clinical grounds, as children with mesenchymal hamartoma are usually asymptomatic. A simple hepatic cyst can be excluded on size criteria, as such lesions are usually small and unilocular (Fig. 39-5). A choledochal cyst can be

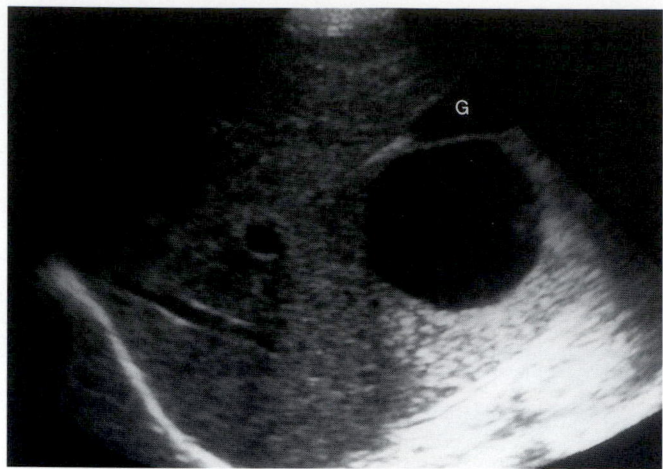

FIGURE 39–5. Hepatic cyst. Longitudinal view through the liver shows a well-circumscribed, rounded, anechoic lesion posterior to the gallbladder (G), representing a simple hepatic cyst.

excluded if it is confirmed that the lesion arises from hepatic parenchyma and not the porta hepatis. Additionally, many choledochal cysts will have associated biliary tract dilatation. Although there is some overlap between a mesenchymal hamartoma and vascular hepatic lesions such as a large hemangioma and a hemangioendothelioma, the latter two lesions can usually be distinguished, as they are typically entirely or predominantly solid and more highly vascular than mesenchymal hamartoma.

References

Barnhart DC, Hirschl RB, Garver KA: Conservative management of mesenchymal hamartoma of the liver. *J Pediatr Surg* 32: 1495–1498, 1997.

Giyanani VL, Meyers PC, Wolfson JJ: Mesenchymal hamartoma of the liver: Computed tomography and ultrasonography. *J Comput Assist Tomogr* 10:51–54, 1986.

Kaufman RA: Is cystic mesenchymal hamartoma of the liver similar to infantile hemangioendothelioma on dynamic computed tomography? *Pediatr Radiol* 22:582–583, 1992.

Ros PR, Goodman ZD, Ishak KG, et al: Mesenchymal hamartoma of the liver: Radiologic-pathologic corrrelations. *Radiology* 158:619–624, 1986.

Stanley P, Hall TR, Wooley MM, et al: Mesenchymal hamartomas of the liver in childhood: Sonographic and CT findings. *AJR* 147:1035–1039, 1986.

Wholey MH, Wojno KJ: Pediatric hepatic mesenchymal hamartoma demonstrated on plain film, ultrasound and MRI, and correlated with pathology. *Pediatr Radiol* 24:143–144, 1994.

40

Figure 40-1 shows a 6-year-old boy with chronic liver disease. What do you see? What are the diagnostic considerations?

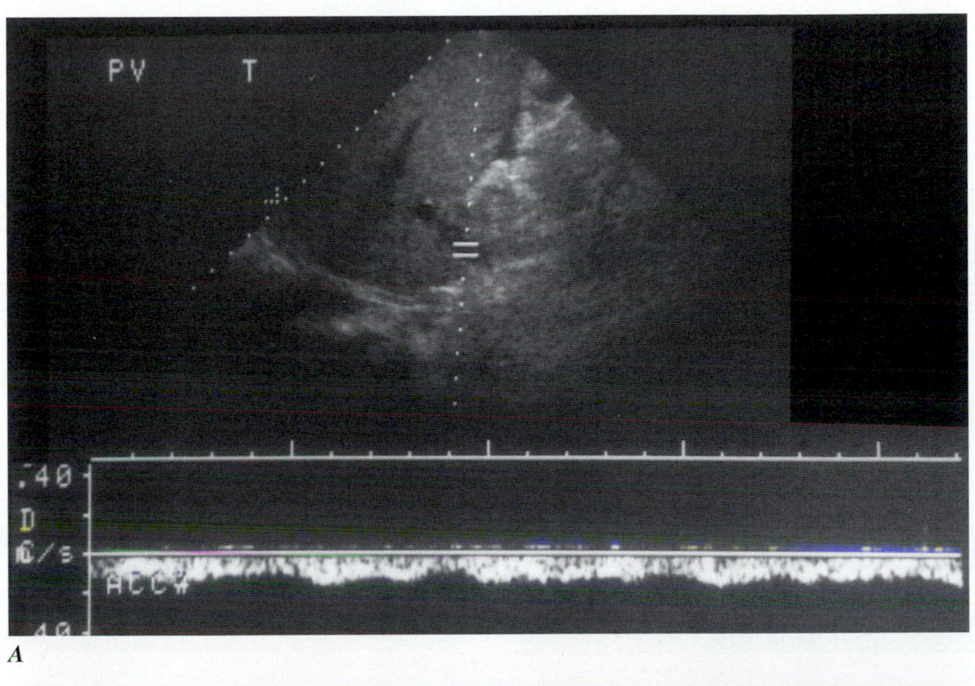

A

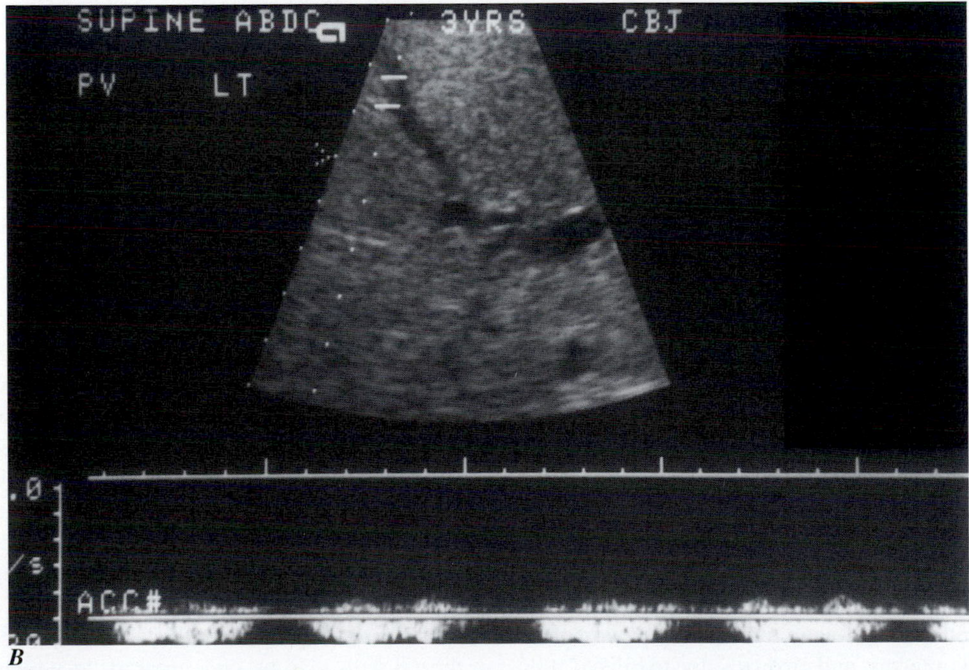

B

FIGURE 40–1. Transverse views through the porta hepatis *(A)* and the left *(B)* portal vein.

CHAPTER 40

Portal Hypertension

CARLOS J. SIVIT

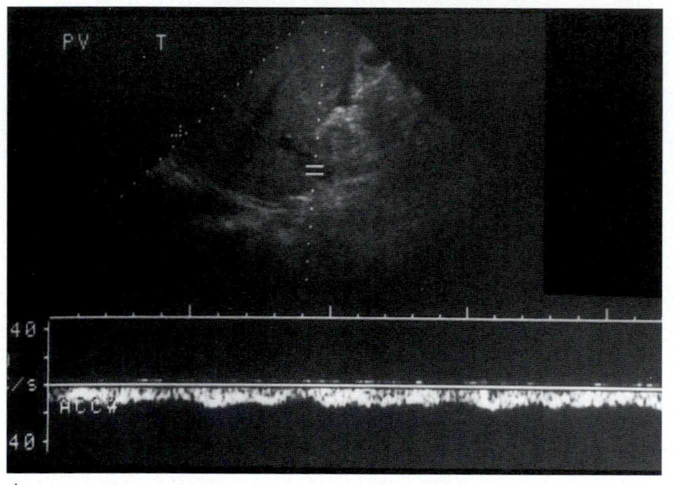

A

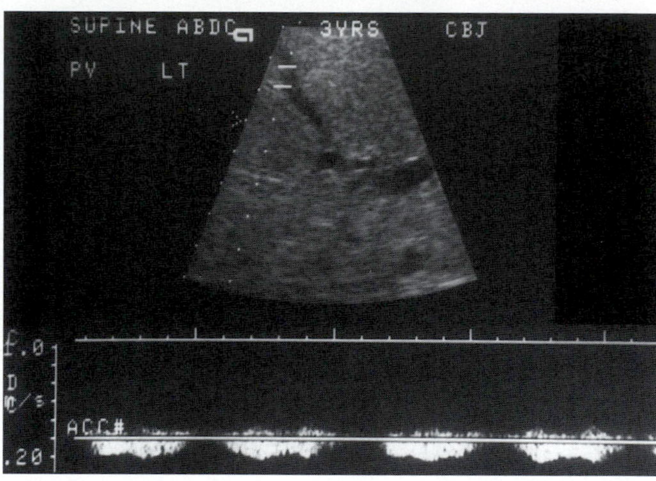

B

FIGURE 40–2. Hepatofugal, or reversed, flow in main and left portal veins secondary to portal hypertension. Transverse views through the main portal vein *(A)* and left portal vein *(B)* demonstrate hepatofugal flow, or flow reversal, in the portal venous system.

The portal vein, which originates from the confluence of the superior mesenteric vein and the splenic vein, normally accounts for approximately three-quarters of hepatic perfusion. It predominantly supplies the hepatic sinusoids, while the hepatic artery supplies the connective tissues and biliary ducts of the portal triads. Portal hypertension develops when there is increased resistance to portal blood flow as a result of extrahepatic or intrahepatic portal venous obstruction (Fig. 40-2). Recent evidence indicates that increased splanchnic blood flow also contributes to elevated portal venous pressures in patients with chronic liver disease.

Predisposing conditions associated with portal hypertension in children include omphalitis, hepatic vein thrombosis (Budd-Chiari syndrome), portal vein thrombosis, pancreatitis, trauma, periportal neoplasms, and cirrhosis due to biliary atresia, α_1-antitrypsin deficiency, Wilson disease, cystic fibrosis, and chronic active hepatitis. Extrahepatic portal obstruction is more common than intrahepatic obstruction in children. The liver is typically normal in children with extrahepatic portal obstruction. Conversely, hepatic parenchymal abnormalities, including abnormal hepatic parenchymal echotexture and contour, are common in children with intrahepatic portal obstruction, since that condition is often associated with chronic liver disease. In children with extrahepatic portal obstruction, portal blood may reach the liver through collateral channels in the suspensory ligaments and hepatorenal and hepatocolic veins. Intrahepatic portal obstruction may be intrinsic or extrinsic, and partial or complete. Intrinsic obstruction is most commonly due to thrombus, while extrinsic obstruction is primarily due to cirrhosis. When there is complete intrahepatic portal obstruction, a condition called cavernous transformation of the portal vein may be encountered, in which the normal portal vein is replaced by a number of thin-walled, tortuous collateral veins (Fig. 40-3).

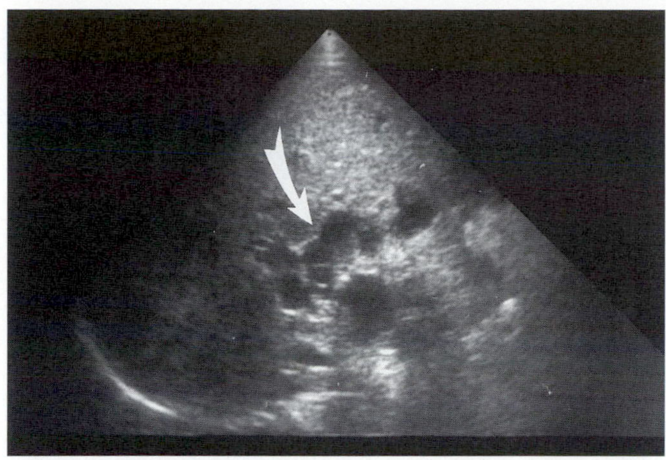

A

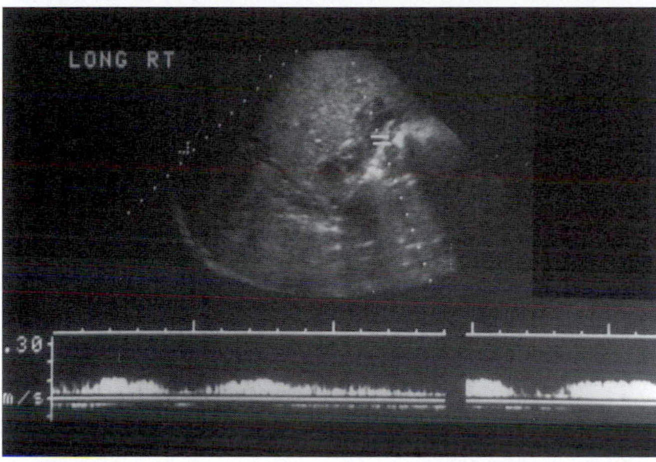

B

FIGURE 40–3. Cavernous transformation of the portal vein. ***A.*** Transverse view through the porta hepatis demonstrates replacement of the main portal vein by a network of small, tortuous vessels representing portal vein cavernous transformation (*arrows*). ***B.*** Duplex Doppler through the same region in the same patient shows hepatopedal venous flow through the small collateral venous channels.

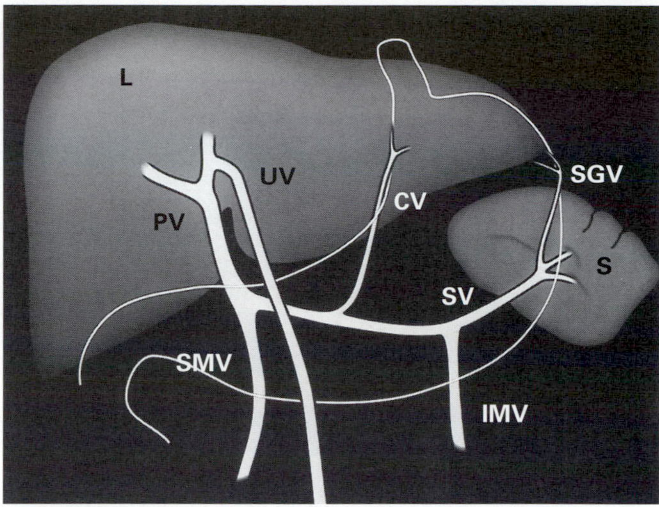

FIGURE 40–4. Diagram of the common portosystemic venous pathways in portal hypertension. PV = portal vein, SMV = superior mesenteric vein, SV = splenic vein, CV = coronary vein, SGV = short gastric vein, UV = umbilical vein, L = liver, S = spleen.

Portal hypertension may be complicated by the development of portal venous flow reversal, or hepatofugal flow, in the portal venous system and through a number of portosystemic shunts (Fig. 40-4). The latter condition leads to dilatation and varicosities of a number of veins that are typically very small. The most common collateral pathway involves the coronary vein, which extends from the portal venous system to the distal esophagus. This can lead to massive upper gastrointestinal tract bleeding from distal esophageal varices, which can be life-threatening. Recanalization of the umbilical vein also develops in a small subset of children with portal hypertension (Fig. 40-5; see also Color Plate 13). The umbilical vein communicates inferiorly with several paraumbilical veins, which can be seen on physical examination as a cluster of diverging midline veins extending to the umbilicus; this has been labeled caput medusae. Hemorrhoids may also develop.

The majority of children with portal hypertension have normal flow direction (hepatopedal flow) in the portal ve-

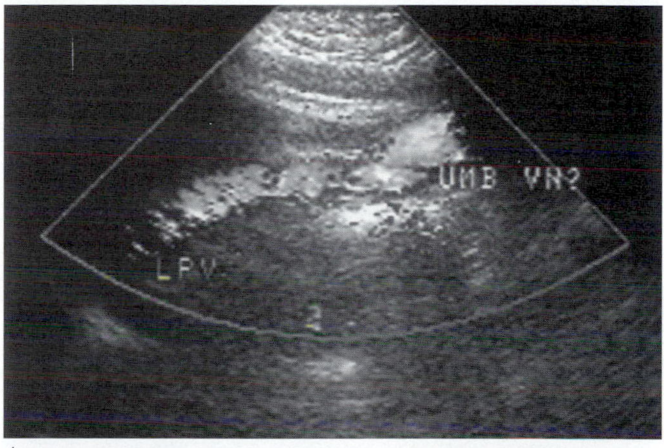

A

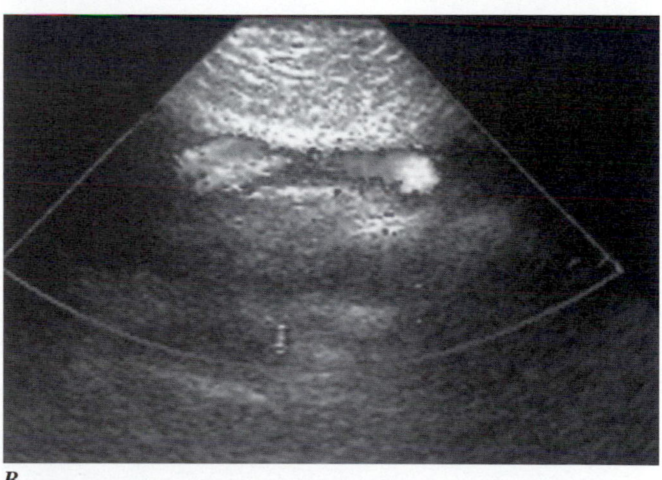

B

FIGURE 40–5. Recanalized umbilical vein associated with portal hypertension. ***A.*** Longitudinal view through the left lobe of the liver in a child with portal hypertension demonstrates flow in the left portal vein (LPV), communicating with a recanalized umbilical vein (UMB VN). ***B.*** Longitudinal midline view through the abdomen in the same patient demonstrates flow in the recanalized umbilical vein. (See Color Plate 13.)

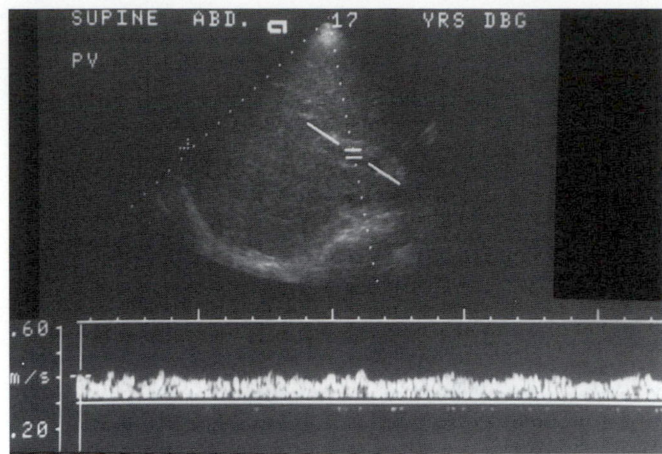

FIGURE 40–6. Normal portal vein waveform. Transverse view through the porta hepatis demonstrates flow toward the liver (hepatopedal flow) with a monophasic waveform.

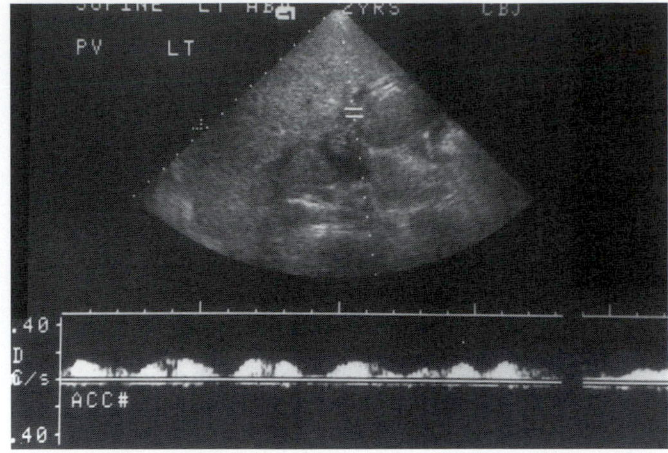

FIGURE 40–8. Pulsatile portal vein flow associated with portal hypertension. Transverse view through the left lobe of the liver in a child with portal hypertension demonstrates pulsatile flow in the left portal vein.

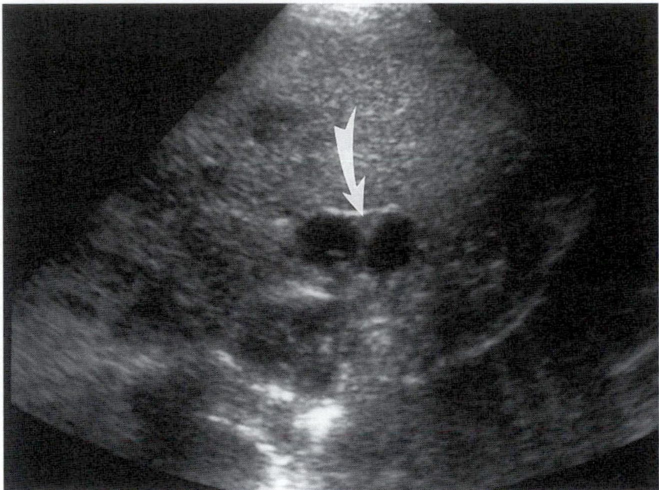

A

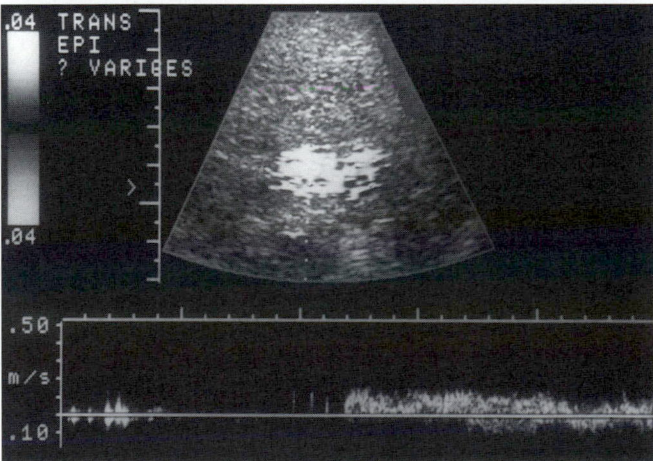

B

FIGURE 40–7. Esophageal varices associated with portal hypertension. ***A.*** Transverse midline view through the epigastrum demonstrates multiple serpiginous collateral vessels posterior to the left lobe of the liver, representing distal esophageal varices (*arrow*). ***B.*** Duplex Doppler through these vessels shows a venous waveform.

nous system. Portal venous flow reversal in children with portal hypertension may be seen in a single vein, or it may be generalized (Fig. 40-1). Portal venous flow reversal is seen more frequently in the right and left portal veins than in the main portal vein. When there is reversal of flow in the main portal vein, intrahepatic portal venous blood flow originates from the hepatic artery via arterioportal shunts. As portal venous flow decreases, arterial flow increases as a homeostatic mechanism to maintain hepatic perfusion. The arteriovenous shunting occurs at the sinusoidal level between hepatic arterioles and portal venules.

Sonography is a reliable, noninvasive method to evaluate children with chronic liver disease and suspected portal hypertension. Doppler sonography has replaced angiography in the assessment of patency and flow direction in the hepatic vasculature of these children. Normal portal venous flow is directed toward the liver and is relatively monophasic (Fig. 40-6). Spectral analysis will show only minor flow fluctuations associated with cardiac or respiratory motion in normal individuals. Findings on sonography in children with portal hypertension include dilatation of the coronary vein (to >6 mm in diameter) with hepatofugal flow; recanalization of the umbilical vein with hepatofugal flow extending into dilated paraumbilical collateral veins (Fig. 40-5); multiple tortuous esophageal varices (Fig. 40-7); pulsatile (phasic) (Fig. 40-8), bidirectional (Fig. 40-9), or hepatofugal flow (Fig. 40-2) in the portal and splenic veins; thickening of the lesser omentum due to venous and lymphatic congestion (Fig. 40-10); splenomegaly (Fig. 40-11); and multiple small serpiginous vessels in the porta hepatis if there is cavernous transformation (Fig. 40-3). If the portosystemic shunt is large, there may be absence of flow in the portal vein.

Imaging of the portal vasculature and portosystemic shunts requires attention to proper technique. The main and right portal veins are best imaged using a right longitudinal intercostal approach, whereas the left portal vein is best imaged through an oblique subcostal approach. The splenic vein is best seen in a midline transverse orientation. The coronary

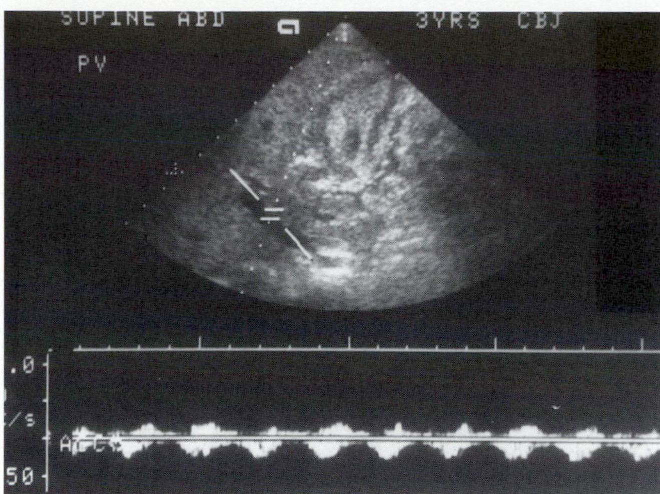

FIGURE 40–9. Bidirectional portal vein flow associated with portal hypertension. Transverse view through the porta hepatis in a child with portal hypertension demonstrates bidirectional flow in the main portal vein.

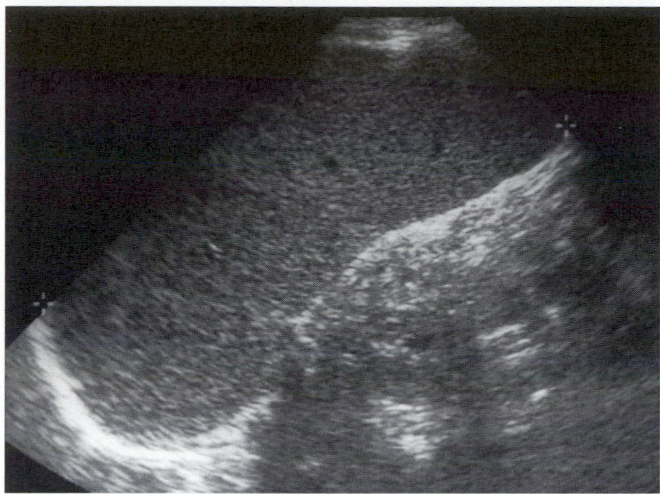

FIGURE 40–11. Splenomegaly associated with portal hypertension. Longitudinal view through the left upper quadrant in a child with portal hypertension shows splenic enlargement.

vein is best imaged in the longitudinal plane, using the left hepatic lobe as a window. This vein drains the distal esophagus and proximal stomach, courses through the lesser omentum, and has a variable connection with the portal venous system, ranging from the portal vein to the splenic vein. The umbilical vein runs in the falciform ligament from the left branch of the portal vein to the anterior abdominal wall and is connected to the superior and inferior epigastric veins. It may be imaged within the liver coursing anteriorly from the left portal vein or along the midline in the anterior abdominal wall extending to the umbilicus (Fig. 40-5). The lesser omentum is imaged in the longitudinal plane between the left lobe of the liver and the aorta at the level of the celiac axis. Thickening of the lesser omentum in children with portal hypertension is probably due to a large tortuous coronary vein and its varicose collaterals coursing through the region or to accompanying lymphatic stasis (Fig. 40-10). The ratio of lesser omental thickness to anteroposterior diameter of the aorta is less than 1.7:1 in "normal" children, whereas it exceeds 2:1 in approximately one-half of children with portal hypertension.

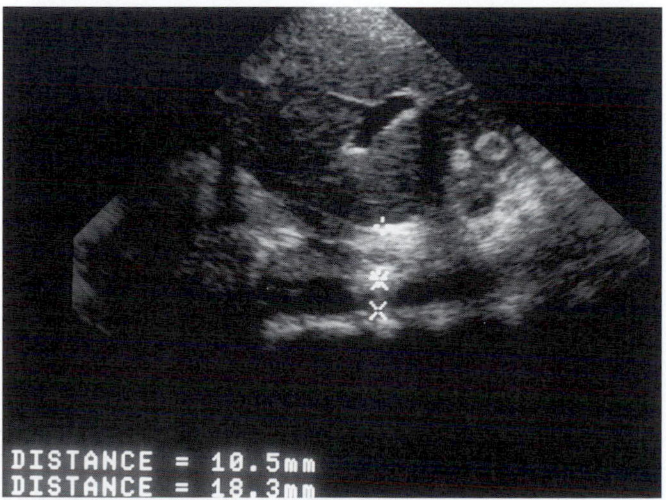

FIGURE 40–10. Thickening of the lesser omentum in a child with portal hypertension. Longitudinal view through the left lobe of the liver shows thickening of the lesser omentum (*between electronic calipers*) immediately anterior to the abdominal aorta.

References

Frider B, Marin AM, Goldberg A: Ultrasonographic diagnosis of portal vein cavernous transformation in children. *J Ultrasound Med* 8:445–449, 1989.

Gibson RN, Gibson PR, Donlan JD, et al: Identification of a patent paraumbilical vein by using doppler sonography: Importance in the diagnosis of portal hypertension. *AJR* 153:513–516, 1989.

Grant EG, Schiller VL, Millener P, et al: Color doppler imaging of the hepatic vasculature. *AJR* 159:943–950, 1992.

Grant EG, Tessler FN, Gomes AS, et al: Color doppler imaging of portosystemic shunts. *AJR* 154:393–397, 1990.

Kane RA, Katz SG: The spectrum of sonographic findings in portal hypertension: A subject review and new observations. *Radiology* 142:453–458, 1982.

Mostbeck GH, Wittich GR, Herold C, et al: Hemodynamic significance of the paraumbilical vein in portal hypertension: Assessment with duplex US. *Radiology* 170:339–342, 1989.

Patriquin H, Lafortune M, Burns PN, et al: Duplex doppler examination in portal hypertension: Technique and anatomy. *AJR* 149:71–76, 1987.

Patriquin H, Tessler G, Grignon A, et al: Lesser omental thickness in normal children: Baseline for detection of portal hypertension. *AJR* 145:693–696, 1985.

Ralls PW: Color doppler sonography of the hepatic artery and portal venous system. *AJR* 155:517–525, 1990.

Subramanyam BR, Balthazar EJ, Madamba MR, et al: Sonography of portosystemic venous collaterals in portal hypertension. *Radiology* 146:161–166, 1983.

Wachsberg RH, Obolevich AT: Blood flow characteristics of vessels in the ligamentum teres fissure at color doppler sonography: Findings in healthy volunteers and in patients with portal hypertension. *AJR* 164:1403–1405, 1995.

Wachsberg RH, Simmons MZ: Coronary vein diameter and flow direction in patients with portal hypertension: Evaluation with duplex sonography and correlation with variceal bleeding. *AJR* 162:637–641, 1994.

Weltin G, Taylor KJW, Carter AR, Taylor CR: Duplex doppler: Identification of cavernous transformation of the portal vein. *AJR* 144:999–1001, 1985.

Westra SJ, Zaninovic AC, Vargas J, et al: The value of portal vein pulsatility on duplex sonograms as a sign of portal hypertension in children with liver disease. *AJR* 165:167–172, 1995.

Zwiebel WJ, Mounford RA, Halliwell MJ, et al: Splanchnic blood flow in patients with cirrhosis and portal hypertension: Investigation with duplex doppler US. *Radiology* 194:807–812, 1995.

41

Figure 41-1 shows a 2-week-old girl with vomiting. What do you see? What are the diagnostic considerations?

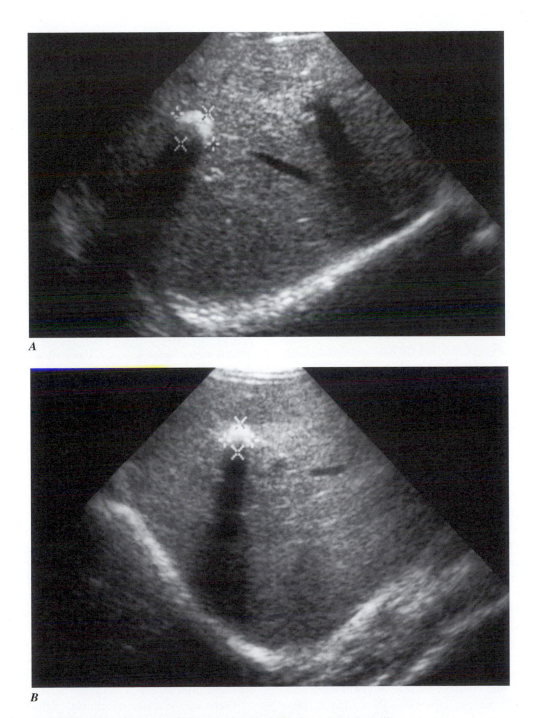

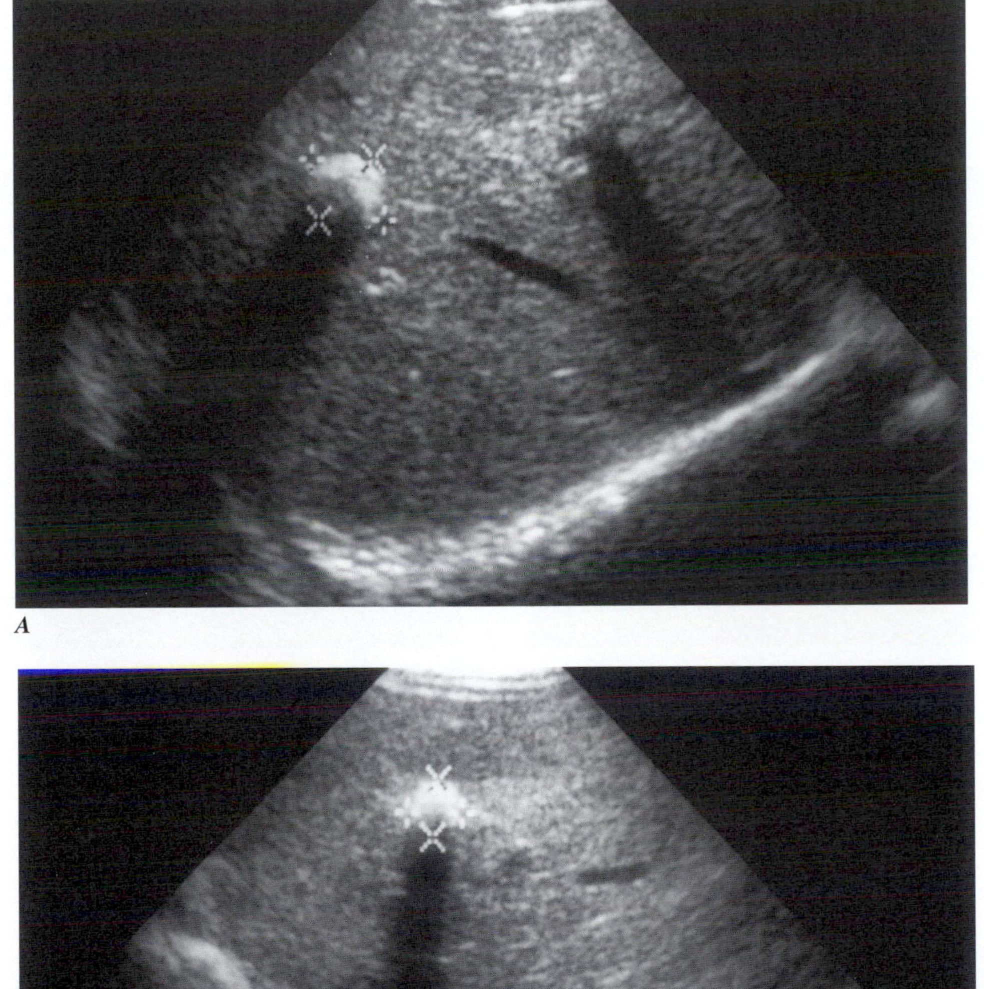

A

B

FIGURE 41–1. Transverse *(A)* and longitudinal *(B)* views through the liver.

CHAPTER 41

Neonatal Hepatic Calcification

CARLOS J. SIVIT

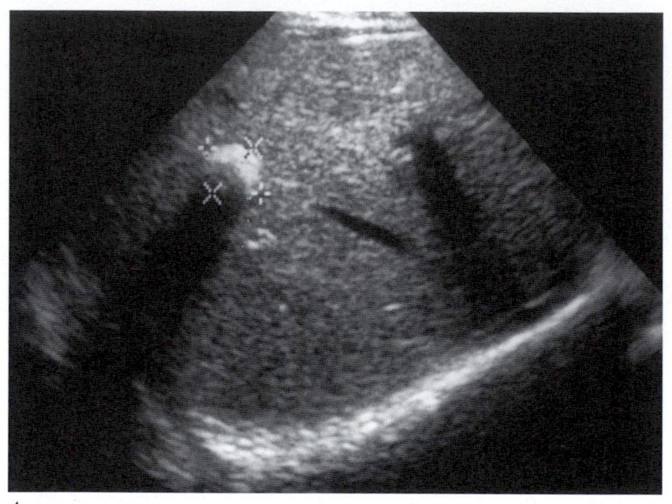

A

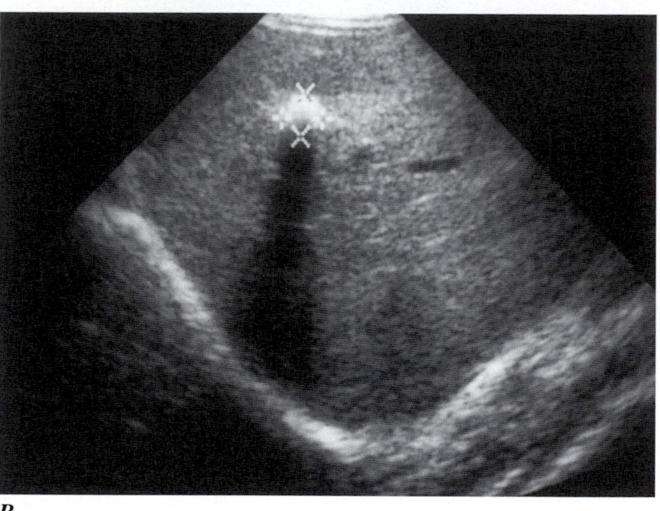

B

FIGURE 41–2. Hepatic parenchymal calcification. Transverse ***(A)*** and longitudinal ***(B)*** views through the right lobe of the liver show a curvilinear hyperechoic parenchymal focus (*between electronic calipers*) with acoustic shadowing representing a hepatic parenchymal calcification.

Neonatal hepatic calcification may be solitary (Fig. 41-2) or diffuse and multifocal (Fig. 41-3). The calcification may arise from hepatic parenchymal or vascular structures. Hepatic parenchymal calcification may arise from infectious, ischemic, and neoplastic conditions. It has also been reported in association with trisomy 18. In the majority of cases, there is no identifiable etiology, and the calcification is considered idiopathic. A variety of congenital infections, including syphilis, cytomegalovirus, toxoplasmosis, rubella, echovirus, and herpes simplex, have been associated with hepatic calcification, probably secondary to an in utero fetal hepatitis. In these cases, calcification often involves multiple abdominal organs. Conditions that result in hepatic ischemia may also lead to dystrophic hepatic calcification. These include placental insufficiency, fetal vascular abnormality, and fetofetal transfusion. Hepatic calcification may develop in the common primary hepatic tumors seen in young children, including hemangioma, hemangioendothelioma, and hepatoblastoma. It may also be seen in metastatic neuroblastoma. When calcification is seen in association with a hepatic tumor, the appearance will be that of a calcified mass, not of isolated calcification. Hepatic vascular calcification may result from thromboemboli in the portal vein, the hepatic vein, or the ductus venosus (Fig. 41-4). The latter vessel shunts blood from the left portal vein to the inferior vena cava in fetuses and usually closes during the first 24 h postnatally. Most cases of calcified hepatic vascular thrombi are associated with prior umbilical vein catheterization.

There are typically no clinical signs and symptoms directly associated with hepatic calcification, although there

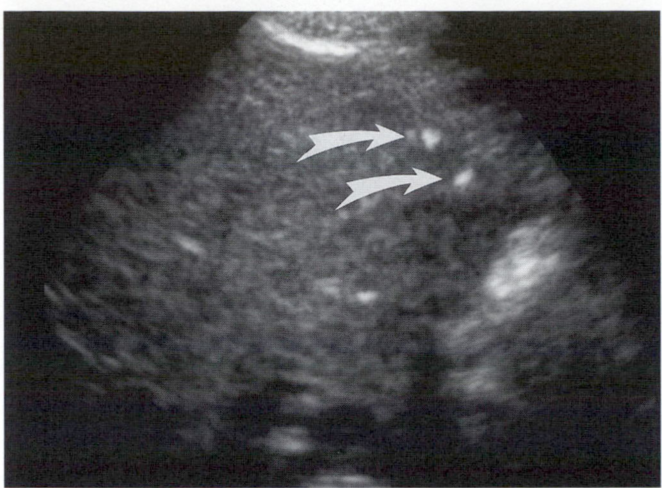

A

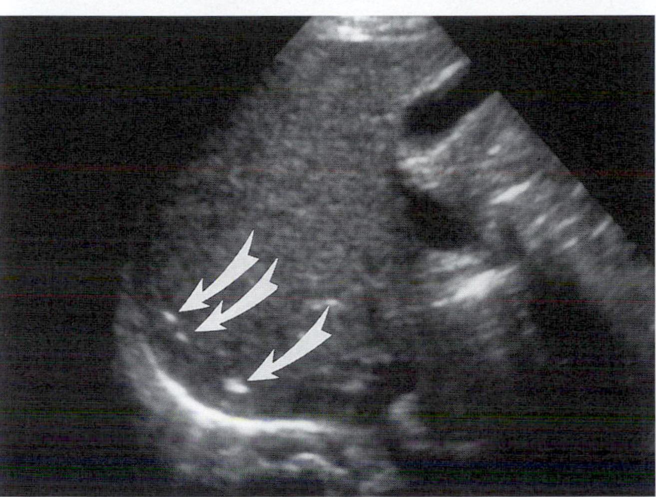

B

FIGURE 41–3. ***A.*** Small peripheral subcapsular hepatic calcifications without acoustic shadowing. Transverse view through the liver demonstrates two small punctate calcifications (*arrows*) in the periphery of the left lobe of the liver. Note the absence of acoustic shadowing due to the small size of the calcifications. ***B.*** Small peripheral subcapsular hepatic calcifications without acoustic shadowing. Transverse view through the liver demonstrates three small rounded calcifications (*arrows*) in the periphery of the posterior segment of the right lobe of the liver. Note the absence of acoustic shadowing due to the small size of the calcifications.

may be clinical manifestations associated with the underlying condition that results in the calcification. In most cases, hepatic calcification in neonates is noted as an incidental finding on conventional radiography or abdominal sonography.

In infants, the liver should be imaged with a 5-MHz sector transducer. A systematic approach is essential, or small lesions such as calcifications can be missed. The gain setting should be adjusted so that the hepatic parenchyma appears homogeneous throughout. Hepatic parenchymal calcifications appear as hyperechoic foci within the hepatic parenchyma that usually demonstrate acoustic shadowing on sonography (Fig. 41-2). They have a rounded, linear, or curvilinear shape. Acoustic shadowing is dependent on the

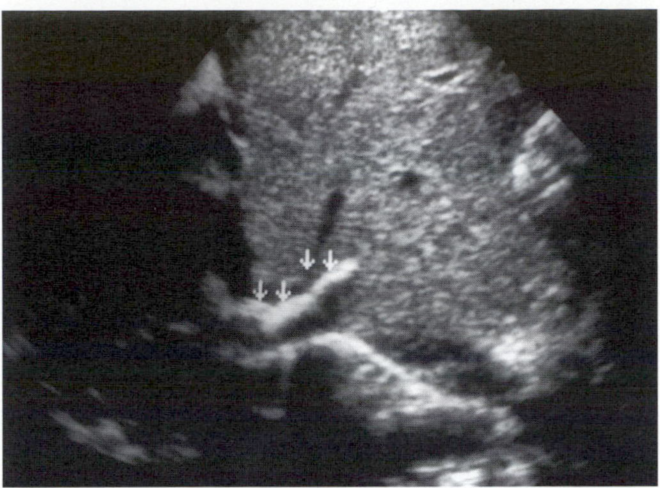

FIGURE 41–4. Hepatic vascular calcification. Longitudinal view through the left lobe of the liver demonstrates a curvilinear calcification within the ductus venosus (*arrows*) extending into the inferior vena cava and right atrium.

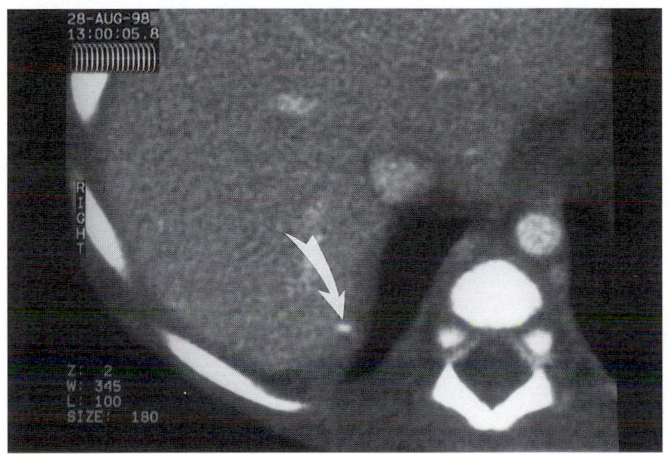

A

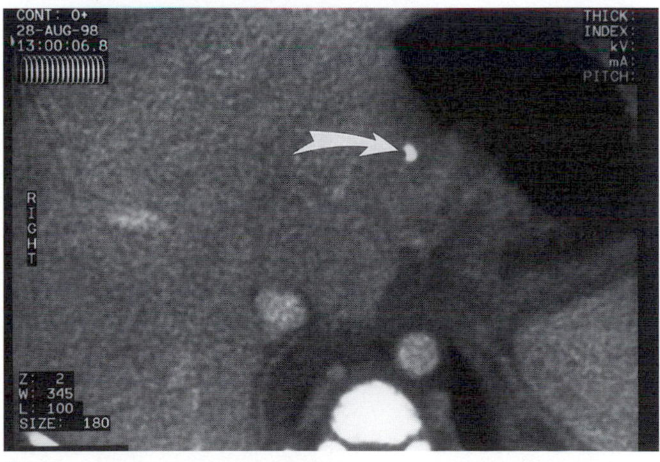

B

FIGURE 41–5. ***A.*** Subcapsular hepatic calcification. Contrast-enhanced computed tomography (CT) scan through the liver in the same patient as in Fig. 41-3 demonstrates a punctate, peripheral subcapsular calcification posteriorly in the right hepatic lobe (*arrow*). ***B.*** Subcapsular hepatic calcification. Contrast-enhanced CT scan through the liver 2 cm below *A* shows another punctate, peripheral subcapsular calcification in the left hepatic lobe (*arrow*).

size of the calcification; therefore, small lesions may not demonstrate any shadowing (Fig. 41-3). Dystrophic calcification associated with global hepatic ischemia is often multifocal and seen peripherally in a subcapsular location (Fig. 41-3).

Hepatic vascular calcifications usually have a characteristic appearance, with a linear configuration and intraluminal location. Flow may still be present around the calcification if the associated thrombus is not completely occlusive. Calcification within the portal vein will appear either as a linear intraluminal calcification or calcified thrombus within the porta hepatis or as a peripherally located linear calcification in an intrahepatic location. Calcification of the ductus venosus has the appearance of an obliquely oriented, paravertebral, linear or curvilinear calcification within the left lobe of the liver (Fig. 41-4). Hepatic vein calcification will also be linear in appearance and may extend to the inferior vena cava. Hepatic vascular calcification may be seen to extend from the portal venous system through the ductus venosus and hepatic vein into the inferior vena cava and right atrium in some patients (Fig. 41-4).

A computed tomography (CT) scan is often performed to exclude the presence of an associated hepatic mass lesion (Fig. 41-5). Preliminary scanning should be performed through the liver without intravenous contrast adminstration to assess for the presence and distribution of calcifications. This should be followed by scanning with the administration of intravenous contrast. Contrast-enhanced CT scan is essential for the determination of an associated hepatic mass lesion.

References

de Filippi G, Betta PG: Vascular liver calcification in infants. *Pediatr Radiol* 18:413–415, 1988.

Friedman AP, Haller JO, Boyer B, et al: Calcified portal vein thromboemboli in infants: Radiography and ultrasonography. *Radiology* 140:381, 1981.

Hawass ND, El Badawi MG, Fatani JA, et al: Foetal hepatic calcification. *Pediatr Radiol* 20:528–535, 1990.

Kogutt MS: Hepatic calcifications presumably due to congenital syphilis. *AJR* 156:634–635, 1991.

Nguyen DL, Leonard JC: Ischemic hepatic necrosis: A cause of fetal liver calcification. *AJR* 147:596–597, 1986.

Richter E, Globi H, Holthusen W, et al: Intrahepatic calcifications in infants and children following umbilical vein catheterization. *Ann Radiol* 27:117–124, 1984.

Rizzo AJ, Haller JO, Mulvihill DM, et al: Calcification of the ductus venosus: A cause of right upper quadrant calcification in the newborn. *Radiology* 173:89–90, 1989.

Stein B, Bromley B, Michlewitz H, et al: Fetal liver calcifications: Sonographic appearance and postnatal outcome. *Radiology* 197:489–492, 1995.

42

Figure 42-1 shows a 10-year-old girl with fever, rash, conjunctivitis, and generalized lymphadenopathy. What is the abnormality? What is the most likely diagnosis?

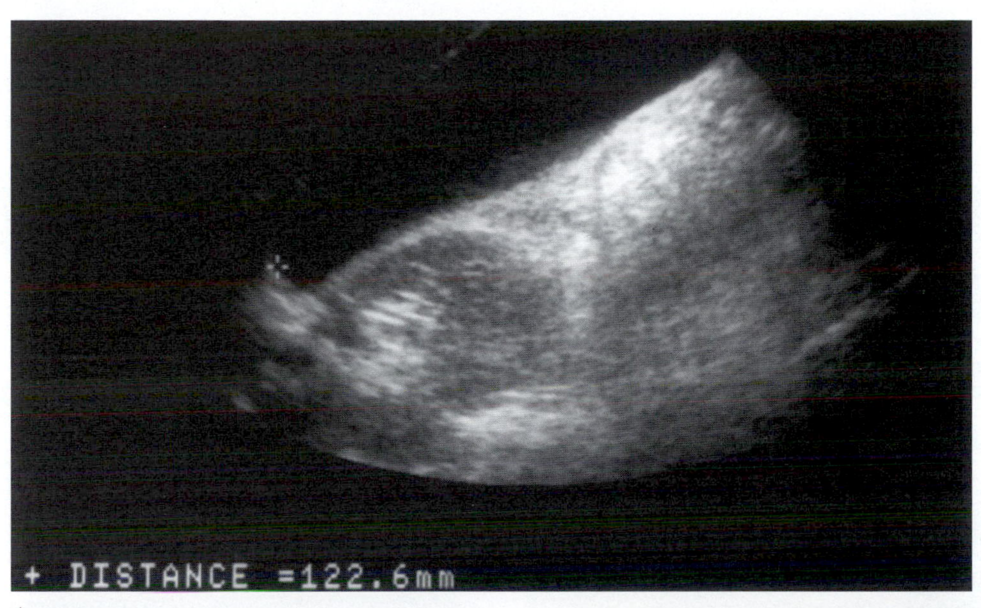

A

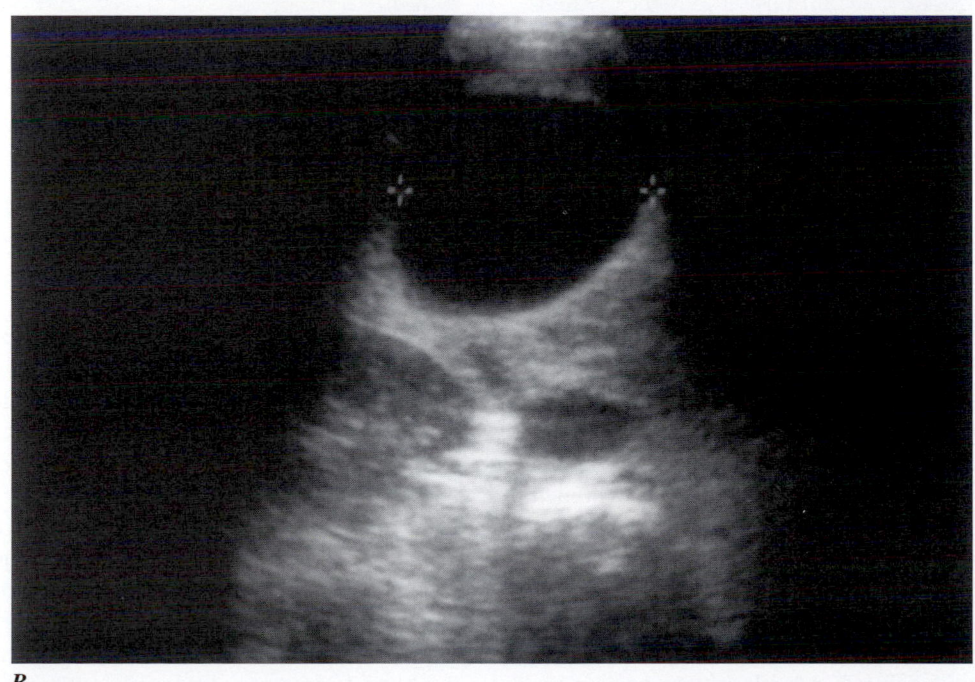

B

FIGURE 42–1. Longitudinal *(A)* and transverse *(B)* views of the gallbladder.

CHAPTER 42

Hydrops of Gallbladder

CHARLES J. CHUNG

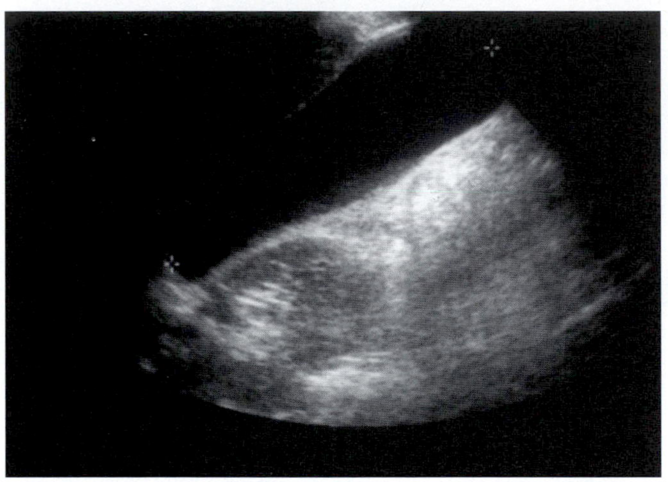

A

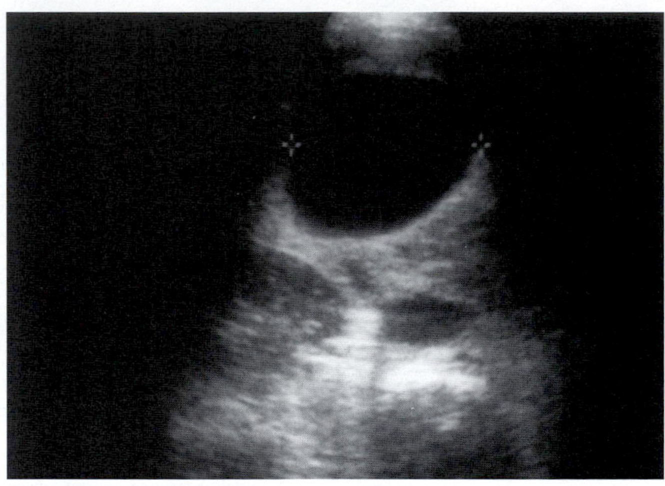

B

FIGURE 42–2. Gallbladder hydrops associated with Kawasaki syndrome. Longitudinal ***(A)*** and transverse ***(B)*** views through the right upper quadrant demonstrate an enlarged gallbladder (*between electronic calipers*) measuring over 12 cm in the longitudinal plane, consistent with hydrops of the gallbladder. There was no associated gallbladder wall thickening, pericholecystic fluid, biliary dilatation, or gallstones.

Acute gallbladder hydrops, or massive distention of the gallbladder by serous fluid, uncommonly occurs in children (Fig. 42-2). It may be seen in association with systemic illness, infection, trauma, or prolonged fasting. Specific conditions that have been associated with gallbladder hydrops include Kawasaki syndrome, Wilson's disease, Henoch-Schönlein purpura, scarlet fever, metachromatic leukodystrophy, familial Mediterranean fever, leptospirosis, typhoid fever, Epstein-Barr virus, Lyme disease, ehrlichiosis, total parenteral nutrition, and generalized sepsis. Gallbladder hydrops has also been reported in neonates in association with partial duodenal obstruction due to either duodenal web or duodenal stenosis. There are also reported cases of gallbladder hydrops without identifiable underlying etiology.

The most common condition associated with hydrops of the gallbladder in children is mucocutaneous lymph node syndrome, otherwise known as Kawasaki syndrome (Fig. 42-2). This condition is a systemic illness of unknown etiology. Recent immunologic evidence suggests that superantigens may be responsible for this illness. The diagnosis of Kawasaki syndrome is made on the basis of clinical criteria. These include fever accompanied by four of the following findings: conjunctivitis, oral mucosal lesions, swelling of the palms and soles with desquamation of the fingertips, erythematous skin rash, and cervical lymphadenopathy. Gallbladder hydrops in these children is felt to arise as a result of a generalized vasculitis that can involve the common bile duct and cystic duct or secondary to external compression of those

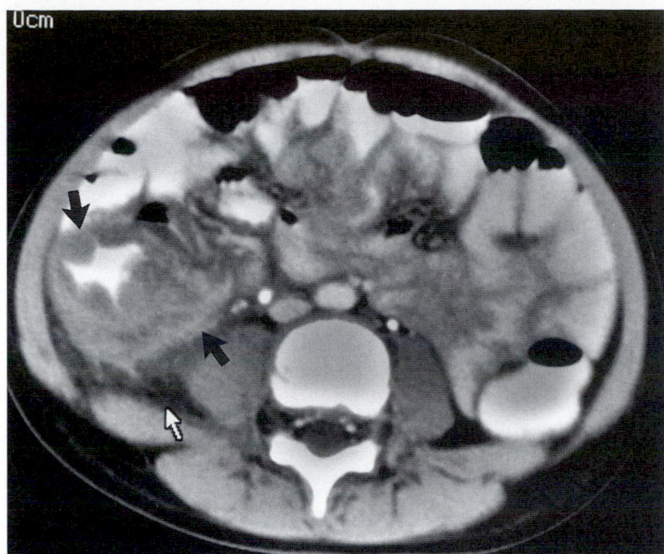

FIGURE 42–3. Bowel wall thickening associated with Kawasaki syndrome. Contrast-enhanced computed tomography scan through the lower abdomen in a child with Kawasaki syndrome demonstrates bowel wall thickening of the ascending colon (*black arrow*), indicative of associated colitis. Also note the stranding of adjacent mesenteric fat (*white arrow*).

structures by enlarged lymph nodes, resulting in a transient obstruction of bile flow. Gallbladder hydrops in children with Kawasaki syndrome usually resolves spontaneously. However, abnormal gallbladder ejection fraction may persist beyond resolution of other clinical symptoms. Rarely, percutaneous drainage or cholecystectomy may become necessary.

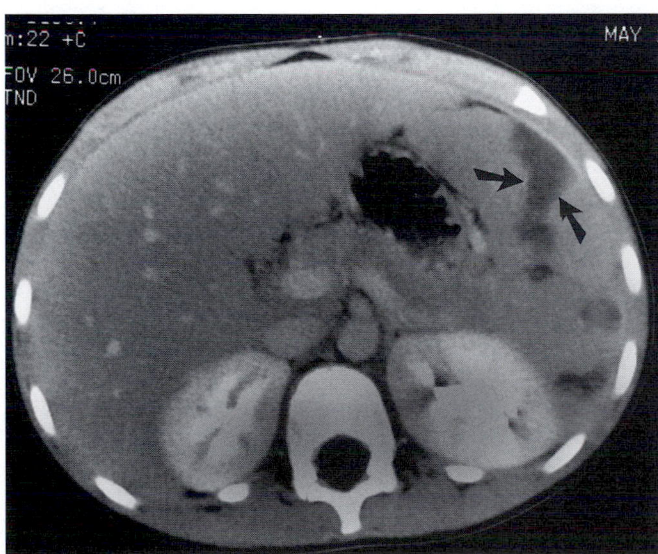

FIGURE 42–4. Splenic infarct associated with Kawasaki syndrome. Contrast-enhanced computed tomography scan through the upper abdomen in a child with Kawasaki syndrome demonstrates multiple peripheral, wedge-shaped defects in the spleen resulting from segmental splenic infarcts. The largest segmental splenic infarct is denoted by arrows.

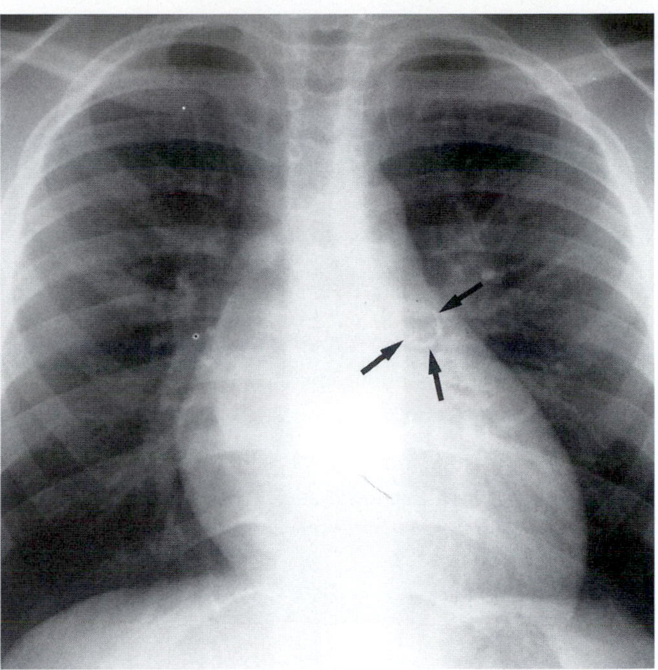

FIGURE 42–5. Coronary calcification associated with Kawasaki syndrome. Chest radiograph of a young adult who had Kawasaki syndrome as a child demonstrates a ring calcification (*arrows*) due to a calcified coronary aneurysm. Cardiac calcifications are seen in approximately one-third of adults with a history of prior Kawasaki syndrome

A variety of associated intraabdominal abnormalities may be noted in children with Kawasaki syndrome. Most of these abnormalities probably result from the systemic vasculitis. They include nephritis, pancreatitis, colitis (Fig. 42-3), lymphadenopathy, splenic infarction (Fig. 42-4), and ascites. Serious intraabdominal complications such as gallbladder perforation or abscess formation are extremely rare. The vast majority of the morbidity and mortality associated with Kawasaki syndrome is due to cardiac and coronary involvement, which may result in coronary aneurysms as well as cardiac dysfunction (Fig. 42-5).

The characteristic sonographic finding associated with gallbladder hydrops is marked distention of the gallbladder without gallbladder wall thickening or calculi (Fig. 42-2). Sludge may be seen within the gallbladder in some cases. The size of the normal gallbladder is variable in children. In fasting infants under 1 year of age, the gallbladder is typically less than 3 cm in length; in fasting older children, it should be less than 7 cm in length. In addition to size criteria, hydrops of the gallbladder may also be associated with a change in gallbladder shape. The normal gallbladder is ovoid in shape, while in gallbladder hydrops the gallbladder may assume a more rounded shape. It should be noted that gallbladder distention is not pathognomonic for gallbladder hydrops. An enlarged gallbladder may also be seen in association with acute cholecystitis, and rarely with gallbladder torsion along the cystic duct. These two conditions are seen more commonly in adults than in children.

References

Bader-Meunier B, Hadchouel M, Fabre M, et al: Intrahepatic bile duct damage in children with Kawasaki disease. *J Pediatr* 120:750–752, 1992.

Barton L, Luisiri A, Dawson J: Hydrops of the gallbladder in childhood infections. *Pediatr Infect Dis J* 14:163–164, 1995.

Choi Y, Sharma B: Gallbladder hydrops in mucocutaneous lymph node syndrome. *South Med J* 82:397–398, 1989.

Chung CJ, Rayder S, Meyers W, et al: Kawasaki disease presenting as focal colitis. *Pediatr Radiol* 26:455–457, 1996.

Cohen E, Stringer D, Smith C, et al: Hydrops of the gallbladder in typhoid fever as demonstrated by sonography. *JCU* 14:633–635, 1986.

Crankson S, Nazer H, Jacobsson B: Acute hydrops of the gallbladder in childhood. *Eur J Pediatr* 151:318–320, 1992.

Dinulos J, Mitchell D, Egerton J, et al: Hydrops of the gallbladder associated with Epstein-Barr virus infection. *Pediatr Infect Dis J* 13:924–929, 1994.

el-Shafie M, Mah C: Transient gallbladder distention in sick premature infants: The value of ultrasonography and radionuclide scintigraphy. *Pediatr Radiol* 16:468–471, 1986.

Horvath M, Weisenbach J: Acute hydrops of the gallbladder in childhood. *Orv Hetil* 135:2829–2832, 1994.

Kim T, Kim I, Kim W, et al: Involvement of the gallbladder in childhood metachromatic leukodystrophy: Ultrasonographic findings. *J Ultrasound Med* 15:821–825, 1996.

McCrindle B, Wood R, Nussbaum A: Henoch-Schonlein syndrome. Unusual manifestations with hydrops of the gallbladder. *Clin Pediatr* 27:254–256, 1988.

Sty J, Starshak R, Goronstein L: Gallbladder perforation in a case of Kawasaki disease: Image correlation. *JCU* 11:381–384, 1983.

Suddleson E, Reid B, Woolley M, et al: Hydrops of the gallbladder associated with Kawasaki syndrome. *J Pediatr Surg* 22:956–959, 1987.

Ziv Y, Feigenberg Z, Dintsman M: Acute inflammation and distension of the gall bladder in infancy. *Aust Paediatr J* 23:53–54, 1987.

43

Figure 43-1 shows a 4-month-old boy with skin lesions. What do you see? What are the diagnostic considerations?

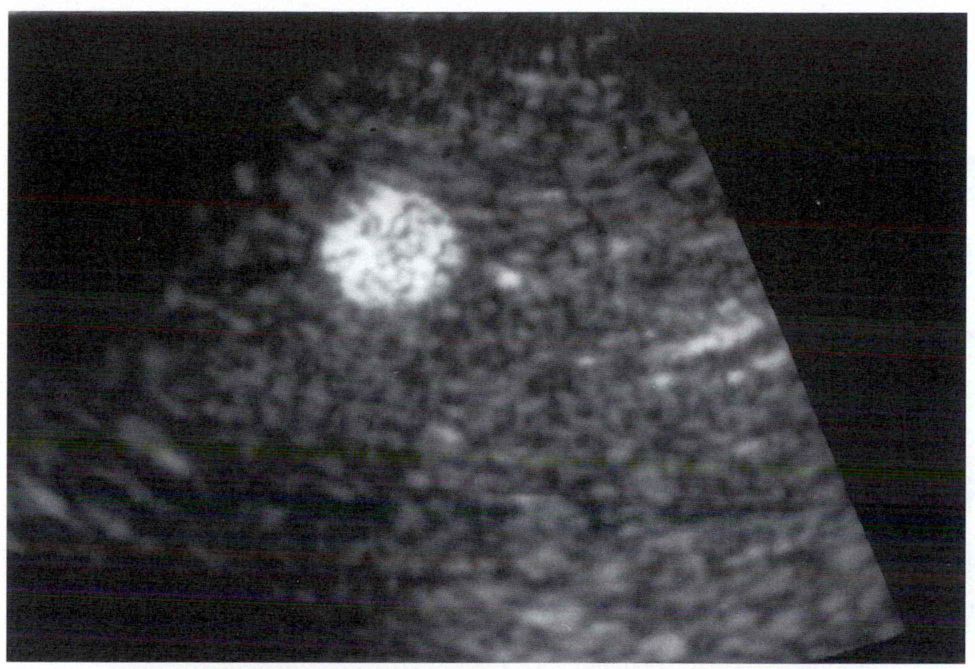

A

B

FIGURE 43–1. Transverse *(A)* and longitudinal *(B)* views through the right lobe of the liver (see Color Plate 14).

CHAPTER 43

Cavernous Hemangioma

CARLOS J. SIVIT

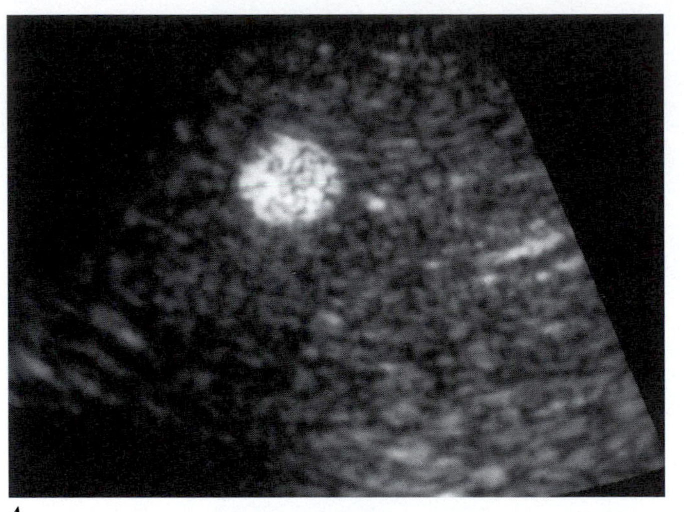

A

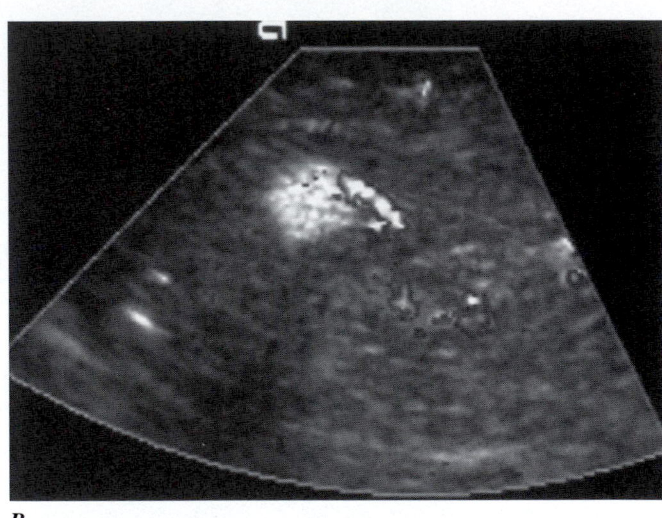

B

FIGURE 43–2. Cavernous hemangioma of the liver. Transverse (***A***) and longitudinal (***B***) demonstrates increased vascularity within the focal hyperechoic hepatic lesion (see Color Plate 15).

Cavernous hemangioma is the most common benign hepatic tumor in children. The tumor is reported to occur in 1 to 2 percent of the general population. Hepatic cavernous hemangioma is usually observed as a solitary mass, but multiple lesions may be noted in 10 percent of patients. There is also an association with hemangiomas at other sites. The tumor is believed to represent a benign congenital hamartoma. Cavernous hemangiomas are composed of large, blood-filled cavernous spaces lined by a single layer of epithelial cells and separated by fibrous septa. This results in a honeycomb appearance on microscopic examination. Cavernous hemangiomas can enlarge in the first year of life. This usually occurs by means of dilatation of existing vascular channels. Subsequently, these tumors typically remain stable in size through adulthood. Large hemangiomas may demonstrate internal hemorrhage, and thrombosis followed by necrosis, fibrosis, and calcification.

Sonography is the principal imaging modality for the assessment of children with suspected cavernous hemangioma of the liver. The lesion is also often identified on sonography as an incidental finding, since most children with this tumor are asymptomatic. The characteristic sonographic appearance of a cavernous hemangioma includes a small mass size (<4 cm in diameter), well-defined margins, and uniform hyperechogenicity (Fig. 43-2; see also Color Plate 15). The increased echogenicity within the tumor results from multiple interfaces within the lesion owing to the internal fibrous septa. Cavernous hemangiomas also commonly demonstrate acoustic enhancement, since the mass is made up of numerous fluid-filled spaces. Most are found in the right lobe of the liver. The tumor is commonly seen in a subcapsular location. Evaluation with color Doppler demonstrates increased vascularity of the center of the tumor (Fig. 43-2). Additionally, enlargement of the celiac artery and decreased diameter of the

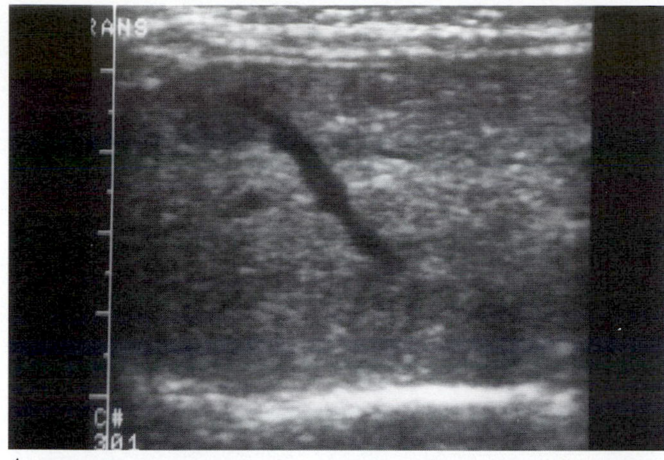

A

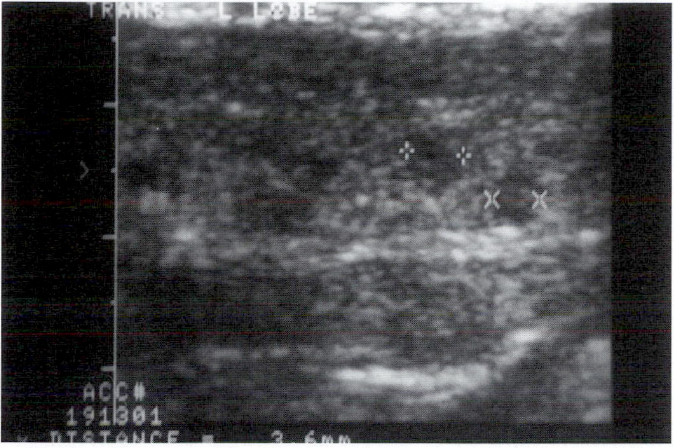

B

FIGURE 43–3. Cavernous hemangioma of the liver. ***A.*** Transverse view through the right lobe of the liver shows a small, well-circumscribed, hypoechoic lesion in a subcapsular location, indicative of a cavernous hemangioma. Note the large feeding vessel. ***B.*** Transverse view through the left lobe of the liver in the same child shows two additional small, hypoechoic lesions (*between electronic calipers*), representing multiple cavernous hemangiomas.

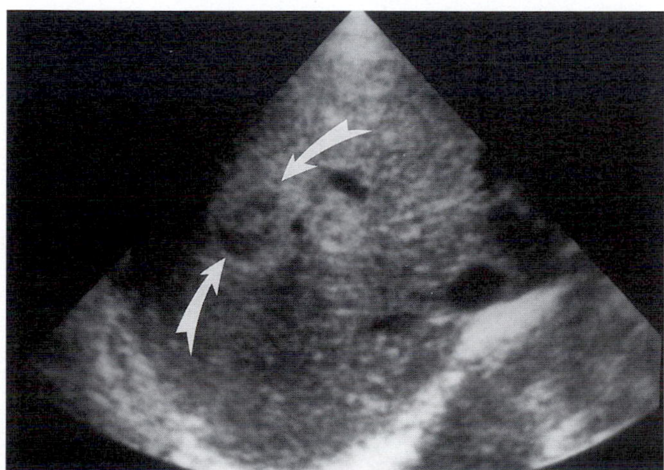

FIGURE 43–4. Cavernous hemangioma of the liver. Transverse view through the right lobe of the liver demonstrates a small, well-circumscribed parenchymal lesion (*arrows*). Note that the mass has a hypoechoic center and a thick echogenic rind.

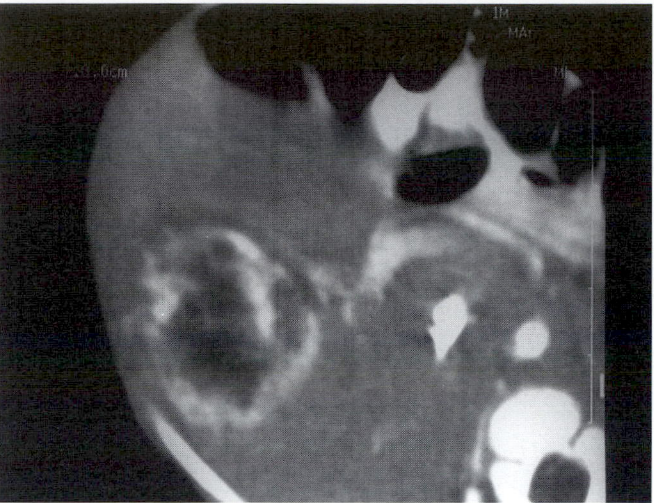

FIGURE 43–5. Cavernous hemangioma of the liver. Contrast-enhanced computed tomography scan through the liver demonstrates a well-circumscribed peripheral lesion in the right hepatic lobe. Note that the mass has a low-attenuation center and intense peripheral contrast enhancement.

abdominal aorta below the celiac artery may be noted on Doppler imaging. The lesions may be multiple. Serial examination may demonstrate an increase in the size of the lesion over the first few months of life. However, there should be little or no change seen after the first year of life.

A small subset of these lesions will have an atypical appearance on sonography. They may occasionally be uniformly hypoechoic (Fig. 43-3) or demonstrate a heterogeneous echotexture. Some have a thick echogenic rind (Fig. 43-4). Additionally, calcification may occasionally be noted. The variability in sonographic appearance is seen more frequently in larger lesions and probably results from the development of previously discussed complications, including hemorrhage, thrombosis, fibrosis, and necrosis.

Cavernous hemangiomas may also be imaged with computed tomography (CT), magnetic resonance imaging (MRI), and nuclear scintigraphy. The characteristic appearance of a cavernous hemangioma on CT is a low-attenuation mass on noncontrast imaging with an enhancement pattern following intravenous contrast administration that is initially peripheral and progressively extends toward the center of the lesion over time (Fig. 43-5). The characteristic appearance of the lesion on MRI is marked hyperintensity on T2-weighted images. Nuclear scintigraphy with technetium-99m red blood cells typically shows decreased activity within the lesion on early dynamic images and progressively increased activity on delayed blood pool images.

References

Bree RL, Schwab RE, Glazer GM, et al: The varied appearances of hepatic cavernous hemangiomas with sonography, computed tomography, magnetic resonance imaging and scintigraphy. *Radiographics* 7:1153–1175, 1987.

Bruneton JN, Drouillard J, Fenart D, et al: Ultrasonography of hepatic cavernous haemangiomas. *Br J Radiol* 56:791–795, 1983.

Gibney RG, Hendin AP, Cooperberg PL, et al: Sonographically detected hepatic haemangiomas: Absence of change over time. *AJR* 149:953–957, 1987.

Itai Y, Ohtomo K, Araki T, et al: Computed tomography and sonography of cavernous hemangioma of the liver. *AJR* 141:315–320, 1983.

McArdle CR: Ultrasonic appearances of a hepatic hemangioma. *JCU* 6:124, 1978.

Mirk P, Rubaltelli L, Bazzocchi M, et al: Ultrasonographic patterns in hepatic haemangiomas. *JCU* 10:373–378, 1982.

Moody AR, Wilson SR: Atypical hepatic hemangioma: A suggestive sonographic morphology. *Radiology* 188:413–417, 1993.

Nelson RC, Chezmar JL: Diagnostic approach to hepatic hemangiomas. *Radiology* 176:11–13, 1990.

Takayasu K, Moriyama N, Shima Y, et al: Atypical radiographic findings in hepatic cavernous hemangioma: Correlation with histologic features. *AJR* 146:1149–1153, 1986.

Tanaka S, Kitamura T, Fujita M, et al: Color doppler flow imaging of liver tumors. *AJR* 154:509–514, 1990.

Tarboury J, Porcel A, Tubiana JM, et al: Cavernous hemangiomas of the liver studied by ultrasound: Enhancement posterior to a hyperechoic mass as a sign of vascularity. *Radiology* 149: 781–785, 1983.

Figure 44-1 shows an 8-year-old boy with fever and acute right upper quadrant pain. What do you see? What are the diagnostic considerations?

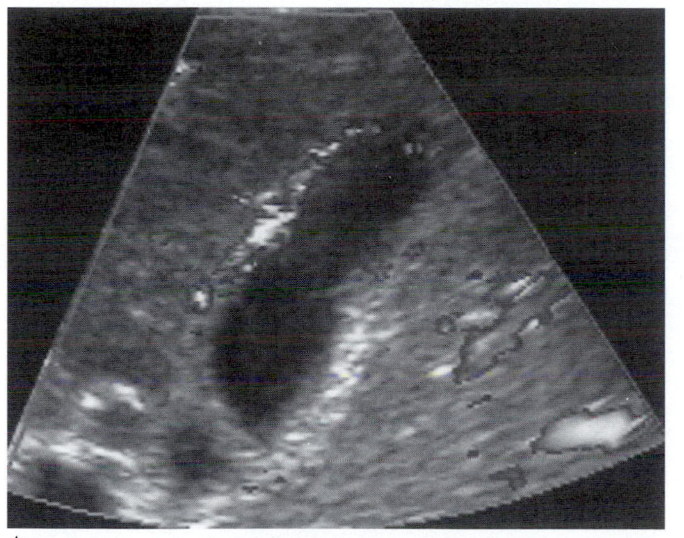

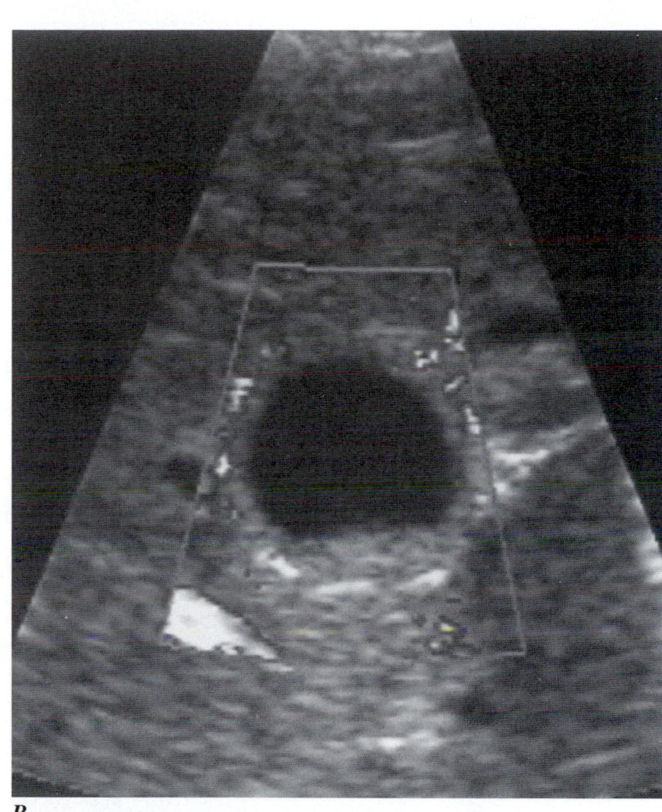

A *B*

FIGURE 44–1. Longitudinal *(A)* and transverse *(B)* views through the gallbladder with color Doppler sonography. (See Color Plate 16.)

CHAPTER 44

Acute Cholecystitis

CARLOS J. SIVIT

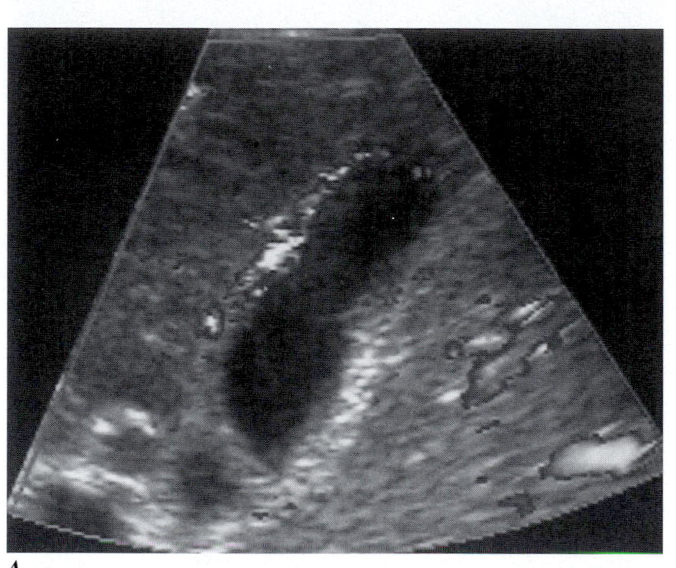
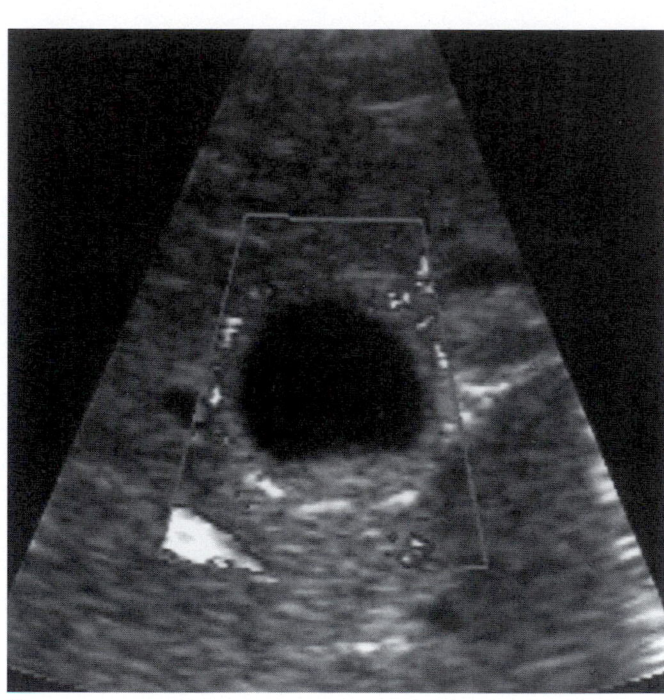

A *B*

FIGURE 44–2. Acute cholecystitis with hypervascularity of the gallbladder. Longitudinal *(A)* and transverse *(B)* views through the gallbladder demonstrate wall thickening and marked hyperemia on color Doppler. (See Color Plate 17.)

Acute cholecystitis may be seen in children, although less frequently than in adults. It can develop secondary to bile stasis associated with persistent calculous obstruction of the cystic duct. This results in local damage to the gallbladder secondary to a change in bile concentration or bile constituents. In children, approximately one-half of cases of acute cholecystitis are not due to cholelithiasis and are therefore referred to as acalculous cholecystitis. This is a far greater percentage than is seen in adults. The principal underlying conditions associated with acalculous cholecystitis in children include recent surgery, fasting states, burns, hyperalimentation, dehydration, systemic illness, and infection due to streptococci, Kawasaki syndrome, and generalized sepsis. There is significant morbidity and mortality associated with acute cholecystitis when the condition is untreated. Serious complications include gallbladder rupture, abscess, and peritonitis. These are very rare in children.

The presenting signs and symptoms of acute cholecystitis vary widely, and the clinical diagnosis may be difficult. This is particularly true in children, since the condition is uncommon. Clinical findings include right upper quadrant pain, nausea, vomiting, and low-grade fever. Focal tenderness over

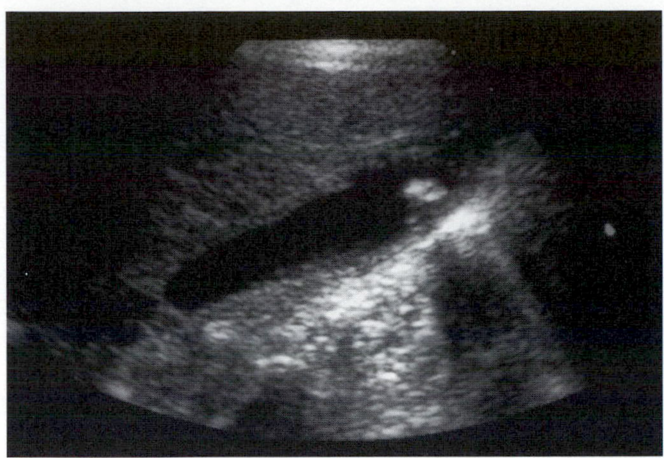

FIGURE 44–3. Cholelithiasis. Longitudinal view through the gallbladder demonstrates a hyperechoic focus with acoustic shadowing, indicative of a gallstone. Also note associated mild gallbladder wall thickening.

the gallbladder (Murphy's sign) may also be present. There is usually elevation of liver enzymes. Jaundice may occasionally be present. As a result of the wide variability in clinical presentation, the imaging assessment of this condition plays an important role in establishing an early diagnosis.

Sonography is commonly utilized in the assessment of children with suspected acute cholecystitis (Fig. 44-2; see also Color Plate 17). Sonography is particularly useful in the evaluation of children with calculous cholecystitis in that it permits assessment of associated biliary tract disease, including cholelithiasis (Fig. 44-3), sludge (Fig. 44-4), and biliary dilatation (Fig. 44-4). Sonographic evaluation of gallstones is dependent on three criteria: hyperechoic foci, acoustic shadowing, and mobility (Fig. 44-3). Gallstones generally respond to gravity and move to the most dependent portion. If the abnormality meets all three criteria, the sensitivity of sonography is greater than 95 percent. However, gallstones may be found in a large number of asymptomatic individuals. The gray-scale sonographic diagnosis of cholecystitis itself is insensitive and nonspecific. Children should be examined in the fasting state to allow for maximal gallbladder distention. Sonographic findings associated with acute cholecystitis include gallbladder wall thickening, defined as wall thickness >3 mm (Fig. 44-5); irregular anechoic areas around the gallbladder wall (Fig. 44-6); pericholecystic fluid; a positive sonographic Murphy's sign, defined as localized tenderness over the gallbladder; and gallbladder distention. Unfortunately, these sonographic findings all lack specificity, as each may be commonly seen in the absence of cholecystitis. Thickening of the gallbladder is seen with a variety of diseases extrinsic to the gallbladder, including congestive heart failure, hypoalbuminemia, hepatitis, and renal failure. Additionally, a normal sonogram does not exclude the diagnosis. The most specific gray-scale sonographic criteria for diagnosing acute cholecystitis are focal gallbladder tenderness in association with calculi.

Color Doppler and power color Doppler sonography have recently been utilized in the diagnosis of acute cholecystitis

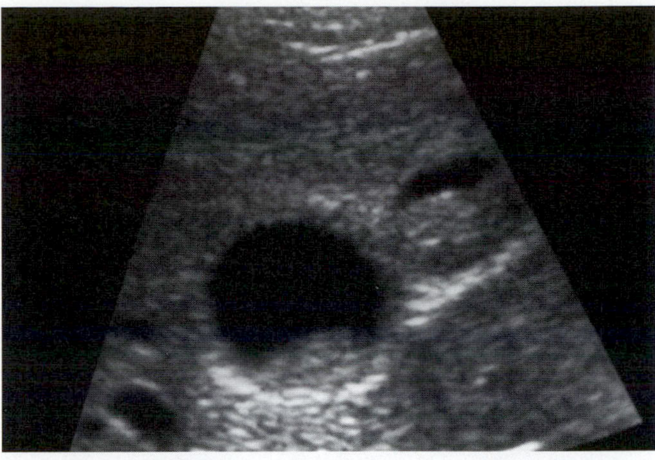

A

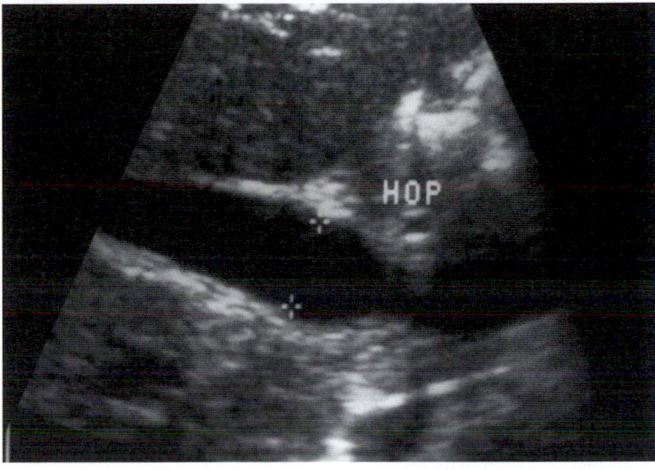

B

FIGURE 44–4. *A.* Sludge in gallbladder. Transverse view through the gallbladder demonstrates intraluminal hypoechoic material without acoustic shadowing, indicative of sludge. ***B.*** Extrahepatic biliary dilatation. Longitudinal view through the head of the pancreas (HOP) in the same child as in ***A*** shows marked dilatation of the distal common bile duct (*between electronic calipers*).

to evaluate flow within the gallbladder wall (Fig. 44-2). The rationale for the use of this technique is based on animal and human studies that show arterial dilatation and extensive venous filling of the gallbladder associated with acute cholecystitis. The use of color Doppler and power color Doppler sonography has resulted in increased specificity in the diagnosis of acute cholecystitis over conventional gray-scale sonography, utilizing gallbladder wall hyperemia as the diagnostic criterion for the condition. However, it should be noted that gallbladder wall hyperemia may also be noted in the absence of acute cholecystitis.

Hepatobiliary radionuclide imaging is also commonly used in the evaluation of children with suspected acute cholecystitis. Children are usually evaluated in the fasting state to facilitate visualization of the gallbladder. Scintigraphic visualization of the gallbladder excludes the diagnosis of calculous cholecystitis with a high degree of accuracy, since the condition is related to cystic duct obstruction. The hallmark finding of calculous cholecystitis on scintigraphy is visual-

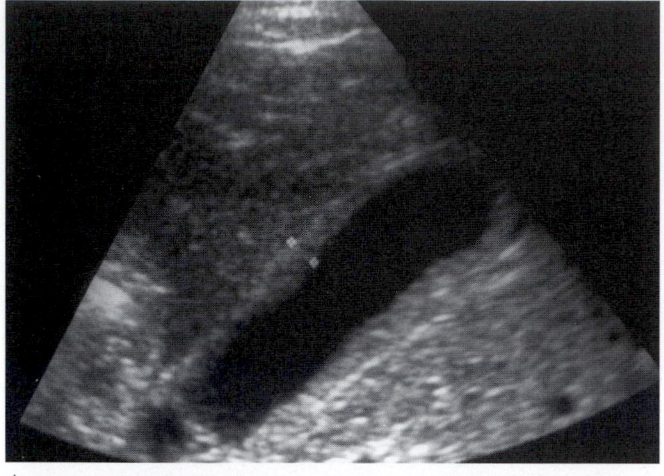

A

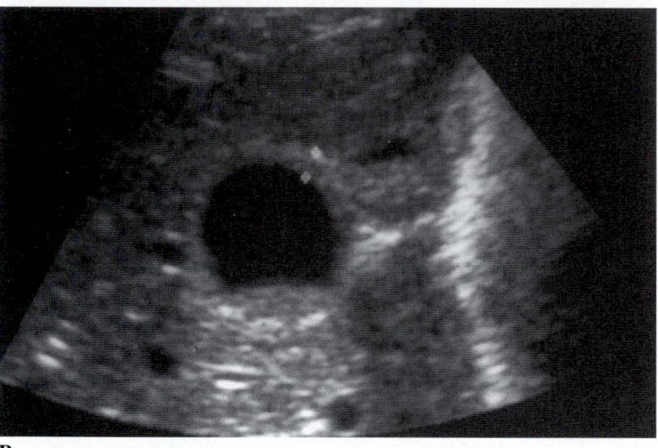

B

FIGURE 44–5. Acute cholecystitis with gallbladder wall thickening. Longitudinal ***(A)*** and transverse ***(B)*** views through the gallbladder in a child with acute cholecystitis demonstrate thickening of the gallbladder wall (*between electronic calipers*).

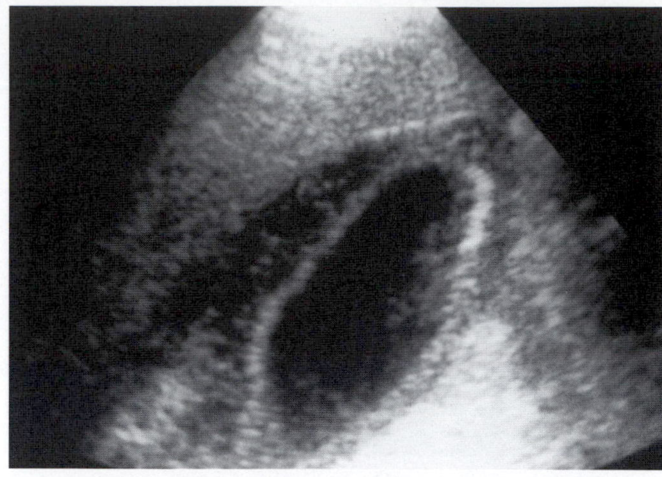

A

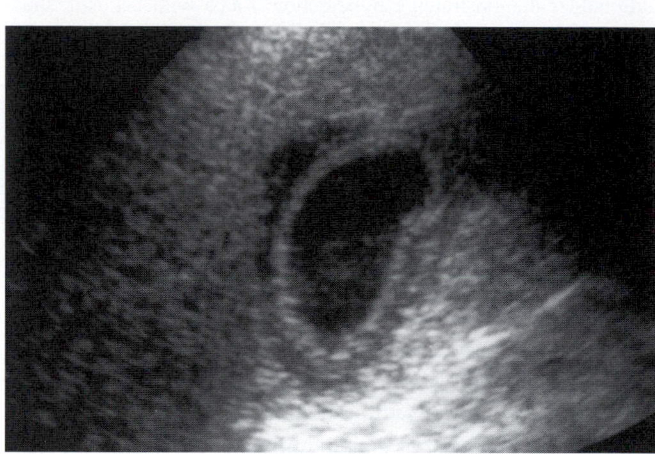

B

FIGURE 44–6. Acute cholecystitis with irregular anechoic areas around the gallbladder wall. Longitudinal (***A***) and transverse (***B***) views through the gallbladder demonstrate thickening of the gallbladder wall. Note that the thickened gallbladder wall demonstrates hypoechoic and anechoic regions.

ization of radioisotope within the common bile duct and proximal small bowel with absence of gallbladder visualization. However, the gallbladder may be visualized in the presence of acalculous cholecystitis.

References

Haller JO: Sonography of the biliary tract in infants and children. *AJR* 157:1051–1058, 1991.

Jeffrey RB, Sommer FG: Follow-up sonography in suspected acalculous cholecystits: Preliminary clinical experience. *J Ultrasound Med* 4:183–187, 1993.

Lee FT, DeLone DR, Bean DW, et al: Acute cholecystitis in an animal model: Findings on color doppler sonography. *AJR* 165: 85–90, 1995.

Martinez A, Bona X, Velasco M, et al: Diagnostic accuracy of ultrasound in acute cholecystitis. *Gastrointest Radiol* 11:334–338, 1986.

Patriquin HB, DiPietro M, Barber FE, et al: Sonography of thickened gallbladder wall: Causes in children. *AJR* 141:57–60, 1983.

Paulson EK, Kliewer MA, Hertzberg BS, et al: Diagnosis of acute cholecystitis with color doppler sonography: Significance of arterial flow in thickened gallbladder wall. *AJR* 162:1105–1108, 1994.

Ralls PW, Colletti PM, Lapin SA, et al: Real-time sonography in suspected acute cholecystitis: Prospective evaluation of primary and secondary signs. *Radiology* 155:767–771, 1985.

Shaler WJ, Leopold GR, Scheible FW: Sonography of the thickened gallbladder wall: A nonspecific finding. *AJR* 136:337–339, 1981.

Simeone JF, Brink JA, Mueller PR, et al: The sonographic diagnosis of acute gangrenous cholecystitis: Importance of the Murphy sign. *AJR* 152:289–290, 1989.

Teefey SA, Baron RL, Bigler SA: Sonography of the gallbladder: Significance of striated (layered) thickening of the gallbladder wall. *AJR* 156:945–947, 1991.

Uggowitzer M, Kugler C, Schramayer G, et al: Sonography of acute cholecystitis: Comparison of color and power color doppler sonography in detecting hypervascularized gallbladder wall. *AJR* 168:707–712, 1997.

Wegener M, Borsch G, Schneider J, et al: Gallbladder wall thickening: A frequent finding in various nonbiliary disorders—a prospective ultrasonographic study. *JCU* 15:307–312, 1987.

45

Figure 45-1 shows a 12-year-old boy with right upper quadrant pain. What do you see? What are the diagnostic considerations?

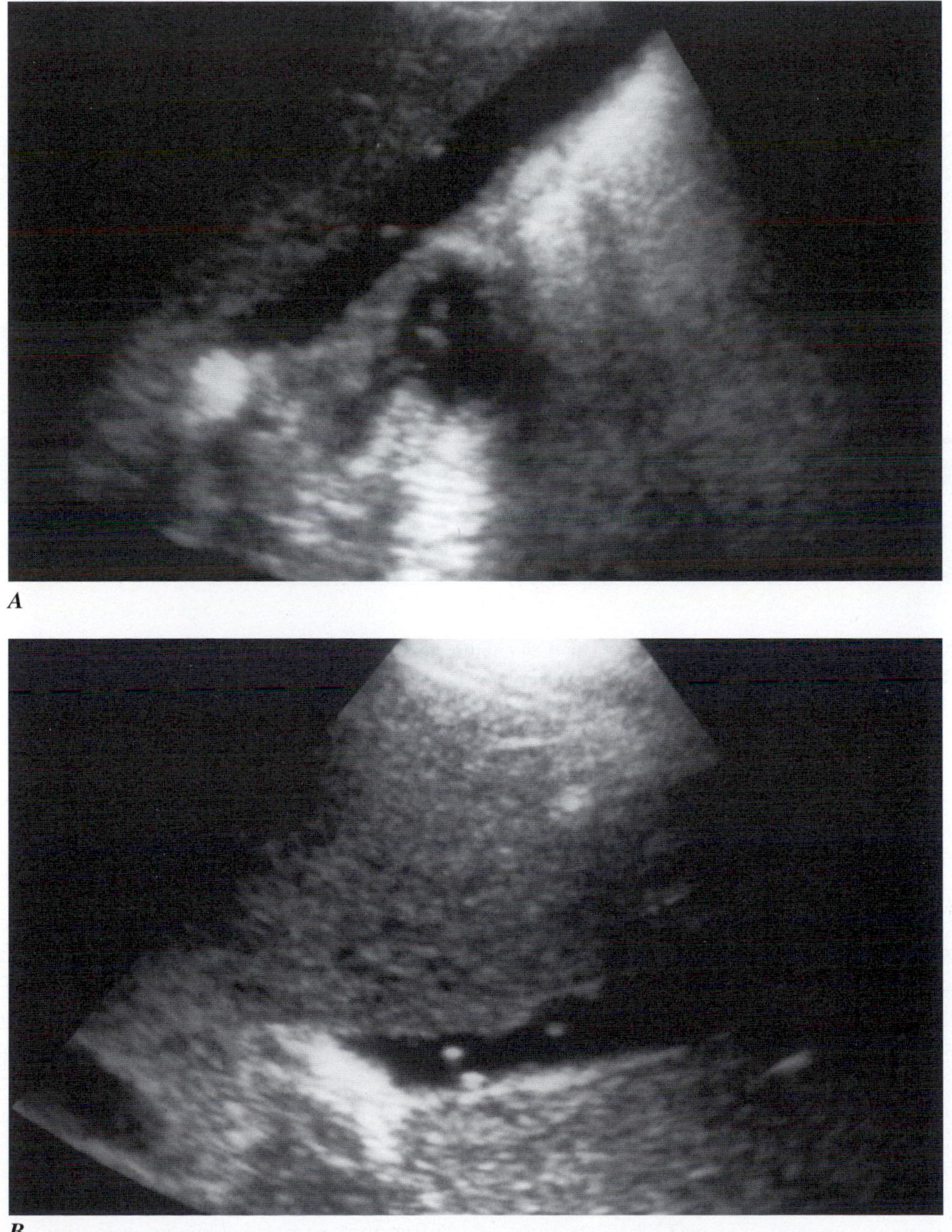

FIGURE 45–1. Supine longitudinal *(A)* and lateral decubitus longitudinal *(B)* views through the gallbladder.

CHAPTER 45

Cholesterosis

CARLOS J. SIVIT

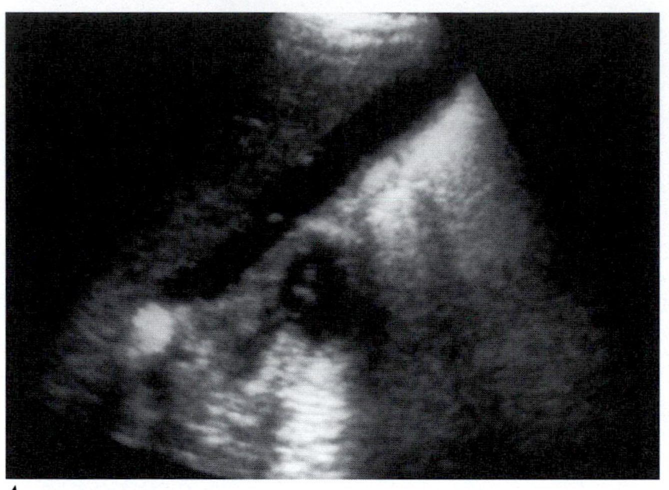

A

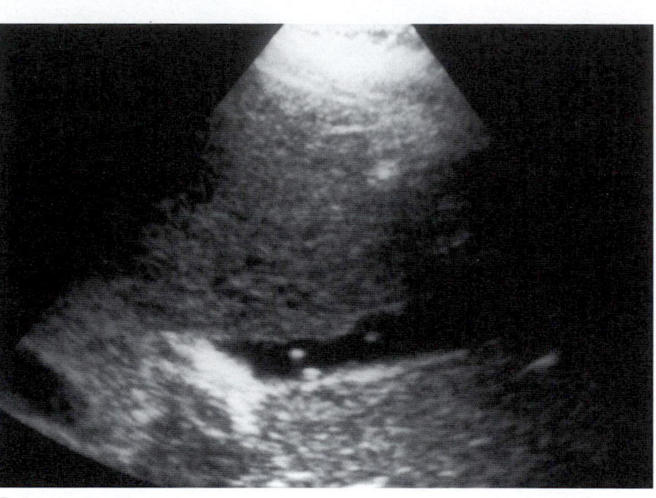

B

FIGURE 45–2. Cholesterosis. Supine longitudinal *(A)* and decubitus longitudinal *(B)* views through the gallbladder show several small, echogenic, nonshadowing masses projecting into the gallbladder lumen. There was no movement of these lesions following decubitus positioning.

Cholesterosis involves abnormal deposition of lipid droplets in the submucosa of the gallbladder wall. It is felt to result from excessive consumption of exogenous cholesterol. The chronic consumption of large amounts of alcohol may be another risk factor in its development. The condition develops secondary to excessive lipid deposition in macrophages. Subsequently, these lipid-laden macrophages become too large and rigid to pass through the endothelium of lymph vessels, resulting in accumulation of these foam cells in the submucosa of the gallbladder wall.

Cholesterosis may be seen in conjunction with cholelithiasis but is more commonly seen in the absence of gallstones. It is unclear whether cholesterosis results in any clinical signs or symptoms. The condition is occasionally observed on sonography in patients imaged because of acute right upper quadrant pain. However, cholesterosis typically persists on follow-up examination in these patients even after they become asymptomatic. In addition, the condition has been observed at autopsy in approximately 1 percent of individuals who were never symptomatic. Therefore, cholesterosis may simply be an incidental finding on sonography.

The sonographic appearance of cholesterosis includes single or multiple adherent, small, echogenic masses that project into the gallbladdder lumen (Fig. 45-2). They are differentiated from gallstones by their lack of mobility with a change in patient positioning and by the absence of acoustic shadowing. Small gallstones may not shadow but should move to the most dependent portion of the gallbladder. Additionally, cholesterosis typically does not change in size over time. The differential diagnosis of fixed, nonshadowing gallbladder wall lesions on sonography includes adenomas, papillomas, inflammatory polyps, mucus retention cysts, and segmental gallbladder wall thickening secondary to adenomyomatosis. All of these lesions are extremely rare in the pediatric population.

References

Alekse RO, Aleksis OT, Il'ina TP: Ultrasonic diagnosis of polypoid formations of the gallbladder. *Ter Arkh* 62:103–108, 1990.

Koga A: Fine structure of the human gallbladder with cholesterosis with special reference to the mechanism of lipid accumulation. *Br J Exp Pathol* 66:605–611, 1985.

CHAPTER 46

Focal Fatty Infiltration of the Liver

CARLOS J. SIVIT

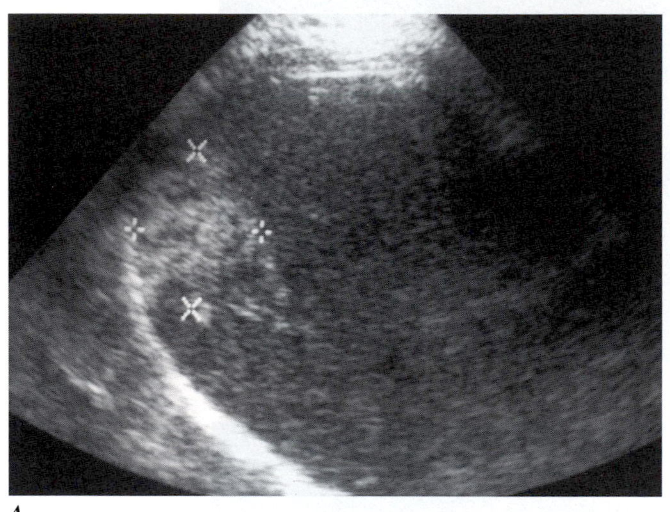

A

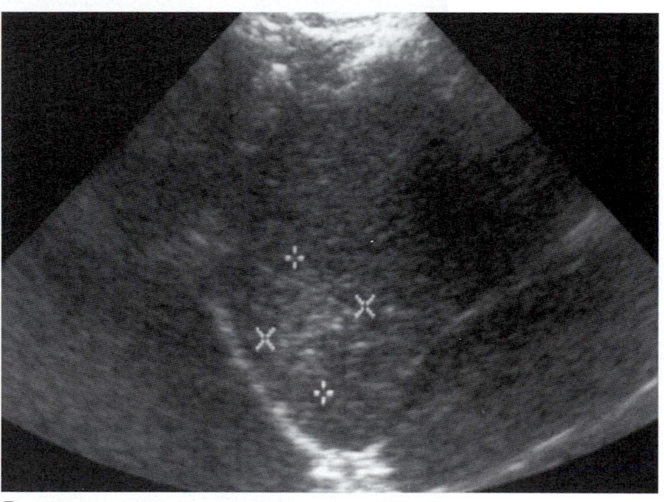

B

FIGURE 46–2. Focal fatty infiltration of the liver. Transverse *(A)* and longitudinal *(B)* views through the right lobe of the liver demonstrate a focal, hyperechoic, peripheral lesion with irregular margins (*between electronic calipers*), representing focal fatty infiltration.

Fatty changes in the liver involve increased triglycerides in the form of droplets in hepatocytes. This results in overloading of previously healthy cells with excess fat. The condition usually follows tissue hypoxia and hepatocellular damage that result in increased fat mobilization within the liver, or is seen in association with enzyme deficiency syndromes in which fat cannot be mobilized out of the liver. Fatty infiltration of the liver has been associated with a variety of conditions, including obesity; hyperlipidemia; diabetes mellitus; metabolic disorders, including galactosemia and fructose intolerance; Reye's syndrome; steroid therapy; malnutrition; hyperalimentation; hepatotoxic drugs; hepatitis; pregnancy; and alcohol abuse. Occasionally, the condition has been reported in otherwise healthy children. Fatty changes can be seen within 3 weeks following an insult. These fatty changes are generally reversible and may resolve as early as 1 week after initial development. Fatty infiltration of the liver is generally diffuse, but occasionally it may be focal in its distribution.

Focal fatty infiltration of the liver has a characteristic appearance on sonography. Normal hepatic parenchyma should have a homogeneous echotexture. The normal liver is slightly hyperechoic relative to the right kidney and slightly hypoechoic relative to the normal spleen. Small echogenic areas

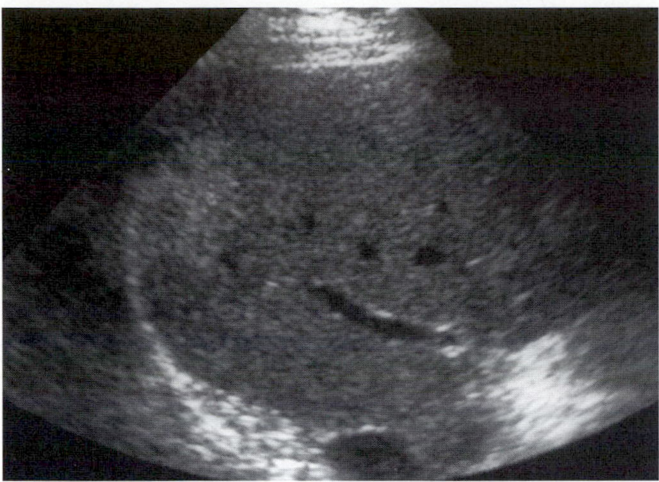

FIGURE 46–3. Focal fatty infiltration of the liver. Transverse view through the right lobe of the liver shows a focal, fan-shaped, hyperechoic lesion, representing focal fatty infiltration.

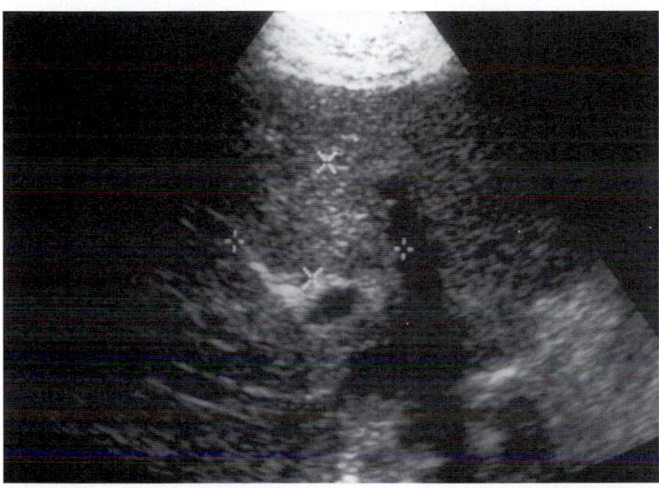

A

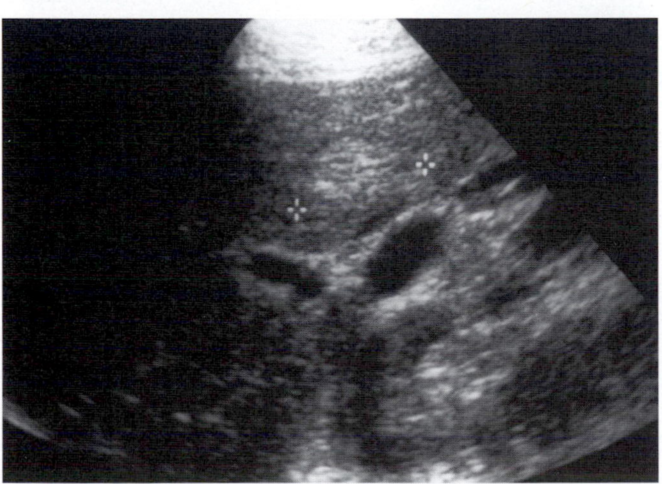

B

FIGURE 46–4. Focal fatty infiltration of the liver mimicking a nodular mass lesion. Transverse (***A***) and longitudinal (***B***) views through the left lobe of the liver demonstrate a focal, rounded, hyperechoic lesion (*between electronic calipers*), representing focal fatty infiltration.

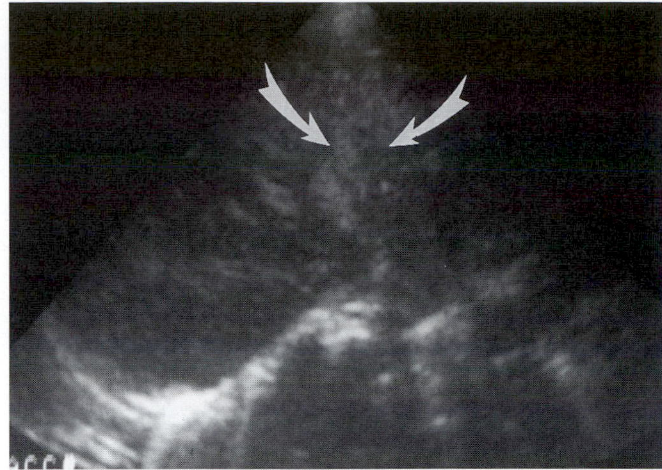

A

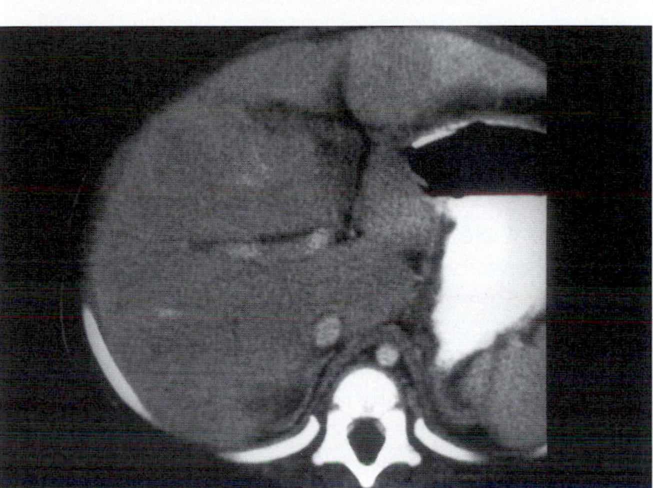

B

FIGURE 46–5. *A.* Focal fatty infiltration of the liver adjacent to the falciform ligament. Transverse view of the left lobe of the liver in a child with prior segmental hepatic infarction demonstrates a focal, hyperechoic region with irregular margins (*arrows*) in the medial segment of the left hepatic lobe adjacent to the falciform ligament. ***B.*** Focal fatty infiltration of the liver adjacent to the falciform ligament. Contrast-enhanced computed tomography scan through the liver in the same child as in Fig. 46-5*A* demonstrates a focal, fan-shaped low-attenuation region in the medial segment of the left hepatic lobe adjacent to the falciform ligament.

representing fibrofatty tissue are normally noted in the hepatic periportal regions. Focal fatty infiltration of the liver is seen as a focal, geographic hyperechoic lesion without mass effect on adjacent vascular structures (Fig. 46-2). It may be fan-shaped with sharp, angulated margins (Fig. 46-3) or have irregular margins (Fig. 46-2). Occasionally, it can have a nodular configuration and mimic a hepatic mass lesion (Fig. 46-4). Focal fatty infiltration has been shown in some cases to follow hepatic infarction. In such instances, focal fatty changes may be seen in watershed areas of hepatic blood supply, such as adjacent to the falciform ligament (Fig. 46-5). Multifocal areas of fatty infiltration may also be seen. When fatty infiltration is extensive and multifocal, areas of normal surrounding hepatic tissue may be mistaken for a mass lesion

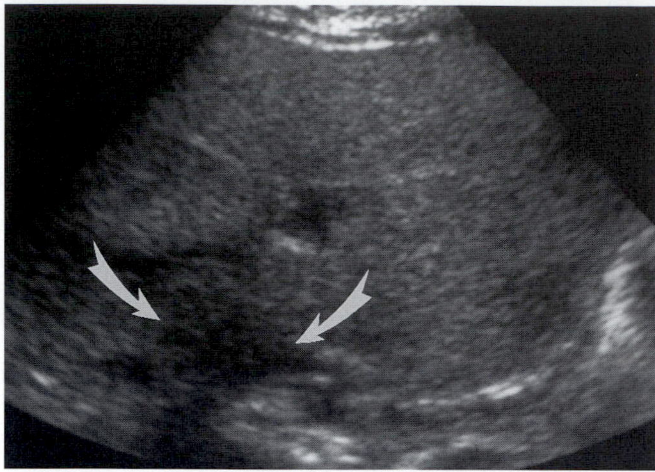

FIGURE 46–6. Extensive multifocal fatty infiltration of the liver. Transverse view through the left lobe of the liver shows multifocal areas of increased hepatic parenchymal echogenicity. A focal area of hepatic tissue demonstrating normal echotexture has the appearance of a focal hypoechoic lesion (*arrows*).

(Fig. 46-6). There is typically sparing of the caudate lobe of the liver when fatty infiltration is extensive and multifocal.

Computed tomography (CT) is also utilized in the evaluation of focal fatty infiltration of the liver when there is a suspicion of a hepatic neoplasm on sonography. Contrast-enhanced CT scan typically shows a geographic area or multifocal areas of decreased attenuation relative to normal hepatic parenchyma without significant displacement of adjacent hepatic or portal veins (Fig. 46-5). However, like sonography, CT may be unable to differentiate between focal fatty infiltration and a true mass. Serial imaging or biopsy may be required for confirmation of the diagnosis. Follow-up examination of focal fatty infiltration demonstrates either resolution or no interval change in the abnormality.

References

Aubin B, Denys A, Lafortune M, et al: Focal sparing of liver parenchyma in steatosis: Role of the gallbladder and its vessels. *J Ultrasound Med* 14:77–80, 1995.

El-Hassan AY, Ibrahim EM, Al-Mulhim FA, et al: Fatty infiltration of the liver: Analysis of prevalence, radiological and clinical features and influence on patient management. *Br J Radiol* 65:774–778, 1992.

Chong VF, Fan YF: Ultrasonographic hepatic pseudolesions: Normal parenchyma mimicking mass lesions in fatty liver. *Clin Radiol* 49:326–329, 1994.

Clain JE, Stephens DH, Charboneau YW: Ultrasonography and computed tomography in focal fatty liver. *Gastroenterology* 87:948–952, 1984.

Henschke CI, Goldman H, Teele RL: The hyperechogenic liver in children: Cause and sonographic appearance. *AJR* 138:841–846, 1982.

Jain KA, McGahan JP: Spectrum of CT and sonographic appearance of fatty infiltration of the liver. *Clin Imaging* 17:162–168, 1993.

Kawashima A, Suehiro S, Murayama S, et al: Focal fatty infiltration of the liver mimicking a tumor: Sonographic and CT features. *J Comput Assist Tomogr* 10:329–331, 1986.

Labuski MR, Eggli KD, Boal DK, et al: Focal fatty infiltration of the liver in a healthy child. *Pediatr Radiol* 22:281–282, 1992.

Quinn SF, Gosnik BB: Characteristic sonographic signs of hepatic fatty infiltration. *AJR* 145:753–755, 1985.

Scatarige JC, Scott WW, Donovan PJ, et al: Fatty infiltration of the liver: Ultrasonographic and computed tomographic correlation. *J Ultrasound Med* 3:9–14, 1984.

Scott WW, Saunders RC, Siegelman SS: Irregular fatty infiltration of the liver: Diagnostic dilemmas. *AJR* 135:67–71, 1980.

Wang SS, Chiang JH, Tsai YT, et al: Focal hepatic fatty infiltration as a cause of pseudotumors: Ultrasonographic patterns and clinical presentation. *JCU* 18:401–409, 1990.

Yoshikawa J, Mastsui O, Takashima T, et al: Focal fatty change of the liver adjacent to the falciform ligament: CT and sonographic findings in five surgically confirmed cases. *AJR* 149:491–494, 1987.

47

Figure 47-1 shows an 18-month-old girl who was injured by a falling television. What are the findings? What is your diagnosis?

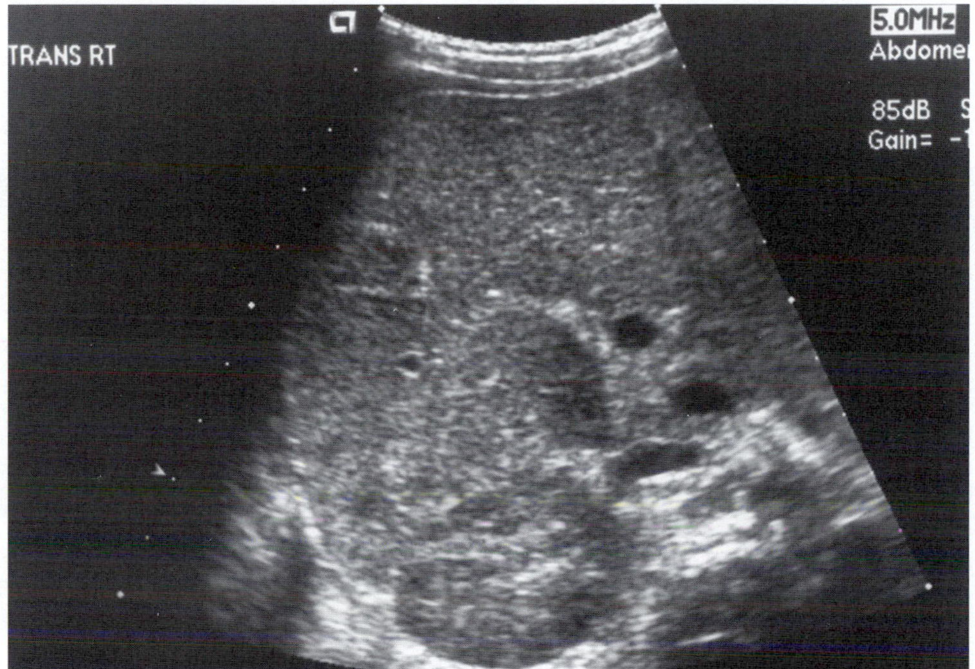

FIGURE 47–1. Transverse view through the right lobe of the liver.

CHAPTER 47

Hepatic Trauma

ELLEN C. BENYA

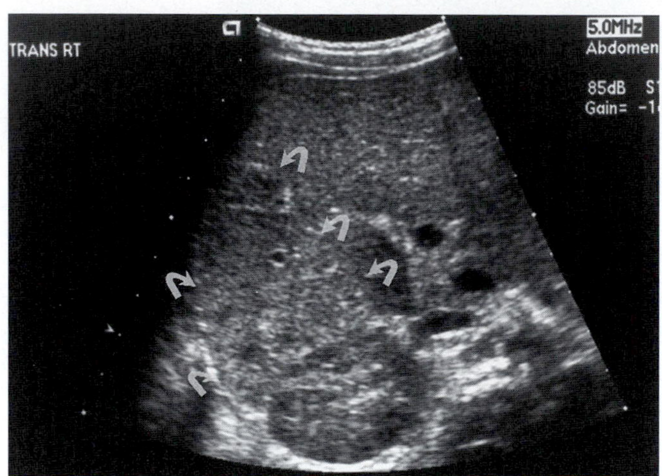

FIGURE 47–2. Hepatic laceration with associated intraparenchymal hematoma. Transverse view through the right lobe of the liver shows a focal heterogeneous area in the posterior segment (*arrows*), representing a hepatic laceration and associated intraparenchymal hematoma.

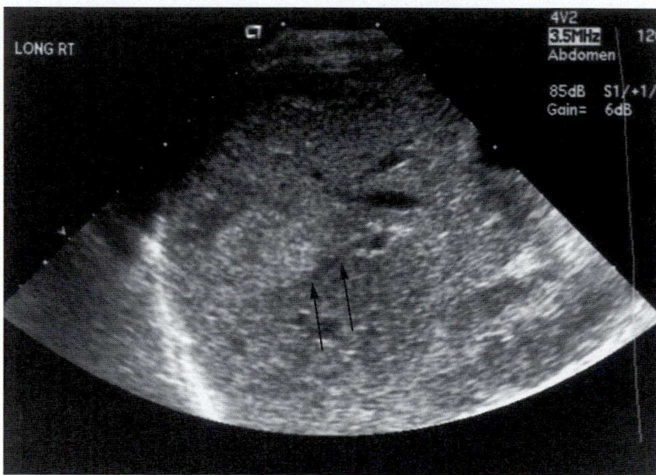

FIGURE 47–3. Intraparenchymal hepatic hematoma demonstrating mass effect on hepatic vasculature. Transverse view of the liver in a child struck by a motor vehicle while riding his bike shows an intraparenchymal hepatic hematoma displacing the hepatic veins (*arrows*).

Hepatic injury is common in children following blunt abdominal trauma. The liver is the viscus either most commonly or second most commonly injured in children, depending upon the specific series. The spectrum of hepatic injury includes parenchymal contusion, laceration, and devascularizing injury. Parenchymal laceration may be simple or complex. Hematoma is commonly associated with hepatic injury. The hematoma may be parenchymal, subcapsular, or perihepatic. Hemoperitoneum is also frequently observed. Diagnostic imaging plays an important role in the initial assessment of injured children, as physical examination and laboratory findings cannot reliably detect injury.

Computed tomography (CT) has traditionally been the examination of choice for the assessment of possible visceral injury in the hemodynamically stable child following blunt abdominal trauma. However, in recent years sonography has been advocated by some as the preferred examination in this setting. Advantages of the use of sonography, compared to CT, in acutely injured children include the ability to perform the examination rapidly at the bedside, the absence of ionizing radiation, the high sensitivity and specificity in the detection of hemoperitoneum, and the lower cost. Disadvantages of the use of sonography are that it is extremely operator-dependent and has decreased sensitivity and specificity for the detection of solid viscus injury compared with CT.

Acute hepatic injury has a variable appearance on sonography. Hepatic laceration typically has a hypoechoic appearance, while associated intraparenchymal hematoma may appear hypoechoic or hyperechoic relative to normal hepatic parenchyma. The intraparenchymal hematoma often has a heterogeneous appearance on sonography (Fig. 47-2). Occasionally, the region of injury is isoechoic relative to adjacent hepatic parenchyma. In these cases, it may be quite difficult to identify the injury on the basis of gray-scale differences in

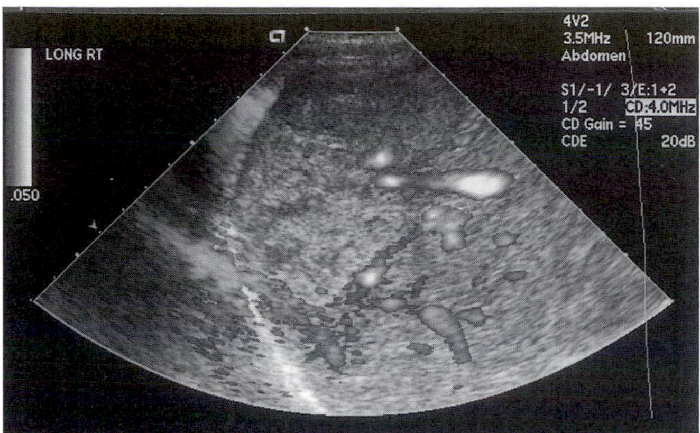

FIGURE 47–4. Color Doppler sonography demonstrating absence of flow in the region of an intraparenchymal hepatic hematoma. Longitudinal view through the liver with color Doppler sonography shows absence of blood flow at the site of the intraparenchymal hematoma (*arrows*). (See Color Plate 18.)

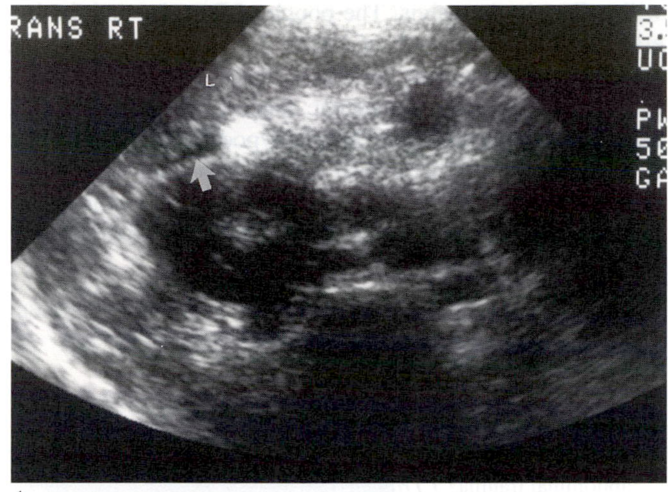

A

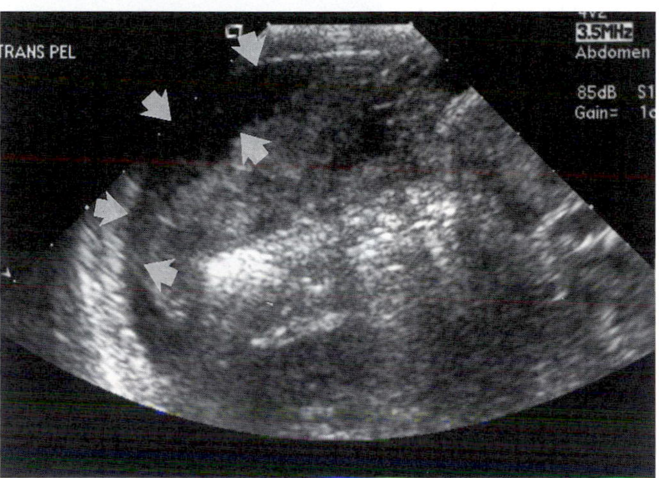

B

FIGURE 47–6. Hemoperitoneum secondary to hepatic injury. ***A.*** Transverse view through the right upper quadrant demonstrates a small amount of fluid in Morison's pouch (*arrow*). L = liver. ***B.*** Transverse view through the right lower quadrant in the same child demonstrates a large amount of fluid in the right paracolic gutter (*arrows*).

hepatic echotexture. Assessment of the hepatic vasculature with gray-scale and color Doppler sonography often provides helpful clues to possible injury. There is often associated displacement of the hepatic vessels secondary to a mass effect from intraparenchymal hematoma (Fig. 47-3). Color Doppler sonography is useful in the assessment of possible hepatic injury, as it demonstrates focal avascular regions within the liver associated with intraparenchymal hematoma (Fig. 47-4; see also Color Plate 18) or surrounding the periphery of the liver in the presence of subcapsular hematoma.

Further evaluation with CT may be necessary in some children who were initially screened with sonography. The advantages of CT relative to sonography include a higher sensitivity and specificity for the detection of solid viscus injury, the ability to more precisely characterize the extent of solid viscus injury (Fig. 47-5), and the ability to detect hollow viscus and bony injury, both of which are not detectable by sonography. Assessment of the abdomen with CT in injured children should be performed with intravenous contrast administration.

The sonographic evaluation of the acutely injured child should include assessment of all solid viscera. Additionally, the entire abdomen and pelvis should be evaluated for the presence of associated peritoneal fluid (Fig. 47-6). Peritoneal fluid detected following blunt trauma is typically hemoperitoneum. Approximately 75 percent of all hepatic injuries will be associated with hemoperitoneum. Hepatic injury will not be associated with hemoperitoneum if there is absence of capsular disruption or if the injury extends to the bare area in the posteromedial aspect of the liver, which is devoid of peritoneal covering. The majority of associated hemoperitoneum

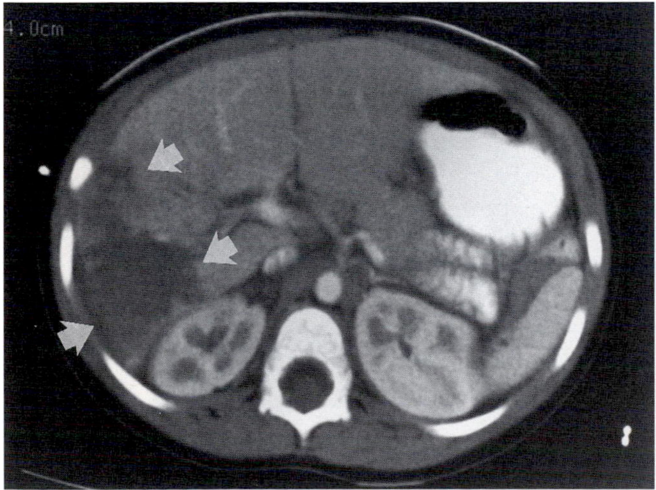

FIGURE 47–5. Hepatic laceration with associated intraparenchymal hematoma on computed tomography (CT). Contrast-enhanced CT scan through the liver in the same child as in Fig. 47-1 demonstrates a focal area of decreased attenuation in the posterior segment of the right lobe of the liver, indicative of hepatic intraparenchymal hematoma (*arrows*).

CHAPTER 48

Choledochal Cyst

CARLOS J. SIVIT

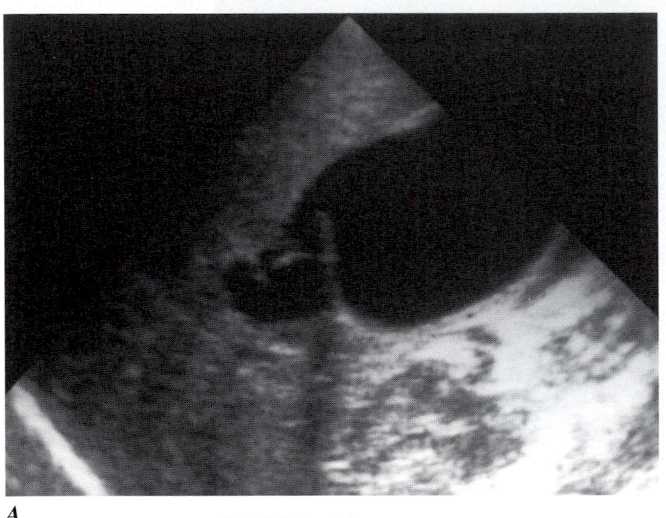

A

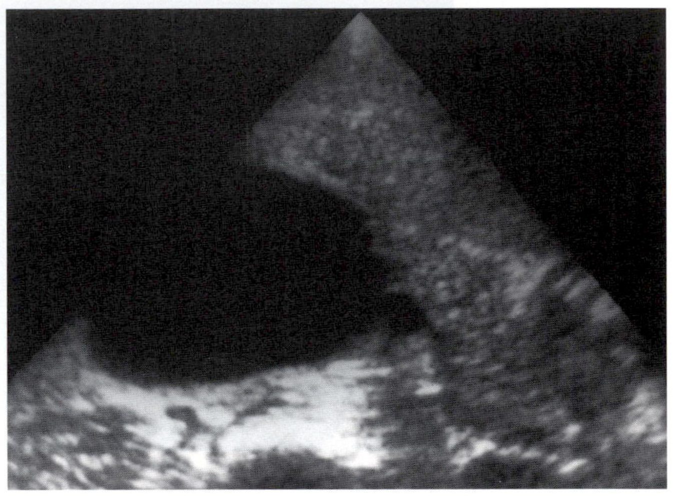

B

FIGURE 48–2. Choledochal cyst. Longitudinal *(A)* and transverse *(B)* views through the liver show a large fusiform mass in the porta hepatis in continuity with the biliary tree. At surgery, the lesion was found to be a choledochal cyst. P = pancreas.

Cystic dilatation of the extra- or intrahepatic biliary tree, also known as choledochal cyst, is an uncommon condition that usually manifests in infants and young children (Fig. 48-2). It should be noted, however, that nearly one-third of patients present after the age of 6 years. Choledochal cyst in the neonate is probably a different entity from that which presents in older children. There is considerable debate concerning the underlying etiology of choledochal cysts. In infants, the focal biliary dilatation may develop as a result of an inherent weakness in the biliary tree in its developmental stages. In a small subgroup of infants, choledochal cysts develop as part of a spectrum of infantile obstructive cholangiopathy that includes neonatal hepatitis and biliary atresia. This condition results in fibrotic scarring of the biliary tract, leading to the sclerotic changes of biliary atresia, and may also result in extrahepatic biliary obstruction, producing cystic dilatation of the extrahepatic bile duct. Focal cystic dilatation of the extrahepatic duct is noted in approximately 10 percent of infants with biliary atresia. One prevailing theory for the development of choledochal cysts in older children is that they represent an acquired condition resulting from an anomaly of the pancreaticobiliary ductal junction due to faulty budding of the primitive pancreatic duct. The ventral pancreatic bud is felt to originate from a more proximal position closer to the liver, resulting in a long common channel that drains both the biliary and pancreatic systems. Typically, the common bile duct and pancreatic duct unite within the sphincter of Oddi to form a common channel, the pancreaticobiliary duct, that opens into the duodenum. This common channel is normally very short, on average measuring 0.5 cm in length. A longer common channel may lead to chronic reflux of pancreatic juice into the bile duct, since the maximum

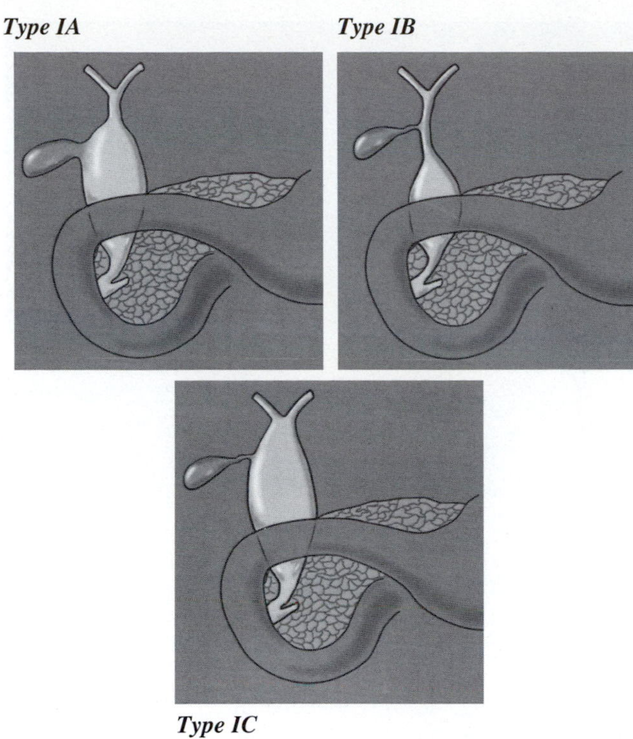

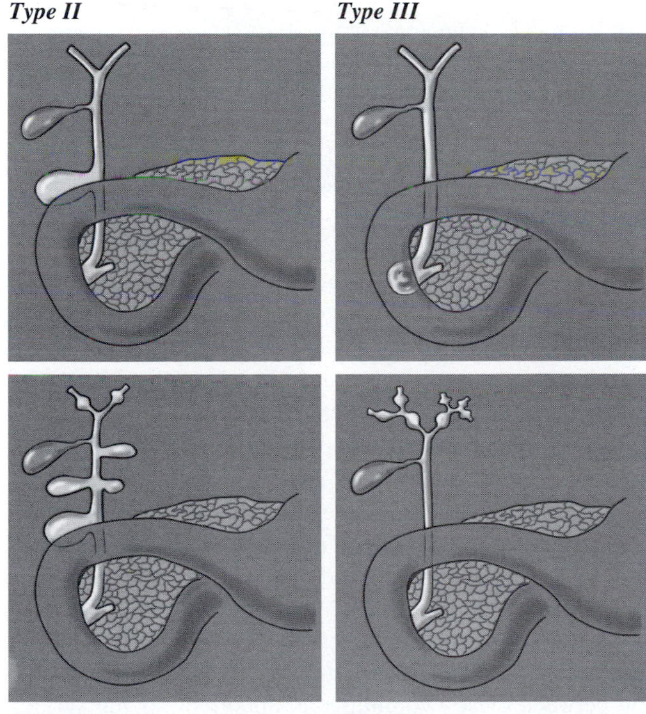

FIGURE 48–3. Diagram of the types of choledochal cysts based on the Todani classification.

pressure in the pancreatic duct exceeds that in the bile duct. This, in turn, results in chronic biliary tract inflammation, mucosal destruction, and fibrosis. Additional features that may influence the development and appearance of choledochal cysts include (1) a right-angled (rather than acute-angled) distal pancreaticobiliary union, (2) the presence or absence of a dilated common channel, and (3) the presence or absence of a patent accessory pancreatic duct. A right-angled pancreaticobiliary union usually results in focal, cystic dilatation of a segment of the common bile duct, while an acute-angled union is associated with fusiform dilatation of the common bile duct.

The clinical presentation of patients with a choledochal cyst is variable. Infants typically present with cholestatic symptoms, including jaundice and acholic stools, that may be indistinguishable from those of biliary atresia. Older patients may present with intermittent jaundice, abdominal pain, or a palpable abdominal mass. Only approximately one-third of older patients demonstrate all three components of the triad. The clinical presentation in older children is usually related to the anatomic features of the cyst. Patients with cystic dilatation of the common bile duct typically present with a palpable mass or jaundice, whereas patients with fusiform dilatation of the common bile duct usually present with abdominal pain. Additionally, patients with a dilated common channel or an accessory pancreatic duct are prone to recurrent pancreatitis.

Choledochal cysts are classified based on their location, cholangiographic morphology, and number of intrahepatic and extrahepatic bile duct cysts. The most widely utilized classification system is by Todani (Fig. 48-3). The most common form, accounting for approximately 80 percent of cases, is type I, which involves dilatation of the extrahepatic biliary tree. Type I choledochal cysts are further classified according to the morphology and location of the affected segment. A type IA cyst involves part or all of the extrahepatic biliary tree. The gallbladder arises directly from the cyst. A type IB cyst involves segmental dilatation of the distal common bile duct, while a type IC cyst involves fusiform dilatation of the common bile duct and common hepatic duct. A type II cyst is a choledochal diverticulum, and a type III cyst involves only the intraduodenal portion of the common bile duct and is described as a choledochocele (Fig. 48-4). A type IV cyst is the second most common type, accounting for approximately 20 percent of cases. It involves multiple cysts of the intra- and extrahepatic biliary tree. A type V cyst involves dilatation of one or several segments of the intrahepatic bile ducts without dilatation of the common bile duct. A type V cyst is in fact a distinct disease entity called Caroli's disease, which, although included in the spectrum of choledochocal cysts, has a different underlying etiology. Caroli's disease is a rare condition inherited as an autosomal recessive trait. Two types have been described. One form is characterized by sacular dilatation of the intrahepatic bile duct, calculus formation, and cholangitis. The second form is characterized by minimal intrahepatic ductal dilatation and is associated with congenital hepatic fibrosis.

Sonography is the imaging method of choice in the evaluation of choledochal cysts. It is utilized to evaluate the size and location of the cyst and to image the entire intra- and extrahepatic biliary tree. Choledochal cysts are anechoic on sonography. The appearance ranges from that of a focal, rounded cyst (Fig. 48-5) to that of fusiform dilatation of the common bile duct and possibly the common hepatic duct (Fig. 48-2). The dilated segment of the extrahepatic biliary tree may be eccentric in appearance relative to the adjacent

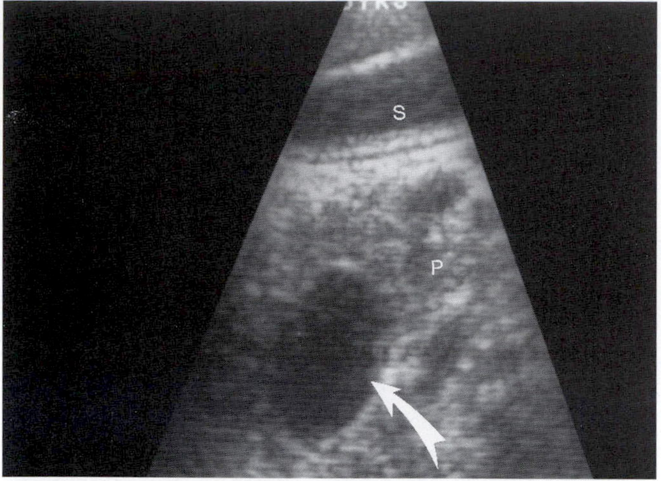

A

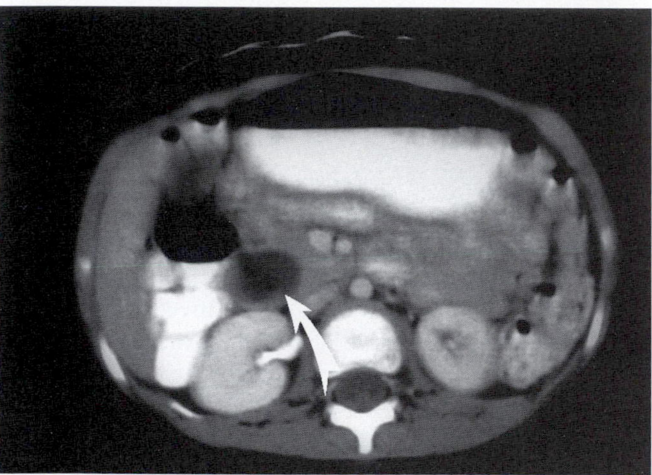

B

FIGURE 48–4. *A.* Type III choledochal cyst (choledochocele). Transverse sonogram through the upper abdomen shows a cystic lesion (*arrow*) in the head of the pancreas. At surgery, this was proven to be a choledochocele. P = pancreas, S = stomach. ***B.*** Type III choledochal cyst (choledochocele). Contrast-enhanced CT scan through the upper abdomen in the same patient as in *A* again demonstrates a focal, cystic lesion (*arrow*) in the head of the pancreas.

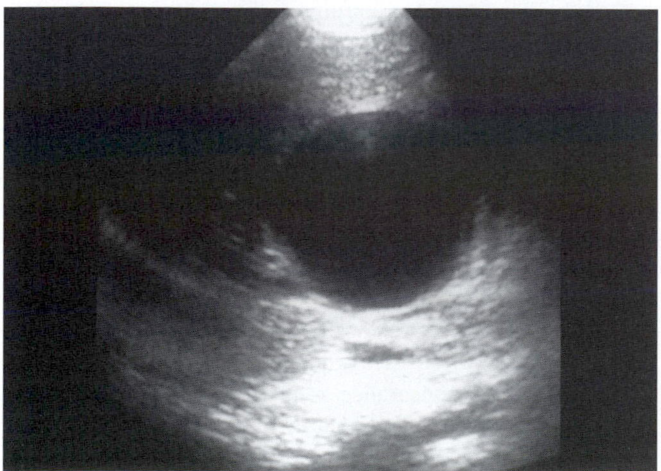

FIGURE 48–5. Choledochal cyst. Transverse view through the porta hepatis shows a focal large cyst.

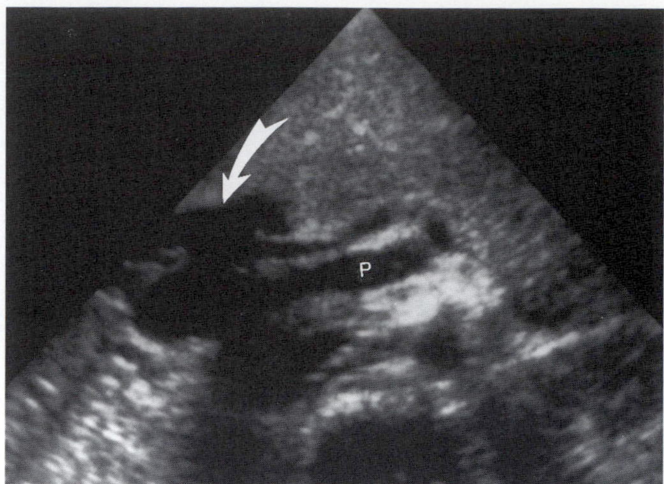

FIGURE 48–6. Choledochal cyst with eccentric, segmental biliary dilatation. Transverse view through the porta hepatis in a patient with a choledochal cyst shows eccentric focal saccular dilatation of the common bile duct (*arrow*). P = portal vein.

ductal system (Fig. 48-6). Choledochal cysts contain a thin wall. In type IV and type V choledochal cysts, there may also be dilatation of segments of the intrahepatic biliary tree that may be focal, segmental, or fusiform and may range from mild to severe (Fig. 48-7). The dilated segments of intrahepatic ducts are typically limited to the central portions of the right and left main hepatic ducts in type IV choledochal cysts, while diffuse multifocal dilatation is noted in type V choledochal cysts. When there is involvement of both the intra- and extrahepatic biliary tree in type IV choledochal cysts, extrahepatic dilatation is usually more severe. However, occasionally there may be marked intrahepatic dilatation as well (Fig. 48-7). Type V choledochal cyst, or Caroli's disease, will also be associated with cystic renal disease on sonography.

There are several sonographic features that are useful in differentiating infants with an isolated choledochal cyst from those with a choledochal cyst associated with biliary atresia. Infants with an isolated choledochal cyst typically have a large cyst size (>6 cm in length), frequent intrahepatic ductal dilatation, and a normal-sized gallbladder. Infants with a choledochal cyst associated with biliary atresia have a smaller cyst size (<3 cm in length), absence of intrahepatic ductal dilatation, and an absent or small gallbladder. Distinction between these two entities is important, as the surgical approach and prognosis with these two conditions differ greatly. Children with an isolated choledochal cyst undergo cyst excision and choledochojejunostomy, while those with associated biliary atresia undergo complete excision of the extrahepatic bile duct and Roux-en-Y portoenterostomy. Infants with an isolated choledochal cyst have a good long-term prognosis, while those with associated biliary atresia have progressive hepatic dysfunction and eventually require liver transplantation.

Computed tomography (CT) is also useful in imaging choledochal cysts. It is helpful in better defining the biliary origin of the cyst, particularly with large lesions. Addition-

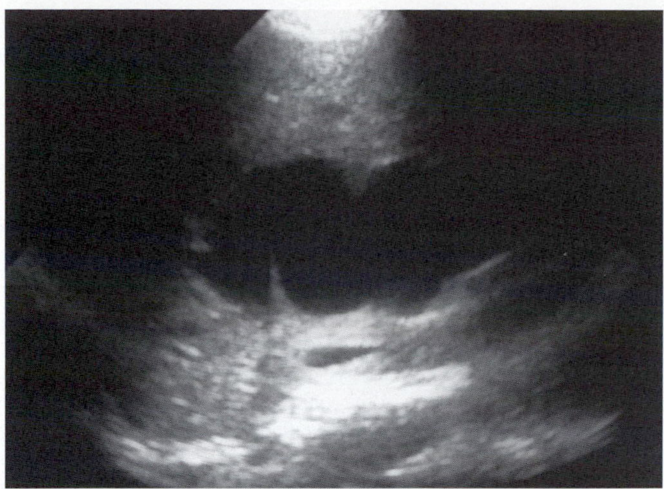

A

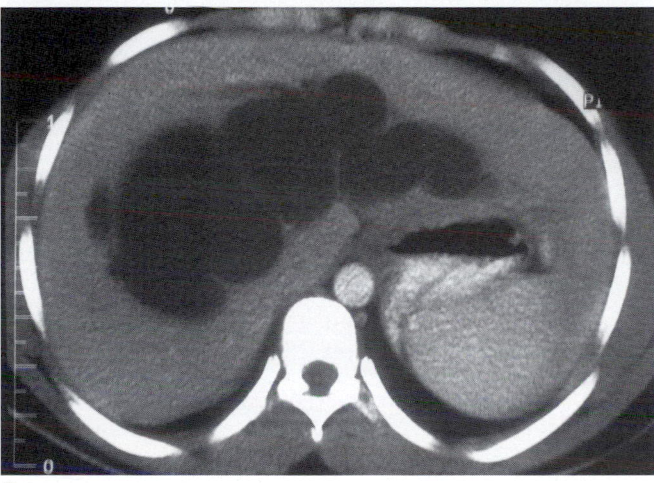

B

FIGURE 48–7. ***A.*** Type IV choledochal cyst with marked fusiform intrahepatic dilatation. Transverse view through the liver demonstrates marked dilation of the intrahepatic biliary tree. ***B.*** Type IV choledochal cyst with marked intrahepatic dilatation. Contrast-enhanced computed tomography scan through the liver in the same patient as in *A* shows marked dilatation of the intrahepatic biliary tree.

ally, CT can precisely define the relationship between the cyst, the pancreatic head (Fig. 48-4), and the porta hepatis and can assess associated intrahepatic biliary dilatation (Fig. 48-7). The appearance on CT of a choledochal cyst is that of a focal, low-attenuation rounded lesion (Fig. 48-4) or fusiform biliary dilatation (Fig. 48-7).

Hepatobiliary scintigraphy is also useful in the evaluation of suspected choledochal cyst to confirm that the mass communicates with the biliary system and to determine the presence of distal obstruction. Additionally, in neonates, the hepatobiliary scan is useful in excluding biliary atresia associated with choledochal cyst. The administered radioisotope is normally excreted into the biliary tract and should reach the duodenum within 1 h of administration. The choledochal cyst will initially appear photopenic on scintigraphy and will gradually fill with radionuclide on delayed imaging

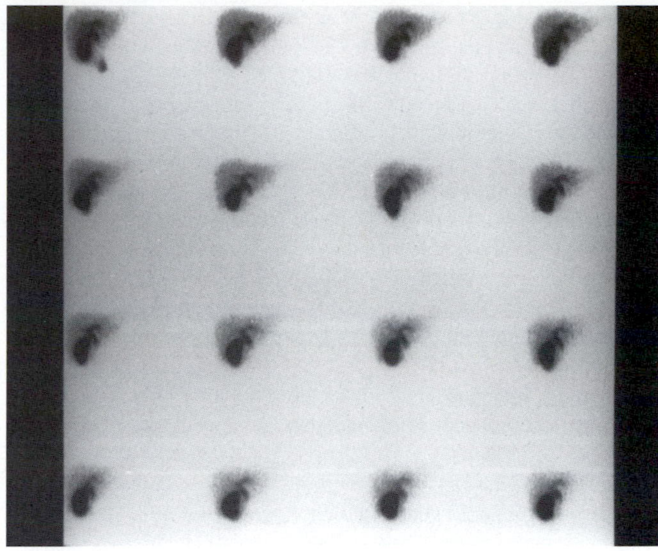

FIGURE 48–8. Choledochal cyst. Hepatobiliary scintigraphy shows normal hepatic uptake of the tracer and retention of the tracer within the choledochal cyst.

(Fig. 48-8). If there is associated biliary atresia, absence of radionuclide in the intestinal tract will be noted on delayed imaging.

The differential diagnosis includes other abdominal cystic lesions, including mesenteric cyst, enteric duplication cyst, and ovarian cyst, since it may not be possible to localize the lesion to the porta hepatis. These other diagnoses can be excluded by confirming the biliary origin of the lesion. That can usually be accomplished through the use of the hepatobiliary scan, which will show accumulation and stasis of the radionuclide in the choledochal cyst, confirming the biliary origin of the lesion.

The most common complication associated with choledochal cysts is biliary stone disease. Additional, uncommon complications reported include ascending cholangitis, spontaneous cyst rupture with bile peritonitis, and malignancy. The risk of developing malignancy, typically carcinoma of the common bile duct or gallbladder, increases with advancing age. It is rare in the first decade of life. The removal of the cyst does not eliminate the possibility of carcinoma developing in the intrahepatic ducts. Therefore, these patients should receive long-term follow-up even after removal of the choledochal cyst.

References

Chaudhary A, Dhar P, Sachdev A, et al: Choledochal cysts—differences in children and adults. *Br J Surg* 83:186–188, 1996.

Haller JO: Sonography of the biliary tract in infants and children. *AJR* 157:1051–1058, 1991.

Han BK, Babcock DS, Gelfand MH: Choledochal cyst with bile duct dilatation: Sonography and 99m-Tc-IDA cholescintigraphy. *AJR* 136:1075–1079, 1981.

Kim OH, Chung HJ, Choi BG: Imaging of the choledochal cyst. *Radiographics* 15:69–88, 1995.

Kim WS, Kim IO, Yeon KM, et al: Choledochal cyst with or without biliary atresia in neonates and young infants: US differentiation. *Radiology* 209:465–469, 1998.

Lin WY, Lin CC, Changlai SP, et al: Comparison of technetium Tc-99m disofenin cholescintigraphy with ultrasonography in the differentiation of biliary atresia from other forms of neonatal jaundice. *Pediatr Surg Int* 12:30–33, 1997.

Papanicolaou N, Abramson SJ, Teele RL, et al: Specific preoperative diagnosis of choledochal cysts by combined sonography and hepatobiliary scintigraphy. *Ann Radiol* 28:276–282, 1985.

Rizzo RJ, Szucs RA, Turner MA: Congenital abnormalities of the pancreas and biliary tree in adults. *Radiographics* 15:49–68, 1995.

Savader SJ, Benenati JF, Venbrux AC, et al: Choledochal cysts: Classification and cholangiographic appearance. *AJR* 156: 327–331, 1991.

Stringer MD, Dhawan A, Davenport M, et al: Choledochal cysts: Lessons from a 20 year experience. *Arch Dis Child* 73:528–531, 1995.

Todani T, Watanabe Y, Narusue M, et al: Congenital bile duct cysts: Classification, operative procedures, and review of thirty-seven cases including cancer arising from choledochal cyst. *Am J Surg* 134:263–269, 1977.

Torrisi JM, Haller JO, Velcek FT: Choledochal cyst and biliary atresia in the neonate: Imaging findings in five cases. *AJR* 155: 1273–1276, 1990.

Yoshida H, Itai Y, Minami M, et al: Biliary malignancies occurring in choledochal cysts. *Radiology* 173:389–392, 1989.

Young W, Blane C, White SJ, et al: Congenital biliary dilatation: A spectrum of disease detailed by ultrasound. *Br J Radiol* 63: 333–336, 1990.

Young WT, Thomas GV, Blethyn AJ, et al: Choledochal cyst and congenital anomalies of the pancreatico-biliary junction: The clinical findings, radiology, and outcome in nine cases. *Br J Radiol* 65:33–38, 1992.

Figure 49-1 shows a 2-year-old boy with persistent fever and abdominal pain following a ruptured appendix. What do you see? What are the diagnostic considerations?

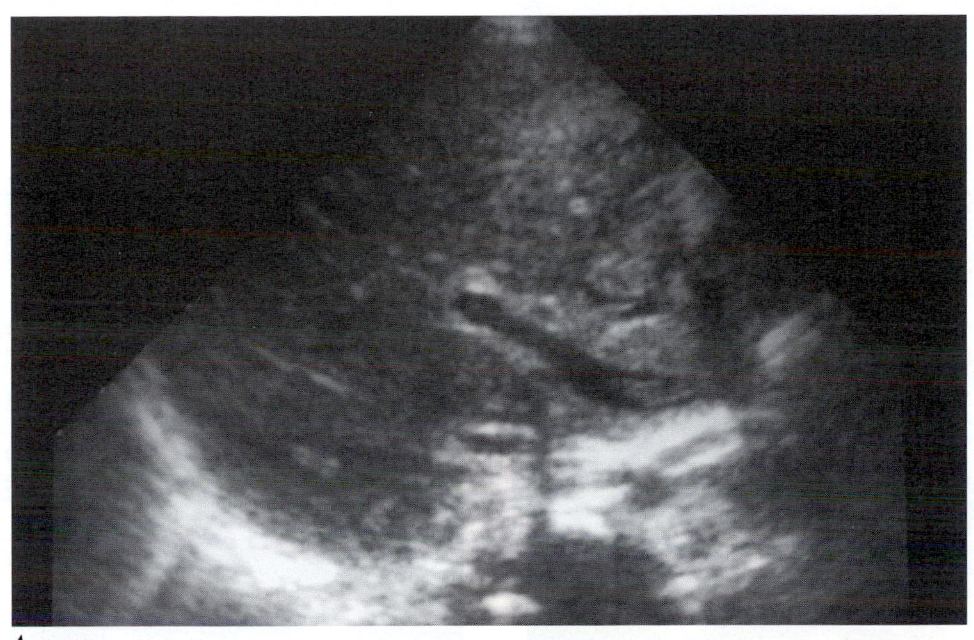

A

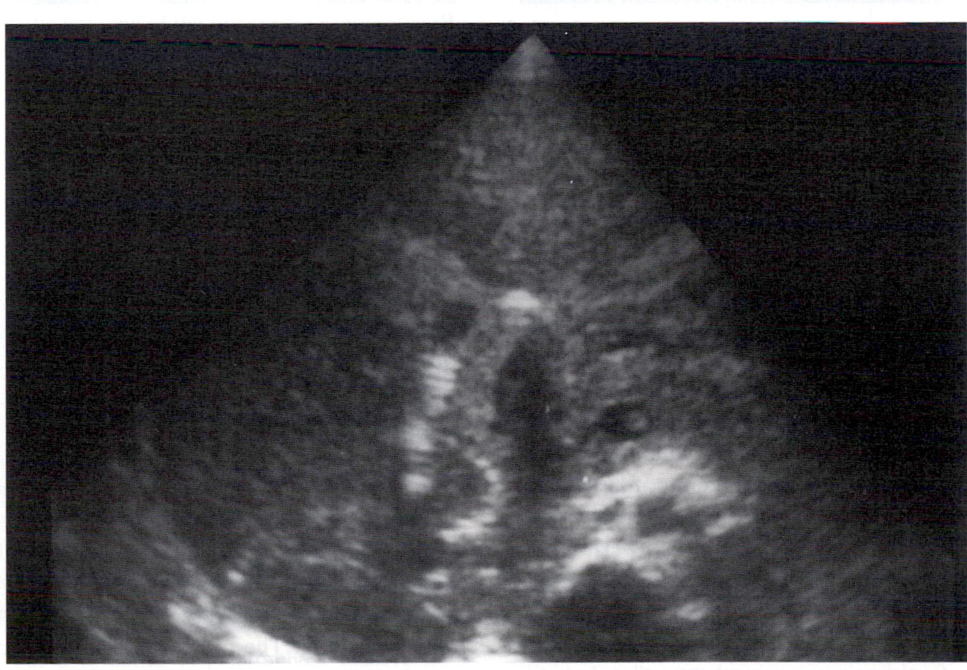

B

FIGURE 49–1. Transverse views through the porta hepatis *(A)* and head of the pancreas *(B).*

is complete occlusion of the portal vein by thrombus, marked dilatation of periportal collaterals may develop, a condition referred to as cavernous transformation of the portal vein. This results in visualization of multiple small vascular channels in the porta hepatis on sonography and lack of visualization of the normal portal vein (Fig. 49-6).

References

Babcock DS: Ultrasound disgnosis of protal vein thrombosis as a complication of appendicitis. *AJR* 119:57–62, 1979.

Farin P, Paajanen H, Miettinen P: Intraoperative US diagnosis of pyelephlebitis (portal vein thrombosis) as a complication of appendicitis: A case report. *Abdom Imaging* 22:401–408, 1997.

Kauzlaric D, Petrovic M, Barmeir E: Sonography of cavernous transformation of the portal vein. *AJR* 142:383–384, 1984.

Schwartz DS, Getner PA, Konstantino MM, et al: Umbilical venous catheterization and the risk of portal vein thrombosis. *J Pediatr* 131:760–762, 1997.

Slovis TL, Haller JO, Cohen HL, et al: Complicated appendiceal inflammatory disease in children: Pyelephlebitis and liver abscess. *Radiology* 171:823–825, 1989.

Ueno N, Sasaki A, Tomiyomo T: Color Doppler ultrasonography in the diagnosis of cavernous transformation of the portal vein. *JCU* 25:227–233, 1997.

Uno A, Ishida H, Konno K, et al: Portal hypertension in childhood and young adults: Sonographic and color Doppler findings. *Abdom Imaging* 22:72–78, 1997.

Van Gansbeke D, Avni EF, Delcour C, et al: Sonographic features of portal vein thrombosis. *AJR* 144:749–752, 1985.

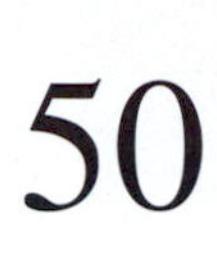

Figure 50-1 shows a 9-year-old boy who recently had a liver transplantation. What do you see? What is your diagnosis?

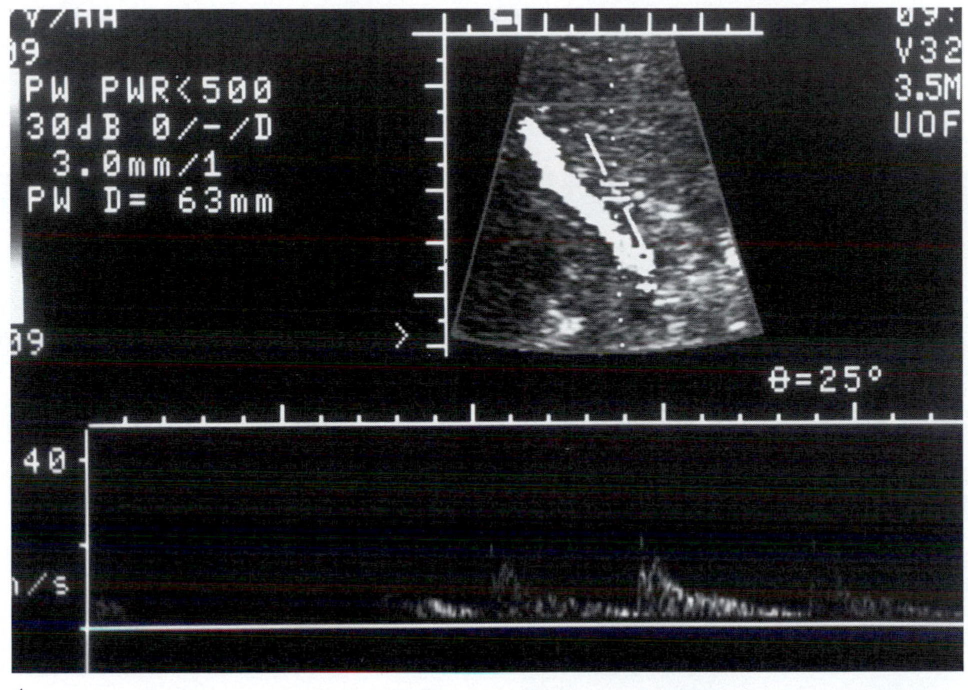

A

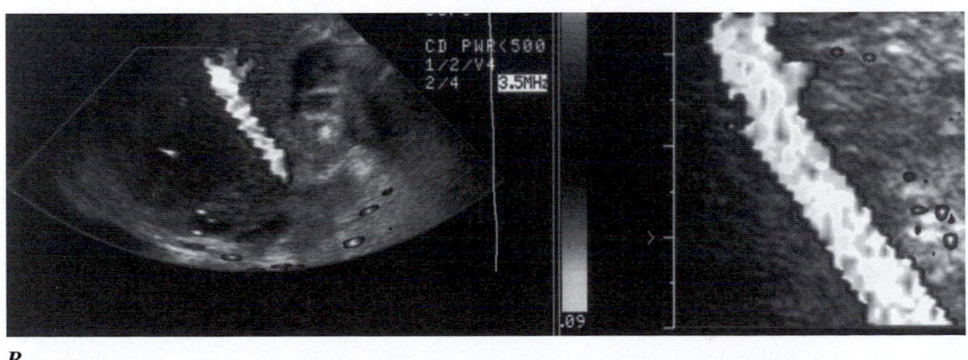

B

FIGURE 50–1. Transverse view through the liver hilum with duplex Doppler sonography on the first day following liver transplantation ***(A)*** and on the third day following transplantation ***(B)***.

CHAPTER 50

Hepatic Artery Thrombosis

ELLEN C. BENYA

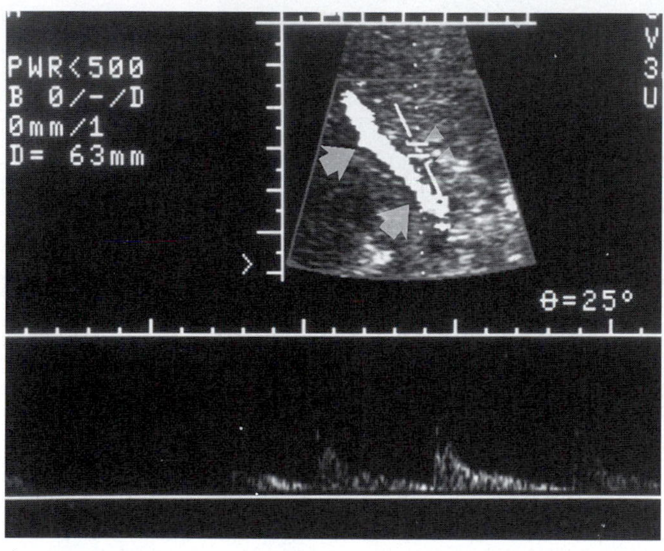

A

B

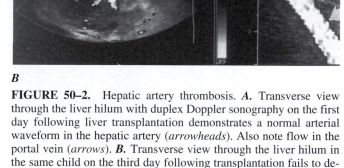

FIGURE 50–2. Hepatic artery thrombosis. ***A.*** Transverse view through the liver hilum with duplex Doppler sonography on the first day following liver transplantation demonstrates a normal arterial waveform in the hepatic artery (*arrowheads*). Also note flow in the portal vein (*arrows*). ***B.*** Transverse view through the liver hilum in the same child on the third day following transplantation fails to detect flow in the hepatic artery. Flow is still noted in the portal vein (*arrows*).

Liver transplantation may have a number of complications that can result in significant morbidity and mortality. These include thrombosis, stenosis, or pseudoaneurysm of the hepatic artery, portal vein, hepatic veins, or inferior vena cava. Hepatic artery thrombosis is the most frequent vascular complication in these patients. It occurs more commonly in children than in adults. The reported incidence of hepatic artery thrombosis following liver transplantation in children ranges from 10 to 40 percent. Typically, hepatic arterial thrombosis occurs within the first 2 months following transplantation. The clinical presentation is variable, ranging from no symptoms or mild elevation of liver enzymes to biliary sepsis or fulminant hepatic necrosis. When thrombosis or occlusion of the hepatic artery occurs in the early posttransplant period, rapid diagnosis is essential, as it may allow surgical revascularization and avoid the need for retransplantation.

Sonography allows for noninvasive serial evaluation of the liver transplant and its vasculature. Sonographic evaluation of the transplant should include gray-scale, color, and pulsed Doppler evaluation of the liver and spleen. The diagnosis of hepatic arterial thrombosis can be made if there is failure to detect hepatic arterial blood flow on color or pulsed Doppler imaging at the hilum of the liver near the location of the portal vein and within the hepatic parenchyma (Fig. 50-2). The reported accuracy of sonography for the detection of hepatic arterial occlusion is variable. The addition of color Doppler imaging has greatly increased the sensitivity and specificity for the diagnosis of hepatic arterial occlusion. Therefore, sonography is now the principal method for assessing possible hepatic arterial thrombosis posttransplantation, replacing angiography.

The assessment of hepatic arterial flow by Doppler sonography requires attention to detail. Low-velocity hepatic arterial flow may occur in the absence of vascular occlusion. It has been reported in association with sepsis and hepatic necrosis. Thus, care should be taken to select optimal velocity and gain settings for both duplex and color Doppler in order to avoid a false-positive diagnosis of arterial occlusion

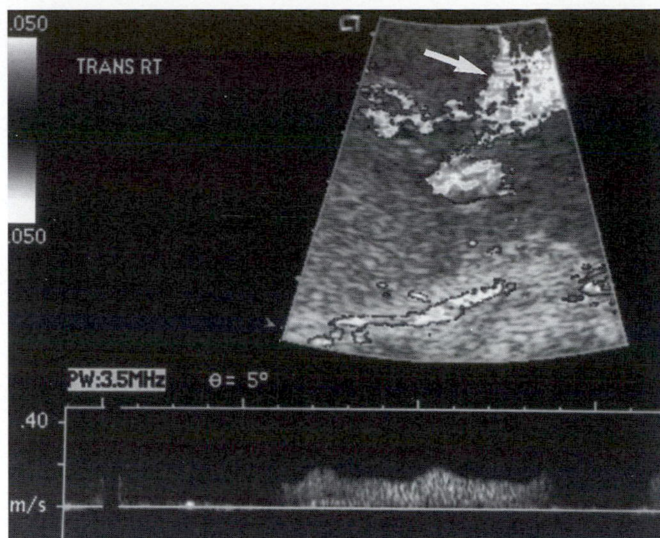

A

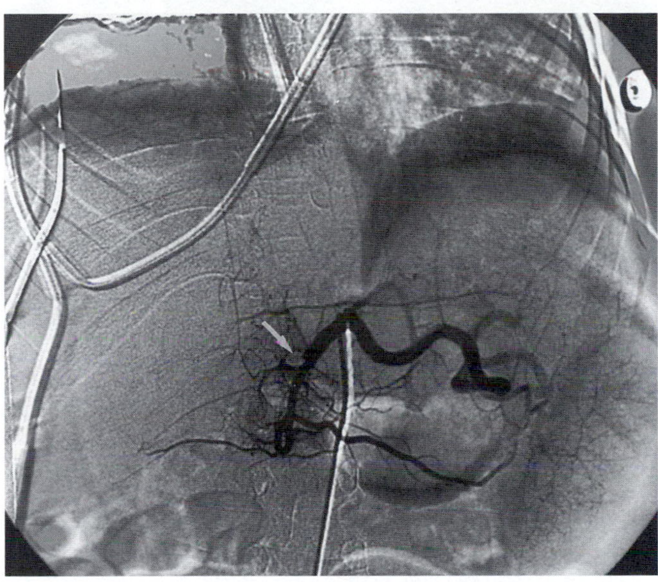

B

FIGURE 50–3. Hepatic arterial occlusion with associated extrahepatic arterial collaterals. ***A.*** Transverse view through the liver hilum with duplex Doppler in a 5-year-old boy following liver transplantation demonstrates multiple extrahepatic arterial collaterals (*arrow*) with a low peak systolic velocity, delayed systolic acceleration, and increased diastolic flow. ***B.*** Celiac arteriography in the same child performed the following day reveals complete occlusion of the hepatic artery (*arrow*).

in children with low-velocity flow. A condition that may lead to a false-negative diagnosis of hepatic arterial occlusion on sonography is the formation of extrahepatic arterial collaterals. These vessels may reconstitute the intrahepatic arterial blood flow when hepatic arterial thrombosis has occurred. These collaterals more commonly form in children than in adults, particularly following a Roux-en-Y choledochojejunostomy. Extrahepatic arterial collaterals can be differentiated from the normal hepatic artery on the basis of their low peak systolic velocity, increased diastolic flow, and prolonged systolic acceleration times (Fig. 50-3). The diagnosis can be confirmed with arteriography.

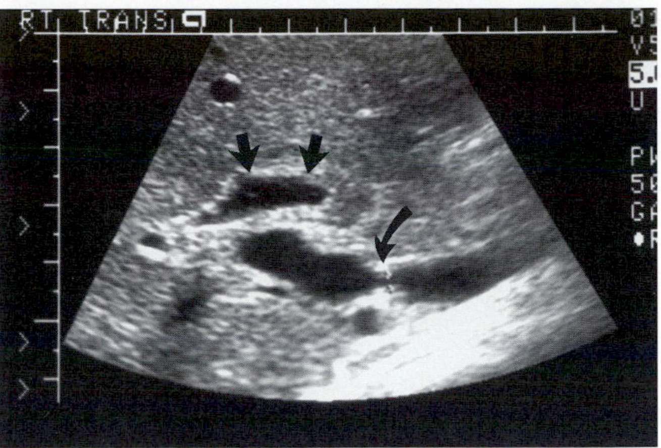

FIGURE 50–4. Biliary dilatation secondary to biliary stricture associated with hepatic artery thrombosis and portal vein stenosis. Transverse view though the porta hepatis following liver transplantation in a 6-year-old boy demonstrates dilatation of the common bile duct (*arrows*). The child had known hepatic arterial occlusion. Also noted is portal vein stenosis (*curved arrow*).

There are several biliary complications that may coexist with hepatic arterial occlusion, since the biliary ducts receive their blood supply solely from the hepatic artery. These include biliary stricture, biliary necrosis, bile leak, biliary infection, and hepatic abscess (Fig. 50-4). The presence of biliary complications or hepatic abscess on gray-scale sonography or computed tomography (CT) examination should prompt careful assessment of the hepatic artery for possible occlusion.

Portal venous occlusion may also occur following liver transplantation. This may be secondary to portal vein thrombosis or stenosis. Portal vein thrombosis occurs less commonly than hepatic artery thrombosis. It has been reported in approximately 5 to 7 percent of children following liver transplantation. Portal vein thrombosis may be discovered during routine imaging surveillance following liver transplantation or following the development of portal hypertension. The diagnosis is made with sonography when there is failure to visualize blood flow in the portal vein on duplex and color Doppler evaluation. Occasionally, echogenic material may be seen filling the portal vein.

Portal vein stenosis is an uncommon vascular complication following liver transplantation in children (Fig. 50-5). It is seen in less than 1 percent of cases. It should be noted that there is frequently a size discrepancy between the donor and recipient portal veins at the time of liver transplantation. Therefore, a decrease in the caliber of the portal vein associated with turbulent blood flow at the site of anastomosis is at times to be expected and is not necessarily diagnostic of portal vein stenosis. Portal vein stenosis is difficult to reliably diagnose by sonography. Therefore, confirmation with portal venography is often required. Sonographic criteria for the diagnosis of portal vein stenosis include a portal vein diameter of less than 2 mm with increased maximal systolic velocity at the site of the stricture (Fig. 50-5). Another sonographic sign

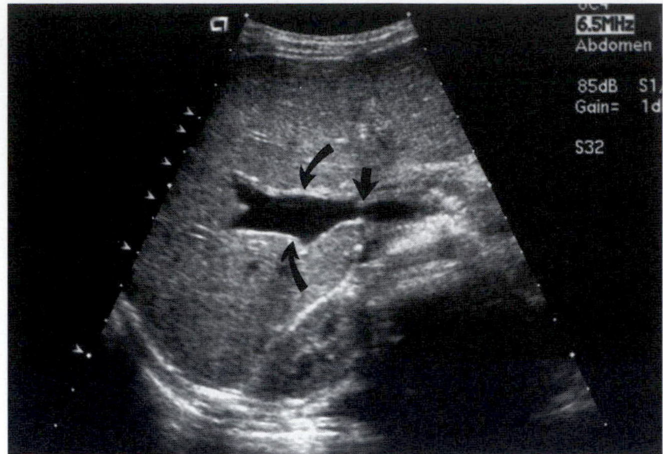

A

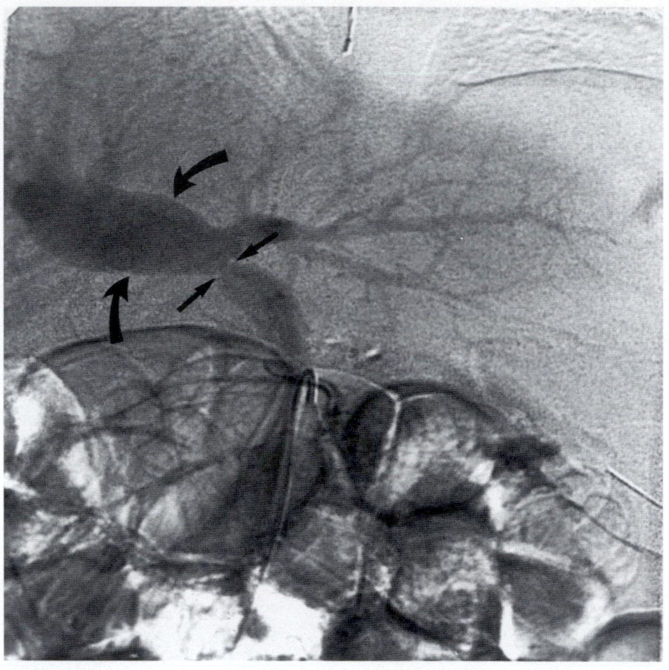

B

FIGURE 50–5. Portal vein stenosis. ***A.*** Transverse view through the porta hepatis shows focal stenosis of the main portal vein (*straight arrow*) with associated poststenotic dilatation (*curved arrows*). ***B.*** Portal venogram performed on the same child confirms the stenosis (*straight arrows*) and poststenotic dilatation (*curved arrows*) of the main portal vein.

associated with portal vein stenosis is postanastomotic dilatation of the portal vein (Fig. 50-5). Portal vein stenosis can usually be managed nonoperatively by percutaneous venoplasty or metallic stenting.

References

Dodd GD, Memel DS, Zajko AB, et al: Hepatic artery stenosis and thrombosis in transplant recipients: Doppler diagnosis with resistive index and acceleration time. *Radiology* 192:657–661, 1994.

Funaki B, Rosenblum J, Leef JA, et al: Angioplasty treatment of portal vein stenosis in children with segmental liver transplants: Mid-term results. *AJR* 169:551–554, 1997.

Hall TR, McDiarmid SV, Grant EG, et al: False-negative duplex Doppler studies in children with hepatic artery thrombosis after liver transplantaion. *AJR* 154:573–575, 1990.

Hellinger A, Roll C, Stracke A, et al: Impact of colour Doppler sonography on detection of thrombosis of the hepatic artery and the portal vein after liver transplantation. *Langenbecks Arch Chir* 381:182–185, 1996.

Kok T, Peeters PMPG, Hew JM, et al: Doppler-ultrasound and angiography of the vasculature of the liver in children after orthotopic liver transplantation: A prospective study. *Pediatr Radiol* 25:517–524, 1995.

Lallier M, St.-Vil D, Dubois J, et al: Vascular complications after pediatric liver transplantation. *J Pediatr Surg* 30:1122–1126, 1995.

Lomas DJ, Britton PD, Farman P, et al: Duplex Doppler ultrasound for the detection of vascular occlusion following liver transplantation in children. *Clin Radiol* 46:38–42, 1992.

McDiarmid SV, Hall TR, Grant EG, et al: Failure of duplex sonography to diagnose hepatic artery thrombosis in a high-risk group of pediatric liver transplant recipients. *J Pediatr Surg* 26: 710–713, 1991.

Pinna AD, Smith CV, Furukawa H, et al: Urgent revascularization of liver allografts after early hepatic artery thrombosis. *Transplantation* 62:1584–1587, 1996.

Rollins NK, Timmons C, Superina RA, et al: Hepatic artery thrombosis in children with liver transplants: False positive findings at Doppler sonography and arteriography in four patients. *AJR* 160:291–294, 1993.

Rollins NK, Sheffeld EG, Andrews WS: Portal vein stenosis complicating liver transplantation in children: Percutaneous transhepatic angioplasty. *Radiology* 182:731–734, 1992.

51

Figure 51-1 shows a 9-year-old girl with HIV infection and elevated liver enzymes. What do you see? What are the diagnostic considerations?

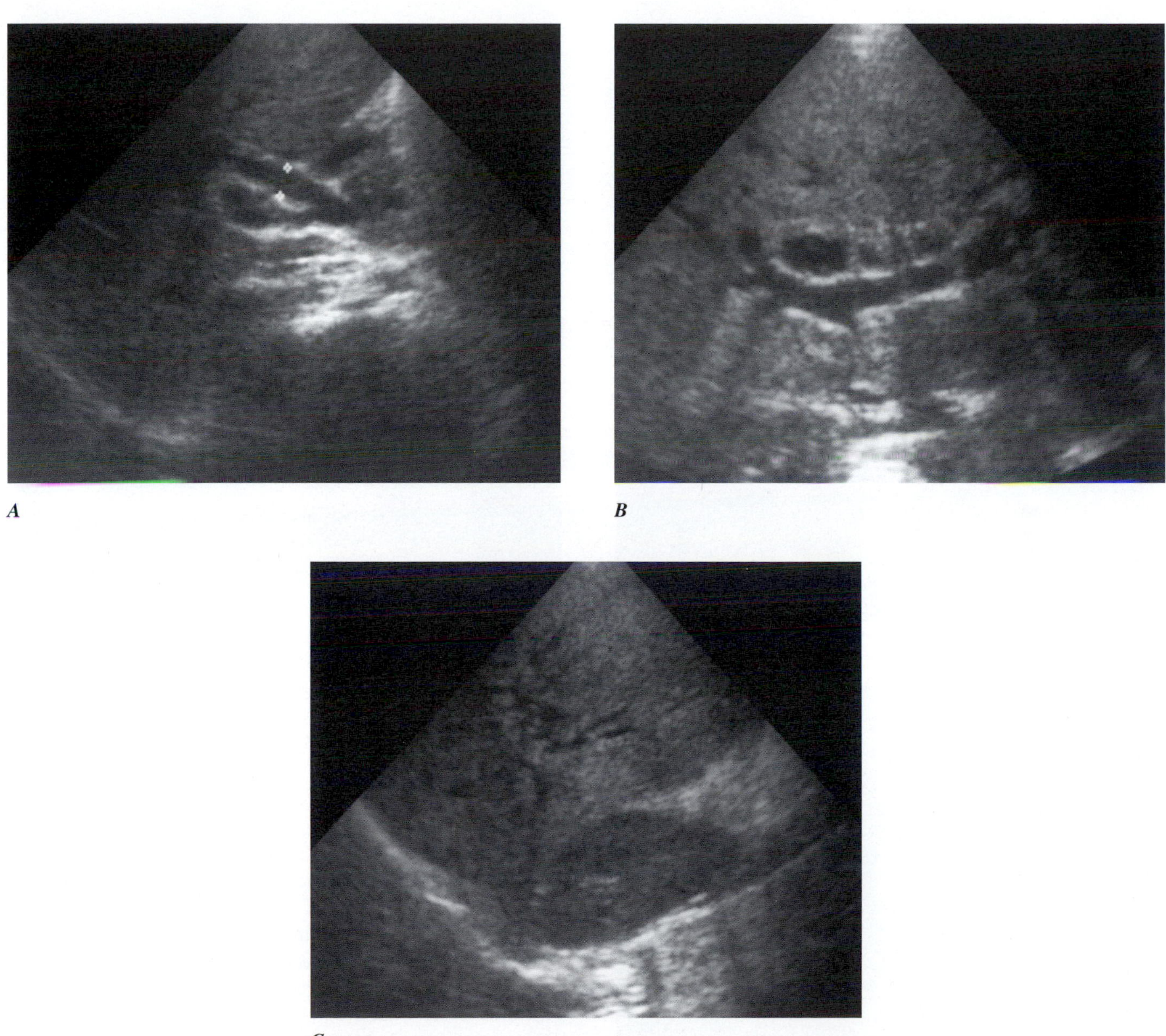

A *B* *C*

FIGURE 51–1. Longitudinal *(A)* and transverse *(B)* views through the porta hepatis. Longitudinal view through the right lobe of the liver *(C)*.

CHAPTER 51

AIDS-related Cholangitis

CARLOS J. SIVIT

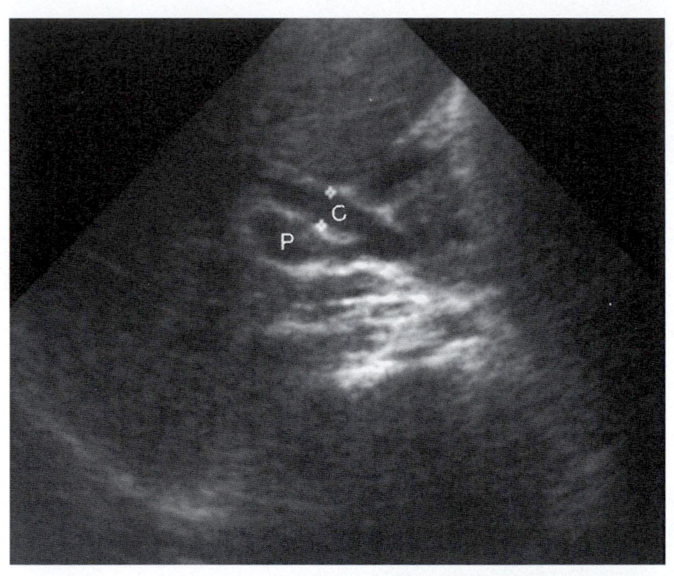

A

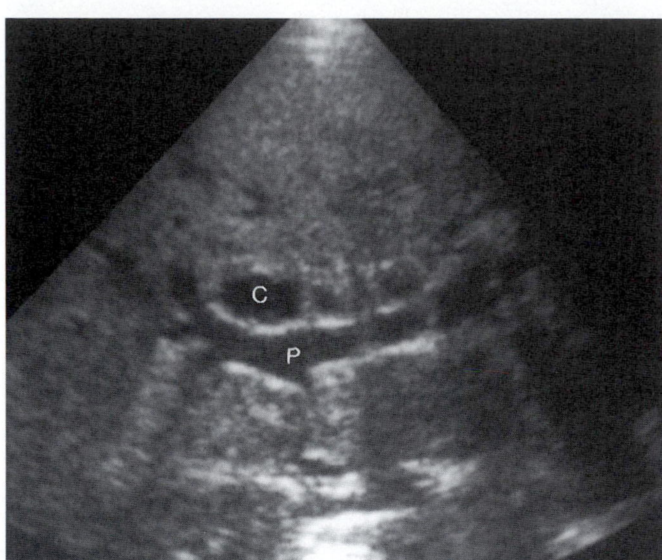

B

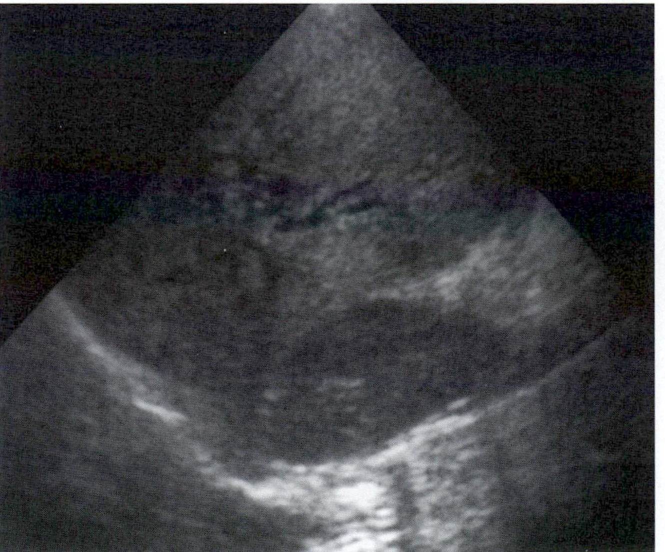

C

FIGURE 51–2. AIDS-related cholangitis. Longitudinal *(A)* and transverse *(B)* views through the porta hepatis demonstrate dilatation of the common bile duct (C). Note the beaded appearance on transverse view. Longitudinal view through the right lobe of the liver *(C)* shows dilatation of the intrahepatic ducts. P = portal vein.

AIDS-related cholangitis is an uncommon condition in children. It has been reported more frequently in adult AIDS patients. Proposed causes of the condition include biliary inflammation due to the immune deficiency itself, direct infiltration of the bile duct mucosa by HIV, and secondary infection by opportunistic organisms that frequently affect the gastrointestinal tract in individuals with AIDS, including *Cryptosporidium*, cytomegalovirus, and *Candida albicans.* Clinical features associated with AIDS-related cholangitis are nonspecific and include right upper quadrant abdominal pain, abdominal tenderness, fever, hepatomegaly, and a cholestatic pattern of liver function test abnormalities, characterized by disproportionate elevation of serum levels of al-

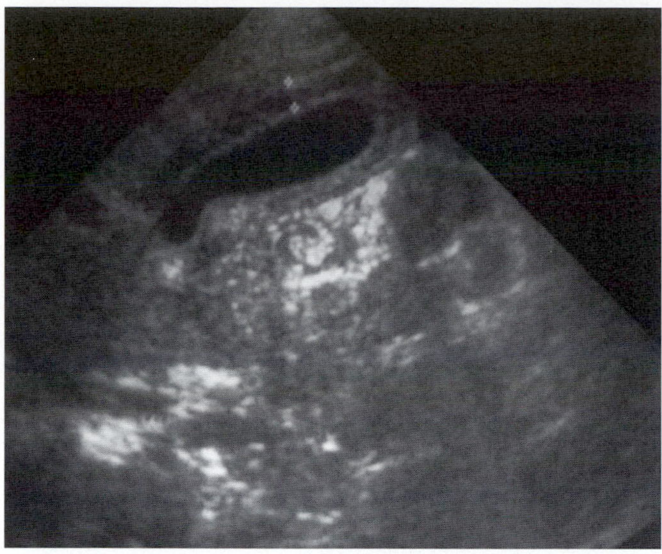

A

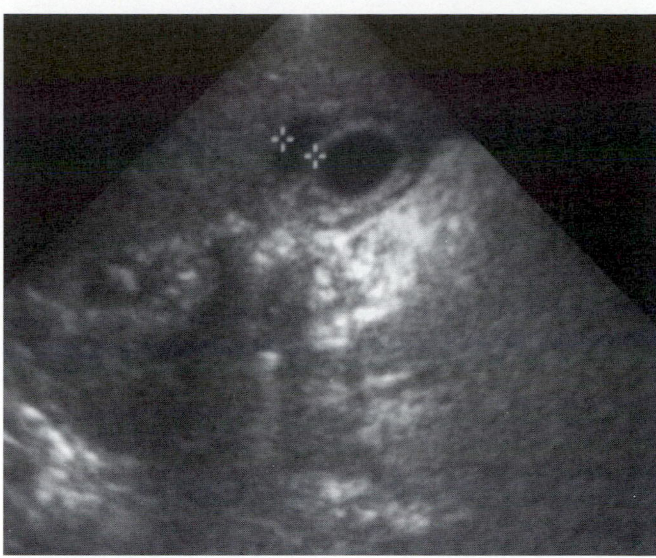

B

FIGURE 51–3. Gallbladder wall thickening associated with AIDS-related cholangitis. Longitudinal ***(A)*** and transverse ***(B)*** views through the liver in a child with AIDS-related cholangitis demonstrate thickening of the gallbladder wall (*between electronic calipers*).

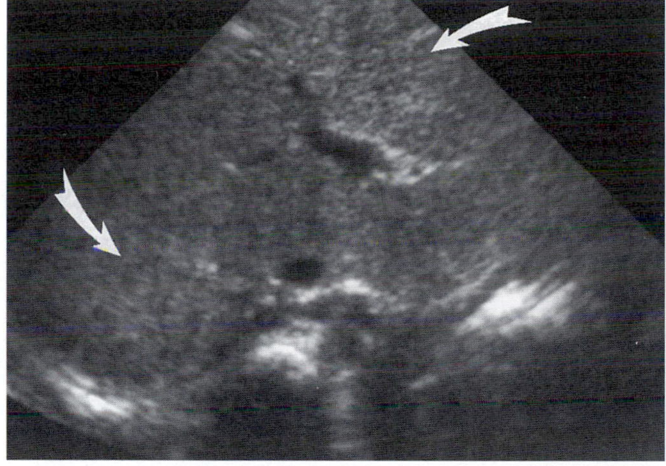

FIGURE 51–4. Abnormal hepatic parenchymal echotexture associated with AIDS-related cholangitis. Transverse view through the liver in a child with AIDS-related cholangitis shows areas of increased hepatic parenchymal echotexture (*arrows*).

kaline phosphatase and total bilirubin levels relative to the transaminase levels.

Hepatobiliary dysfunction is common in children with AIDS. Most cases are not directly due to the HIV infection, but rather are secondary to chemotherapy, chronic hyperalimentation, or malnutrition-induced hepatic tissue damage. Hepatic tissue sampling in these children often demonstrates nonspecific histopathologic abnormalities associated with chronic illness. Many children demonstrate multiple hepatobiliary abnormalities at histopathology. Additionally, there may be direct involvement of the hepatic parenchyma and the biliary tree by HIV-specific opportunistic infections or neoplasms.

Sonography provides a noninvasive method for evaluating the hepatobiliary tract in children with AIDS and is often used as the primary mode of evaluation in children with suspected hepatic or biliary abnormalities. Sonographic findings associated with AIDS-related cholangitis include dilatation, irregularity, and stricture of the intra- and extrahepatic bile ducts (Fig. 51-2) and dilatation and wall thickening of the gallbladder (Fig. 51-3). An echogenic nodule may be noted in the distal common bile duct, representing edema of the papilla of Vater. Hepatic parenchymal abnormalities may also be noted on sonography, including diffuse hyperechogenicity of the hepatic parenchyma and periportal hyperechogenicity (Fig. 51-4). In severe cases, suppurative cholangitis can result in hepatic abscess formation. It should be noted that hepatobiliary abnormalities are commonly seen in children with AIDS in the absence of cholangitis. Additionally, sonography may be normal in some children with cholangitis. Therefore, sonography lacks sensitivity and specificity in establishing the diagnosis. The precise characterization of biliary abnormalities associated with AIDS-related cholangitis usually requires cholangiography. Findings at cholangiog-

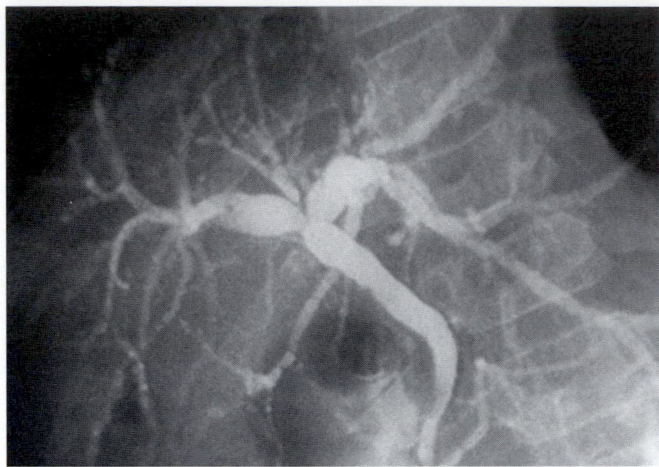

FIGURE 51–5. AIDS-related cholangitis. Spot film from an endoscopic retrograde cholangiopancreatography examination in a child with AIDS-related cholangitis shows marked tortuosity of the intrahepatic biliary tree, with regions of alternating strictures and sacculations, resulting in a beaded appearance. Note that the extrahepatic ducts are mildly dilated.

raphy in this condition include papillary stenosis and focal strictures with intervening segments of normal and increased ductal caliber (Fig. 51-5).

The prognosis of AIDS-related cholangitis is variable and is primarily related to the stage of HIV infection and other associated abnormalities. Treatment of the underlying opportunistic infection is a hallmark of the management of this condition, since the majority of cases are associated with chronic gastrointestinal tract infection. Additionally, endoscopic sphincterotomy often provides pain relief in patients with associated papillary stenosis.

References

Chung CJ, Sivit CJ, Rakusan TA, et al: Hepatobiliary abnormalities on sonography in children with HIV infection. *J Ultrasound Med* 13:205–210, 1994.

Da Silva F, Boudghene F, Lecomte I, et al: Sonography in AIDS-related cholangitis: Prevalence and cause of an echogenic nodule in the distal end of the common bile duct. *AJR* 160:1205–1207, 1993.

Daly CA, Padley SP: Sonographic prediction of a normal or abnormal ERCP in suspected AIDS related sclerosing cholangitis. *Clin Radiol* 51:618–621, 1996.

Delfalque D, Menu Y, Girard PM, et al: Sonographic diagnosis of cholangitis in AIDS patients. *Gastrointest Radiol* 14:143–147, 1989.

Dolmatch BL, Laing FC, Federle MP, et al: AIDS-related cholangitis: Radiographic findings in nine patients. *Radiology* 163: 313–316, 1987.

McCarty M, Choudhri AH, Helbert M, et al: Radiologic features of AIDS related cholangitis. *Clin Radiol* 40:582–585, 1989.

Nash JA, Cohen SA: Gallbladder and biliary tract disease in AIDS. *Gastroenterol Clin North Am* 26:323–335, 1997.

Rusin JA, Sivit CJ, Rakusan TA, et al: AIDS-related cholangitis in children: Sonographic findings. *AJR* 159:626–627, 1992.

52

Figure 52-1 shows a 2-week-old boy with fever and leukocytosis following an episode of necrotizing enterocolitis. What do you see? What are the diagnostic considerations?

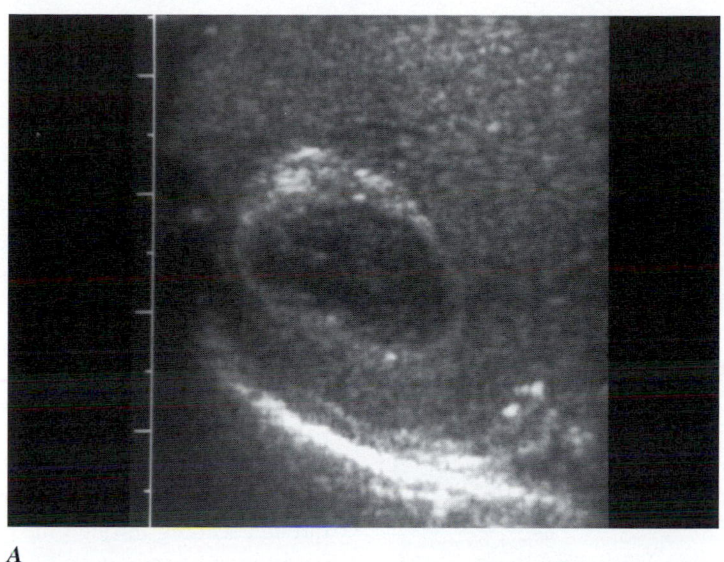

A

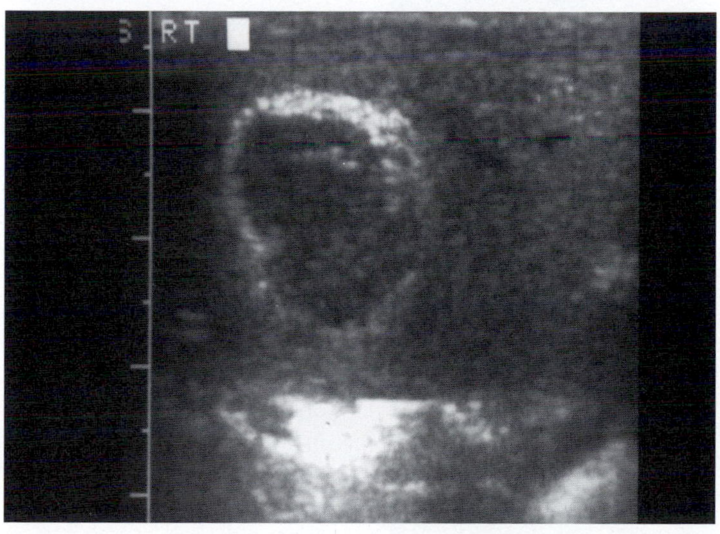

B

FIGURE 52–1. Transverse *(A)* and longitudinal *(B)* views through the liver.

CHAPTER 52

Hepatic Abscess

CARLOS J. SIVIT

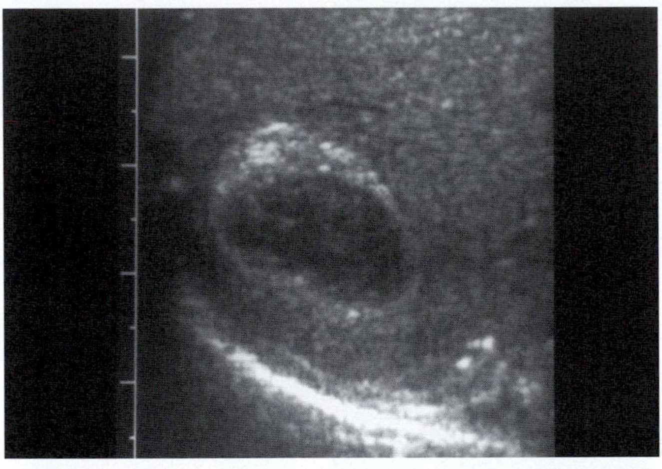

A

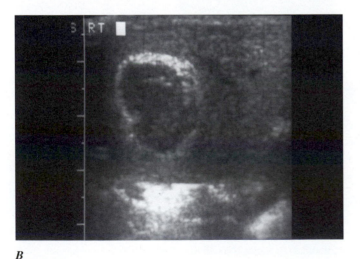

B

FIGURE 52–2. Hepatic abscess. Transverse ***(A)*** and longitudinal ***(B)*** views through the liver in an infant with a hepatic abscess demonstrate a focal hypoechoic hepatic parenchymal lesion with a thick hyperechoic center, indicative of a hepatic abscess.

Hepatic abscess is uncommon in children. It may be noted in infants as a complication of necrotizing enterocolitis or following umbilical vein catheterization. In older children, it is most frequently observed in the immunocompromised, including those with chronic granulomatous disease, those with acquired immunodeficiency syndrome, and those who have had bone marrow transplantation. In immunocompromised patients, infection usually reaches the liver through the blood vessels or lymphatics. Hepatic abscess may also result from contiguous spread of infection in suppurative cholangitis or through seeding through the portal venous system following perforation of the appendix. The clinical features of hepatic abscess are nonspecific. They include fever, leukocytosis, hepatomegaly, and abdominal pain.

Hepatic abscess in immunocompromised patients may be due to bacterial or fungal infection, while in nonimmunocompromised patients it usually results from bacterial infection. *Escherichia coli* is the most common bacterial organism resulting in hepatic abscess in infants, while *Staphylococcus aureus* is the most common organism in older children. Bacterial infection of the liver typically results in a single abscess. The exception to this is in disseminated cat-scratch disease, which is caused by *Bartonella henselae,* a gram-negative organism, which may result in multiple hepatic and splenic lesions. *Candida albicans* is the most common fungal organism resulting in hepatic abscess. Hepatic involvement in these patients usually occurs in the face of systemic involvement. The spectrum of hepatic disease seen with *Candida* infection ranges from a solitary lesion to multiple microabscesses.

Sonography is a useful modality for assessing children with suspected hepatic abscess (Fig. 52-2). The ability to perform the examination at the bedside is useful, as these patients may be too sick to travel to the radiology suite. The most common sonographic appearance of a pyogenic hepatic abscess is that of a solitary, uniformly hypoechoic, or cystic lesion (Fig. 52-3). Another common appearance is that of a lesion with a thick hyperechoic outer zone surrounding a hy-

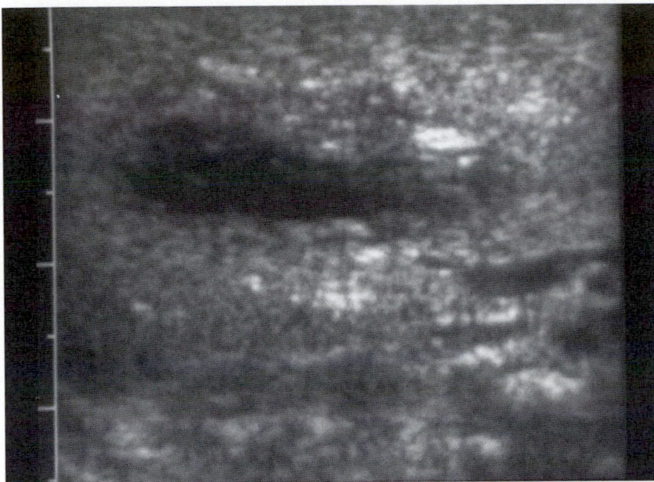

FIGURE 52–3. Hepatic abscess. Transverse view through the liver in a child with a hepatic abscess shows a focal, oval-shaped, uniformly hypoechoic parenchymal lesion.

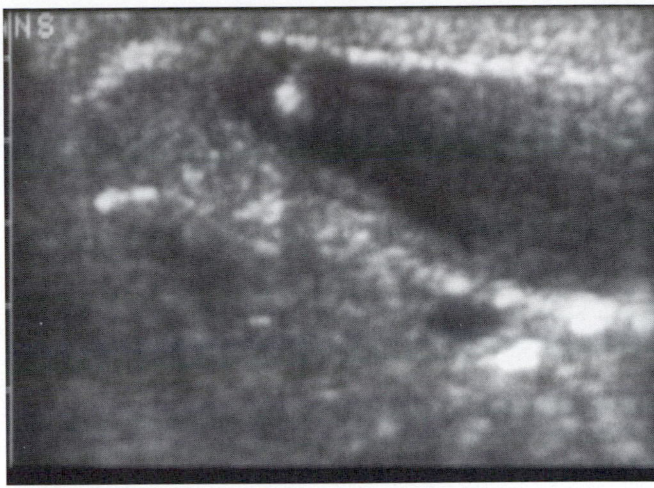

FIGURE 52–5. Hepatic abscess with calcification. Transverse view through the liver in a child with a hepatic abscess demonstrates an oval-shaped hypoechoic parenchymal lesion with a punctate calcification, resulting in acoustic shadowing.

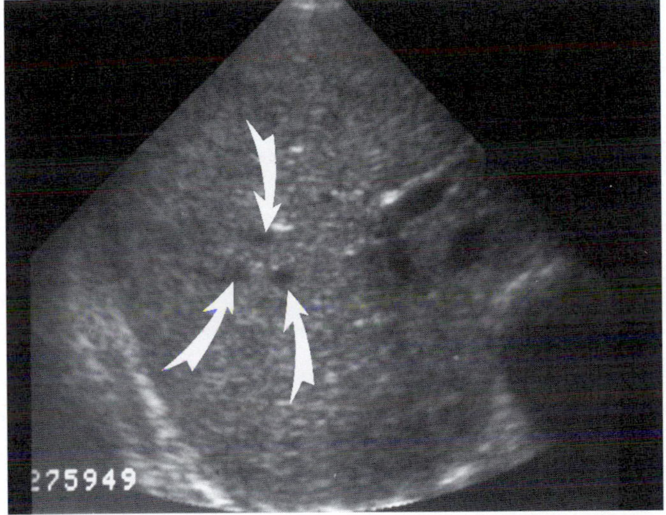

FIGURE 52–4. Hepatic microabscesses due to fungal infection. Transverse view through the liver demonstrates several small, hypoechoic lesions (*arrows*), representing hepatic microabscesses.

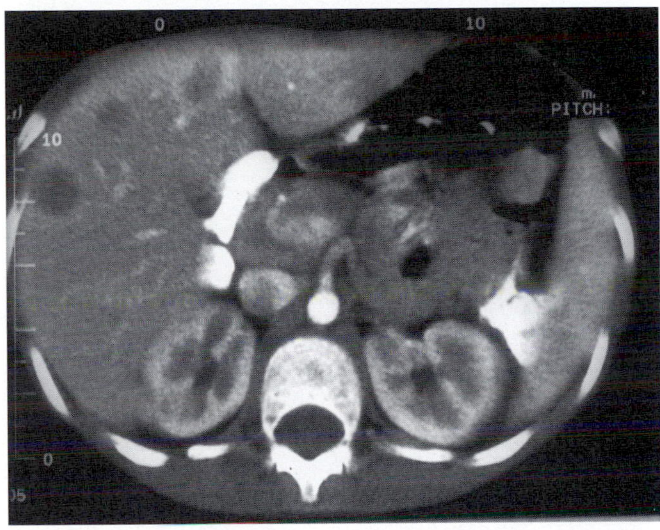

FIGURE 52–6. Multiple small hepatic abscesses. Contrast-enhanced computed tomography scan through the upper abdomen in a child with disseminated cat-scratch disease demonstrates multiple low-attenuation lesions within the liver, representing multiple small abscesses.

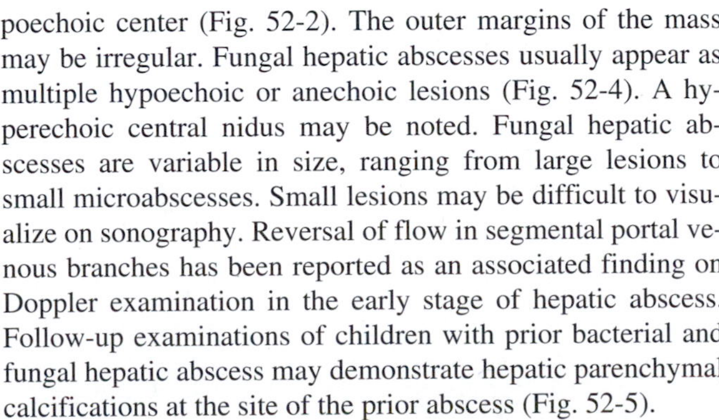

poechoic center (Fig. 52-2). The outer margins of the mass may be irregular. Fungal hepatic abscesses usually appear as multiple hypoechoic or anechoic lesions (Fig. 52-4). A hyperechoic central nidus may be noted. Fungal hepatic abscesses are variable in size, ranging from large lesions to small microabscesses. Small lesions may be difficult to visualize on sonography. Reversal of flow in segmental portal venous branches has been reported as an associated finding on Doppler examination in the early stage of hepatic abscess. Follow-up examinations of children with prior bacterial and fungal hepatic abscess may demonstrate hepatic parenchymal calcifications at the site of the prior abscess (Fig. 52-5).

Contrast-enhanced computed tomography (CT) scan is also useful for the evaluation of hepatic abscess, as CT can delineate the location and extent of the abscess more precisely than can sonography. Additionally, CT can identify other organ system involvement. It is particularly useful in the evaluation of fungal abscess or disseminated lesions secondary to cat-scratch disease, since the lesions are typically small and multiple. Additionally, there is often involvement of other organs, primarily the spleen and kidneys. The most common CT appearance of a hepatic abscess is that of a low-attenuation lesion with or without an enhancing rim (Fig. 52-6). Magnetic resonance imaging (MRI) has also been utilized to assess hepatic abscesses. The characteristic appearance on MRI is that of high signal intensity on T2-weighted imaging.

References

Dewbury KC, Joseph AEA, Milward Sadler GH, et al: Ultrasound in the diagnosis of the early liver abscess. *Br J Radiol* 53: 1160–1165, 1980.

Halvorsen RA, Korobkin M, Foster WL, et al: The variable CT appearance of hepatic abscesses. *AJR* 142:941–946, 1984.

Kawamoto S, Soyer PA, Fishman EK, et al: Nonneoplastic liver disease: Evaluation with CT and MR imaging. *Radiographics* 18:827–848, 1998.

Laurin S, Kaude JV: Diagnosis of liver-spleen abscesses in children—with emphasis on ultrasound for the initial and follow-up examination. *Pediatr Radiol* 14:198–204, 1984.

Lin ZY, Wang JH, Wang LY, et al: Changes in intrahepatic portal hemodynamic in early stage hepatic abscesses. *J Ultrasound Med* 15:595–598, 1996.

Oleszczuk-Raszke K, Cremin BJ, Fisher RM, et al: Ultrasonic features of pyogenic and amoebic abscess. *Pediatr Radiol* 19: 230–233, 1989.

Pastakia B, Shawker TH, Thaler M, et al: Hepatosplenic candidiasis: Wheels within wheels. *Radiology* 166:417–421, 1988.

Ralls PW: Focal inflammatory disease of the liver. *Radiol Clin North Am* 36:377–389, 1998.

Slovis TL, Haller JO, Cohen HL, et al: Complicated appendiceal inflammatory disease in children: Pyelophlebitis and liver abscess. *Radiology* 171:823–825, 1989.

Sty JR, Starshak RJ: Comparative imaging in the evaluation of hepatic abscesses in immunocompromised children. *JCU* 11: 11–15, 1983.

Zinzindohoue F, Guiard-Schmid JB, La Scola B, et al: Portal triad involvement in cat-scratch disease. *Lancet* 348:1178–1179, 1996.

53

Figure 53-1 shows a 4-month-old boy with elevated liver enzymes. What do you see? What are the diagnostic considerations?

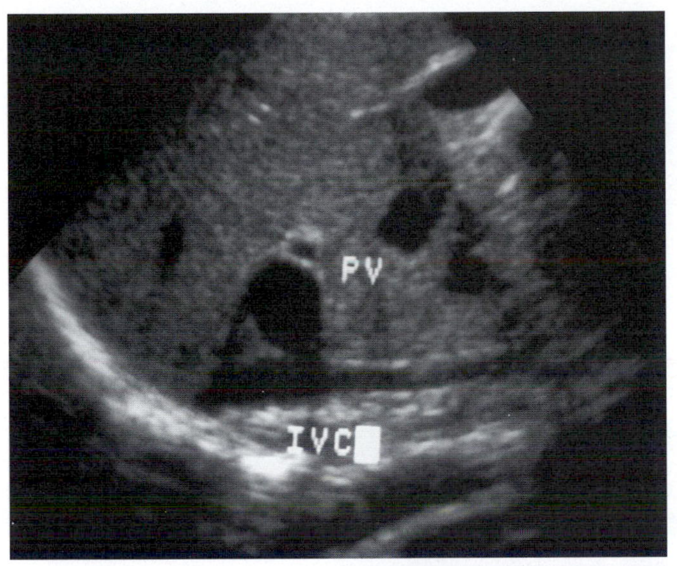

A

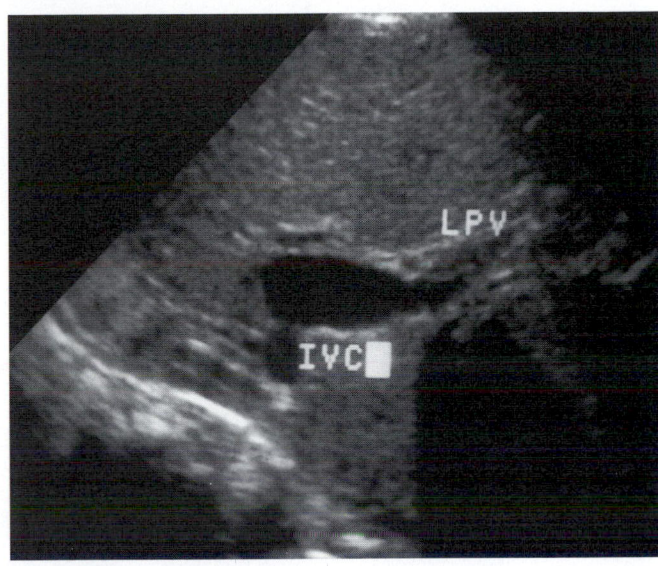

B

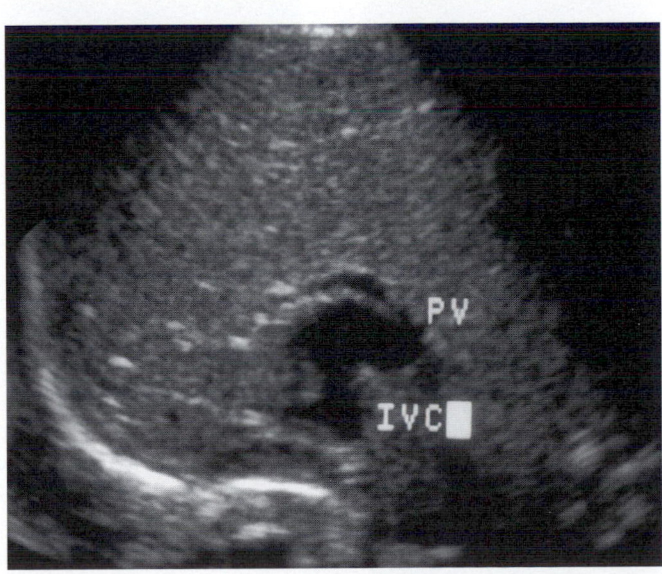

C

FIGURE 53–1. Longitudinal *(A)* and transverse *(B, C)* views through the liver.

CHAPTER 53

Persistent Ductus Venosus

CARLOS J. SIVIT

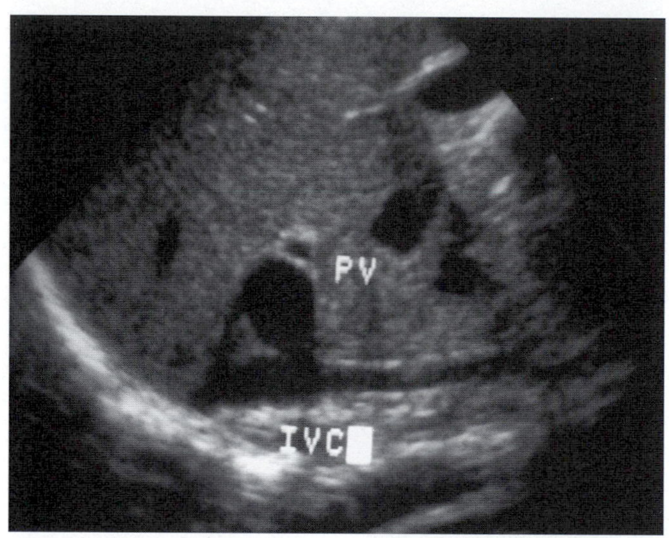

A

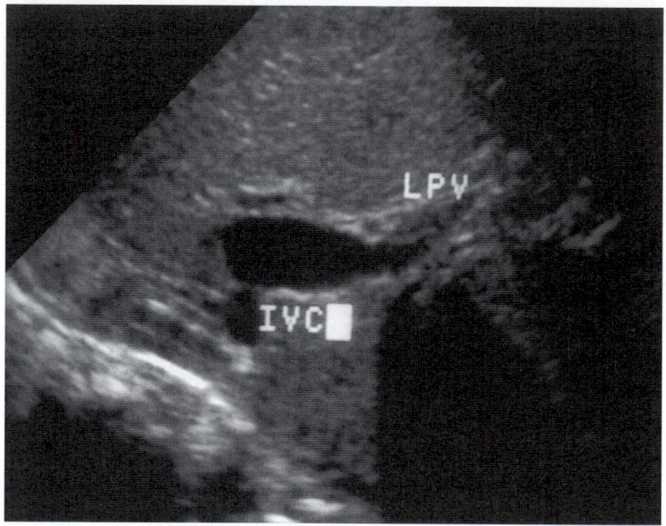

B

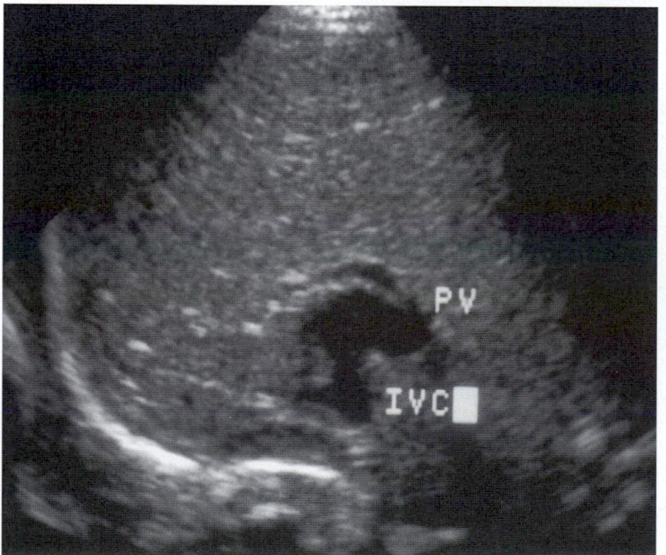

C

FIGURE 53–2. Persistent ductus venosus. Longitudinal *(A)* and transverse *(B, C)* views through the liver demonstrate a short vascular channel extending from the left portal vein (PV) to the inferior vena cava (IVC), representing a persistent ductus venosus.

The ductus venosus is a circulatory shunt unique to fetal life. In fetuses, it is the continuation of the umbilical vein. It originates from the left portal vein and extends to the left hepatic vein near the confluence of the hepatic veins and the inferior vena cava. During fetal life, the ductus venosus provides a low-resistance bypass of the portal venous system for blood returning through the umbilical vein, allowing oxygenated umbilical venous blood to reach the systemic circulation. Flow through the ductus venosus gradually decreases postnatally following cessation of umbilical vein flow. The ductus venosus closes in one-half of all infants by 1 week of age, and in approximately 90 percent of infants by 3 weeks of age. Following its postpartum closure, the ductus venosus undergoes fibrosis, becoming the ligamentum venosum. This thin, fibrous remnant is usually not visible on sonography. However, the fissure in which it is located is visible as a linear,

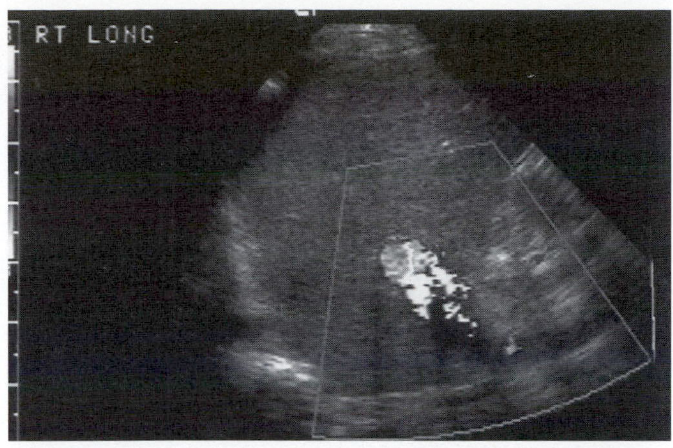

A

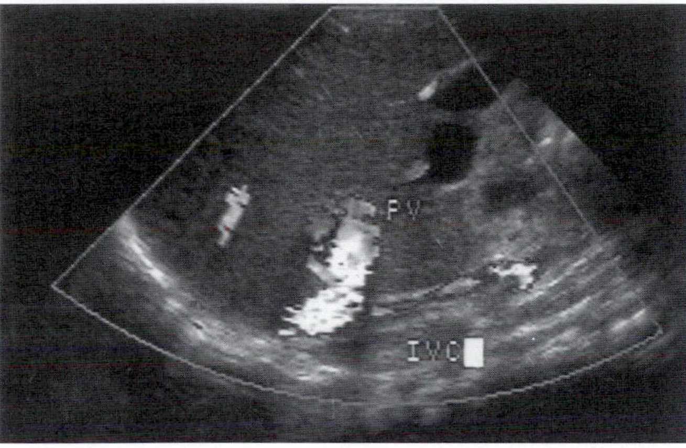

B

FIGURE 53–3. ***A.*** Persistent ductus venosus. Longitudinal view through the liver in the same child as in Fig. 53-1 with color Doppler demonstrates normal hepatopedal flow (toward the liver) in the main portal vein. ***B.*** Persistent ductus venosus. Longitudinal view through the liver in the same child as in ***A*** shows that the direction of flow through the ductus venosus is from the left portal vein (PV) to the inferior vena cava (IVC). (See Color Plate 19.)

hyperechoic area between the caudate lobe and the medial segment of the left hepatic lobe and extending from the posterior and superior surface of the liver to the hilum.

Reports of the persistence of the ductus venosus, resulting in a congenital portosystemic shunt, are rare. The condition has been associated with progressive hepatic dysfunction and encephalopathy. Persistence of the ductus venosus may occur as a response to severe hepatic dysfunction and the development of portal hypertension or as a primary vascular abnormality that may be the cause of the progressive hepatic dysfunction. In cases associated with portal hypertension, it has been postulated that persistence of the ductus venosus follows severe perinatal hepatic dysfunction that results in elevation of portal venous pressures early in life, leading to recruitment of the ductus venosus as a collateral pathway. Thus, persistence of the ductus venosus may be indicative of neonatal hemodynamic compromise. There have also been reports of patency of the ductus venosus associated with normal portal venous pressures. Therefore, persistence of the ductus venosus may be a primary abnormality that results in hepatic dysfunction. In such cases, it is felt that blood chronically bypassing the liver deprives hepatocytes of nutrients, thus impairing hepatocyte function, including protein synthesis and detoxification of ammonia. Reported histopathologic changes in the liver in cases of persistent patency of the ductus venosus include cirrhosis, partial nodular transformation, steatosis, and hypoplasia of the intrahepatic portal venous system. The hepatic abnormalities and associated encephalopathy have been shown in an animal model to be reversible following ligation of the ductus venosus.

Sonography is commonly utililized to evaluate children with hepatic dysfunction. The sonographic evaluation of the liver in these children should include a complete assessment of the hepatic vasculature, including the hepatic veins and portal venous system. A persistent ductus venosus is identified on sonography as a short vascular channel originating from the left portal vein and extending to the left hepatic vein or inferior vena cava (Fig. 53-2). It is approximately 2 cm in length. The direction of flow within the ductus venosus is from the left portal vein toward the inferior vena cava, which can be demonstrated on color or duplex Doppler (Fig. 53-3; see also Color Plate 19). The direction of flow in the main portal vein, right portal vein, and left portal vein proximal to the ductus venosus is typically in the normal hepatopedal direction (Fig. 53-3). There is usually hepatofugal, or reversed, flow in the left portal vein distal to the patent ductus venosus. This indicates the presence of a significant shunt through the ductus venosus. Additionally, there may be associated hypoplasia of the intrahepatic portal venous system. Other sonographic abnormalities, including hepatomegaly, abnormal hepatic echotexture, splenomegaly, and ascites, may also be noted if severe hepatic dysfunction is present.

Computed tomography (CT) may also be useful in the evaluation of persistent ductus venosus in that it can better define the vascular relationships (Fig. 53-4). The CT examination should be performed following intravenous contrast

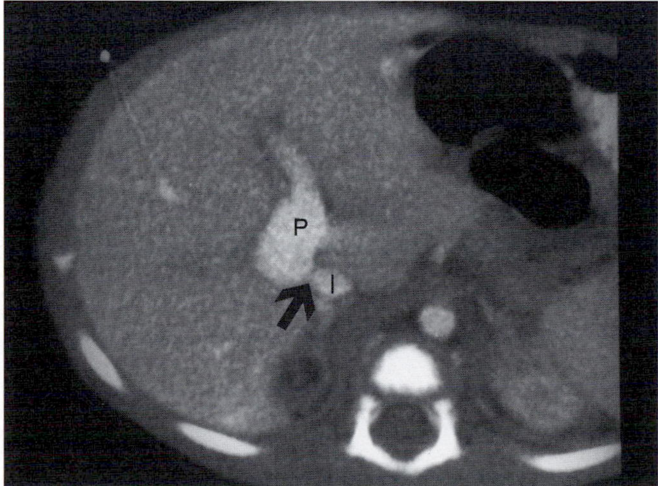

FIGURE 53–4. Persistent ductus venosus with hypoplasia of the intrahepatic portal venous system. Contrast-enhanced computed tomography through the liver in the same child as in Fig. 53-1 demonstrates a persistent ductus venosus (*arrow*) communicating between the left portal vein (P) and the inferior vena cava (I).

media administration. The CT findings in persistent ductus venosus are similar to those on sonography. A short vascular channel originating from the left portal vein and extending to the left hepatic vein or inferior vena cava (Fig. 53-4) is noted.

References

Bellah RD, Hayek J, Littlewood-Teele R: Anomalous portal venous connection to the suprahepatic vena cava: Sonographic demonstration. *Pediatr Radiol* 20:115–117, 1989.

Farrant P, Meire HB, Karani J: Ultrasound diagnosis of portocaval anastomosis in infants—a report of eight cases. *Br J Radiol* 69:389–393, 1996.

Gitzelmann R, Arbenz UV, Willi UV: Hypergalactosemia and portosystemic encephalopathy due to persistence of the ductus venosus Arantii. *Eur J Pediatr* 151:564–568, 1992.

Loberant N, Barak M, Gaitini D: Closure of the ductus venosus in neonates: Findings on real-time gray-scale, color-flow doppler, and duplex doppler sonography. *AJR* 159:1083–1085, 1992.

Maisawa S, Takasago Y, Oyake Y, et al: Patent ductus venosus with hypoplastic right hepatoportal system in a young child born with symmetric intra-uterine growth retardation. *Eur J Pediatr* 151:569–572, 1992.

Mori K, Dohi T, Yamamoto H, et al: An enormous shunt between the portal and hepatic veins associated with multiple coronary artery fistulas. *Pediatr Radiol* 21:66–68, 1990.

Strouse PJ, DiPietro MA: Persistent patency of the ductus venosus: Consequence of portal hypertension in an infant? *J Ultrasound Med* 16:559–561, 1997.

Uchino T, Endo F, Ikeda S, et al: Three brothers with progressive hepatic dysfunction and severe hepatic steatosis due to a patent ductus venosus. *Gastroenterology* 110:1964–1968, 1996.

Wanless IR, Lentz JS, Roberts EA: Partial nodular transformation of liver in an adult with persistent ductus venosus. *Arch Pathol Lab Med* 109:427–432, 1985.

Section C
SPLEEN

54

Figure 54-1 shows a 9-year-old girl with increasing abdominal pain 2 days after being injured in a motor vehicle crash. What are the findings? What is your diagnosis?

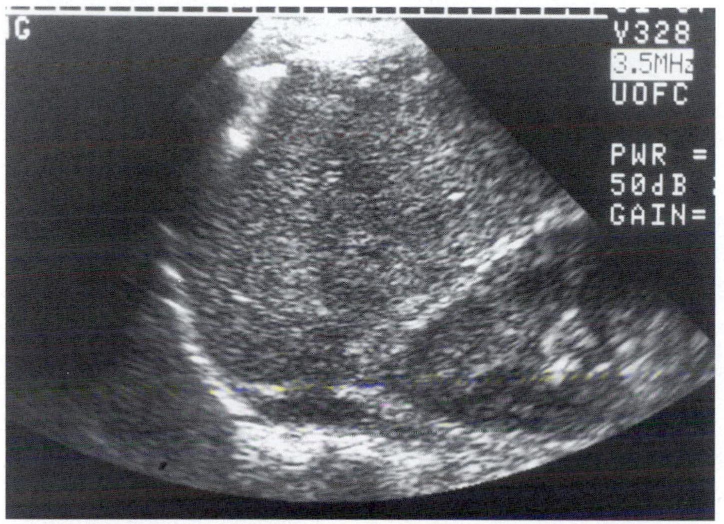

A

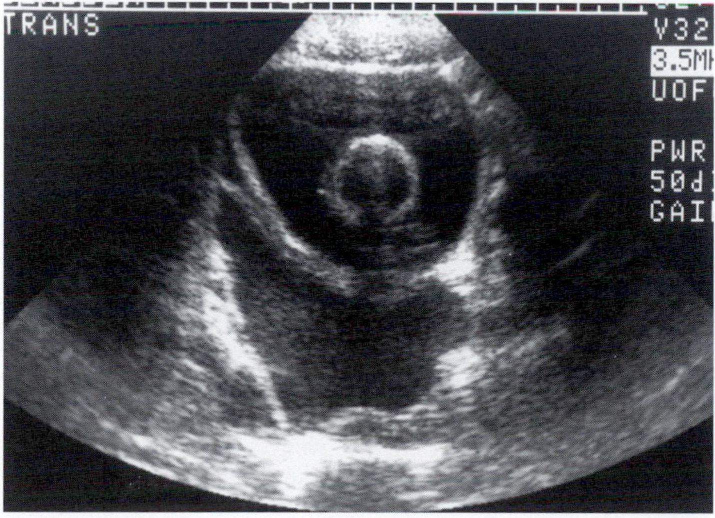

B

FIGURE 54–1. ***A.*** Longitudinal view through the spleen. ***B.*** Transverse view through the pelvis.

CHAPTER 54

Splenic Trauma

ELLEN C. BENYA

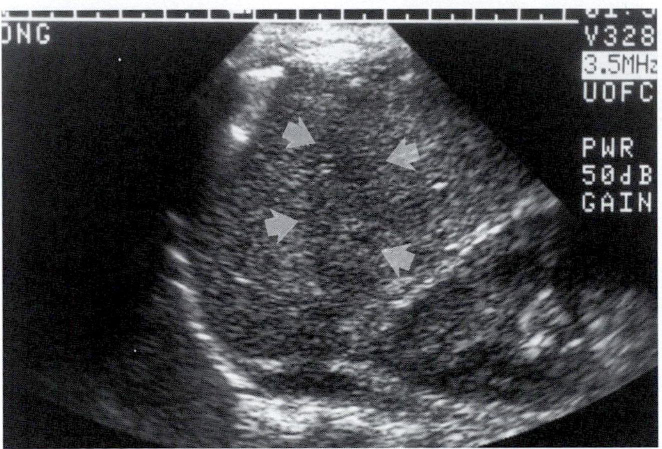

A

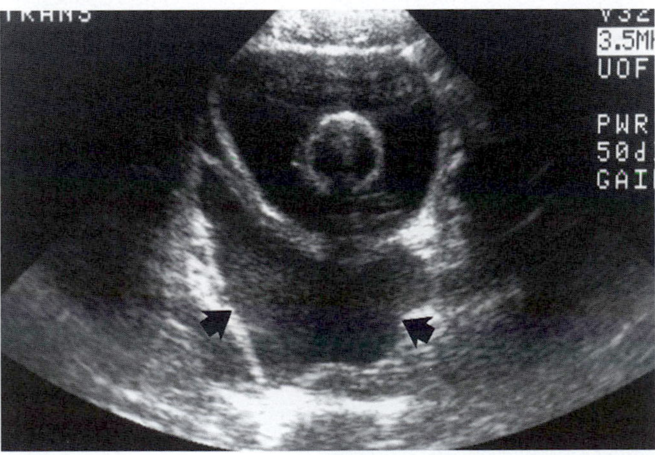

B

FIGURE 54–2. Splenic laceration associated with intraparenchymal hematoma and hemoperitoneum. ***A.*** Longitudinal view through the spleen shows a focal heterogeneous area within the spleen (*arrows*), representing a splenic laceration and associated intraparenchymal hematoma. ***B.*** Transverse view through the pelvis in the same child shows a moderate amount of hypoechoic fluid in the pouch of Douglas (*arrows*), presumed to be associated hemoperitoneum.

Splenic injury is common in children following blunt abdominal trauma. The spleen is the viscus either most commonly or second most commonly injured in children, depending upon the specific series. The spectrum of splenic injury includes parenchymal contusion, laceration, and devascularizing injury. Parenchymal laceration may be simple or complex. A complex laceration typically results in a shattered or fragmented spleen as a result of the small size of the organ. Splenic injury often results in associated hematoma, which may be parenchymal, subcapsular, or perisplenic. Hemoperitoneum is also frequently observed. Diagnostic imaging plays an important role in the initial assessment of injured children, as physical examination and laboratory findings cannot reliably detect injury.

Computed tomography (CT) has traditionally been the examination of choice for the assessment of possible visceral injury in the hemodynamically stable child following blunt abdominal trauma. However, in recent years sonography has been advocated by some as the preferred examination in this setting. Advantages of the use of sonography, compared to CT, in acutely injured children include the ability to perform the examination rapidly at the bedside, the absence of ionizing radiation, the high sensitivity and specificity in the detection of hemoperitoneum, and the lower cost. Disadvantages of the use of sonography are that it is extremely operator-dependent and has decreased sensitivity and specificity for the detection of solid viscus injury compared with CT.

Acute splenic injury has a variable appearance on sonography. Splenic injury will usually result in the loss of the normal homogeneous echotexture of the spleen (Fig. 54-2). Splenic laceration typically has a hypoechoic appearance (Fig. 54-3), while associated intraparenchymal hematoma may appear hypoechoic or hyperechoic relative to normal splenic parenchyma. The intraparenchymal hematoma often has a heterogeneous appearance on sonography (Figs. 54-2 and 54-3). Occasionally, the region of injury is isoechoic relative to adjacent splenic parenchyma. In these cases, it may be quite difficult to identify the injury on the basis of gray-scale differences in splenic echotexture. Assessment of the

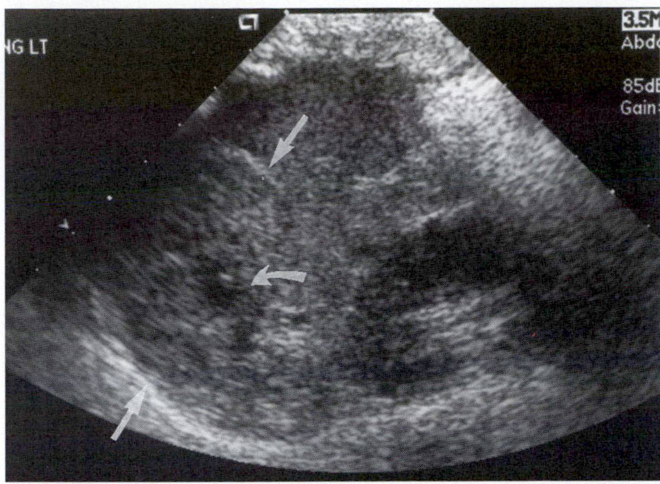

A

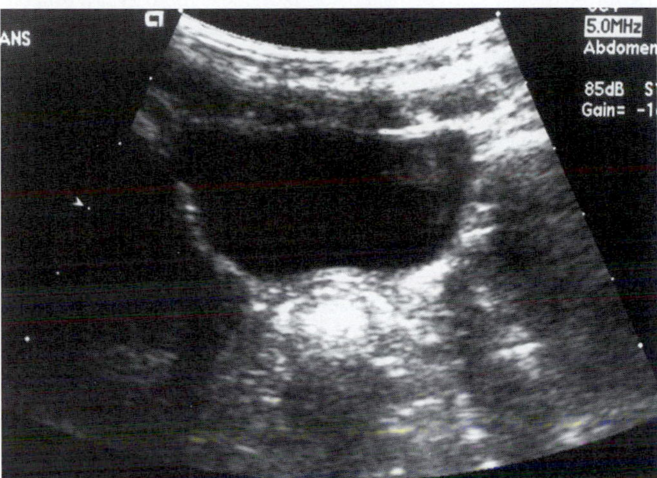

B

FIGURE 54–3. Splenic laceration associated with intraparenchymal hematoma. ***A.*** Longitudinal view through the spleen demonstrates a linear hypoechoic region (*curved arrow*), representing a splenic laceration associated with an adjacent area of parenchymal heterogeneity (*straight arrows*) representing an intraparenchymal hematoma. ***B.*** Transverse view through the pelvis in the same child demonstrates absence of associated peritoneal fluid. There were no fluid pockets noted anywhere in the abdomen or pelvis.

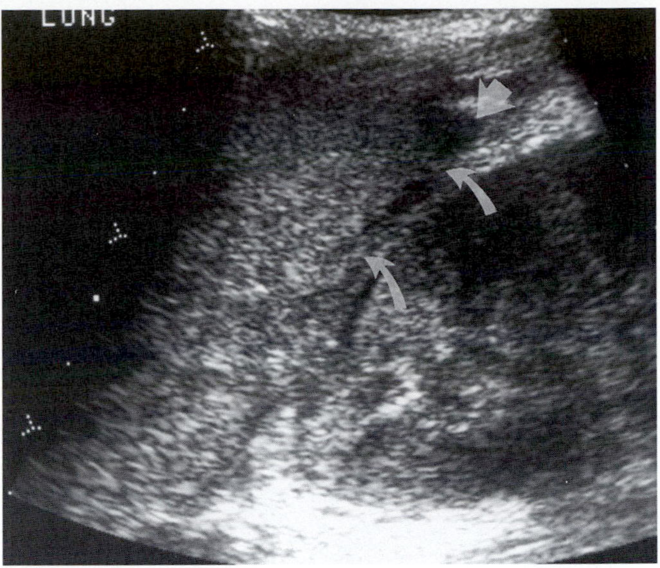

FIGURE 54–4. Splenic injury associated with an ill-defined splenic margin and perisplenic fluid. Longitudinal view through the spleen in a child with splenic injury demonstrates an ill-defined margin of the inferior aspect of the spleen (*curved arrows*). Also note a small amount of associated perisplenic fluid (*straight arrow*).

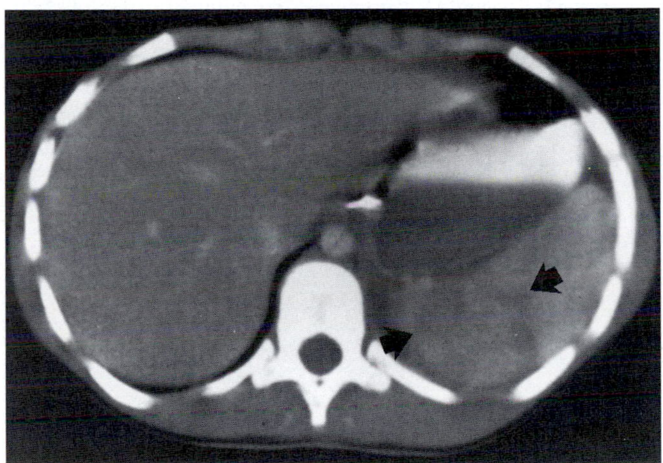

FIGURE 54–5. Splenic laceration on computed tomography (CT). Contrast-enhanced CT scan through the upper abdomen in the same child as in Fig. 54-1 demonstrates a linear area of decreased attenuation in the spleen, indicative of a splenic laceration (*arrow*).

splenic vasculature with color Doppler sonography often provides helpful clues to possible injury, as it demonstrates focal avascular regions within the spleen associated with intraparenchymal hematoma or surrounding the periphery of the spleen in the presence of subcapsular hematoma. Additionally, the presence of perisplenic fluid or an ill-defined splenic margin may also help identify splenic injury (Fig. 54-4).

Further evaluation with CT may be necessary in some children who were initially screened with sonography. The advantages of CT relative to sonography include a higher sensitivity and specificity for the detection of solid viscus injury, the ability to more precisely characterize the extent of solid viscus injury (Fig. 54-5), and the ability to detect hollow viscus and bony injury, neither of which is detectable by sonography. Assessment of the abdomen with CT in injured children should always be performed with intravenous contrast administration.

The sonographic evaluation of the acutely injured child should include assessment of all solid viscera. Additionally, the entire abdomen and pelvis should be evaluated for the presence of associated peritoneal fluid. Peritoneal fluid detected following blunt trauma is typically blood, or hemoperitoneum. The sonographic assessment of possible splenic injury should not depend solely on the identification of hemoperitoneum, since approximately one-fifth of all splenic injuries are not associated with free peritoneal blood (Fig.

54-3). Splenic injury will not be associated with hemoperitoneum if there is absence of capsular extension of the laceration or absence of capsular disruption. Even in cases associated with capsular disruption, the hemorrhage may be contained in a perisplenic hematoma. If associated hemoperitoneum is present, the majority will collect in the pelvis. The pouch of Douglas and the lateral pelvic recesses, both of which are located in the pelvis, are the most dependent peritoneal spaces. Acute hemoperitoneum typically has an anechoic appearance on sonography. Occasionally, the fluid may have a hypoechoic appearance. It is not possible to distinguish hemoperitoneum from other types of fluid in the greater peritoneal cavity, including preexisting ascites, third-space fluid losses, or extravasated bowel or bladder contents.

References

Adler DA, Blane CE, Coran AG, et al: Splenic trauma in the pediatric patient: The integrated roles of ultrasound and computed tomography. *Pediatrics* 78:576–580, 1986.

Akgur FM, Aktug T, Olguner M, et al: Can ultrasonography replace computed tomography in the assessment of children with blunt abdominal trauma? *J Trauma* 42:626–628, 1997.

Filiatraut D, Longpre D, Patriquin H, et al: Investigation of childhood blunt trauma: A practical approach using ultrasound as the initial diagnostic modality. *Pediatr Radiol* 17:373–379, 1987.

Katz S, Lazar L, Rathams V, et al: Can ultrasonography replace computed tomography in the initial assessment of children with blunt abdominal trauma? *J Pediatr Surg* 31:649–651, 1996.

Kaufman RA, Towbin R, Babcock DS, et al: Upper abdominal trauma in children: Imaging evaluation. *AJR* 142:449–460, 1984.

Krupnick AS, Teitelbaum JD, Geiger JD, et al: Use of abdominal ultrasonography to assess pediatric splenic trauma. Potential pitfalls in the diagnosis. *Ann Surg* 225:408–414, 1997.

Luks FI, Lemire A, St.-Vil D, et al: Blunt abdominal trauma in children: The practical value of ultrasonography. *J Trauma* 34: 607–610, 1993.

McKenney KL, Nunez DB, McKenney MG, et al: Sonography as the primary screening technique for blunt abdominal trauma: Experience with 899 patients. *AJR* 170:979–985, 1998.

Taylor GA, Guion CJ, Potter BM, et al: CT of blunt abdominal trauma in children. *AJR* 153:555–559, 1989.

Taylor GA, Sivit CJ: Computed tomography of abdominal trauma in children. *Semin Pediatr Surg* 1:253–259, 1992.

Taylor GA, Sivit CJ: Post traumatic peritoneal fluid: Is it a reliable indicator of intraabdominal injury in children? *J Pediatr Surg* 30:1644–1648, 1995.

VanSonnenberg E, Simeone JF, Mueller PR, et al: Sonographic appearance of hematoma in liver, spleen and kidney: A clinical, pathological and animal study. *Radiology* 147:507–510, 1983.

55

Figure 55-1 shows a 15-year-old girl with sore throat, fever, fatigue, and vague abdominal pain. What do you see? What is your diagnosis?

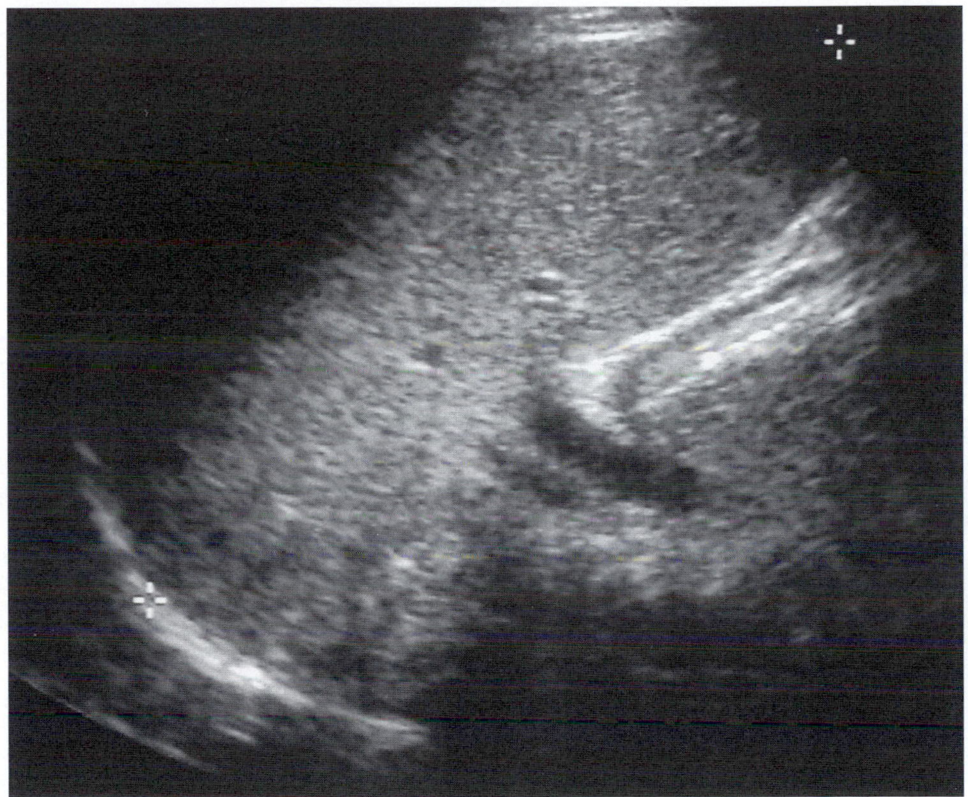

FIGURE 55–1. Longitudinal view through the spleen. The distance between the electronic calipers is 20 cm.

CHAPTER 55

Splenomegaly

LYNN ANSLEY FORDHAM

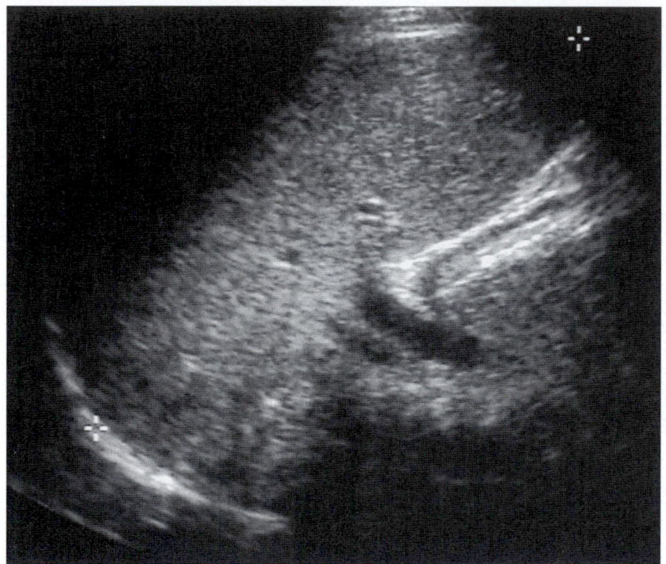

FIGURE 55–2. Splenomegaly. Longitudinal view through the splenic hilum shows a markedly enlarged, homogeneous spleen without focal parenchymal abnormality. The splenic length measured 20 cm. The monospot was positive, diagnostic of infectious mononucleosis.

The spleen is composed of red pulp and white pulp. The red pulp contains mononuclear phagocytic cells, and the white pulp contains lymphoid cells. The spleen serves two functions: filtering blood and participating in the immune response. Therefore, it plays a role similar to that of lymph nodes in the lymphatic system. The spleen also serves as a storage site or source of lymphoreticular cells, hematopoietic cells, and platelets.

Splenomegaly is commonly encountered in children. It is associated with a large number of underlying conditions (Table 55-1). The most common disorders associated with splenomegaly in children are portal hypertension; infection, including cat-scratch disease, Epstein-Barr virus, and systemic candidiasis; hemoglobinopathies; leukemia; and lymphoma. Splenic enlargement occurs in portal hypertension as a result of congestion, whereas splenomegaly associated with infection and malignancy is due to diffuse splenic infiltration by the infectious or neoplastic process. Splenomegaly associated with Epstein-Barr infection can be massive. It may rarely be complicated by splenic rupture.

Sonography is the principal modality utilized in the assessment of children with suspected splenomegaly. Sonography is useful both in establishing the diagnosis of splenomegaly and in evaluating for possible underlying etiology. It is particularly helpful in establishing a diagnosis when there is uncertainty as to whether a mass that is palpable in the left abdomen is an enlarged spleen or a separate mass. A 5-MHz transducer is used in infants and small children; a 3.5-MHz transducer may be needed in larger children. Massive splenomegaly is obvious on sonography, as the left kidney is dwarfed by the large spleen (Fig. 55-2). Measurement of splenic length is required when splenic enlargement is less severe. The splenic length is measured in the coronal plane at the level of the splenic hilum. Age-specific maximal values for normal splenic length have been established by Rosenberg et al. The upper limit of normal for splenic length increases from 6 cm in a newborn to 8 cm at age 2 years and 12 cm at age 12 years. Another method of assessing splenomegaly is by determining the ratio of the splenic–to–left kidney length.Using this method, splenomegaly is diagnosed if the spleen is more than 1.25 times the length of the left kidney.

Sonography is also useful for evaluating conditions associated with splenic enlargement. Although splenomegaly is a nonspecific finding, there are often additional abnormalities that suggest a specific diagnosis. The sonographic evaluation of a child with splenomegaly should include a thorough assessment of the splenic and hepatic parenchyma for possible focal lesions or signs of chronic liver disease. The hepatic vasculature, particularly the hepatic and portal veins, should be evaluated with duplex and color Doppler techniques to

TABLE 55-1
Differential Diagnosis of Splenomegaly

Infections
Brucellosis
Candida*
Cat-scratch disease
Epstein-Barr virus
Hepatitis
Histoplasmosis
Kala-azar
Malaria
Rickettsia
Septicemia
Typhoid
Tuberculosis
Storage diseases
Gaucher's disease
Mucopolysaccharidoses
Neimann-Pick disease
Hemolytic anemias
Hemoglobinopathies
Hereditary spherocytosis
Splenic sequestration
Extramedullary hematopoesis
Immunologic/inflammatory
Rheumatoid arthritis
Sarcoid
Systemic lupus erythematosus
Congestion
Portal hypertension
Right heart failure
Splenic or portal vein thrombosis
Neoplasms
Benign mesenchymal tumors
Hodgkin's lymphoma
Leukemia
Non-Hodgkin's lymphoma
Miscellaneous conditions
Congenital epidermoid cysts
Posttraumatic cysts
Splenic infarction
Splenic torsion

*More common conditions are in bold type.

assess for possible hepatic vein thrombosis or portal hypertension. Sonographic assessment should also include the retroperitoneum and mesentery for possible lymphadenopathy, which would be suggestive of lymphoma.

The normal splenic parenchyma is homogeneous and slightly more echogenic than the adjacent renal cortex. Focal abnormalities in the enlarged spleen may be hyperechoic, hypoechoic, or anechoic relative to normal splenic tissue. The most common focal hyperechoic abnormality in the enlarged spleen is dystrophic calcification from prior granulomatous infection. Focal hypoechoic areas associated with splenomegaly may be due to a variety of infections, including cat-scratch disease (Fig. 55-3) and systemic candidiasis. Hypoechoic splenic lesions may also be associated with lymphoma or early splenic infarction. Focal anechoic splenic lesions include parasitic cysts; splenic pseudocysts, which include posttraumatic splenic cysts and liquefying splenic tissue following segmental splenic infarct (Fig. 55-4); and true splenic cysts, otherwise called congenital or epidermoid cysts

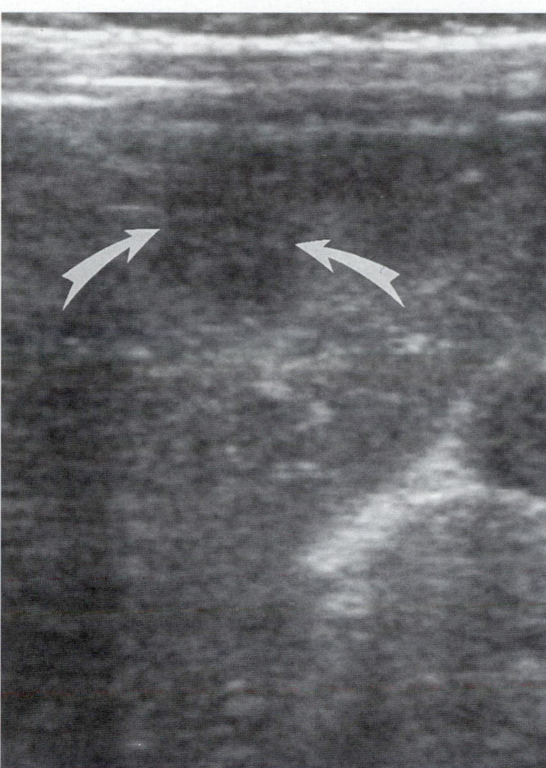

FIGURE 55–3. Splenomegaly associated with focal parenchymal lesion. Magnified transverse view obtained with a linear transducer demonstrates a focal hypoechoic area in the periphery of the spleen (*arrows*). The child had cat-scratch disease.

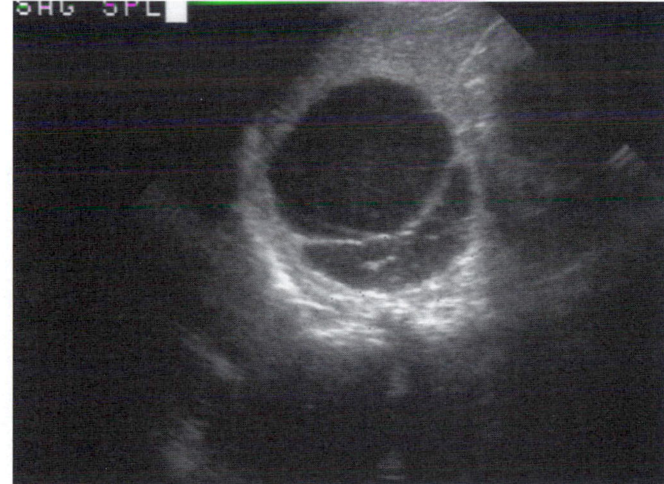

FIGURE 55–4. Splenic infarction. Coronal view through left upper quadrant in a child with sickle cell disease presenting with acute left upper quadrant pain demonstrates a peripherally located, complex cystic area near the dome of the spleen, indicative of prior splenic infarction. The anechoic region represents liquefaction of splenic tissue. On follow-up imaging, the spleen was smaller than expected for the child's age, consistent with prior splenic infarction.

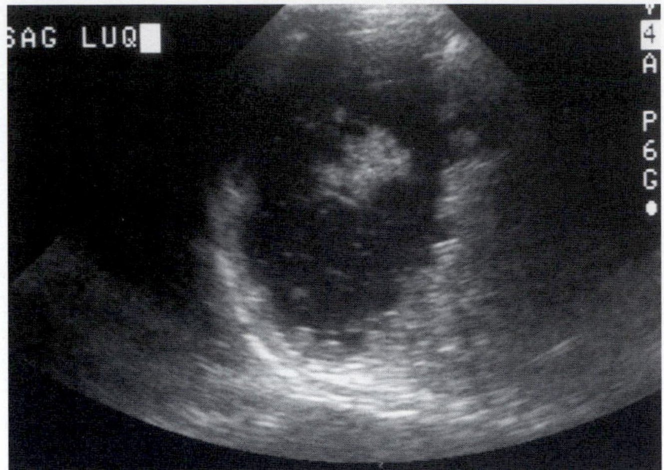

FIGURE 55–5. Splenic epidermoid cyst. Coronal view through the left upper quadrant demonstrates a complex cyst within the spleen. Note the acoustic enhancement, indicating that the lesion is cystic. Also note the septations and internal echoes within the lesion.

(Fig. 55-5). The splenic pseudocysts do not have an epithelial lining, whereas the true cysts are lined by epithelium and surrounded by a fibrous wall. The three types of cyst are indistinguishable from one another on sonography.

References

Dachman AH, Ros PR, Muran PJ, et al: Nonparasitic splenic cysts: A report of 52 cases with radiologic-pathologic correlation. *AJR* 147:537–542, 1986.

Daneman A, Martin DJ: Congenital epithelial splenic cysts in children. *Pediatr Radiol* 12:119–125, 1982.

Goerg C, Schwerk WB, Goerg K: Sonography of focal lesions of the spleen. *AJR* 156:949–953, 1991.

Keder R, Merchant S, Malde H, et al: Multiple reflective channels in the spleen: A sonographic sign of portal hypertension. *Abdom Imaging* 19:453–458, 1994.

Loftus WK, Meterweli C: Ultrasound assessment of mild splenomegaly: Spleen/kidney ratio. *Pediatr Radiol* 28:98–100, 1998.

O'Reilly RA: Splenomegaly in 2,505 patients at a large university medical center from 1913 to 1995 – 1963 to 1995: 449 patients. *West J Med* 169:88–97, 1998.

Rosenberg HK, Markowitz RI, Kolberg H, et al: Normal splenic size in infants and children: Sonographic measurements. *AJR* 157:119–121, 1991.

Urrutia M, Mergo PJ, Ros LH, et al: Cystic masses of the spleen. *Radiographics* 16:107–129, 1996.

Section D
PANCREAS

56

Figure 56-1 shows a 14-year-old boy with underlying chronic disease, nausea, vomiting, and abdominal pain. What are the findings? What is the underlying chronic disease?

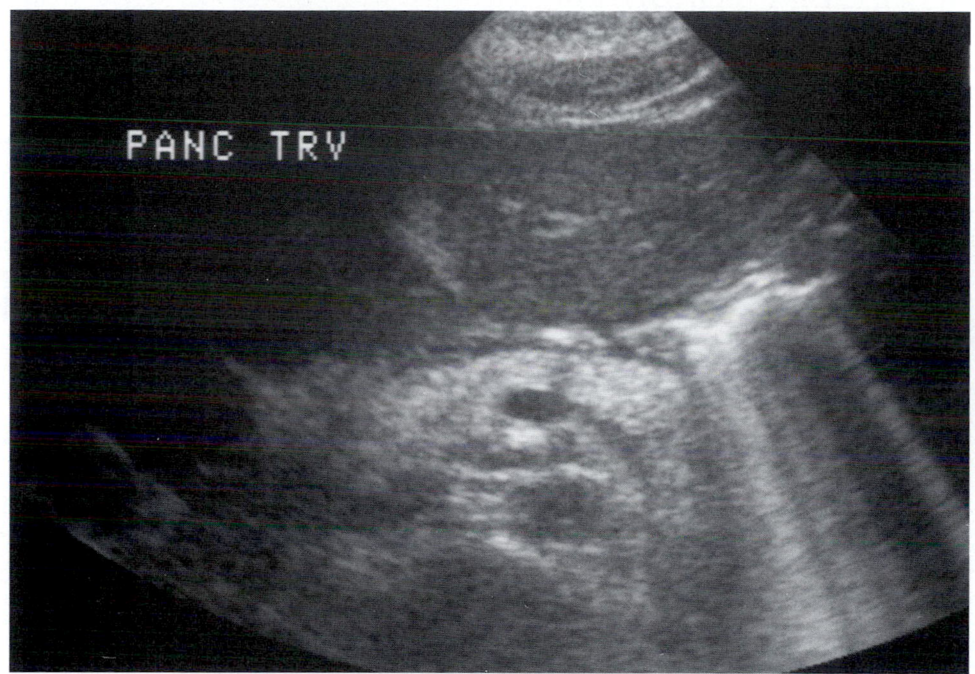

FIGURE 56–1. Transverse view through the upper abdomen.

CHAPTER 56

Fatty Replacement of the Pancreas in Cystic Fibrosis

LYNN ANSLEY FORDHAM

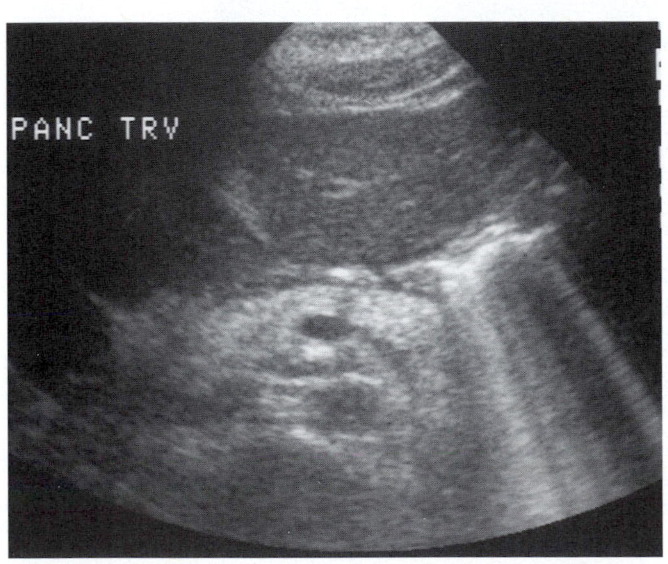

FIGURE 56–2. Increased pancreatic echogenicity associated with cystic fibrosis. Transverse view through the upper abdomen demonstrates a diffusely echogenic pancreas. Note the increased pancreatic echogenicity relative to the left lobe of the liver anterior to the pancreas. The splenic vein is seen coursing posterior to the pancreas.

Cystic fibrosis is the most common lethal autosomal recessive disease in Caucasian populations, occurring in approximately 1 in 2500 live births. The disease results in abnormally thick secretions, resulting in obstruction of ducts and hollow organs. The thick, obstructing secretions are due to an underlying abnormality in chloride transfer in the cell membrane. The most common cause of morbidity and mortality in cystic fibrosis is pulmonary disease. In the respiratory system, obstruction of the airways leads to chronic pneumonia, bronchiectasis, and respiratory failure. Chronic sinusitis and obstructive azospermia are nearly universal. Cystic fibrosis affects the liver, biliary tract, gastrointestinal tract, and pancreas, leading to obstruction and dysfunction. An increased risk of gastrointestinal malignancies has also been reported.

Cystic fibrosis is caused by a variety of mutations in a gene on the long arm of chromosome 7. The product of that gene is a protein termed cystic fibrosis transmembrane conductance regulator (CFTR), which regulates chloride transfer across epithelial membranes. The most frequent mutation is delta F 508, which is present in approximately two-thirds of individuals with cystic fibrosis. More than 500 associated mutations have been reported. One in 20 Caucasians carries a cystic fibrosis mutation. In some individuals the pulmonary disease dominates the clinical picture, while in others hepatobiliary disease is predominant. Attempts have been made to correlate the clinical manifestations of disease with the underlying genetic defects. There is no correlation between genotype and phenotype in pulmonary disease. Conversely, genotype predicts phenotype in pancreatic disease. A minority of individuals with cystic fibrosis produce sufficient pancreatic enzymes, and these patients have mutations that mildly decrease either the function or the amount of CFTR. The majority of individuals with cystic fibrosis have pancreatic insufficiency and require pancreatic enzyme replacement.

Cystic fibrosis is the most common cause of pancreatic insufficiency in individuals under 30 years of age. Exocrine pancreatic insufficiency results in malabsorption, fat intolerance, and steatorrhea. Abnormally thick pancreatic secretions lead to duct obstruction, acinar atrophy, and mild inflammation.

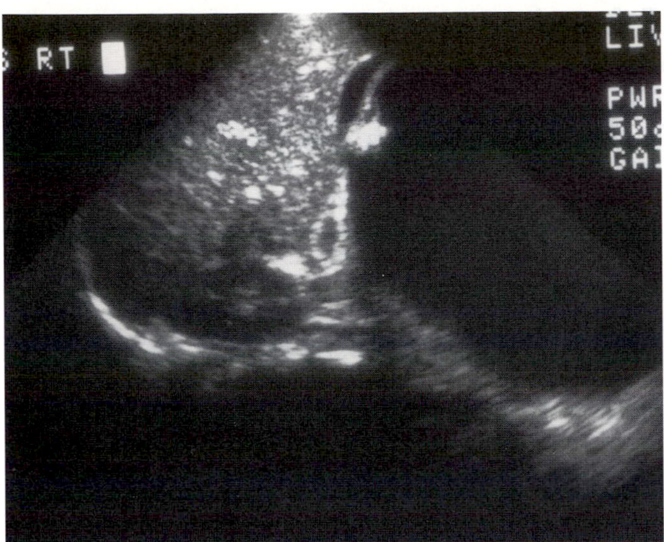

FIGURE 56–3. Large pancreatic cyst associated with cystic fibrosis. Transverse view through the upper abdomen in a child with cystic fibrosis demonstrates a large cyst originating in the tail of the pancreas. (*Courtesy of Gail Lonergan, MD.*)

These result in progressive pancreatic fibrosis and fatty replacement, ductal ectasia, cyst formation, and calcification. Endocrine pancreatic dysfunction is less common than exocrine dysfunction. Some 30 to 50 percent of individuals with cystic fibrosis have some level of glucose intolerance, but diabetes is present in only 1 to 2 percent. The CFTR protein has not been identified in pancreatic islet cells, and therefore endocrine dysfunction is probably secondary to pancreatic fibrosis.

Sonography is usually the initial imaging modality of choice in children with suspected pancreatic disease. The pancreas can be succesfully visualized by sonography in the majority of children. The pancreas is usually better visualized in fasting individuals, since gas and food in the stomach following a meal may limit the examination. The head and body of the pancreas are best scanned through the left lobe of the liver, while the tail of the pancreas is best viewed utilizing the spleen as a window.

Sonographic abnormalities of the pancreas are seen in nearly all individuals with cystic fibrosis. The most common sonographic finding in children with cystic fibrosis is increased echogenicity of the pancreas (Fig. 56-2). The normal pancreas should be slightly more echogenic than the liver or spleen. Increased pancreatic echogenicity in children with cystic fibrosis is due to fatty replacement and/or fibrosis of the pancreas. As a result of the hyperechogenicity of the pancreas, the pancreatic margins may be difficult to delineate. The pancreas may blend in with the surrounding retroperitoneal fat and not be identified on sonography. Pancreatic ductal obstruction can lead to ductal and acinar dilatation, manifested by intraductal calcification and cyst formation. Pancreatic cysts associated with cystic fibrosis are felt to develop when functional secretory capacity is maintained despite ductal obstruction. The resultant pancreatic cysts are usually quite small. Rarely, they may reach a large size (Fig. 56-3). Ductal obstruction can also result in atrophy of the gland. Therefore, the pancreas in these children is typically small in size.

Hepatobiliary abnormalities are commonly noted on sonography in children with cystic fibrosis. These include sludge, cholelithiasis, a small or absent gallbladder, and abnormalities of hepatic contour and echotexture if biliary cirrhosis is present. Cirrhosis in these patients typically follows a pericholangitis that develops as a result of mechanical obstruction of the biliary ducts. Portal hypertension is rarely seen. It develops in approximately 2 percent of patients with cystic fibrosis.

Computed tomography (CT) scan of the abdomen is occasionally performed in children with cystic fibrosis. The pancreas in these children will typically appear small in size and demonstrate diffuse parenchymal low attenuation due to fatty replacement (Fig. 56-4). Computed tomography is more useful than sonography in precisely evaluating the presence of ductal calcification. Additionally, CT allows for enhanced localization of cystic lesions seen in the upper abdomen as intrapancreatic or extrapancreatic (Fig. 56-5).

Increased pancreatic echogenicity may also be noted with fatty replacement or fibrosis of the pancreas associated with chronic pancreatitis or following pancreatic necrosis in severe acute pancreatitis. Pancreatic cysts may also be noted in association with acute or chronic pancreatitis. Congenital pancreatic cysts may also be seen. These are typically associated with von Hippel–Lindau disease or autosomal dominant polycystic kidney disease.

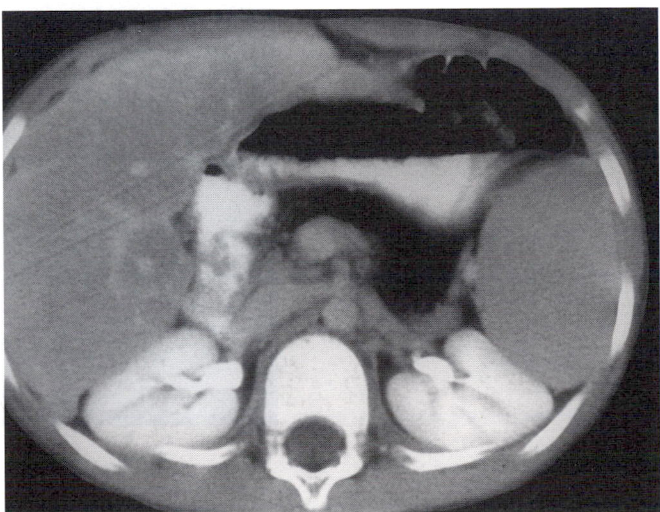

FIGURE 56–4. Fatty replacement of the pancreas at computed tomography (CT). Contrast-enhanced CT scan through the upper abdomen in a child with cystic fibrosis demonstrates diffuse low attenuation through the pancreas, diagnostic of fatty replacement.

CHAPTER 57

Acute Pancreatitis

CARLOS J. SIVIT

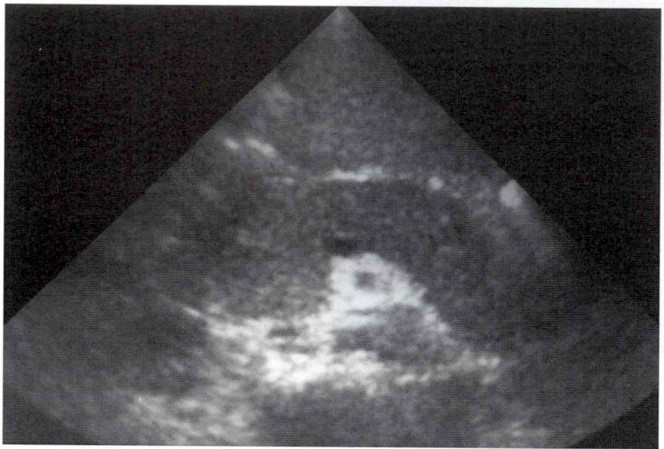

A

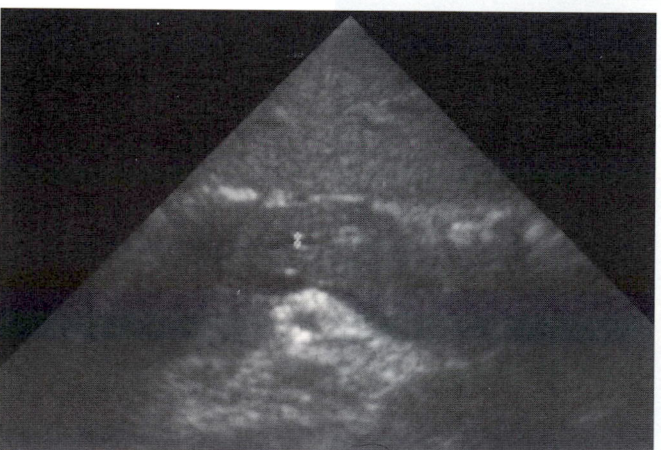

B

FIGURE 57–2. Acute pancreatitis. *A.* Transverse view through the pancreas in a child with clinical pancreatitis demonstrates diffuse gland enlargement. Note that the gland still has a normal homogeneous echotexture. ***B.*** Transverse view through the pancreas slightly caudal to *A* shows dilatation of the main pancreatic duct (*between electronic calipers*).

The most common cause of acute pancreatitis in children is pancreatic injury following blunt abdominal trauma. Pancreatic injury typically results from direct compression of the pancreatic head or body against the vertebral column. In children, this injury most commonly occurs following a motor vehicle crash or related to a collision with bicycle handlebars. Acute pancreatitis may also have a variety of nontraumatic causes, including infection, drug toxicity, obstruction at the ampulla of Vater, pancreas divisum, cystic fibrosis, and hereditary pancreatitis. The infection that most commonly results in pancreatitis is mumps. Pancreatitis has also been reported with other viral infections, including measles and rubella. Drugs associated with the development of acute pancreatitis include steroids, L-asparaginase, hydrochlorothiazide, and azothioprine. The most common obstructive cause is choledocholithiasis with obstruction at the ampulla of Vater. Pancreas divisum is a developmental anomaly of the pancreas in which the dorsal and ventral pancreatic ducts fail to fuse. The dorsal duct drains via the accessory duct of Santorini into the minor duodenal papilla, while the ventral duct drains via the common bile duct into the papilla of Vater. In these individuals, pancreatitis results if the duct of Santorini and the accessory papilla are too small to transmit the volume of pancreatic secretions that must flow through them. This, in turn, leads to pooling of pancreatic secretions. Pancreatitis in children with cystic fibrosis results from ductal obstruction and leakage of pancreatic enzymes. Approximately 1 percent of children with cystic fibrosis develop pancreatitis. Hereditary pancreatitis is an autosomal dominant disease characterized by recurrent attacks of acute pancreatitis.

Clinical findings of acute pancreatitis include upper abdominal pain that may localize to the epigastric region and radiate to the back, abdominal tenderness, vomiting, and fever. Levels of pancreatic enzymes, amylase and lipase, are elevated in blood and urine. Acute pancreatitis is classified as mild or severe on the basis of clinical and pathologic changes. Mild acute pancreatitis is characterized by minimal

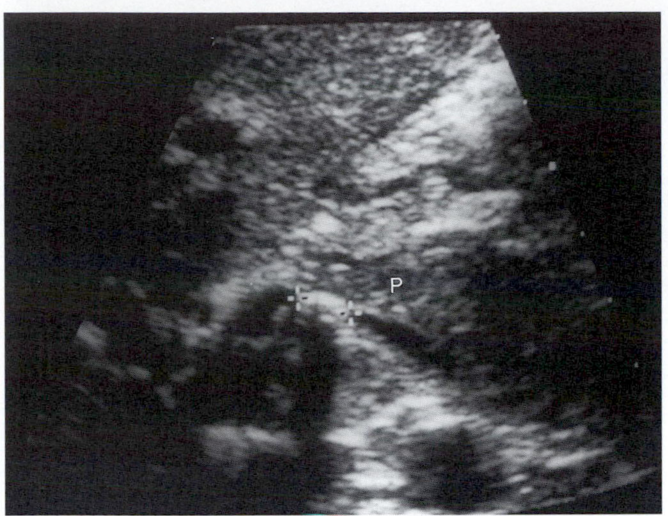

A

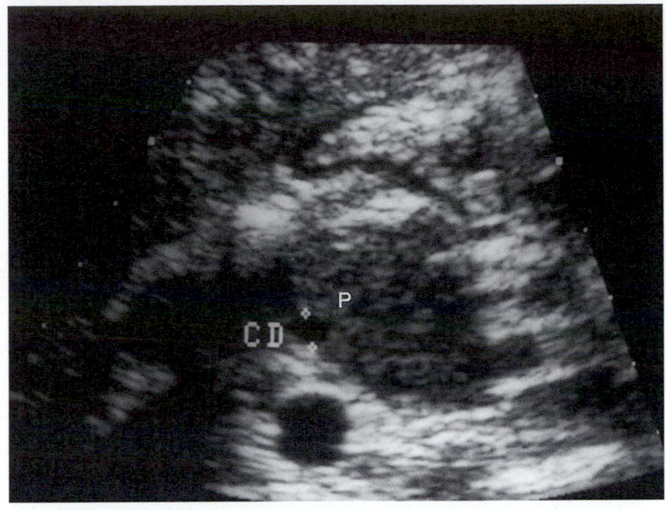

B

FIGURE 57–3. Dilatation of the distal common bile duct associated with choledocholithiasis and acute pancreatitis. ***A.*** Transverse view through the head of the pancreas (P) shows a hyperechoic focus in the distal common bile duct with acoustic shadowing, consistent with a distal common bile duct stone. ***B.*** Transverse view through the head of the pancreas (P) in the same child slightly cephalad to the view showing the distal common bile duct stone shows dilatation of the distal common bile duct (*between electronic calipers*).

systemic signs and rapid response to medical therapy. There is usually an improvement in physical signs and laboratory values within 48 to 72 h. Mild acute pancreatitis is characterized pathologically by interstitial edema. Rarely, microscopic foci of acinar cell necrosis may be noted. Severe acute pancreatitis is characterized by more severe clinical findings, including shock, renal failure, gastrointestinal tract bleeding, and pulmonary insufficiency. The development of pancreatic pseudocysts and abscesses is common. The clinical distinction between acute and severe pancreatitis is usually evident early in the course of the disease. Progression from mild to severe disease is rare.

Sonography is the principal modality utilized in the initial assessment of children with suspected nontraumatic acute pancreatitis (Fig. 57-2). The pancreas is an extraperitoneal organ located in the anterior pararenal space. Immediately anterior to the anterior pararenal space is the lesser sac, an intraperitoneal compartment. There are several important imaging landmarks in the evaluation of the pancreas. The inferior vena cava lies posterior to the pancreatic head. The pancreatic neck, which is located at the junction of the pancreatic head and body, is directly anterior to the origin of the portal vein at the confluence of the superior mesenteric vein and the splenic vein. The body and tail of the pancreas are directly anterior to the splenic vein and caudal to the splenic artery. The pancreas should be imaged with a high-frequency sector or linear array transducer. It can be visualized in the majority of children. The most difficult portion of the pancreas to visualize is the tail. The pancreas should demonstrate a homogeneous echotexture that is isoechoic to liver and spleen.

Sonography should be used not in the diagnosis of pancreatitis, as it has a low sensitivity and specificity for diagnosis of the condition, but rather to evaluate for possible complications of pancreatitis or for associated predisposing conditions. Sonography is particularly useful for the evaluation of associated extrapancreatic fluid collections. Additionally, sonography is useful in the evaluation of choledocholithiasis, which may be associated with acute pancreatitis (Fig. 57-3). The pancreas may appear normal on sonography, particularly in cases of mild pancreatitis. Sonographic findings observed in acute pancreatitis include focal or diffuse gland enlargement (Fig. 57-2), pancreatic ductal dilation (Fig. 57-2), increased or decreased pancreatic parenchymal echotexture, and free or focal extrapancreatic fluid collections. Pancreatic enlargement in acute pancreatitis is felt to be due to diffuse gland edema. The diagnosis of pancreatic enlargement is made on the basis of the anteroposterior diameter of the gland on transverse view (Fig. 57-4). The gland will vary in size with the age of the individual. As a general rule, the normal anteroposterior diameter of the pancreatic head and tail should not exceed 2 cm in children, regardless of age, and the anteroposterior diameter of the pancreatic body should not exceed 1 cm.

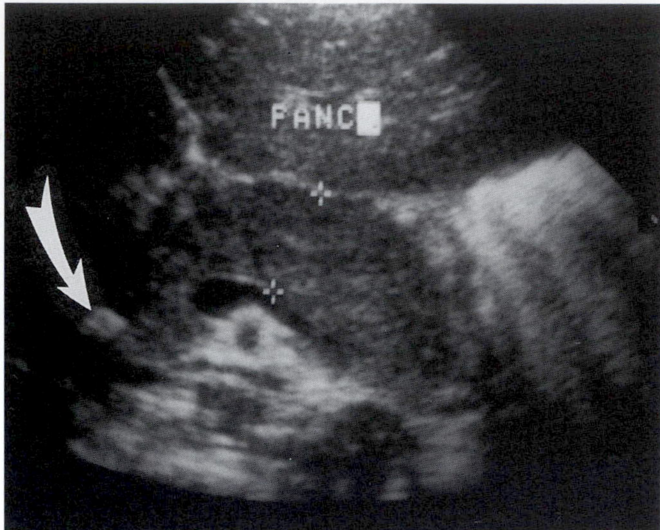

FIGURE 57–4. Acute pancreatitis with enlargement of the body of the pancreas. Transverse view through the body of the pancreas demonstrates increased anteroposterior diameter (*between electronic calipers*), indicative of pancreatic enlargement. Note the associated gallstone in the distal common bile duct (*arrow*).

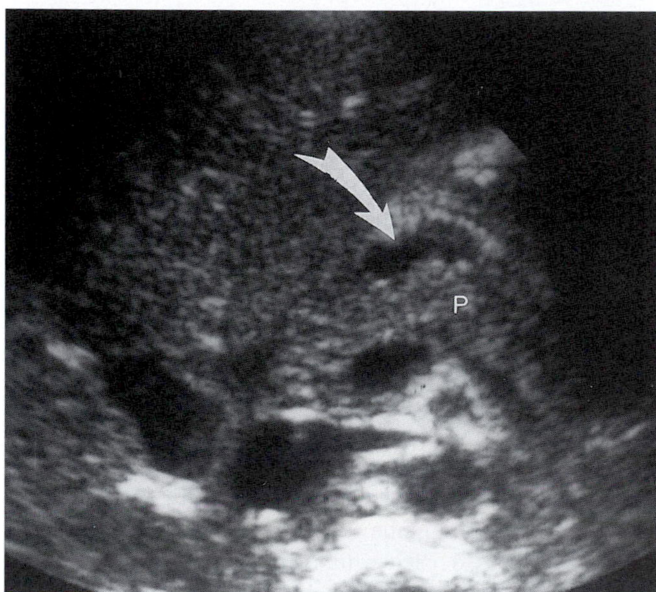

FIGURE 57–5. Pancreatic laceration. Transverse view through the neck of the pancreas demonstrates a partial-thickness defect (*arrow*) representing a laceration. P = pancreas.

In acute pancreatitis secondary to pancreatic injury, sonography may demonstrate the associated pancreatic laceration (Fig. 57-5) or fracture (Fig. 57-6). A pancreatic laceration will appear sonographically as a partial-thickness hypoechoic or anechoic linear defect, usually in the neck or body of the pancreas (Fig. 57-5). The sonographic diagnosis may be difficult, as there may be minimal separation of the pancreatic fragments. If there is a fracture or complete transection of the pancreas, a full-thickness defect through the pancreas will be noted (Fig. 57-6). There is typically greater separation of the fractured fragments.

Acute fluid collections associated with pancreatitis represent pancreatic juice that spreads throughout the connective tissue surrounding the pancreas, since the pancreas does not have a well-developed capsule. The fluid collections will assume the shape of the intraperitoneal or extraperitoneal space in which they are located. The most common locations for these fluid collections are the anterior pararenal space, lesser sac, lesser omentum, and transverse mesocolon. These collections will appear anechoic or hypoechoic with increased through transmission on sonography. Most acute peripancreatic fluid collections resolve completely within a few weeks. A minority will evolve into pseudocysts. Formation of a pseudocyst requires at least 4 weeks following the onset of acute pancreatitis. Pseudocysts are round or oval in shape and are surrounded by a thin capsule containing fibrous tissue. They may be anechoic (Fig. 57-7) or contain internal echoes due to necrotic debris or hemorrhage (Fig. 57-8). They are typically found in close proximity to the pancreas. Sonogra-

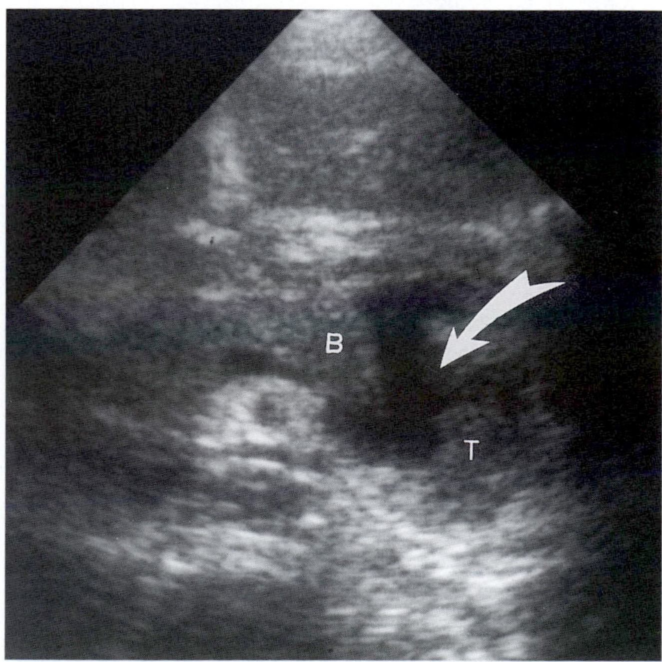

FIGURE 57–6. Pancreatic transection. Transverse view through the junction of the body and tail of the pancreas demonstrates a pancreatic transection (*arrow*). Note the separation between the pancreatic body (B) and tail (T).

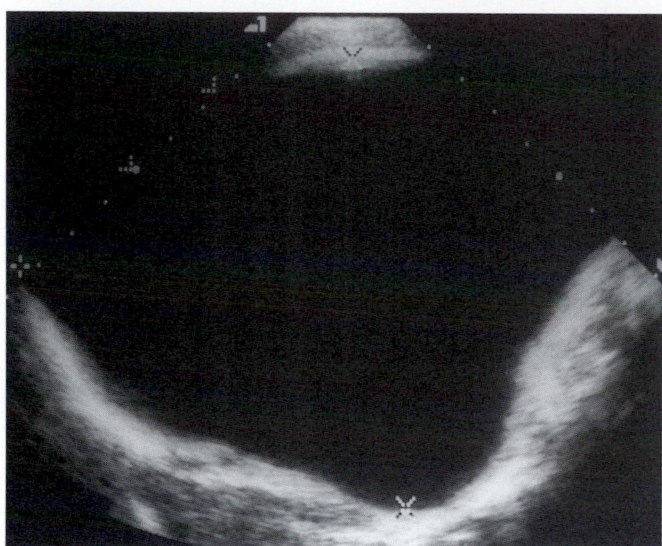

FIGURE 57–7. Pancreatic pseudocyst. Longitudinal view through the upper abdomen in a child with prior pancreatitis demonstrates a large anechoic cyst, representing a pancreatic pseudocyst.

phy is the preferred modality for the follow-up evaluation of extrapancreatic fluid collections, including pseudocysts (Fig. 57-8). A pseudocyst may spontaneously resolve or may persist and require intraoperative or percutaneous drainage.

Computed tomography (CT) is the preferred method for the initial evaluation of suspected pancreatic injury associated with acute pancreatitis (Fig. 57-9). Direct signs of injury may be difficult to identify, owing to the small size of the gland, the paucity of surrounding fat, and the minimal separation of fracture fragments. Signs of pancreatic injury on CT are listed in Table 57-1. The best predictor of pancreatic injury on CT is unexplained peripancreatic fluid (fluid in the anterior pararenal space or lesser sac). Computed tomography is also the examination of choice for the initial assessment of extrapancreatic fluid collections, as it is superior to sonography for defining the extent of these lesions. Additionally, CT is the best modality for assessing possible pancreatic necrosis and pancreatic abscess, which are complications of severe pancreatitis (Fig. 57-10). Pancreatic necrosis is characterized by zones of nonviable or devitalized pancreatic parenchyma, while pancreatic abscess is an intraabdominal collection of purulent material located in close proximity to

TABLE 57-1
CT Findings in Children with Pancreatic Injury

Direct visualization of injury
Focal or diffuse gland enlargement
Fluid in anterior pararenal space
Fluid separating splenic vein and pancreas
Lesser scan fluid
Free peritoneal fluid
Thickened anterior renal fascia

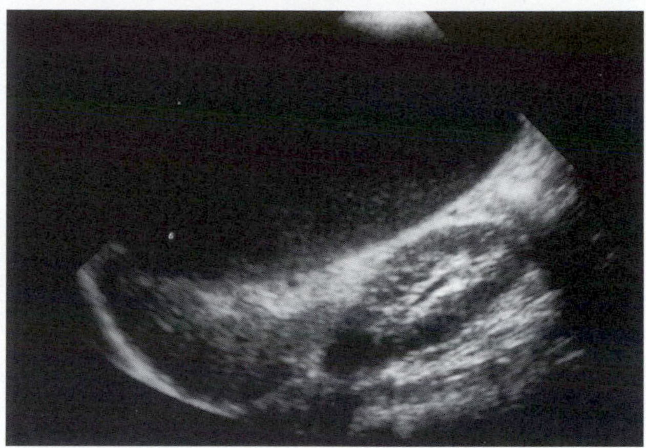

A

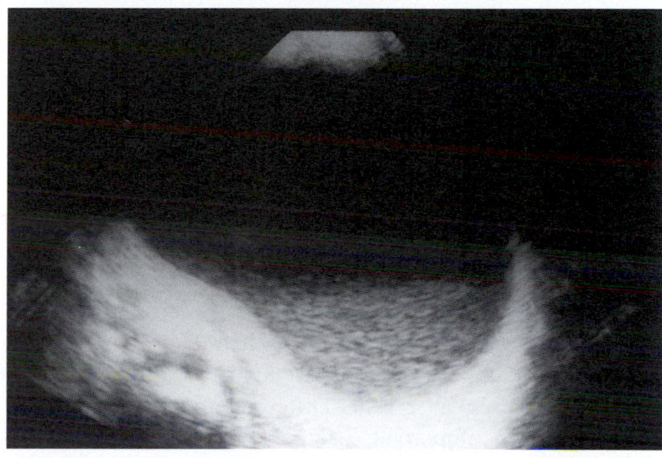

B

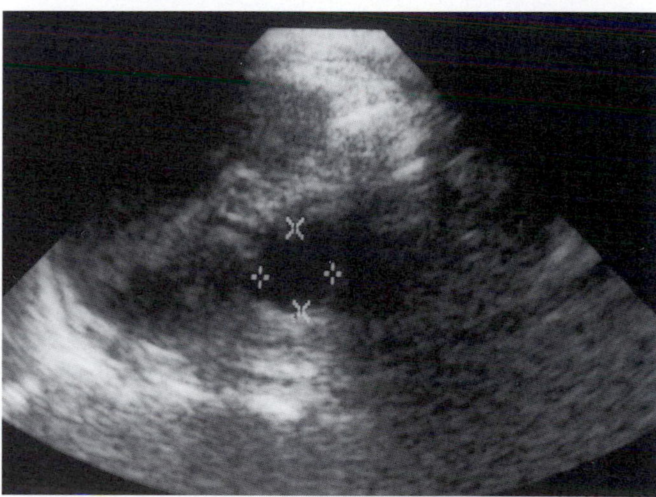

C

FIGURE 57–8. Pancreatic pseudocyst. Longitudinal *(A)* and transverse *(B)* views through the left upper quadrant in a child with prior pancreatitis show a large, oval-shaped, cystic lesion anterior to the left kidney. Note that the lesion contains internal echoes, probably representing debris with a fluid-debris level. ***C.*** Longitudinal view through the left upper quadrant in the same child 3 weeks after the initial exam shows a marked decrease in cyst size (*between electronic calipers*).

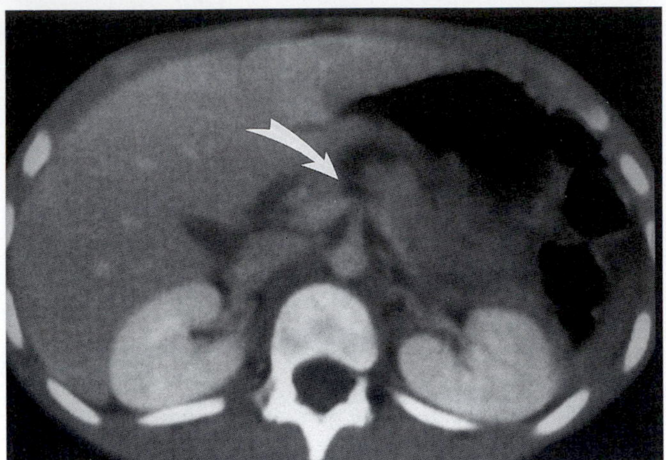

FIGURE 57–9. Pancreatic laceration. Contrast-enhanced computed tomography scan through the upper abdomen in a child evaluated following blunt abdominal trauma demonstrates a low-attenuation laceration through the neck of the pancreas (*arrow*).

the pancreas containing little or no necrosis. The CT appearance of pancreatic necrosis is that of a well-circumscribed area of decreased or absent parenchymal enhancement that is larger than 3 cm in diameter or involves 30 percent or more of the area of the pancreas (Fig. 57-10). A pancreatic abscess will appear on CT as a focal fluid collection with near-water attenuation and a relatively thick wall. The wall may demonstrate variable enhancement. Differentiation between these two processes is important, as a pancreatic abscess can typically be drained percutaneously, whereas pancreatic necrosis may require surgical debridement.

References

Balthazar EJ, Freeny PC, Van Sonnenberg E: Imaging and intervention in acute pancreatitis. *Radiology* 193:297–306, 1994.

Balthazar EJ, Robinson DL, Megibow AJ, et al: Acute pancreatitis: Value of CT in establishing prognosis. *Radiology* 174:331–336, 1990.

Coleman BG, Arger PH, Rosenberg HK, et al: Gray-scale sonographic assessment of pancreatitis in children. *Radiology* 146: 145–150, 1983.

Fleischer AC, Parker P, Kirchner SG, et al: Sonographic findings of pancreatitis in children. *Radiology* 146:151–155, 1983.

Jeffrey RB: Sonography in acute pancreatitis. *Radiol Clin North Am* 27:5–17, 1989.

Jeffrey RB, Laing FC, Wing VW: Extrapancreatic spread of acute pancreatitis: New observations with real-time US. *Radiology* 159:707–711, 1986.

King LR, Siegel MJ, Balfe DM: Acute pancreatitis in children: CT findings of intra- and extrapancreatic fluid collections. *Radiology* 195:196–200, 1995.

Siegel MJ, Martin KW, Worthington JL: Normal and abnormal pancreas in children: US studies. *Radiology* 165:15–18, 1987.

Siegel MJ, Sivit CJ: Pancreatic emergencies. *Radiol Clin North Am* 35:815–830, 1997.

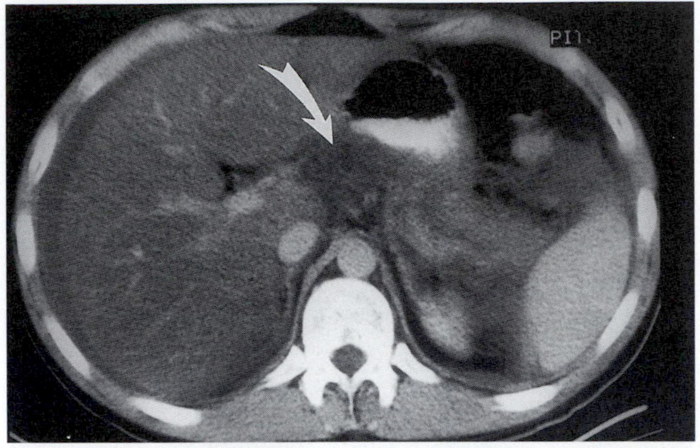

A

B

C

FIGURE 57–10. Pancreatic necrosis. ***A.*** Contrast-enhanced computed tomography (CT) scan through the pancreas in a child with severe acute pancreatitis demonstrates a focal area of decreased parenchymal enhancement in the neck of the pancreas (*arrow*), indicative of pancreatic necrosis. ***B.*** Contrast-enhanced CT scan through the pancreas in the same child 3 weeks later shows diffuse low attenuation throughout the pancreatic parenchyma. The findings are indicative of liquefaction following extensive pancreatic necrosis. ***C.*** Transverse view through the pancreas in the same child 2 weeks after the CT scan in ***B*** shows a diffusely hypoechoic pancreas with poorly defined margins, indicative of organ liquefaction following pancreatic necrosis.

Section E
ADRENAL GLAND

58

Figure 58-1 shows a 15-month-old girl with a palpable abdominal mass. What do you see? What are the diagnostic considerations?

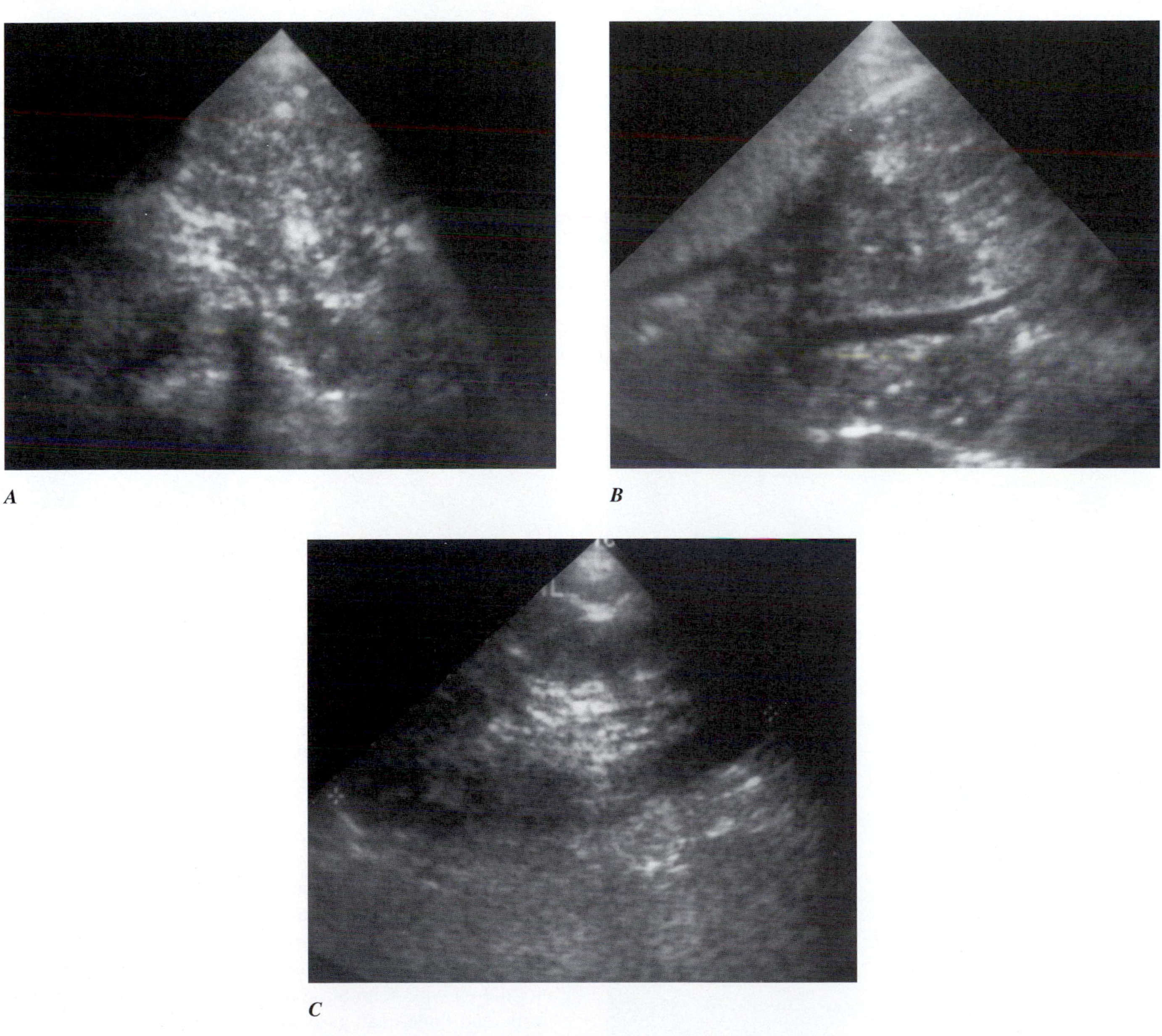

FIGURE 58–1. Transverse *(A)* and longitudinal *(B)* views through the right suprarenal region. Longitudinal view through the right kidney *(C)*.

CHAPTER 58

Neuroblastoma

CARLOS J. SIVIT

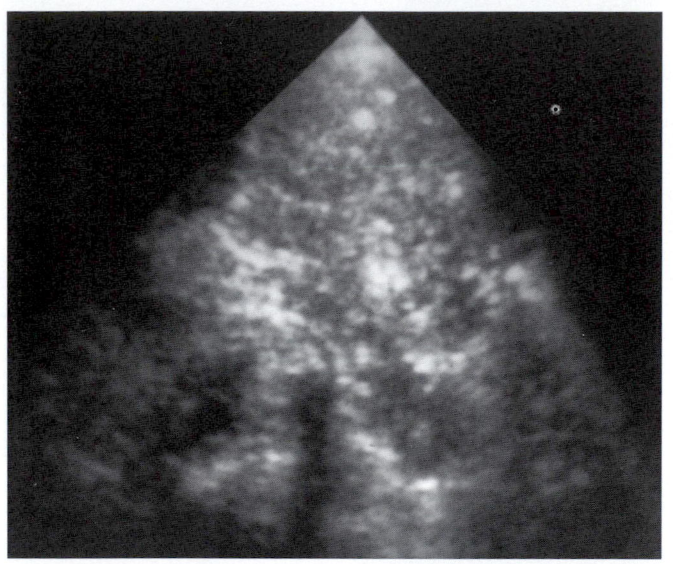

A

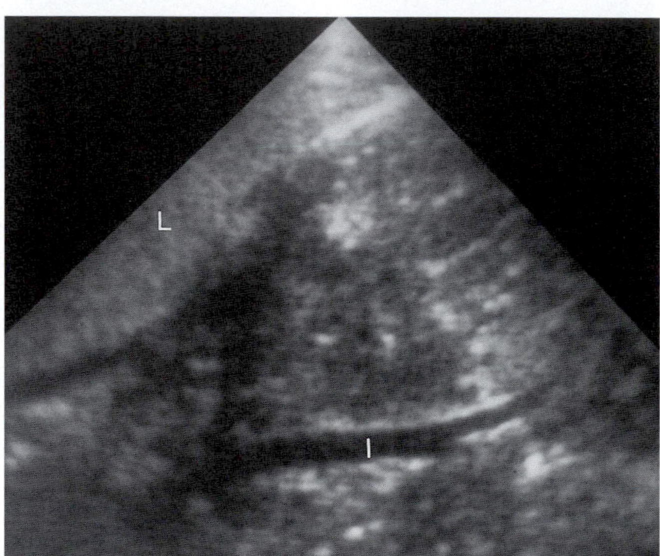

B

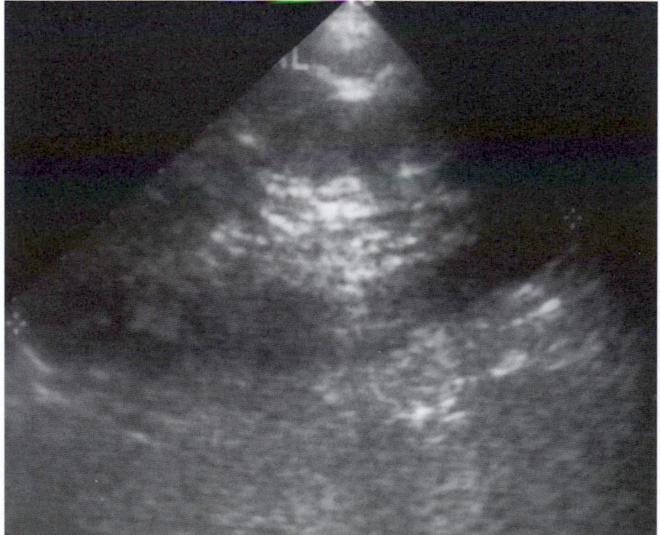

C

FIGURE 58–2. Neuroblastoma. Transverse *(A)* and longitudinal *(B)* views through the right suprarenal region demonstrate a large, solid, heterogeneous mass. Note the punctate hyperechoic regions, which probably represent calcifications. Longitudinal view through the right kidney *(C)* demonstrates a normal appearance, indicating that this mass is of adrenal origin. L = liver, I = inferior vena cava.

Neuroblastoma is the most common extracranial solid malignant tumor and the third most common malignancy in children, surpassed in incidence only by leukemia and primary brain tumors. Neuroblastoma accounts for 10 percent of all pediatric neoplasms and approximately 15 percent of all deaths due to neoplasms in children. Approximately one-half of children with neuroblastoma present prior to the age of 2 years, and three-quarters prior to the age of 4 years. Long-term survival for most children with neuroblastoma remains elusive. Children presenting under the age of 1 year generally have a good prognosis, while those presenting above the age

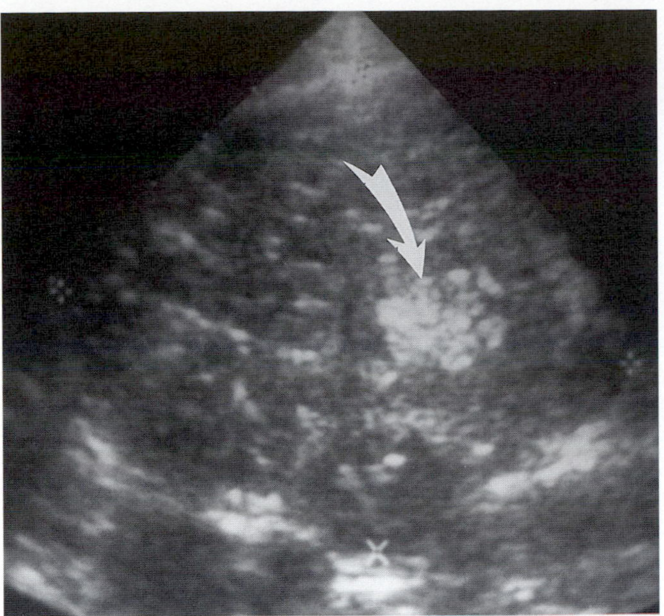

FIGURE 58–3. Neuroblastoma with hyperechoic region. Longitudinal view through the right suprarenal region demonstrates a large, solid, heterogeneous mass (*between electronic calipers*). Note the rounded echogenic region (*arrow*), which probably represents calcification or hemorrhage.

of 1 year present with metastatic disease and have an extremely poor prognosis. There is increasing evidence that complete surgical resection of the primary tumor improves long-term survival.

Neuroblastoma and its more differentiated forms, ganglioneuroblastoma and ganglioneuroma, arise from primitive sympathetic neuroblasts of the embryonic neural crest. The three neural crest tumors are differentiated by the degree of cellular maturation. Neuroblastoma is the most common of the three. The majority of neuroblastomas are adrenal, but they may also originate from other organs derived from neural crest cells, such as the sympathetic paraspinal, mesenteric, and perivesical ganglia. Microscopically, the tumor consists of small, round cells that are similar to those of lymphoma and Ewing's sarcoma.

Abdominal neuroblastoma presents most frequently as a palpable abdominal mass. It may also present with signs and symptoms due to metastatic disease and paraneoplastic syndromes, including myoclonus, opsoclonus, and intractable watery diarrhea associated with hypokalemia. Other nonspecific signs and symptoms associated with neuroblastoma include fever, weight loss, hypertension, and anemia. Approximately two-thirds of children with neuroblastoma have metastatic disease at the time of presentation. Common sites of metastatic involvement include bone, bone marrow, liver, and lymph nodes.

Sonography is often the initial imaging modality performed in children with neuroblastoma. A normal examination is useful in excluding an abdominal mass lesion. Approximately two-thirds of abdominal neuroblastomas arise from the adrenal gland. Therefore, the most frequent sonographic appearance is that of a solid, suprarenal mass (Fig. 58-2). It is typically heterogeneous in echotexture, with areas that are hyperechoic relative to normal hepatic and renal parenchyma intermixed with hypoechoic areas (Fig. 58-3). The more echogenic areas may represent hemorrhage or calcification. Calcifications are noted in approximately two-thirds of these tumors. Cystic areas representing tumor necrosis may also be noted (Fig. 58-4). Neuroblastoma is an infiltrating neoplasm; therefore, the tumor margins are usually poorly defined. Metastatic involvement of hepatic

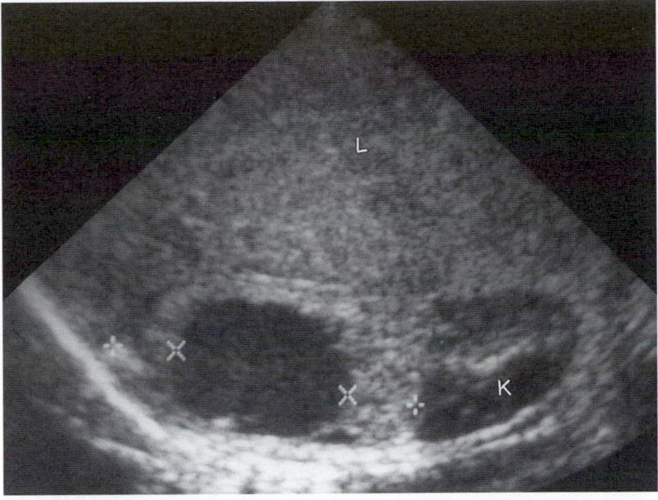

A

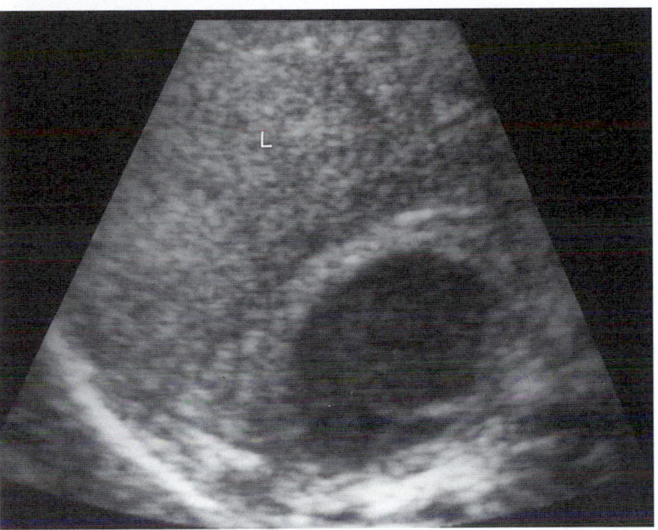

B

FIGURE 58–4. Neuroblastoma with anechoic region. Transverse ***(A)*** and longitudinal ***(B)*** views through the right upper abdomen demonstrate a right adrenal mass with a central anechoic region that probably represents liquefaction necrosis. L = liver, K = right kidney.

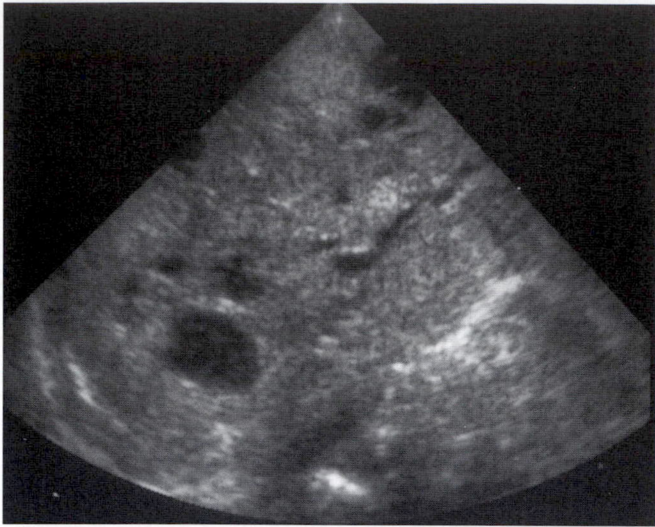

FIGURE 58–5. Neuroblastoma with hepatic metastases. Longitudinal view through the liver in an infant with stage IV-S neuroblastoma show multiple hypoechoic lesions, representing multiple hepatic parenchymal metastases. R = right kidney.

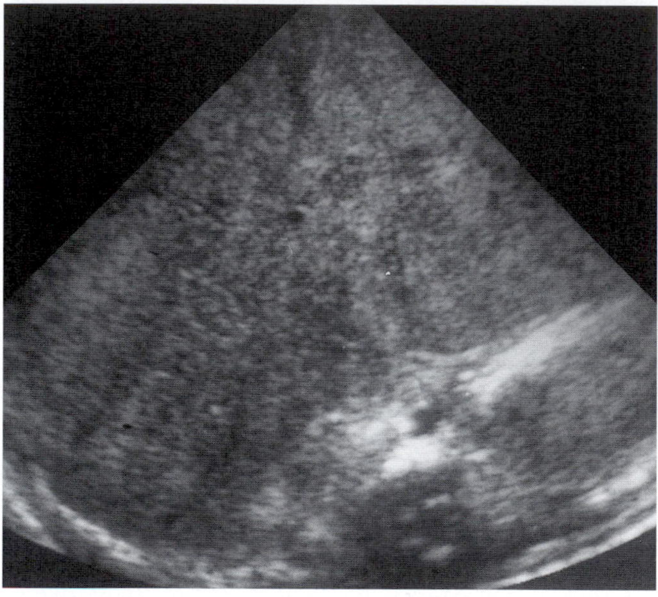

FIGURE 58–6. Neuroblastoma with hepatic metastases. Transverse view through the liver in an infant with stage IV-S neuroblastoma demonstrates a diffusely heterogeneous hepatic parenchymal appearance.

parenchyma will appear as discrete hypoechoic lesions (Fig. 58-5) or as heterogeneity of the parenchyma (Fig. 58-6).

Cross-sectional imaging with computed tomography (CT) or magnetic resonance imaging (MRI) is the primary means of evaluating and staging neuroblastoma and determining surgical resectability. This is very important, as complete resection of the primary tumor improves survival. The tumor is poorly encapsulated and infiltrative. Thus, it has a tendency to encase retroperitoneal blood vessels and infiltrate through the spinal foramina into the extradural space of the spinal canal (Fig. 58-7); MRI is superior to CT in the evaluation of extension into the spinal canal. Stage I neuroblastoma is confined to the organ of origin. In stage II, there is local tumor extension that does not cross the midline, while in stage III tumors there is extension across the midline or the presence of contralateral lymph node involvement. Stage IV neuroblastoma is disseminated to the liver, bone, bone marrow, and central nervous system. Stage IV-S refers to localized (stage I or II) tumor with dissemination limited to liver, skin, or bone marrow. It is primarily noted in very young children (<1 year) and has a good prognosis (similar to that for stage I or II).

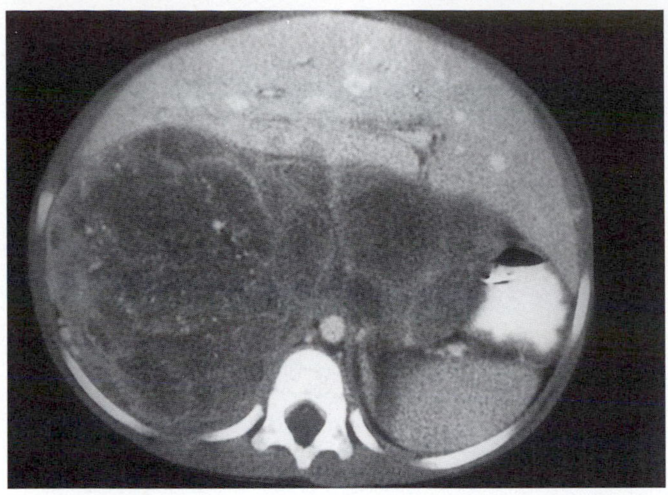

A

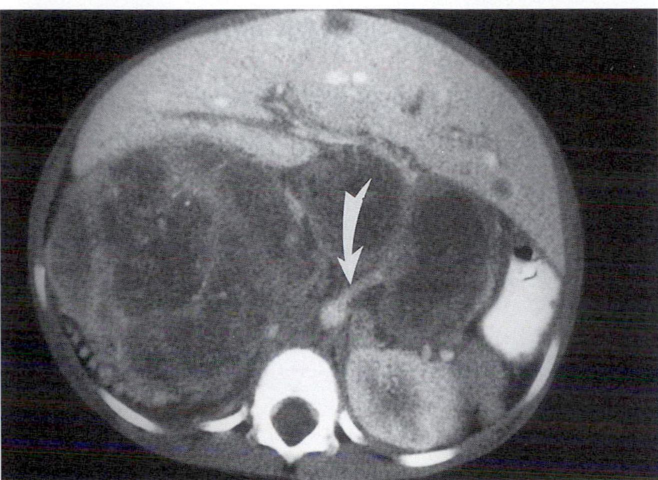

B

FIGURE 58–7. Infiltrative neuroblastoma. ***A.*** Contrast-enhanced computed tomography (CT) scan through the upper abdomen demonstrates a large, solid mass that crosses the midline and contains multiple punctate areas of calcification. ***B.*** Image on CT 2 cm below ***A*** shows the mass completely encircling the celiac axis (*arrow*). ***C.*** Image on CT 2 cm below ***B*** shows the mass encasing the left renal vein (*arrow*).

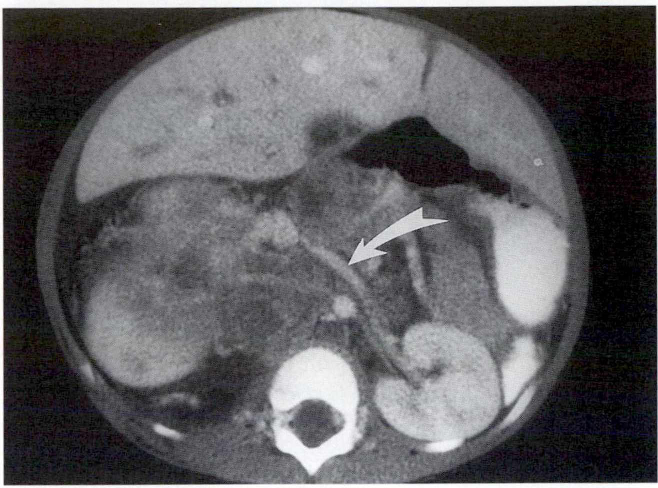

C

References

Amundson GM, Trevenen CL, Mueller DL, et al: Neuroblastoma: A specific sonographic tissue pattern. *AJR* 148:943–945, 1987.

Atkinson GO, Zaatari GS, Lorenzo RL, et al: Cystic neuroblastoma in infants: Radiographic and pathologic features. *AJR* 146: 113–117, 1986.

Bousvaros A, Kirks DR, Grossman H: Imaging of neuroblastoma: An overview. *Pediatr Radiol* 16:89–106, 1986.

Daneman A: Adrenal neoplasms in children. *Semin Roentgenol* 23:205–215, 1988.

David R, Lamki N, Fan S, et al: The many faces of neuroblastoma. *Radiographics* 9:859–882, 1989.

Foglia R, Fonkalstrud E, Feig S, et al: Accuracy of diagnostic imaging as determined by delayed operative intervention for advanced neuroblastoma. *J Pediatr Surg* 24:708–711, 1989.

Kornreich G, Horev C, Kapinsky N, et al: Neuroblastoma: Evaluation with contrast enhanced MR imaging. *Pediatr Radiol* 21:566–569, 1991.

Lowe RE, Cohen MD: Computed tomographic evaluation of Wilms tumor and neuroblastoma. *Radiographics* 4:915–928, 1984.

Westra SJ, Zaninovic AC, Hall TR, et al: Imaging of the adrenal gland in children. *Radiographics* 14:1323–1340, 1994.

59

Figure 59-1 shows a 2-year-old girl with virilization. What do you see? What are the diagnostic considerations?

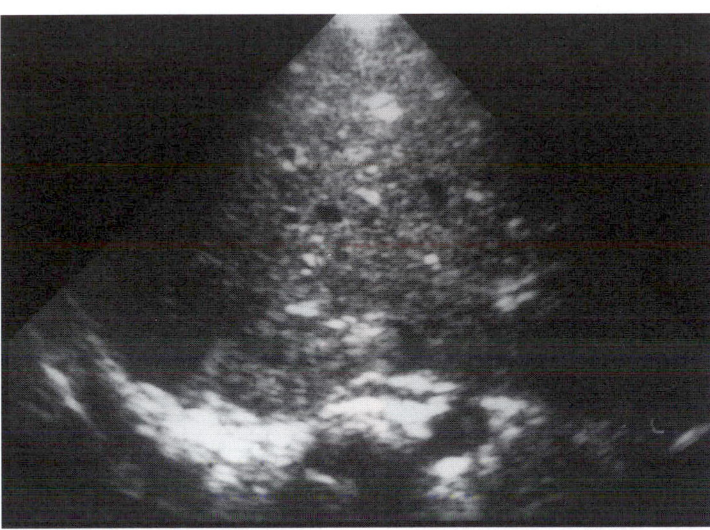

A

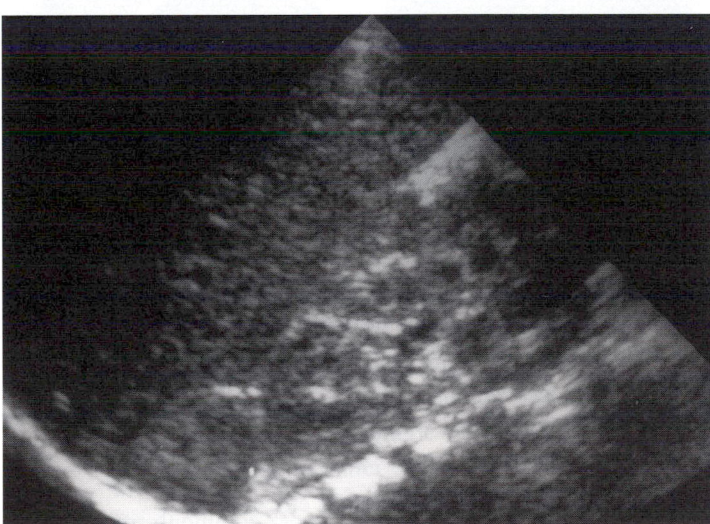

B

FIGURE 59–1. Transverse *(A)* and longitudinal *(B)* views through the right suprarenal region.

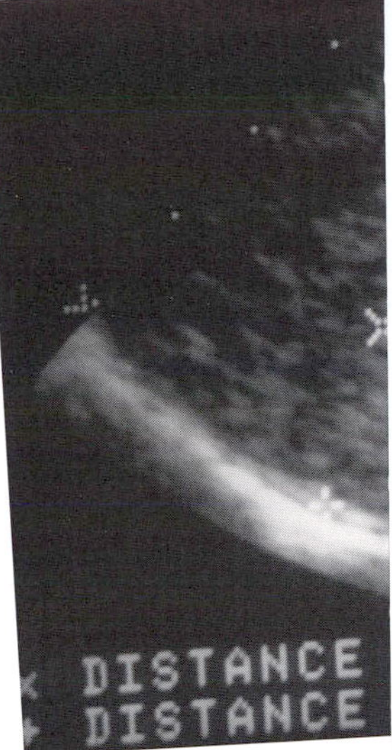

FIGURE 59–3. Small
view through the right su
syndrome demonstrates a
(between electronic calipe
carcinoma at surgery. Nc
2 cm in maximum diamet

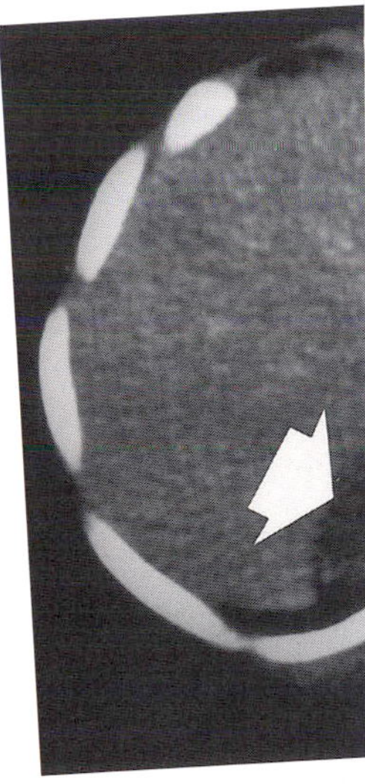

FIGURE 59–5. Ad
computed tomography
child as in Fig. 59-1 d
right adrenal mass (*str*
into the inferior vena c

In adults, adren
than adrenocortica
number adenomas
are rare in childho
adrenocortical car
hormonally active
carcinomas are t
there is overlap in

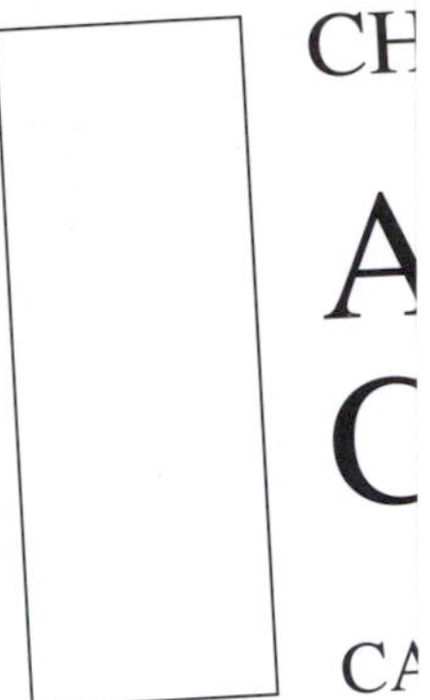

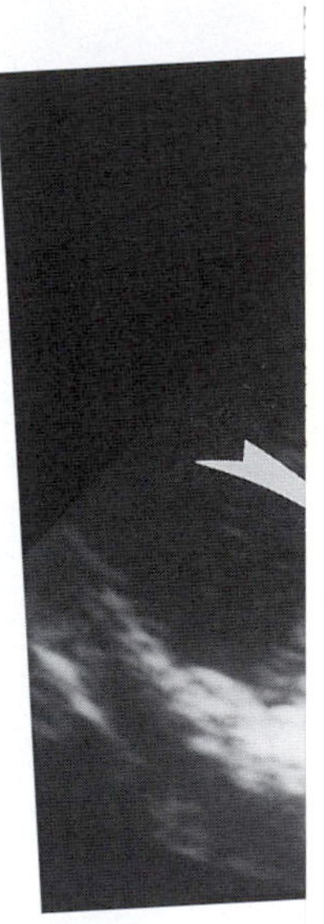

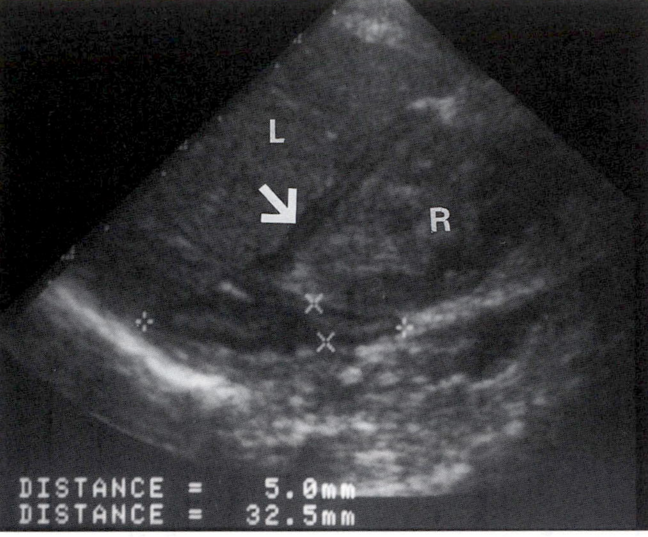

FIGURE 61–7. Enlarged adrenal gland associated with congenital adrenal hyperplasia. Long-axis view through the right adrenal gland demonstrates an enlargement in adrenal length and width. Note the electronic calipers measuring the length and width of the posterior right adrenal limb. The anterior right adrenal limb is also visualized (*arrow*). R = right kidney, L = liver.

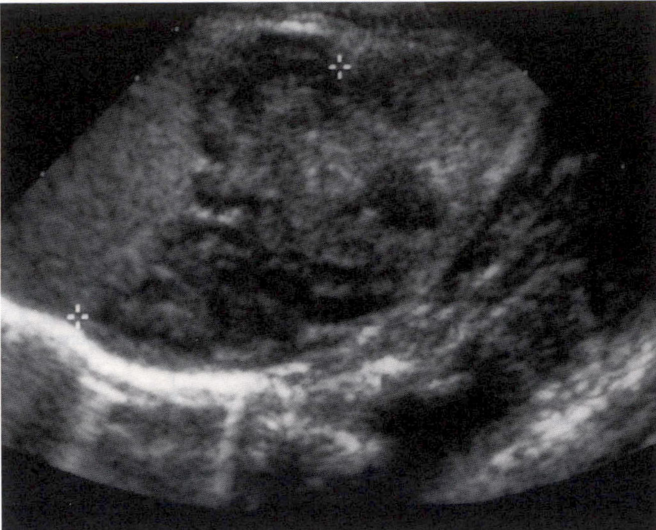

FIGURE 61–8. Cerebriform appearance of enlarged adrenal gland in an infant with congenital adrenal hyperplasia. Longitudinal image through the left suprarenal region shows an enlarged left adrenal with a wavy, cerebriform appearance. The electronic calipers denote the superior and inferior margins of the anterior adrenal limb.

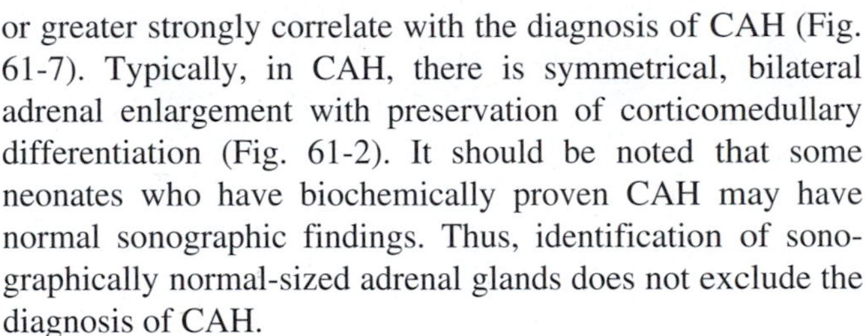

or greater strongly correlate with the diagnosis of CAH (Fig. 61-7). Typically, in CAH, there is symmetrical, bilateral adrenal enlargement with preservation of corticomedullary differentiation (Fig. 61-2). It should be noted that some neonates who have biochemically proven CAH may have normal sonographic findings. Thus, identification of sonographically normal-sized adrenal glands does not exclude the diagnosis of CAH.

Adrenal enlargement associated with CAH may demonstrate a cerebriform pattern, which has been reported as being specific to this disease even if the adrenal glands do not appear enlarged. The cerebriform pattern consists of a wrinkled surface that evokes some similarities to brain gyri, in contrast to the normal straight or slightly convex surface of the adrenal glands (Fig. 61-8).

Adrenal enlargement associated with CAH has characteristics that permit differentiation of CAH from other neonatal adrenal conditions. Adrenal hemorrhage is characterized by a different clinical presentation and, on sonography, enlargement of the adrenal gland that is asymmetric and masslike, with associated loss of the normal corticomedullary differentiation. Rare adrenal tumors also would result in unilateral or asymmetric adrenal enlargement, with loss of the normal adrenal architecture.

References

Avni EF, Rypens F, Smet MH, et al: Sonographic demonstration of congenital adrenal hyperplasia in the neonate: The cerebriform pattern. *Pediatr Radiol* 23:88–90, 1993.

Bryan PJ, Caldamone AA, Morrison SC, et al: Ultrasound findings in the adreno-genital syndrome. *J Ultrasound Med* 7:675–679, 1988.

Ghiacy S, Dubbins PA, Baumer H: Ultrasound demonstration of congenital adrenal hyperplasia. *JCU* 13:419–420, 1985.

Hauffa BP, Menzel D, Stolecke H: Age related changes in adrenal size during the 1st years of life in normal newborns, infants and patients with CAH due to 21-hydroxylase deficiency: Comparison of US and hormonal parameters. *Eur J Pediatr* 148:43–49, 1988.

Oppenheimer DA, Carroll BA, Yousem S: Sonography of the normal neonatal adrenal gland. *Radiology* 146:157–160, 1983.

Scott EM, Thomas A, McGarrigle HG, et al: Serial adrenal ultrasonography in normal neonates. *J Ultrasound Med* 9:279–283, 1990.

Sivit CJ, Hung W, Taylor GA, et al: Sonography in neonatal congenital adrenal hyperplasia. *AJR* 156:141–143, 1991.

Section F
URINARY TRACT

62

Figure 62-1 shows a 1-year-old girl with a history of prior urinary tract infection. What do you see? What are the diagnostic considerations?

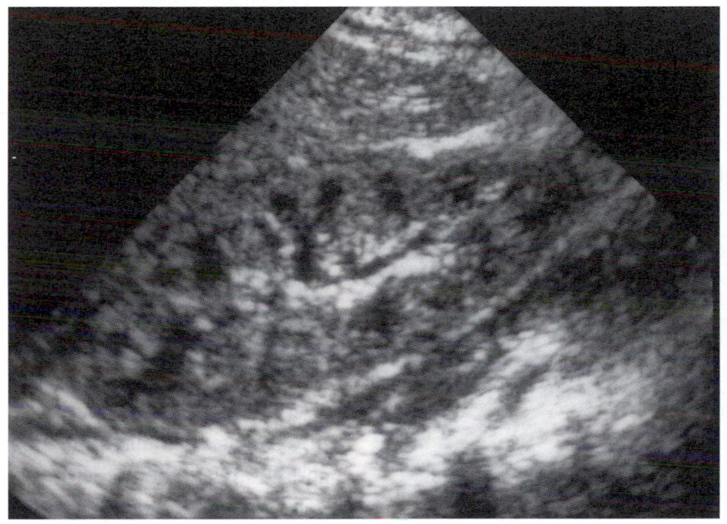

A

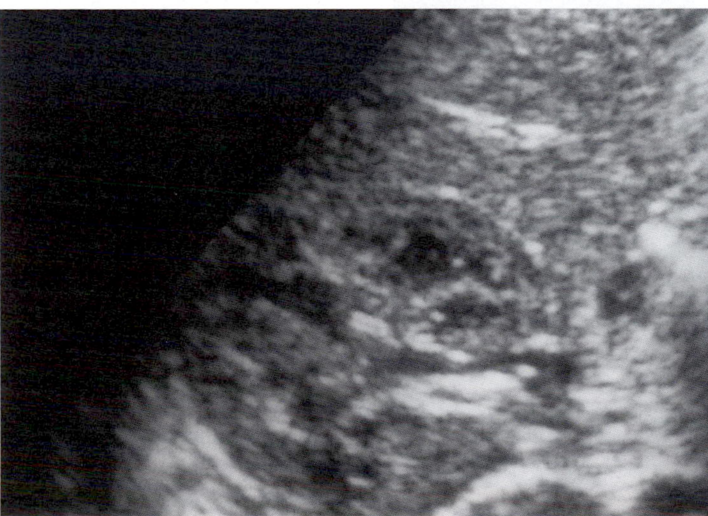

B

FIGURE 62–1. Longitudinal *(A)* and transverse *(B)* views through the right kidney.

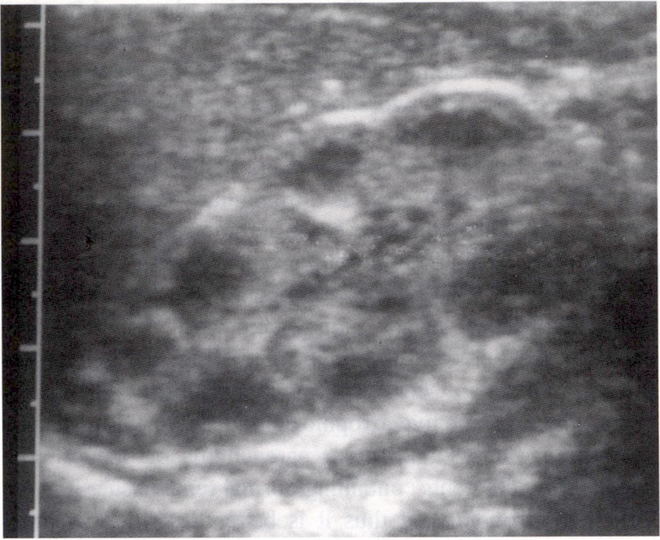

FIGURE 62–7. Neonatal kidney. Longitudinal view through the right kidney in a 2-day-old infant demonstrate a renal cortex that is slightly hyperechoic to the liver. Also note the large, well-defined, hypoechoic renal pyramids and the paucity of renal sinus fat.

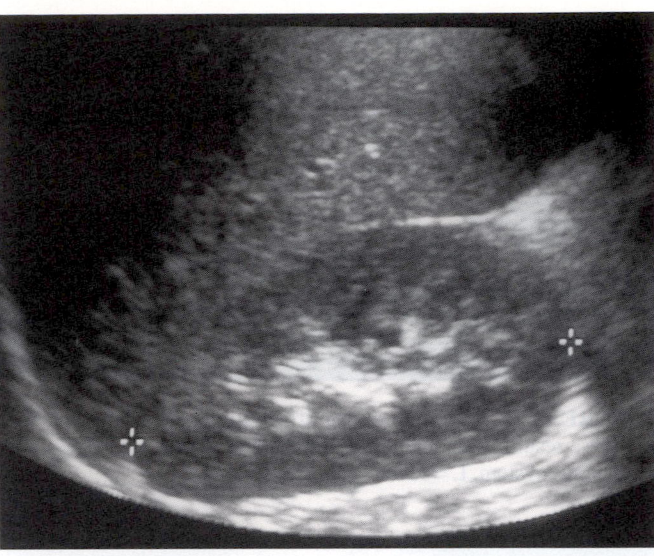

FIGURE 62–8. Normal kidney in older child, demonstrating increased renal sinus fat. Longitudinal view through a normal right kidney in a 6-year-old child demonstrates increased echogenicity centrally relative to Figs. 62-1 and 62-5, indicative of increased renal sinus fat.

junctional parenchyma on the basis of (1) location at the site of metanephric element fusion, (2) being bordered by a junctional parenchymal defect, and (3) the presence of renal cortex that is continuous with adjacent cortex.

There are several important differences between the sonographic appearance of the normal kidney in neonates and that in older children and adults. One difference in the appearance of the neonatal kidney involves the echogenicity of the renal cortex (Fig. 62-7). The normal neonatal renal cortex is more echogenic than the renal cortex in older children and adults. The neonatal renal cortex is often isoechoic and occasionally hyperechoic (in premature infants) relative to the liver and spleen (Fig. 62-7). This has been attributed to several factors, including (1) a greater proportion of glomeruli in the cortex, (2) a greater cellular component of the glomeruli, and (3) a greater proportion of the loops of Henle being in the cortex. These factors result in a greater number of acoustical interfaces in the renal cortex, thus increasing the echogenicity. This neonatal cortical pattern persists until approximately 2 to 4 months of age. A second difference in the appearance of the neonatal kidney involves the medullary pyramids. The normal neonatal renal pyramids are larger, better defined, and more hypoechoic than those in older children and adults, with accentuation of the corticomedullary junction (Fig. 62-7). Thus, they may be confused with a dilated collecting system or renal cysts. The renal pyramids remain prominent through the first few years of life. A third difference in the appearance of the neonatal kidney is that the renal sinus contains a paucity of fat, and therefore it is not as echogenic as in older children or adults. There is a gradual increase in the amount of renal sinus fat through adolescence (Fig. 62-8).

References

Gross GW, Thornburg AJ, Bellinger MF: Normal renal growth in children with myelodysplasia. *AJR* 146:615–617, 1986.

Haller JO, Berdon WE, Friedman AP: Increased renal cortical echogenicity: A normal finding in neonates and infants. *Radiology* 142:173–174, 1982.

Han BK, Babcock DS: Sonographic measurement and appearance of normal kidneys in children. *AJR* 145:611–616, 1985.

Hayden CK, Santa-Cruz FR, Amparo EG, et al: Ultrasonographic evaluation of renal parenchyma in infancy and childhood. *Radiology* 152:413–417, 1984.

Hricak H, Slovis TL, Callen CW, et al: Neonatal kidneys: Sonographic anatomic correlation. *Radiology* 147:699–702, 1983.

Rosenbaum DM, Korngold E, Teele RL: Sonographic assessment of renal length in normal children. *AJR* 142:467–469, 1984.

Schlesinger AE, Hernandez RJ, Zerin JM, et al: Interobserver and intraobserver variations in sonographic renal length measurements in children. *AJR* 156:1029–1032, 1991.

Yeh H, Halton KP, Shapiro RS, et al: Junctional parenchyma: Revised definition of hypertrophied column of Bertin. *Radiology* 185:725–732, 1992.

Zerin JM, Blane CE: Sonographic assessment of renal length in children: A reappraisal. *Pediatr Radiol* 24:101–106, 1994.

63

Figure 63-1 shows a 3-week-old girl with a urinary tract infection. What do you see? What are the diagnostic considerations?

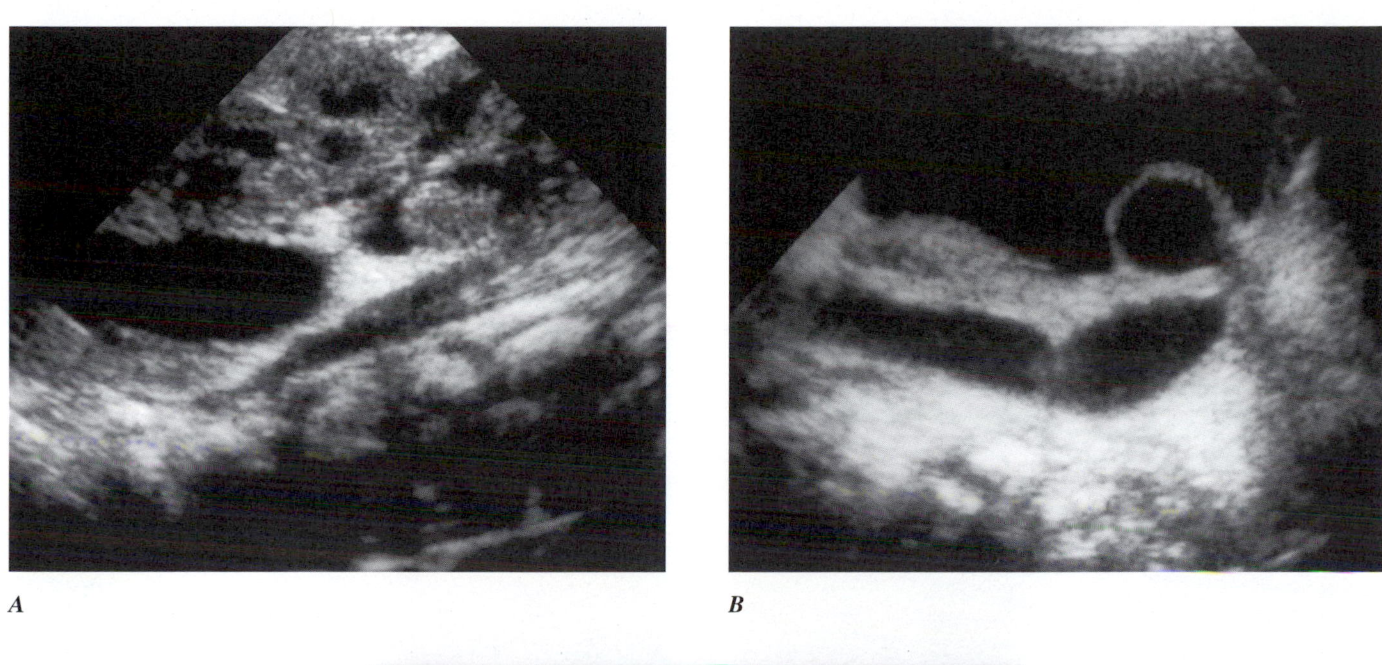

A *B*

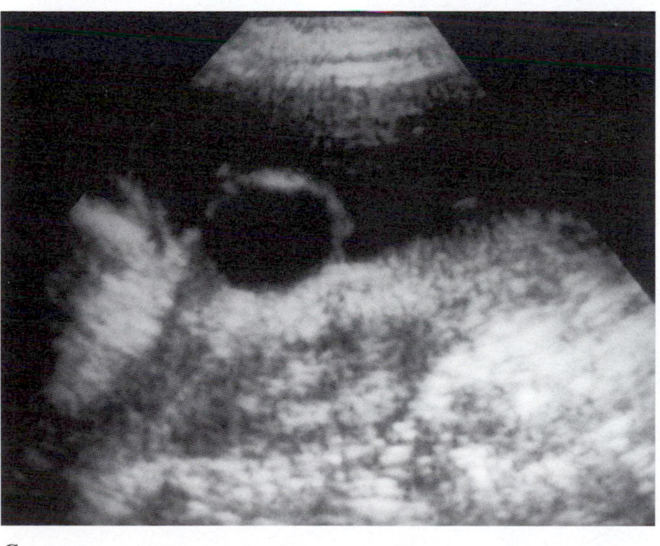

C

FIGURE 63–1. Longitudinal view through the right kidney *(A)*. Longitudinal *(B)*, and transverse *(C)* views through the bladder.

CHAPTER 63

Ureterocele

CARLOS J. SIVIT

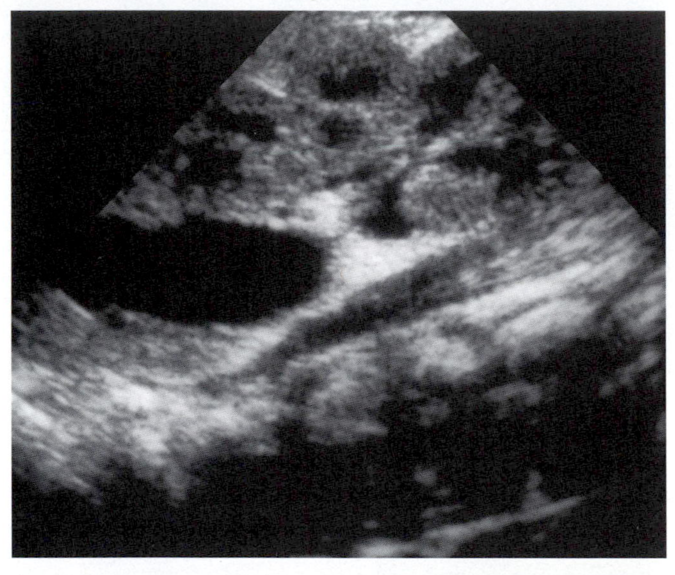

A

B

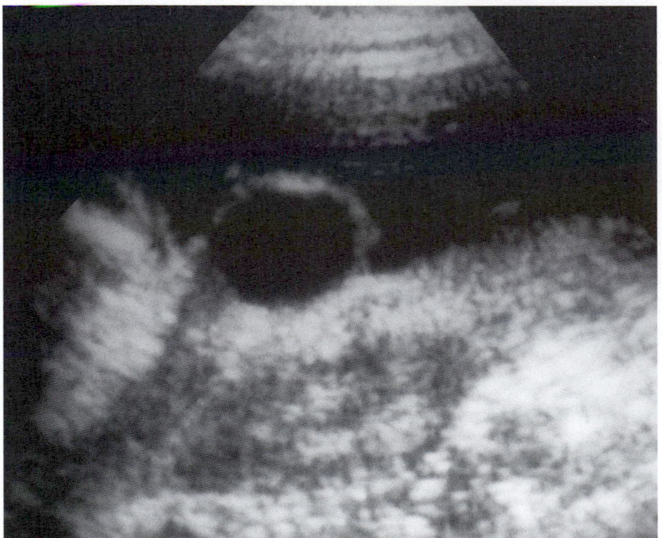

C

FIGURE 63–2. Ureterocele associated with a duplex ureter. ***A.*** Longitudinal view through the right kidney demonstrates a duplex collecting system with dilatation of the upper-pole moiety. ***B.*** Longitudinal view through the bladder demonstrates dilatation of a right distal ureter and an oval-shaped, anechoic lesion with a thin echogenic rim within the bladder, indicative of a ureterocele. Transverse ***(C)*** views through the bladder also demonstrate the ureterocele.

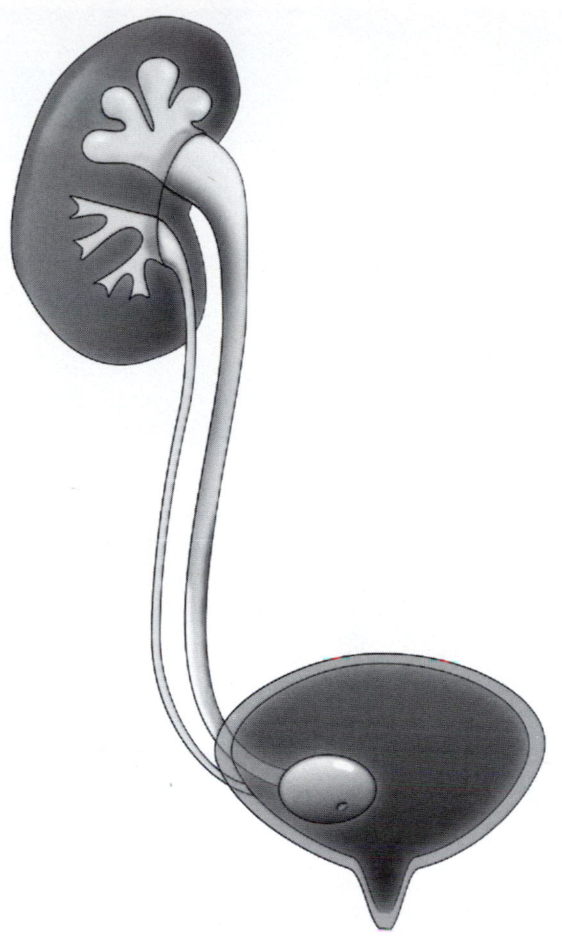

FIGURE 63–3. Diagram of a duplex collecting system with a ureterocele involving the upper-pole ureter, which inserts into the bladder ectopically, medial and inferior to the orifice of the lower-pole ureter.

A ureterocele represents a cystic dilatation of the intravesical segment of the distal ureter (Fig. 63-2). Ureteroceles vary greatly in size. Several theories have been proposed regarding their etiology. These include (1) ureteral meatal obstruction, (2) incomplete muscularization of the distal ureter, and (3) excessive dilatation of the distal ureter as it is absorbed into the bladder. A ureterocele may be associated with either a single ureter or a duplex ureter. Ureteroceles associated with a duplex ureter are far more common than single-ureter ureteroceles. Ureteroceles associated with a single ureter usually arise from a normally positioned ureteral orifice near the bladder trigone. They are occasionally associated with obstruction of the involved ureter. In ureteroceles associated with a duplex ureter, the ureterocele typically involves the ureter draining the upper renal pole. The ureteral orifice of the upper-pole moiety in a duplex collecting system will lie medial and inferior to the orifice of the lower-pole ureter (Fig. 63-3). This is referred to as the Weigert-Meyer rule. Ectopic ureteroceles are more common in females than in males. There is often ureteral obstruction associated with a ureterocele related to a duplex ureter. Additionally, there is often scarring, with diminished renal function and varying degrees of dysplasia involving the upper-pole renal moiety drained by the ectopic ureter. The ureter draining the lower renal pole often demonstrates vesicoureteral reflux.

Most ureteroceles are detected during sonographic evaluation of the urinary tract following a urinary tract infection. Occasionally, if the ureterocele reaches a large size, it may be palpated as a pelvic mass. With the widespread utilization of prenatal sonographic screening, the presence of a ureterocele is often detected on prenatal sonography. It appears that this increased prenatal detection of ureterocele associated with a duplex ureter has allowed for the improved preservation of upper-pole renal moieties in these children through earlier diagnosis and urologic referral prior to deterioration of renal function.

Sonography is the principal imaging modality utilized in the assessment of a ureterocele. The typical sonographic appearance of a ureterocele is that of a rounded or oval-shaped anechoic lesion with a thin echogenic rim (Fig. 63-2). Visualization of the ureterocele is enhanced when the bladder is only partially filled. The increased intravesicular pressure that develops at large bladder volumes may result in effacement of the ureterocele. Simple ureteroceles, defined as ureteroceles arising from a normally positioned ureteral orifice, tend to be smaller than ectopic ureteroceles. The ureter and pelvicaliceal system above the simple ureterocele may be dilated or of normal caliber. Occasionally, simple ureteroceles in males may prolapse into the urethra and result in a bladder outlet obstruction. Typically, the ureter and pelvicaliceal system above a ureterocele associated with a duplex ureter are dilated (Fig. 63-2). A ureterocele associated with a duplex ureter may be large enough to obstruct the bladder outlet and both the ipsilateral and contralateral ureters (Fig. 63-4). The ipsilateral lower-pole ureter may also appear dilated on sonography in the absence of obstruction secondary to vesicoureteral reflux.

Ureteroceles are typically treated with endoscopic incision. The principal complication of surgical treatment is the development of secondary vesicoureteral reflux. On postoperative sonography, a variety of appearances may be noted within the bladder, including focal mucosal thickening (Fig. 63-5), a pseudomass (Fig. 63-6), a residual ureterocele decreased or unchanged in size (Fig. 63-7), or no residual abnormality. The postoperative sonographic appearance has not been found to correlate with long-term outcome.

The ureterocele may also be demonstrated through voiding cystourethrography. The ureterocele is best seen during early bladder filling with contrast material (Fig. 63-8). The increased intravesicular pressure that develops at large bladder volumes may result in effacement of the ureterocele. Rarely, the ureterocele can evert and simulate a bladder diverticulum. The voiding cystourethrogram may also show associated vesicoureteral reflux into the lower-pole ureter in children with a duplex-ureter ureterocele.

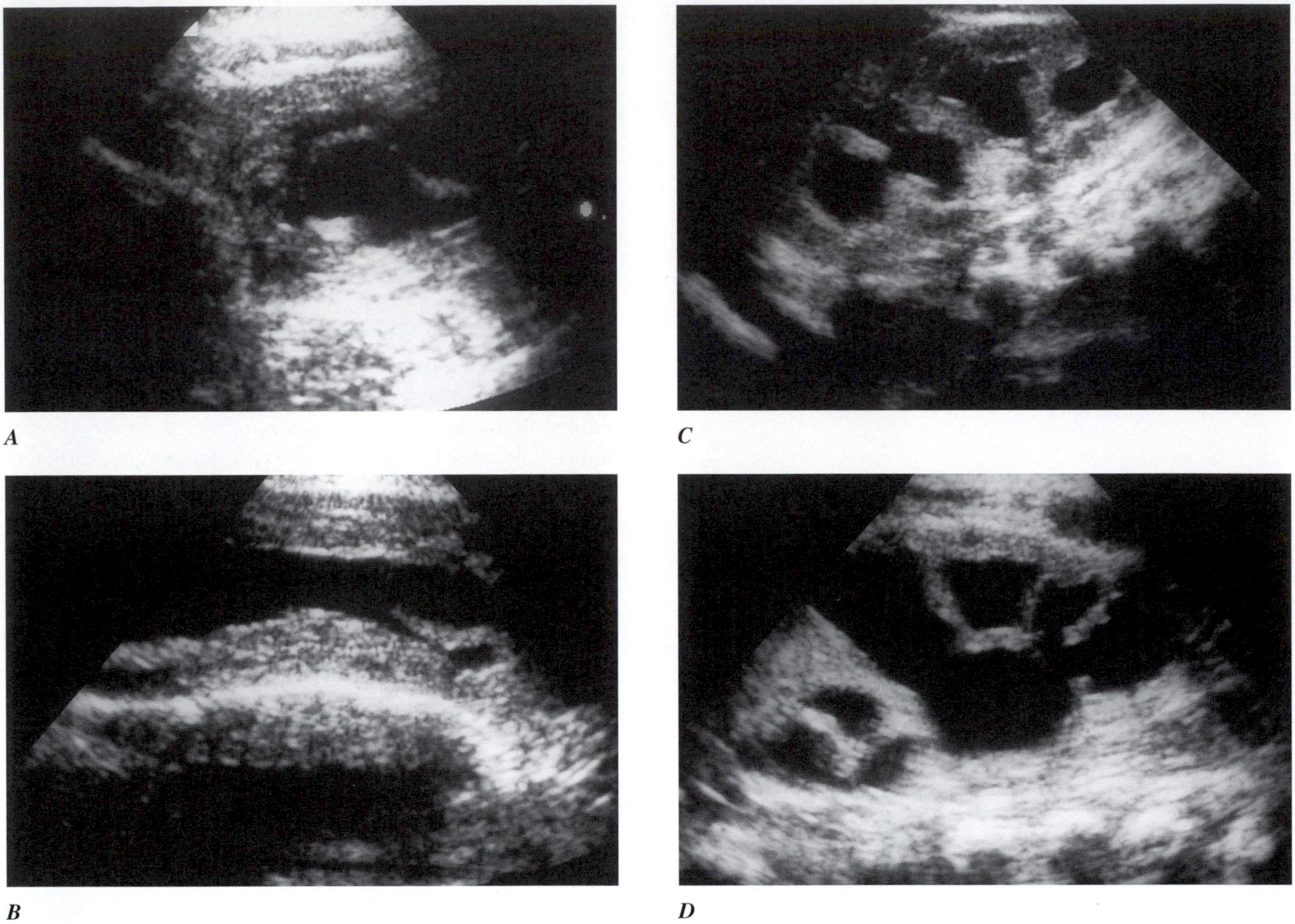

A *C*

B *D*

FIGURE 63–4. Large ureterocele resulting in bladder outlet obstruction and bilateral hydronephrosis. ***A.*** Transverse view through the base of the bladder demonstrates a large ureterocele. ***B.*** Longitudinal view through the bladder in the same child demonstrates bladder wall thickening secondary to bladder outlet obstruction. Longitudinal views through the right ***(C)*** and left ***(D)*** kidneys demonstrate bilateral hydronephrosis.

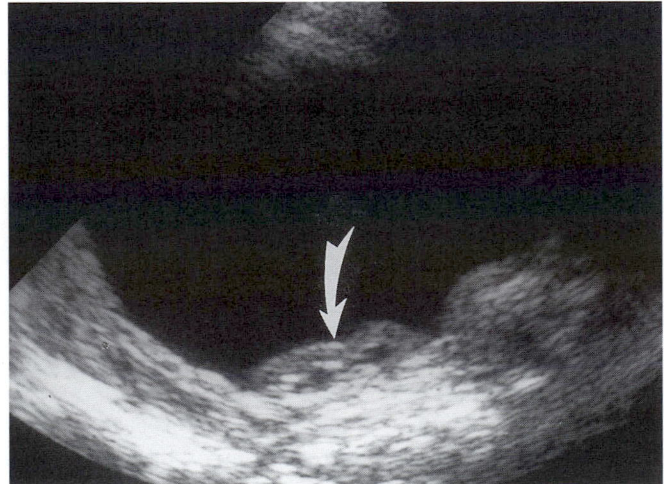

FIGURE 63–5. Ureterocele with focal mucosal thickening following endoscopic incision. Longitudinal view through the bladder in a child with prior endoscopic incision of a ureterocele demonstrates focal mucosal thickening (*arrow*).

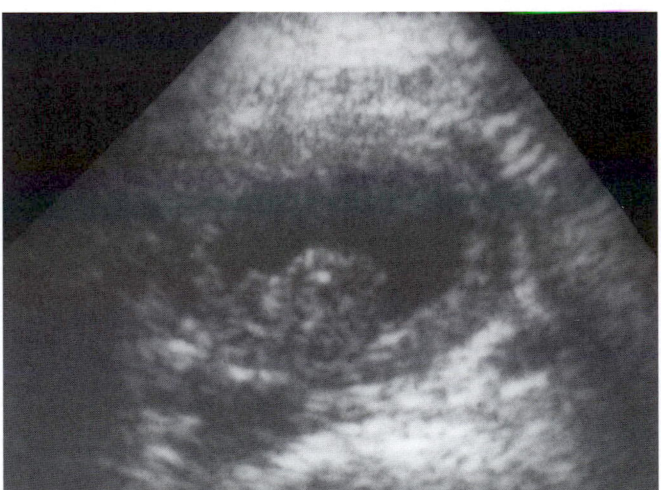

FIGURE 63–6. Ureterocele with a pseudomass appearance following endoscopic incision. Transverse view through the bladder in a child who had previously undergone endoscopic incision of a ureterocele shows a pseudomass at the right ureterovesical junction.

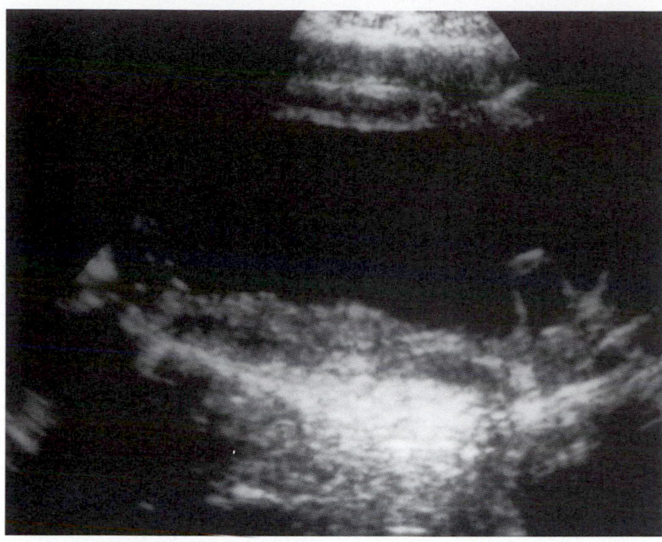

FIGURE 63–7. Ureterocele that decreased in size following endoscopic incision. In the same child as in Fig. 63-4, transverse view through the bladder following endoscopic ureterocele incision demonstrates a residual ureterocele that has decreased in size since the preoperative examination.

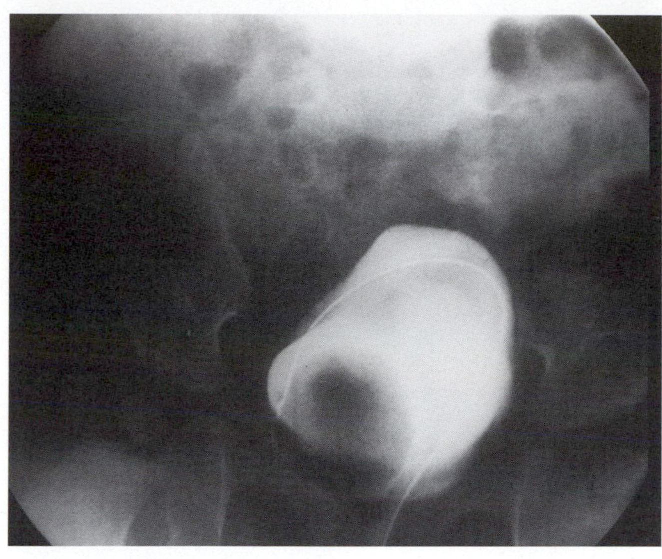

FIGURE 63–8. Ureterocele. Oblique spot radiograph from a voiding cystourethrogram demonstrates a large filling defect within the bladder, indicative of a ureterocele.

References

Abel C, Lendon M, Gough DC: Histology of the upper pole in complete urinary duplication—does it affect surgical management? *Br J Urol* 80:663–665, 1997.

Bellah RD, Long FR, Canning DA: Ureterocele eversion with vesicoureteral reflux in duplex kidneys: Findings at voiding cystourethrography. *AJR* 165:409–413, 1995.

Blane CE, Ritchey ML, DiPietro MA, et al: Single system ectopic ureters and ureteroceles associated with dysplastic kidney. *Pediatr Radiol* 22:217–220, 1992.

Fernbach SK, Feinstein KA: Abnormalities of the bladder in children: Imaging findings. *AJR* 162:1143–1150, 1994.

Fernbach SK, Feinstein KA, Spencer K, et al: Ureteral duplication and its complications. *Radiographics* 17:109–127, 1997.

Friedman AP, Haller JO, Schulze G, et al: Sonography of vesical and perivesical abnormalities in children. *J Ultrasound Med* 2:385–390, 1983.

Keesling CA, O'Hara SM, Chavez DR, et al: Sonographic appearance of the bladder after endoscopic incision of ureteroceles. *AJR* 170:759–763, 1998.

Nussbaum AR, Dorst JP, Jeffs RD, et al: Ectopic ureter and ureterocele: Their varied sonographic manifestations. *Radiology* 159: 227–235, 1986.

Rypens F, Avni EF, Bank WO, et al: The ureterovesical junction in children: Sonographic findings after surgical or endoscopic treatment. *AJR* 158:837–842, 1992.

Share JC, Lebowitz RL: Ectopic ureterocele without ureteral and calyceal dilatation (ureterocele disproportion): Findings on urography and sonography. *AJR* 152:567–571, 1989.

Van Savage JG, Mesrobian HG: The impact of prenatal sonography on the morbidity and outcome of patients with renal duplication anomalies. *J Urol* 153:768–770, 1995.

64

Figure 64-1 shows a newborn with palpable enlarged kidneys on physical examination. What do you see? What are the diagnostic possibilities?

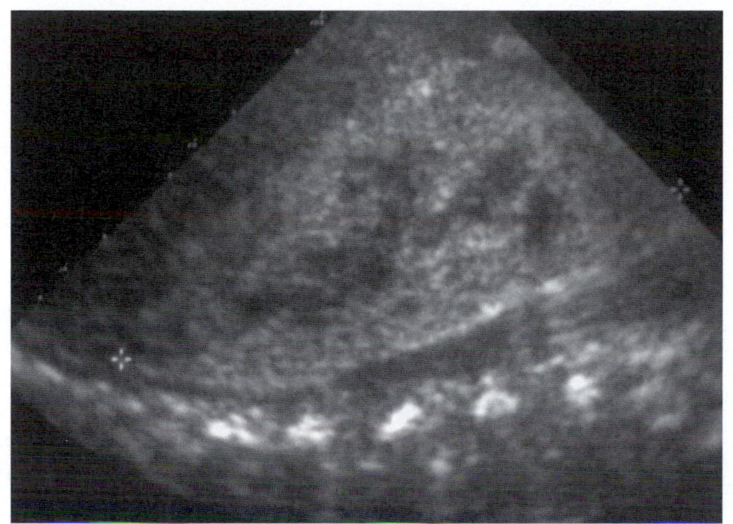

A

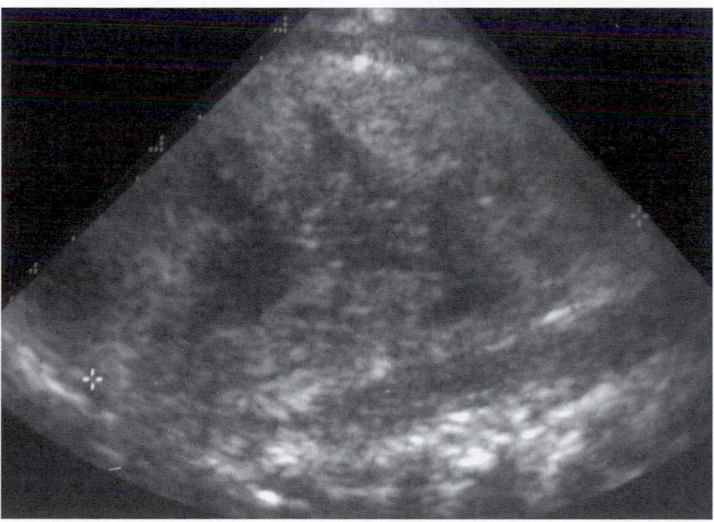

B

FIGURE 64–1. Longitudinal views through the right *(A)* and left *(B)* kidneys.

CHAPTER 64

Autosomal Recessive Polycystic Kidney Disease

STUART C. MORRISON

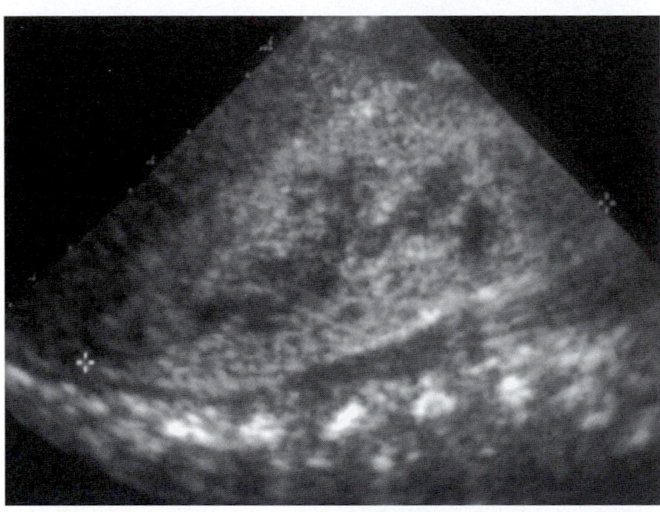

A

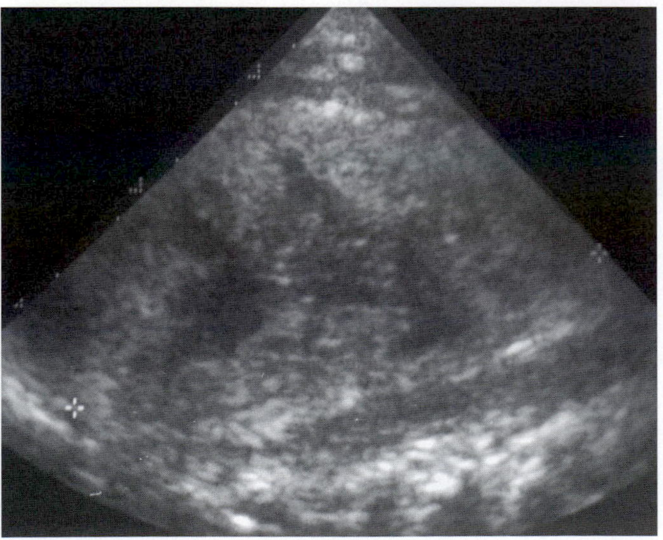

B

FIGURE 64–2. Autosomal recessive polycystic kidney disease. Longitudinal views through the right *(A)* and left *(B)* kidneys demonstrate bilateral renal enlargement. Note that the kidneys demonstrate increased parenchymal echogenicity, with loss of the normal corticomedullary differentiation. The normal reniform shape is maintained. There are no visible macrocysts.

Autosomal recessive polycystic kidney disease (ARPKD) is an inherited disorder characterized by nephromegaly, microscopic or macroscopic cystic dilatation of the renal collecting tubules, and periportal hepatic fibrosis. The renal abnormalities are seen early in life, while the liver pathology becomes predominant with increasing age. The age of initial clinical presentation is sometimes used as an artificial classification system, dividing the disease into perinatal, neonatal, infantile, and juvenile forms. However, there is much overlap between these four types, which represent different phenotypic manifestations of the same genetic abnormality. Histopathologic findings of ARPKD consist of cystic dilatation of the renal collecting tubules with the nephrons remaining normal. Cystic dilatation of the bile ducts and periportal hepatic fibrosis are also present. The remaining hepatic parenchyma remains normal.

Infants with ARPKD typically present with palpable renal masses or with renal insufficiency. They may also present with respiratory distress or with spontaneous pneumothorax due to associated pulmonary hypoplasia. The condition is being increasingly diagnosed in utero as a result of the widespread use of prenatal sonographic screening.

The characteristic sonographic appearance of ARPKD includes enlarged, hyperechoic kidneys bilaterally (Fig. 64-2). Renal enlargement is usually symmetrical in appearance. The cysts are typically too small to be visualized on sonography. However, the multiple interfaces associated with the cystic dilatation of the renal collecting ducts result in increased renal parenchymal echogenicity. The dilated collecting ducts

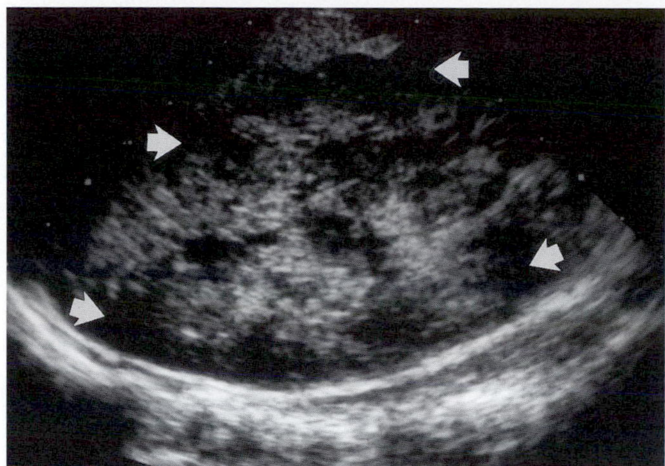

FIGURE 64–3. Autosomal recessive polycystic kidney disease (ARPKD). Longitudinal view through the right kidney in an infant with ARPKD demonstrates renal enlargement and loss of the normal corticomedullary differentiation. Note the sonolucent rim around the periphery of the kidney (*white arrows*), which is characteristic of the condition.

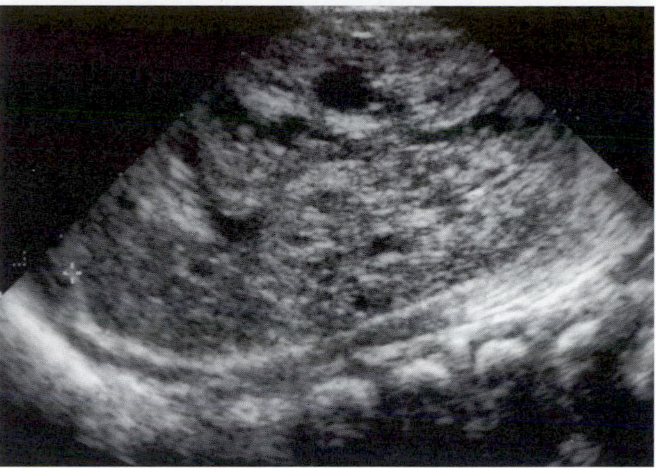

FIGURE 64–4. Autosomal recessive polycystic kidney disease (ARPKD) with associated macrocysts. Longitudinal view through the right kidney in a 5-year-old boy with ARPKD demonstrates renal enlargement and poor corticomedullary differentiation. Note that there are multiple scattered macrocysts throughout the kidney.

extend from the cortex through the medulla, so that the normal sharp distinction between echogenic renal cortex and sonolucent pyramids is lost. Therefore, the kidneys demonstrate poor corticomedullary differentiation. A peripheral sonolucent rim may be present (Fig. 64-3) and is considered by some to be pathognomonic for the disorder. The etiology of this finding is poorly understood. The sonolucent rim may be due to compressed normal renal cortex without cysts, or it may represent thin-walled, fluid-filled cystic spaces resulting from severe tubular dilatation. The radial array of the ectatic tubules may be visible in the renal medulla with the use of a high-frequency transducer. Occasionally, renal macrocysts are identified on sonography in infants and children with ARPKD. The cysts are typically small, usually 2 to 3 mm in maximum diameter (Fig. 64-4). Rarely, larger cysts, which may be several centimeters in diameter, may be identified. The cysts may occur in both the cortex and the medulla. Calcifications may develop in older children with ARPKD. This is felt to result either from urine stagnation in the dilated collecting tubules, resulting in precipitation of stone material, or from decreased excretion of urinary citrate. Most surviving children with this disorder demonstrate a decrease in renal size and echotexture over time. The renal size may be normal for age in surviving older children with ARPKD.

The liver typically appears normal on sonography in infants and young children with ARPKD. In older children with the disease, cystic dilatation of the bile ducts may be noted (Fig. 64-5). The bile ducts, although dilated, are not

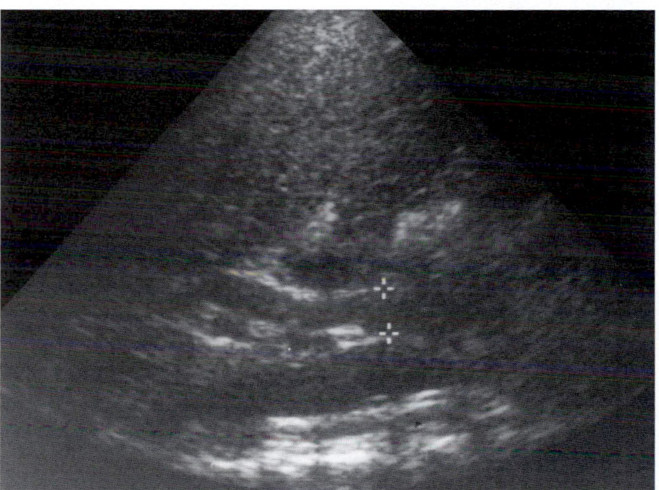

A

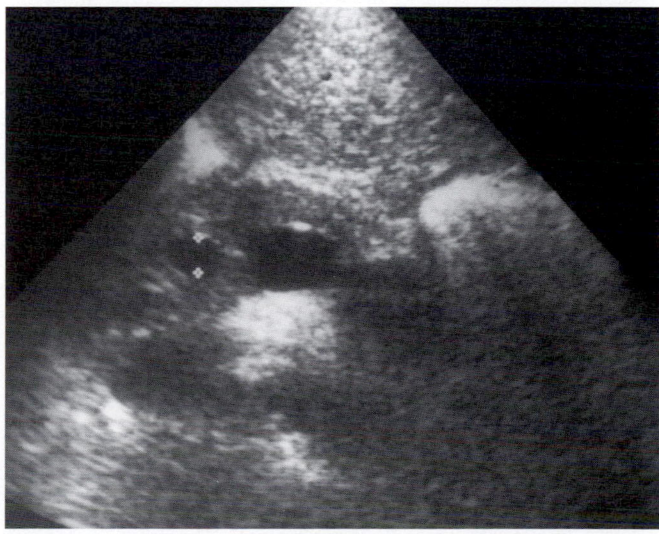

B

FIGURE 64–5. Common bile duct dilatation associated with hepatic fibrosis and autosomal recessive polycystic kidney disease (ARPKD). ***A.*** Longitudinal view through the porta hepatis in a 14-year-old boy with ARPKD demonstrates marked dilatation of the common bile duct (*between the calipers*). ***B.*** Transverse view through the head of the pancreas in the same child shows dilatation of the distal common bile duct (*between the calipers*).

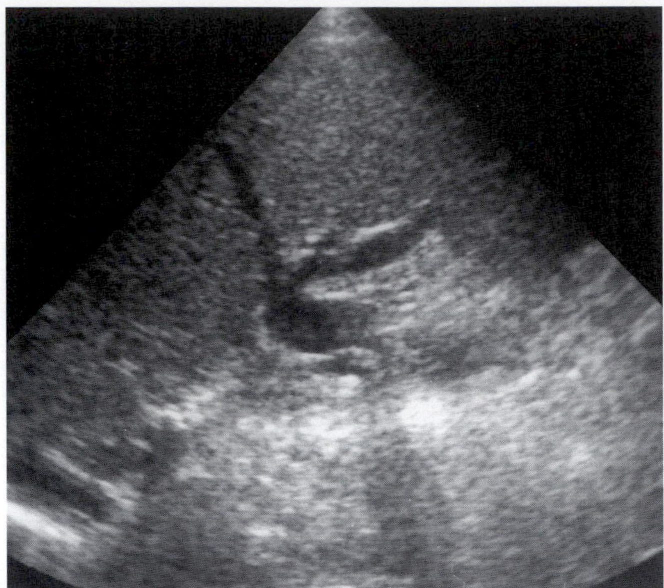

FIGURE 64–6. Splenomegaly associated with hepatic fibrosis and autosomal recessive polycystic kidney disease. Longitudinal view through the spleen in the same child as in Fig. 64-5 shows an enlarged spleen.

obstructed. This condition has some overlap with Caroli's disease. There may be associated bulbar protrusion of the bile duct wall into the portal vein, a finding referred to as the central dot sign. Additionally, sonographic findings associated with portal hypertension, including portosystemic collaterals, reversal of portal venous flow, and splenomegaly, may be noted (Fig. 64-6).

The diagnosis of ARPKD is often initially made in utero. Findings on fetal sonography include symmetrical, bilateral renal enlargement (Fig. 64-7). The fetal kidneys may not appear enlarged until the third trimester. The fetal kidneys also demonstrate increased echogenicity. The renal surface usually remains smooth, and the kidneys typically maintain a normal reniform shape. The urinary bladder is usually small. Oligohydramnios is a frequent associated finding, resulting from decreased fetal urine production.

The differential diagnosis of enlarged echogenic kidneys that may contain cysts in infants and young children also includes autosomal dominant polycystic kidney disease (formerly called adult-type polycystic kidney disease) (Figs. 64-8 and Fig. 64-9) and glomerulocystic renal disease (Fig. 64-10). Autosomal dominant polycystic kidney disease rarely presents in young children. It results in cystic dilatation of the nephrons and collecting ducts. The condition typically presents with renal failure in young adults. Most individuals initially become symptomatic between the third and fifth decades. The kidneys typically appear normal on sonography in early childhood. However, the diagnosis is occasionally made in infants and fetuses. Autosomal dominant polycystic kidney disease is characterized by multiple, bilateral renal macrocysts with intervening normal renal parenchyma (Fig. 64-8). The cysts are of varying size. They are randomly arranged throughout the cortex and medulla. As the cysts enlarge, they distort adjacent renal parenchyma (Fig. 64-9). There is associated bilateral renal enlargement due to the presence of multiple large cysts. Autosomal dominant polycystic kidney disease may also result in hepatic, pancreatic, and seminal vesicle cysts. These cysts are typically not seen in childhood. Additionally, the condition is associated with cerebral aneurysms.

Glomerulocystic disease is a rare cystic disease of childhood. It is characterized by cystic dilatation of Bowman's space and the initial segment of the proximal convoluted

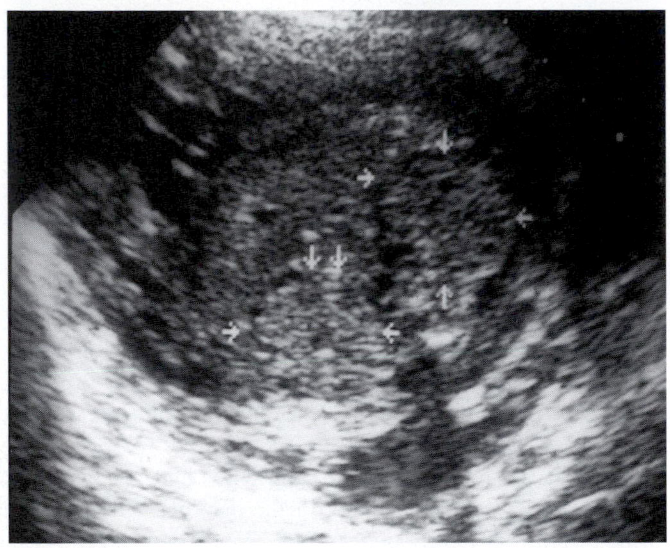

A

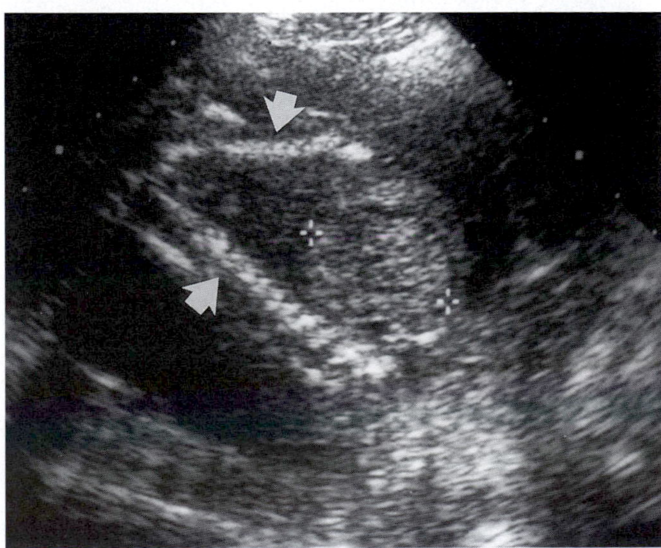

B

FIGURE 64–7. Autosomal recessive polycystic kidney disease (ARPKD) on prenatal sonography. ***A.*** Transverse view through the upper fetal abdomen at 19 weeks gestation shows bilateral renal enlargement (*arrows*). Note the absence of amniotic fluid surrounding the fetus. ***B.*** Longitudinal view of the same fetus through the fetal abdomen shows an enlarged, echogenic kidney (*between cursors*) adjacent to the spine. Also note the narrowed thorax. The chest has a triangular appearance (*between white arrowheads*) due to associated pulmonary hypoplasia. The diagnosis of ARPKD was confirmed after birth.

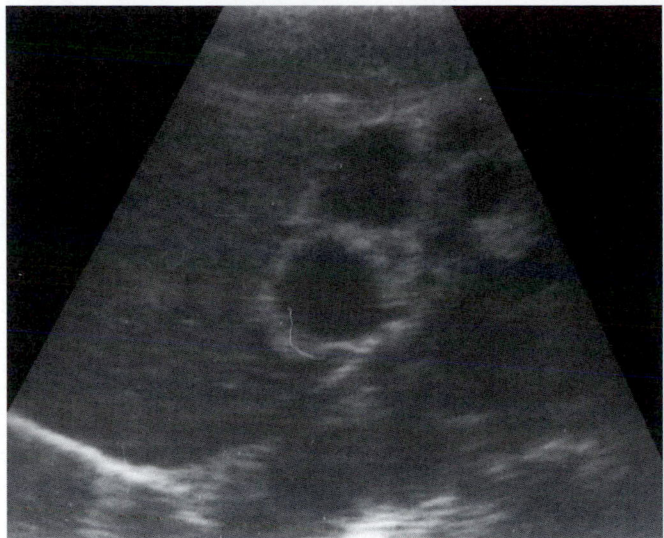

FIGURE 64–8. Autosomal dominant polycystic kidney disease in a neonate. Longitudinal view through the right kidney in an infant with autosomal dominant polycystic kidney disease demonstrates multiple large cysts. Also note the echogenic renal parenchyma relative to the adjacent liver. The left kidney also demonstrated multiple cysts.

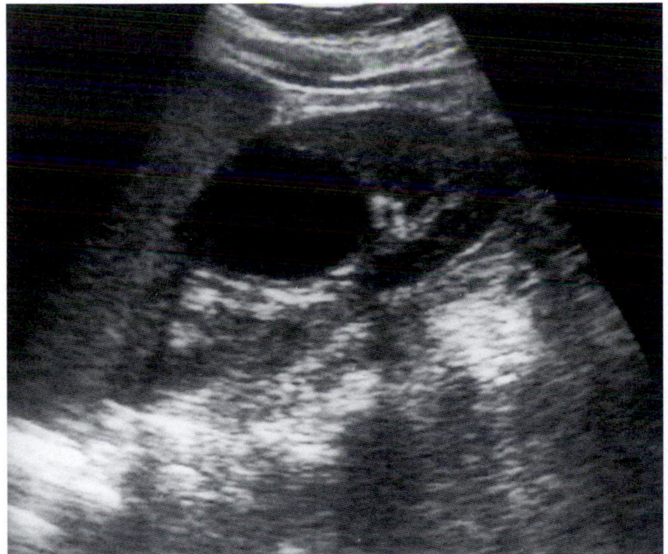

FIGURE 64–9. Autosomal dominant polycystic kidney disease in an older child. Longitudinal view through the right kidney in a 12-year-old boy with autosomal dominant polycystic kidney disease demonstrates a large macrocyst distorting the adjacent renal parenchyma. Note that the renal parenchymal echotexture is normal. There is also normal corticomedullary differentiation. Additional cysts were noted in the left kidney.

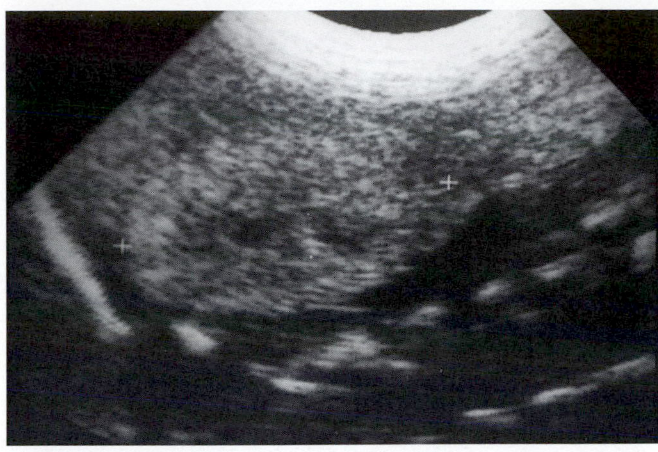

A

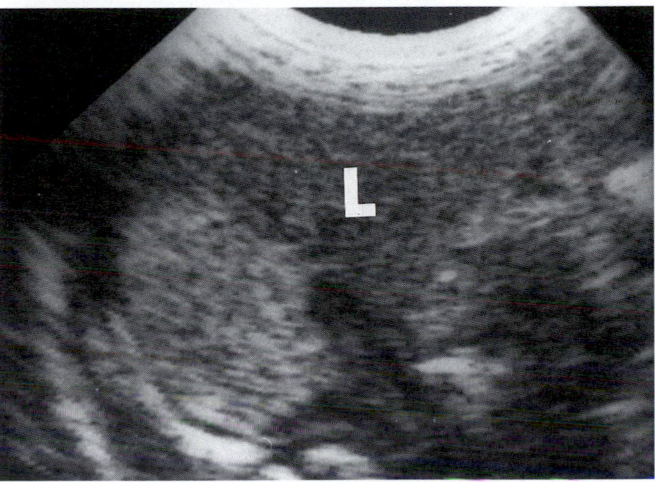

B

FIGURE 64–10. Glomerulocystic disease. Longitudinal *(A)* and transverse *(B)* views through the right kidney in a 1-week-old infant demonstrate increased renal echogenicity, with loss of corticomedullary differentiation. The left kidney had a similar appearance. The normal reniform appearance is maintained. The diagnosis of glomerulocystic disease was established at renal biopsy. L = liver.

tubule. Glomerulocystic disease can occur in otherwise normal infants or be associated with various syndromes, including Zellweger syndrome and renal retinal dysplasia. The cysts are present only in the cortex. There are no cysts in the medulla, as the loop of Henle and the collecting ducts are spared. The cysts may be microscopic and not be visible on sonography. However, there will be increased renal parenchymal echogenicity due to the reflections of the sound beam by the multiple interfaces of the small cysts (Fig. 64-10).

Autosomal recessive polycystic kidney disease often has a poor outcome. There is a high mortality rate in the neonatal period associated with this condition. The principal early causes of death are respiratory failure secondary to pulmonary hypoplasia and renal insufficiency. Most patients who survive early childhood will eventually develop chronic liver disease, resulting in hepatic dysfunction and portal hypertension. There are few adult survivors with this condition.

References

Anton PA, Abramowsky CR: Adult polycystic renal disease presenting in infancy: A report emphasizing the bilateral involvement. *J Urol* 128:1290–1291, 1982.

Bear JC, McManamon P, Morgan J, et al: Age at clinical onset and at ultrasonographic detection of adult polycystic kidney disease: Data for genetic counselling. *Am J Med Genet* 18:45–53, 1984.

Blickman JG, Bramson RT, Herrin JT: Autosomal recessive polycystic kidney disease: Long-term sonographic findings in patients surviving the neonatal period. *AJR* 164:1247–1250, 1995.

Blyth H, Ockenden BG: Polycystic disease of kidneys and liver presenting in childhood. *J Med Genet* 8:257–284, 1971.

Currarino G, Stannard MW, Rutledge JC: The sonolucent cortical rim in infantile polycystic kidneys: Histologic correlation. *J Ultrasound Med* 8:571–574, 1989.

Fitch SJ, Stapleton FB: Ultrasonographic features of glomerulocystic disease in infancy: Similarity to infantile polycystic kidney disease. *Pediatr Radiol* 16:400–402, 1986.

Hayden CK, Swischuk LE: Renal cystic disease. *Semin Ultrasound, CT, MR* 12:361–373, 1991.

Jain M, LeQuesne GW, Bourne AJ, Henning P: High-resolution ultrasonography in the differential diagnosis of cystic diseases of the kidney in infancy and childhood: Preliminary experience. *J Ultrasound Med* 16:235–240, 1997.

Keenan JF, Rifkin MD: Ultrasonographic diagnosis of seminal vesicle cysts in polycystic kidney disease. *J Ultrasound Med* 15:343–344, 1995.

Lucaya J, Enriquez G, Nieto J, et al: Renal calcifications in patients with autosomal recessive polycystic kidney disease: Prevalence and causes. *AJR* 160:359–362, 1993.

MacDonald RA, Avner ED: Inherited polycystic kidney disease in children. *Semin Nephrol* 11:632–642, 1991.

Marchal GJ, Desmet VJ, Proesmans C, et al: Caroli disease: High-frequency US and pathologic findings. *Radiology* 158:507–511, 1986.

65

Figure 65-1 shows a 1-day-old boy with prenatal hydronephrosis. What do you see? What are the diagnostic considerations?

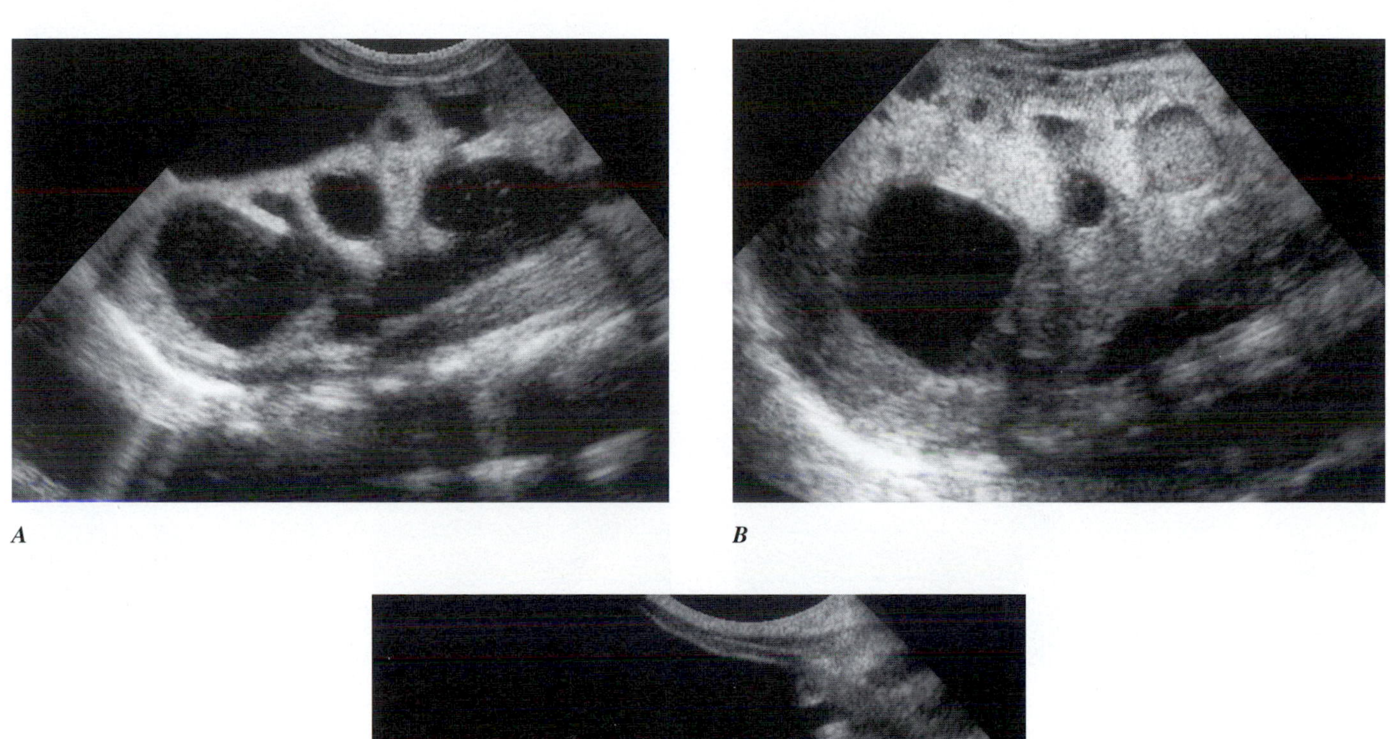

FIGURE 65–1. Longitudinal views through the right kidney ***(A)***, left kidney ***(B)***, and bladder ***(C)***.

CHAPTER 65

Posterior Urethral Valves

DOROTHY I. BULAS

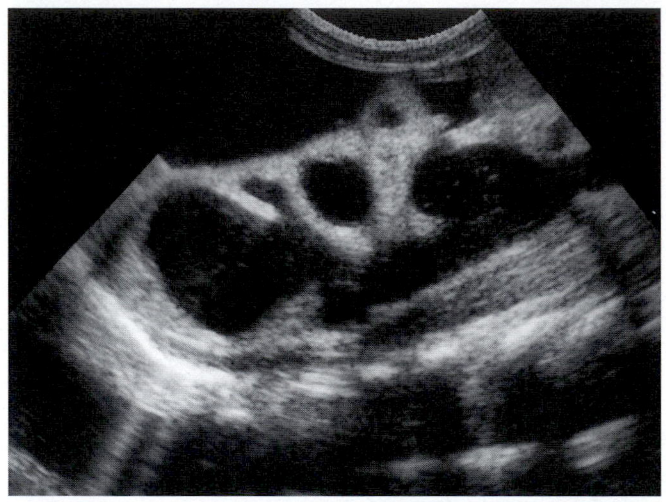

A

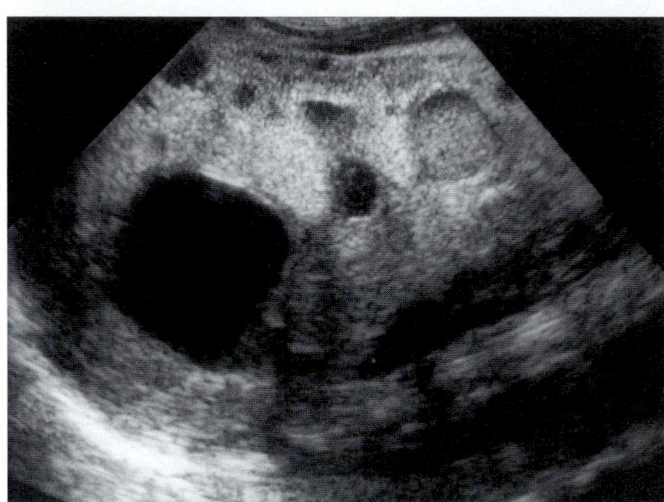

B

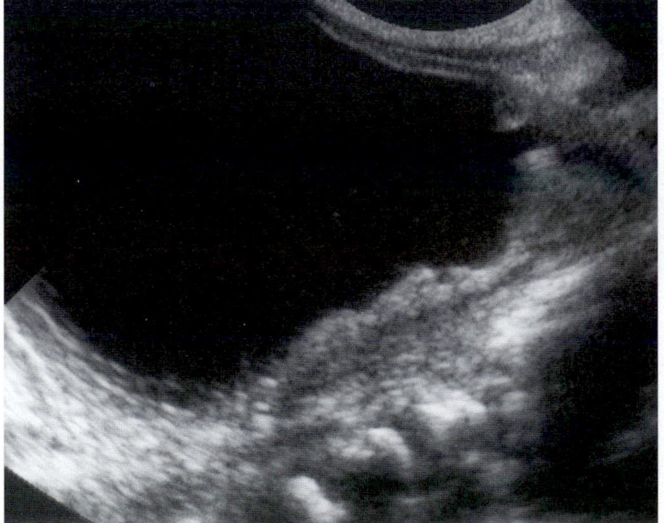

C

FIGURE 65–2. Posterior urethral valve (PUV). Longitudinal views through the right *(A)* and left *(B)* kidneys in an infant with PUV demonstrate moderate to severe dilatation of the intrarenal collecting systems. There is debris within the left intrarenal collecting system. Also note that the renal parenchyma is abnormally echogenic, indicative of secondary renal dysplasia. Longitudinal view through the pelvis *(C)* demonstrates bladder dilatation.

Posterior urethral valve (PUV) is a malformation complex consisting of valve obstruction of the posterior urethra. It is the most common cause of urethral obstruction in boys. The condition results in secondary bladder obstruction and hypertrophy (Fig. 65-2). Bladder obstruction leads to ureteral, renal pelvic, and caliceal dilatation and to vesicoureteral reflux (Fig. 65-2). The degree of renal collecting system dilatation ranges from mild to severe. Severe obstruction developing early in the prenatal period can result in renal dysplasia. The condition may be associated with oligohy-

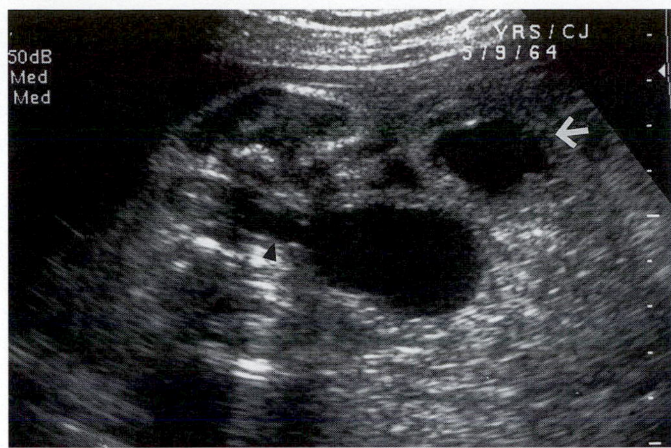

A

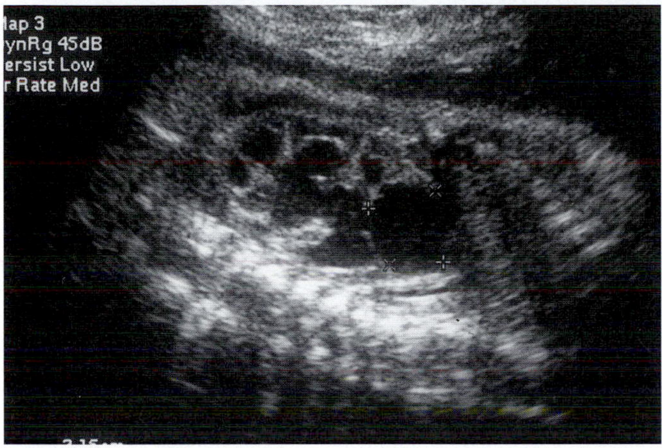

B

FIGURE 65–3. Posterior urethral valve. ***A.*** Coronal view through the fetal abdomen demonstrates a dilated bladder. At the bladder base, there is a dilated linear structure, consistent with a dilated posterior urethra (*arrowhead*). Superior to the bladder is a markedly dilated left renal pelvis (*white arrow*). ***B.*** Coronal view through the right kidney in the same fetus demonstrates dilated calices and renal pelvis. The renal cortex is thinned diffusely. A 2-cm lower-pole cortical cyst is demarcated by the cursors.

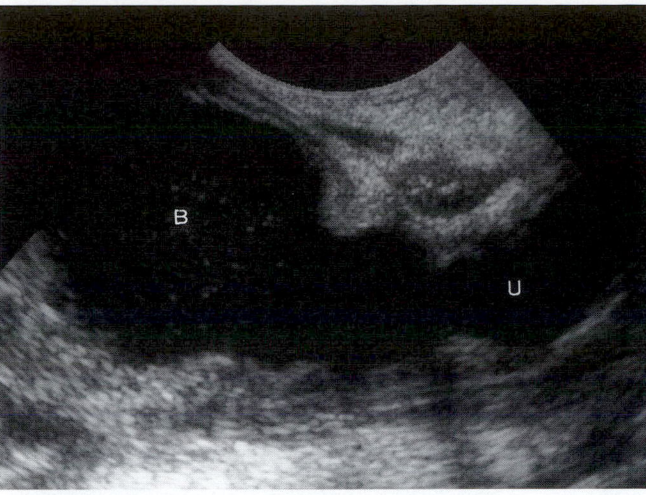

FIGURE 65–4. Dilated posterior urethra secondary to posterior urethral valve (PUV). Perineal scan in an infant with PUV demonstrates a dilated posterior urethra (U). B = bladder.

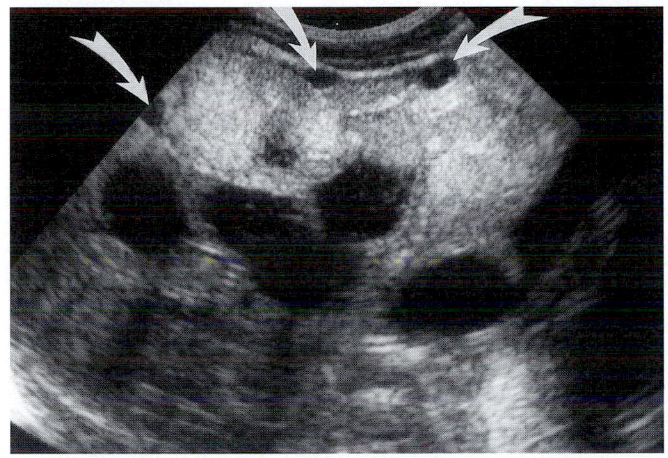

FIGURE 65–5. Renal dysplasia secondary to posterior urethral valve (PUV). Longitudinal view through the left kidney in an infant with PUV demonstrates echogenic renal parenchyma and cortical cysts (*arrows*), indicative of secondary renal dysplasia.

dramnios and pulmonary hypoplasia. If severe oligohydramnios is present, the mortality rate is greater than 90 percent. Prenatal vesicoamniotic shunting may benefit some cases of PUV.

Children with PUV present most frequently in the newborn period with palpable flank masses secondary to associated hydronephrosis. The two most common abdominal masses in a newborn are of renal origin: hydronephrosis and multicystic dysplastic kidney. Infants may also present with decreased or absent urine output, or with respiratory distress secondary to associated pulmonary hypoplasia. Older infants and children may present following urinary tract infection or secondary to failure to thrive. In the past decade, with the widespread development of fetal screening, the diagnosis of PUV is often made on prenatal sonographic evaluation (Fig. 65-3).

Sonographic findings associated with PUV in the newborn period include bladder dilatation (Fig. 65-2), bladder wall thickening, posterior urethral dilatation (Fig. 65-4), bilateral ureteral dilatation and redundancy, renal pelvis and caliceal dilatation with renal parenchymal thinning (Fig. 65-2), and urinary ascites. Debris secondary to urinary stasis may be noted within the renal collecting system (Fig. 65-2). The renal collecting system dilatation is typically bilateral but can be asymmetric. Renal cortical cysts or echogenic renal parenchyma may be noted if there is secondary renal dysplasia (Fig. 65-5). These two latter findings indicative a poor prognosis, with progressive deterioration of renal function.

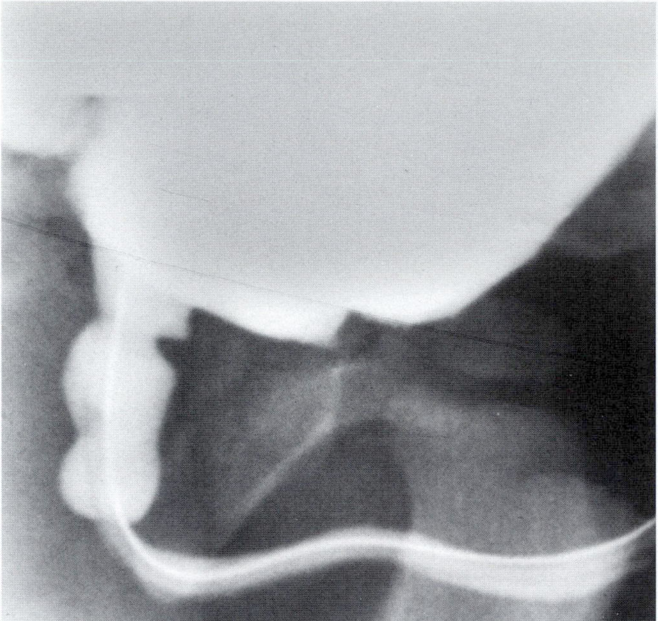

FIGURE 65–6. Dilated posterior urethra secondary to posterior urethral valve (PUV). Spot radiograph from a voiding cystourethrogram shows a dilated posterior urethra, indicative of PUV.

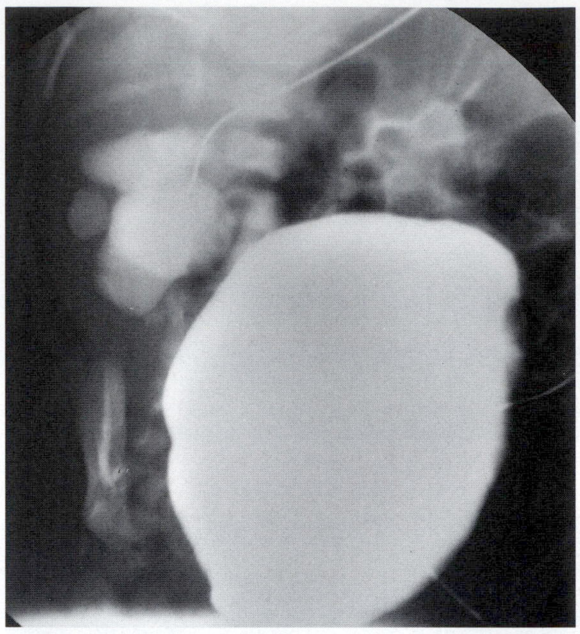

FIGURE 65–7. Prune-belly syndrome. Voiding cystourethrogram in an infant with prune-belly syndrome demonstrates an enlarged bladder and right-sided vesicoureteral reflux. Note that there is moderate dilatation of the right renal collecting system.

The diagnosis of PUV has traditionally been confirmed by a voiding cystourethrogram through the demonstration of a dilated posterior urethra (Fig. 65-6). The voiding cystourethrogram is also essential to demonstrate associated vesicoureteral reflux. The dilated posterior urethra can also be well shown on sonography through transperineal scanning with a high-frequency transducer (Fig. 65-4).

The differential diagnosis of a male infant with bilateral collecting system dilatation includes prune-belly syndrome, bilateral vesicoureteral reflux, and primary megaureter. The latter two conditions can be distinguished from PUV on the basis of the absence of posterior urethral dilatation. Prune-belly, or Eagle-Barrett, syndrome consists of the triad of hypotonic abdominal wall, large hypotonic bladder with dilated ureters, and cryptorchidism (Fig. 65-7). There is also associated dilatation of the posterior urethra. This condition can be distinguished from PUV on the basis of the associated abdominal wall hypotonia. In addition, a patent urachus may be present. The etiology of prune-belly syndrome is poorly defined. Some consider it to represent a mesenchymal defect, while others feel it is the result of transient urethral obstruction, leading to bladder and ureteral distention and resultant pressure atrophy of the abdominal musculature. The bladder distention is felt to interfere with testicular descent, resulting in cryptorchidism.

References

Avni EF, Rodesch F, Schulman CC: Fetal uropathies: Diagnostic pitfalls and management. *J Urol* 134:921–925, 1985.

Burton BK, Dillard RG: Prune-belly syndrome: Observations supporting the hypothesis of abdominal overdistension. *Am J Med Genet* 17:669–672, 1984.

Cohen HL, Susman M, Haller JO, et al: Posterior urethral valve: Transperineal US for imaging and diagnosis in male infants. *Radiology* 192:261–264, 1994.

Cremin BJ: A review of ultrasonic appearance of posterior urethral valve and ureteroceles. *Pediatr Radiol* 16:357–364, 1986.

King LR, Hatcher PA: Natural history of fetal and neonatal hydronephrosis. *Pediatr Urol* 34:433, 1994.

Macpherson RI, Leitheser RE, Gordon L, et al: Posterior urethral valves: An update and review. *Radiographics* 6:753–791, 1986.

McMahon RA, Renou PM, Scheckleton PA, et al: Severe urethral obstruction diagnosed at 14 weeks gestation: Variability of outcome with and without drainage. *Fetal Diagn Ther* 10:343–348, 1995.

Parkhouse HF, Barratt TM, Dillon MJ, et al: Long-term outcome of boys with posterior urethral valves presenting at birth. *J Pediatr Surg* 62:59–62, 1988.

Stephens FD, Gupta D: Pathogenesis of prune-belly syndrome. *J Urol* 152:2328–2331, 1994.

Young JJ, Frontz WA, Baldwin JC: Congenital obstruction of the posterior urethra. *J Urol* 3:289–365, 1991.

66

Figure 66-1 is an image of the left kidney of an 8-day-old full-term neonate who presented with a reddening of the soft tissues of his lower anterior abdominal wall and abdominal distention. Figure 66-2 is a longitudinal image of the left lower quadrant. You are worried about obstruction of the genitourinary system and would like to use this exam to rule out the possibility of posterior urethral valve (PUV). The transvesicle bladder views showed questionable bladder wall thickening but no posterior urethral dilatation. What do you note on the unknown image? Are you still worried about PUV? What other ultrasound (US) technical maneuver can be used to help make the diagnosis?

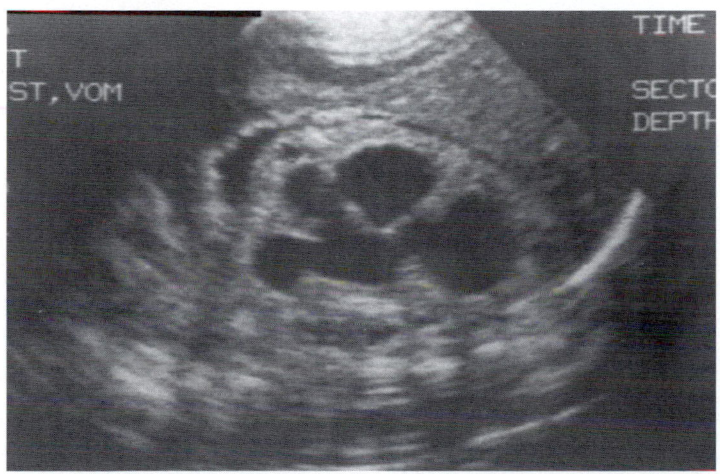

FIGURE 66–1. Kidney. Longitudinal plane. The spleen and superior are on the reader's right.

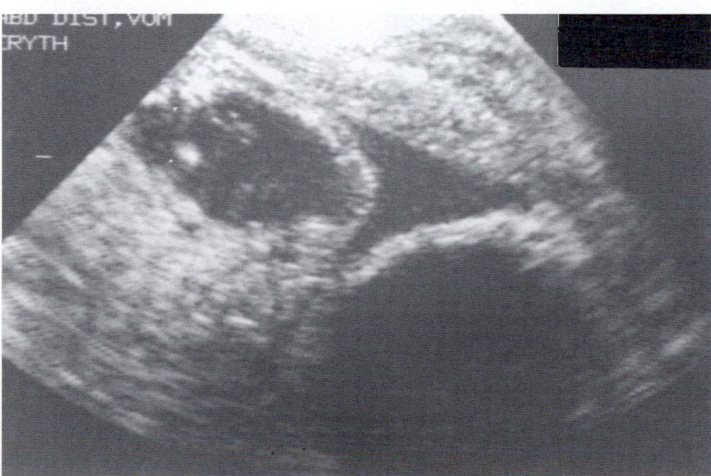

FIGURE 66–2. Left lower quadrant. Longitudinal plane.

CHAPTER 66

Forniceal Rupture and Urinary Ascites from Posterior Urethral Valve

HARRIS L. COHEN

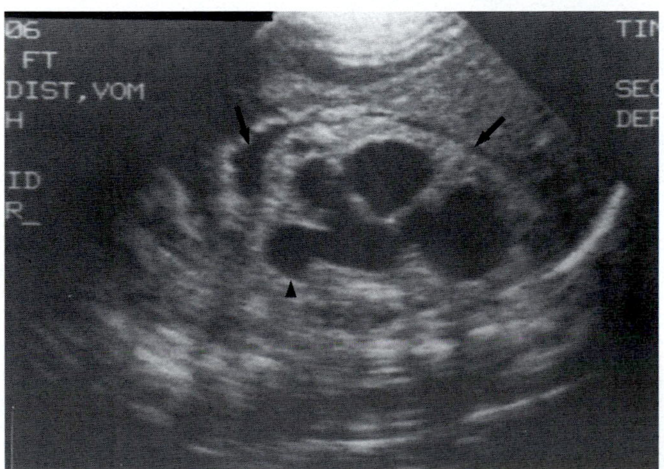

FIGURE 66–3. Annotated version of Fig. 66-1. Posterior urethral valve causing hydronephrosis and forniceal rupture. Kidney. Longitudinal plane. The spleen and superior are on the reader's right. There is moderate pyelocaliceal system dilatation. Some proximal ureteral dilatation is noted (*arrowhead*). Forniceal rupture is responsible for the perirenal fluid/urine (*arrows*). This was the source of urinary ascites, which serendipitously led to the reddening of the skin of the child's abdominal wall.

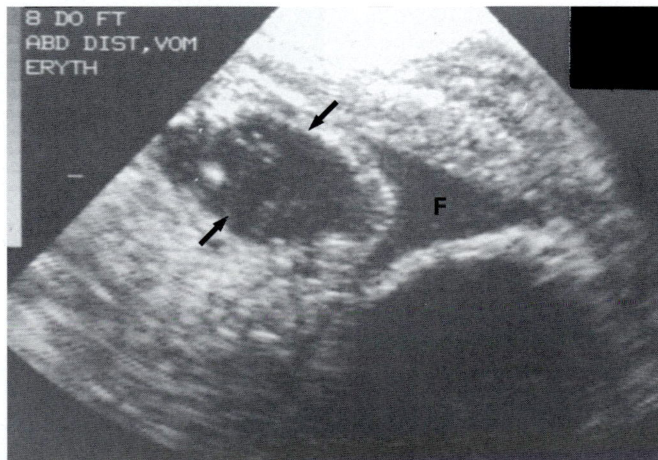

FIGURE 66–4. Annotated version of Fig. 66-2. Urinary ascites. Left lower quadrant. Longitudinal plane. A triangle of free fluid (F), proven to be urinary ascites, was noted in the left lower quadrant, inferior to contained fluid in the left kidney's perirenal space (*arrows*). The urinary ascites accumulated from the forniceal rupture of a left pyelocaliceal system obstructed by a posterior urethral valve.

Figure 66-3, the annotated version of Fig. 66-1, shows moderate hydronephrosis with a small amount of perirenal fluid. This perirenal fluid is urine that has leaked from rupture of a caliceal fornix, an area of weakness in an obstructed genitourinary system. The fluid leaked into the peritoneum, and the patient presented because of urinary ascites. The urinary ascites is seen in Fig. 66-4, the annotated version of Fig. 66-2. Because an obstructing PUV is a major consideration in hydronephrosis, especially when associated with urinary ascites in a newborn, an attempt was made on the US exam to prove PUV. Previous chapters in this text have discussed PUV. Most individuals attempt to image the relatively pathognomonic dilated posterior urethra of PUV patients by transvesicle US. This case is presented to highlight the fact that one may find this information using a transperineal approach.

WHAT IS PUV?

To recapitulate briefly, PUV is a relatively common congenital anomaly in which redundant tissue, an obliquely placed diaphragm or mucosal fold, found within the posterior urethra and usually related to the verumontanum, obstructs urinary outflow. Cremin and Aaronson highlighted the fact that the valve is a single and not a paired structure. Posterior urethral valve occurs in one of every 5000 to 8000 boys. It is the most common cause of urinary tract obstruction and the leading cause of end-stage renal disease in boys. Renal dysfunction can, it is hoped, be reduced by early diagnosis and treatment.

Clinical findings include a palpable kidney or bladder. Ultrasound findings include bladder hypertrophy, posterior urethral dilatation from obstruction, and—if there is vesicoureteral reflux—ureteral and pyelocaliceal system dilatation. As in this case, the force of the refluxing and obstructed urine within the pyelocaliceal system may lead to rupture at the caliceal fornix, although urinary ascites can also be seen with other obstructions, such as ureteropelvic junction (UPJ) obstruction. The presence of a dilated ureter, as seen during the examination but shown only proximally in these images (Fig. 66-3), would go against UPJ as a possibility. Other possible manifestations of leaking urine include urinoma and urothorax.

ULTRASOUND FOR PUV

In 1982, Gilsanz et al suggested the use of transvesicle US to identify dilatation and elongation of the posterior urethra and thereby differentiate between a neurogenic cause of bladder outlet obstruction and PUV. Imaging a dilated posterior urethra to confirm the diagnosis of PUV (although rarer possibilities such as congenital urethra strictures may also cause similar images) is not always possible using the fluid-filled bladder as an ultrasound window. Blumhagen was unable to note posterior urethral dilatation in 50 percent of his proven cases of PUV evaluated through a fluid-filled bladder. Although his work was done in the early 1980s, his facts ring true today. In a review of five of our cases, we were unable to see the dilated urethra in three of them using a transvesicle approach. McAlister has suggested the use of a Credé maneuver—i.e., pressing on the patient's bladder—as a method of forcing urine from the bladder to the posterior urethra and perhaps allowing better transvesicle imaging and diagnosis. We have had a 6-year-old patient with a dilated bladder and significant hydronephrosis bilaterally void while the transducer was placed transperineally to note how his posterior urethra, unable to be evaluated when empty, looked in a distended state, when voiding. We also used this method to see if we could denote valve tissue in his urethra. The posterior urethra looked normal, and we saw no PUV. A voiding cystourethrogram (VCU) performed later confirmed our US results.

THE TRANSPERINEAL TECHNIQUE FOR EVALUATING PUV

The transperineal technique (Fig. 66-5) consists of placing a transducer between the scrotum and the anus. We usually glove the transducer, placing gel in the glove or condom and on top of the skin of the perineum. The technique dates back to 1983, when Cremin and Aaronson reported using perineal sagittal US views to image a dilated posterior urethra and diagnose PUV. They noted posterior urethral dilatation in eight

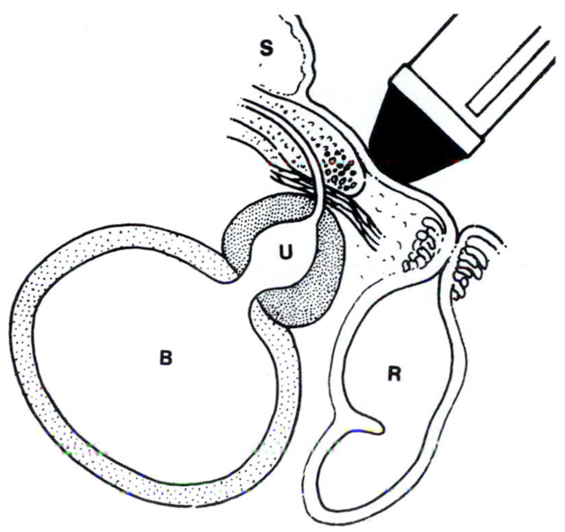

A

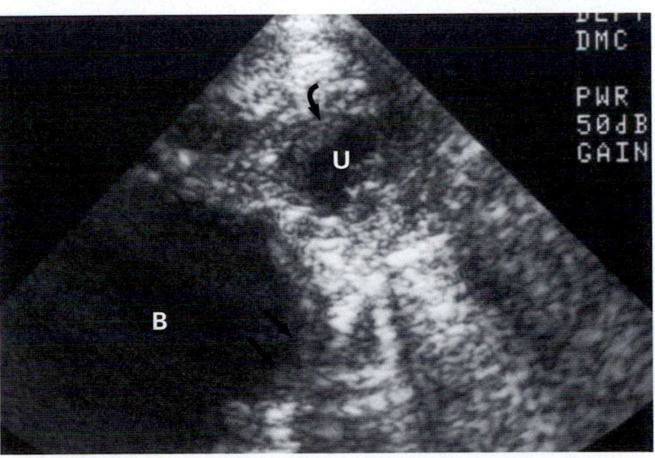

B

FIGURE 66–5. Transperineal technique for posterior urethral valve (PUV) diagnosis. ***A.*** Schematic line drawing. Longitudinal plane. The transducer is on the perineum. The urethra (U) is dilated as a result of PUV. The bladder (B) wall is thickened. S = symphysis pubis, R = rectum. ***B.*** Ultrasound. Longitudinal (sagittal) plane. A dilated urethra (U) is seen distal to (and therefore closer to the transducer than) a distended bladder (B). The walls (*curved arrow*) of the urethra appear thickened. The bladder wall is thickened (*arrows*). (*From Cohen et al 1994, with permission.*)

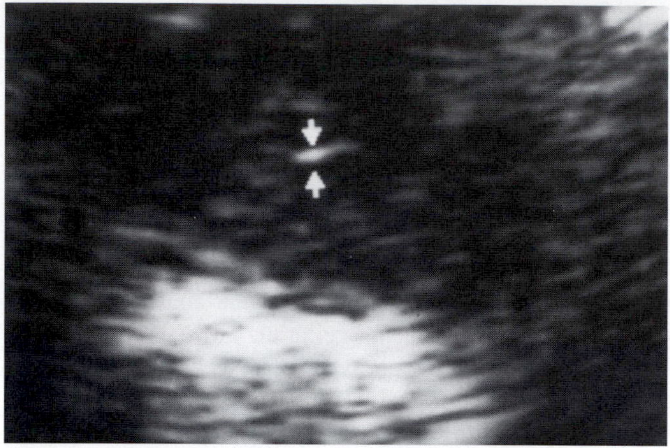

A

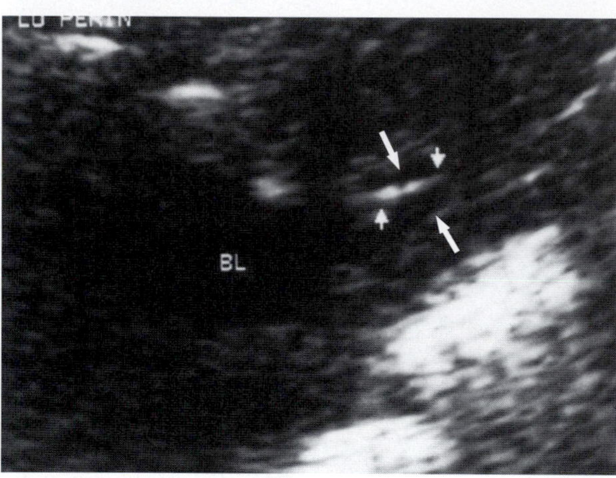

B

FIGURE 66–6. Transperineal imaging of posterior urethral valve (PUV) and actual valve tissue. ***A.*** Transverse perineal view. Arrows point to an echogenic line within a dilated posterior urethra. It was diagnosed as, and proved to be, actual valve tissue in a neonate with PUV. The urethra was not imaged on the transvesicle view of this neonate. ***B.*** Longitudinal perineal view. In this orthogonal projection, the bladder (BL) is distended. Its wall, hard to see on this darkened image, is thickened. Of note is dilatation of the posterior urethra (*long arrows*). Small arrows point to the linear echogenicity running obliquely through the distended posterior urethra, which is consistent with and proved to be valve tissue. (*From Cohen et al 1994, with permission.*)

children with known bladder distention who proved to have PUV at VCU and cystoscopy. They found, and we later confirmed, that posterior urethral dilatation is better imaged using this perineal technique than using a transvesicle approach. From a logical point of view, the nearer the structure of concern is to a well-focused transducer, the better it will be imaged. This has been most elegantly demonstrated in the analysis of the ovary when it is in its usual position in the lower pelvis. This seems to also hold true with transperineal US work to rule out PUV.

In 1994, we reported improved posterior urethral imaging when an orthogonal view—i.e., the transverse perineal view (Fig. 66-6)—was added. We were able, probably because of improved US machinery, to see not only dilatation of the posterior urethra in several patients but also heretofore unreported contained echogenic lines that were later proven to be actual valve tissue. We were also able to note what appeared to be urethral wall thickening. As seems to be the case with all US information that can be obtained before or after birth, what is learned with regard to one group (e.g., the neonate) can be used in the analysis of the other (e.g., the fetus).

In 1998, we reported the imaging of dilated thickened urethras containing valve tissue in fetuses later proven to have PUV. We are cautious in diagnosing PUV when we see urethral wall thickening alone, as this may have other causes. We hope that our understanding will increase with time and experience.

FINAL POINT

If you are worried about the possibility of PUV in a patient and would like to look from another vantage point, please consider transperineal views. They can be most helpful.

References

Blumhagen J: Echographic findings in posterior urethral valves. Presented at the 26th annual meeting of the Society for Pediatric Radiology, Atlanta, GA, 1983.

Cohen HL, Susman M, Haller J, et al: Posterior urethral valve: Transperineal US for imaging and diagnosis in male infants. *Radiology* 192:261–264, 1994.

Cohen HL, Zinn H, Patel A, et al: Prenatal sonographic diagnosis of posterior urethral valves: Identification of valves and thickening of the posterior urethral wall. *JCU* 26:366–370, 1998.

Cremin B, Aaronson I: Ultrasonic diagnosis of posterior urethral valve in neonates. *Br J Radiol* 56:435–438, 1983.

Gilsanz V, Miller J, Reid B: Ultrasonic characteristics of posterior urethral valves. *Radiology* 145:143–145, 1982.

Macpherson R, Leithiser R, Gordon L, Turner W: Posterior urethral valves: An update and review. *Radiographics* 6:753–791, 1986.

McAlister W: Demonstration of the dilated prostatic urethra in posterior urethral valve patients. *J Ultrasound Med* 3:189–190, 1984.

67

Figure 67-1 shows an 18-month-old boy with a palpable abdominal mass. What do you see? What are the diagnostic considerations?

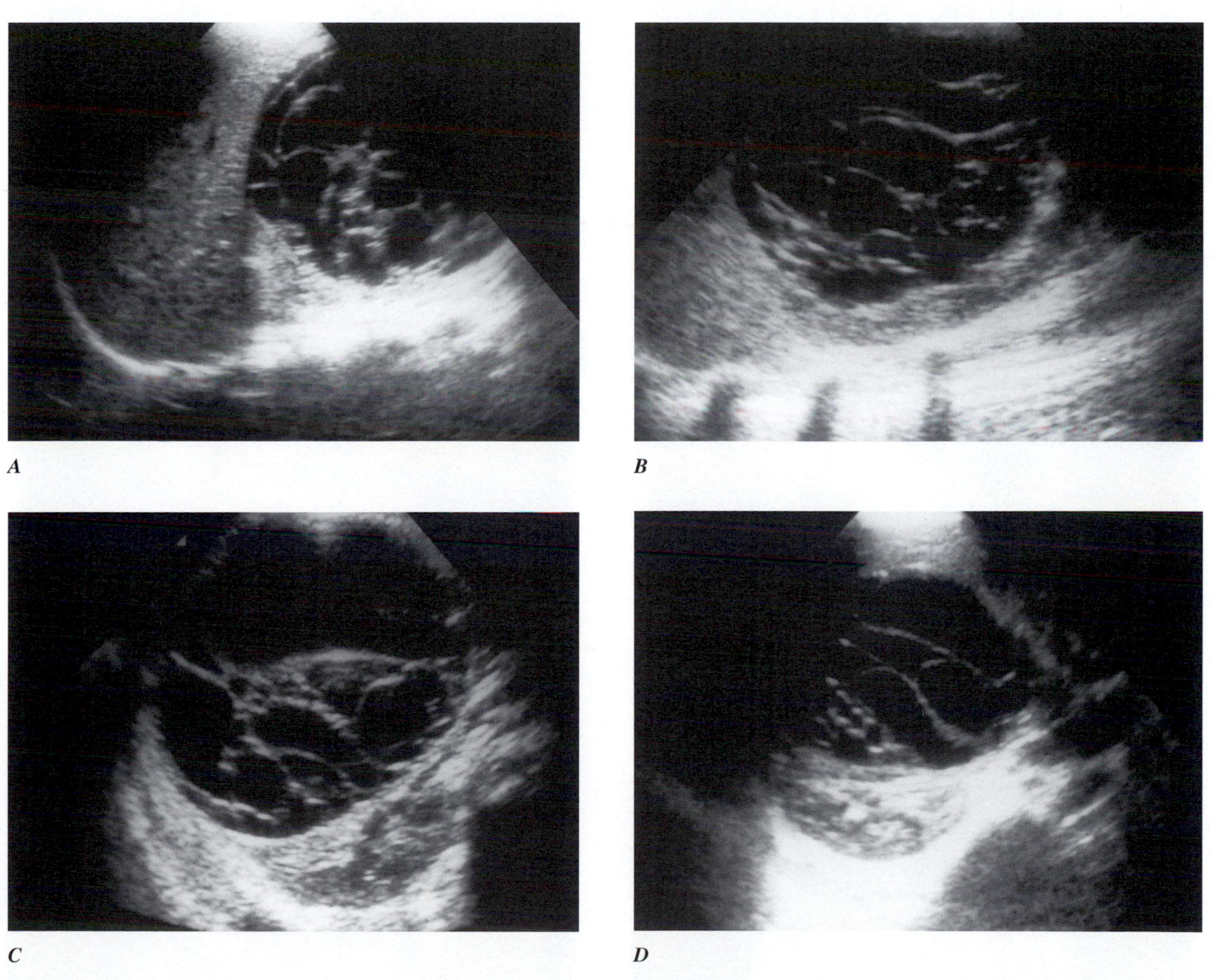

FIGURE 67–1. Longitudinal *(A, B)* and transverse *(C, D)* views through the right flank.

CHAPTER 67

Multilocular Cystic Renal Tumor

CARLOS J. SIVIT

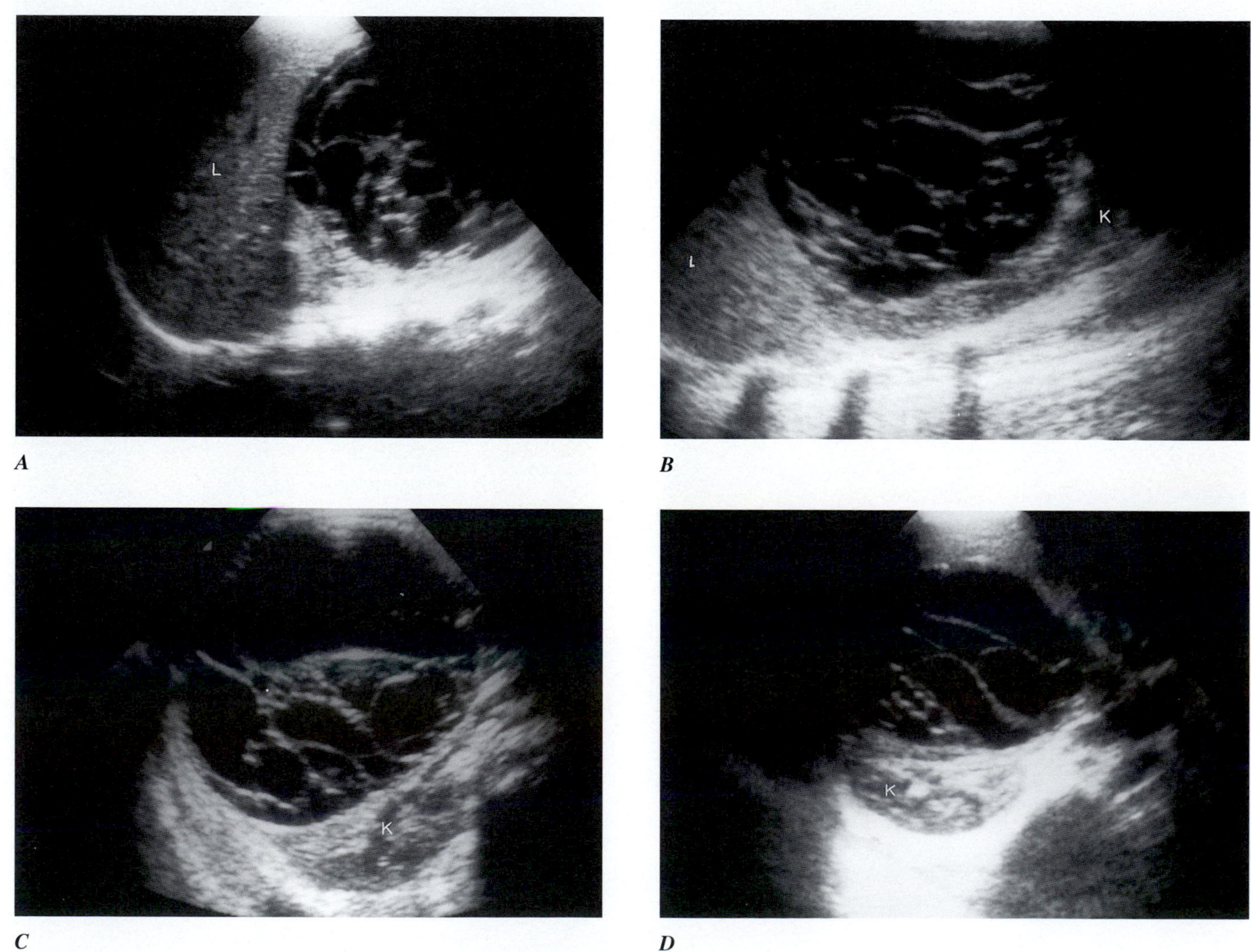

A *B* *C* *D*

FIGURE 67–2. Multilocular cystic renal tumor. Longitudinal ***(A, B)*** and transverse ***(C, D)*** views through the right flank demonstrate a well-circumscribed cystic mass with numerous septations, originating in the right kidney (K). Note the rim of normal right renal tissue surrounding the mass (*arrow*). L = liver.

Multilocular cystic renal tumor refers to two types of uncommon, predominantly benign renal lesions with an occasional propensity for malignancy. These lesions, cystic nephroma and cystic poorly differentiated nephroblastoma, are histologically distinct but grossly indistinguishable. These entities were previously called multilocular cystic nephroma. The tumor is predominantly unilateral, although bilateral cases have been reported. The gross appearance is that of a large, well-circumscribed focal renal tumor that involves only a part of the kidney. The remaining portion of the kidney usually functions normally. Occasionally, the tumor can prolapse into the renal pelvis and cause obstruction of the collecting system. The tumor contains a thick capsule and numerous cysts of varying sizes that do not communicate with one another. These cysts are lined with epithelium. There are intervening septa between the cysts. The only difference between the two types of multilocular cystic renal tumor is that in cystic nephroma the septa are fibrous and may contain well-differentiated tubular structures, while in cystic poorly differentiated nephroblastoma the septa contain blastemal cells with or without embryonal stromal cells. There are no solid elements other than the septae in this lesion, which differentiates the entity from Wilms' tumor.

Multilocular cystic renal tumor is often an incidental finding on imaging examination. These tumors are seen primarily in young children. There is a male predominance of 2:1. Two-thirds of cases are noted in children under the age of 2 years. The tumor is also seen in adults, primarily in females over the age of 30 years. Children with multilocular cystic renal tumor are often asymptomatic. Occasionally, they may present with a palpable abdominal mass or with hematuria. There are no specific clinical signs or symptoms associated with this lesion.

The two subtypes of multilocular cystic renal tumor cannot be differentiated on imaging examination. The sonographic appearance is that of a well-circumscribed cystic renal mass (Fig. 67-2). Multiple anechoic or hypoechoic cysts of varying sizes with intervening septa are noted. Some of the cysts may contain internal echoes if there has been prior hemorrhage. The cysts demonstrate acoustic enhancement. There are no solid elements in this lesion. However, the presence of multiple small cysts may result in numerous acoustic interfaces, which can mimic solid areas. There is typically replacement of a segment of the involved kidney. However, usually a segment of normal renal tissue can also be identified. This may appear as a crescent rim of renal tissue surrounding the mass (Fig. 67-2). There may be associated dilatation of the intrarenal collecting system if the tumor has prolapsed into the renal pelvis. Rarely, cystic lesions may be noted in the contralateral kidney if bilateral metachronous tumors are present (Fig. 67-3).

Computed tomography (CT) and magnetic resonance imaging (MRI) are useful for delineating the extent of renal involvement and evaluating possible metastatic disease. The CT appearance is that of a focal, well-circumscribed, multicystic renal lesion (Fig. 67-4). Solid areas representing septal elements may be also noted. The septa demonstrate variable enhancement following intravenous contrast administration.

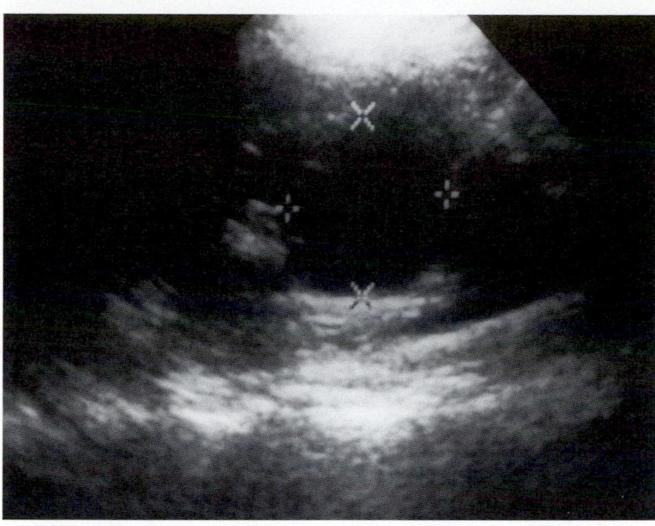

FIGURE 67–3. Bilateral metachronous multilocular cystic renal tumor. Longitudinal view through the left kidney in the same child as in Fig. 67-1 show a well-circumscribed cystic mass originating from the lower pole.

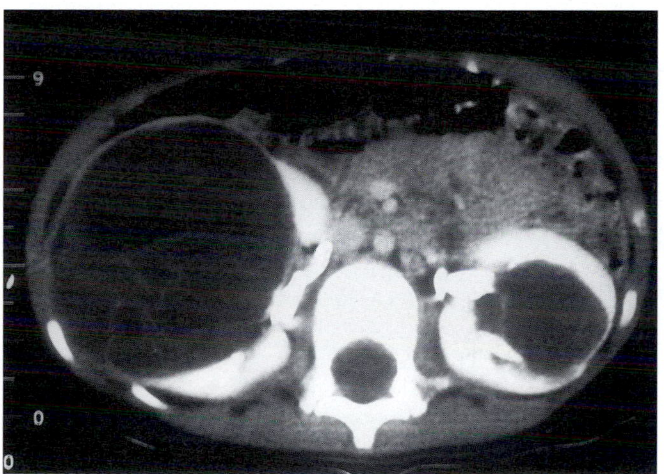

FIGURE 67–4. Multilocular cystic renal tumor. Contrast-enhanced CT scan through the upper abdomen 2 cm below shows bilateral cystic renal masses.

There is typically only partial replacement of the involved kidney, and areas of normal renal parenchyma are also identified. Calcifications within this lesion are rare. On MRI, an encapsulated multilocular renal mass is demonstrated. The capsule demonstrates low signal intensity on all pulse sequences, while the cysts demonstrate high signal intensity on both T1-weighted and T2-weighted images.

Multilocular cystic renal tumor is treated with surgical resection. If the tumor is unilateral, a nephrectomy is usually performed. When there are bilateral metachronous tumors, a partial nephrectomy may be attempted. Chemotherapy is usually given if elements of nephroblastoma are noted at the time of surgical resection or if metastatic disease is present at the time of diagnosis. The prognosis for this neoplasm is excellent, as associated metastatic disease is rare.

References

Agrons FA, Wagner BJ, Davidson AJ, et al: Multilocular cystic renal tumor in children: Radiologic-pathologic correlation. *Radiographics* 15:653–669, 1995.

Banner MP, Pollack HM, Chatten J, et al: Multilocular renal cysts: Radiologic-pathologic correlation. *AJR* 136:239–247, 1981.

Cohen MD: Genitourinary tumors, in *Imaging of Children with Cancer,* Cohen MD (ed). St. Louis, Mosby–Year Book, 1992.

Dalla-Palma L, Pozzi-Mucelli F, di Donna A, et al: Cystic renal tumors: US and CT findings. *Urol Radiol* 12:67–73, 1990.

Garrett A, Carty H, Pilling D: Multilocular cystic nephroma: Report of three cases. *Clin Radiol* 38:55–57, 1987.

Geller E, Smergel EM, Lowry PA: Renal neoplasms of childhood. *Radiol Clin North Am* 35:1391–1413, 1997.

Madewell JE, Goldman SM, Davis CJ, et al: Multilocular cystic nephroma: A radiographic-pathologic correlation of 58 patients. *Radiology* 146:309–321, 1983.

Thijssen AM, Carpenter B, Jimenez C, et al: Multilocular cyst (multilocular cystic nephroma) of the kidney: A report of 2 cases with an unusual mode of presentation. *J Urol* 142:346–348, 1989.

68

Figure 68-1 shows a 2-day-old infant with a two-vessel umbilical cord. What do you see? What are the diagnostic considerations?

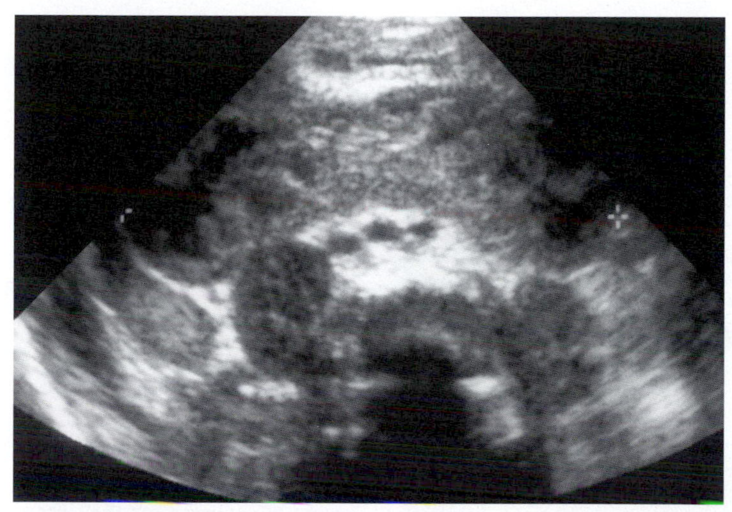

A

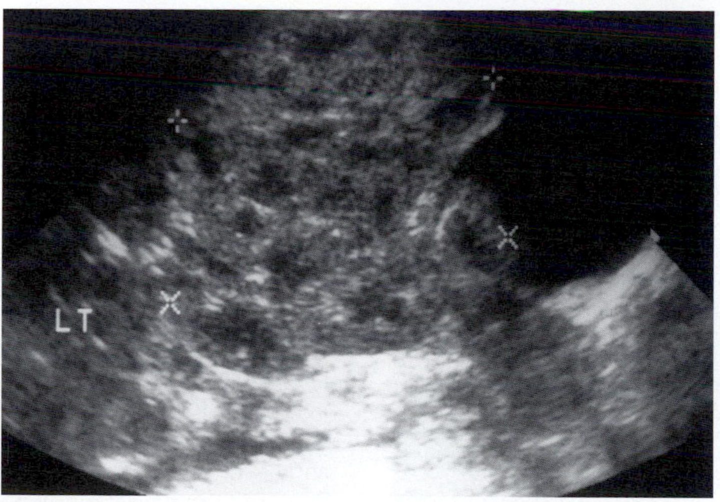

B

FIGURE 68–1. Transverse *(A)* and longitudinal *(B)* views through the midabdomen.

CHAPTER 68

Horseshoe Kidney

CARLOS J. SIVIT

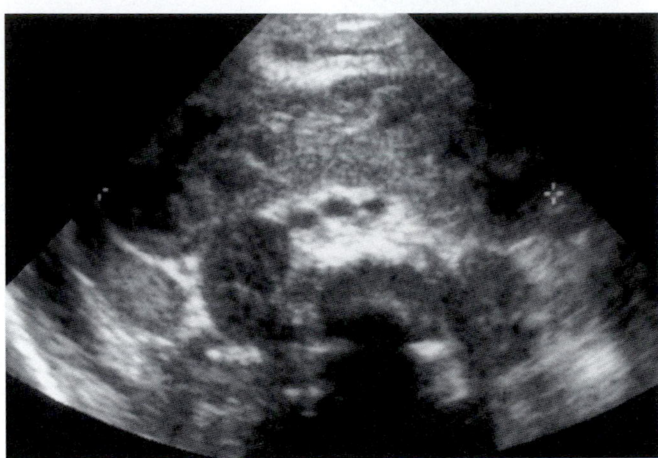

A

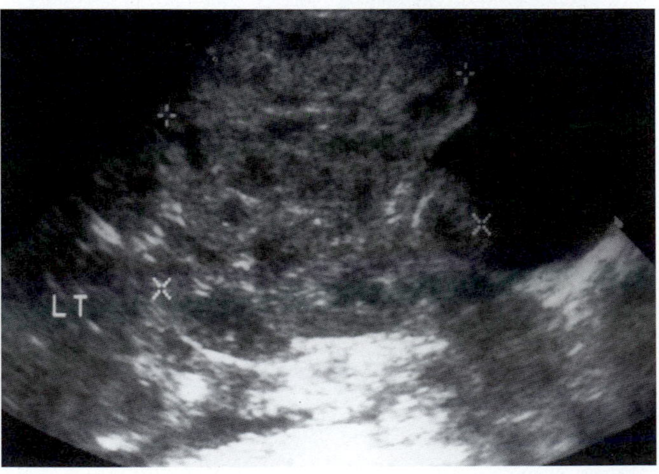

B

FIGURE 68–2. Horseshoe kidney. Transverse *(A)* and longitudinal *(B)* views through the midabdomen demonstrate the horseshoe kidney. Note the isthmus crossing the midline anterior to the great vessels on the transverse view. Also note the close apposition of the kidneys on the coronal view and their lower than expected location. The lower renal poles are noted to terminate immediately above the bladder.

Renal ectopy and fusion abnormalities are felt to develop during the process of renal ascent from the pelvis in early fetal life. Failure of the fetal kidney to complete a normal ascent is felt to be due to a variety of factors, including abnormalities of the ureteral bud or metanephric blastema, genetic causes, teratogenic causes, or anomalous vasculature that creates a barrier to ascent. Simple renal ectopy refers to a kidney that remains in the ipsilateral retroperitoneal space, while crossed renal ectopy refers to a kidney that crosses the midline. When crossed renal ectopy develops, the kidneys may remain separate, or they may fuse. The nephrogenic masses may fuse in the midline during renal ascent, resulting in a horseshoe kidney. Conversely, one kidney may ascend slightly ahead of the other. If this occurs and the inferior pole of one kidney comes in contact with the superior pole of the trailing kidney, crossed fused ectopia results. Crossed fused ectopia may also develop if a single nephrogenic mass is induced by ureteral buds from both sides.

Horseshoe kidney is the most common renal fusion abnormality. The reported prevalence ranges from 1 in 400 to 1 in 1800. The abnormality is more common in males than in females. The renal fusion in this condition occurs along the lower poles, resulting in an isthmus crossing the midline (Figs. 68-2 and 68-3). The composition of the isthmus is parenchymal or fibrous. The horseshoe kidney is typically positioned low in the abdomen, with the isthmus lying just below the junction of the inferior mesenteric artery and the aorta. The ureters typically cross anterior to the isthmus and descend from the anteriorly positioned renal pelves. The condition is associated with trisomy 18, Turner's syndrome, and neural tube defects. Approximately one-third of children with horseshoe kidney also have genitourinary, gastrointestinal, cardiovascular, and skeletal abnormalities. Horseshoe kidney is associated with an increased risk of obstruction, vesicoureteral reflux, infection, urolithiasis, and malignancy. The uteropelvic junction is the most common site of obstruction. The presence of horseshoe kidney does not adversely affect survival. Approximately one-third of individuals with the condition remain undiagnosed prior to death.

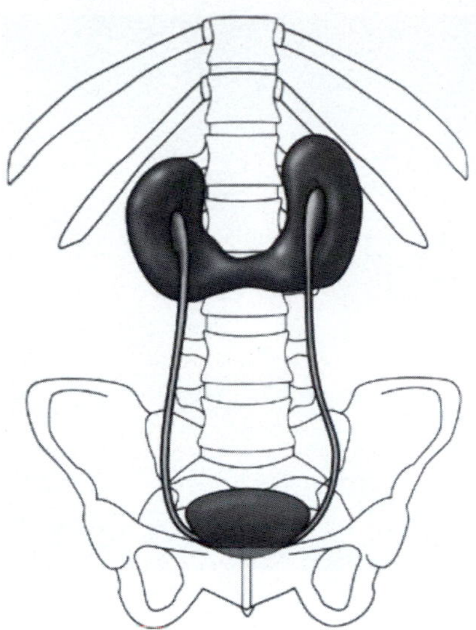

FIGURE 68–3. Diagram of horseshoe kidney.

Crossed renal ectopia is the second most common renal fusion abnormality, after horseshoe kidney. The crossed ectopic kidney crosses the midline to lie on the opposite side from the ureteral insertion into the bladder. There are four varieties of crossed renal ectopia (Figs. 68-4 to 68-7). Crossed renal ectopia may occur with fusion (Fig. 68-4), without fusion (Fig. 68-5), as a solitary kidney (Fig. 68-6), or as a bilateral process (Fig. 68-7). Approximately 85 percent of cases of crossed renal ectopia occur with fusion, while 10 percent occur without fusion. Solitary and bilateral crossed ectopia are very rare. The relationship of the fused kidneys in crossed fused ectopia varies widely. The most common type involves fusion of the upper pole of the crossed kidney with the lower pole of the normally positioned kidney. The renal pelves typically remain in an anterior position.

The diagnosis of horseshoe kidney can be accurately established by sonography. The sonographic appearance of horseshoe kidney is characterized by medially oriented inferior

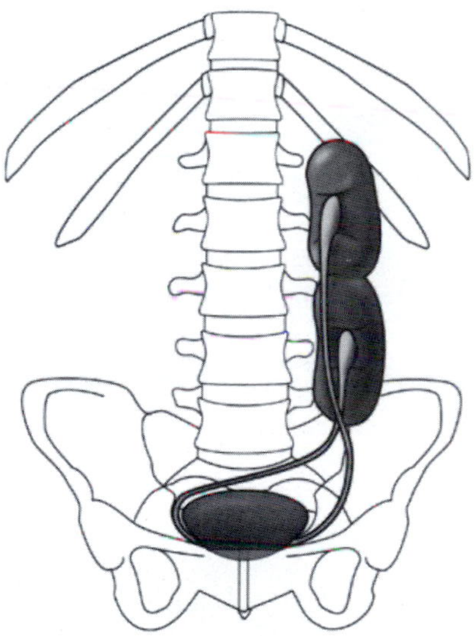

FIGURE 68–4. Diagram of crossed fused renal ectopia.

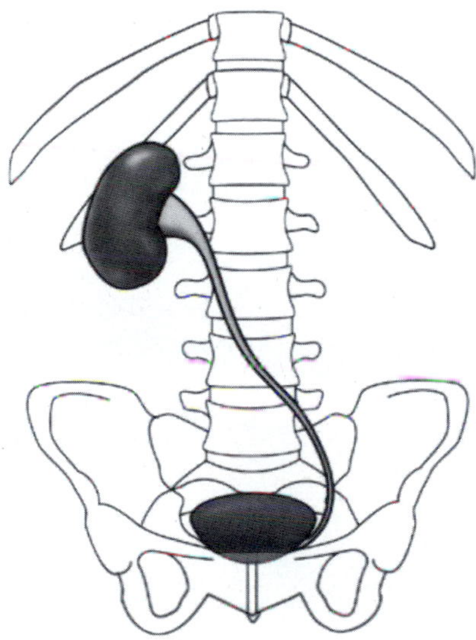

FIGURE 68–6. Diagram of solitary crossed renal ectopia.

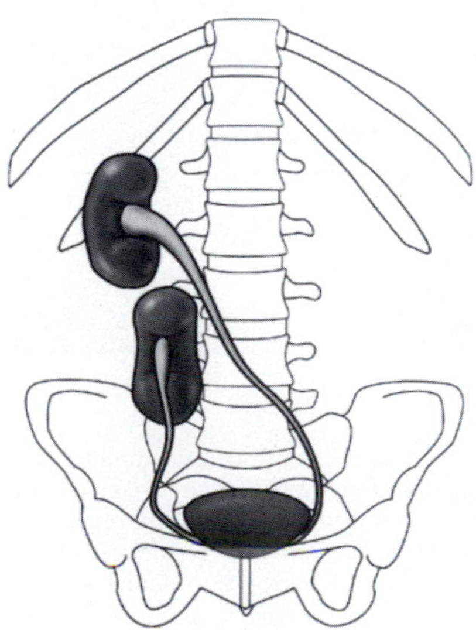

FIGURE 68–5. Diagram of crossed renal ectopia without fusion.

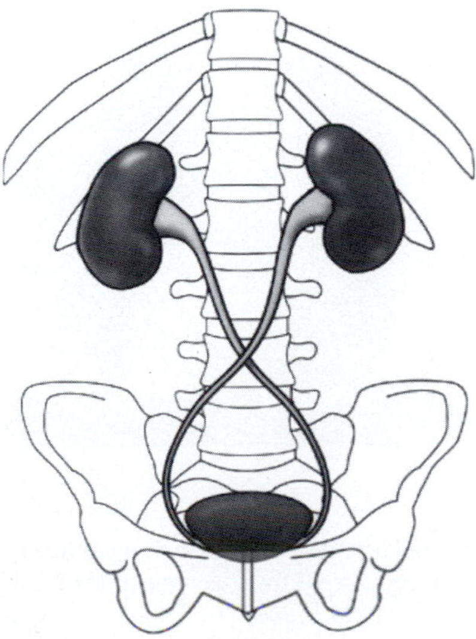

FIGURE 68–7. Diagram of bilateral crossed renal ectopia.

poles and an isthmus crossing the midline and connecting the inferior poles (Fig. 68-2). The isthmus usually lies anterior to the aorta and inferior vena cava. Occasionally, it may be positioned posterior to those vessels. The proximal ureters will be seen to pass anterior to the isthmus. The isthmus may occasionally be difficult to demonstrate on sonography. In these instances, the diagnosis is suggested by the medial orientation of the inferior renal poles. Sonography can also aid in the evaluation of possible coexisting renal abnormalities, including obstructive uropathy, renal dysplasia, and urolithiasis (Fig. 68-8).

Sonography is also useful in the assessment of crossed fused ectopia. The diagnosis can be excluded if separate kidneys are noted on the two sides of the midline. The sonographic appearance of crossed fused ectopia varies widely; it may resemble a mass lesion connected to the kidney. Sonographic findings that are useful in establishing the diagnosis of crossed fused ectopia include extension of the mass anterior to the spine, absence of a kidney in the contralateral renal fossa, and presence of reniform elements within the "mass" (Fig. 68-9). Coexisting urinary tract abnormalities, including

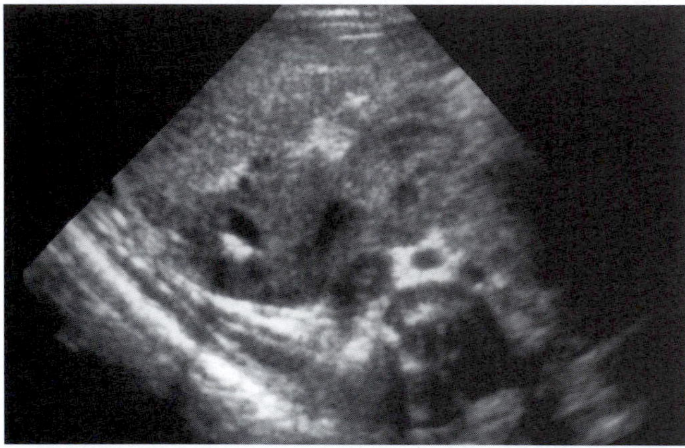

A

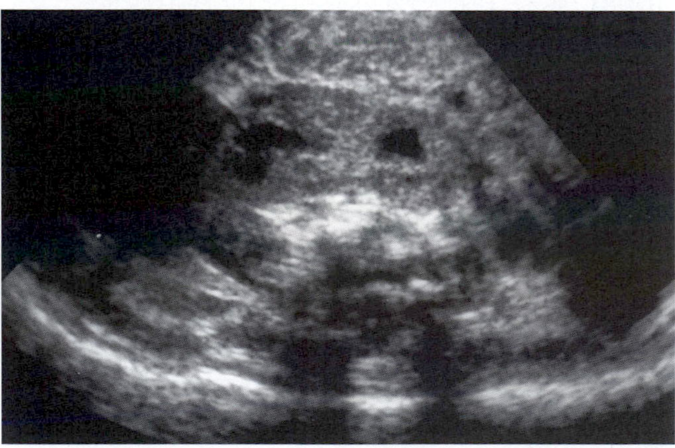

B

FIGURE 68–8. Horseshoe kidney with associated urolithiasis. ***A.*** Transverse view through the right renal fossa demonstrates a calculus within the upper pole of the right kidney. ***B.*** Transverse midline view inferior to ***A*** demonstrates the isthmus, diagnostic of horseshoe kidney.

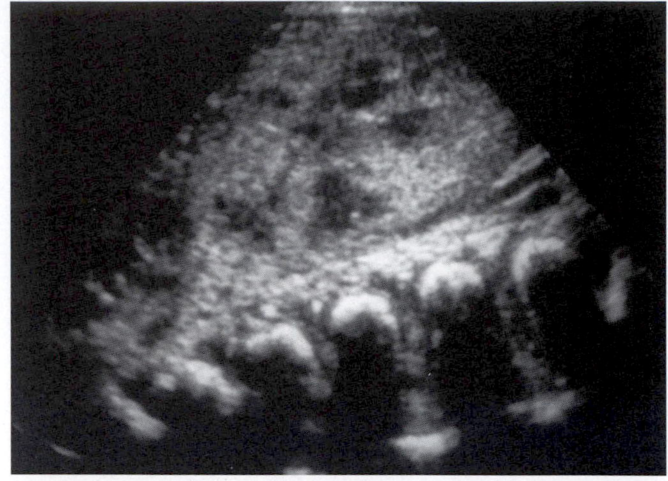

A

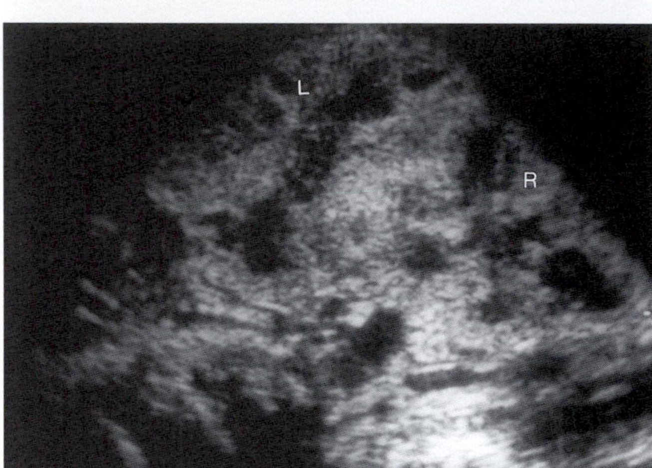

B

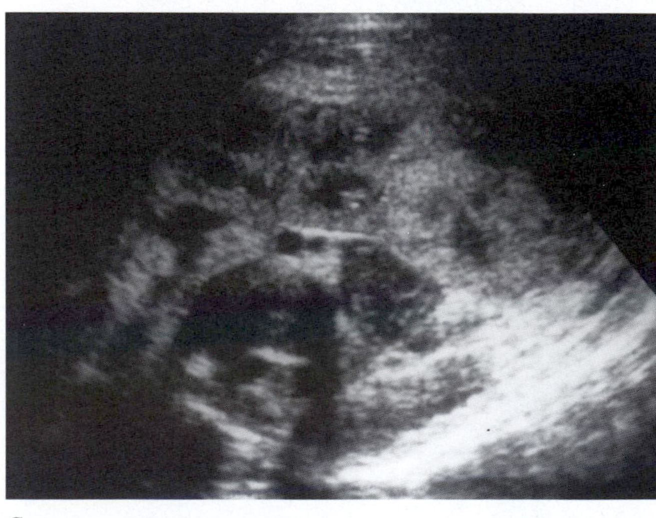

C

FIGURE 68–9. Crossed fused renal ectopia. ***A.*** Longitudinal view through the left renal fossa demonstrates a left kidney oriented in the longitudinal plane. ***B.*** Longitudinal view through the left renal fossa inferior to ***A*** shows fusion of the inferior pole of the left kidney (L) with the superior pole of the right kidney (R). Note that the normal reniform appearance of both kidneys is still present. ***C.*** Transverse view through the midline inferior to ***B*** shows that the inferior kidney is positioned with its long axis in the transverse plane.

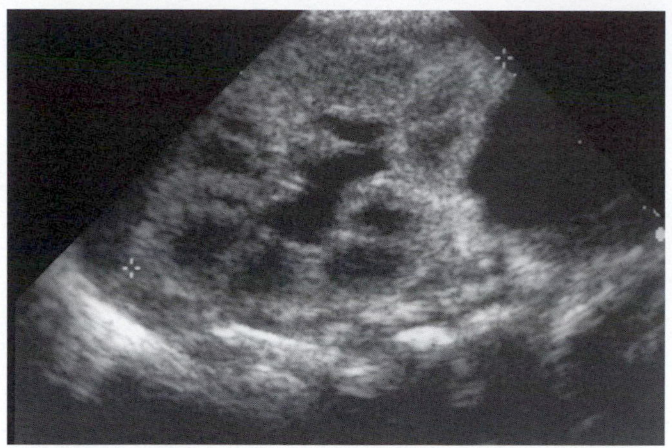

A

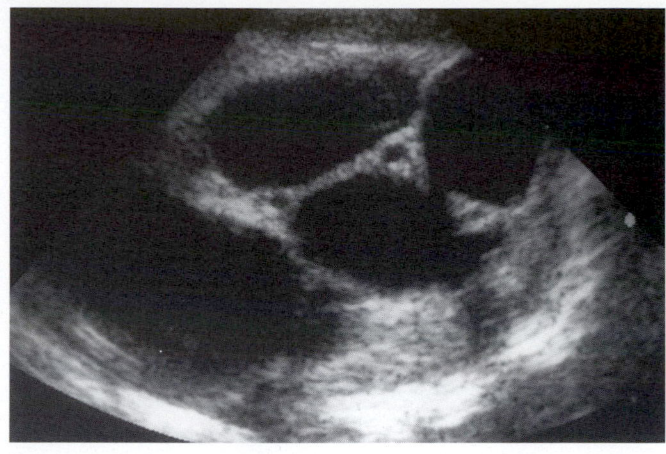

B

FIGURE 68–10. Crossed fused renal ectopia with associated multicystic dysplastic kidney. ***A.*** Longitudinal view through the right renal fossa demonstrates a normal-appearing kidney superiorly (*between electronic calipers*). Note the large cyst inferiorly. ***B.*** Longitudinal view of the right renal fossa inferior to ***A*** demonstrates multiple renal cysts that do not communicate, indicative of multicystic dysplastic kidney of the fused lower renal unit.

obstructive uropathy, renal dysplasia, and urolithiasis, will also be seen more commonly in children with crossed fused ectopia than in the general population (Fig. 68-10).

References

Banerjee B, Brett I: Ultrasound diagnosis of horseshoe kidney. *Br J Radiol* 64:898–900, 1991.

Benchekroun A, Lachkar A, Soumana A, et al: Pathological horseshoe kidney. 30 case reports. *Ann Urol* 32:279–282, 1998.

Boullier J, Chehval MJ, Purcell MH: Removal of a multicystic half of a horseshoe kidney: Significance of preoperative evaluation in identifying abnormal surgical anatomy. *J Pediatr Surg* 27:1244–1246, 1992.

Goodman JD, Norton KI, Carr L, et al: Crossed fused renal ectopia: Sonographic diagnosis. *Urol Radiol* 8:13–16, 1986.

Hohenfellner M, Schultz-Lampel D, Lampel A, et al: Tumor in the horseshoe kidney: Clinical implications and review of embryogenesis. *J Urol* 147:1098–1102, 1992.

Lubat E, Hernanz-Schulman M, Genieser NB, et al: Sonography of the simple and complicated ipsilateral fused kidney. *J Ultrasound Med* 8:109–114, 1989.

McCarthy S, Rosenfeld AT: Ultrasonography in crossed renal ectopia. *J Ultrasound Med* 3:107–112, 1984.

Van Every MJ: In utero detection of horseshoe kidney with unilateral multicystic dysplasia. *Urology* 40:435–437, 1992.

69

Figure 69-1 shows a 1-day-old boy with a palpable abdominal mass. What do you see? What are the diagnostic considerations?

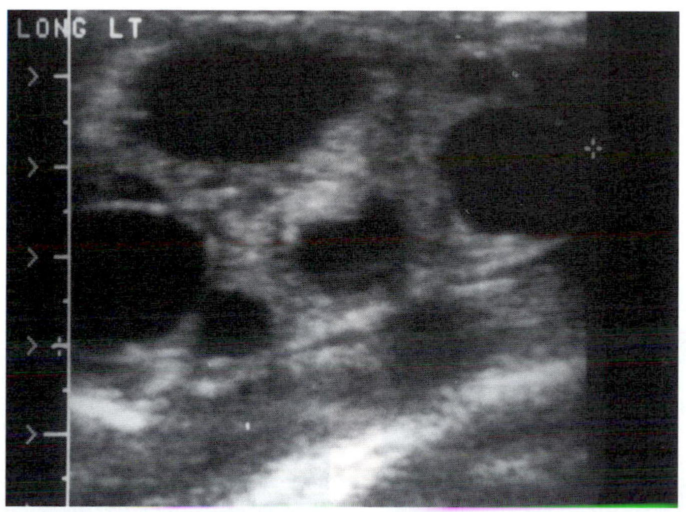

A

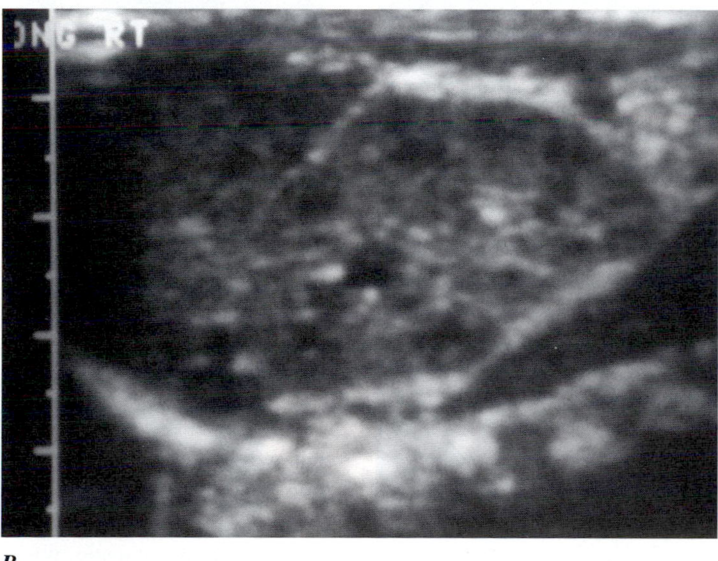

B

FIGURE 69–1. Longitudinal views through the left *(A)* and right *(B)* kidneys.

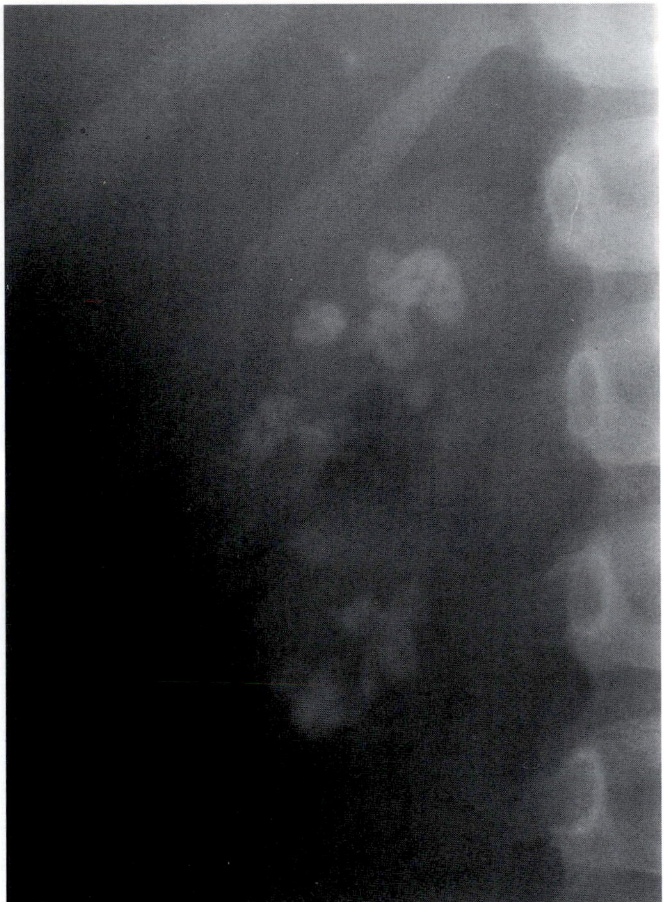

FIGURE 71–6. Medullary nephrocalcinosis on conventional radiography. Magnified spot radiograph of the right abdomen demonstrates severe medullary nephrocalcinosis of the right kidney.

medullary nephrocalcinosis, the abnormality can be seen on abdominal radiography (Fig. 71-6).

Sonography is the modality of choice for monitoring premature infants on furosemide therapy for the development of medullary nephrocalcinosis. Sonographic monitoring is important, since patients will usually be asymptomatic and the condition can be succesfully reversed with treatment (Fig. 71-7). Infants are typically screened at monthly intervals beginning at 4 to 6 weeks of age. The primary treatment of medullary nephrocalcinosis due to furosemide therapy is discontinuation of the furosemide. In some instances a thiazide diuretic is added, which decreases urinary calcium excretion.

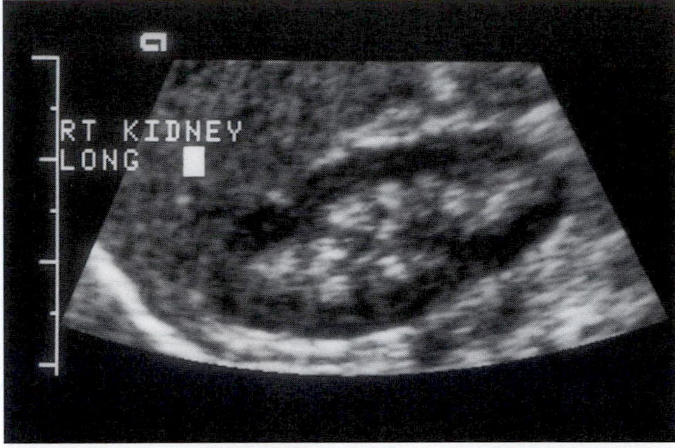

A

B

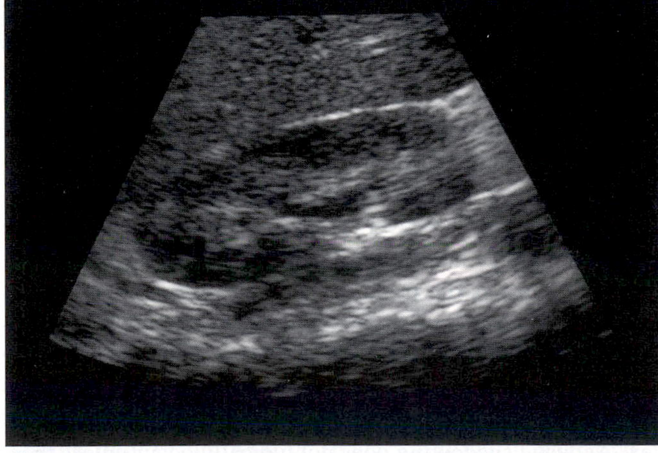

C

FIGURE 71–7. Resolution of medullary nephrocalcinosis. ***A.*** Longitudinal view through the right kidney in a 4-month-old premature infant demonstrates medullary nephrocalcinosis. ***B.*** Longitudinal view through the right kidney on follow-up examination 2 months later demonstrates improvement in the medullary nephrocalcinosis. ***C.*** Longitudinal view through the right kidney on follow-up examination 3 months following the examination in ***B*** shows complete resolution of the medullary nephrocalcinosis.

References

Adams ND, Rowe JC: Nephrocalcinosis. *Clin Perinatol* 19: 179–195, 1992.

Fischer AF, Parker BR, Stevenson DK: Nephrolithiasis following in utero diuretic exposure: An unusual case. *Pediatrics* 81: 712–714, 1988.

Glasier CM, Stoddard RA, Ackerman NB Jr., et al: Nephrolithiasis in infants: Association with chronic furosemide therapy. *AJR* 140:107–108, 1983.

Hernanz-Schulman M: Hyperechoic renal medullary pyramids in infants and children. *Radiology* 181:9–11, 1991.

Hufnagle KG, Khan SN, Penn D, et al: Renal calcifications: A complication of long-term furosemide therapy in preterm infants. *Pediatrics* 70:360–363, 1982.

Jacinto JS, Mondanlou HD, Crade M, et al: Renal calcification incidence in very low weight infants. *Pediatrics* 81:31–35, 1988.

Katz ME, Karlowicz MG, Adelman RD: Nephrocalcinosis in very low birth weight neonates: Sonographic patterns, histologic characteristics and clinical risk factors. *J Ultrasound Med* 13: 777–782, 1994.

Malek RS, Kelalis PP: Pediatric nephrolithiasis. *J Urol* 113: 545–551, 1975.

Matsumoto J, Han BK, de Rovetto CR, Welch TR: Hypercalciuric Bartter syndrome: Resolution of nephrocalcinosis with indomethacin. *AJR* 152:1251–1253, 1989.

Patriquin H, Robitaille P: Renal calcium deposition in children: Sonographic demonstration of the Anderson-Carr progression. *AJR* 146:1253–1256, 1986.

Shultz PK, Strife JL, Strife CF, et al: Hyperechoic renal medullary pyramids in infants and children. *Radiology* 181:163–167, 1991.

Toyoda K, Miyamoto Y, Ida M, et al: Hyperechoic medulla of the kidneys. *Radiology* 173:431–434, 1989.

72

Figure 72-1 shows a 6-year-old girl with acute flank pain. What do you see? What are the diagnostic considerations?

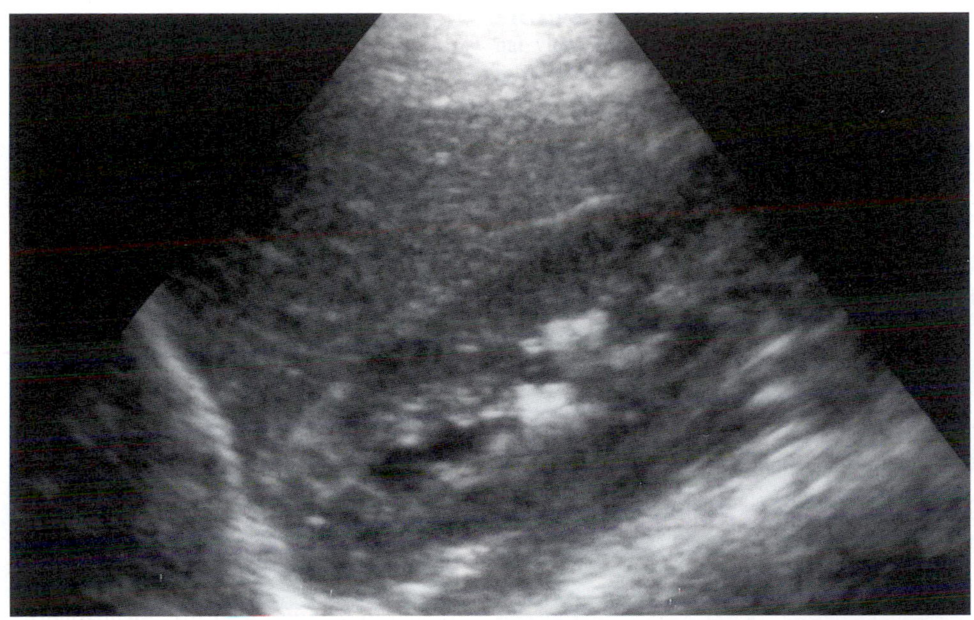

A

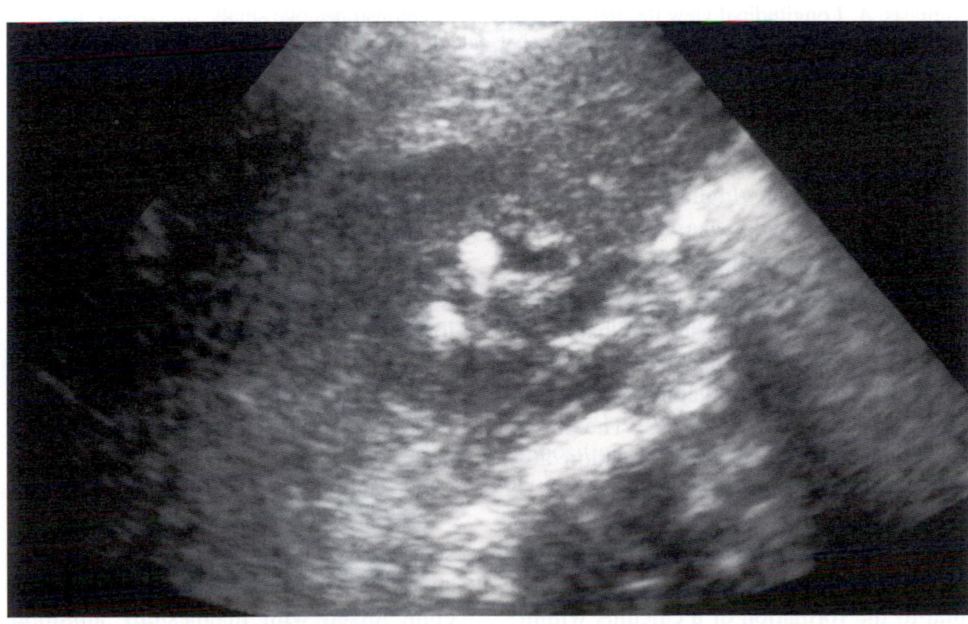

B

FIGURE 72–1. Longitudinal *(A)* and transverse *(B)* views through the right kidney.

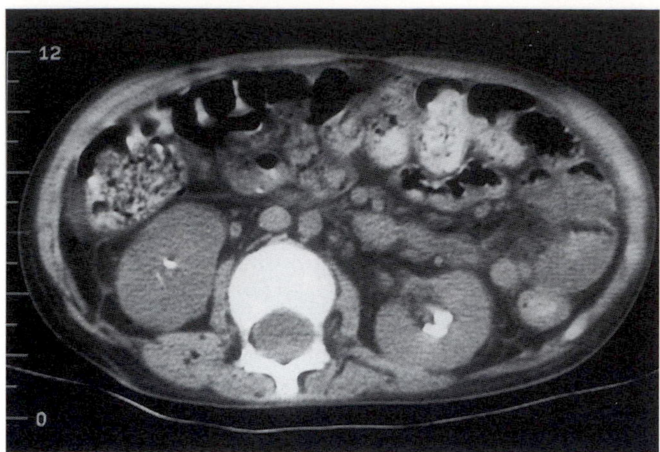

FIGURE 72–6. Unenhanced helical computed tomography (CT) scan of urolithiasis. Unenhanced helical CT through the kidneys demonstrates bilateral calculi.

ment of the obstruction. Additionally, sonography may underestimate partial obstruction if the child is dehydrated.

In recent years, unenhanced helical computed tomography (CT) has been shown to be valuable in the assessment of children with suspected urolithiasis. Computed tomography has become the examination of choice in children with acute flank pain in whom a diagnosis is uncertain. It can accurately determine the presence of renal, ureteral, or bladder calculi (Fig. 72-6). The high sensitivity and specificity of CT in the detection of ureteral calculi is particularly appealing, as the ureter is a difficult area to examine with sonography. Additionally, CT allows for the assessment of extraurinary causes of acute flank pain.

References

Banner MP, Pollack HM: Urolithiasis in the lower urinary tract. *Semin Roentgenol* 17:140–148, 1982.

Dyer RB, Chen MY, Zagoria RJ: Abnormal calcifications in the urinary tract. *Radiographics* 18:1405–1424, 1998.

Erwin BC, Carroll BA, Sommer FG: Renal colic: The role of ultrasound in initial evaluation. *Radiology* 152:147–150, 1984.

Gros DA, Thakkar RN, Lakshmanan Y, et al: Urolithiasis in spina bifida. *Eur J Pediatr Surg* 8:68–69, 1998.

Haddad M, Sharif HS, Shahed MS, et al: Renal colic: Diagnosis and outcome. *Radiology* 184:83–88, 1992.

Kronner KM, Casale AJ, Cain MP, et al: Bladder calculi in the pediatric augmented bladder. *J Urol* 160:1096–1098, 1998.

Remer EM, Herts BR, Streem SB, et al: Spiral noncontrast CT versus combined plain radiography and renal US after extracorporeal shock wave lithotripsy: Cost-identification analysis. *Radiology* 204:33–37, 1997.

Saita H, Matsukawa M, Fukushima H, et al: Ultrasound diagnosis of ureteral stones: Its usefulness with subsequent excretory urography. *J Urol* 140:28–31, 1988.

Santos-Victoriano M, Brohard BH, Cunningham RJ: Renal stone disease in children. *Clin Pediatr* 37:583–599, 1998.

Smith RC, Verga M, McCarthy S, et al: Diagnosis of acute flank pain: Value of unenhanced helical CT. *AJR* 166:97–101, 1996.

Sommer FG, Jeffrey RB, Rubin GD, et al: Detection of ureteral calculi in patients with suspected renal colic: Value of reformatted noncontrast helical CT. *AJR* 165:509–513, 1995.

Sperrin MW, Rogers K: The architecture and composition of uroliths. *Br J Urol* 82:781–784, 1998.

Terai A, Ueda T, Kakehi Y, et al: Urinary calculi as a late complication of the Indiana continent urinary diversion: Comparison with the Kock pouch procedure. *J Urol* 155:66–68, 1996.

Van Arsdalen KN: Pathogenesis of renal calculi. *Urol Radiol* 6:65–73, 1984.

73

Figure 73-1 shows a 1-month-old male with a urinary tract infection. What do you see? What are the diagnostic considerations?

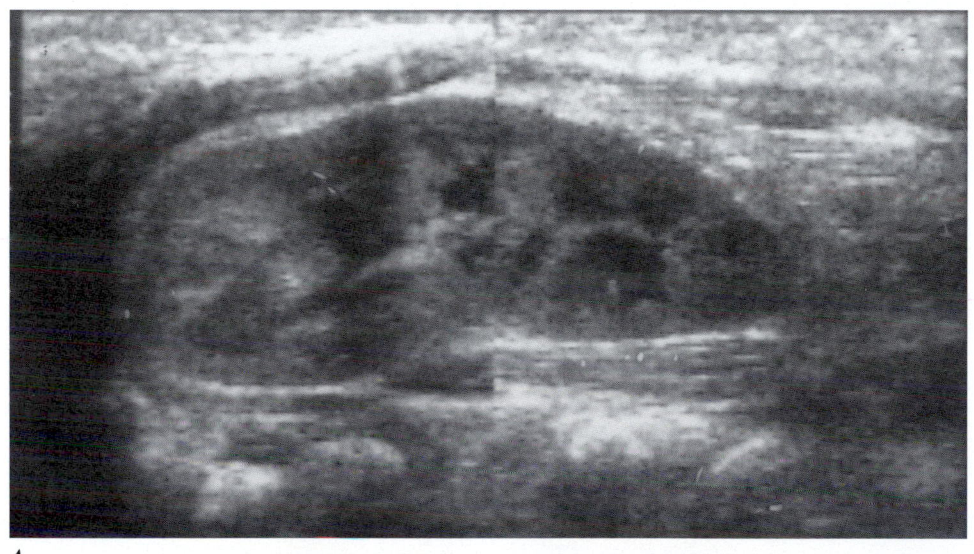

A

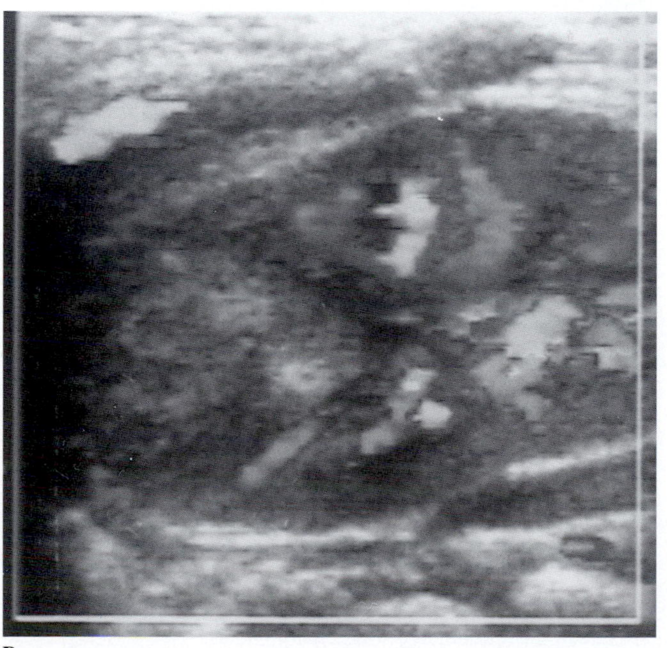

B

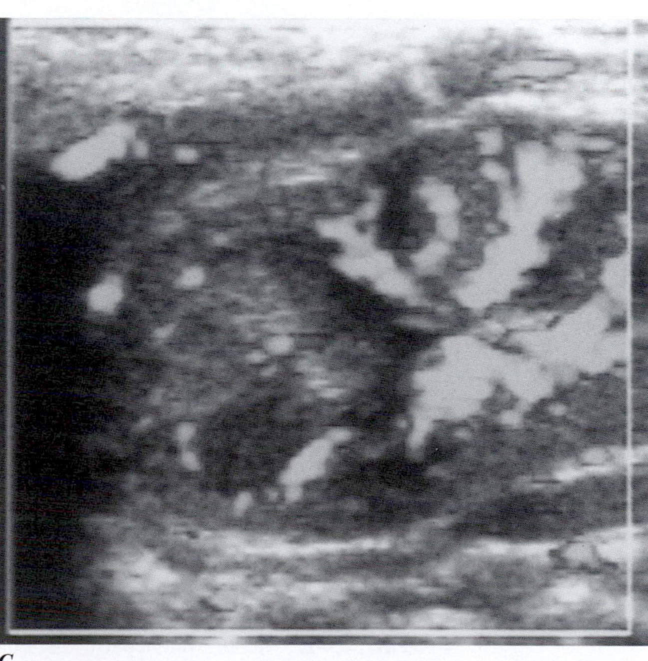

C

FIGURE 73–1. Longitudinal views of the left kidney with gray-scale sonography ***(A),*** color Doppler sonography ***(B),*** and power color Doppler sonography ***(C).*** (See Color Plate 20.)

CHAPTER 73

Acute Pyelonephritis

LYNNE RUESS

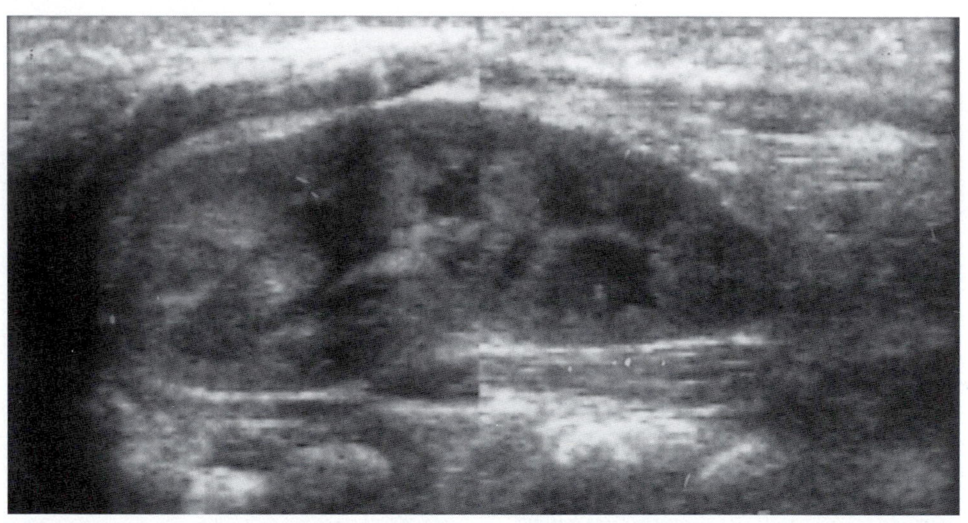

A

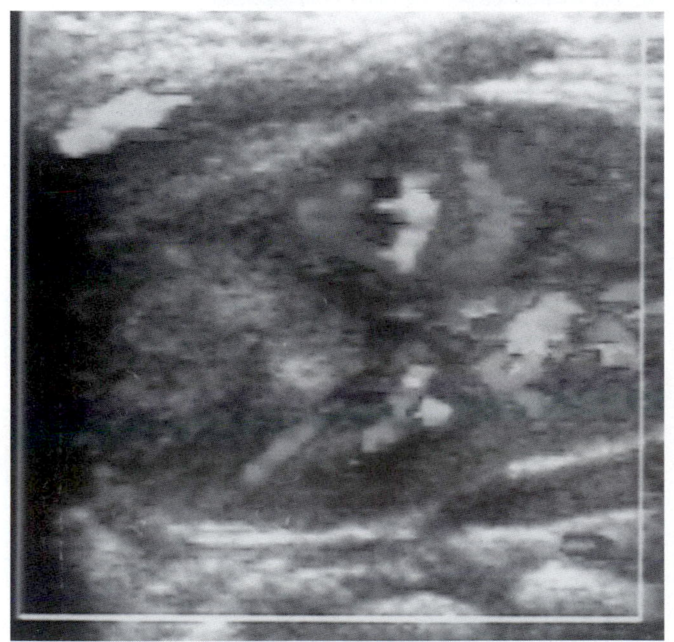

B

C

FIGURE 73–2. Acute pyelonephritis. ***A.*** Longitudinal view of the left kidney shows enlargement of the left upper pole, with increased echogenicity and loss of normal corticomedullary differentiation. ***B.*** Longitudinal view of the left kidney in the same patient with color Doppler shows decreased vascularity in the left upper pole. ***C.*** Longitudinal view of the left kidney in the same patient with power Doppler also shows decreased vascularity in the left upper pole, consistent with acute pyelonephritis. (See Color Plate 21.)

Urinary tract infection (UTI) is common in children. The imaging evaluation of a child with a UTI typically includes sonography of the urinary tract, including the kidneys and bladder. Sonography is performed in children with a UTI primarily to demonstrate structural anomalies that can predispose to infection, including obstructive uropathy and other congenital abnormalities. Sonography also can demonstrate acute renal parenchymal infection (acute pyelonephritis) (Fig. 73-2; see also Color Plate 21) and complications of acute renal infection, such as pyonephrosis, renal abscess formation, and perinephric spread of infection. This has clinical relevance, since the diagnosis of acute pyelonephritis on the basis of clinical and laboratory findings alone can be difficult. There are gray-scale sonographic abnormalities that suggest pyelonephritis; however, sonography is a less sensitive imaging modality for the diagnosis than renal cortical scintigraphy or computed tomography (CT). Therefore, renal cortical scintigraphy or CT is the preferred modality for the evaluation of this condition. Gray-scale sonography allows detection of acute pyelonephritis in less than half the cases. The addition of color Doppler and power Doppler imaging increases the sensitivity of sonography for the diagnosis of acute pyelonephritis (Fig. 73-2). However, sonography utilizing the Doppler technique still remains relatively insensitive for the diagnosis, missing approximately one-third to one-fourth of cases of acute pyelonephritis.

Acute bacterial pyelonephritis is characterized by focal, multifocal, or generalized renal involvement. The infection of renal parenchyma results in edema and obstruction of collecting tubules in inflamed areas. Consequently, this is associated with intense vasoconstriction of peripheral arterioles in these areas. The resultant regional decrease in renal cortical perfusion is thought to be the explanation for areas of decreased flow on color Doppler sonography (Fig. 73-2; see also Color Plate 21), photopenia on renal cortical scintigraphy (Fig. 73-3) and decreased parenchymal enhancement on contrast-enhanced CT examination in children with acute pyelonephritis (Fig. 73-4).

The areas of edema that characterize acute bacterial pyelonephritis may result in increased renal size, abnormal echotexture, and decreased corticomedullary differentiation on sonography (Fig. 73-2). These changes result from the edema that accompanies acute pyelonephritis. Increased renal size may be focal or diffuse. A diffuse increase in renal size may be quantified on sonography by measuring renal length or renal volume and comparing the obtained values with age-specific tables. The renal echotexture may be focally increased or decreased relative to normal parenchyma in acute pyelonephritits (Fig. 73-2).

Color and power Doppler imaging increase the sensitivity for detecting pyelonephritis by detecting segmental renal perfusion abnormalities. Color and power Doppler imaging allow evaluation of regional blood flow in the interlobar and interlobular arteries. In acute pyelonephritis, there is decreased Doppler signal in the inflamed regions of the kidney, consistent with the relative hypoperfusion of the affected renal cortex (Fig. 73-2). The affected area or areas often have a wedge, or triangular, shape.

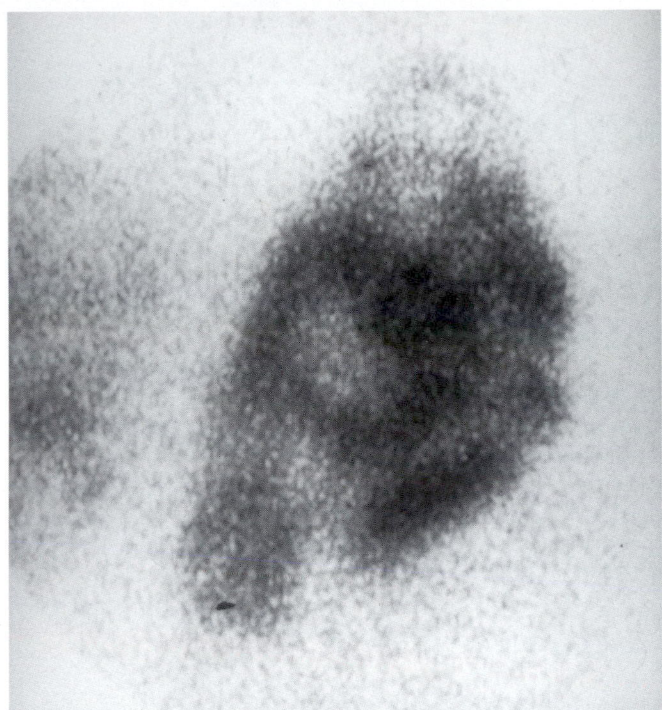

A

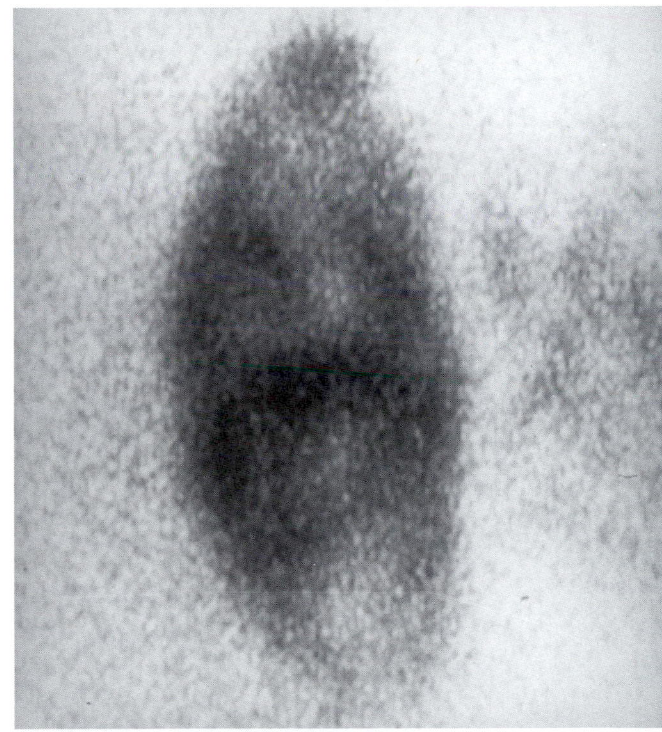

B

FIGURE 73–3. Acute multifocal pyelonephritis. Posterior oblique views of the left *(A)* and right *(B)* kidneys from a dimercaptosuccinic acid (DMSA) scan demonstrate multiple photopenic defects, consistent with multifocal pyelonephritis.

The renal parenchyma rapidly returns to normal following treatment of acute pyelonephritis (Fig. 73-5). One series reported a normalization of renal length in an average of 11 days. Another report demonstrated a reduction in renal

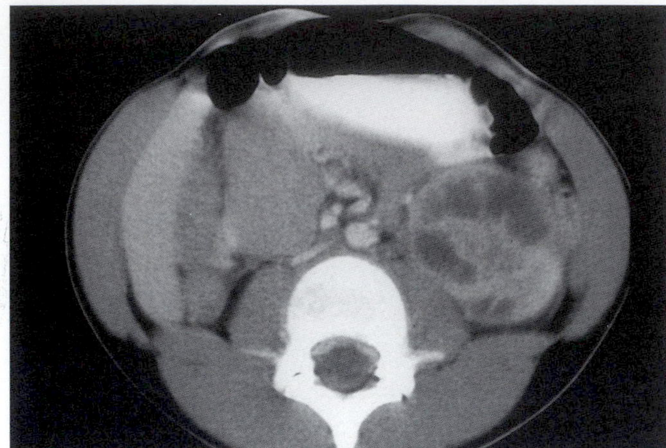

FIGURE 73–4. Acute multifocal pyelonephritis. Contrast-enhanced computed tomography scan through the left kidney demonstrates multiple peripheral low-attenuation areas, indicative of multifocal pyelonephritis.

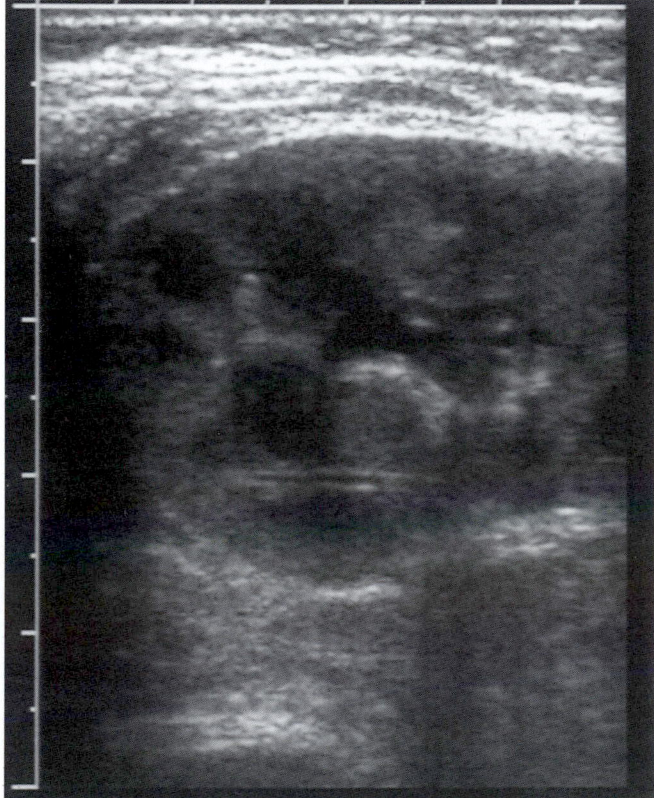

FIGURE 73–5. Resolving pyelonephritis. Follow-up evaluation 2 weeks later of the left kidney in the same patient as in Fig. 73-1. Longitudinal view of the left kidney now shows a normal-appearing kidney. Color and power Doppler imaging of this kidney were also normal.

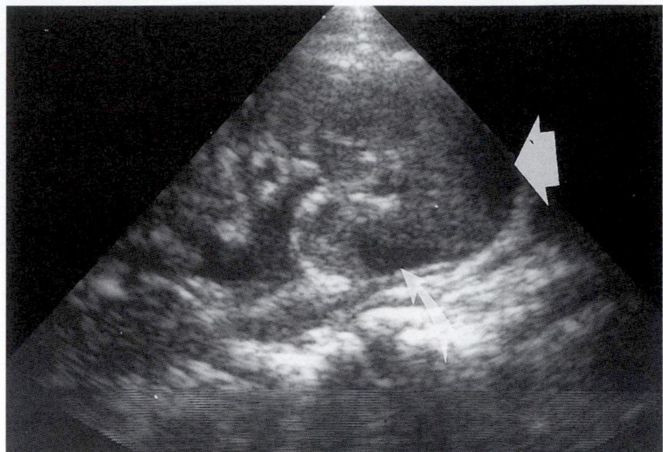

A

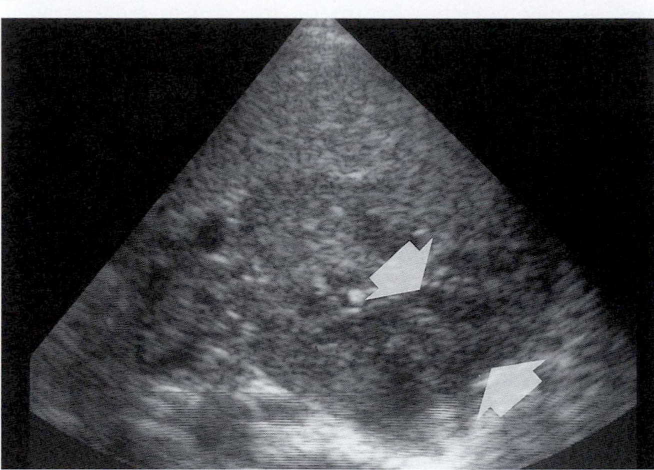

B

FIGURE 73–6. Renal abscess. Longitudinal ***(A)*** and transverse ***(B)*** views of the left kidney demonstrate focal enlargement of the lower pole, indicative of acute pyelonephritis (*straight arrows*). The area of abnormality is relatively hypoechoic relative to normal renal parenchyma. However, note the small triangular anechoic area, indicative of a small abscess (*curved arrow*).

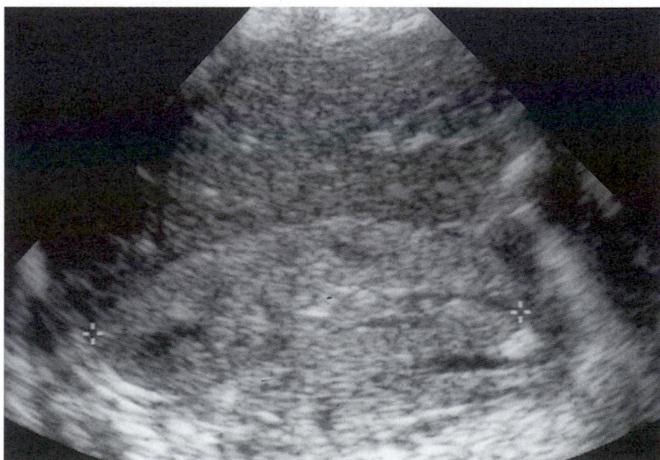

FIGURE 73–7. Acute pyelonephritis due to *Candida albicans*. Longitudinal view of the right kidney in an immunosuppressed patient demonstrates a diffusely enlarged, echogenic kidney with loss of normal corticomedullary differentiation. Blood and urine cultures were positive for *C. albicans*. Note that the right kidney is hyperechoic relative to the hepatic parenchyma.

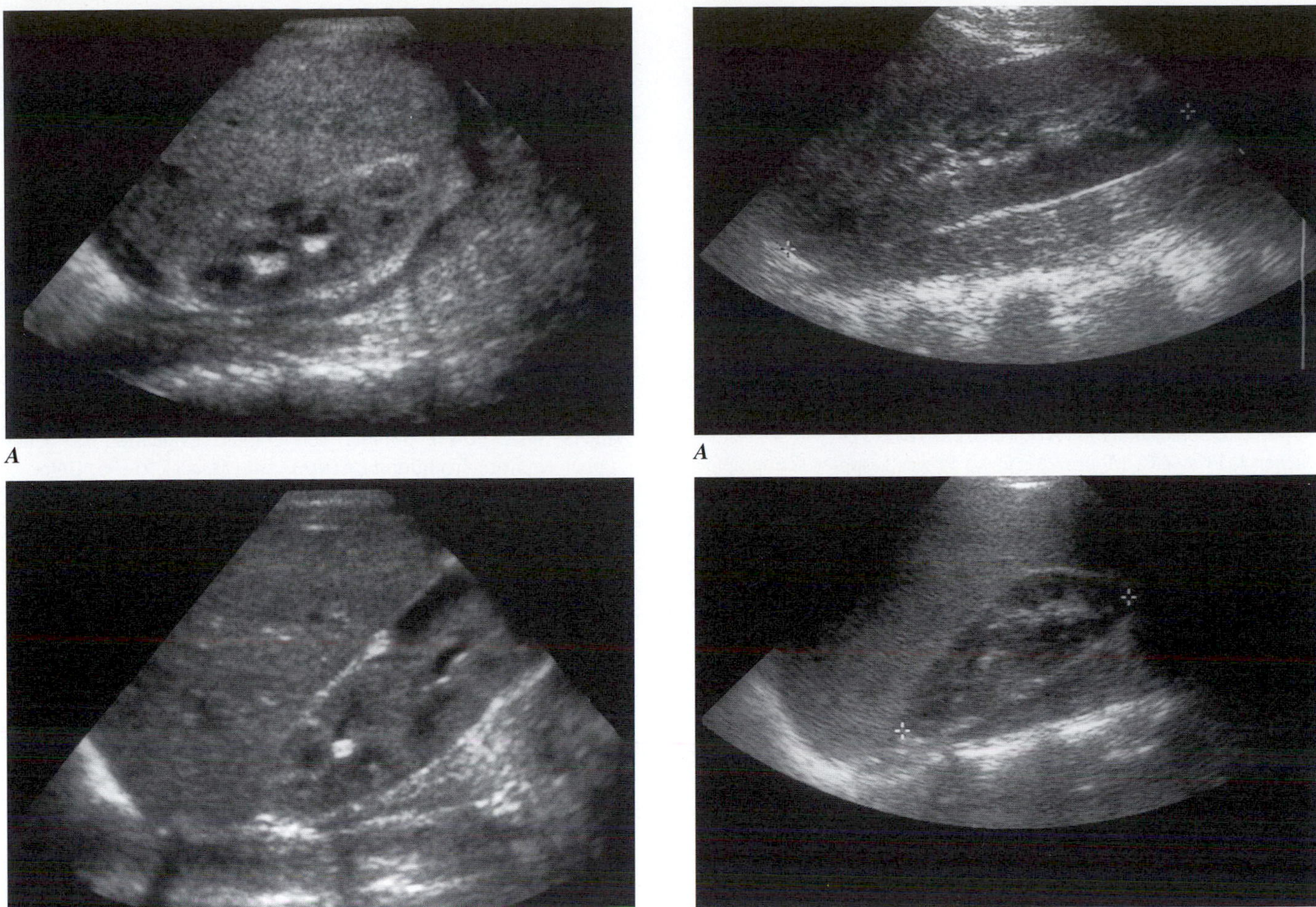

FIGURE 73–8. Fungal abscess ("fungus ball") in renal collecting system. ***A.*** Longitudinal view through the right kidney in a child with disseminated *Candida* infection demonstrates two echogenic foci within the right intrarenal collecting system, consistent with fungus balls or small fungal abscesses. ***B.*** Longitudinal view through the right kidney in the same child 1 month later demonstrates calcification of one of the previously seen fungus balls. Note the acoustic shadowing posteriorly. The other lesion is no longer identified.

FIGURE 73–9. Global renal scarring. Longitudinal views through the right ***(A)*** and left ***(B)*** kidneys demonstrate discrepant renal sizes. The left kidney is significantly smaller than the right kidney, which is normal for the child's age. The child has had several prior episodes of left-sided pyelonephritis that resulted in severe renal scarring.

volume by approximately 60 percent within 2 weeks. The renal parenchymal echotexture also rapidly returns to normal (Fig. 73-5). Rapid resolution of hypoperfusion defects on color and power Doppler imaging has also been observed, with normalization of flow to the renal cortex in involved areas.

The distinction between acute pyelonephritis and renal abscess can occasionally be difficult on sonography. Both acute pyelonephritis and renal abscess will demonstrate an area of decreased vascularity on color Doppler examination. On gray-scale sonographic examination, a renal abscess typically has a complex appearance. It may demonstrate anechoic areas (Fig. 73-6) or debris, and occasionally has debris-fluid levels. However, there may be some overlap between the two conditions, and CT may be needed to make the distinction between acute pyelonephritis and smaller renal abscesses.

Diffuse renal involvement is often seen in children with acute pyelonephritis due to infection by fungi such as *Candida*. Renal involvement in fungal infection is typically diffuse, with multiple microabscesses in the renal cortex, interstitium, and tubules. On sonography, diffusely enlarged, echogenic kidneys may be identified (Fig. 73-7). Additionally, there may be development of fungal abscesses or "fungus balls" in the renal pelvis or the bladder (Fig. 73-8).

Children are at increased risk for developing renal scarring after upper urinary tract infection. Approximately one-half of children with acute pyelonephritis will develop renal scars. The scars develop solely at sites of prior acute pyelonephritis. The development of renal scarring correlates with the severity of the initial infection. It is also age-dependent. Renal scarring is more likely to develop following acute pyelonephritis in younger children. New areas of scarring are uncommon after the age of 6 years. Renal scintigraphy is the preferred method of evaluating for renal scars. Sonography is relatively insensitive for the identification of renal scarring unless the scarring is extensive. Renal scarring is identified on sonography as a focal area of cortical loss. The kidney may also be smaller than anticipated for age and show less than expected growth when compared to earlier studies in the same child or compared to the contralateral kidney (Fig. 73-9).

References

Bjorgvinsson E, Majd M, Eggli KD: Diagnosis of acute pyelonephritis in children: Comparison of sonography and 99m-Tc-DMSA scintigraphy. *AJR* 157:539–543, 1991.

Clautice-Engle T, Jeffrey RB Jr: Renal hypoperfusion: Value of power Doppler imaging. *AJR* 168:1227–1231, 1997.

Dacher J, Pfister C, Monroc M, et al: Power Doppler sonographic pattern of acute pyelonephritis in children: Comparison with CT. *AJR* 166:1451–1455, 1996.

Dinkle E, Orth S, Dittirch M, et al: Renal sonography in the differentiation of upper from lower urinary tract infection. *AJR* 146:775–780, 1986.

Eggli KD, Eggli D: Color Doppler sonography in pyelonephritis. *Pediatr Radiol* 22:422–425, 1992.

Kirpeker M, Abiri MM, Hilfer C, et al: Ultrasound in the diagnosis of systemic candidiasis (renal and cranial) in very low birth weight premature infants. *Pediatr Radiol* 16:17–20, 1986.

Lavocat MP, Granjon D, Allard D, et al: Imaging of pyelonephritis. *Pediatr Radiol* 27:159–165, 1997.

Pickworth FE, Carlin JB, Ditchfield MR, et al: Sonographic measurement of renal enlargement in children with acute pyelonephritis and time needed for resolution: Implications for renal growth assessment. *AJR* 165:405–408, 1995.

Roberts JA: Etiology and pathophysiology of pyelonephritis. *Am J Kidney Dis* 17:1–9, 1991.

Siegel MJ, Glasier CM: Acute focal bacterial nephritis in children: Significance of ureteral reflux. *AJR* 137:257–260, 1981.

Winters WD: Power doppler sonographic evaluation of acute pyelonephritis in children. *J Ultrasound Med* 15:91–96, 1996.

74

Figure 74-1 shows a 10-month-old boy with a palpable left flank mass. What do you see? What are the diagnostic considerations?

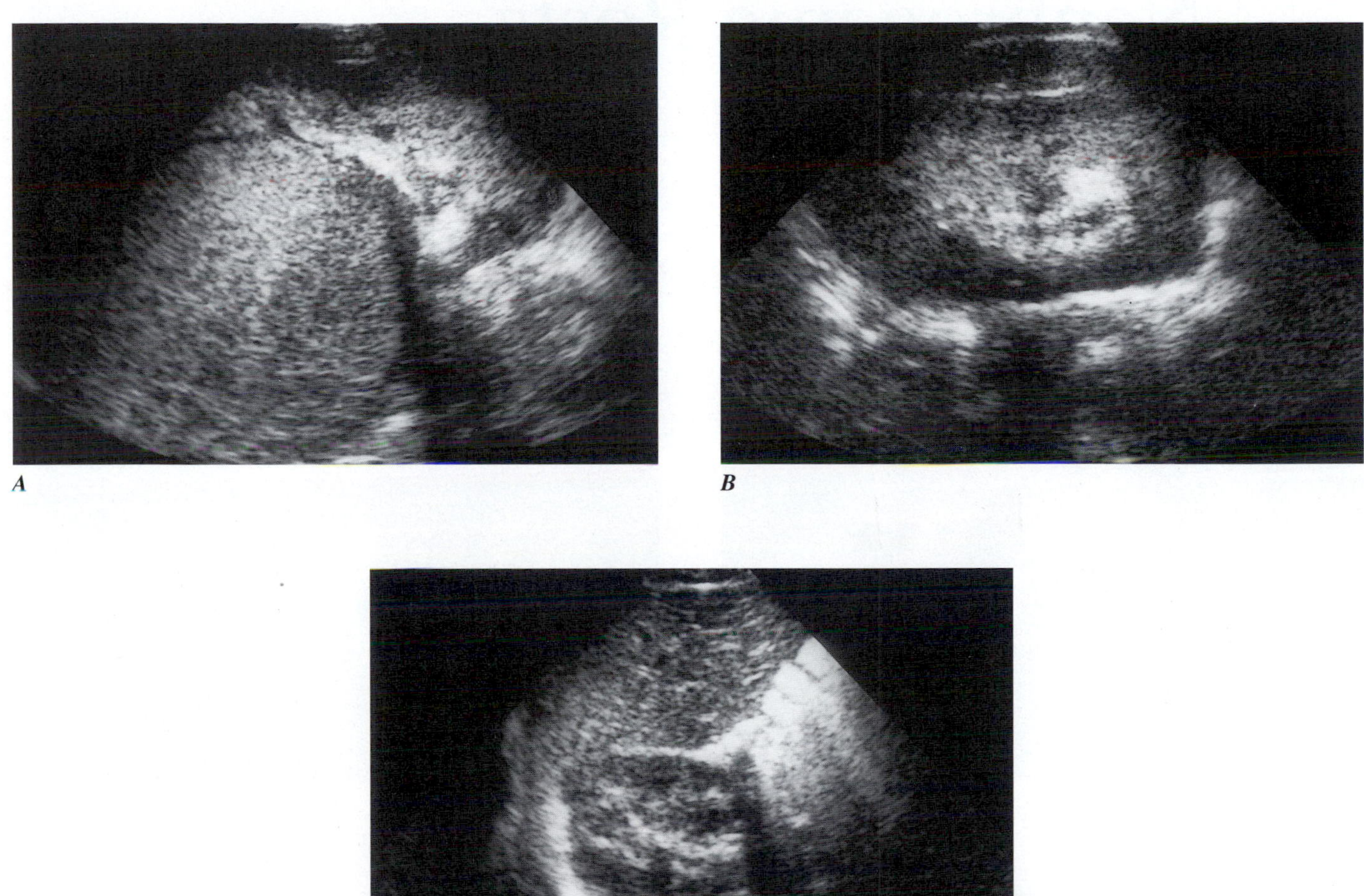

FIGURE 74–1. Longitudinal views through the medial *(A)* and lateral *(B)* regions of the left kidney and a transverse view through the right kidney *(C)*.

CHAPTER 74

Wilms' Tumor with Bilateral Nephrogenic Rests

MELISSA T. MYERS

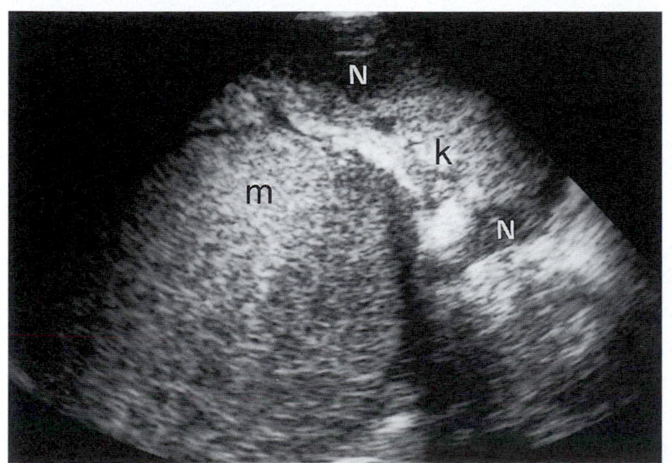

A

B

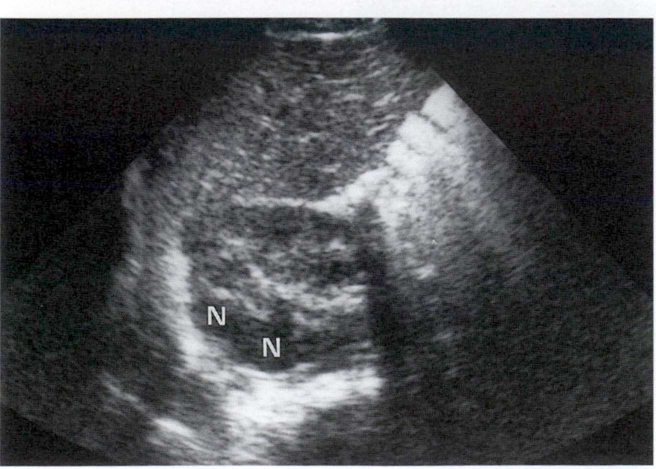

C

FIGURE 74–2. Wilms' tumor with bilateral nephrogenic rests. ***A.*** Longitudinal view through the medial portion of the left kidney shows a large, well-defined, echogenic mass (m) arising from the medial aspect of the left kidney (k). Inferior to the large mass is a smaller rind of hypoechoic tissue (N), representing perilobar nephrogenic rests. ***B.*** Longitudinal view through the lateral portion of the same kidney also demonstrates a rind of hypoechoic tissue, representing perilobar nephrogenic rests (N). ***C.*** Transverse view of the right kidney shows subtle hypoechoic lesions at the periphery of the kidney, representing additional nephrogenic rests. Note that these lesions are smaller and less confluent than those on the left.

Wilms' tumor is the most common renal tumor in childhood. It is seen primarily in young children, with the mean age at presentation being between 2 and 3 years. The occurrence of

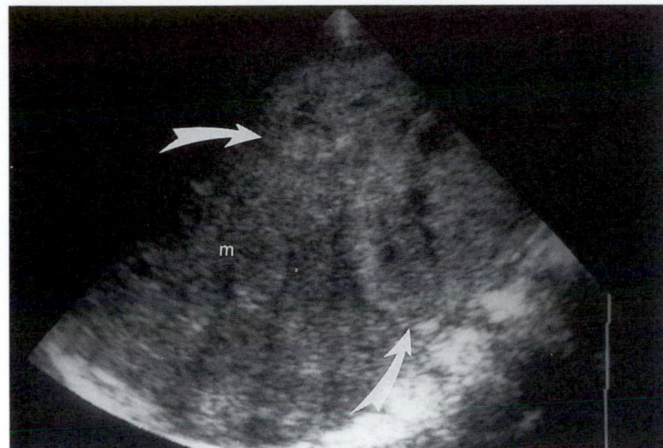

FIGURE 74–3. Wilms' tumor with the "claw" sign. Transverse view through the right kidney demonstrates a large intrarenal mass (m). Note the rim of renal parenchyma anteriorly and posteriorly (*arrows*).

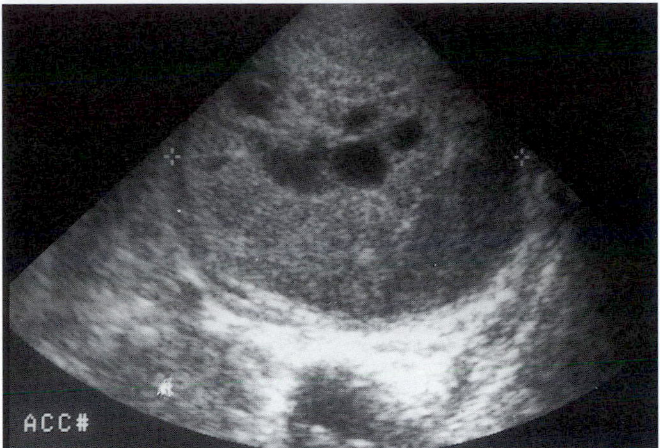

A

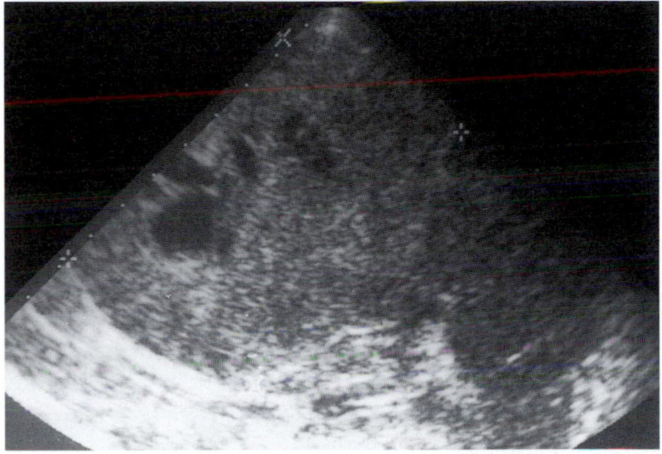

B

FIGURE 74–4. Wilms' tumor with internal anechoic regions indicative of necrosis. Transverse ***(A)*** and longitudinal ***(B)*** views through the left kidney demonstrate a complex renal mass (*between electronic calipers*) with anechoic regions that represent areas of liquefaction necrosis.

Wilms' tumor is associated with various congenital anomalies, including hemihypertrophy, Beckwith-Wiedemann syndrome (consisting of macroglossia, omphalocele, and visceromegaly), sporadic aniridia, Drash syndrome, Bloom syndrome, and trisomy 18. A Wilms' tumor is usually large at the time of initial diagnosis. The neoplasm may be bilateral. It is noted in both kidneys in approximately 10 percent of cases. Bilateral tumors are usually synchronous but may be metachronous.

Wilms' tumor is an embryonal neoplasm that arises from persistent metanephric blastemal cells, known as nephrogenic rests. Nephrogenic rests can be separated into two distinct types based upon their location within the kidney. Anatomically, the kidney is divided into lobes that constitute a medullary pyramid and its associated renal cortical mantle. Perilobar nephrogenic rests are located at the periphery of the renal lobe (Fig. 74-2), while intralobar nephrogenic rests are located anywhere within the renal lobe. Nephrogenic rests are presumed to be potential precursors to the development of Wilms' tumor, although the rests themselves are not malignant. It is felt that some nephrogenic rests remain dormant, others regress, and still others grow and have the potential to degenerate into Wilms' tumors. Multiple sites of macroscopic nephrogenic rests distributed throughout the kidneys are also referred to as nephroblastomatosis. Nephrogenic rests are found in approximately 1 percent of autopsies on newborns. However, it is rare to find them beyond infancy in normal individuals. Conversely, they are found in approximately 40 percent of children with unilateral Wilms' tumor and nearly all of those children with bilateral Wilms' tumor. When nephrogenic rests are noted in association with Wilms' tumor, they are observed either adjacent to the tumor or distributed throughout the kidneys.

Children with Wilms' tumor present most frequently with a palpable abdominal mass. Occasionally, they may manifest systemic signs, including abdominal pain, malaise, anorexia, weight loss, and fever. Hematuria is observed in approximately one-fourth of children with Wilms' tumor at the time of initial presentation. Gross hematuria is suggestive of tumor invasion of the renal pelvis or renal vein. Hypertension may also be present due to increased renin production by the tumor.

Sonography is often the initial imaging modality performed in children with neuroblastoma. A normal sonographic examination in a child with a suspected abdominal mass is useful in excluding a mass lesion. The characteristic sonographic finding in Wilms' tumor is that of a large, solid mass with a well-defined margin or pseudocapsule (Fig. 74-2). The intrarenal location of the mass is confirmed by demonstrating a rim of normal renal tissue surrounding the lesion (Fig. 74-3). This is referred to as the "claw" sign. The mass may be homogeneous in echotexture or heterogeneous due to hemorrhage or necrosis within it. Cystic areas representing tumor necrosis are occasionally noted within the mass (Fig. 74-4). Calcifications are uncommonly noted. Wilms' tumor may extend to regional lymph nodes or into the renal vein and inferior vena cava. Therefore, these vessels

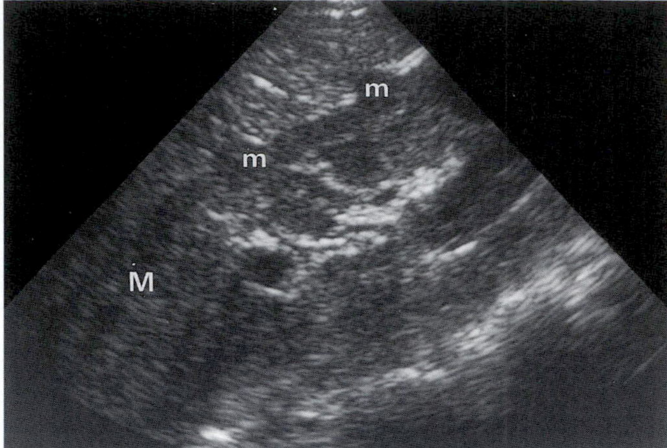

FIGURE 74–5. Nephrogenic rests. Longitudinal view through the right kidney demonstrates multiple small nephrogenic rests. Note the larger rest in the upper pole (M) and the smaller rests in the mid and lower poles (m).

should be closely scrutinized for the presence of tumor thrombus.

The imaging evaluation of a child with suspected Wilms' tumor should also include careful assessment of the contralateral kidney for associated tumor or nephrogenic rests. Perilobar nephrogenic rests will appear on sonography as small, peripheral hypoechoic masses (Fig. 74-2), while intralobar rests will be distributed throughout the renal parenchyma. The lesions may be isoechoic and difficult to detect on sonography (Fig. 74-5). The only finding may be a nodular or scalloped renal surface.

Contrast-enhanced computed tomography (CT) is used to stage patients with Wilms' tumor because it provides an overview of the intraabdominal extent of the tumor and also

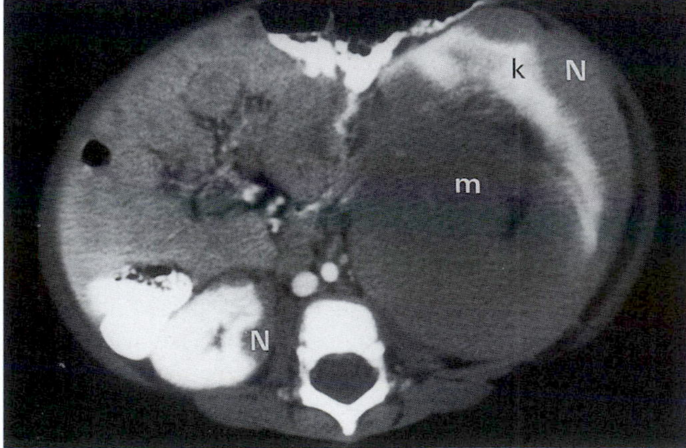

FIGURE 74–6. Wilms' tumor and nephrogenic rests on computed tomography (CT). Contrast-enhanced CT scan demonstrates a large, heterogeneous mass, representing a Wilms' tumor (m) at the medial aspect of the left kidney (k), and a homogeneous, low-attenuation rind laterally, representing nephrogenic rests (N). Note the compressed functioning renal tissue sandwiched in between. There are also nephrogenic rests (N) in the medial aspect of the right kidney.

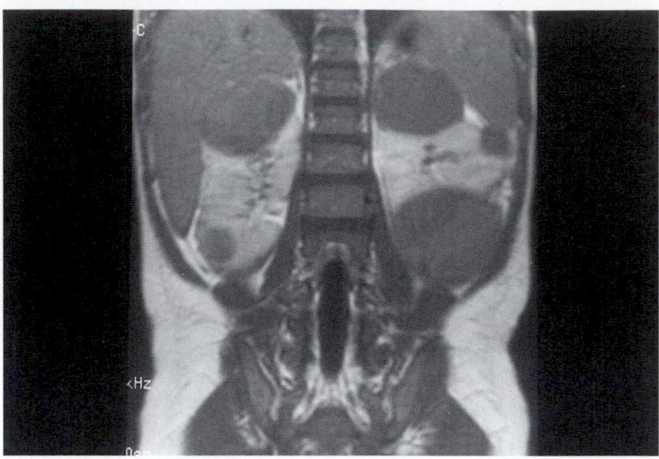

FIGURE 74–7. Bilateral Wilms' tumors and nephrogenic rests. Magnetic resonance imaging shows one large mass and one small mass in the right kidney and two large masses and one small mass in the left kidney. At biopsy, the three large renal masses were noted to be Wilms' tumors, while the smaller lesions were noted to be nephrogenic rests.

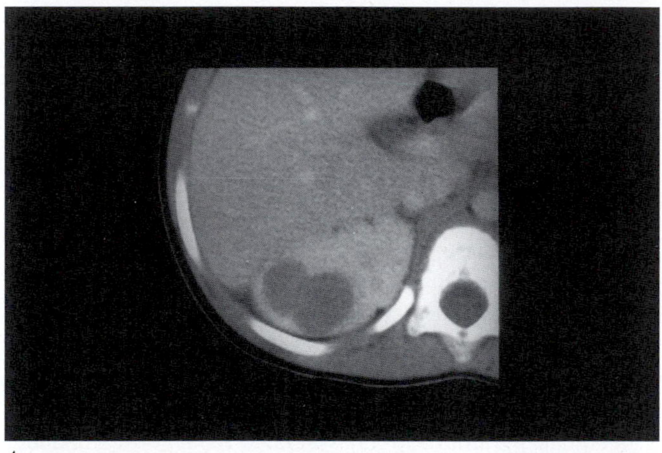

A

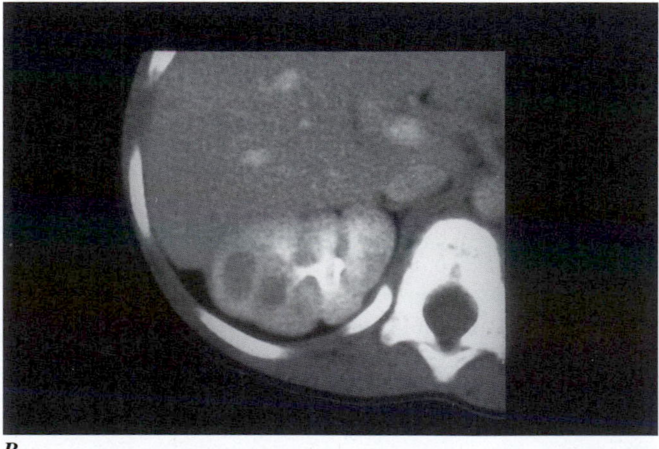

B

FIGURE 74–8. Size regression of nephrogenic rests. ***A.*** Magnified view of a contrast-enhanced computed tomography (CT) section through the right kidney demonstrates two rounded, homogeneous, low-attenuation lesions. Biopsy of one of the lesions demonstrated that these were intralobar nephrogenic rests. ***B.*** Magnified view of a contrast-enhanced CT section through the right kidney in the same child 9 months later shows interval size regression of both lesions.

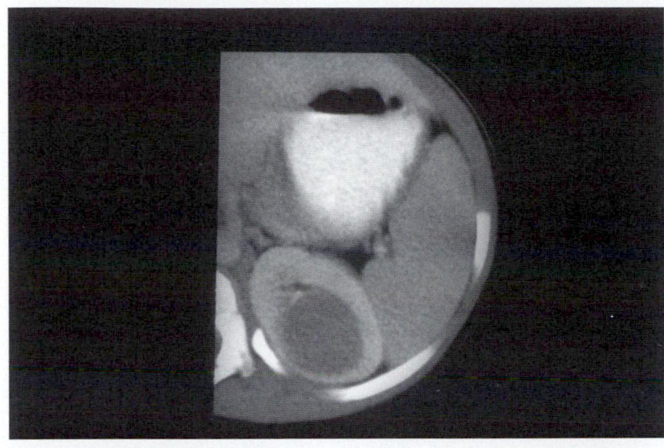

A

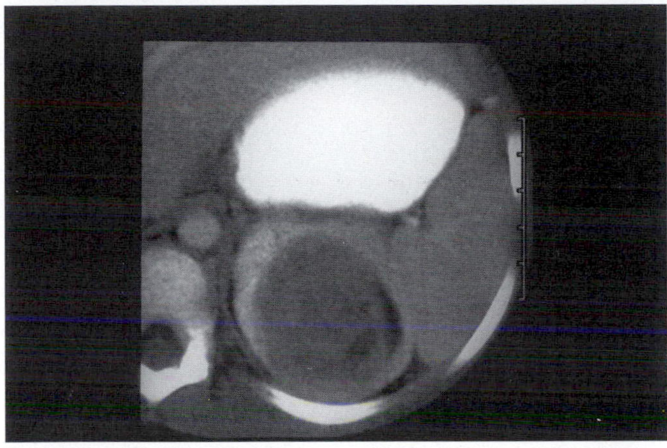

B

FIGURE 74–9. Degeneration of nephrogenic rest into Wilms' tumor. ***A.*** Magnified view of a contrast-enhanced computed tomography (CT) section through the left kidney demonstrates a rounded, homogeneous, low-attenuation mass that at biopsy was noted to be a nephrogenic rest. ***B.*** Magnified view of a contrast-enhanced CT section through the left kidney in the same child 6 months later demonstrates interval growth of the lesion. Additionally, note that the mass now has heterogeneous attenuation. At biopsy, Wilms' tumor was noted.

detects pulmonary metastatic deposits. In addition, CT is more sensitive and specific than sonography for identifying nephrogenic rests. Following the intravenous administration of contrast, there is rapid enhancement of normal, functioning renal tissue, while Wilms' tumor and nephrogenic rests enhance to a lesser extent (Fig. 74-6). Wilms' tumor is typically large and heterogeneous in appearance, whereas nephrogenic rests tend to be small, ovoid or plaque-like lesions. They typically demonstrate homogeneous enhancement with decreased attenuation relative to normal renal parenchyma. Magnetic resonance imaging (MRI) with gadolinium enhancement is also useful in evaluating children with Wilms' tumor and nephrogenic rests (Fig. 74-7). It allows for accurate assessment of potential vascular invasion and is highly sensitive in the detection of small nephrogenic rests.

The treatment and follow-up of children with Wilms' tumor and associated nephrogenic rests has several important goals: (1) eradication of the primary tumor, (2) screening for and prevention of the development of a second malignancy, which can arise from the nephrogenic rests, and (3) maintenance of adequate renal function. Preoperative chemotherapy is often administered in order to reduce the size of the dominant tumor prior to segmental, nephron-sparing resection. Chemotherapy may also reduce the malignant potential of the other precursor lesions.

Children with nephrogenic rests must be closely monitored for malignant degeneration of one of the rests into a metachronous tumor. Repeated surgical intervention with biopsy is impractical and may cause unacceptable renal damage, so serial cross-sectional imaging plays an important role. Imaging follow-up may detect interval regression of nephrogenic rests (Fig. 74-8), growth of hyperplastic rests, or growth of a new malignant tumor (Fig. 74-9). Unfortunately, it may be difficult to distinguish a hyperplastic nephrogenic rest from a small Wilms' tumor by either imaging or histology. Several imaging criteria are helpful, however. The development of a large, dominant mass suggests malignancy, whereas multiple small masses of similar size are presumed to represent nephrogenic rests. Heterogeneity within the lesion also indicates likely malignancy. Since hyperplastic rests reflect the growth of multiple cells, they tend to be plaque-like, ovoid, or irregular in shape, while malignant Wilms' tumors tend to be spherical.

References

Beckwith JB: Precursor lesions of Wilms' tumor: Clinical and biological implications. *Med Pediatr Oncol* 21:158–168, 1993.

Beckwith JB, Kiviat NB, Bonadio JF: Nephrogenic rests, nephroblastomatosis, and the pathogenesis of Wilms' tumor. *Pediatr Pathol* 10:1–36, 1990.

Clericuzio CL, Johnson C: Screening for Wilms' tumor in high-risk individuals. *Hematol Oncol Clin North Am* 9:1253–1265, 1995.

Fernbach SK, Feinstein KA, Donaldson JS, et al: Nephroblastomatosis: Comparison of CT with US and urography. *Radiology* 166:153–156, 1988.

Gylys-Morin V, Hoffer FA, Kozalewich H, Shamberger RC: Wilms' tumor and nephroblastomastosis: Imaging characteristics at gadolinium-enhanced MR imaging. *Radiology* 188:517–521, 1993.

Newsham I, Cavenee W: Tumors and developmental anomalies associated with Wilms' tumor. *Med Pediatr Oncol* 21:199–204, 1993.

Regalado JJ, Rodriguez MM, Toledano S: Bilaterally multicentric synchronous Wilms' tumor: Successful conservative treatment despite persistence of nephrogenic rests. *Med Pediatr Oncol* 25:420–423, 1997.

Reiman TAH, Siegel MJ, Shackelford GD: Wilms' tumor in children: Abdominal CT and US evaluation. *Radiology* 160: 501–505, 1986.

Sharpe CR, Franco EL: Etiology of Wilms' tumor. *Epidemiol Rev* 17:415–432, 1995.

White KS, Kirks DR, Bove KE: Imaging of nephroblastomatosis: An overview. *Radiology* 182:1–5, 1992.

75

Figure 75-1 shows a newborn infant with a prenatal diagnosis of hydronephrosis. What do you see? What is the differential diagnosis?

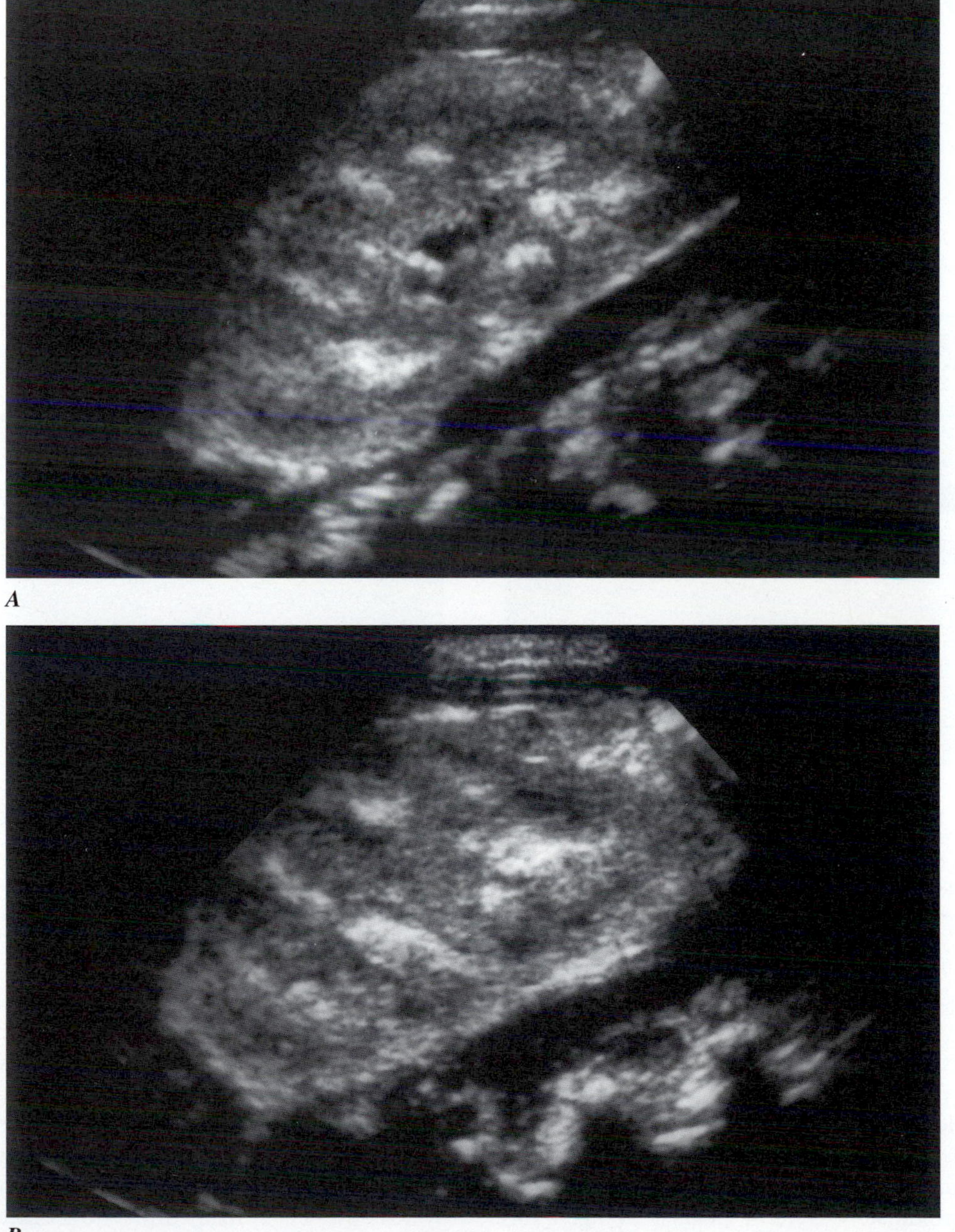

FIGURE 75–1. Longitudinal views through the right *(A)* and left *(B)* kidneys.

CHAPTER 75

Transient Increased Medullary Echogenicity of the Newborn

KAREN E. BASILE

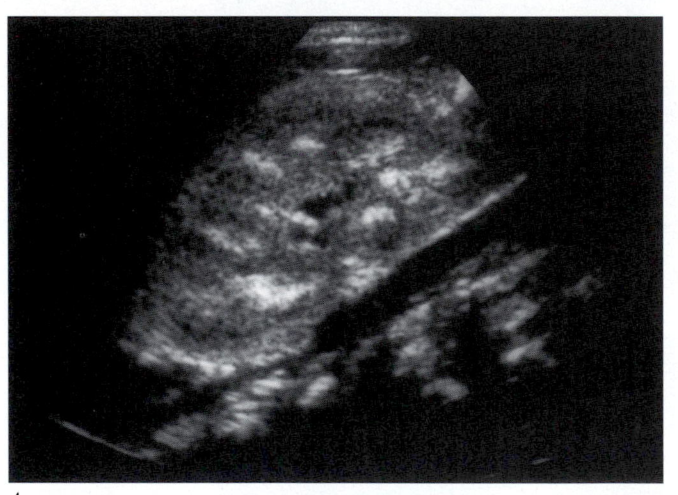

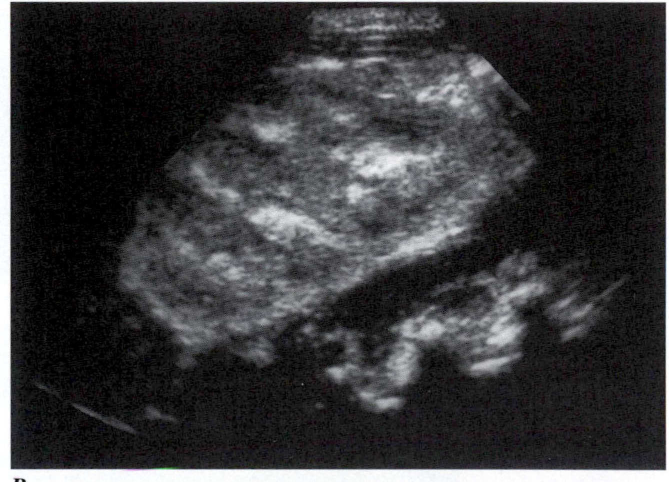

A *B*

FIGURE 75–2. Transient renal medullary hyperechogenicity of the newborn. Longitudinal views through the right *(A)* and left *(B)* kidneys demonstrate hyperechogenicity at the periphery of the renal pyramids diffusely. The renal echotexture is otherwise normal.

The sonographic appearance of the normal kidney in neonates differs from that in older children and adults. The normal neonatal renal cortex is more echogenic than the renal cortex in older children and adults. In infants, the renal cortex is often isoechoic and occasionally hyperechoic relative to the normal liver and spleen. This neonatal cortical pattern persists until approximately 2 to 4 months of age. The medullary pyramids of the kidney in newborns also differ in appearance from those in older children and adults. The medullary pyramids are larger, better defined, and more hypoechoic in infants than in older children. Finally, the neonatal kidney contains a paucity of renal sinus fat. Therefore, the renal sinus is not as echogenic as the sinus in the older child.

In recent years, an increasing number of neonates are being evaluated by sonography. This is in large part due to the widespread practice of prenatal sonographic screening, which now detects many urinary tract abnormalities in utero. Many neonates who have suspected urinary tract abnormalities on prenatal sonography undergo follow-up scanning shortly after birth. As a result of the increased use of renal

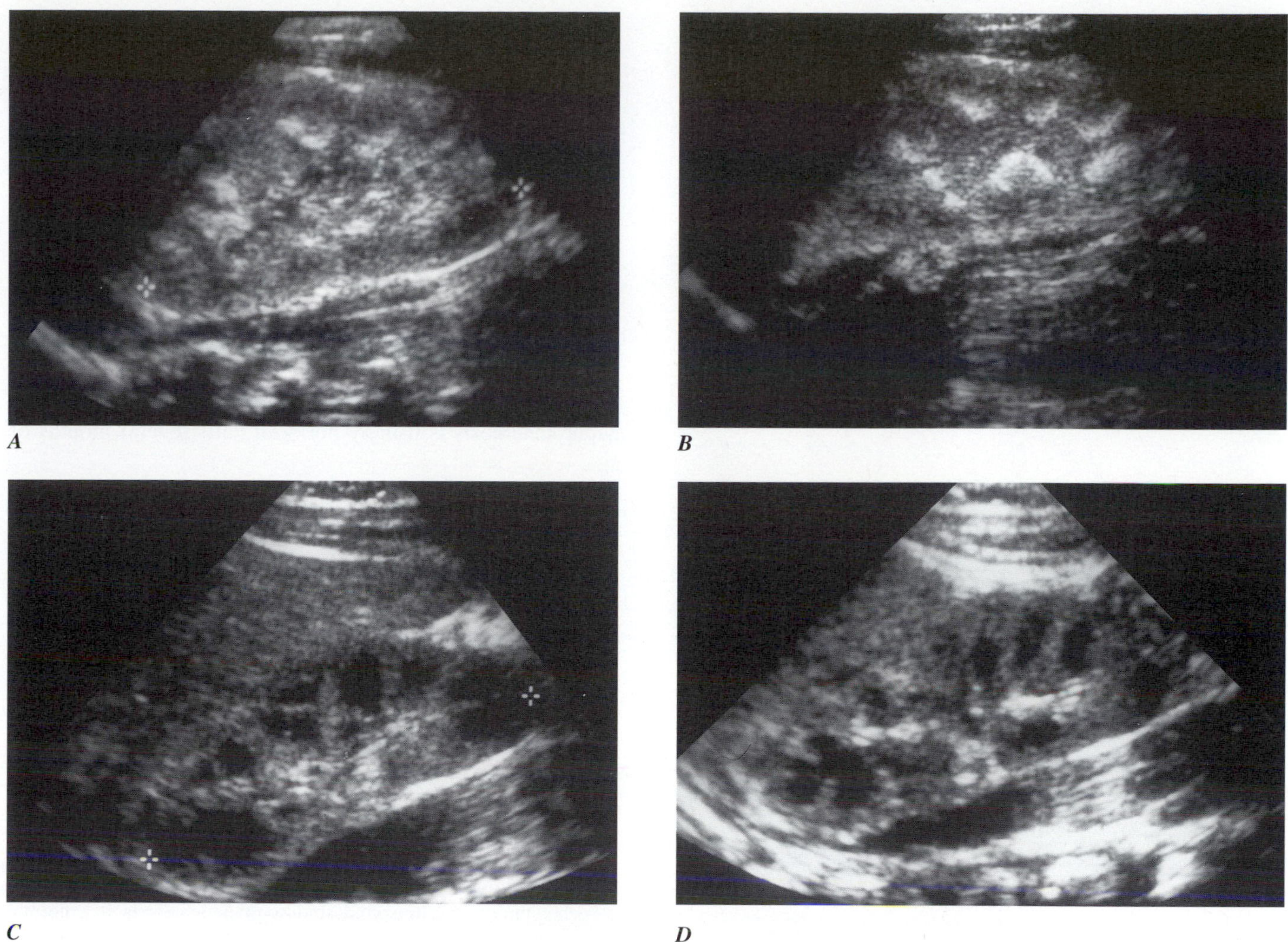

FIGURE 75–3. Resolution of transient renal medullary hyperechogenicity of the newborn. Longitudinal views through the right *(A)* and left *(B)* kidneys in a 2-day-old infant demonstrate echogenic renal pyramids bilaterally. Follow-up longitudinal views through the right *(C)* and left *(D)* kidneys 3 weeks later show complete resolution of the increased medullary echogenicity. Both kidneys now demonstrate a normal echotexture, with prominent hypoechoic medullary pyramids.

sonography in neonates over the past decade, there have been increasing reports of transient increases in the hyperechogenicity of the renal medulla in this population (Fig. 75-2). In the original reports, this finding occurred in oliguric or anuric infants. Therefore, the sonographic finding was initially felt to be associated with transient renal insufficiency in newborns. More recent reports have shown that increased echogenicity is frequently observed in the renal pyramids of normal infants in the absence of any renal pathology. Controversy persists as to whether or not infants with medullary hyperechogenicity have increased urinary protein excretion.

The most likely etiology for transient medullary hyperechogenicity of the newborn is transient tubular stasis. The exact cause of the increased medullary echogenicity is unclear. It is important to recognize that the sonographic finding typically resolves by 1 to 2 weeks of age and is not associated with long-term renal dysfunction (Fig. 75-3). Transient renal medullary hyperechogenicity has also been called stasis nephropathy and Tamm-Horsfall proteinuria. The alternative names are not appropriate because most infants with this finding do not have symptoms of renal insufficiency and Tamm-Horsfall is simply a common urine protein that is not associated with this finding.

Transient renal medullary hyperechogenicity of the newborn is typically associated with normal renal size and shape on sonographic evaluation. The increased medullary echogenicity is typically seen diffusely throughout both kidneys. However, the finding may occasionally be unilateral. Additionally, the medullary hyperechogenicity may be seen only within a focal portion of the kidney. The hyperechoic region may be seen thoughout the entire renal pyramids (Fig. 75-3) or may involve only the tips of the pyramids (Fig. 75-4). The hyperechoic regions gradually become smaller over the first 2 weeks of life. Approximately 85 percent of neonates with

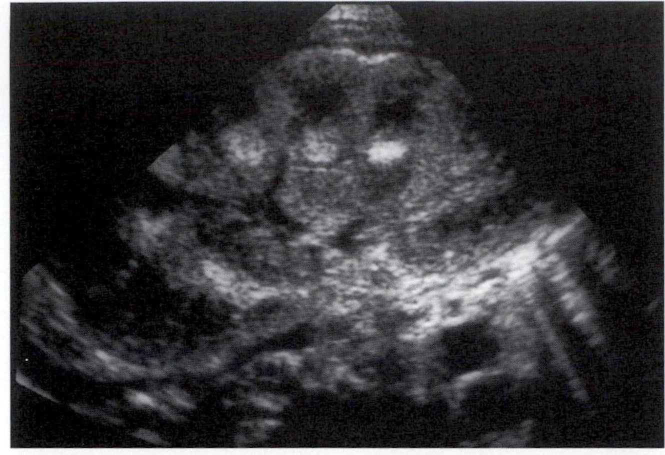

A

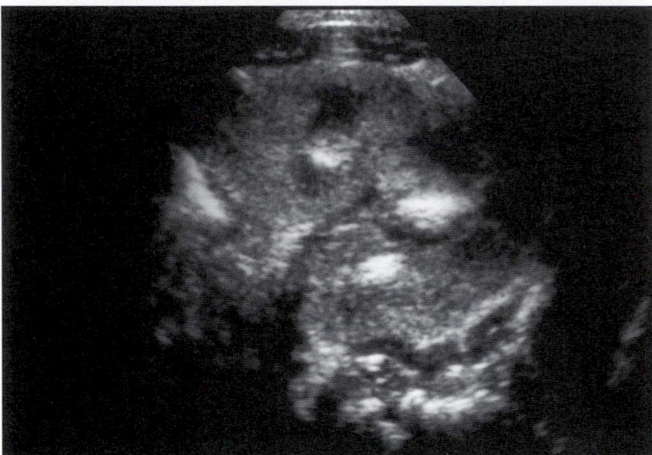

B

FIGURE 75–4. Transient renal medullary hyperechogenicity of the newborn involving only the tips of the renal pyramids. Longitudinal *(A)* and transverse *(B)* views through the right kidney in a 5-day-old infant demonstrate increased echogenicity involving the tips of the medullary pyramids. Note that the remainder of the renal pyramids appears hypoechoic.

this finding have normal-appearing kidneys by 1 week of age. With progressive improvement, the abnormality is primarily visible in a paracaliceal detection until it eventually resolves.

The differential diagnosis of transient medullary hyperechogenicity of the newborn includes conditions resulting in medullary nephrocalcinosis, including hypercalcemic states, distal renal tubular acidosis, chronic furosemide therapy, and oxalosis. Transient medullary hyperechogenicity of the newborn can be distinguished from medullary nephrocalcinosis on the basis of the age of the patient and confirmed on sonographic follow-up. Transient medullary hyperechogenicity of the newborn will typically be identified in the first week of life and should resolve by 2 weeks of age, whereas medullary nephrocalcinosis is usually not seen until several months of age.

References

Hijazi Z, Keller MS, Gaudio KM, et al: Transient renal dysfunction of the neonate. *Pediatrics* 82:929–930, 1988.

Howlett DC, Greenwood KL, Jarosz JM, et al: The incidence of transient renal medullary hyperechogenicity in neonatal ultrasound examination. *Br J Radiol* 70:140–143, 1997.

Jequier A, Kaplan BS: Echogenic renal pyramids in children. *JCU* 19:283–287, 1991.

Paivansalo MJ, Kallioinen MJ, Merikanto JS, et al: Hyperechogenic "rings" in the periphery of renal medullary pyramids as a sign of renal disease. *JCU* 19:283–287, 1991.

Riebel TW, Abraham K, Wartner R, et al: Transient renal medullary echogenicity in ultrasound studies of neonates: Is it a normal phenomenon and what are the causes? *JCU* 21:25–31, 1993.

Shultz PK, Strife JL, Strife CF, et al: Hyperechoic renal medullary pyramids in infants and children. *Radiology* 181:163–167, 1991.

Starinsky R, Vardi O, Batash D, et al: Increased renal medullary echogenicity in neonates. *Pediatr Radiol* 25:543–545.

76

Figure 76-1 shows a 4-year-old boy with decreased renal function. What do you see? What are the diagnostic considerations?

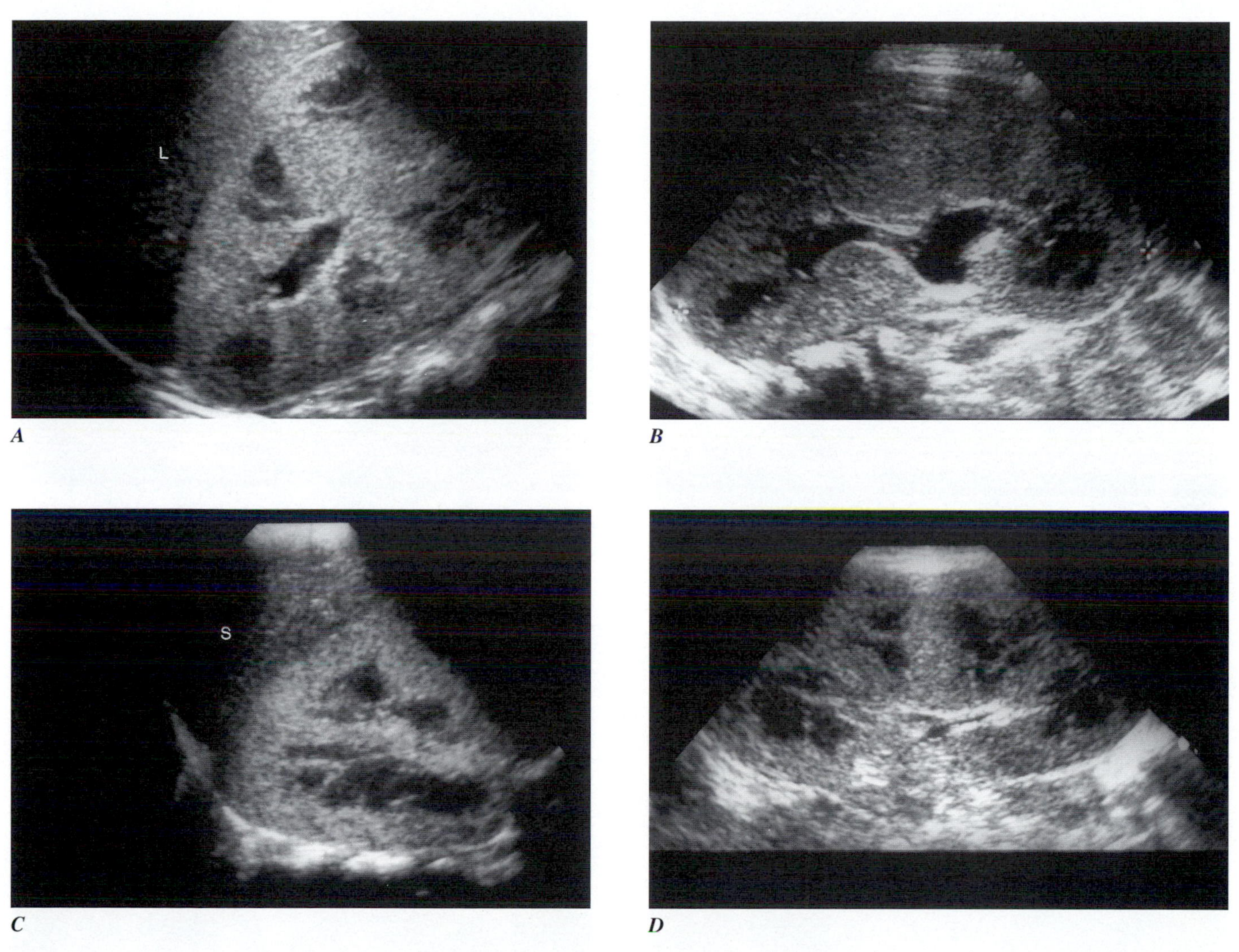

FIGURE 76–1. Longitudinal views through the right kidney *(A, B).* Longitudinal views through the left kidney *(C, D).*

CHAPTER 76

Medical Renal Disease

CARLOS J. SIVIT

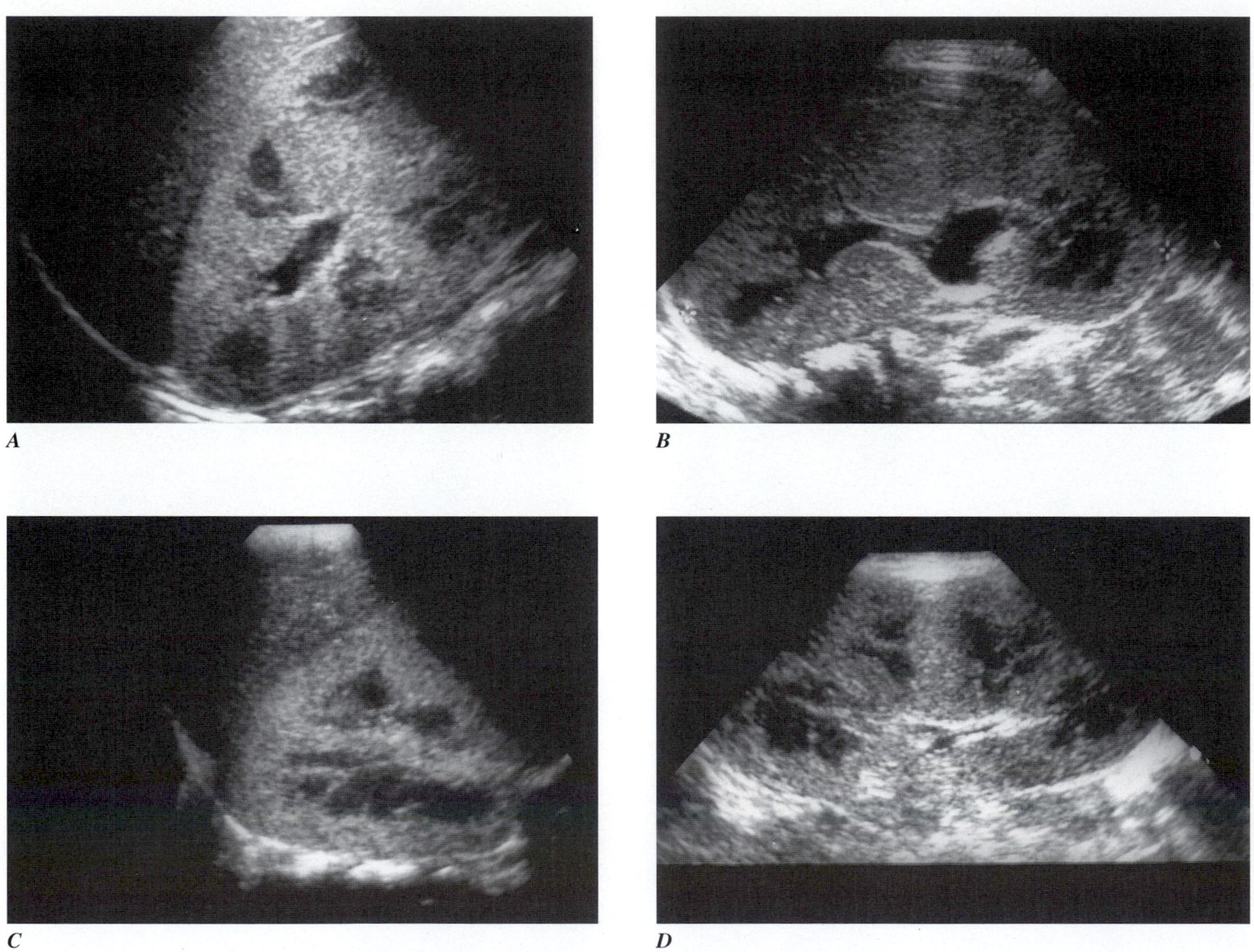

FIGURE 76–2. Increased renal parenchymal echogenicity associated with lymphoma. Longitudinal views through the right *(A, B)* and left *(C, D)* kidneys show diffusely increased renal parenchymal echogenicity bilaterally. Note that the kidneys are hyperechoic relative to the liver (L) and spleen (S). There is also diffuse bilateral renal enlargement.

The normal renal cortex in children over the age of 4 months is usually hypoechoic relative to the liver or spleen. Occasionally, the renal cortex may be isoechoic relative to those adjacent organs. It has been shown that renal echogenicity equal to the echogenicity of the liver and spleen is not a good indicator of renal disease. However, in normal children, other than preterm infants, the echotexture of the renal parenchyma should not be greater than that of liver and spleen.

The sonographic finding of diffuse, bilateral increased renal parenchymal echogenicity is a nonspecific finding indicative of diffuse renal parenchymal disease that may involve glomerular, tubular, interstitial, or vascular abnormalities (Fig. 76-2). It may also be seen with renal involvement in lymphoma or leukemia. The entity is generally described as medical renal disease. Increased renal parenchymal echogenicity is found in between one-third and two-thirds of chil-

TABLE 76-1
Conditions Associated with Increased Renal Parenchymal Echogenicity

Acute glomerulonephritis
Acute tubular necrosis
Glycogen storage disease
Hemolytic uremic syndrome
HIV nephropathy
Leukemia
Lymphoma
Nephrotic syndrome
Renal failure
Sickle cell anemia

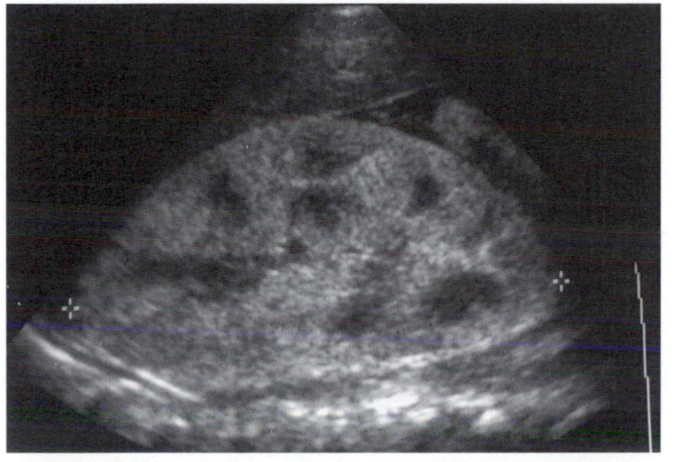
A

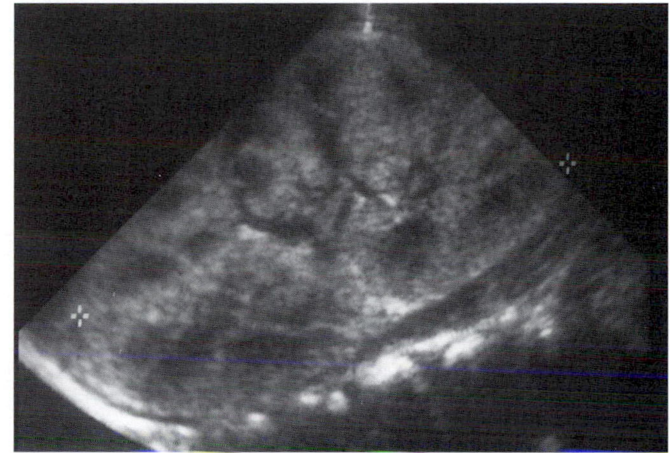
B

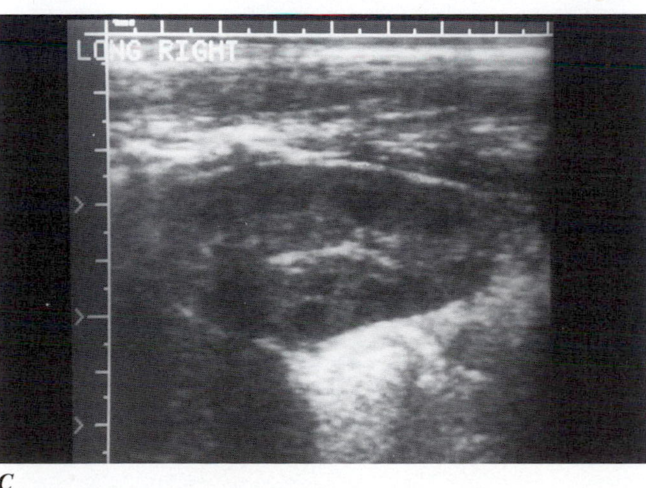

C

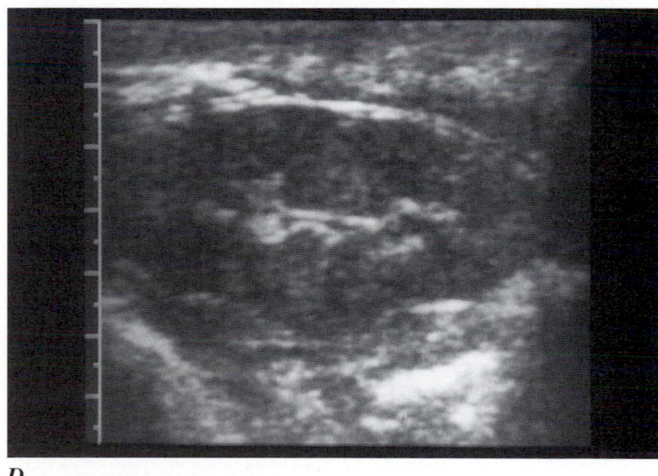
D

FIGURE 76–3. Reversible medical renal disease. Longitudinal views of the right *(A)* and left *(B)* kidneys in a child with acute renal failure due to acute tubular necrosis show enlarged, hyperechoic kidneys bilaterally. Longitudinal views of the right *(C)* and left *(D)* kidneys in the same child 10 months later, following normalization of renal function, show normal renal size and normal renal parenchymal echotexture.

dren with known renal disease. Some of the common causes of increased renal parenchymal echogenicity in children are listed in Table 76-1. Renal size ranges from normal to increased in all of these conditions. Sonography cannot be used to discriminate among these conditions.

The sonographic finding of increased renal parenchymal echogenicity is significant in that it indicates the presence of renal disease that is usually associated with decreased renal function. Correlation has been shown between increased renal parenchymal echogenicity and elevated blood urea nitrogen and serum creatinine values. However, sonography cannot discriminate between reversible and irreversible renal insufficiency. Improvement in renal parenchymal echogenicity is often seen with improvement in renal function (Fig. 76-3).

References

Brenbridge AN, Chevalier RL, Kaiser DL: Increased renal cortical echogenicity in pediatric disease: Histopathologic correlations. *JCU* 14:595–600, 1986.

Choyke PL, Grant EG, Hoffer FA, et al: Cortical echogenicity in the hemolytic uremic syndrome: Clinical correlation. *J Ultrasound Med* 7:439–442, 1988.

Hamper UM, Goldblum LE, Hutchins GM, et al: Renal involvement in AIDS: Sonographic-pathologic correlation. *AJR* 150: 1321–1325, 1988.

Hricak J, Cruz C, Romanski R, et al: Renal parenchymal disease: Sonographic-histologic correlation. *Radiology* 144:141–147, 1982.

Kay CJ: Renal diseases in patients with AIDS: Sonographic findings. *AJR* 159:551–554, 1992.

Kenney PJ, Brinsko RE, Patel DV, et al: Sonography of the kidneys in hemolytic uremic syndrome. *Invest Radiol* 21:547–550, 1986.

Kraus RA: Increased renal parenchymal echogenicity: Causes in pediatric patients. *Radiographics* 10:1009–1018, 1990.

Krensky AM, Reddish JM, Teele RL: Causes of increased renal echogenicity in pediatric patients. *Pediatrics* 72:840–846, 1983.

Platt JF, Rubin JM, Bowerman RA, et al: The inability to detect kidney disease on the basis of echogenicity. *AJR* 151:317–319, 1988.

77

Figure 77-1 shows an 8-year-old boy with leukemia who has had a bone marrow transplant. What do you see? What are the diagnostic considerations?

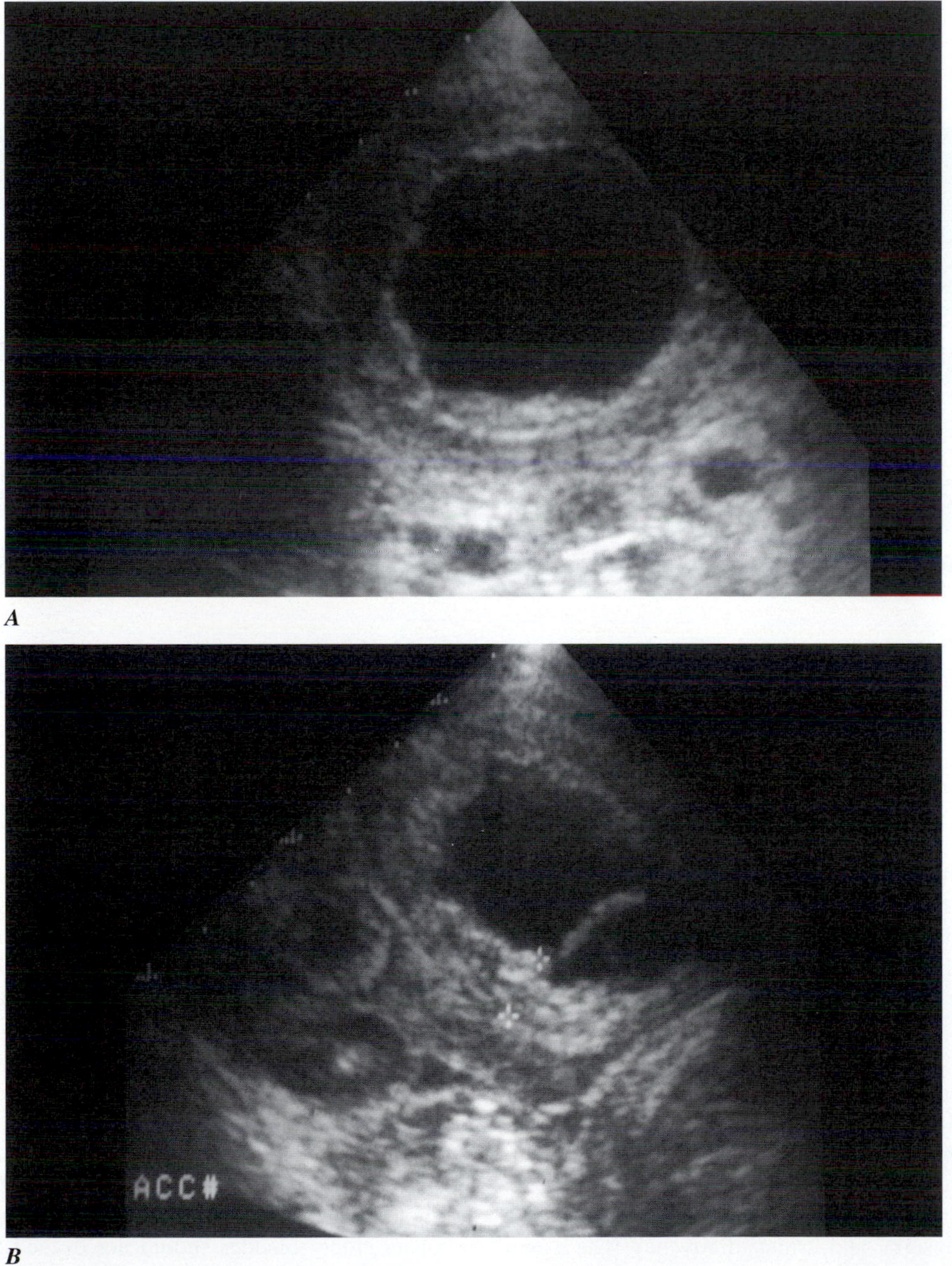

FIGURE 77–1. Transverse *(A)* and longitudinal *(B)* views through the bladder.

CHAPTER 77

Hemorrhagic Cystitis

CARLOS J. SIVIT

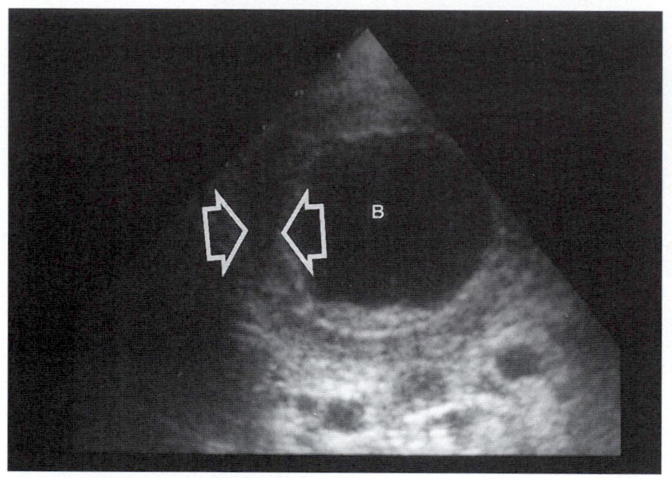

A

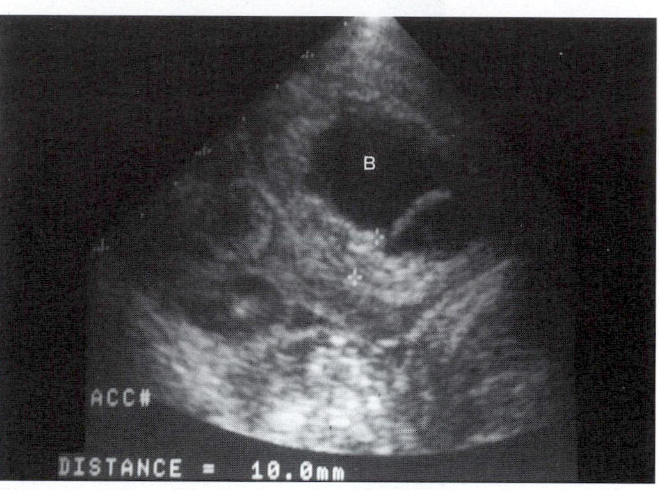

B

FIGURE 77–2. Hemorrhagic cystitis. ***A.*** Transverse view through the bladder demonstrates marked circumferential bladder wall thickening (*arrows*). ***B.*** Longitudinal view through the bladder in the same child as in ***A*** shows circumferential bladder wall thickening (*between electronic calipers*). Note septation within the bladder lumen that is probably the residual of prior blood clots. B = bladder.

Hemorrhagic cystitis results from diffuse bleeding of the endothelial lining of the bladder. The etiology may be multifactorial. The condition has been associated with drugs, infection, and toxins. Chemotherapeutic agents, particularly cyclophosphamide and busulfan, are the drugs most commonly associated with the condition. It has been most frequently reported following bone marrow transplantation, particularly in younger children. It has been reported as early as 1 week and as late as 4 months following transplantation. Infectious organisms associated with hemorrhagic cystitis include *Escherichia coli* and adenovirus.

Children with hemorrhagic cystitis typically present with gross hematuria, dysuria, and urinary frequency. The extent of hemorrhage can be severe, and the condition may be life-threatening. Treatment usually involves bladder irrigation, blood transfusions, and the maintenance of adequate hydration. Endoscopic removal of blood clots in the bladder is sometimes required, as the clots may result in bladder outlet obstruction.

Sonography is a useful modality for assessing the extent of bladder involvement in hemorrhagic cystitis. It is also useful for monitoring the response to therapy. The sonographic findings noted in children with hemorrhagic cystitis include focal, multifocal, or circumferential bladder wall thickening (Fig. 77-2). The bladder wall thickness varies with the state of bladder filling. The wall of a well-distended bladder should not exceed 3 mm in maximal diameter, and the wall of an empty bladder should not exceed 5 mm in diameter. Bladder wall thickening associated with hemorrhagic cystitis is usually most pronounced in the hypoechoic muscularis

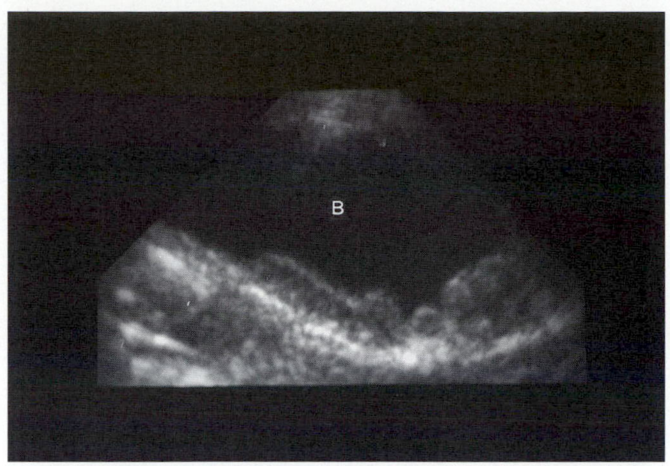

FIGURE 77–3. Hemorrhagic cystitis with a polypoid appearance on sonography. Longitudinal view through the bladder in a child with hemorrhagic cystitis demonstrate irregular bladder wall thickening that has a nodular or polypoid appearance. B = bladder.

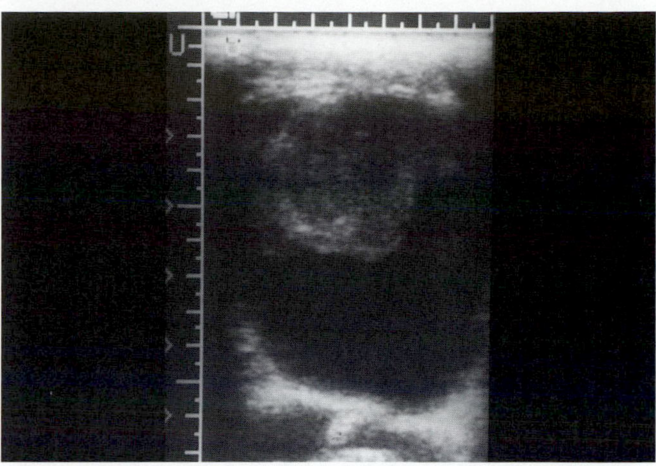

FIGURE 77–4. Non-Hodgkin's lymphoma of bladder wall. Transverse view through the bladder shows a focal bladder wall mass. The mass did not change in appearance with bladder filling. Lymphoma of the bladder wall was noted at surgery.

layer. The echogenic mucosal and submucosal layers are less involved. The thickening may be polypoid in appearance, with circumscribed thickened bladder wall projecting into the bladder lumen (Fig 77-3). Thus, it may resemble a bladder wall mass. Echogenic blood clots may be noted within the bladder lumen. The bladder may have a reduced capacity. In severe cases, there may be complete contraction of the bladder without a visualized lumen.

Hemorrhagic cystitis may resemble a focal bladder mass. The most common primary bladder wall malignant neoplasm in children is rhabdomyosarcoma. Other malignant neoplasms include undifferentiated sarcoma, lymphoma, and leiomyosarcoma. Benign tumors are rare and include hemangioma, neurofibroma, fibroma, fibromatous polyp, papilloma, and leiomyoma. One finding that is helpful in distinguishing hemorrhagic cystitis from a true bladder wall mass is that bladder wall thickening associated with hemorrhagic cystitis will usually change in contour and thickness with increasing bladder filling, whereas a true bladder wall mass will not change (Fig. 77-4). Follow-up sonographic examination is also useful in distinguishing between hemorrhagic cystitis and a bladder wall mass. In hemorrhagic cystitis, there should be resolution of the bladder wall thickening with improvement of clinical symptoms. Thus, persistence of focal bladder wall abnormality on follow-up sonographic evaluation should prompt evaluation for possible mass lesion.

References

Benya EC, Sivit CJ, Quinones RR: Abdominal complications after bone marrow transplantation in children: Sonographic and CT findings. *AJR* 161:1023–1027, 1993.

Cartoni C, Arcese W, Avvisati G, et al: Role of ultrasonography in the diagnosis and follow-up of hemorrhagic cystititis after bone marrow transplantation. *Bone Marrow Transplant* 12:463–467, 1993.

Dohmen K, Harada M, Ishibashi H, et al: Ultrasonographic studies on abdominal complications in patients receiving marrow-ablative chemotheraphy and bone marrow or blood stem cell transplantation. *JCU* 19:321–333, 1991.

Jequier S, Rousseau O: Sonographic measurements of the normal bladder wall in children. *AJR* 149:563–566, 1987.

Rosenberg HK, Eggli KD, Zerin JM, et al: Benign cystitis in children mimicking rhabdomyosarcoma. *J Ultrasound Med* 13: 921–932, 1994.

Yang CC, Hurd DD, Case LD, et al: Hemorrhagic cystitis in bone marrow transplantation. *Urology* 44:322–328, 1994.

78

Figure 78-1 shows a 5-year-old boy with fever and abdominal pain. What do you see? What are the diagnostic considerations?

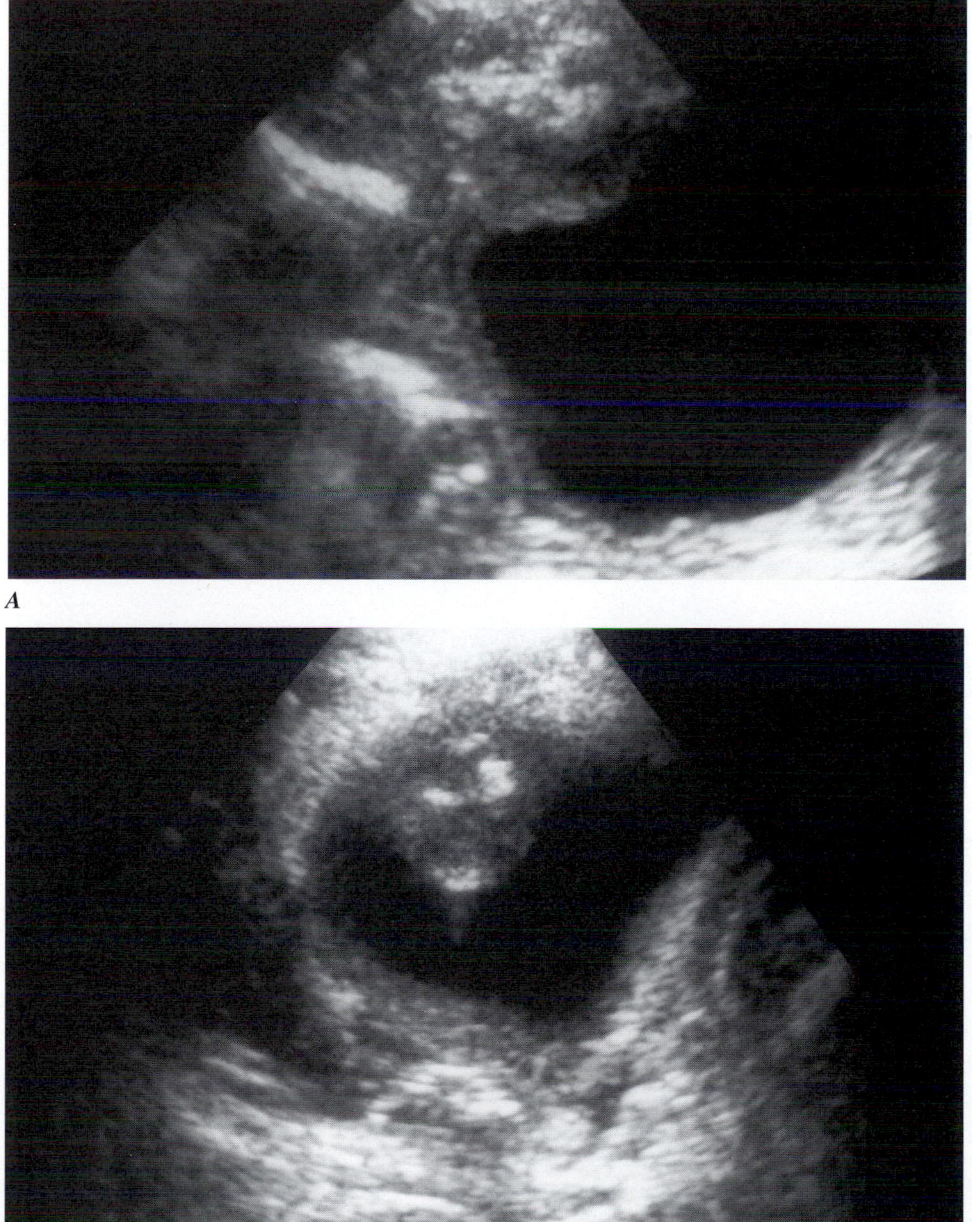

FIGURE 78–1. Longitudinal *(A)* and transverse *(B)* views through the pelvis in the midline.

CHAPTER 78

Infected Urachal Remnant

CARLOS J. SIVIT

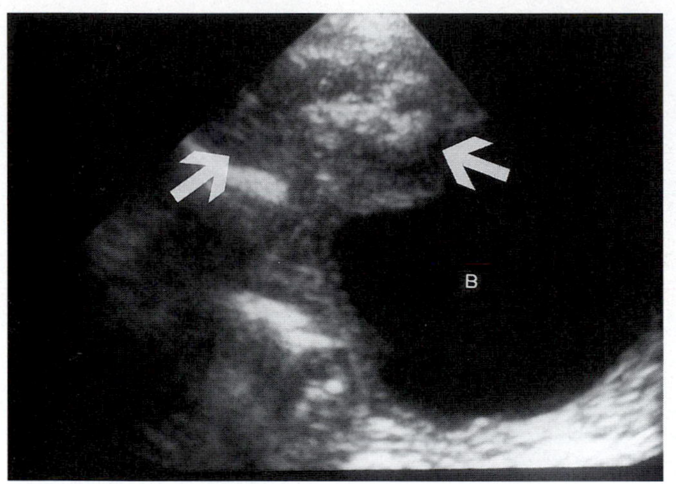

A

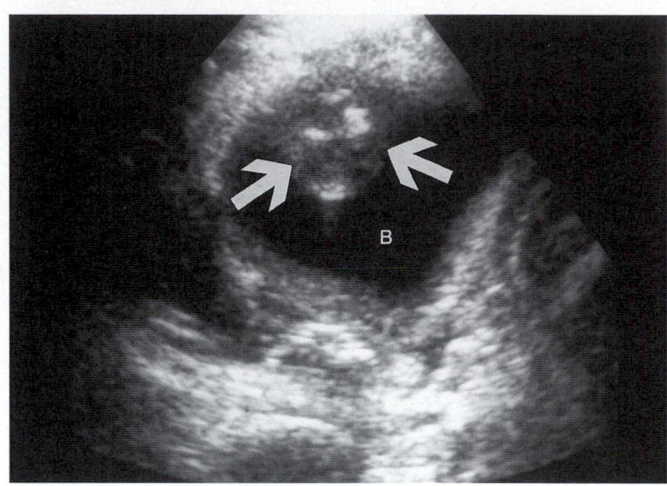

B

FIGURE 78–2. Infected urachal remnant. Longitudinal *(A)* and transverse *(B)* views through the pelvis show a complex midline mass (*arrows*) above the dome of the bladder (B). Note the mass effect on the bladder. At surgery, an infected urachal remnant was noted.

The urachus is an allantoic remnant located in the midline between the umbilicus and the dome of the bladder (Fig. 78-2). It lies in the space of Retzius behind the transversalis fascia and anterior to the peritoneum. The urachal lumen is typically obliterated during fetal life or early in the neonatal period, and the remnant is reduced to a fibrous cord that extends from the dome of the bladder to the umbilicus and is also known as the median umbilical ligament. This normal structure may be visible in young children as a small, elliptical, hypoechoic structure on the anterosuperior surface of the urinary bladder (Fig. 78-3). Occasionally, there is failure of all or a portion of the urachal lumen to be obliterated. Such abnormalities are characterized as urachal remnant abnormalities.

There are four types of urachal remnant abnormalities: (1) patent urachus, (2) urachal sinus, (3) urachal diverticulum, and (4) urachal cyst. A patent urachus results from failure of the allantoic lumen to close, leading to a tubular connection between the anterosuperior aspect of the bladder and the umbilicus (Figs. 78-4 and 78-5). This abnormality typically results in leakage of urine through the umbilicus. Patent urachus has been reported in association with prune-belly syndrome. The latter condition consists of deficient abdominal musculature, urinary tract abnormalities, and cryptorchidism. The sonographic appearance of a patent urachus is that of a hypoechoic or anechoic tubular midline tract extending from the umbilicus to the dome of the bladder. The lumen may be collapsed and not visible on sonography.

There may be failure to close of only a portion of the urachus. When only a portion of the urachus adjacent to the abdominal wall remains patent, it forms a urachal sinus (Fig. 78-6). This also usually results in periodic umbilical discharge. This is more difficult to demonstrate on sonography,

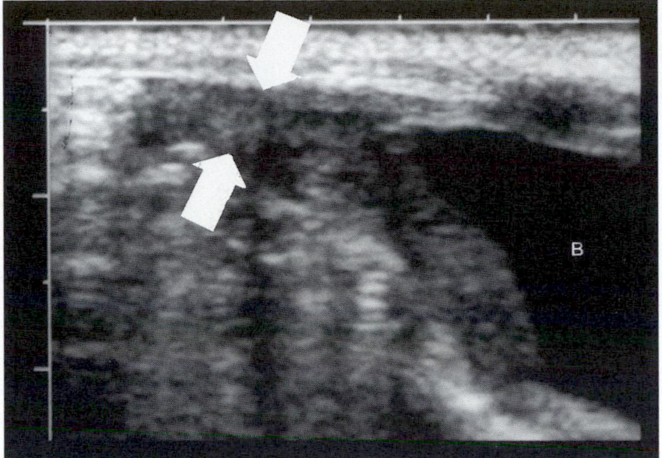

FIGURE 78–3. Normal urachal remnant. Longitudinal view through the pelvis shows a small, hypoechoic structure (*arrows*) anterior and superior to the bladder dome. This is the characteristic sonographic appearance and location for a normal urachal remnant. B = bladder.

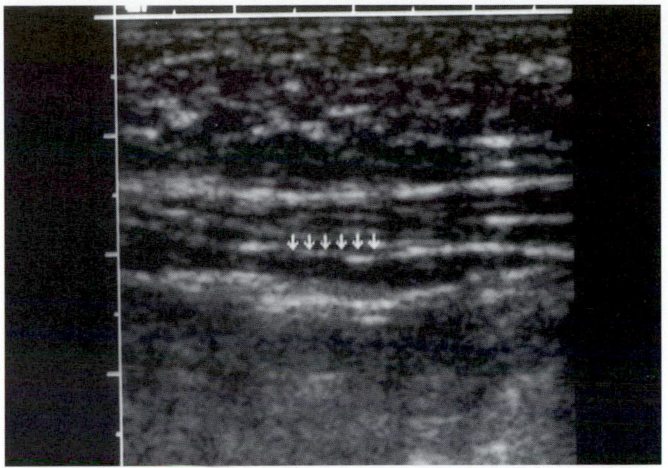

A

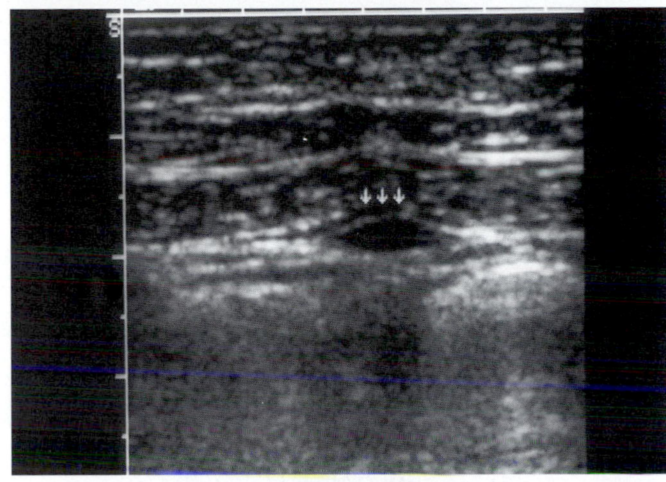

B

FIGURE 78–5. Patent urachus. ***A.*** Longitudinal view through the lower abdomen below the umbilicus in a child with umbilical drainage shows a hypoechoic, tubular midline tract (*arrows*). ***B.*** Transverse midline view through the lower abdomen demonstrates the hypoechoic midline tract (*arrows*).

as the tract can be short, and the lumen may be collapsed. When only a portion of the urachus adjacent to the bladder remains open, it forms a urachal diverticulum (Fig. 78-7). This is the least common of the urachal remnant abnormalities. This condition usually does not produce symptoms unless there is urinary stasis, which may lead to infection. Additionally, there may be failure to close of an isolated segment of the midportion of the urachus with obliteration at both ends, resulting in a urachal cyst (Fig. 78-8). This is the most common urachal remnant. The sonographic appearance is that of an anterior, midline cyst located between the umbilicus and the bladder.

Voiding cystourethrography (VCU) is also useful in the evaluation of a possible urachal abnormality. A patent urachus may occasionally fill with contrast during a VCU. If it fills with contrast, the patent urachus will appear as a midline tract extending from the bladder dome to the umbilicus. However, the majority of lesions will not be identified on VCU, as they will not fill with contrast. A urachal

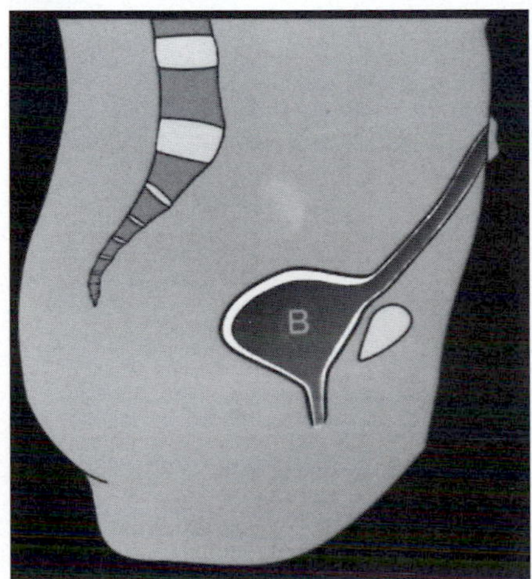

FIGURE 78–4. Diagram of a patent urachus (P). B = bladder.

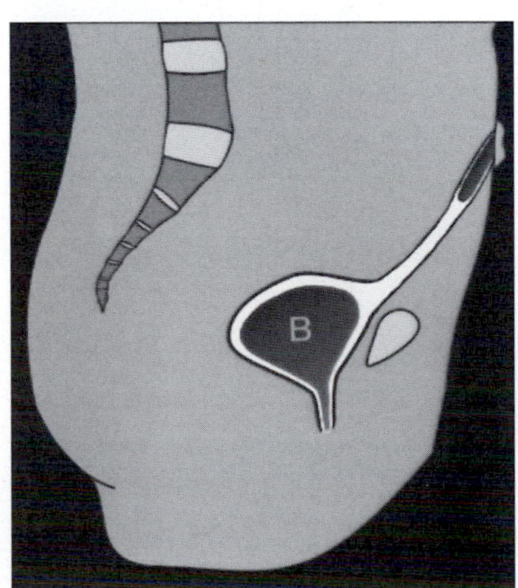

FIGURE 78–6. Diagram of a urachal sinus (S). B = bladder.

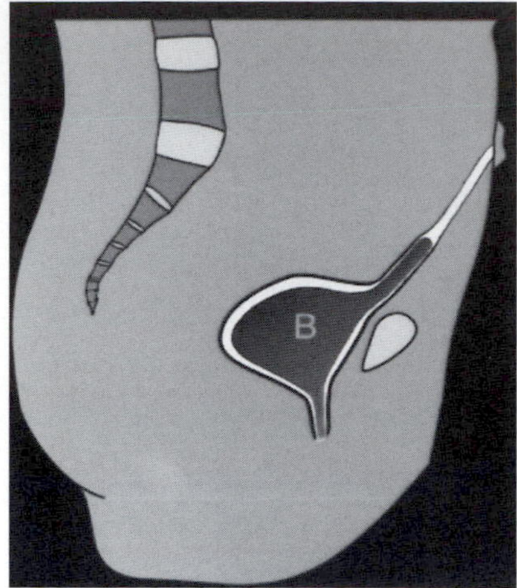

FIGURE 78–7. Diagram of a urachal diverticulum. B = bladder.

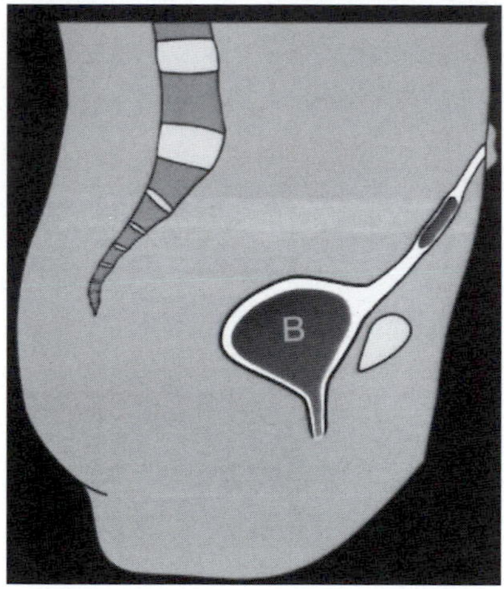

FIGURE 78–8. Diagram of a urachal cyst. B = bladder.

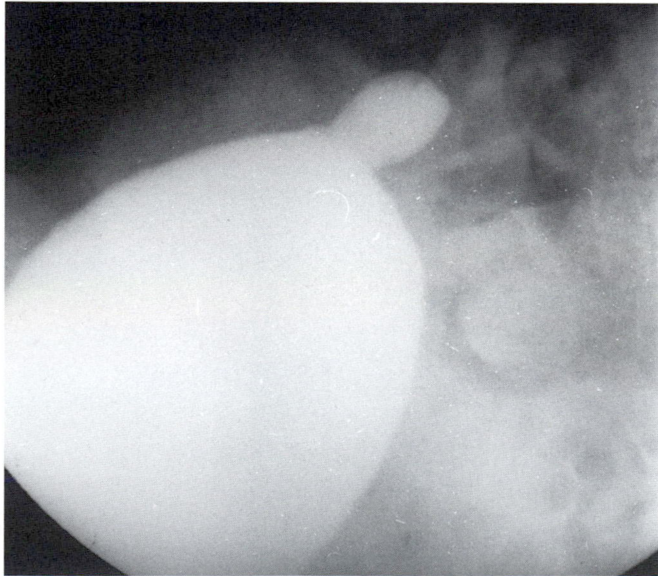

FIGURE 78–9. Urachal diverticulum. Lateral view of the bladder during a voiding cystourethrogram demonstrates a contrast-filled urachal diverticulum originating from the bladder anteriorly and superiorly.

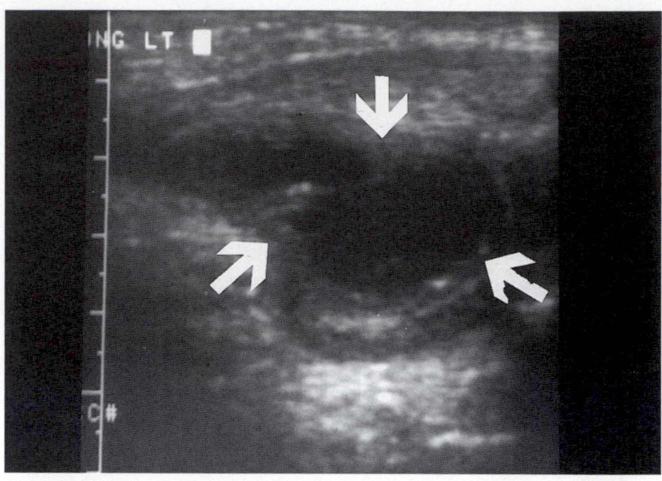

A

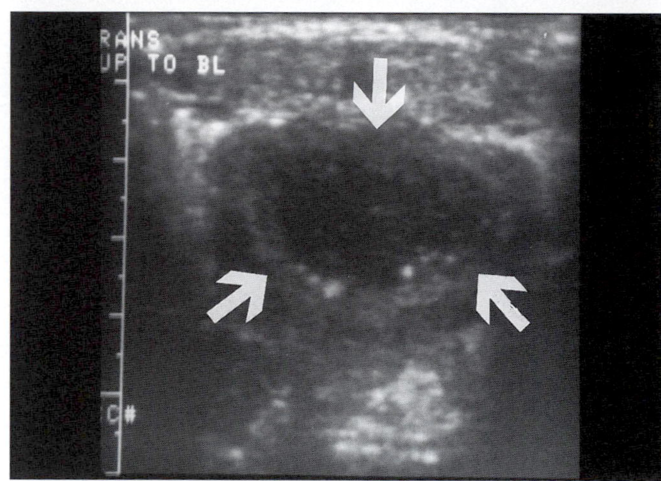

B

FIGURE 78–10. Infected urachal remnant. Longitudinal *(A)* and transverse *(B)* midline views through the upper pelvis show a spherical, thick-walled, complex midline mass (*arrows*). At surgery, an infected urachal remnant was noted.

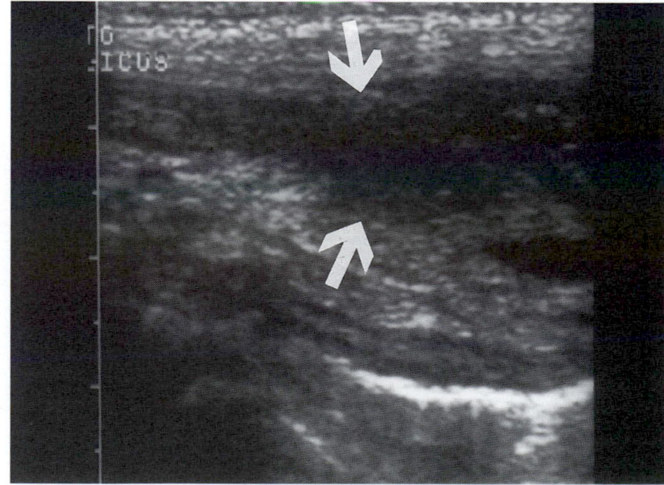

FIGURE 78–11. Infected urachal remnant. Longitudinal midline view through the upper pelvis shows a complex tubular mass (*arrows*) extending from the umbilicus to the dome of the bladder. This was noted to be an infected urachal remnant at surgery.

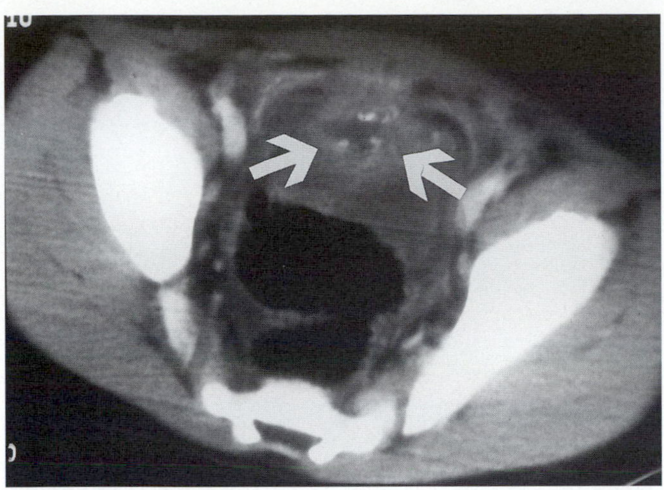

FIGURE 78–12. Computed tomography (CT) scan of infected urachal remnant. Contrast-enhanced CT scan through the pelvis shows a complex midline mass (*arrows*) immediately above the bladder. At surgery, an infected urachal remnant was noted.

diverticulum typically does fill with contrast and is seen as a midline outpouching originating from the bladder dome (Fig. 78-9).

Urachal remnants may become infected, resulting in enlargement of the structure (Fig. 78-2). On sonography, a complex midline mass is noted between the umbilicus and the dome of the bladder (Fig. 78-10). A tubular component to the lesion can usually be identified (Fig. 78-11). This latter finding is important, as it allows differentiation of urachal remnants from other processes that result in an abdominal abscess. Computed tomography may provide improved definition of the extent of the abscess and enhanced delineation of the anatomic relationship of the abscess to the bladder (Fig. 78-12).

References

Avni EF, Matos C, Diard F, et al: Midline omphalovesical anomalies in children: Contribution of US imaging. *Urol Radiol* 10:189–194, 1988.

Boyle G, Rosenberg HK, O'Neill J: An unusual presentation of an infected urachal cyst. *Clin Pediatr* 27:130–134, 1988.

Cacciarelli AA, Kass EJ, Yang SS: Urachal remnants: Sonographic demonstration in children. *Radiology* 174:473–475, 1990.

DiSantis DJ, Siegel MJ, Katz ME: Simplified approach to umbilical remnant abnormalities. *Radiographics* 11:59–66, 1991.

Khati NJ, Enquist EG, Javitt MC: Imaging of the umbilicus and periumbilical region. *Radiographics* 18:413–431, 1998.

Zieger B, Sokol B, Rohrschneider WK, et al: Sonomorphology and involution of the normal urachus in asymptomatic newborns. *Pediatr Radiol* 28:156–161, 1998.

79

Figure 79-1 shows a 2-year-old boy with urinary retention and hematuria. What is the abnormality? What is the most likely diagnosis?

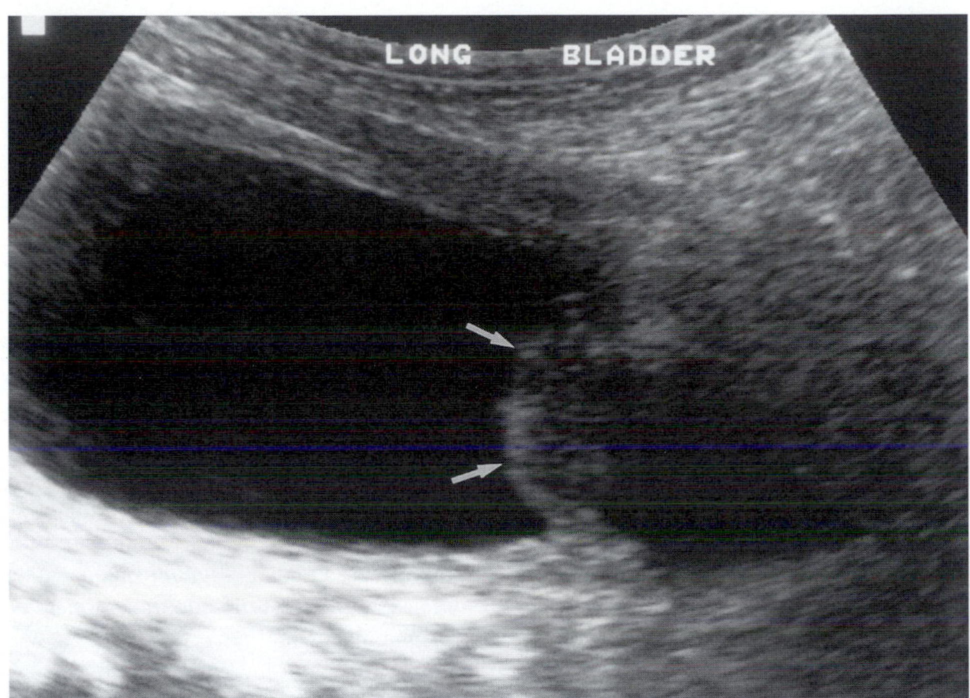

FIGURE 79–1. Longitudinal view through the bladder.

CHAPTER 79

Rhabdomyosarcoma of the Bladder

CHARLES J. CHUNG

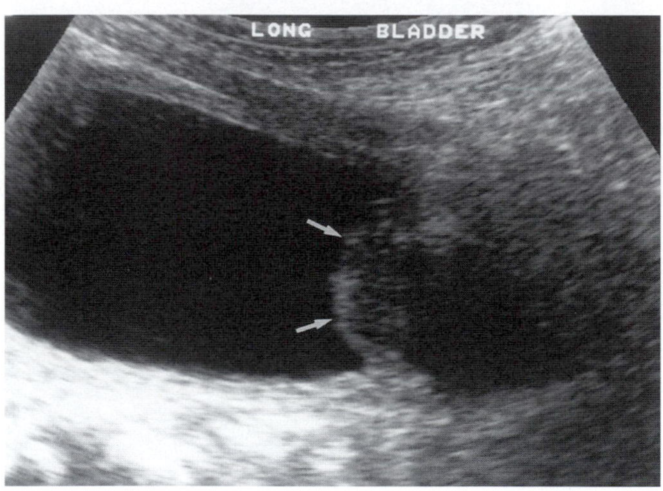

FIGURE 79–2. Bladder rhabdomyosarcoma. Longitudinal view through the bladder demonstrates a rounded soft tissue mass arising from the bladder base (*arrows*). The lesion is isoechoic relative to adjacent musculature. Note that it contains areas of decreased echotexture.

Embryonal rhabdomyosarcoma is the most common malignant neoplasm of the bladder in children (Fig. 79-2). Approximately 20 to 30 percent of all rhabdomyosarcomas arise from the genitourinary tract. Most of these originate from the bladder base. In males, the tumor also frequently involves the prostate gland, and the organ of origin cannot be precisely determined. The most common clinical finding associated with these tumors is urinary retention. Additional signs and symptoms may include hematuria, constipation, abdominal or pelvic pain, or a palpable mass.

On sonography, rhabdomyosarcoma of the bladder typically appears as a solid, polypoid mass that projects into the bladder lumen (Fig. 79-2). These tumors are usually large. Cystic areas representing tumor necrosis or hemorrhage may be noted within the lesion. Infiltrating tumors demonstrate irregular bladder wall thickening. The bladder capacity may be markedly diminished when the tumor reaches a large size. There may also be associated dilatation of the upper urinary tract due to partial ureteral obstruction.

A number of other malignant or benign primary bladder neoplasms may be noted in childhood. All of these tumors are quite rare. Malignant tumors are more common than benign ones. Other malignant bladder neoplasms that may be seen in childhood include transitional cell carcinoma, adenocarcinoma, lymphoma (Fig. 79-3), leukemia, leiomyosarcoma, pheochromocytoma, endodermal sinus tumor, and Ewing's sarcoma. These malignant lesions can reach a large size (Fig. 79-3). It is not possible to differentiate them from rhabdomyosarcoma on the basis of the sonographic appearance. Benign bladder neoplasms in children include hemangioma, papilloma, fibroepithelial polyp (Fig. 79-4), and the pseudosarcomatous myofibroblastic tumor. The typical sonographic appearance of the benign lesions is that of focal bladder wall thickening or a soft tissue mass projecting into the bladder lumen (Fig. 79-4).

Inflammatory, infectious, and posttraumatic lesions may result in focal bladder wall thickening that may simulate a neoplasm. Inflammatory or infectious cystitis may cause areas of irregular bladder wall thickening (Fig. 79-5). If the bladder demonstrates reduced capacity and circumferential isoechoic wall thickening with intact mucosa in the setting of hematuria, dysuria, and urinary frequency, an inflammatory lesion should be considered more likely. A follow-up ultrasound in 2 weeks will probably demonstrate resolution of the focal mass, thus distinguishing the lesion from a neoplasm. In endemic regions, schistosomiasis can also result in bladder wall thickening that may be focal and simulate a mass lesion (Fig. 79-6). A bladder hematoma associated with prior

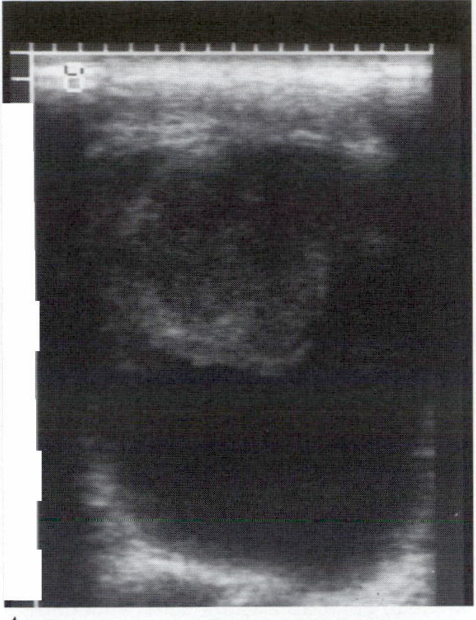

A

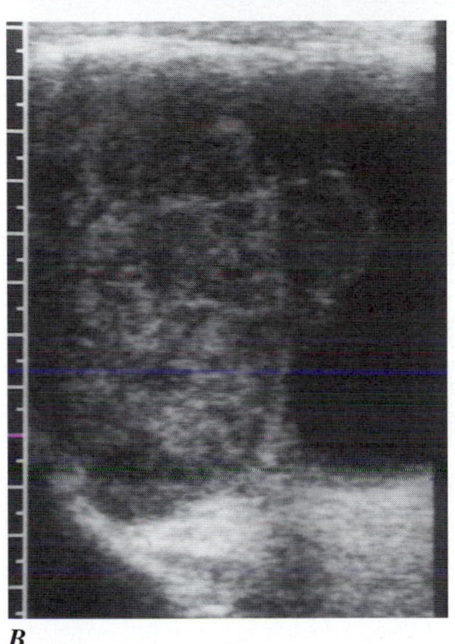

B

FIGURE 79–3. Non-Hodgkin's lymphoma involving the bladder wall. Transverse *(A)* and longitudinal *(B)* views through the bladder demonstrate a large, lobulated bladder wall mass.

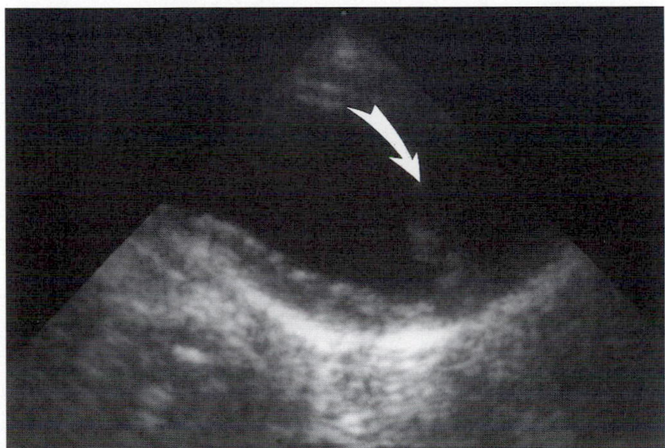

FIGURE 79–4. Fibroepithelial polyp. Longitudinal view through the bladder demonstrates a small soft tissue mass (*arrow*) originating from the bladder wall and protruding into the lumen.

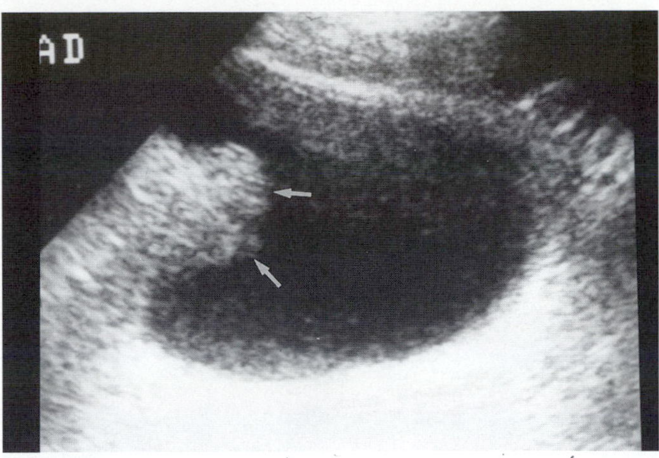

FIGURE 79–5. Cystitis mimicking a bladder neoplasm. Transverse view of the bladder demonstrates focal lateral bladder wall thickening (*arrows*) that has the appearance of a bladder wall mass. The child had a history of long-term bladder catheter placement. Follow-up sonography in 2 weeks demonstrated resolution of the abnormality.

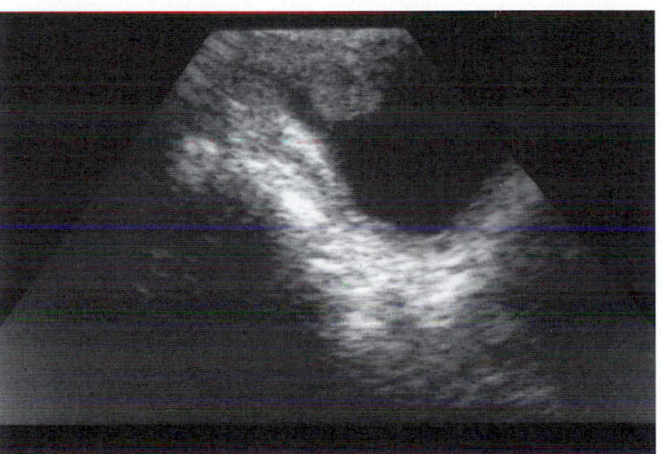

A

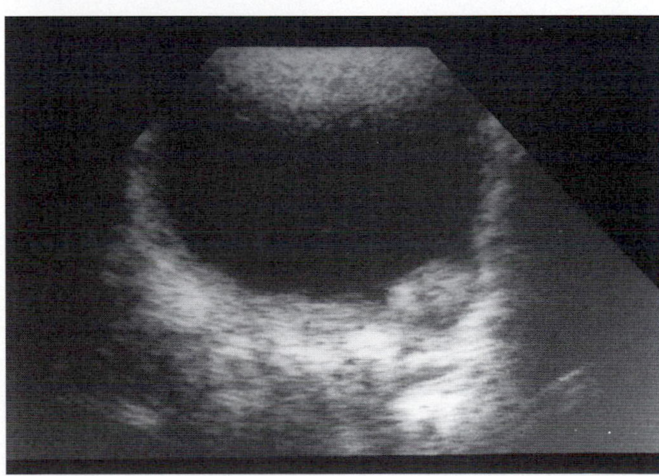

B

FIGURE 79–6. Bladder wall thickening secondary to schistosomiasis. Longitudinal *(A)* and transverse *(B)* views through the bladder demonstrate focal bladder wall thickening that resembles a mass.

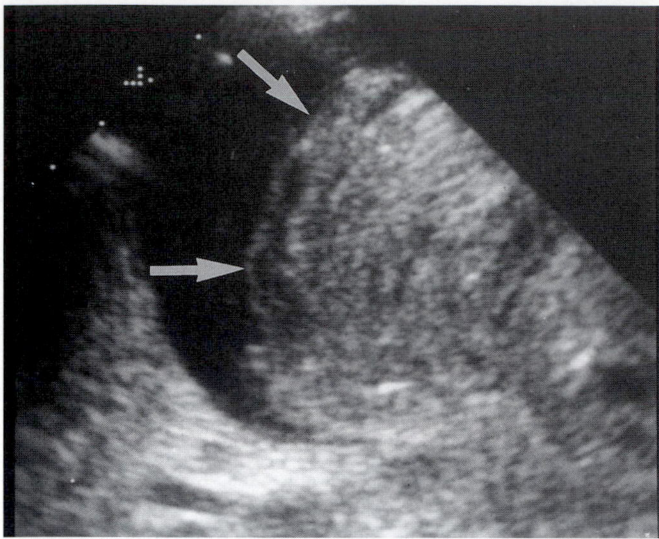

FIGURE 79–7. Bladder hematoma due to hemorrhagic cystitis mimicking a bladder neoplasm. Longitudinal view through the bladder demonstrates a large, laminated mass *(arrows)* that nearly replaces the entire bladder lumen. The mass could not be separated from the bladder wall. The child had a clinical history consistent with hemorrhagic cystitis. Follow-up sonography 1 month following the examination demonstrated resolution of the abnormality.

trauma or hemorrhagic cystitis may also simulate a bladder neoplasm (Fig. 79-7). A hematoma can be distinguished from neoplasm on the basis of resolution on follow-up sonography.

References

Agrons G, Wagner B, Lonergan G, et al: Genitourinary rhabdomyosarcoma in children: Radiologic-pathologic correlation. *Radiographics* 17:919–937, 1997.

Crecelius S, Bellah R: Pheochromocytoma of the bladder in an adolescent: Sonographic and MR imaging findings. *AJR* 165:101–103, 1995.

Fernbach S, Feinstein K: Abnormalities of the bladder in children: Imaging findings. *AJR* 162:1143–1150, 1994.

Hoenig D, McRae S, Chen S, et al: Transitional cell carcinoma of the bladder in the pediatric patient. *J Urol* 156:203–205, 1996.

Hojo H, Newton WJ, Hamoudi A, et al: Pseudosarcomatous myofibroblastic tumor of the urinary bladder in children: A study of 11 cases with review of the literature. *Am J Surg Pathol* 19:1224–1236, 1995.

Musselman P, Kay R: The spectrum of urinary tract fibroepithelial polyps in children. *J Urol* 136:476–477, 1986.

O'Sullivan P, Daneman A, Chan H, et al: Extragonadal endodermal sinus tumors in children: A review of 24 cases. *Pediatr Radiol* 13:249–257, 1983.

Poddenvin F, Bayart M: Urothelial tumor of the bladder in children. *J Urol* 101:191–194, 1995.

Rosenberg H, Eggli K, Zerin J, et al: Benign cystitis in children mimicking rhabdomyosarcoma. *J Ultrasound Med* 13:921–932, 1994.

Royal S, Hedlund G, Galliani C: Rhabdomyosarcoma of the dome of the urinary bladder: A difficult imaging diagnosis. *AJR* 167:524–525, 1996.

Williams M, Ibrahim S, Rickwood A: Hamartoma of the urinary bladder in an infant with Beckwith-Wiedemann syndrome. *Br J Urol* 65:106–107, 1990.

Section G
GASTROINTESTINAL TRACT, MESENTERY, AND PERITONEAL CAVITY

80

Figure 80-1 shows a 6-year-old boy with hemihypertrophy. What do you see? What are the diagnostic considerations?

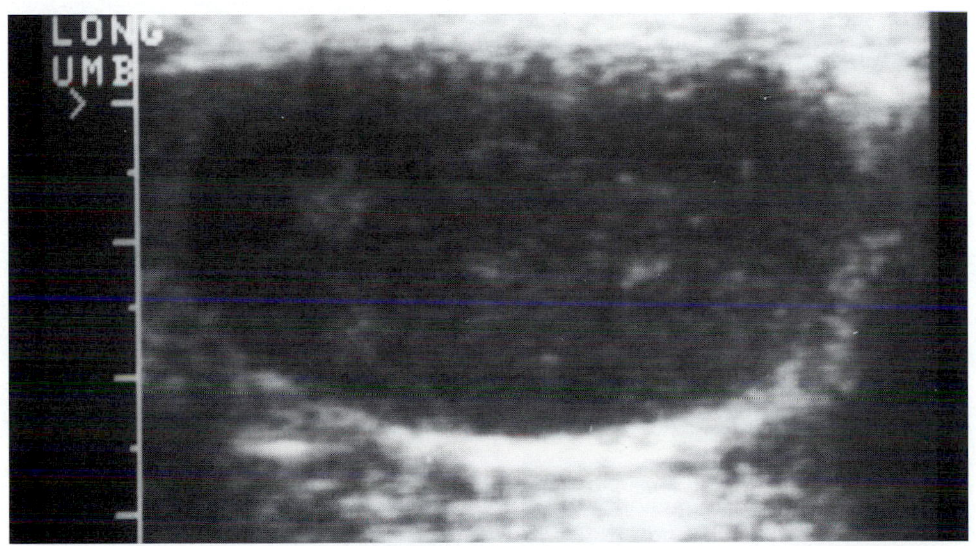

A

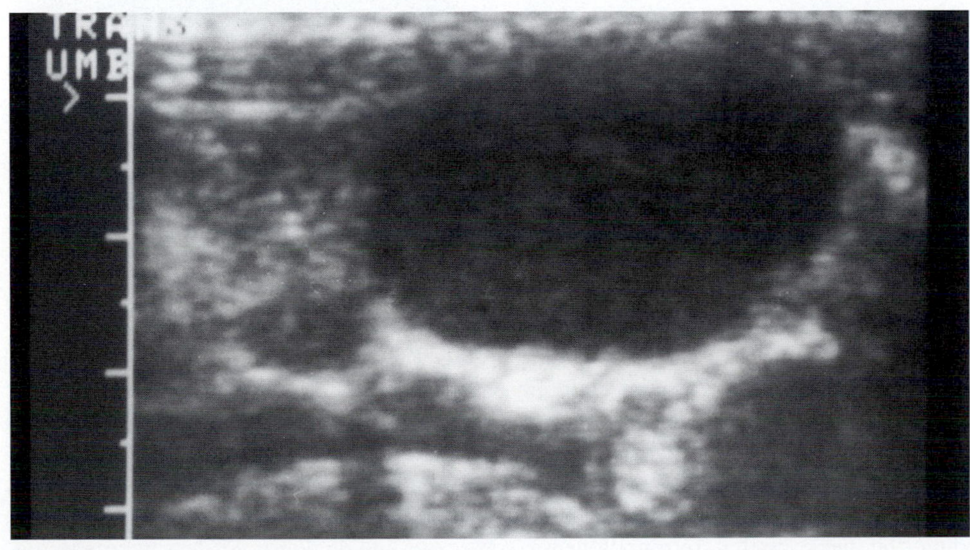

B

FIGURE 80–1. Longitudinal *(A)* and transverse *(B)* views through the lower abdomen.

CHAPTER 80

Castleman Disease of the Mesentery

CARLOS J. SIVIT

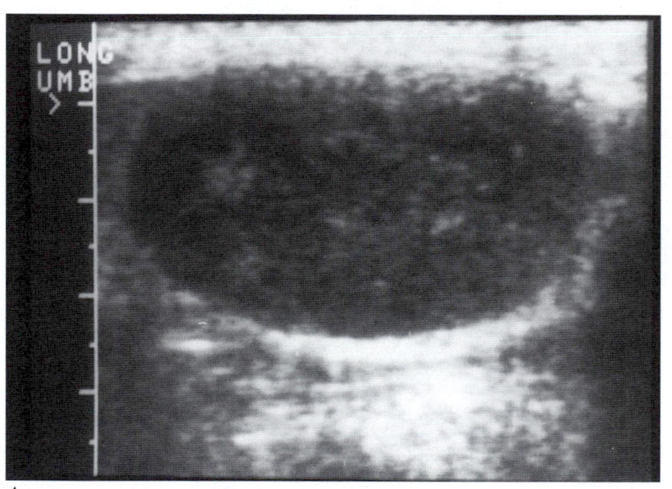

A

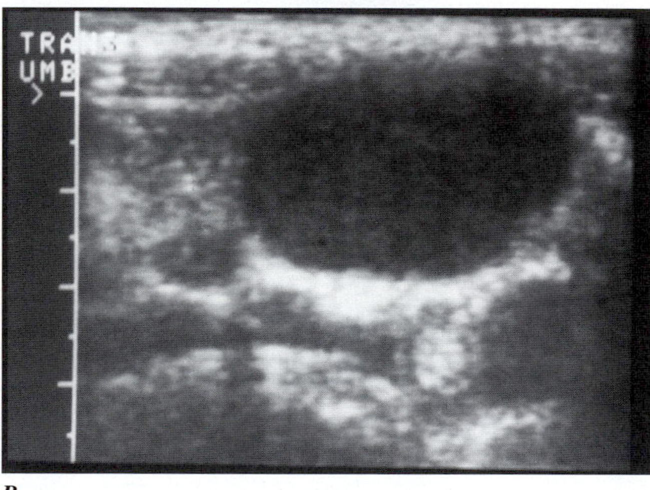

B

FIGURE 80–2. Castleman tumor of the mesentery. Longitudinal *(A)* and transverse *(B)* views through the right lower quadrant of the abdomen demonstrate a markedly enlarged, oval-shaped mesenteric lymph node. It is slightly hypoechoic relative to the anterior abdominal musculature. Note the homogeneous echotexture within the enlarged lymph node. At surgery, Castleman tumor of the mesentery was noted.

Castleman disease, also known as giant lymph node hyperplasia and angiofollicular lymph node hyperplasia, is a rare benign condition characterized by massive lymph node enlargement. It has been reported primarily in older children and young adults. The etiology of the disease is unknown. The condition is generally confined to a limited part of the body. It primarily involves the mediastinum but has also been reported to involve extrathoracic sites containing lymphoid tissue, including the neck, axilla, retroperitoneum, mesentery, and pelvis. Castleman tumor of the mesentery is very rare. The local form of Castleman disease has no malignant potential. Therefore, it is definitively treated with local excision.

There are two histologic types of Castleman disease. The more common is the hyaline-vascular type, which accounts for approximately 90 percent of cases. This type is highly vascular. It is characterized by the presence of small hyaline follicles and by intrafollicular capillary proliferation. The less common plasma cell type accounts for 10 percent of cases and demonstrates less hypervascularity, larger follicles, and more plasma cells. A widespread or multicentric form of Castleman disease has also been described. This form, which

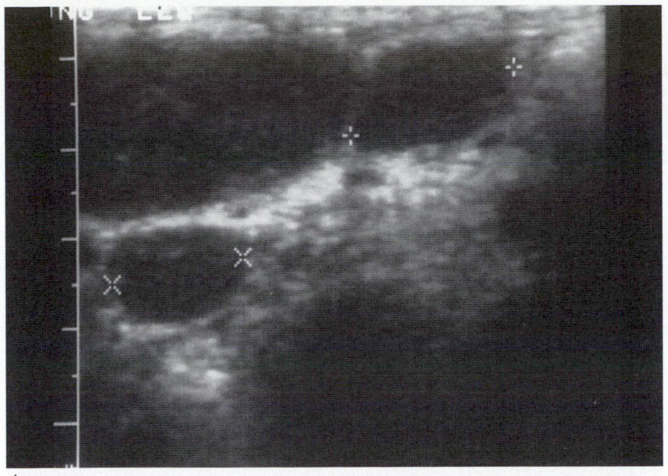

A

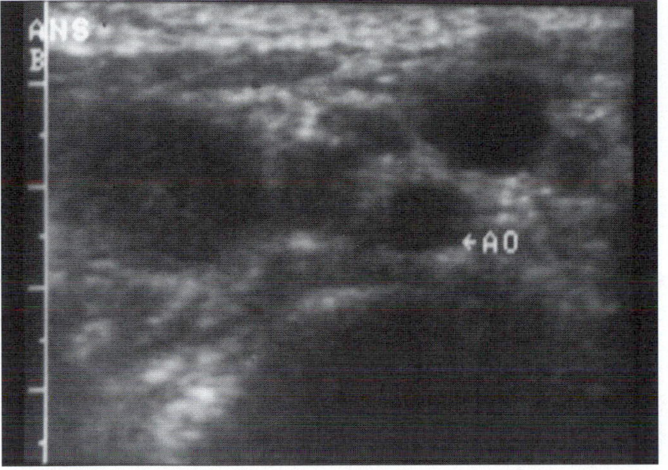

B

FIGURE 80–3. Castleman tumor of the mesentery. ***A.*** Longitudinal view through the left upper quadrant in the same child as in Fig. 80-1 shows additional enlarged mesenteric lymph nodes. ***B.*** Transverse view through the midabdomen in the same child shows additional enlarged mesenteric lymph nodes anterior to the abdominal aorta (AO).

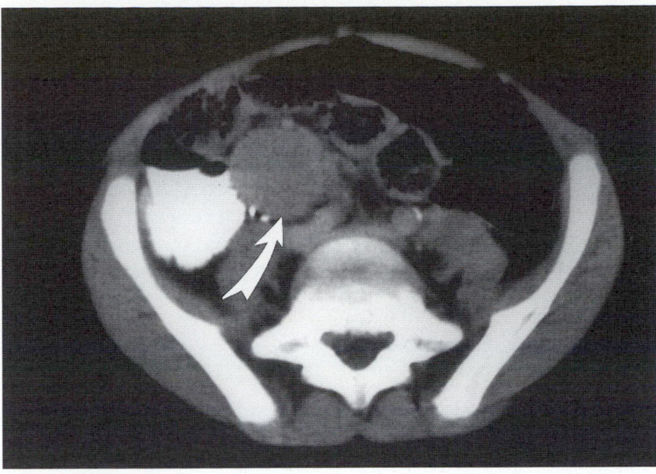

FIGURE 80–4. Castleman tumor of the mesentery. Contrast-enhanced computed tomography (CT) scan through the lower abdomen in the same child as in Fig. 80-1 demonstrates a large, rounded soft tissue mass (*arrow*), representing massive mesenteric lymph node enlargement in the right lower quadrant medial to the cecum.

is far less common than the localized form, is very aggressive. It results in hepatomegaly, splenomegaly, anemia, hypergammaglobulinemia, and generalized lymphadenopathy. The generalized form of Castleman tumor is often fatal.

Castleman tumor of the mesentery is usually recognized on sonography as an incidental finding, as the children are usually asymptomatic. In children, the mesentery is best assessed on sonography with a high-frequency linear transducer utilizing the graded compression technique. Overlying bowel loops can be compressed through the use of graded compression.

The appearance of Castleman tumor of the mesentery on sonography is that of massively enlarged mesenteric lymph nodes (Fig. 80-2) surrounded by smaller lymph nodes (Fig. 80-3). The enlarged lymph nodes have an oval shape, although they may appear somewhat flattened on examination with graded compression sonography (Fig. 80-2). The enlarged lymph nodes have a homogeneous appearance on sonography and are isoechoic or hypoechoic relative to surrounding tissues and muscles. They may be noted anywhere along the small-bowel mesentery, which extends from the left upper quadrant obliquely downward to the right sacroiliac joint (Fig. 80-2). The more common hyaline-vascular form of Castleman tumor shows pronounced vascularity on color Doppler imaging.

Computed tomography (CT) provides better delineation of the origin and extent of the lesion than sonography and is therefore essential for preoperative planning. Additionally, CT is useful in excluding involvement of other abdominal organs. The CT examination should be performed following the use of intravenous and oral contrast. The oral contrast is necessary in order to distinguish unopacified bowel loops from mesenteric pathology. The CT of Castleman tumor demonstrates large, round or oval masses in the small-bowel mesentery (Fig. 80-4). The mass demonstrates soft tissue attenuation. Moderate enhancement may be seen within the mass following the administration of intravenous contrast.

Castleman tumor of the mesentery can be distinguished from mesenteric lymphadenopathy due to a variety of infectious or neoplastic conditions on the basis of the size of the enlarged lymph nodes. Mesenteric lymph node enlargement associated with Castleman tumor is massive, with the anteroposterior lymph node diameter usually being greater than 4 cm. Conversely, mesenteric lymphadenopathy associated with other abdominal or pelvic inflammatory and infectious conditions rarely results in a lymph node with diameter of greater than 2 cm.

References

Barki Y, Shadked G, Levy I: Mesenteric Castleman disease: Sonographic diagnosis. *JCU* 20:486–488, 1992.

Ferreiros J, Leon NG, Mata I, et al: Computed tomography in abdominal Castleman's disease. *J Comput Assist Tomogr* 13: 433–436, 1989.

Garber SJ, Shaw DG: Case report: The ultrasound and computed tomography appearance of mesenteric Castleman disease. *Clin Radiol* 43:429–430, 1991.

Iida E, Kohno A, Mikami T, et al: Mesenteric Castleman tumor. *J Comput Assist Tomogr* 7:338–340, 1983.

Libson E, Fields S, Strauss S, et al: Widespread Castleman disease: CT and US findings. *Radiology* 166:753–755, 1988.

Olscamp G, Weisbrod G, Sanders D, et al: Castleman disease: Unusual manifestations of unusual disorders. *Radiology* 135:43–48, 1980.

Ruess L, Frazier AA, Sivit CJ: CT of the mesentery, omentum, and peritoneum in children. *Radiographics* 15:89–104, 1995.

Sivit CJ, Newman KD, Chandra RS: Visualization of enlarged mesenteric lymph nodes at US examination: Clinical significance. *Pediatr Radiol* 23:471–475, 1993.

81

Figure 81-1 shows a 16-year-old girl with chronic abdominal pain. What do you see? What are the diagnostic considerations?

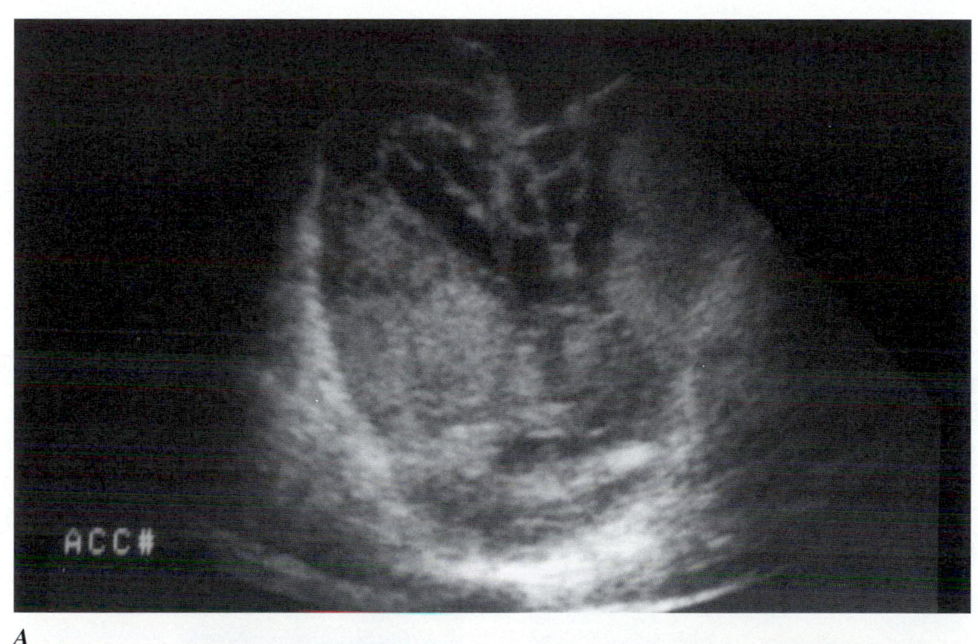

A

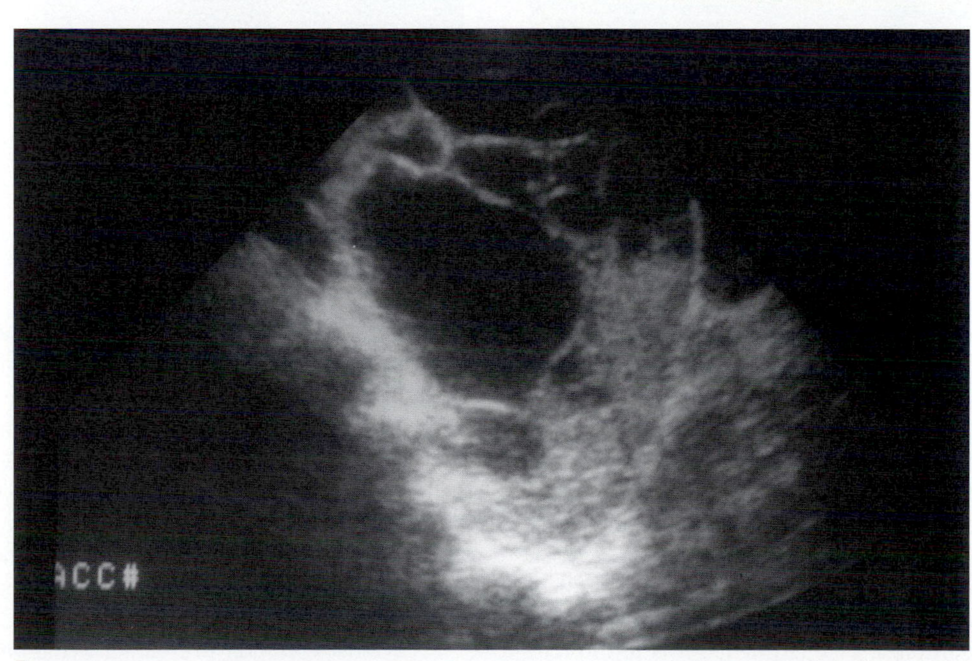

B

FIGURE 81–1. Transverse *(A)* and longitudinal *(B)* views through the lower abdomen.

CHAPTER 81

Cystic Peritoneal Mesothelioma

CARLOS J. SIVIT

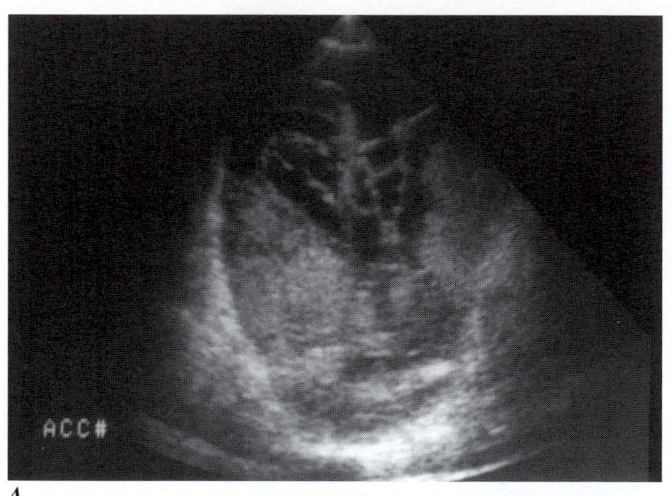

A

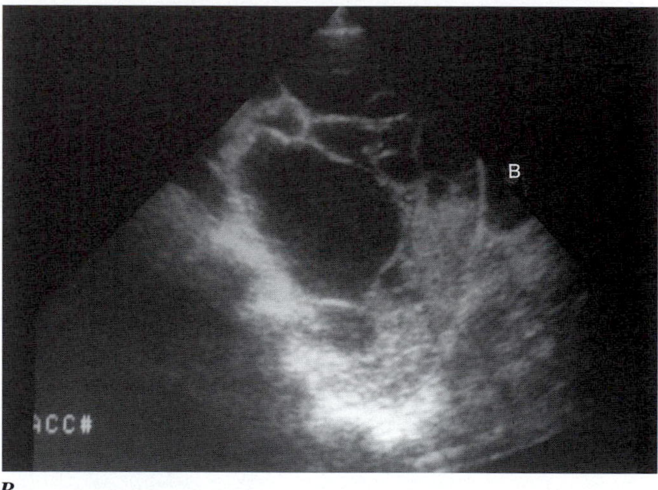

B

FIGURE 81–2. Cystic peritoneal mesothelioma. Transverse *(A)* and longitudinal *(B)* views through the pelvis demonstrate a complex cystic mass, with multiple cysts of varying sizes and solid elements. B = bladder.

Cystic mesothelioma is a very rare primary neoplasm of the peritoneal cavity in older children and adults. It is seen almost exclusively in females. The hallmark of the lesion is multiple thin-walled cysts, lined with mesothelial cells, that contain clear serous or straw-colored fluid, with intervening connective tissue. It is a diffuse or multifocal lesion involving the peritoneum, omentum, and pelvic and abdominal viscera. It has a predilection for the surfaces of the pelvic viscera. Cystic mesothelioma is part of the spectrum of mesenchymal neoplasms that can arise from the pleura and from the pericardial and peritoneal compartments. It is felt to represent an intermediate form between two neoplasms of the abdomen that have a mesothelial origin, the benign adenomatoid tumor and the malignant peritoneal mesothelioma, which is a more common neoplasm in adults. There are two important differences between cystic peritoneal mesothelioma and malignant mesothelioma. First, cystic mesothelioma is not related to prior asbestos exposure, unlike malignant mesothelioma. Second, cystic peritoneal mesothelioma does not have malignant potential. It does not metastasize, although there frequently are local recurrences. These lesions can usually be resected from neighboring peritoneal surfaces with little difficulty. However, they are difficult to eradicate completely as a result of their frequent multifocal origin.

The most common presenting symptom in patients with cystic peritoneal mesothelioma is chronic or intermittent abdominal pain. Other reported symptoms include early satiety, weight loss, urgency, frequency, and dysfunctional uterine

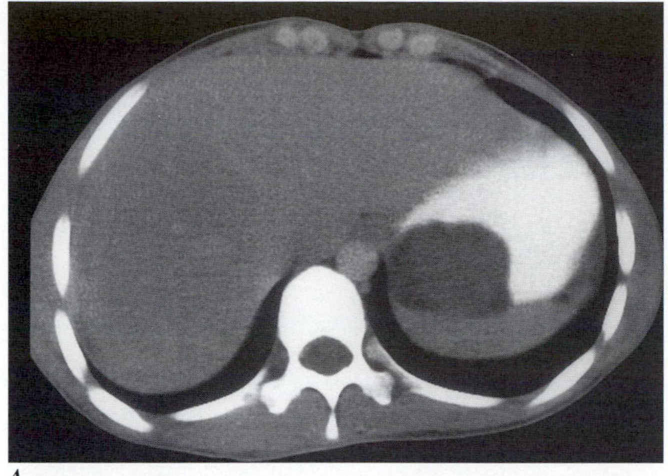

A

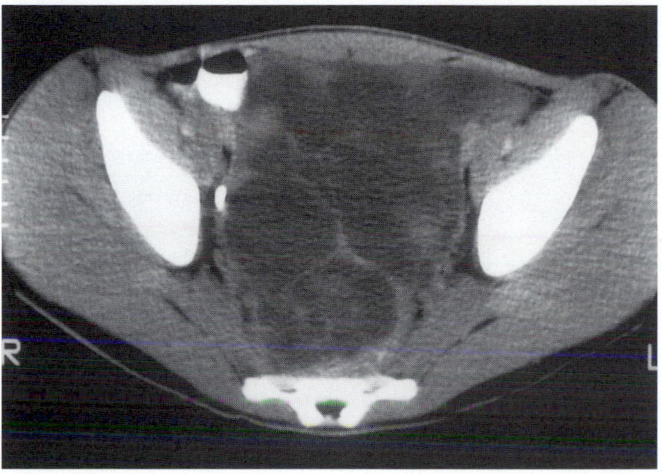

B

FIGURE 81–3. Cystic peritoneal mesothelioma. ***A.*** Contrast-enhanced computed tomography (CT) scan through the upper abdomen in the same patient as in Fig. 81-1 demonstrates a low-attenuation peritoneal mass immediately anterior to the spleen displacing the greater curvature of the stomach. ***B.*** Contrast-enhanced CT scan through the pelvis in the same patient as in ***A*** demonstrates a large, well-circumscribed, multiseptated, cystic mass.

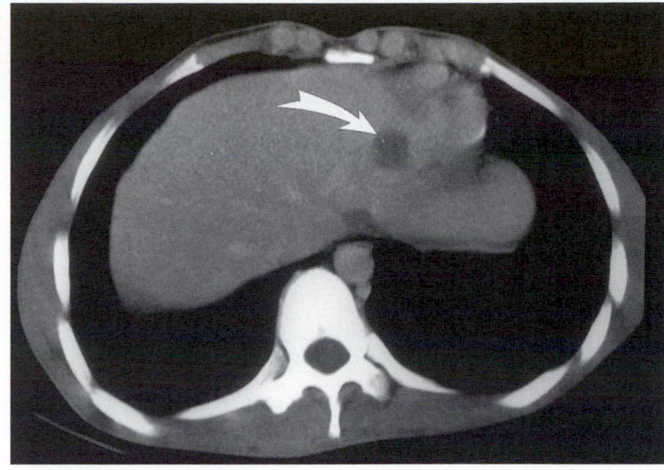

FIGURE 81–4. Recurrence of cystic peritoneal mesothelioma. Contrast-enhanced computed tomography (CT) scan through the upper abdomen in the same patient as in Fig. 81-3, 6 months after the CT examination in Fig. 81-3 and after the patient had undergone primary resection, demonstrates a low-attenuation peritoneal subphrenic mass (*arrow*), representing recurrence of cystic peritoneal mesothelioma. Note that secondary to the partial volume effect, the mass appears surrounded by hepatic parenchyma, although it is in a suprahepatic location.

bleeding. An abdominal or pelvic mass may be palpated on physical examination. However, frequently there are no abnormal findings on physical examination, and the neoplasm is initially observed as an incidental finding on imaging examination.

The characteristic sonographic finding of peritoneal mesothelioma is that of a large multicystic mass (Fig. 81-2) in the lower abdomen or pelvis. It is usually difficult to identify the ovaries as separate structures, given the size of these lesions and their primary pelvic origin. Masses as large as 25 cm in diameter have been reported. The cysts are uniformly anechoic and range from several millimeters to several centimeters in diameter. The septations between the cysts are thin. Solid elements may be noted as well (Fig. 81-2). These solid areas within the mass may represent the increased interfaces of small microcysts that are below the resolution of the transducer or may represent thickened peritoneum, mesentery, or omentum. Calcifications within these masses have not been reported. Multiple lesions may be noted throughout the peritoneal cavity.

Computed tomography (CT) and magnetic resonance imaging (MRI) are also commonly utilized to image this neoplasm. These modalities are helpful in defining the location and extent of the lesion for preoperative planning and for postoperative surveillance. This is particularly useful when the mass is multifocal in various widely separated peritoneal locations (Fig. 81-3) or to assess for recurrent disease (Fig. 81-4). The appearance of this lesion on CT is that of a large, well-circumscribed, multilocular cystic mass (Fig. 81-3). The cyst walls are thin and do not enhance following intravenous contrast administration. On MRI, there typically is low signal intensity on T1-weighted images and intermediate or high signal intensity on proton density and T2-weighted images.

The differential diagnosis includes other large cystic abdominal and pelvic lesions, including mesenteric cyst, ovarian cyst, ovarian cystadenoma or adenocarcinoma, and ovarian or mesenteric teratoma. It may be difficult to distinguish cystic peritoneal mesothelioma from a mesenteric cyst if the lesion is entirely cystic. Both lesions are typically quite large and contain numerous septations. A mesenteric cyst will not contain solid areas. Differentiation from ovarian lesions can be made if normal ovaries can be identified separate from the lesion. However, this may be difficult, as most cystic peritoneal mesotheliomas are very large and often arise from the surface of pelvic viscera. Usually the ovaries cannot be identified separate from the mass on imaging examination. Teratomas can be usually be distinguished from cystic peritoneal mesothelioma, since they often contain fat or calcification.

References

Moriwaki Y, Kobayashi S, Harada H, et al: Cystic mesothelioma of the peritoneum. *J Gastroenterol* 31:868–874, 1996.

O'Neil JD, Ros PR, Storm BL, et al: Cystic mesothelioma of the peritoneum. *Radiology* 170:333–337, 1989.

Ruess L, Frazier AA, Sivit CJ: CT of the mesentery, omentum, and peritoneum in children. *Radiographics* 15:89–104, 1995.

Schneider JA, Zelnick EJ: Benign cystic peritoneal mesothelioma. *JCU* 13:190–192, 1985.

Sivit CJ: CT scan of mesentery-omentum peritoneum. *Radiol Clin North Am* 34:863–884, 1996.

82

A 5-week-old boy presents with projectile nonbilious vomiting for 3 days. Figures 82-1 and 82-2 were obtained during an ultrasound (US) study. What is his diagnosis?

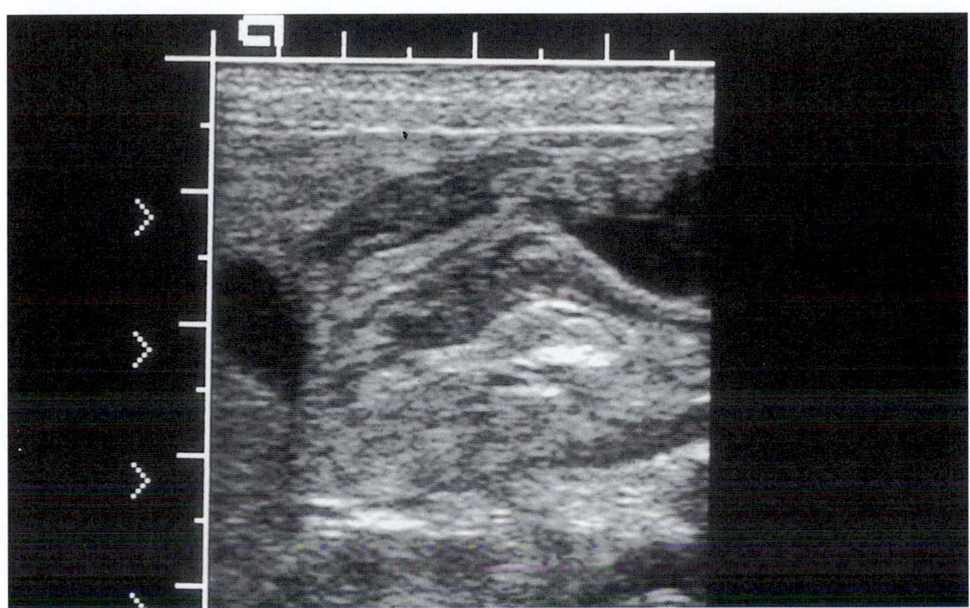

FIGURE 82–1. Longitudinal image of antropyloric region.

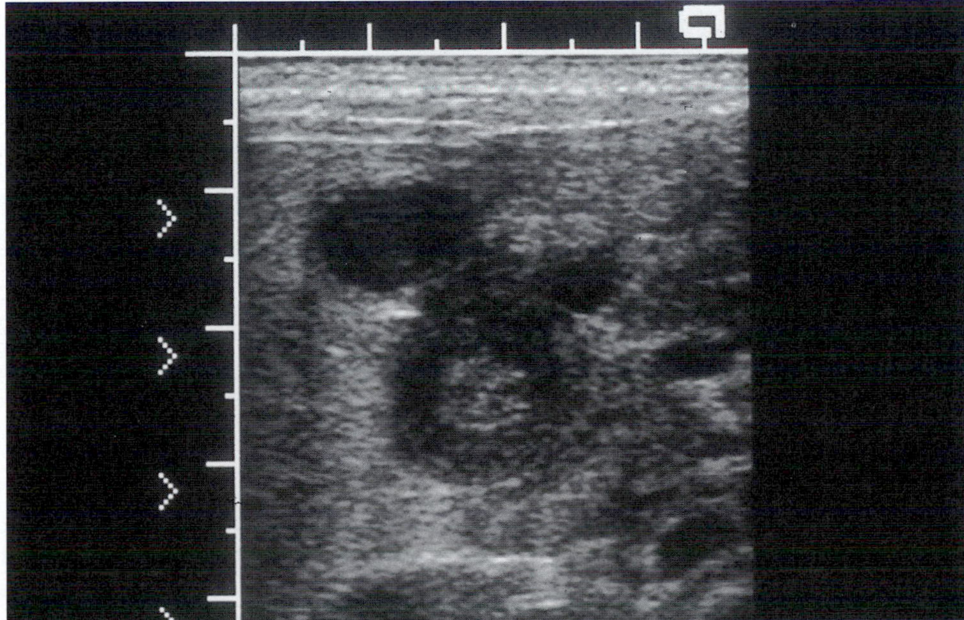

FIGURE 82–2. Transverse image of antropyloric region.

CHAPTER 82

Hypertrophic Pyloric Stenosis

HARRIS L. COHEN

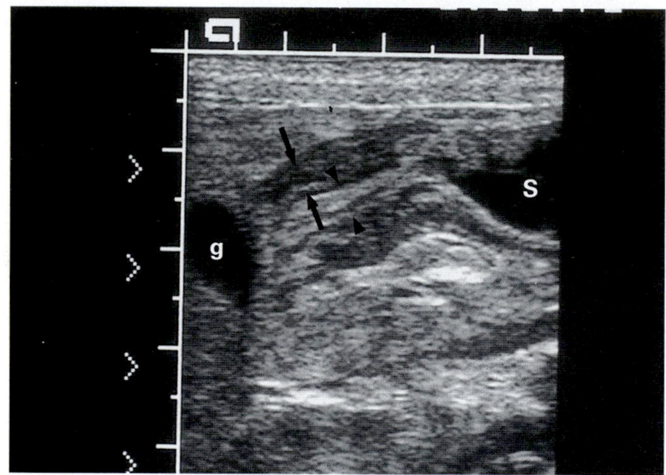

FIGURE 82–3. Annotated version of Fig. 82-1. Hypertrophic pyloric stenosis. Longitudinal image of antropyloric region and pylorus. Fluid is seen in the stomach antrum (S) proximal to the pylorus. The muscle walls of the pylorus—those on the more superficial surface (*arrow*) as well as the deeper surface—are echopenic. In the center of the pylorus is a linear echogenicity (*arrowheads*), which represents the more echogenic mucosa. The pylorus was consistently 20 mm long and its muscle wall 4 mm thick. This allowed a diagnosis of HPS. One can see the gallbladder (g) just distal to the pylorus. The close relationship of the gallbladder to the duodenal bulb can occasionally help in finding the pyloric region.

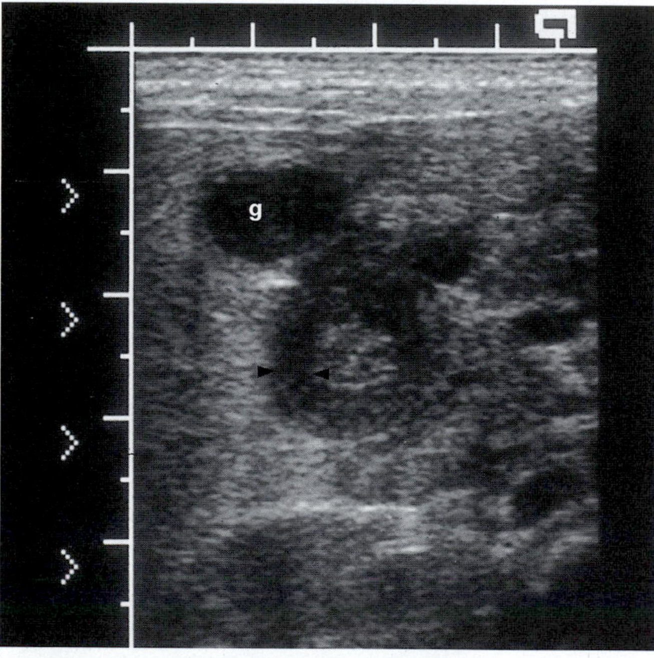

FIGURE 82–4. Annotated version of Fig. 82-2. Hypertrophic pyloric stenosis. Transverse image through pylorus. The echopenic pyloric muscle (*arrows*) is thick, measuring 4 mm or greater at various positions around this "bagel" or "doughnut." The echogenic mucosa is seen centrally. G = gallbladder.

Figure 82-3, the annotated version of Fig. 82-1, shows a thickened pyloric muscle and elongated pyloric canal. Figure 82-4, the annotated version of Fig. 82-2, confirms the thickening of the pyloric muscle by showing the classic "doughnut" or "bagel" sign of this abnormality. This 6-week-old, who has been vomiting over 3 days, has hypertrophic pyloric stenosis (HPS).

These classic abnormal images are far different from what is seen in the perfectly normal patient. The normal pyloric channel either is not imaged as fluid crosses it from the stomach antrum to the duodenal bulb and descending duodenum or is seen to be short in length (Fig. 82-5), shorter than is required to make the diagnosis of HPS. The muscle wall of a normal pylorus is thin.

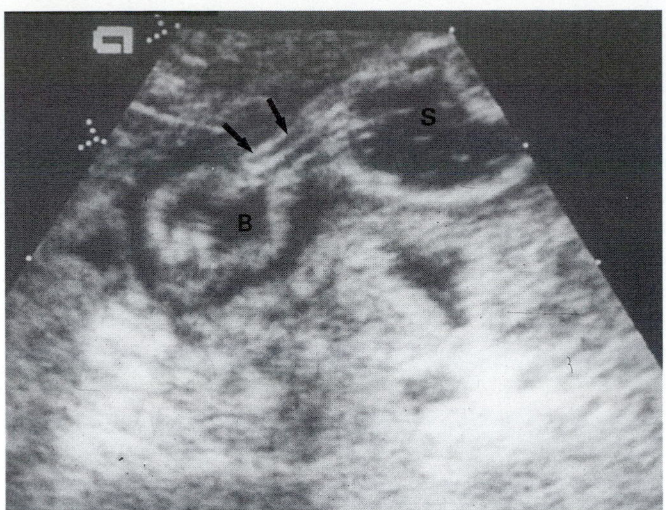

FIGURE 82–5. Normal pylorus. Longitudinal plane through pylorus. ***A.*** Water in the stomach antrum (S) and duodenal bulb (d) is essentially echoless, with a few bright echoes due to some residual and normal aeration of water that the patient drank. The pylorus (*arrows*) is only a few millimeters long. The echopenic muscle around the pylorus was not thick enough to diagnose HPS on this image.

WHAT IS HYPERTROPHIC PYLORIC STENOSIS?

Hypertrophic pyloric stenosis is an idiopathic thickening of the circular muscles of the pylorus. The abnormality classically presents in a previously healthy infant who develops vomiting as a result of the relative obstruction of the egress of gastric contents into the duodenum by the hypertrophied muscle. With this obstruction, the pylorus elongates (Fig. 82-6). The vomiting is usually described as *projectile,* i.e., occurring with force.

Patients classically present at 6 weeks of age but certainly can present earlier, even in the first days of life. The vomiting is nonbilious and therefore does not evoke fear of midgut volvulus, which usually presents as bilious vomiting in the first days of life. Among patients with HPS, boys outnumber girls. First-born children and those with positive family histories of HPS, particularly on the mother's side, are at greatest risk. It is important for the clinician to note whether there is an electrolyte disturbance from the vomiting. A history of weight loss is more suggestive of true abnormality rather than a neonate who is "spitting up" [i.e., has gastroesophageal reflux (GER)]. The presence of a pyloric mass or "olive" on physical examination allows a ready clinical diagnosis, and the patient can be treated with surgical pyloromyotomy. Without a definitive clinical diagnosis, the patient will undergo an imaging workup. Ultrasound is the gold standard for the diagnosis of HPS and can help rule out other clinical concerns.

VOMITING FOR THE FIRST TIME AT SEVERAL WEEKS OF LIFE—CLINICAL AND IMAGING CONSIDERATIONS

The most common causes of nonbilious vomiting or regurgitation in the nonseptic child during the first 3 months of life are GER, hypertrophic pyloric stenosis, and pylorospasm. A septic child may have gastroenteritis. Regurgitation, or GER, is a very common finding in the first 3 months of a neonate's life. Vomiting, or the forceful extrusion of gastric contents, in the neonate can be a more significant clinical problem. The differentiation between vomiting and regurgitation may be clinically difficult. All three of these conditions may lead to projectile "vomiting," with that in the case of GER often due to overfeeding. Gastroesophageal reflux may be diagnosed from the medical history, by watching an actual feeding, or monitoring for esophageal acidity. Less often, clinicians will request an upper gastrointestinal (UGI) series or US examination (Fig. 82-7) to "rule out reflux."

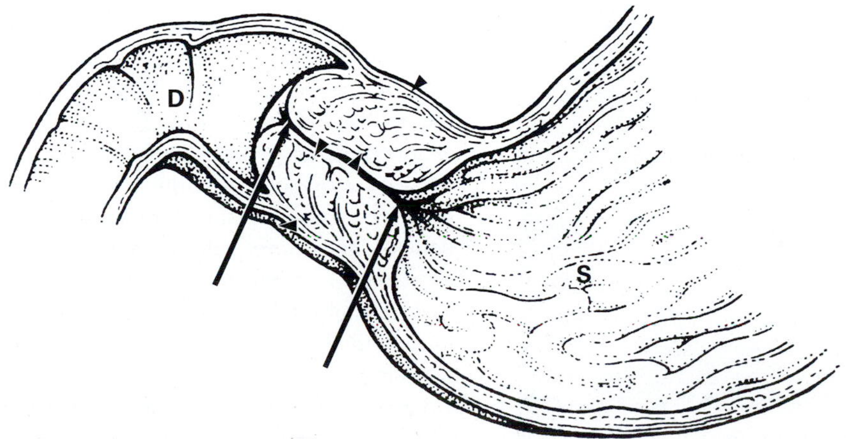

FIGURE 82–6. Hypertrophic pyloric stenosis. Schematic drawing of longitudinal plane through pylorus. The pyloric channel (*arrows*) is elongated. Note the thickened muscle of the pylorus (*arrowheads*). S = stomach antrum, D = duodenum. (*From Haller JO, Cohen HL: Hypertrophic pyloric stenosis: Diagnosis using US.* Radiology *161:335–339, 1986, with permission.*)

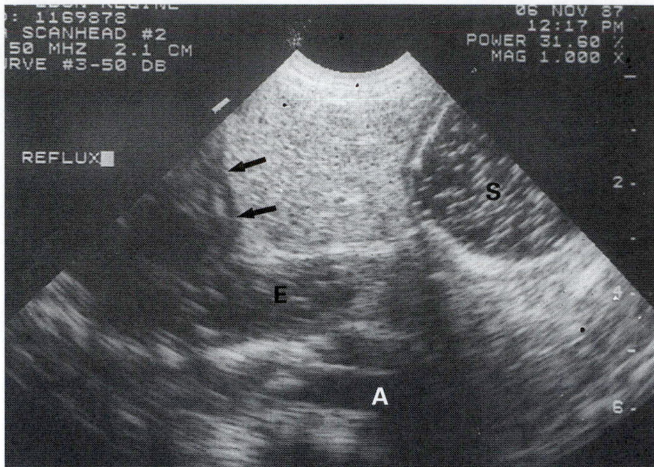

FIGURE 82–7. Gastroesophageal reflux. Ultrasound. Longitudinal plane through aorta, angling slightly to the left. Fluid with echogenic debris from water with normal aeration (milk products may also appear echogenic) is seen in the stomach (S). Fluid was seen to enter the esophagus from the stomach, consistent with gastroesophageal reflux. The esophageal fluid is seen above and below the diaphragm (*arrows*). A = aorta.

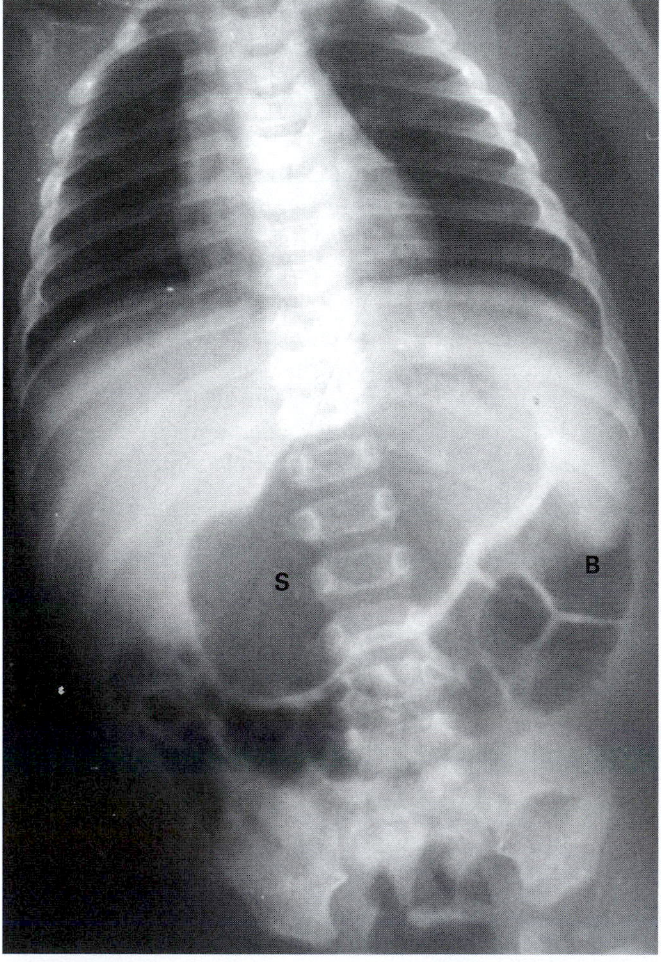

FIGURE 82–8. Hypertrophic pyloric stenosis (HPS)—caterpillar sign. Plain film. Chest/abdomen. Anteroposterior view. The stomach (S) peristalsing against a pyloric obstruction, as in this patient with HPS, looks like a caterpillar viewed from above and walking to the right lower quadrant. Obviously, the obstruction cannot be a complete one because there is air in the large and small bowel. B = splenic flexure of large colon.

HYPERTROPHIC PYLORIC STENOSIS

Imaging Findings

If a patient is thought to have HPS, we immediately suggest an US examination. As with other clinical problems, knowledge of what other modalities show or have shown when used in the past has been helpful in determining diagnostic criteria using US.

Plain-film abdominal radiography (Fig. 82-8) may show gastric distention. On occasion, a mass impression of the thickened pyloric muscle on an air-filled gastric antrum may be noted. However, radiographs are most often *not* helpful in the diagnosis of HPS and are usually nonspecific in cases of GER or gastroenteritis.

The conventional UGI series is excellent for diagnosing obstructive causes of vomiting. In cases of HPS (Fig. 82-9), one can note the mass impression of the hypertrophied pyloric muscle on the barium-filled antrum ("shoulder sign"), or the filling of the proximal pylorus ("beak sign") or the entire elongated pylorus ("string sign") with barium. The UGI series allows ready diagnosis of GER as well as less likely causes of obstruction, such as midgut volvulus, gastric volvulus, or annular pancreas. The UGI series is certainly a viable alternative to US for the diagnosis of HPS. However, only US provides a rapid diagnosis without raising worries about radiation exposure. We know that US can be used to effectively rule out HPS and the other diagnoses of concern, i.e., GER and pylorospasm. Contrary to what some groups have reported in the literature, we rarely need to go to a second exam such as the UGI series to rule out HPS or its differential diagnostic considerations.

Ultrasound Findings

Ultrasound has become a standard and highly sensitive, specific, and accurate method for diagnosing HPS since its introduction for this diagnosis in 1977 by Teele and Smith. Ultrasound allows the direct visualization of the pylorus and reveals the thickened circular muscle and an elongated pyloric length in patients with HPS. It can show US equivalents of the historically reported UGI signs, e.g., the mass impression of muscle on antrum (Fig. 82-10), the string sign, and the double track sign (Fig. 82-11). Measurements of pyloric channel length, pyloric diameter, and muscle thickness have been used by several authors for diagnosis. The overlap of transverse pyloric diameter measurements between normal patients and those with HPS has caused us and others to abandon this criterion. Measurements of pyloric length and muscle wall thickness are key. Blumhagen and Noble found muscle thickness to be the most discriminating and accurate measurement, noting it as 4.8 ± 0.6 mm in HPS patients and 1.8 ± 0.4 mm in normal patients. Measurements of 4 mm are considered positive for HPS, with measurements between 3 and 4 mm a gray zone, particularly in the younger or smaller neonate. Muscle thickness measurement may be obtained on transverse or longitudinal views of the pylorus. Wilson and Vanhoutte considered a 2-cm pyloric length to be definitively abnormal. Stunden et al felt that pyloric canal length was the

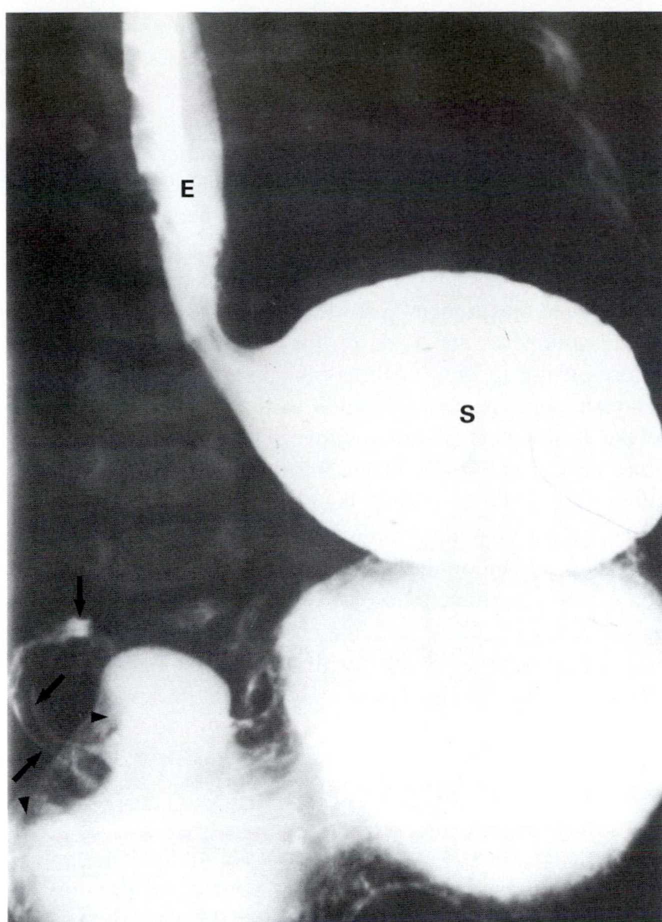

FIGURE 82–9. Hypertrophic pyloric stenosis. Upper gastrointestinal series. Contrast is seen in the stomach (S) as well as an elongated pylorus (*arrows*) whose muscle's mass impression (shoulder sign) (*arrowheads*) is seen as mass effect on the contrast-filled antrum. The esophagus (E) is also filled with contrast due to significant reflux during the procedure. A contrast-filled elongated pyloric channel is evidence of the string sign of HPS.

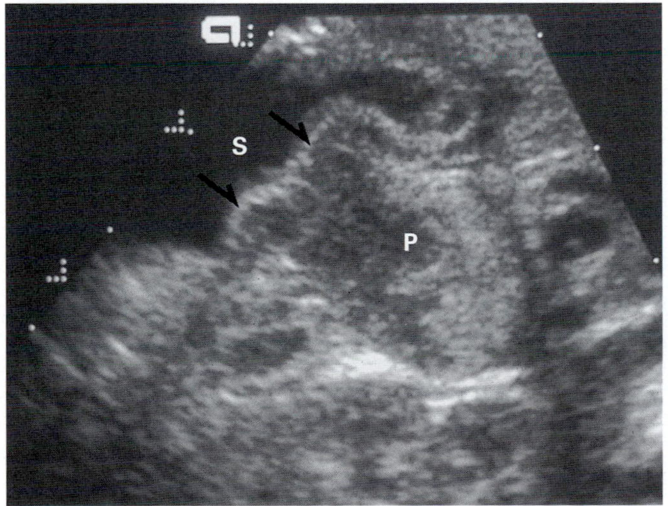

FIGURE 82–10. Hypertrophic pyloric stenosis—shoulder sign. Ultrasound. Longitudinal plane through pylorus. The stomach (S) is fluid-filled. The mass (asterisk) of the proximal thickened pylorus (P) is seen poking into the fluid-filled stomach (*arrows*), a more direct visualization of what is seen with the upper gastrointestinal series. This image of thickened pyloric mass has also been referred to as the cervix sign, because it looks like one.

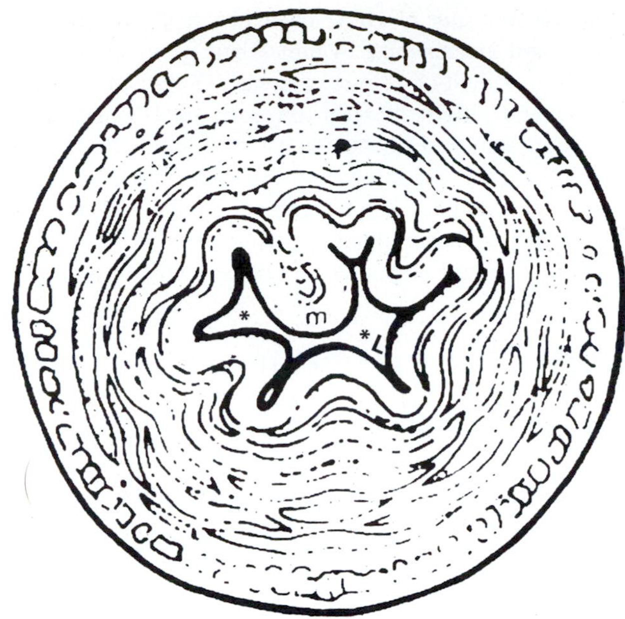

A

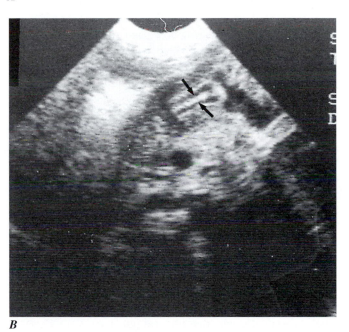

B

FIGURE 82–11. Hypertrophic pyloric stenosis—double-track sign. ***A.*** Schematic drawing. Transverse plane through pylorus. Mass impression of the muscle on the single pyloric channel compresses it into several smaller "channels" (*asterisks*). m = mucosa, L = lumen. (*From Haller JO, Cohen HL, Hypertrophic pyloric stenosis: Diagnosis using US.* Radiology *161:335–339, 1986, with permission.*) ***B.*** Ultrasound (US). Longitudinal plane through pylorus. Mass impression on a fluid-filled pylorus compresses the water in the pylorus into several channels. Two are seen on this image, the US equivalent of the barium double-track sign. (*From Cohen HL, Schechter S, Mestel A, et al: Ultrasonic "double track" sign in hypertrophic pyloric stenosis.* J Ultrasound Med *6:139–143, 1987, with permission.*)

only precise indicator of HPS. Their negative cases had *no* pylorus length greater than 14 mm. Their positive cases all had a pylorus length of 18 mm or greater. Swischuk et al reviewed several pitfalls of HPS diagnosis by US, including the false appearance of thickening of the pyloric muscle wall on tangential views of the pylorus. Keeping the echogenic channel in the middle of the image can prevent this. One must, however, be aware that hypertrophy may be somewhat asymmetric—i.e., the bagel may not be perfectly round.

TECHNIQUE FOR FLUID-AIDED US OF THE UPPER GI TRACT TO "RULE OUT HPS"

My US technique for the diagnosis of HPS in the vomiting infant without bilious vomiting is similar, in many ways, to the methods of performing a neonatal UGI that I was taught when I was a fellow. In many cases a nasogastric tube (8F, 15 in) is placed into the neonate's stomach to remove any gastric contents that may interfere with our US exam, particularly milk products, which are echogenic, and significant air, which can cause ring down and dirty shadowing artifacts. The stomach is then filled with an echoless contrast material (water). Tap water is echoless within minutes of placement into the stomach or after standing in a receptacle (that is, after the initially contained echogenicities due to aeration dissipate). This is less of a concern with other in-hospital bottled fluids (e.g., Pedialyte). The echoless nature of the fluid allows us to follow it into the duodenum and, if we are fortunate, to the ligament of Treitz in normal individuals. It also allows diagnosis of GER, at least into the lower chest. Evaluation of the mid- to upper chest is limited by the air-filled lungs. Some authorities prefer feeding the patient water by bottle. I prefer placement of the water by a nasogastric tube. This allows a rapid exam, less swallowed air from crying and drinking from a bottle, and a more definitive statement with regard to GER. To fill the stomach, 60 mL (a feeding) of fluid is placed through the tube. The tube is immediately pulled to avoid the GER that can occur from a tube's crossing the gastroesophageal junction.

The transducer is first placed just to the right of midline at the top of the abdomen, in the area of the gallbladder and duodenal bulb. If we see an abnormal pylorus that does not change with time, the diagnosis is made and the patient is sent to the operating room. If there is any doubt or if abdominal gas obscures detail, we do the exam with water as a contrast agent. The neonate is then examined in supine and right side down positions, so as to see as much stomach as possible, particularly the gastric antrum, and to note how it handles a fluid load, and to note whether the pylorus opens and fluid flows to the descending duodenum or whether the fluid is held up by a nonchanging, thickened, and elongated pylorus, which would suggest the diagnosis of HPS. At the same time, we can look at the gastroesophageal junction to note whether fluid extends from the stomach to the esophagus above it and through the diaphragm to prove GER. We look at the gastroesophageal junction in the transverse plane angling to the level of the diaphragm and in the longitudinal plane angling slightly to the left of the aorta.

We use a high-frequency transducer, preferably 7.5 MHz or greater. Depending on the machine I am using, I will often use a sector or convex array transducer rather than a linear array transducer because it has a wider field of view and a smaller footprint. If I need to see one area better, or if the pylorus is superficial, I will switch to the linear array. Cineloop has made our work much easier, since we can immediately go back and recapture a "just seen" image.

Measurements are made on the longitudinal view of the pylorus using machine calipers. Calipers are placed on the echopenic muscles (superficial as well as deep in relationship to the transducer) of the pylorus. The length is measured more easily with fluid in the antrum, as this allows exact knowledge of the position of the proximal pylorus. We sometimes use a trace to determine the true measurement when the pylorus is curved on the image. On the transverse image, we obtain muscle thicknesses at various positions about the bagel (or doughnut or, as Teele and Smith first called it, target) of the thickened pylorus with a central echogenic pyloric channel due to contained mucosa.

SOME MEASUREMENT DEBATE

A muscle thickness 4 mm or greater is definitely abnormal. A muscle thickness less than 2 mm is considered definitively normal. There is debate about the significance of measurements between 2 and 4 mm. Individual cases proven at surgery to have HPS have had muscle wall thickness measurements between 3 and 4 mm. We use a 4-mm measurement beyond 4 weeks of age as our positive wall thickness but warn our clinicians about the possibility of lesser measurements in the very young. Errors can be made in measuring muscle thickness because of the subtle nature of the millimeter differences. We luckily also have the pyloric length measurement to help us; if a thickness measurement is 3.5 mm and the length is 18 mm or greater, this is most suggestive of HPS. We obviously discuss these very unusual cases and their diagnostic dilemmas with our clinicians. De-

TABLE 82-1
US Findings Suggesting Hypertrophic Pyloric Stenosis

1. Elongated pylorus (= or >18 mm)
2. Thickened pyloric muscle (= or > 4 mm)
3. Unchangeability of findings 1 and 2 during the study
4. Double track of fluid in pylorus

Caveats:

Patients with pylorospasm may have similar images at some point during their US study. This is true with the double track sign as well.

Abnormal measurements may be lower for the patient who presents at a younger age (4 weeks or less) or is a premature (who at 6 weeks is not truly 6 weeks of age but really only the gestational age at birth plus 6 weeks), as this may allow him or her to have the measurements of a younger patient. For these younger patients, we warn the clinician when wall thicknesses are 3 mm or greater and are rigorous in evaluating change during the study and offering follow-up exams if necessary.

spite all the above, we have not erred in an HPS diagnosis yet. We never "live or die" on the basis of a number, however. The ability to study fluid movement through the pylorus in real time can save an exam by showing change in the pyloric image and suggesting another diagnosis, particularly pylorospasm.

So, I repeat: An unchanging pyloric image that is 4 mm thick and 18 mm long is HPS.

References

Alford B, McIlhenny J: The child with acute abdominal pain and vomiting. *Radiol Clin North Am* 30:441–453, 1992.

Blumhagen JD, Noble HG: Muscle thickness in hypertrophic pyloric stenosis: Sonographic determination. *AJR* 140:221–223, 1983.

Cohen HL, Babcock D: Vomiting in the 0–3 month age group, in *Appropriateness Criteria for Imaging and Treatment Decisions,* ACR Task Force on Appropriateness Criteria (ed). Reston, VA: American College of Radiology, 1995:PD2.1-2.11.

Cohen HL, Haller JO, Mestel A, et al: Neonatal duodenum: Fluid-aided US examination. *Radiology* 164:805–809, 1987.

Cohen HL, Schechter S, Mestel A, et al: Ultrasonic "double track" sign in hypertrophic pyloric stenosis. *J Ultrasound Med* 6: 139–143, 1987.

Cohen HL, Zinn H, Haller J, et al: Ultrasonography of pylorospasm: Findings may simulate hypertrophic pyloric stenosis. *J Ultrasound Med* 17: 705–711, 1998.

Haller JO, Cohen HL: Hypertrophic pyloric stenosis: Diagnosis using US. *Radiology* 161:335–339, 1986.

Haran PJ, Darling DB, Sciammas F: The value of the double-track sign as a differentiating factor between pylorospasm and hypertrophic pyloric stenosis in infants. *Radiology* 86:723–725, 1966.

Hayden CK Jr: Update: Ultrasonography of the gastrointestinal tract in infants and children. *Abdom Imaging* 21:9–20, 1996.

Hernanz-Schulman M, Sells L, Ambrosino M, et al: Hypertrophic pyloric stenosis in the infant without a palpable olive: Accuracy of sonographic diagnosis. *Radiology* 193:771–776, 1994.

Hilton S. The vomiting child, in *Practical Pediatric Radiology,* 2d ed, Hilton S, Edwards D (eds). Philadelphia: Saunders, 1994: 297–299.

Stunden RJ, LeQuesne GW, Little KET: The improved ultrasound diagnosis of hypertrophic pyloric stenosis. *Pediatr Radiol* 16: 200–205, 1986.

Swischuk L, Hayden CK Jr, Stansberry S: Sonographic pitfalls in imaging of the antropyloric region in infants. *Radiographics* 9:437–447, 1989.

Teele RL, Smith EH: Ultrasound in the diagnosis of idiopathic hypertrophic pyloric stenosis. *N Engl J Med* 296:1149–1150, 1977.

Wilson DA, Vanhoutte JJ: The reliable sonographic diagnosis of hypertrophic pyloric stenosis. *JCU* 12:201–204, 1984.

83

A 6-week-old male presented with a history of projectile vomiting. Figure 83-1 is an image taken during a fluid-aided ultrasound (US) exam of the upper gastrointestinal tract. What do you think? Figure 83-2 is an image taken 3 min after the first. What do you think now? What is the diagnosis?

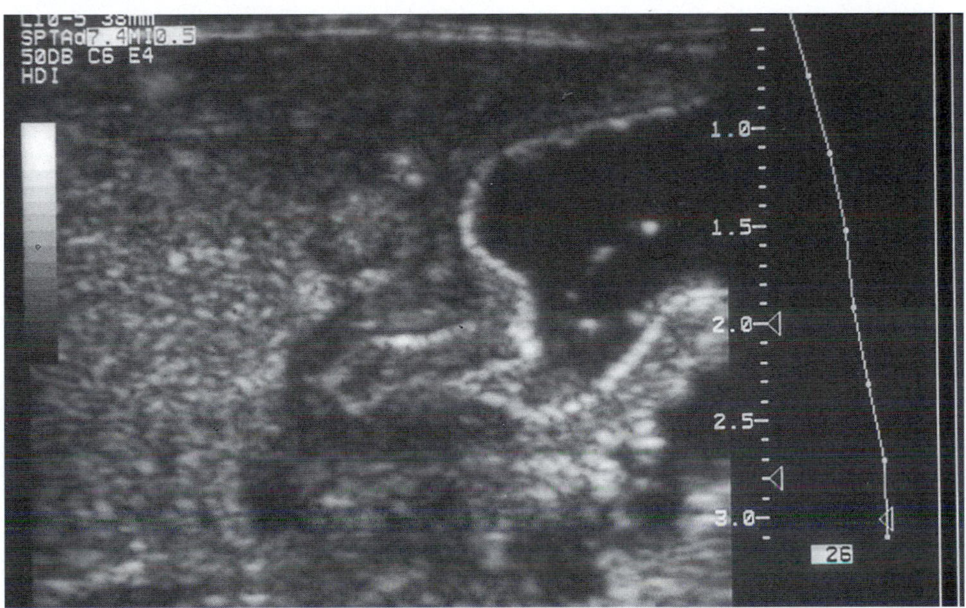

FIGURE 83–1. Ultrasound. Antropyloric region. Longitudinal plane through pylorus.

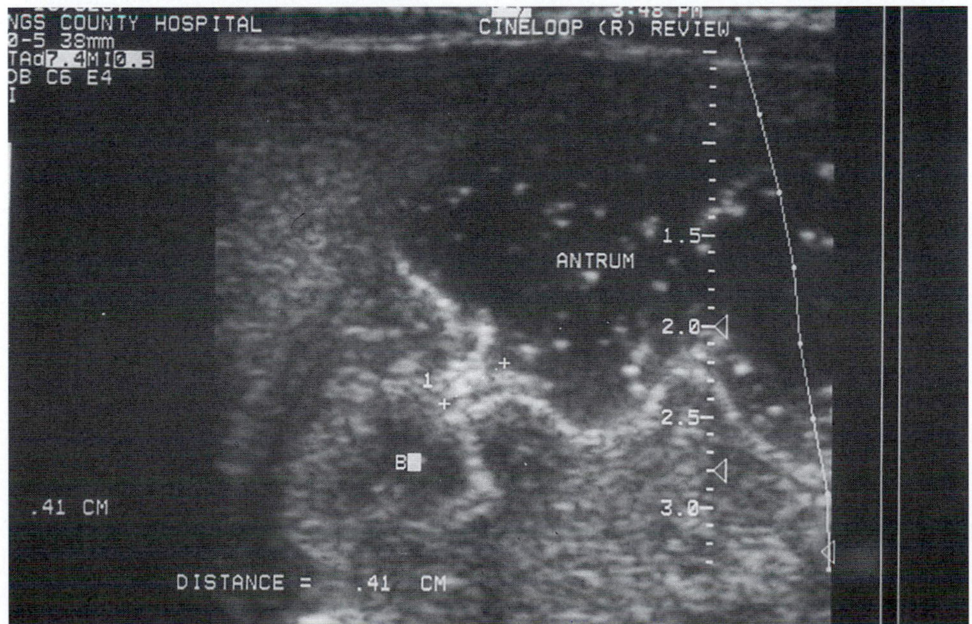

FIGURE 83–2. Ultrasound. Antropyloric region. Longitudinal plane through pylorus, 3 minutes later.

CHAPTER 83

Pylorospasm

HARRIS L. COHEN AND DANIEL L. ZINN

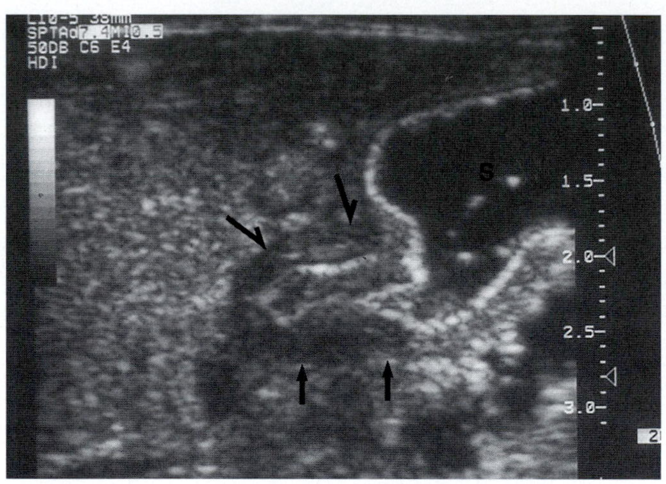

FIGURE 83–3. Annotated version of Fig. 83-1. Pylorospasm. Ultrasound. Antropyloric region. Longitudinal plane through pylorus. Fluid is noted in the stomach (S). The pylorus (*arrows*) appears thick-walled and elongated despite measurements that fall short of a hypertrophic pyloric stenosis (HPS) diagnosis, a length of 13 mm and a width of 3 mm. The image looks like a classic cervix sign of HPS.

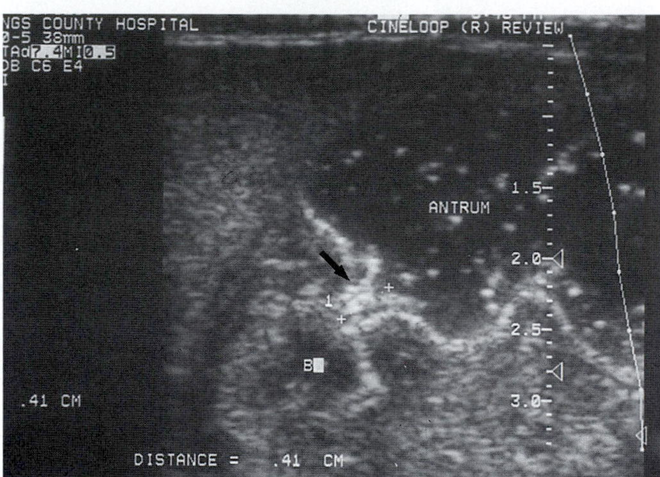

FIGURE 83–4. Annotated version of Fig. 83-2. Pylorospasm. Ultrasound. Antropyloric region. Longitudinal plane through pylorus. The same patient several minutes later has fluid in the stomach (ANTRUM) as well as the duodenal bulb (B), indicating that there has been passage of fluid through the pylorus (*arrow*) . The pyloric length is shorter at 4 mm.

Figure 83-3, the annotated version of Fig. 83-1, shows what looks like the typical elongated and thickened pylorus of hypertrophic pyloric stenosis (HPS). Several minutes later, however, the imaged changed on real-time examination. Figure 83-4, the annotated version of Fig. 83-2, shows a pylorus of normal length and no wall thickening. Another image, Fig. 83-5, taken between those two images, shows significant thickening of a portion of the pylorus but also shows evidence that fluid entered the duodenal bulb. What gives? The patient has pylorospasm. The clinician was told that the patient did not have HPS. We warn clinicians that they should follow such patients carefully. This is primarily because there are few and scattered reports on the subject. Some clinicians will treat the patients with antispasmodics. Others, as in this case, give the patient no medication and the patient does well.

The interpretation of Figs. 83-3 and 83-4 can be confusing. For someone who has learned the classic US images diagnostic for HPS, Fig. 83-3 looks just like them. True, the measurements in this case—3-mm pyloric muscle thickness and 13-mm pyloric length—aren't equal to what we consider positive for HPS (4 mm thick and 18 mm long), but there are published ultrasound tables declaring thicknesses of 3 mm and lengths of 12 mm or greater as positive for HPS. We are also not totally free from confusion. The wall thicknesses in Fig. 83-5 are 3.8 and 4.4 mm; the latter number we would consider definitively positive, at least if the pyloric length was positive as well and there was no changeability of the pyloric image. The fact that Fig. 83-4 shows a pyloric length of only 4 mm and no significant thickening solidifies the impression that this is a case of pylorospasm. Again, these images were obtained within minutes of each other! This

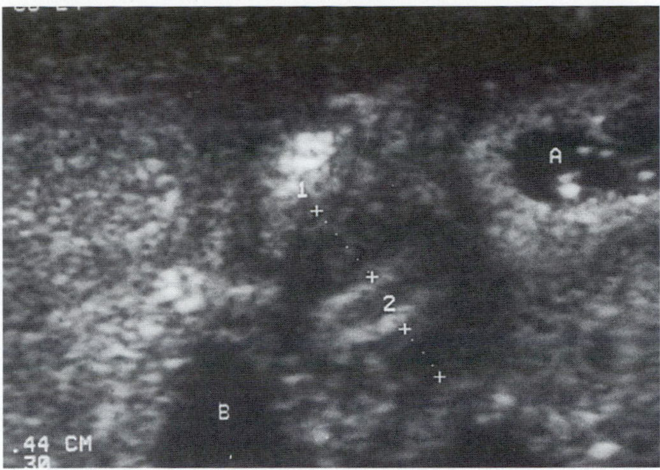

FIGURE 83–5. Pylorospasm. Ultrasound. Antropyloric region. Longitudinal plane through pylorus. This image, taken at a time between those of Figs. 83-3 and 83-4, shows very thick pyloric muscle (measured by crosses), with at least one measurement greater than 4 mm. There is, however, significant fluid in the duodenal bulb, suggesting that fluid has been passing through. This goes moderately against the diagnosis of hypertrophic pyloric stenosis and for the diagnosis of pylorospasm.

change from abnormal to normal suggests the diagnosis of pylorospasm. To some, this is controversial. In our experience, we have avoided more than 40 potential pyloromyotomies by making this diagnosis and following the child clinically, as opposed to sending the patient immediately to surgery.

WHAT IS PYLOROSPASM?

Pylorospasm is a key cause of vomiting, including projectile vomiting, in infants. Not much is said about it, although it is noted to be extremely common in infancy and the most frequent cause of gastric outlet obstruction. Gastric hyperacidity and vagal overstimulation have been suggested by some as causative factors. Vanderwinden et al have theorized that a defect in nitrous oxide production necessary for pyloric relaxation may cause pylorospasm, and that that may lead to HPS. Patients with HPS have been noted to have enlarged enteric nerve fibers in the hypertrophied circular muscle and a lack of diaphorase activity.

No matter what the cause of pylorospasm is, its effect is to at least temporarily limit coordinated gastric emptying, which normally involves a contraction of the gastric antrum, followed by a sequential contraction of the pyloric region and the duodenum. Contractions that prevent early egress of food, in solid form, from the antrum into the duodenum are important normal physiologic actions. Pylorospasm may be an overzealous form of this normal physiologic action, which young infants have and certainly grow out of. Whether this is related to stories of HPS that burned themselves out and did not require surgery is conjecture. We are cautious about diagnosing pylorospasm based on measurements alone, particularly in the first month of life, because we fear that a developing HPS may be missed. It is because of this that younger patients are very closely followed clinically.

PYLOROSPASM—ULTRASOUND FINDINGS THAT OTHERS HAVE TALKED ABOUT

The imaging literature on this condition is sparse. Some authors have had completely different experiences from those that we have had. However, if one looks at the reports carefully, one can cull information that confirms our findings. Although Swischuk's group noted that pylorospasm is clinically common, they typically saw no muscle thickening and warned imagers not to cut the pylorus with a tangential beam and create an erroneously thick pyloric wall. We avoid this possibility by making sure that the pyloric channel is seen and is central in our image of the pylorus. Hernanz-Schulman's group reported seven cases of pylorospasm among a group of patients with projectile vomiting or "rule out HPS" histories. They found pyloric lengths of 10 to 14 mm and muscle wall thicknesses of 1.3 to 2.7 mm among patients they termed as having "pylorospasm or early evolving HPS." Some may see this group's pyloric lengths as positive for HPS. None of their measurements would be called positive by us, and therefore there would appear to be no fear of confusing HPS with pylorospasm on a single US image. Hayden et al discussed unrelenting pylorospasm and delayed gastric emptying associated with gastric ulcer disease in infants. Two of those patients had slight thickening (2 to 3 mm) of the pyloric muscles, which Hayden et al considered reactive hypertrophy, and five had elongated pyloric lengths of 15 to 23 mm. Blumhagen noted a few cases sent to him as possible HPS that had pyloric muscles 3 to 3.5 mm thick but that he called pylorospasm on the basis of occasional brief opening of the pyloric channel with a peristaltic wave.

WHAT IS OUR ULTRASOUND TECHNIQUE?

We reviewed our technique in Chap. 82. We use a nasogastric tube (8F, 15 in) placed into the neonate's stomach. We place 60 mL of water, the equivalent of a feeding, through the tube and use it as an echoless contrast material. We note how the stomach, particularly the antrum, handles this fluid load and whether the pylorus opens and fluid flows to the descending duodenum. If the fluid is held up, the patient will have either HPS or pylorospasm. The trick is in noting (1) whether the muscle wall thickness (MWT) and pyloric channel length measurements do not quite add up to those of HPS (i.e., 4 mm MWT and 18 mm length) and (2) whether there is changeability of the pyloric area, our classic finding in pylorospasm, or the essentially constant obstructing mass of HPS.

Our method confirms Alford and McIlhenny's suggestion that bottle or nasogastric tube feeding be used so as to evaluate gastric peristalsis and its effect on the antrum. This method allows one to note pyloric relaxation and fluid entry into the duodenal bulb and sweep as findings suggestive of

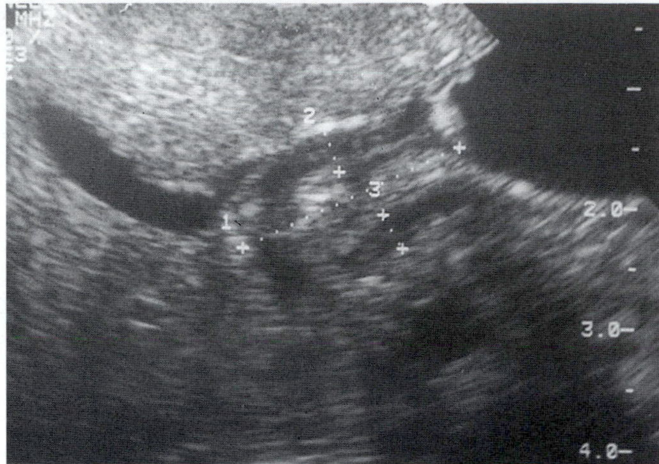

FIGURE 83–6. Pylorospasm—elongated pyloric length. Ultrasound. Antropyloric region. Longitudinal plane through pylorus. The image is a classic one for hypertrophic pyloric stenosis. Pyloric length is 20 mm, which is positive. However, the wall thicknesses are not 4 mm. Still, some might read this as positive but for the fact that it completely disappeared in minutes.

pylorospasm, and an unchanging mass with impression on the antrum as evidence of HPS. Our findings conform with earlier comments of ours and even earlier comments of Blumhagen's that noted the difficulty in differentiating between pylorospasm and HPS and suggested careful observation of the handling of a liquid feeding as well as measurement of pyloric length and muscle wall thickness to differentiate the two entities. Our work shows positive pylorospasm cases with 3 to 3.5 mm and greater thicknesses for at least a portion of the study. Our ability to follow the echoless fluid by US, aided by improvements in currently available US equipment, has allowed us to avoid the necessity for barium studies and therefore fluoroscopy.

TABLE 83-1
Summary of HPS vs. Largest Pylorospasm Measurements

	Mean	Range	Standard deviation
Hypertrophic Pyloric Stenosis (n = 37)			
Wall thickness	5.3 mm	3.0–7.7 mm	0.9 mm
Pyloric length	22.5 mm	14–31 mm	3.6 mm
Pylorospasm (n = 34)			
Wall thickness			
Maximum thickness	3.8 mm	1.5–6.0 mm	1.0 mm
Minimum thickness	0.9 mm	0–2.9 mm	1.0 mm
Pyloric length			
Maximum length	14.4 mm	3.4–27 mm	4.7 mm
Minimum length	3.5 mm	0–15 mm	3.7 mm

SOURCE: *From Cohen HL, Zinn H, Haller J, et al: Ultrasonography of pylorospasm: Findings may simulate hypertrophic pyloric stenosis. 17:705–711, 1998. Used with permission.*

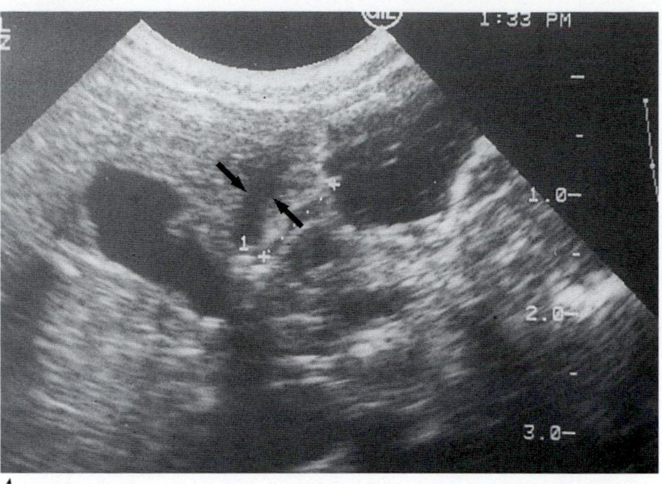

A

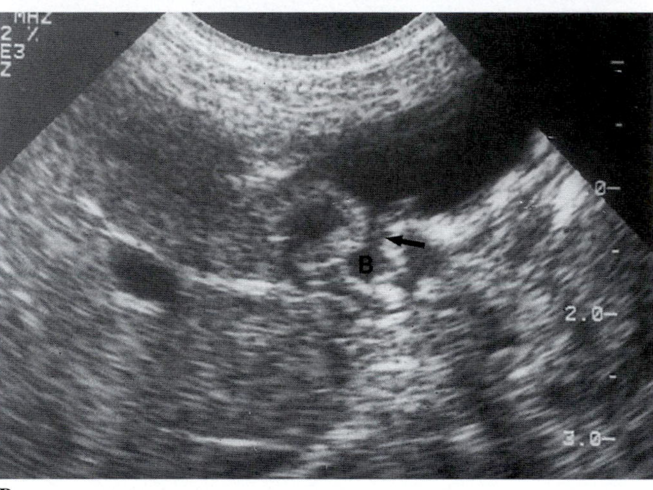

B

FIGURE 83–7. Pylorospasm—significant changeability. Ultrasound. Antropyloric region. Longitudinal plane through pylorus. ***A.*** This image was obtained after one that showed a very elongated pylorus. On this view, the pylorus is only 8 mm long and does not suggest hypertrophic pyloric stenosis. The pyloric muscle (*arrows*) appears thicker than normal. ***B.*** Within minutes, fluid can be seen in the antrum, pyloric channel (*arrow*), and bulb (B). Changeability is a hallmark of pylorospasm, which was the diagnosis.

PYLOROSPASM: ULTRASOUND FINDINGS THAT WE ARE TALKING ABOUT

We studied the US exams of a series of patients sent to us to "rule out HPS." We reviewed the US measurement findings for the 37 with HPS and the 34 labeled as having pylorospasm based on their US findings and confirmed clinically over time. Our measurements are given in Table 83-1. Taking the greatest measurement for length and the widest for muscle thickness obtained during a given US exam, patients with pylorospasm had mean measurements that might suggest HPS—i.e., 14.4 mm pyloric length and 3.8 mm wall thickness. Among the pylorospasm patients, 53 percent had MWTs greater than 4 mm, and 18 percent had pyloric lengths of greater than 18 mm (Fig. 83-6) for some portion of the study. However, the pylorospasm exams showed measurement changeability (Fig. 83-7). At some point in every one of these studies, the measurements were normal. In addition, imaging a pylorus that opened completely suggested pylorospasm. Of note was the fact that we saw double tracking of the pyloric channel and other signs that have long been considered evidence of HPS alone. Obviously, if pylorospasm can simulate the images of HPS, it certainly can simulate some of its imaging signs.

A key point: Pylorospasm may simulate HPS on a given image or for a given measurement at least at some point in a US study. We should take advantage of our radiation-free real-time examinations to watch the pylorus just a little bit longer, particularly as it handles a fluid load. How have my techniques changed? I spend an extra 5 min per exam. I encourage the addition of fluid into the stomach. Try it. It should help you.

References

Alford B, McIlhenny J: The child with acute abdominal pain and vomiting. *Radiol Clin North Am* 30:441–453, 1992.

Blumhagen J: Invited commentary. The role of ultrasonography in the evaluation of vomiting in infants. *Pediatr Radiol* 16:267–270, 1986.

Cohen HL, Babcock D: Vomiting in the 0–3 month age group, in *Appropriateness Criteria for Imaging and Treatment Decisions,* ACR Task Force on Appropriateness Criteria (ed). Reston: American College of Radiology, 1995:PD2.1–2.11.

Cohen HL, Schechter S, Mestel A, et al: Ultrasonic "double track" sign in hypertrophic pyloric stenosis. *J Ultrasound Med* 6:139–143, 1987.

Cohen HL, Zinn H, Haller J, et al: Ultrasonography of pylorospasm: Findings may simulate hypertrophic pyloric stenosis. 17: 705–711, 1998.

Ganong W: *Review of Medical Physiology,* 17th ed. Norwalk, CT, Appleton & Lange, 1995:453.

Haran PJ, Darling DB, Sciammas F: The value of the double-track sign as a differentiating factor between pylorospasm and hypertrophic pyloric stenosis in infants. *Radiology* 86:723–725, 1966.

Hayden CK Jr: Update: Ultrasonography of the gastrointestinal tract in infants and children. *Abdom Imaging* 21:9–20, 1996.

Hayden CK Jr, Swischuk L, Rytting J: Gastric ulcer disease in infants: US findings. *Radiology* 164:131–134, 1987.

Hernanz-Schulman M, Sells L, Ambrosino M, et al: Hypertrophic pyloric stenosis in the infant without a palpable olive: Accuracy of sonographic diagnosis. *Radiology* 193:771–776, 1994.

John S, Swischuk L: The pediatric gastrointestinal tract, in *Diagnostic Ultrasound,* 2d ed, Rumack C, Wilson S, Charboneau J (eds). St Louis, Mosby–Year Book, 1998:1717–1747.

O'Keeffe F, Stansberry S, Swischuk L, Hayden CK Jr: Antropyloric muscle thickness at US in infants: What is normal? *Radiology* 178:827–830, 1991.

Swischuk L, Hayden CK Jr, Stansberry S: Sonographic pitfalls in imaging of the antropyloric region in infants. *Radiographics* 9:437–447, 1989.

Swischuk L, Hayden C Jr, Tyson K: Short segment pyloric narrowing: Pylorospasm or pyloric stenosis? *Pediatr Radiol* 10: 201–205, 1981.

Vanderwinden J-M, Mailleux P, Schiffman S, et al: Nitric oxide synthase activity in hypertrophic pyloric stenosis. *N Engl J Med* 327:511–515, 1992.

84

Figure 84-1 shows a 6-month-old boy with bilious vomiting. What do you see? What are the diagnostic considerations?

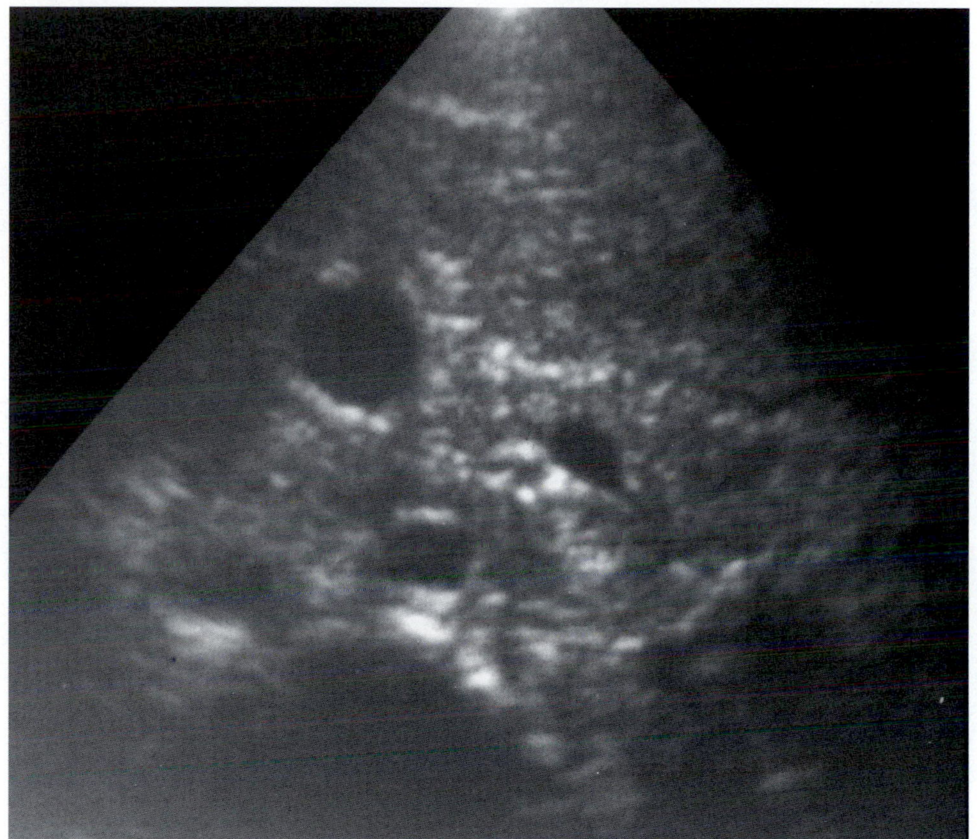

FIGURE 84–1. Transverse view through the upper abdomen.

CHAPTER 84

Midgut Malrotation

CARLOS J. SIVIT

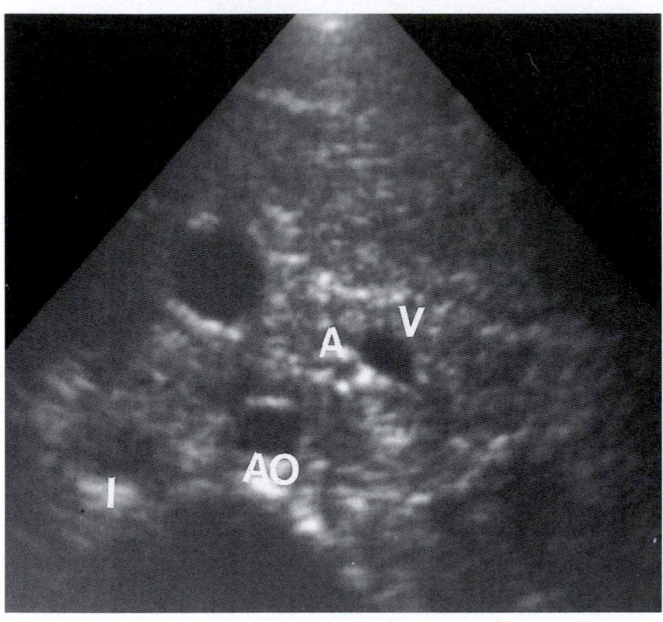

FIGURE 84–2. Midgut malrotation. Transverse image through the upper abdomen demonstrates reversal in the position of the mesenteric vessels. Note that the superior mesenteric vein (V) is to the left of the superior mesenteric artery (A). Midgut malrotation was confirmed on upper gastrointestinal tract examination. AO = aorta, I = IVC.

Malrotation of the small-bowel mesentery around the superior mesenteric artery occurs when the normal process of fetal gut development is arrested. It may result in duodenal obstruction secondary to remnant peritoneal folds that cross the duodenum (Ladd's bands) or in twisting of the shortened mesentery, resulting in midgut volvulus. Approximately 90 percent of patients present in the first month of life, while others present in later life or remain asymptomatic throughout their lifetime. Although midgut malrotation is an uncommon entity, prompt diagnosis is important, since the consequences of delayed diagnosis of a closed-loop obstruction from midgut volvulus may be life-threatening. Midgut malrotation is the diagnosis of exclusion in infants and children with bilious vomiting. The upper gastrointestinal tract examination is the principal imaging modality for evaluating this condition. However, the diagnosis can also be made on sonography. Occasionally, abdominal sonography may be the initial imaging examination performed in children with midgut malrotation. Thus, it is important to recognize the sonographic findings associated with this condition.

The sonographic diagnosis of midgut malrotation is predicated on identifying the relative positions of the superior mesenteric artery (SMA) and superior mesenteric vein (SMV) (Fig. 84-2). The child is examined in a supine position. The exam is performed with a 5.0- or 7.0-MHz sector transducer, depending on patient size. The SMA is identified at its origin at the anterior wall of the abdominal aorta, while the SMV is traced from the portal vein confluence. The relationship of both vessels is evaluated as far caudal as possible. Doppler imaging can be used to confirm which vessel is the artery and which is the vein. The normal situation is for the SMA to be to the left of the SMV (Figs. 84-3, 84-4). In most

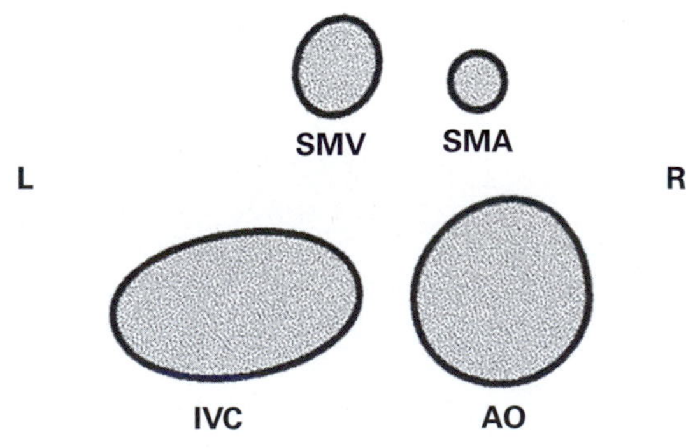

FIGURE 84–3. Diagram showing the normal mesenteric vascular relationship. Note that the superior mesenteric vein is to the right of the superior mesenteric artery.

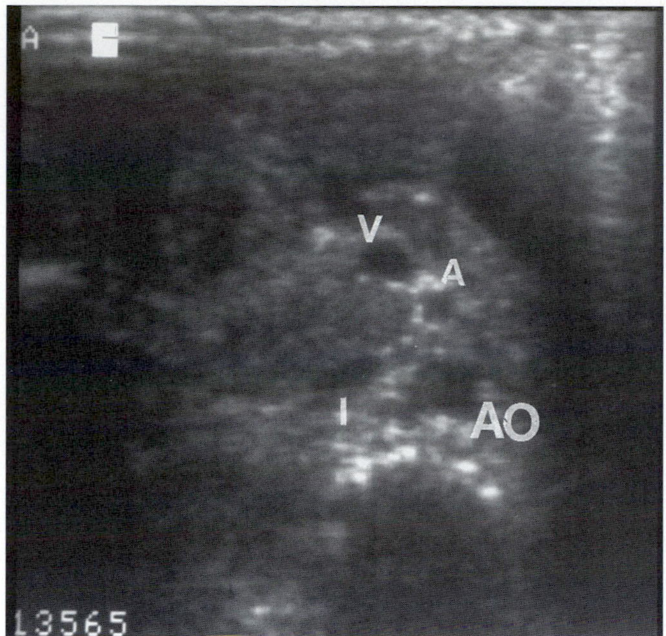

FIGURE 84–4. Normal mesenteric vascular relationship. Transverse view through the upper abdomen demonstrates the normal relationship of the mesenteric vessels. Note that the superior mesenteric vein (V) is to the right of the superior mesenteric artery (A). AO = aorta, I = IVC.

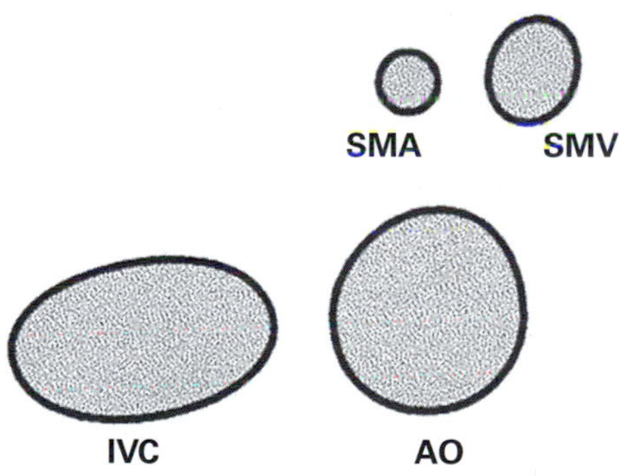

FIGURE 84–5. Diagram showing reversal of the normal mesenteric vascular relationship. Note that the superior mesenteric vein is to the left of the superior mesenteric artery.

children with midgut malrotation, there is reversal of this normal relationship. Thus, the SMV is positioned to the left of the SMA (Figs. 84-2, 84-5). This abnormal orientation may be noted throughout the course of the vessels or through only a segment of their course. If reversal of the mesenteric vasculature is observed on sonography, the diagnosis of midgut malrotation should be confirmed by upper gastrointestinal tract examination. Children with midgut malrotation will demonstrate an abnormal ligament of Treitz on upper gastrointestinal tract examination. In children with midgut malrotation, the ligament of Treitz will be at a lower height than the duodenal bulb and/or to the right of midline (Fig. 84-6). Another reported finding in children with midgut malrotation on sonography or computed tomography is twisting of the mesentery around the artery (Fig. 84-7). In various series, the prevalence of mesenteric vascular reversal in midgut malrotation has ranged from 53 to 87 percent. This range of values is not high enough to allow the use of sonography as the primary means of establishing this diagnosis. Approximately 15 to 20 percent of children with midgut malrotation will have a ventral position of the SMV relative to the SMA

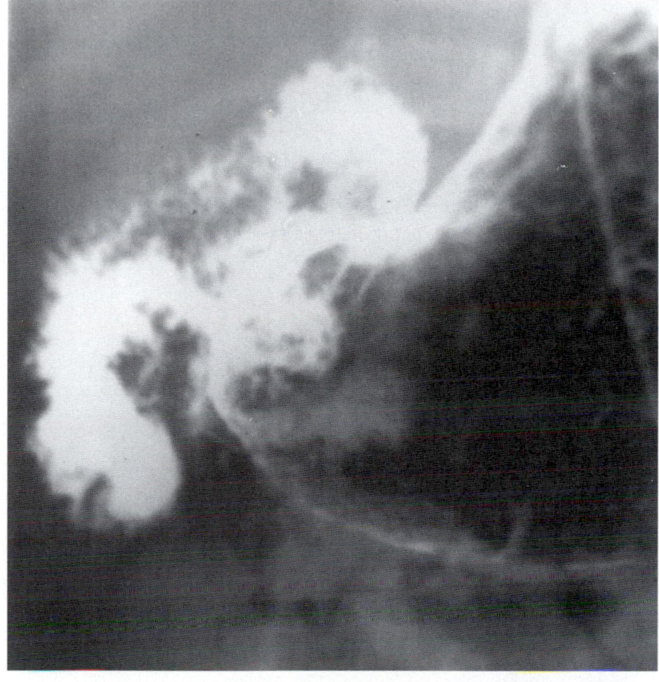

FIGURE 84–6. Midgut malrotation. Upper gastrointestinal tract examination demonstrates the ligament of Treitz located to the right of the spine, a finding diagnostic of midgut malrotation.

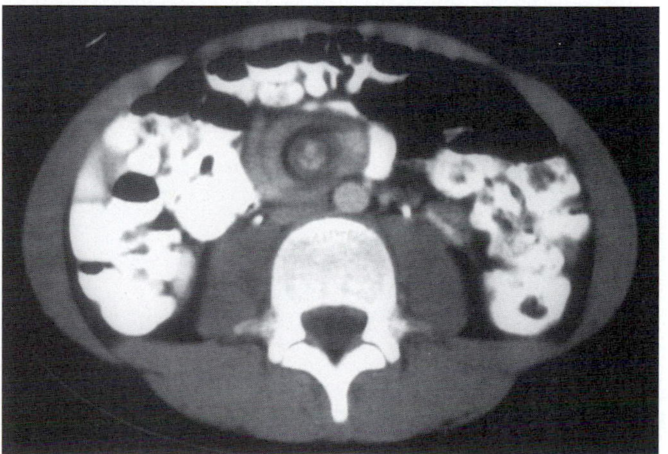

FIGURE 84–7. Twisting of the mesentery around the superior mesenteric artery (SMA) in a "whirlpool" pattern in a child with malrotation and midgut volvulus. Computed tomography scan through the midabdomen demonstrates twisting of the small-bowel mesentery around the SMA. Malrotation with midgut volvulus was confirmed at surgery.

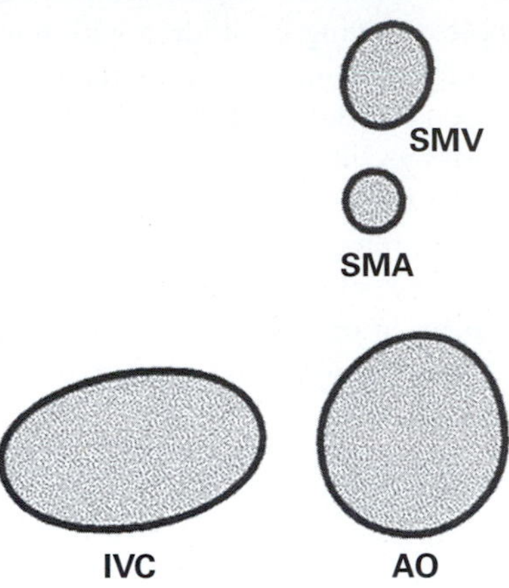

FIGURE 84–8. Diagram showing a ventral position of the superior mesenteric vein (V) relative to the superior mesenteric artery (A). AO = aorta, I = IVC.

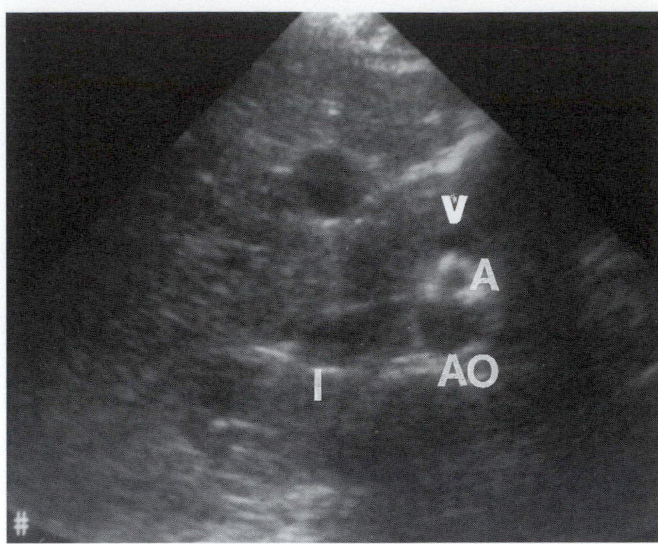

FIGURE 84–9. Ventral position of the superior mesenteric vein (SMV) relative to the superior mesenteric artery (SMA). Transverse image through the upper abdomen demonstrates a ventral position of the SMV (V) relative to the SMA (A). AO = aorta, I = IVC.

(Figs. 84-8 and 84-9), while a small subset will have a normal mesenteric vascular relationship. The ventral position of the SMV relative to the SMA is nonspecific, as it is seen more commonly in normal individuals.

References

Dufour D, Delaet MH, Dassonville M, et al: Midgut malrotation, the reliability of sonographic diagnosis. *Pediatr Radiol* 22:21–23, 1992.

Loyer E, Eggli KD: Sonographic evaluation of superior mesenteric vascular relationship in malrotation. *Pediatr Radiol* 19:173–175, 1989.

Pracros JP, Sann L, Genin G, et al: Ultrasound diagnosis of midgut volvulus: The "whirlpool" sign. *Pediatr Radiol* 22:18–20, 1992.

Shimanuki Y, Aihara T, Takano H, et al: Clockwise whirpool sign at color Doppler US: An objective and definitive sign of midgut volvulus. *Radiology* 199:261–264, 1996.

Weinberger E, Winters WD, Liddell RM, et al: Sonographic diagnosis of intestinal malrotation in infants: Importance of the relative positions of the superior mesenteric artery and vein. *AJR* 159:825–828, 1992.

Zerin JM, DiPietro MA: Mesenteric vascular anatomy at CT: Normal and abnormal appearances. *Radiology* 179:739–742, 1991.

Zerin JM, DiPietro MA: Superior mesenteric vascular anatomy at US in patients with surgically proved malrotation of the midgut. *Radiology* 183:693–694, 1992.

85

Figure 85-1 shows a 2-year-old boy with abdominal pain and vomiting. What do you see? What are the diagnostic considerations?

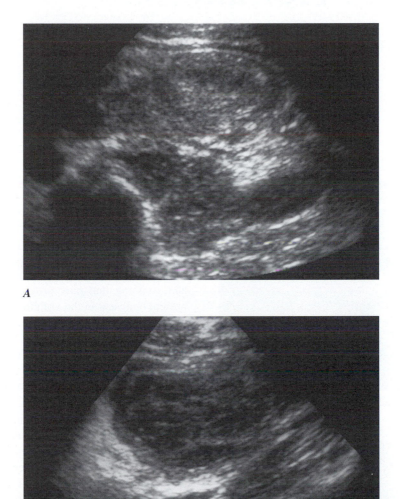

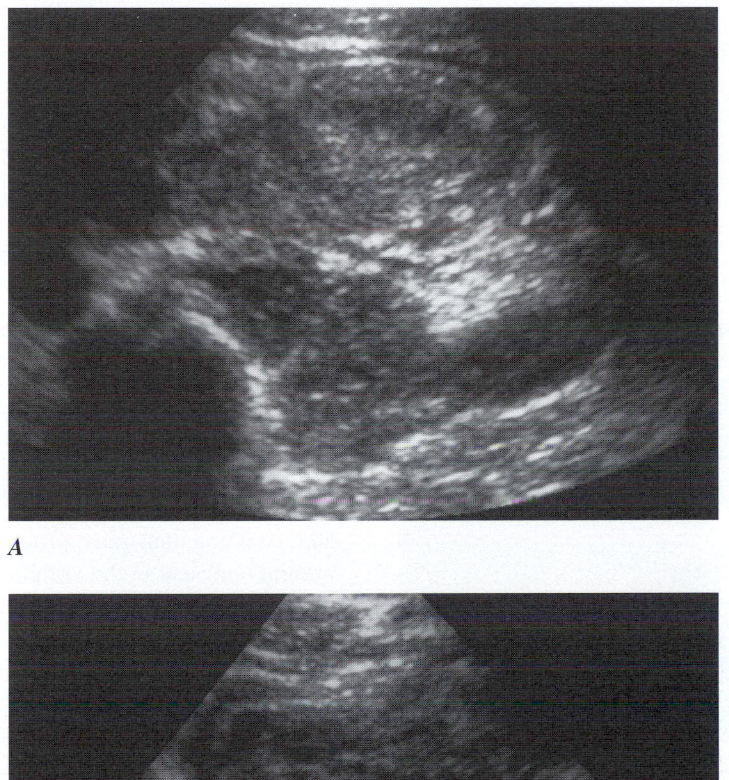

A

B

FIGURE 85–1. Transverse (*A*) and longitudinal (*B*) views through the upper abdomen.

CHAPTER 85

Intramural Bowel Hematoma

CARLOS J. SIVIT

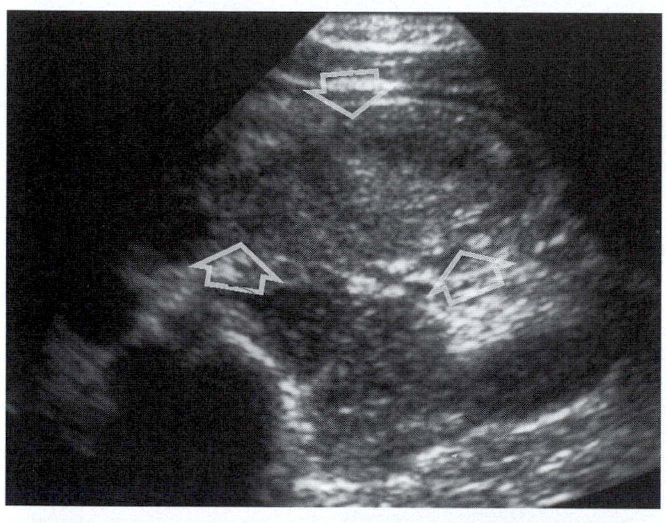

A

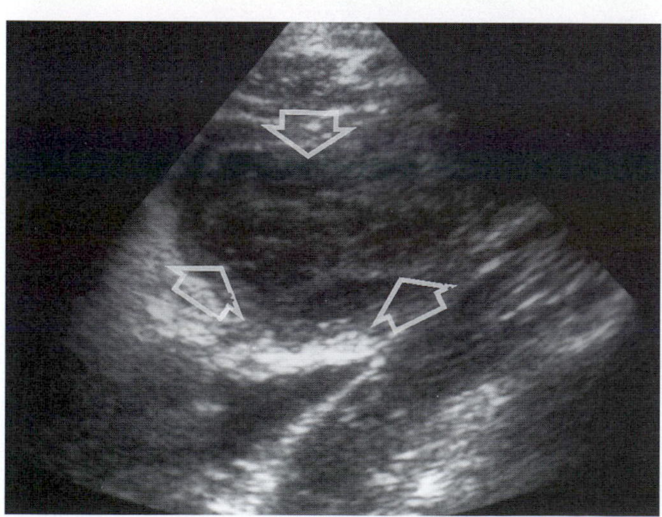

B

FIGURE 85–2. Intramural bowel hematoma of the duodenum. Transverse *(A)* and longitudinal *(B)* views through the upper abdomen show a thickened eccentric segment of duodenal wall (*arrows*). Note that the bowel wall has a heterogeneous echotexture. The bowel lumen is not visualized.

Hemorrhage into the bowel wall most commonly occurs in children following blunt trauma. This results from direct compression of the duodenum against the spine. It may also be associated with a coagulopathy, Henoch-Schönlein purpura, and endoscopic procedures. The most common site for an intramural bowel hematoma is the duodenum. The bowel wall hematoma can constrict or completely obstruct the bowel lumen. Patients typically present with abdominal pain and vomiting that may progressively worsen. Bile may be present or absent in the vomitus, depending on the location of the hematoma relative to the ampulla of Vater. The onset of symptoms may be delayed. One-third of patients become symptomatic more than 48 h following the initial development of an intramural hematoma.

Sonography is a useful modality for assessing children with suspected intramural hematoma, particularly in association with nontraumatic conditions. The examination can be performed using a high-frequency sector scanner or using the graded compression technique with a high-frequency linear transducer. The upper abdomen should be scanned in both the transverse and longitudinal planes. The sonographic appearance of an intramural bowel hematoma is variable. The area of bowel wall thickening is always focal (Fig. 85-2). However, the region of thickening may be diffuse throughout a bowel segment, or it may be eccentric. The thickened segment of bowel wall may be predominantly hyperechoic or have a heterogeneous echotexture on initial sonographic examination (Fig. 85-2). With subsequent liquefaction, anechoic regions may be noted (Fig. 85-3). The involved bowel

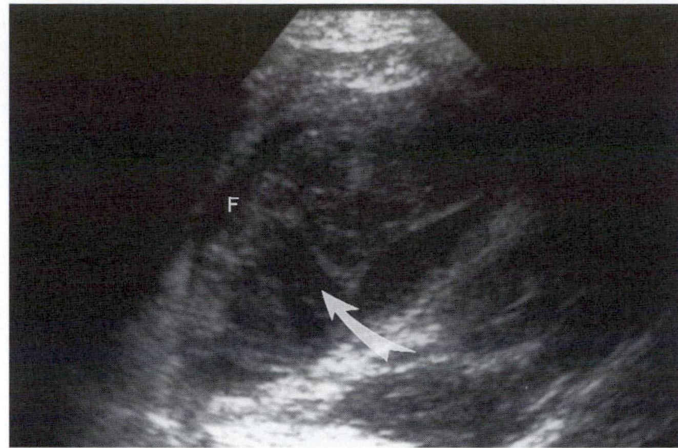

A

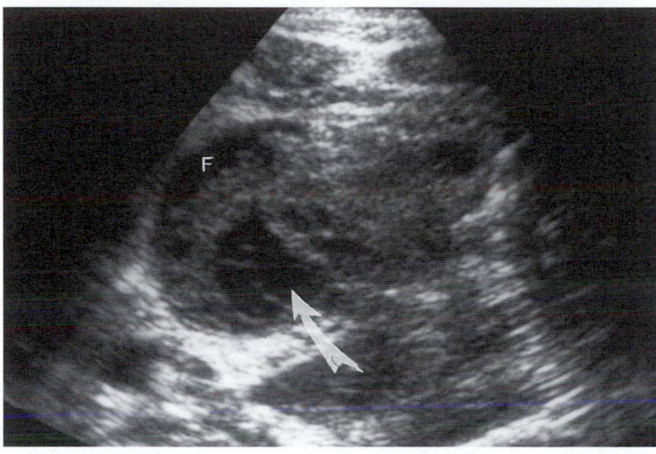

B

FIGURE 85–3. Duodenal hematoma with liquefaction. Transverse ***(A)*** and longitudinal ***(B)*** views through the upper abdomen 7 days later in the same patient as in Fig. 85-1 show anechoic areas within the hematoma (*arrow*), representing liquefaction. Note that fluid can now be observed in the bowel lumen (F).

segment typically demonstrates decreased or absent peristalsis. Additionally, there is often a contiguous segment of proximal fluid-filled dilated bowel due to a partial luminal obstruction at the site of the hematoma.

Computed tomography (CT) remains the primary method for evaluating suspected intramural bowel hematoma following blunt abdominal trauma. Computed tomography can distinguish between an intramural hematoma and bowel rupture and also assess injury to other abdominal viscera. The distinction between an intramural bowel hematoma and bowel rupture is important, as the former condition is usually treated nonoperatively, while the latter requires emergency laparotomy. Findings on CT associated with an intramural bowel hematoma include focal bowel wall thickening and luminal narrowing. The bowel wall thickening can be circumferential or eccentric (Fig. 85-4). Large hematomas can be dumbbell-shaped. The presence of extraluminal oral contrast extravasation or extraluminal air indicates bowel rupture. Moderate to large amounts of peritoneal fluid are also highly suggestive of bowel rupture.

The prognosis for intramural bowel hematoma is excellent. An upper gastrointestional tract examination is usually performed to establish the degree of obstruction and to exclude perforation. The characteristic appearance on contrast examination includes fold thickening, mass effect, and a coiled spring effect (Fig. 85-5). Typically patients are supported with nasogastric suction and parenteral feeding. A repeat contrast examination is performed at 5- to 7-day intervals to assess whether the obstruction has resolved prior to beginning oral feedings. Sonography is also a useful modality for serial evaluation. The sonographic measurement of bowel wall thickness in the involved segment can provide a quantitative measure of improvement. Usually the involved bowel segment appears normal within 1 to 2 weeks following the initial hemorrhage.

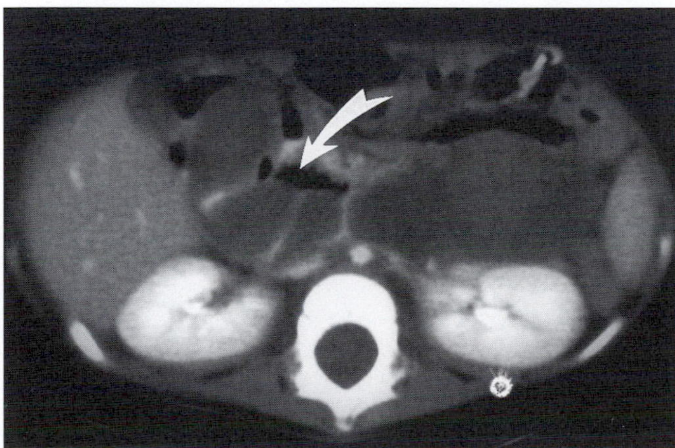

FIGURE 85–4. Computed tomography (CT) of duodenal hematoma. Contrast-enhanced CT scan through the upper abdomen in a child with a large duodenal hematoma demonstrates eccentric bowel wall thickening involving the posterior wall of the duodenum. Note the associated narrowed bowel lumen (*arrow*).

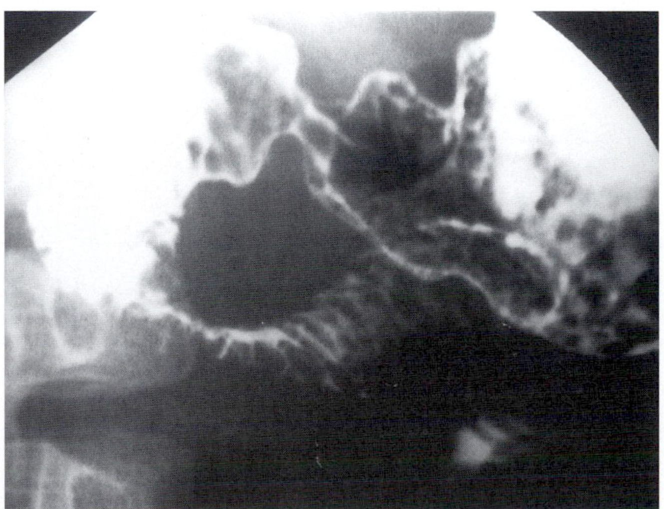

FIGURE 85–5. Duodenal hematoma on upper gastrointestinal tract examination. Upper gastrointestinal tract examination in a child with a duodenal hematoma shows luminal narrowing in the transverse portion of the duodenum due to the mass effect of the hematoma.

There are several conditions that may mimic intramural bowel hematoma on sonography. These include intestinal intussusception and focal bowel wall thickening due to inflammatory bowel disease and infection. An intussusception can usually be differentiated from an intramural hematoma if a "target" or "doughnut" lesion is identified, representing the central invaginating intussusceptum and the outer intussuscipiens. Bowel wall thickening secondary to infection or inflammatory bowel disease usually is distinguished from an intramural hematoma on the basis of the location of the abnormality. Bowel wall thickening due to infection or inflammation most commonly involves the distal small intestine, whereas intramural bowel hematoma typically involves the duodenum.

References

Couture A, Veyrac C, Baud C, et al: Evaluation of abdominal pain in Henoch-Schoenlein syndrome by high frequency ultrasound. *Pediatr Radiol* 22:12–17, 1992.

Hayashi K, Futagawa S, Kozaki S, et al: Ultrasound and CT diagnosis of intramural duodenal hematoma. *Pediatr Radiol* 18: 167–168, 1988.

Hernanz-Schulman L, Genieser NB, Ambrosino M: Sonographic diagnosis of intramural duodenal hematoma. *J Ultrasound Med* 8:273–276, 1989.

Kunin JR, Korobkin M, Ellis JH, et al: Duodenal injuries caused by blunt trauma: Value of CT in differentiating perforation from hematoma. *AJR* 160:1221–1223, 1993.

Miyamoto Y, Fukuda Y, Urushibara K, et al: Ultrasonographic findings in duodenum caused by Schoenlein-Henoch purpura. *JCU* 1:299–303, 1989.

Orel SG, Nussbaum AR, Sheth S, et al: Duodenal hematoma in child abuse: Sonographic detection. *AJR* 151:147–149, 1988.

Sidhu MK, Weinberger E, Healey P: Intramural duodenal hematoma after blunt abdominal trauma. *AJR* 170:38, 1998.

Sivit CJ, Eichelberger MR, Taylor GA: CT in children with rupture of the bowel caused by blunt trauma: Diagnostic efficacy and comparison with hypoperfusion complex. *AJR* 163:1195–1198, 1994.

Vu Nghiem H, Jeffrey RB, Mindelzun RE: CT of blunt trauma to the bowel and mesentery. *AJR* 160:53–58, 1993.

86

Figure 86-1 shows a 15-month-old child with crampy abdominal pain. What do you see? What are the diagnostic considerations?

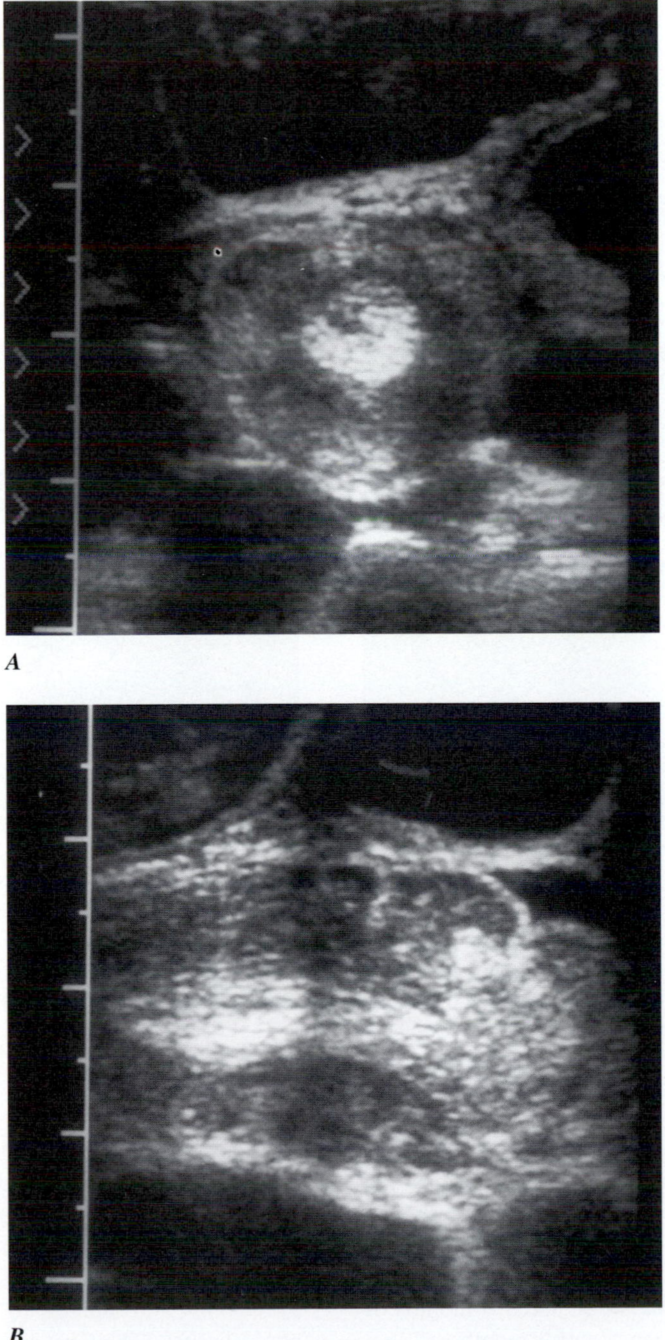

FIGURE 86–1. Longitudinal *(A)* and transverse *(B)* views through the right midquadrant.

CHAPTER 86

Intestinal Intussusception

CARLOS J. SIVIT

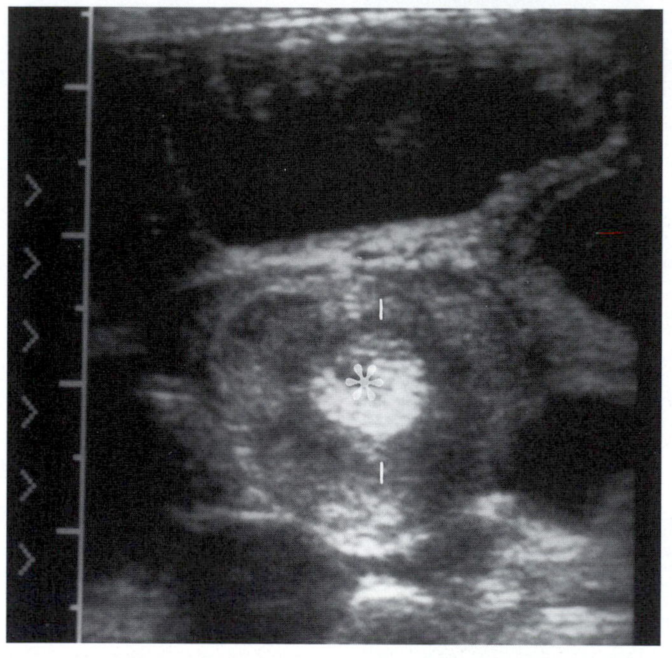

A

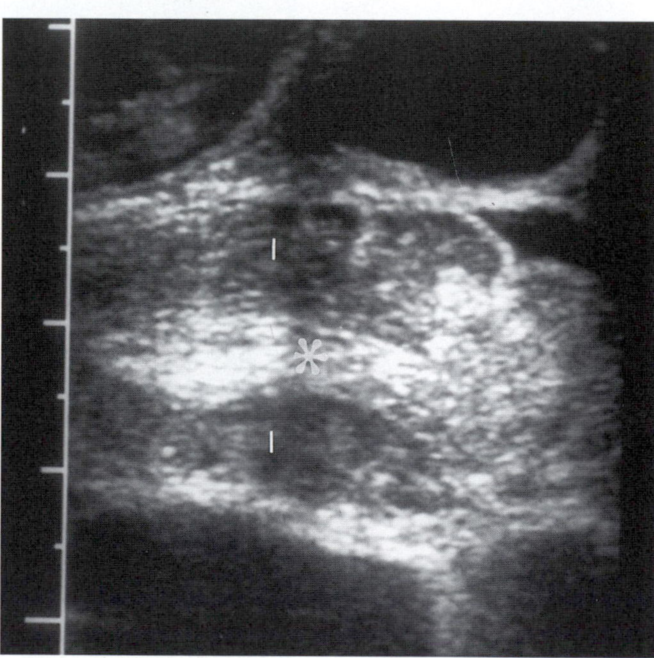

B

FIGURE 86–2. Intestinal intussusception. Longitudinal *(A)* and transverse *(B)* views through the right upper quadrant demonstrate a soft tissue mass, representing an intussusception. There is a hypoechoic outer rim, representing the receiver loop, or intussuscipiens (I). The central echogenic region is the intussusceptum (*). On the transverse view, the mass has a rounded shape and demonstrates a "target" appearance, while in long axis an elongated, tubular appearance is observed. Note the surrounding fluid-filled, dilated small-bowel loops.

Intestinal intussusception is the most common acute abdominal disorder of early childhood (Fig. 86-2). The condition occurs when a portion of the intestine, referred to as the intussusceptum, invaginates into another portion, referred to as the intussuscipiens (Fig. 86-3). Intussusception occurs more frequently in males than in females. It is seen primarily in younger children. The condition is rare under 3 months of age. The peak incidence is between 5 and 9 months of age, and 75 percent of children with this condition are under the age of 2 years. There is a wide spectrum of presenting signs and symptoms in children with intestinal intussusception. The most frequent clinical findings are abdominal pain, currant jelly stools, and a palpable abdominal mass.

The most common type of intussusception is ileocolic, followed by ileoileocolic, ileoileal, and colocolic. Over 95 percent of intussusceptions have no recognizable pathologic lead points and are felt to arise from hypertrophy of lymphoid tissues. They are labeled as being idiopathic. Rarely, recognizable causes for the intussusception are found, including Meckel's diverticulum, intestinal polyp, enteric duplica-

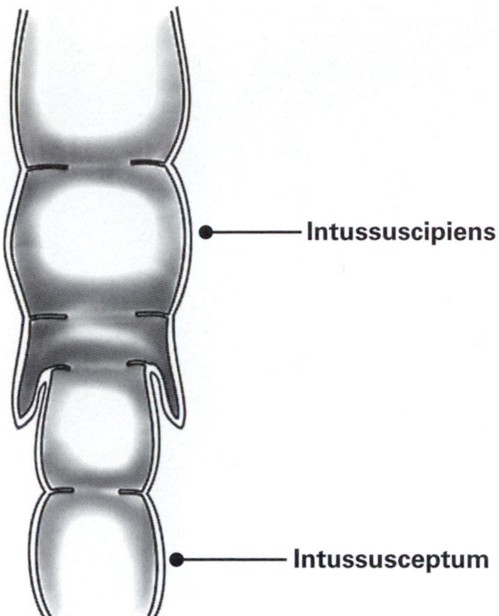

FIGURE 86–3. Diagram of an intussusceptum invaginating into the intussuscipiens.

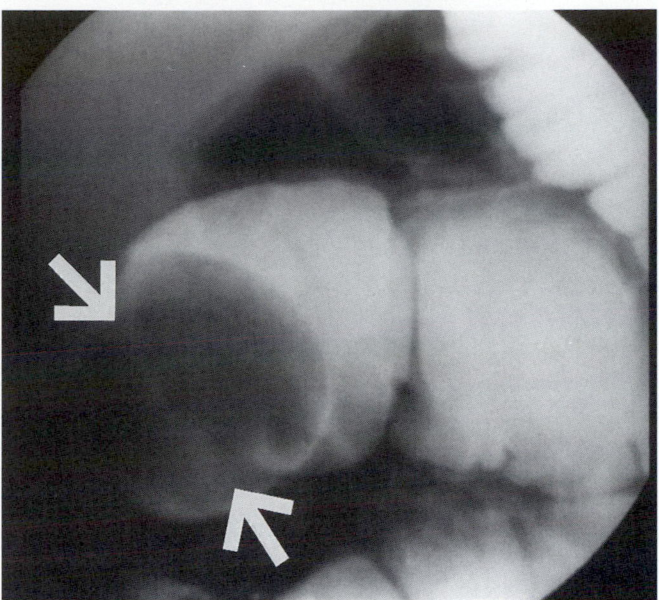

FIGURE 86–4. Intussusception on contrast enema examination. Spot radiograph of the hepatic flexure during a contrast enema examination shows a rounded soft tissue mass at the junction of the ascending colon and the transverse colon (*arrows*), indicative of an intussusception.

tion, intramural hematoma, and lymphoma. Recognizable lead points are commonly noted in children under the age of 3 months or over the age of 3 years.

Until recently, conventional radiography and the contrast enema examination were the principal imaging methods used in North America for the diagnosis and treatment of intussusception. Sonography has now also gained acceptance as a reliable method for the initial screening of children with suspected intussusception. In various large series, sonography has had a sensitivity of 100 percent for the diagnosis of this condition. The use of sonography allows more selective use of contrast enema examinations, only for therapeutic purposes (Fig. 86-4). Sonography has the additional advantage of permitting the diagnosis of other abnormalities that would be overlooked on the enema examination.

A technique of graded compression is used in the sonographic evaluation, with pressure applied with a linear high-frequency transducer. One should follow the colon from right to left, scanning the entire abdomen and pelvis in both longitudinal and axial planes. The sonographic appearance in the transverse plane is that of a mass lesion over 3 cm in maximum diameter. It may demonstrate an outer hypoechoic region surrounding an echogenic center (Fig. 86-2). This has been characterized as a "target" or "doughnut" appearance. Another reported appearance in the transverse plane is that of multiple concentric rings (Fig. 86-5). This variability in sonographic appearance is probably based on the degree of bowel wall edema. The bowel mucosa and submucosa are hyperechoic on sonography, while the muscularis is hypoechoic. Thus, when there is little bowel edema present, multiple hypo- and hyperechoic layers are noted, representing mucosa, submucosa, and muscularis in the intussusceptum and intussuscipiens. With increasing degrees of bowel edema, the hyperechoic mucosal and submucosal echoes are obliterated in the outer intussuceptum, resulting in a more uniform target appearance. On long axis, the hypoechoic layers on each side of an echogenic center may result in a "pseudokidney" appearance (Fig. 86-6).

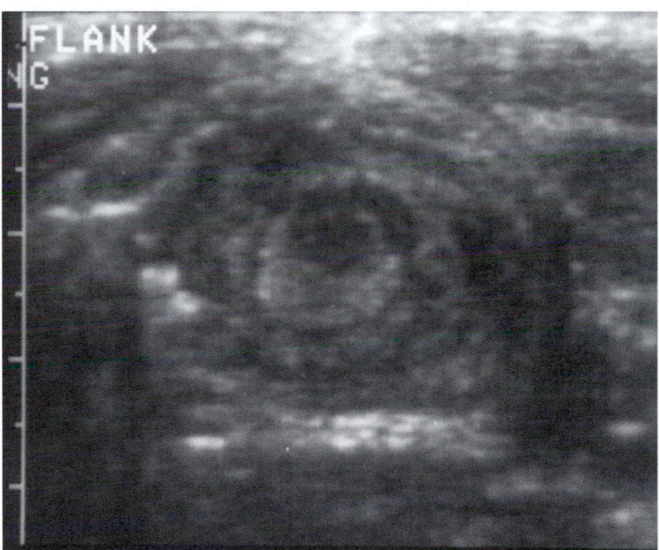

FIGURE 86–5. Intussusception with multiple concentric rings. Transverse view through the right midquadrant demonstrates a rounded mass with multiple concentric hypoechoic and hyperechoic rings. This was proven to be an intussusception on contrast enema.

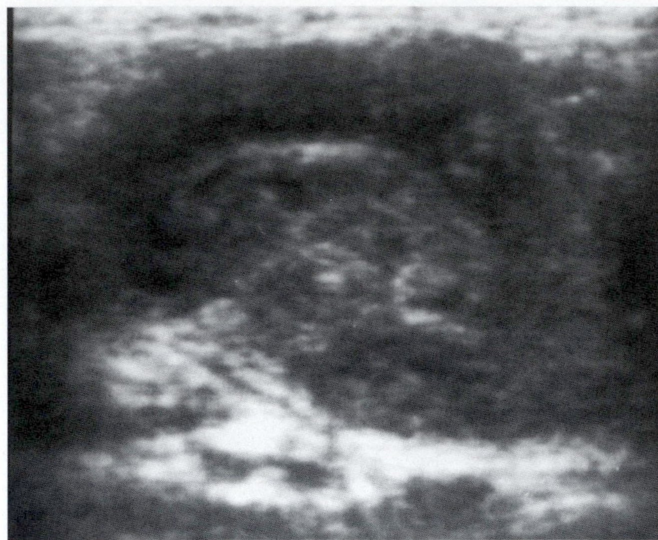

FIGURE 86–6. Pseudokidney appearance of an intussusception. Oblique view through the right midquadrant demonstrates a soft tissue mass that resembles the kidney in shape. An intussusception was confirmed on contrast enema.

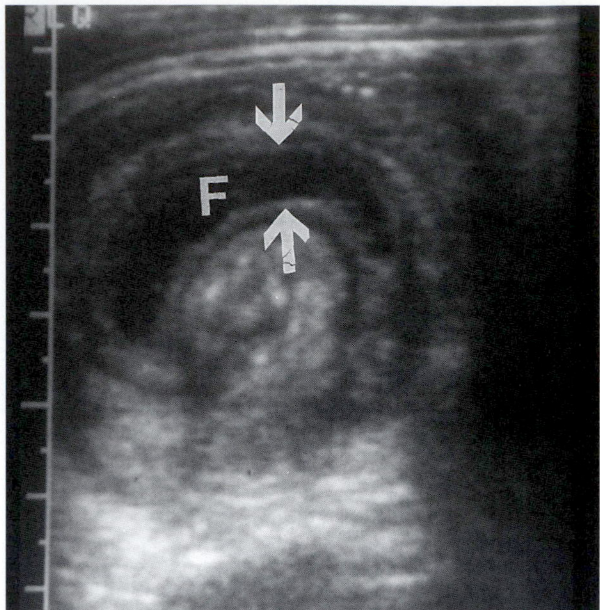

A

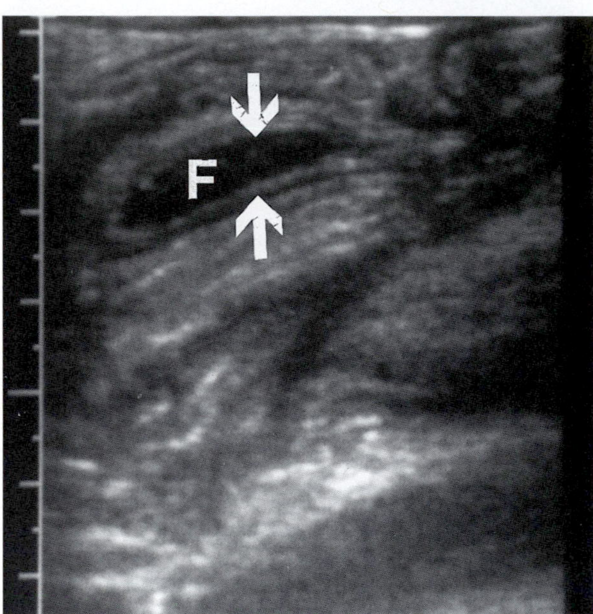

B

FIGURE 86–7. Trapped fluid within an intussusception. ***A.*** Transverse view of an intussusception shows an anechoic crescent (F) between the enfolded limbs of the intussusception, representing trapped fluid limited by the serosal layers of both limbs (*arrows*). ***B.*** Longitudinal view of the same patient shows a spherical collection (F), representing fluid within the serosal layers of both limbs (*arrows*).

Various sonographic findings have been reported to be predictive of the success of hydrostatic reduction of intussusception. These are listed in Table 86-1. The presence of a thick external hypoechoic rim, the presence of substantial amounts of trapped peritoneal fluid within the intussusception (Fig. 86-7), and the absence of flow within the intussusception on color Doppler sonography correlate with decreased success of reduction and potential bowel ischemia. However, these findings do not represent contraindications to attempted reduction. Values for increased thickness of the external rim have ranged from 8 to 16 mm in various studies. The appearance of fluid within the intussusception may represent fluid within the incompletely collapsed lumen of the intussusception, fluid in the lumen of the intussuscipiens, or trapped peritoneal transudate. The latter finding typically appears as a crescent-shaped fluid collection surrounded by a hypoechoic rim that represents the serosal layers of both limbs of the intussusception. When flow within the intussusception is being evaluated, Doppler parameters should be set to detect slow flow by adjusting color sensitivity and threshold settings.

The use of sonography to guide hydrostatic reduction has also been reported, with good results. An enema is administered while the patient is monitored by sonography. The instilled fluid is monitored as it courses through the large bowel until there is complete disappearance of the intussusception from the colon and terminal ileum and retrograde filling of the distal small bowel with fluid.

TABLE 86-1
Sonographic Findings Predictive of Successful Intussusception Reduction by Contrast Enema

Thin external hypoechoic rim
Absence of trapped fluid inside the intussusception
Presence of flow on color Doppler

There are various conditions that may mimic intussusception on sonography, including focal bowel wall thickening due to infection, inflammatory bowel disease, and intramural hematoma. Therefore, the specificity of sonography for the diagnosis of intussusception is not as high as the sensitivity.

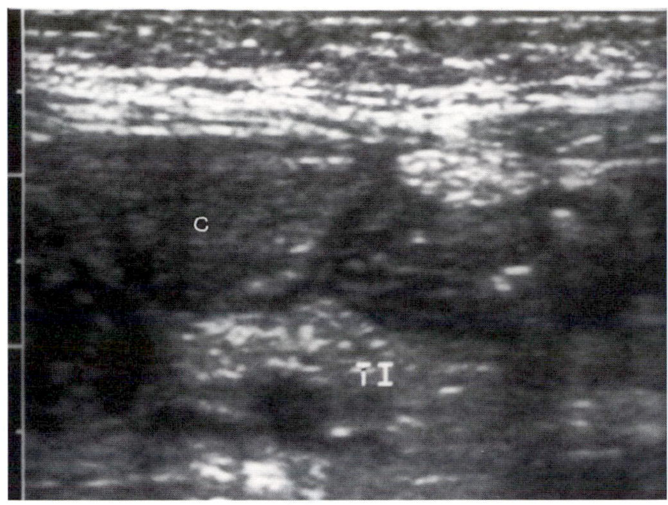

A

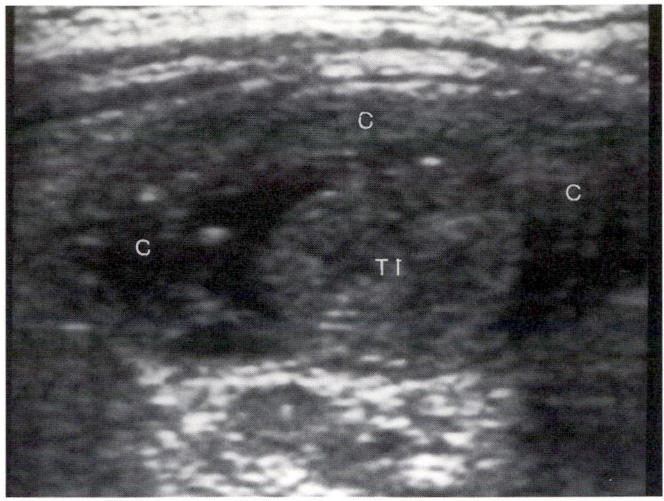

B

FIGURE 86–8. Persistent bowel wall thickening in the ileocecal region following successful intussusception reduction. Transverse *(A)* and longitudinal *(B)* views through the right lower quadrant following successful intussusception reduction demonstrate persistent thickening of the cecum (C) and terminal ileum (TI), mimicking persistence of the intussusception.

Additionally, edema may persist in the ileocecal region following successful intussusception reduction and mimic a persistent intussusception (Fig. 86-8). However, these other conditions can usually be distinguished from intussusception on contrast enema examination.

References

del-Pozo G, Albillos JC, Tejedor D: Intussusception: US findings with pathologic correlation—the crescent-in-doughnut sign. *Radiology* 199:688–692, 1996.

del-Pozo G, Gonzalez-Spinola J, Gomez-Anson B, et al: Intussusception: Trapped peritoneal fluid detected with US—relationship to reducibility and ischemia. *Radiology* 201:379–383, 1996.

Lagalla R, Caruso G, Novara V, et al: Color doppler ultrasonography in pediatric intussusception. *J Ultrasound Med* 13:171–174, 1994.

Lim HK, Bae SH, Lee KH, et al: Assessment of reducibility of ileocolic intussusception in children: Usefulness of color doppler sonography. *Radiology* 191:781–785, 1994.

Pracros JP, Tran-Minh VA, Morin De Finfe CH, et al: Acute intestinal intussusception in children: Contribution of ultrasonography (145 cases). *Ann Radiol* 30:525–530, 1987.

Riebel TW, Nasir R, Weber K: US-guided hydrostatic reduction of intussusception in children. *Radiology* 188:513–516, 1993.

Swischuk LE, Hayden CK, Boulden T: Intussusception: Indications for ultrasonography and an explanation of the doughnut and pseudokidney signs. *Pediatr Radiol* 15:388–391, 1985.

Verschelden P, Filiatrault D, Garel L, et al: Intussusception in children: Reliability of US in diagnosis—a prospective study. *Radiology* 184:741–744, 1992.

Weinberger E, Winters WD: Intussusception in children: The role of sonography. *Radiology* 184:601–602, 1992.

Woo SK, Nim JS, Suh SJ, et al: Childhood intussusception: US-guided hydrostatic reduction. *Radiology* 182:77–80, 1992.

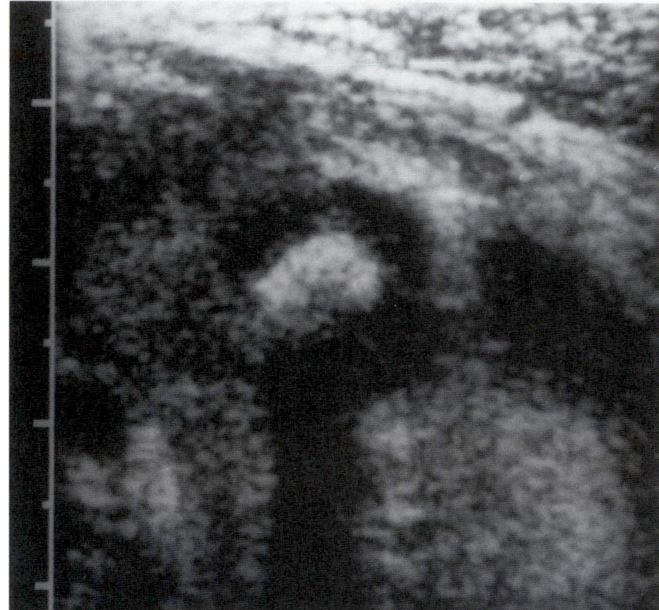

FIGURE 87–5. Acute appendicitis with appendicolith. Transverse view through the appendix shows an enlarged, noncompressible appendix with an echogenic appendicolith. Note the acoustic shadowing caused by the appendicolith.

The criteria for sonographic diagnosis of appendicitis include visualization of an incompressible appendix that has a maximum cross-sectional diameter of at least 6 mm (Fig. 87-1), identification of an appendicolith (Fig. 87-5), or demonstration of a complex mass or focal fluid collection representing a periappendiceal abscess following perforated appendicitis (Fig. 87-6). Appendicoliths appear as echogenic foci with acoustic shadowing (Fig. 87-5). They may be seen within the appendiceal lumen or surrounded by a periappendiceal abscess. Color Doppler sonography is a useful adjunct in confirming the diagnosis of appendicitis. The appendiceal wall will demonstrate marked hyperemia on color Doppler examination in acute appendicitis (Fig. 87-7; see

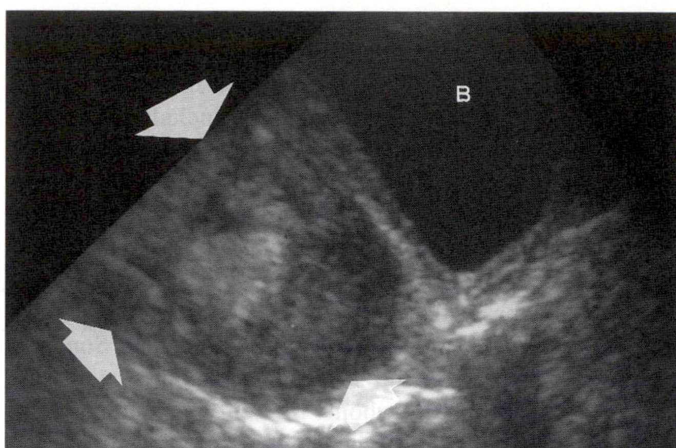

A

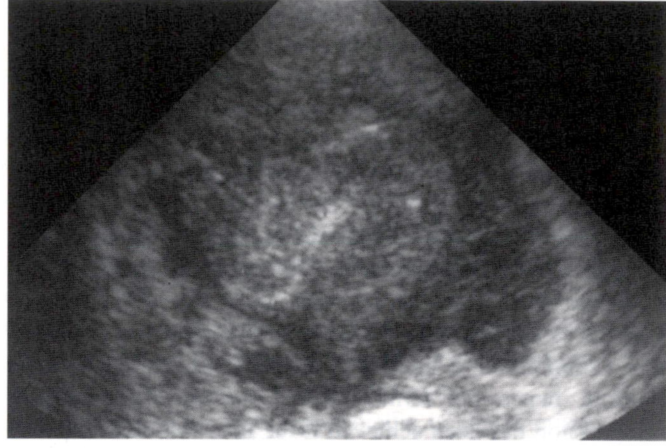

B

FIGURE 87–6. Perforated appendicitis. ***A.*** Longitudinal view through the pelvis shows a complex mass (*arrows*) posterior to the bladder, representing a pelvic abscess secondary to perforated appendicitis. B = bladder. ***B.*** Transverse view through the pelvis in the same patient as in ***A*** demonstrates a well-circumscribed, complex mass, representing a pelvic abscess secondary to perforated appendicitis.

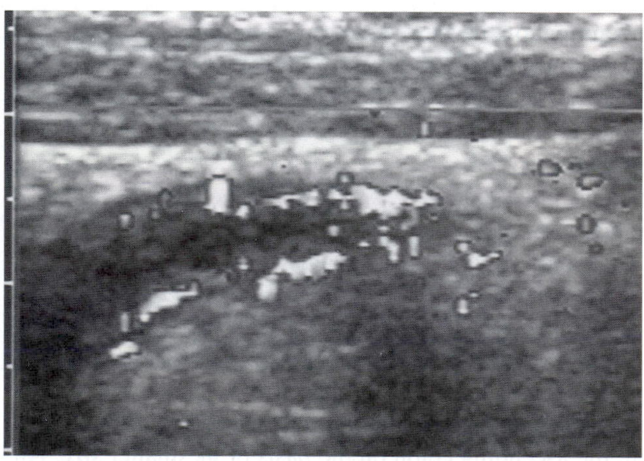

A

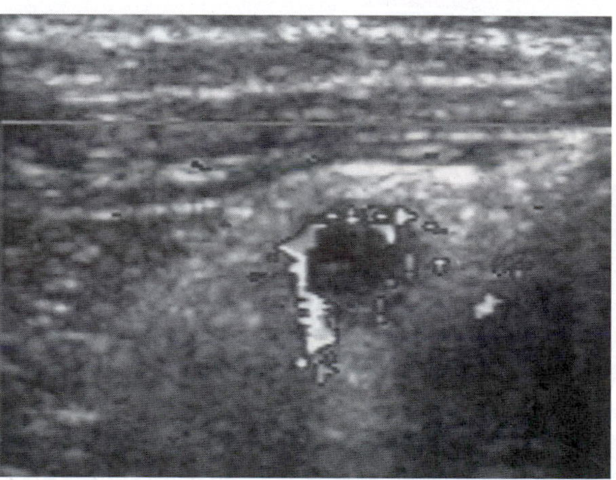

B

FIGURE 87–7. Acute appendicitis on color Doppler sonography. ***A.*** Longitudinal view through the appendix with color Doppler sonography in a child with acute appendicitis demonstrates marked hyperemia in the appendiceal wall. ***B.*** Transverse view through the appendix in the same child as in ***A*** with color Doppler sonography again shows marked appendiceal hyperemia. (See Color Plate 22.)

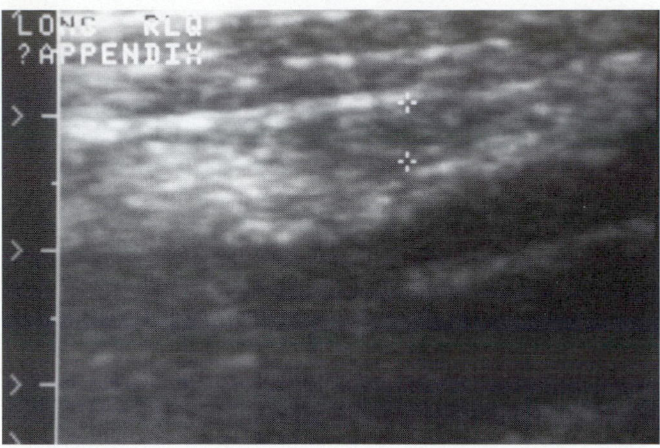

A

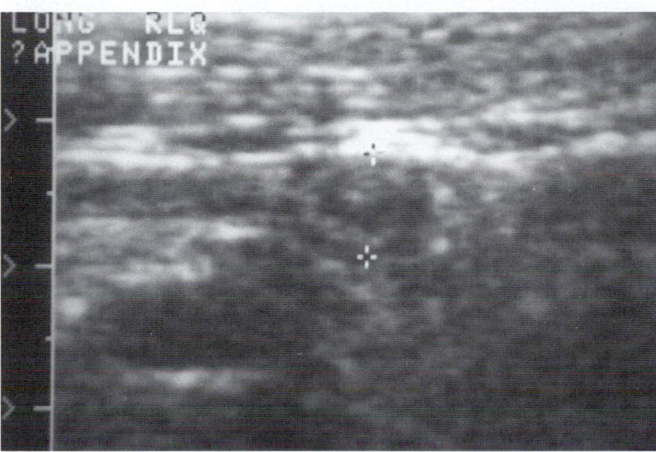

B

FIGURE 87–8. Focal appendicitis. ***A.*** Transverse view through the proximal appendix demonstrates a compressible, normal-sized appendix (*between electronic calipers*). ***B.*** Transverse view through the distal appendix in the same patient as in *A* shows an enlarged distal segment of the appendix (*between electronic calipers*). At surgery, the patient had focal appendicitis restricted to the distal appendix.

also Color Plate 22), while the normal appendix will not demonstrate any flow. Additionally, color Doppler will demonstrate hyperemia within a right lower quadrant or pelvic mass following appendiceal perforation.

The principal pitfalls of the sonographic diagnosis of acute appendicitis occur with focal appendicitis, retrocecal appendicitis, and perforated appendicitis. In focal appendicitis, inflammation may be localized to the distal end (Fig. 87-8). Therefore, it is important to image the entire length of the appendix to avoid false-negative diagnoses. The appendiceal tip can be identified on the basis of its blind termination. A retrocecal appendix may be difficult to visualize, particularly if the ascending colon and distal small bowel contain large amounts of air that cannot be compressed. If the psoas muscle is visualized, however, even a retrocecal appendix should be seen. The appendix may not be recognizable following perforation. Additionally, even if a portion is identified, the diameter may be normal, as the intraluminal pressure has been relieved. Thus, the principal finding in perforated appendicitis is a periappendiceal mass (Fig. 87-6), which may represent thickening of adjacent atonic bowel loops, interloop fluid pockets, phlegmon, or abscess.

Computed tomography (CT) is also useful for evaluating complications of appendicitis, such as perforation with phlegmon or abscess formation. It can delineate the location and extent of associated abdominal and pelvic fluid collections, including interloop abscesses (Fig. 87-9), better than sonography. Additionally, it can determine the relative size of liquefied versus nonliquefied components within the collection. Recently, CT has been gaining increased acceptance for the diagnosis of nonperforated appendicitis (Fig. 87-10). It is particularly useful in children who are difficult to examine because of their large girth, when graded compression is difficult because of extreme abdominal tenderness, or when the sonographic findings are equivocal.

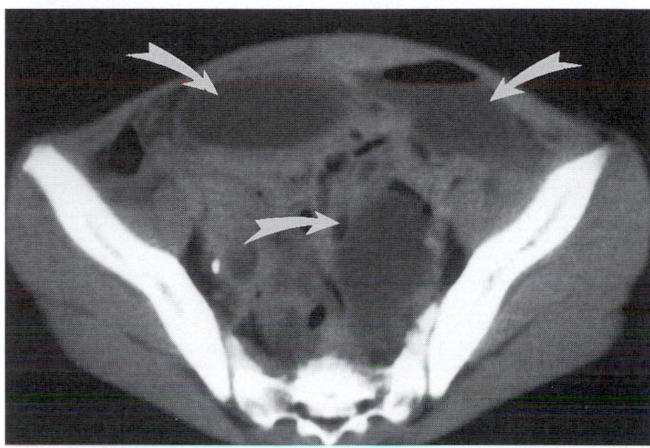

FIGURE 87–9. Perforated appendicitis on computed tomography (CT). A CT scan through the lower abdomen shows multiple low-attenuation collections (*arrows*), representing interloop abscesses following appendiceal perforation.

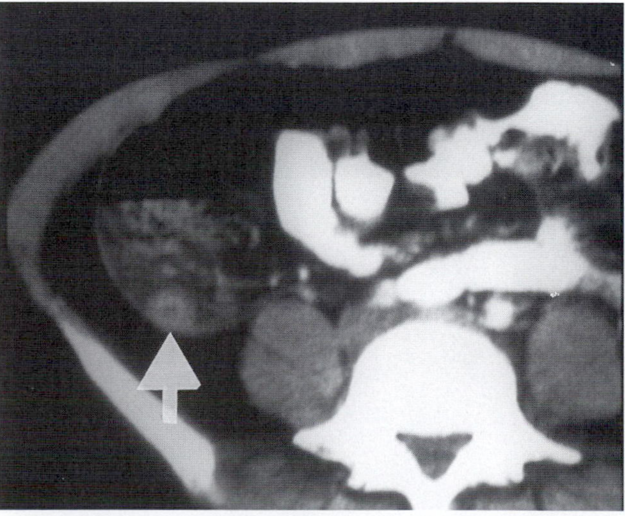

FIGURE 87–10. Nonperforated appendicitis on computed tomography (CT). A CT scan through the lower abdomen demonstrates an enlarged appendix in cross section (*arrow*), with infiltration of surrounding periappendiceal fat.

References

Abu-Yousef MM, Bleicher JJ, James JW, et al: High resolution sonography of acute appendicitis. *AJR* 149:53–58, 1987.

Hayden CK, Kuchelmeister J, Lipscomb TS: Sonography of acute appendicitis in childhood: Perforation versus nonperforation. *J Ultrasound Med* 11:209–216, 1992.

Jeffrey RB, Laing FC, Townsend RR: Acute appendicitis: Sonographic criteria based on 250 cases. *Radiology* 167:327–329, 1988.

Kao SCS, Smith WL, Abu-Yousef M, et al: Acute appendicitis in children: Sonographic findings. *AJR* 153:375–379, 1989.

Larson JM, Peirce JC, Ellinger DM, et al: The validity and utility of sonography in the diagnosis of appendicitis in the community setting. *AJR* 153:687–691, 1989.

Puylaert JCBM: Acute appendicitis: US evaluation using graded compression. *Radiology* 158:355–360, 1986.

Quillin SP, Siegel MJ: Appendicitis in children: Color doppler sonography. *Radiology* 184:745–747, 1992.

Quillin SP, Siegel MJ: Efficacy of color doppler sonography. *Radiology* 191:557–560, 1994.

Quillin SP, Siegel MJ, Coffin CM: Acute appendicitis in children: Value of sonography in detecting perforation. *AJR* 159: 1265–1268, 1992.

Ramachandran P, Sivit CJ, Newman KD, et al: Ultrasound as an adjunct in the diagnosis of acute appendicitis: A four year experience. *J Pediatr Surg* 31:164–169, 1996.

Rao PM, Rhea JT, Novelline RA, et al: Helical CT technique for the diagnosis of appendicitis: Prospective evaluation of a focused appendix CT examination. *Radiology* 202:139–144, 1997.

Siegel MJ, Carel C, Surratt S: Ultrasonography of acute abdominal pain in children. *JAMA* 266:1987–1989, 1991.

Sivit CJ: Diagnosis of acute appendicitis in children: Spectrum of sonographic findings. *AJR* 161:147–152, 1993.

Sivit CJ, Newman KD, Boenning DA, et al: Appendicitis: Usefulness of US in a pediatric population. *Radiology* 185:549–552.

Vignault F, Filiatrault D, Brandt ML, et al: Acute appendicitis in children: Evaluation with US. *Radiology* 176:501–504, 1990.

88

Figure 88-1 shows a 14-year-old boy with acute right lower quadrant pain. What do you see? What are the diagnostic considerations?

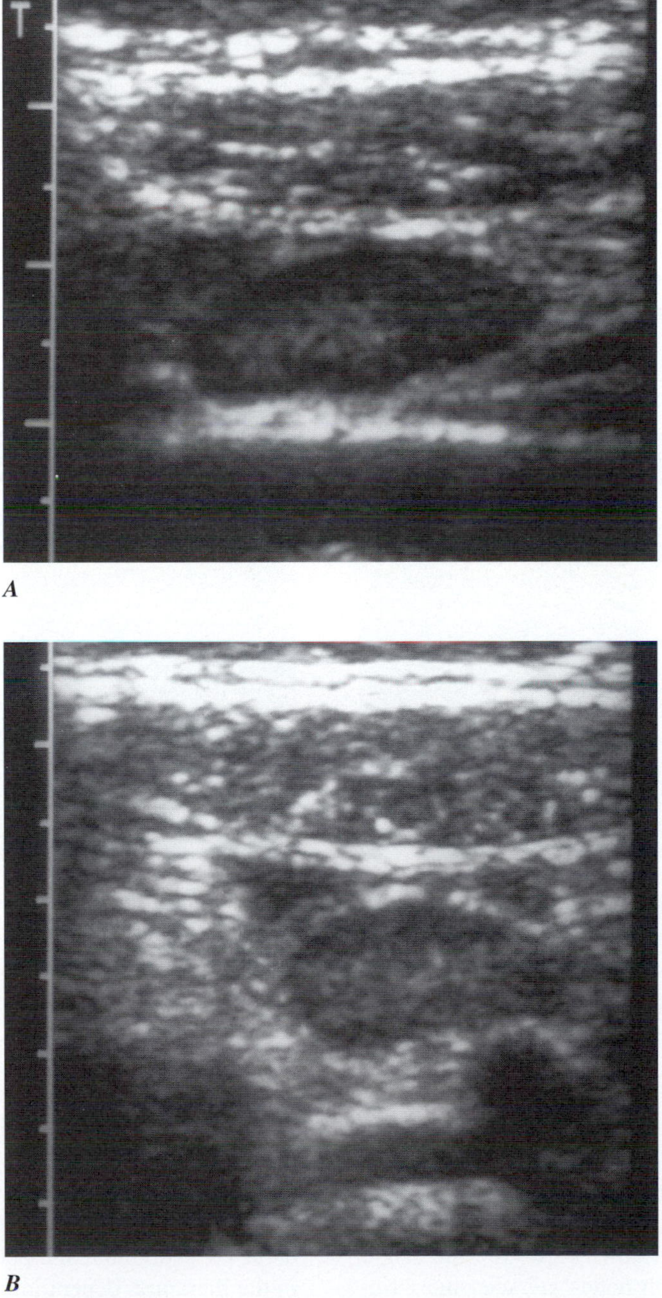

FIGURE 88–1. Longitudinal *(A)* and transverse *(B)* views through the right side of the abdomen.

CHAPTER 88

Mesenteric Lymphadenopathy

CARLOS J. SIVIT

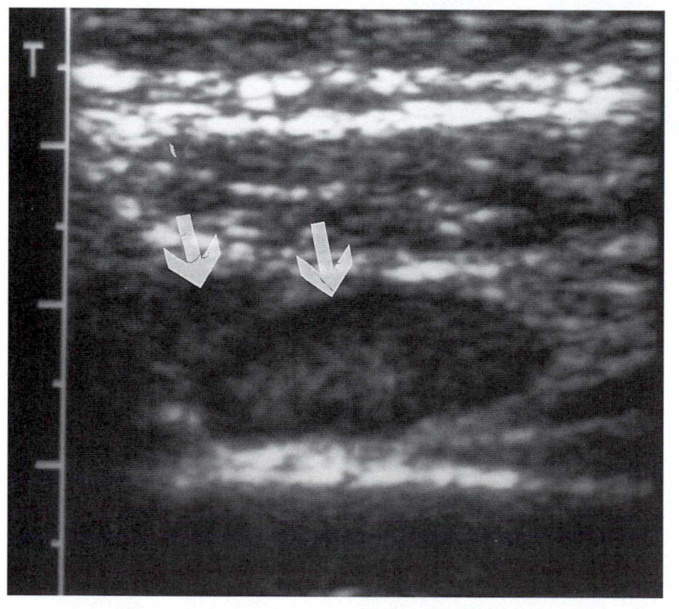

A

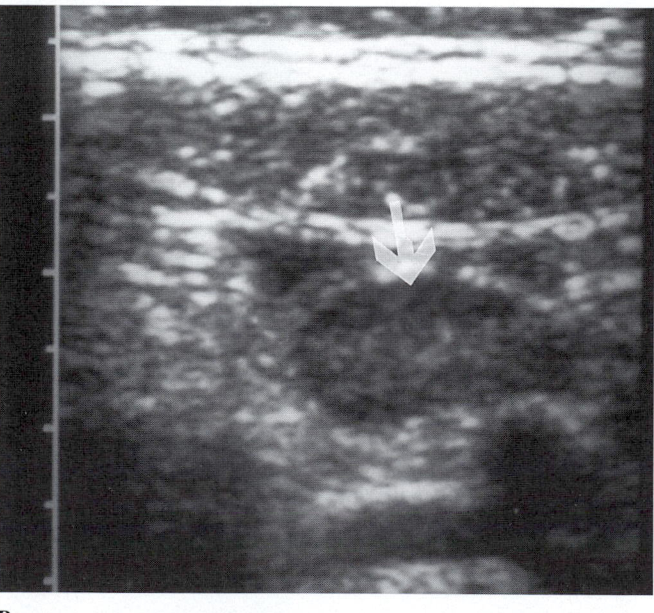

B

FIGURE 88–2. Enlarged mesenteric lymph nodes. Longitudinal *(A)* and transverse *(B)* views through the right lower quadrant obtained utilizing the graded compression technique with a linear high-frequency transducer show several enlarged, oval-shaped mesenteric lymph nodes (*arrows*). Note the relatively homogeneous appearance of the lymph nodes. They appear slightly hypoechoic relative to the anterior abdominal wall muscles.

Mesenteric lymph nodes are located along the ileal and jejunal arteries and the superior mesenteric vein in folds of the small-bowel mesentery. Thus, their expected location extends from the left upper quadrant at the root of the jejunoileal mesentery obliquely downward to the right sacroiliac joint. Mesenteric lymph nodes are seen most frequently on sonography in the right iliac fossa. Enlarged mesenteric lymph nodes have an oval shape, although they may appear somewhat flattened following graded compression examination (Fig. 88-2). The lymph nodes have a homogeneous appearance on sonography and are isoechoic or hypoechoic relative to surrounding tissues and muscles. Standards for abdominal and pelvic lymph node enlargement vary in the literature, depending on the imaging modality. Mesenteric lymph nodes are considered enlarged on graded compression sonography when the maximal anteroposterior

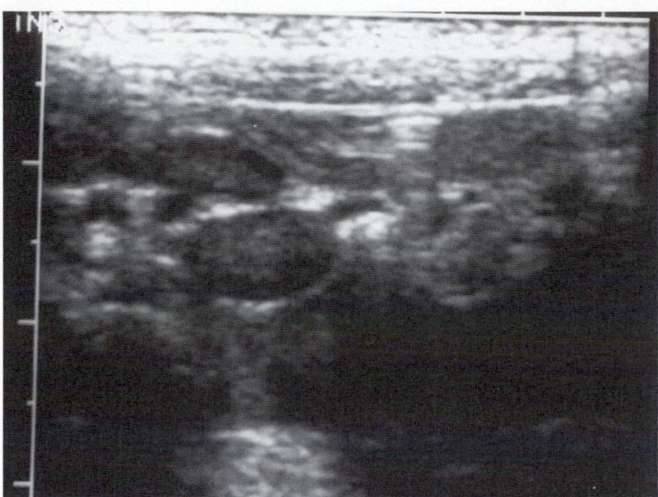

A

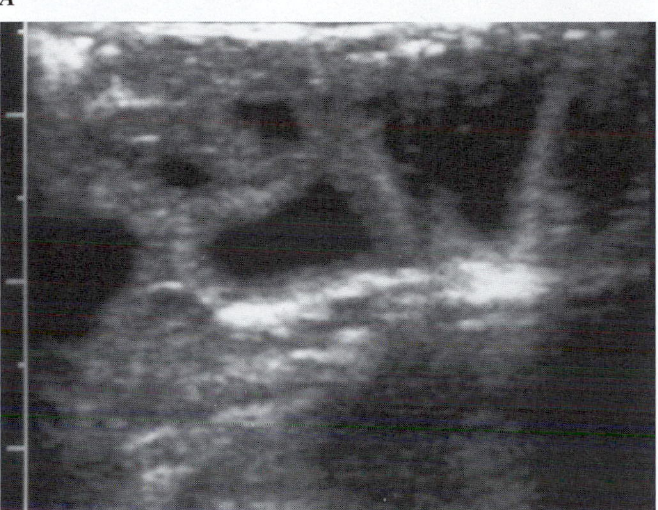

B

FIGURE 88–3. Enlarged mesenteric lymph nodes associated with *Yersinia* terminal ileitis. ***A.*** Transverse view through the right lower quadrant shows several enlarged, oval-shaped mesenteric lymph nodes. ***B.*** Longitudinal view of the right lower quadrant in the same patient demonstrates thickening of distal small-bowel loops. Stool cultures were positive for *Yersinia*

diameter exceeds 4 mm. This measurement represents the shortest diameter, since the lymph nodes assume an oval, flattened shape with graded compression.

It is important to distinguish between the sonographic finding of mesenteric lymph node enlargement and the clinical syndrome of mesenteric lymphadenitis. Mesenteric lymph node enlargement on sonography is a nonspecific finding associated with infection of the gastrointestinal tract by any of a large number of viral, bacterial, mycobacterial, and parasitic organisms (Fig. 88-3). Enlarged mesenteric lymph nodes may also be seen with inflammatory conditions and malignancy. The precise origin of this finding is often not determined. Mesenteric lymphadenitis is a clinical entity whose symptoms are related to benign inflammation of the lymph nodes by infectious or inflammatory processes.

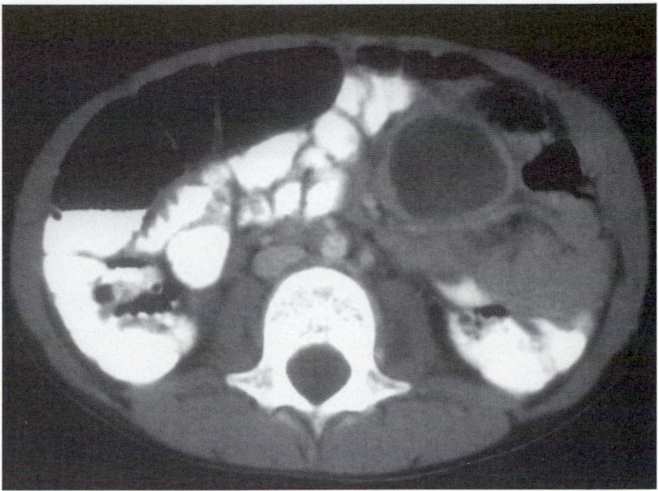

FIGURE 88–4. Suppurative mesenteric lymphadenitis. Computed tomography scan through the lower abdomen shows a rounded, low-density lesion with a thick, enhancing wall (*arrows*). At surgery, this proved to be a suppurative mesenteric lymph node..

Mesenteric lymphadenitis is conservatively treated by nonsurgical means, but often the diagnosis is made at nontherapeutic appendectomy. In several series, mesenteric lymphadenitis has been the most frequent alternative diagnosis in children who underwent surgery because of suspected acute appendicitis and had a normal appendix at surgery. Histology of these lymph nodes typically reveals nonspecific, reactive changes. The clinical syndrome of mesenteric lymphadenitis is therefore felt in some cases to mimic an "acute abdomen." Patients may present with right lower quadrant pain and tenderness, fever, and an elevated white blood cell count. Rarely, mesenteric lymphadenitis may be complicated by abscess formation (Fig. 88-4) or mesenteric venous thrombosis and require surgical intervention.

The widespread utilization of graded compression sonography has resulted in the identification of enlarged mesenteric lymph nodes in children with less severe symptomatology. The graded compression technique utilizes a high-frequency linear transducer to eliminate overlying bowel gas and fluid, thus reducing the distance from the transducer to the region of interest. It has been shown that enlarged mesenteric lymph nodes can be associated with a variety of abdominal and pelvic disorders, including acute appendicitis (Fig. 88-5). Enlarged mesenteric lymph nodes have also occasionally been identified in asymptomatic children. The potential coexistence of enlarged mesenteric lymph nodes visualized on sonography with a large number of associated conditions, including acute appendicitis, indicates that there should be a continued search for additional abdominal or pelvic abnormalities when enlarged lymph nodes are identified.

Enlargement of mesenteric lymph nodes associated with retroperitoneal lymphadenopathy is highly suggestive of malignancy or mycobacterial infection. The most common neoplasm that involves the mesentery in children is non-Hodgkin's lymphoma. In children with acquired immune deficiency syndrome, mesenteric lymphadenopathy associated

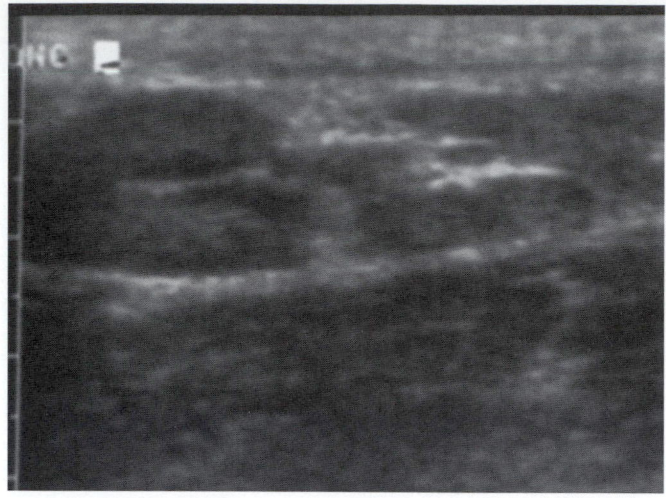

A

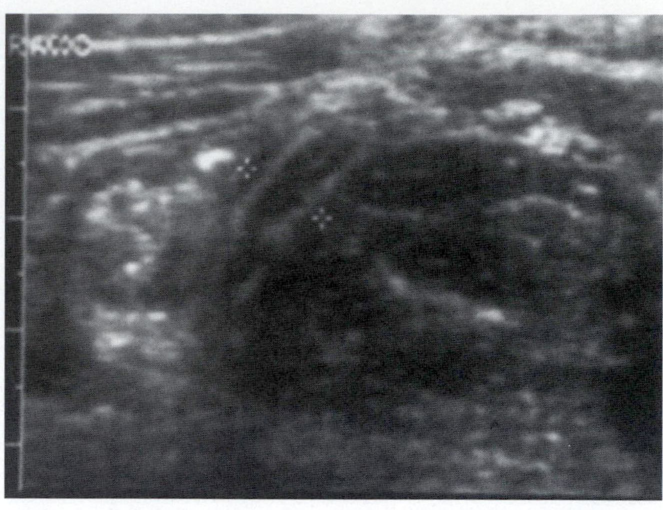

B

FIGURE 88–5. Enlarged mesenteric lymph nodes associated with acute appendicitis. ***A.*** Longitudinal view through the right lower quadrant demonstrates several enlarged, oval-shaped mesenteric lymph nodes. ***B.*** Oblique view through the right lower quadrant in the same patient shows an enlarged appendix (*between calipers*).

with enlargement of other nodal chains is a frequent finding. It is seen in association with *Mycobacterium avium-intracellulare* infection, lymphoma, and diffuse infiltrative lymphocytosis syndrome.

Computed tomography (CT) scan is useful in the evaluation of children with mesenteric lymph node enlargement for associated retroperitoneal lymphadenopathy and solid organ abnormalities if malignancy is suspected and for suppurative mesenteric lymphadenitis and abscess formation (Fig. 88-4). The CT examination in this setting should be performed following the administration of both intravenous and oral contrast media to optimize visualization of solid viscus and gastrointestinal tract pathology.

References

Asch MJ, Amoury RA, Touloukian RJ, et al: Suppurative mesenteric lymphadenitis. *Am J Surg* 115:570–573, 1968.

Chung CJ, Sivit CJ, Rakusan TA: Abdominal lymphadenopathy in children with AIDS. *Pediatric AIDS and HIV infection: Fetus to Adolescent* 5:305–308, 1994.

Kunkel MJ, Brown LG, Banta H, et al: Meningococcal mesenteric adenitis and peritonitis in a child. *Pediatr Infect Dis J* 10: 471–473, 1991.

Lau W, Fan S, Yiu T, et al: Negative findings at appendectomy. *Am J Surg* 148:375–378, 1984.

Liebman WM, St. Geme JW: Enteroviral pseudoappendicitis. *Am J Dis Child* 120:77–78, 1970.

Matsumoto T, Iida M, Sakai T, et al: Yersinia terminal ileitis: Sonographic findings in eight patients. *AJR* 156:965–967, 1991.

Puylaert JBCM: Mesenteric adenitis and terminal ileitis: US evaluation using graded compression. *Radiology* 161:691–695, 1986.

Puylaert JCBM, Lalisang RI, van der Werf SDJ, et al: Campylobacter ileocolitis mimicking acute appndicitis: Differentiation with graded compression US. *Radiology* 166:737–740, 1988.

Rao PM, Rhea JT, Novelline RA: CT diagnosis of mesenteric adenitis. *Radiology* 202:145–149, 1997.

Sivit CJ: Diagnosis of acute appendicitis in children: Spectrum of sonographic findings. *AJR* 161:147–152, 1996.

Sivit CJ, Newman KD, Chandra RS: Visualization of enlarged mesenteric lymph nodes at US examination: Clinical significance. *Pediatr Radiol* 23:471–475, 1993.

Vignault F, Filiatraut D, Brandt ML, et al: Acute appendicitis in children: Evaluation with US. *Radiology* 176:501–504, 1990.

89

Figure 89-1 shows a 5-year-old girl with a palpable abdominal mass. What do you see? What are the diagnostic considerations?

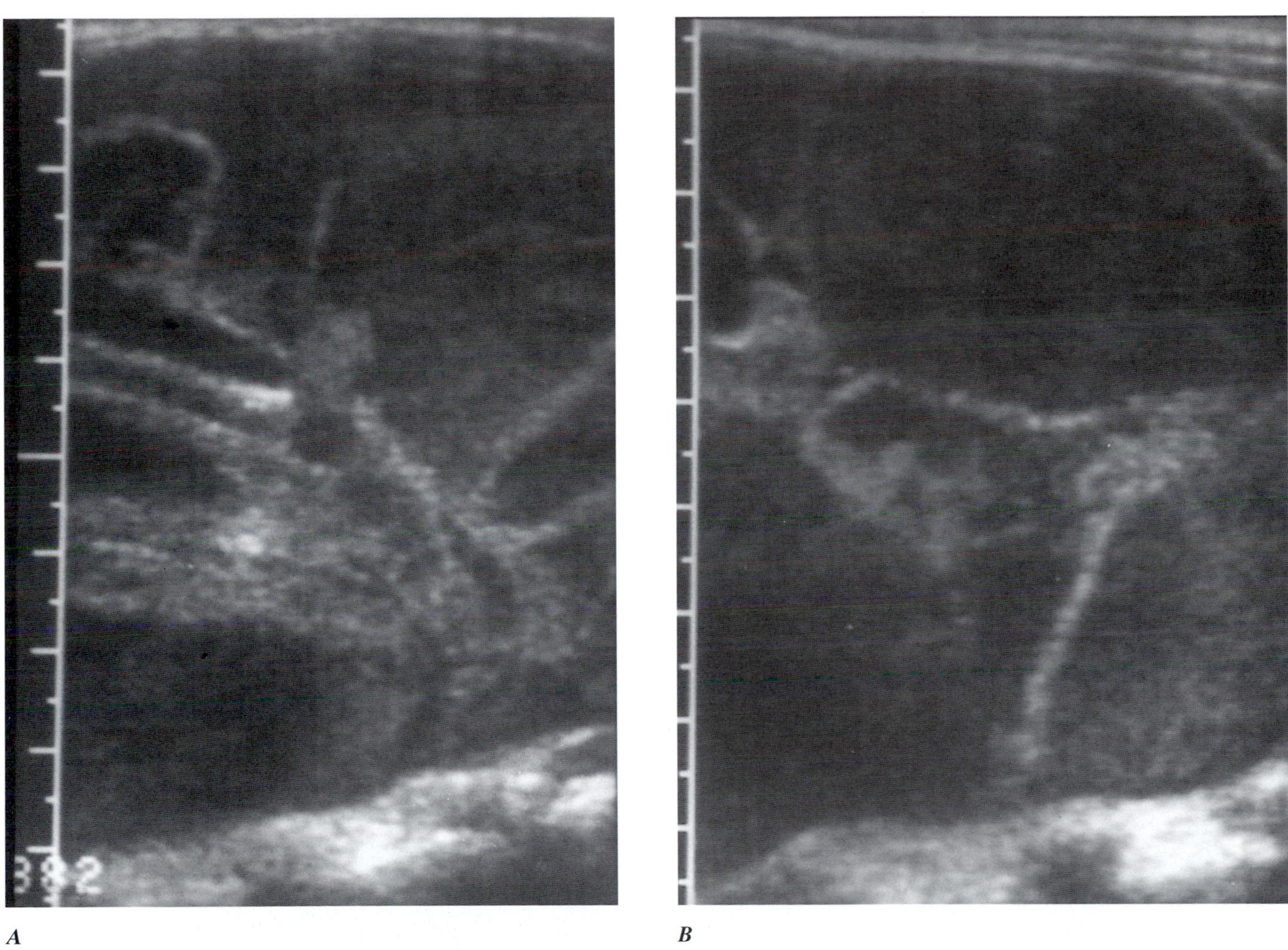

FIGURE 89–1. Longitudinal views through the lower abdomen *(A)* and upper pelvis *(B).*

CHAPTER 91

Neutropenic Typhlitis

CARLOS J. SIVIT

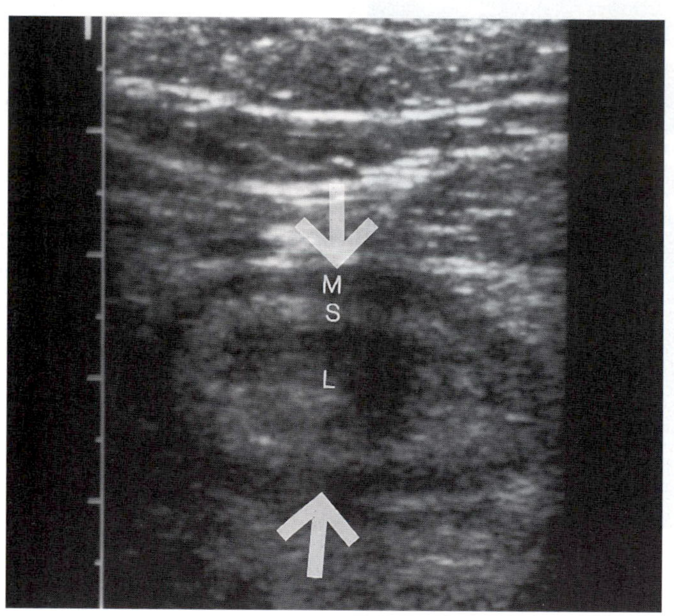

A

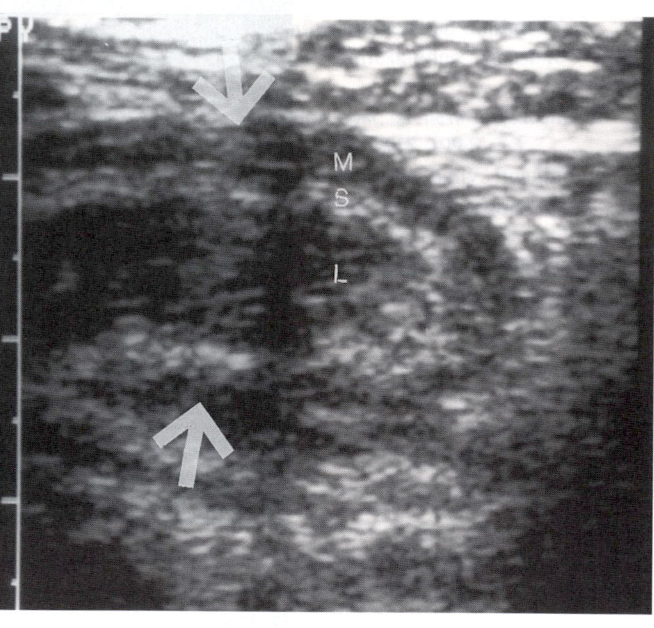

B

FIGURE 91–2. Neutropenic typhlitis. Transverse *(A)* and longitudinal *(B)* views through the right lower quadrant utilizing the graded compression technique demonstrate thickening of the cecum (*arrows*) and appendix. Note the asymmetric thickening of the echogenic mucosal and submucosal layers (S) relative to the muscularis layer (M) in the cecum. L = bowel lumen.

Neutropenic typhlitis is a necrotizing enteropathy of the right colon that develops in the setting of severe neutropenia. Proposed predisposing factors include severe neutropenia and cytotoxic, drug-induced ileus. These factors are felt to lead to colonic stasis, distention, and ischemia. Subsequently, mucosal ulceration and secondary bacterial invasion may develop. This can progress to mucosal and submucosal necrosis accompanied by marked intramural edema and hemorrhage. The histopathologic findings are usually limited to the cecum, ascending colon, appendix, and terminal ileum. The cecum and ascending colon are at greatest risk for involvement because these are areas of relatively greater stasis and distensibility.

Neutropenic typhlitis occurs most commonly in children with leukemia, but it has also been reported in those with a number of other conditions, including lymphoma and aplastic anemia, and following bone marrow transplantation. There has been a marked increase in the number of reported cases of neutropenic typhlitis in recent years. This is probably due to the increasing intensity of chemotherapeutic agents used to treat pediatric malignancy and to the wider availability of sonography and cross-sectional imaging for diagnosis.

Clinical signs and symptoms associated with neutropenic typhlitis vary; they include fever, nausea, vomiting, abdominal pain, and abdominal tenderness that frequently localizes to the right lower quadrant. Diarrhea is common and is often bloody. The condition can usually be successfully managed with supportive medical treatment. However, the disease can be severe, and complications include bowel obstruction, bowel perforation, sepsis, and death.

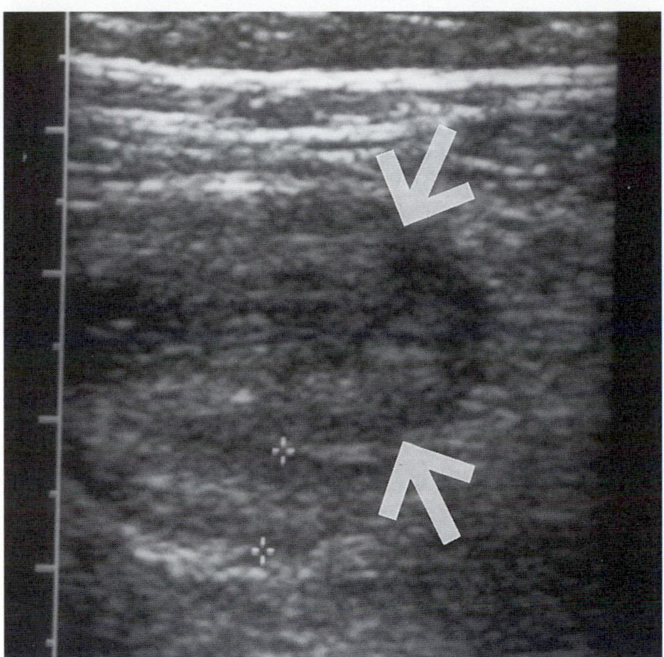

FIGURE 91–3. Neutropenic typhlitis with appendiceal thickening. Longitudinal view through the right lower quadrant in a child with neutropenic typhlitis shows cecal wall thickening (*arrows*) and appendiceal thickening (*between electronic calipers*). Note the primarily echogenic appearance of the cecal wall thickening.

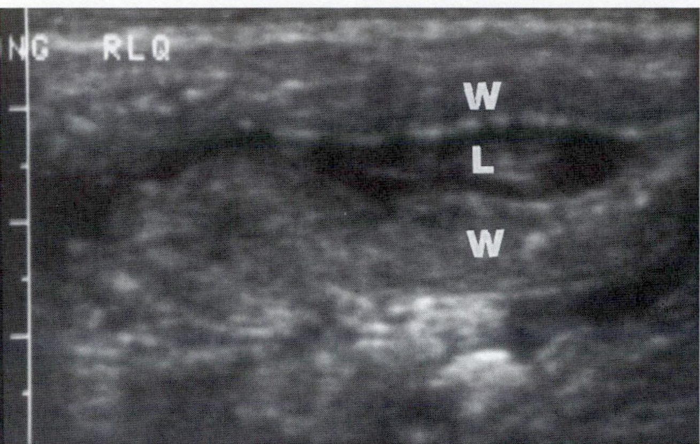

FIGURE 91–4. Neutropenic typhlitis with echogenic cecal wall thickening. Longitudinal view through the right lower quadrant shows cecal thickening. Note that the entire wall appears echogenic. L = bowel lumen, W = bowel wall.

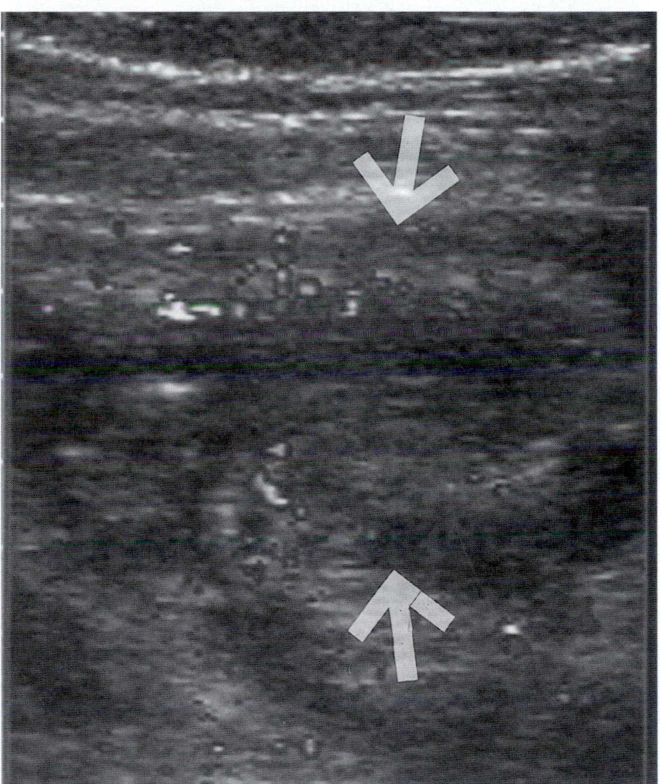

FIGURE 91–5. Neutropenic typhlitis with hyperemia demonstrated on color Doppler examination. Transverse view of the right lower quadrant in a child with neutropenic typhlitis after a bone marrow transplant shows cecal thickening (*arrows*) with pronounced bowel wall hyperemia by color Doppler. Note the thickened hyperechoic mucosal/submucosal layer and the hypoechoic muscularis layer. (See Color Plate 23.)

Sonography is a useful modality for assessing children with suspected neutropenic typhlitis. The ability to perform the examination at the patient's bedside is critical, as often these patients are too sick to travel to the radiology suite. The examination is performed utilizing the graded compression technique with a high-frequency linear transducer. Compression must be applied slowly, since these children are usually quite tender. The colon should be examined in its entirety, imaging from right to left in both transverse and longitudinal planes, but emphasis should be placed on scanning the right lower quadrant, since the disease primarily involves the cecum (Fig. 91-2).

Sonographic findings in neutropenic typhlitis include colonic bowel wall thickening (Fig. 91-2), distal ileal bowel wall thickening, appendiceal wall thickening (Fig. 91-3), and increased echogenicity surrounding the cecum, representing infiltration of the pericecal fat. The normal bowel wall should measure <3 mm in diameter. Involvement of the colon is typically most severe in, or restricted to, the cecum. However, it is not unusual to see associated thickening of the ascending colon, and occasionally the transverse colon may be affected. Colonic bowel wall thickening in typhlitis is a transmural process, but the mucosal and submucosal layers are involved to a greater degree than the muscularis layer. Thus, the thickened colonic segment often appears predominantly echogenic as a result of the asymmetric involvement of the hyperechoic mucosal and submucosal regions (Fig. 91-4; see also Color Plate 23). On color Doppler, marked bowel wall hyperemia may be noted in the involved bowel segment (Fig. 91-5). The secondary involvement of the appendix in neutropenic typhlitis is important to note, as acute appendicitis is usually a differential consideration in these children. Thus, recognition that appendiceal wall thickening associated with cecal thickening can be part of the spectrum of abnormalities observed in neutropenic typhlitis may prevent unnecessary laparotomy for presumed appendicitis. Sonography is also useful for follow-up examination to monitor serial changes in the extent

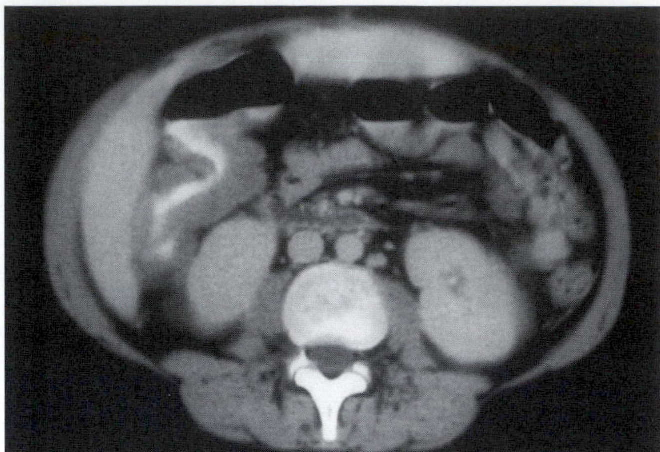

A

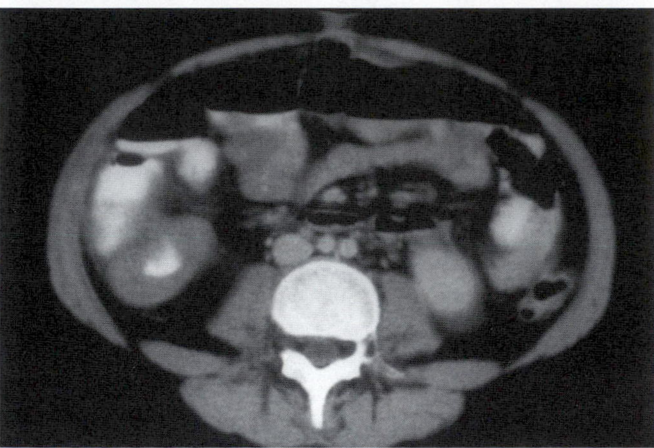

B

FIGURE 91–6. Computed tomographphy (CT) of neutropenic typhlitis. ***A.*** A CT scan through the mid-abdomen in a child with leukemia, neutropenia, and abdominal pain demonstrates focal thickening of the ascending colon at the hepatic flexure. ***B.*** A CT scan through the lower abdomen 2 cm below *A* shows cecal wall thickening.

and severity of disease. Decreasing bowel and appendiceal wall diameters are seen with clinical improvement.

Computed tomography (CT) is also utilized in the evaluation of children with suspected neutropenic typhlitis, as CT can delineate the extent of colonic bowel wall thickening better than sonography (Fig. 91-6). Additional variable findings on CT include stranding of pericecal fat and dilatation of the distal small bowel. Computed tomography is particularly useful in children that are difficult to examine with graded compression sonography because of extreme tenderness, in cases where the sonographic findings are equivocal, and in cases where perforation is suspected.

The differential diagnosis in a neutropenic patient with fever and severe abdominal signs and symptoms also includes acute appendicitis, pseudomembranous colitis, ischemic colitis, intussusception from lymphomatous or leukemic infiltration of the bowel wall, small-bowel obstruction, and bowel perforation. Neutropenic typhlitis can be differentiated from acute appendicitis on sonography by identifying isolated appendiceal enlargement without associated cecal thickening. Distinction of neutropenic typhlitis from pseudomembranous and ischemic colitis can be difficult, as all can involve the right colon. However, pseudomembranous and ischemic colitis usually do not result in predominantly echogenic bowel wall thickening. An intussusception will appear as a focal mass with a "target" or "doughnut" appearance in the transverse plane (Fig. 86-2) and have a "pseudokidney" appearance on longitudinal view (Fig. 86-6).

References

Abramson SJ, Berdon WE, Baker DH: Childhood typhlitis: Its increasing association with acute myelogenous leukemia: Report of five cases. *Radiology* 146:61–64, 1983.

Alexander JE, Williamson SL, Seibert JJ, et al: The ultrasonographic diagnosis of typhlitis (neutropenic colitis). *Pediatr Radiol* 18:200–204, 1988.

Benya EC, Sivit CJ, Quinones RR: Abdominal complications after bone marrow transplantation in children: Sonographic and CT findings. *AJR* 161:1023–1027, 1993.

Glass-Royal MC, Choyke PL, Gootenberg JE, Grant EG: Sonography in the diagnosis of neutropenic colitis. *J Ultrasound Med* 6:671–673, 1987.

Kaste SC, Flynn PM, Furman WL: Acute lymphoblastic leukemia presenting with typhlitis. *Med Pediatr Oncol* 28:209–212, 1997.

McNamara MJ, Chalmers AG, Morgan M, et al: Typhlitis in acute childhood leukemia: Radiological features. *Clin Radiol* 37: 83–86, 1986.

Sloas MM, Flynn PM, Kaste SC: Typhlitis in children with cancer: A 30-year experience. *Clin Infect Dis* 17:484–490, 1993.

Teefey SA, Montana MA, Goldfogel GA, et al: Sonographic diagnosis of neutropenic typhlitis. *AJR* 149:731–733, 1987.

92

Figure 92-1 shows an obese 9-year-old girl with right-sided abdominal pain and low-grade fever. What is the finding? What is the differential diagnosis?

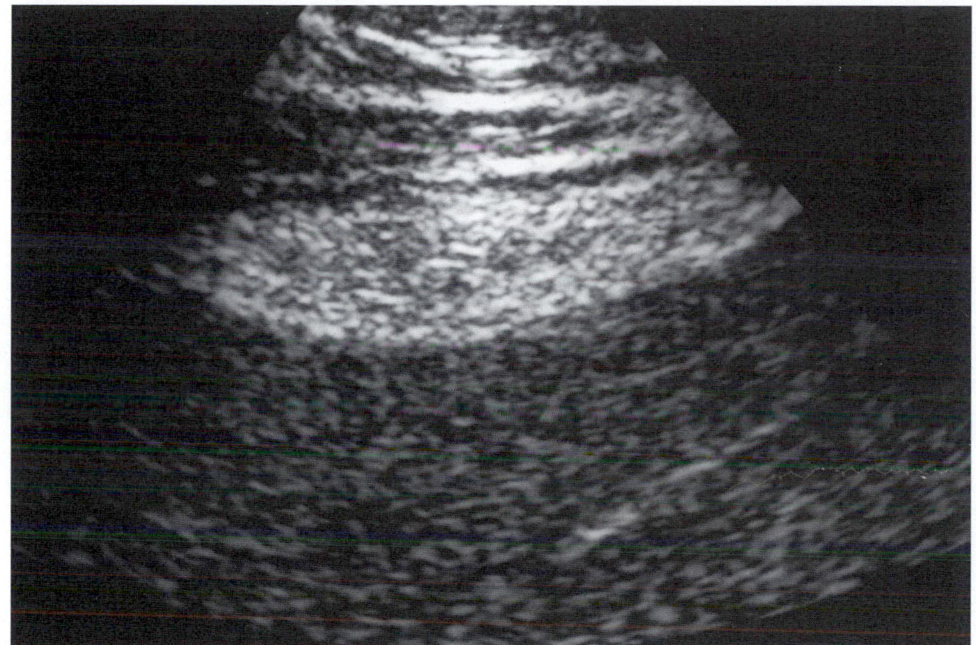

FIGURE 92–1. Transverse view through the right upper abdomen.

CHAPTER 92

Segmental Omental Infarction

MELISSA T. MYERS

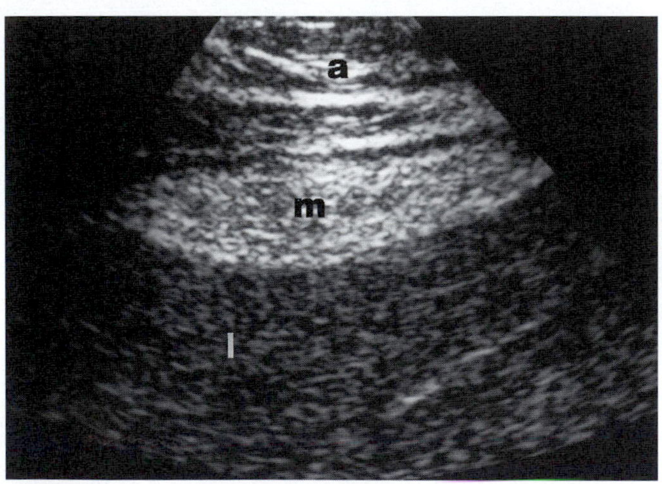

FIGURE 92–2. Segmental omental infarction. Transverse view through the right upper abdomen demonstrates an ovoid, noncompressible echogenic mass (m) anterior to the right lobe of the liver (l) and posterior to the anterior abdominal musculature (a). Note that the lesion demonstrates a mass effect upon the liver.

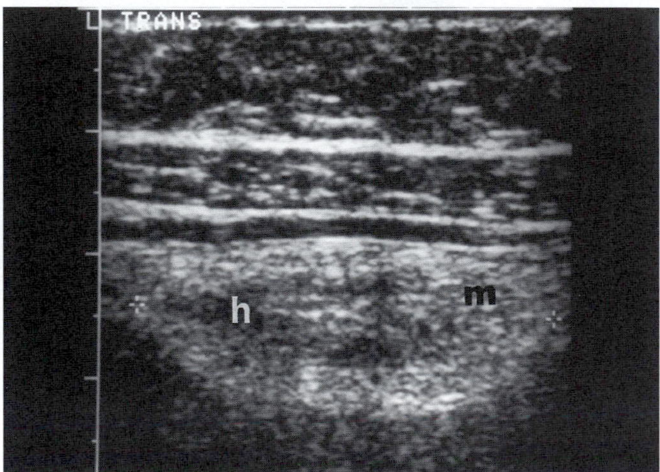

FIGURE 92–3. Segmental omental infarction. Transverse view through the right upper abdomen with a linear high-frequency transducer demonstrates a heterogeneous mass (m) with a hyperechoic periphery and a hypoechoic center (h).

Segmental omental infarction is a rare condition that may result in acute abdominal pain in both children and adults. Approximately 15 percent of cases occur in the pediatric age group. The youngest reported case is in a 3-year-old child. The infarction of omental fat may be primary or secondary. The primary form is idiopathic, while the secondary form may be caused by torsion of the omentum, vasculitis, or hypercoagulation. Trauma or overeating may induce venous infarction in predisposed individuals. Obesity may also be contributory, although not all patients with this entity are obese.

Segmental omental infarction occurs in the anterolateral aspect of the peritoneum at or just above the level of the umbilicus. Therefore, it is thought to be due to a congenital vascular anomaly in the venous circulation of the greater omentum. In the embryo, the greater omentum is derived from the dorsal mesogastrium, and the lesser omentum is derived from the ventral mesogastrium. Occasionally, the right lateral aspect of the greater omentum is derived from an abnormal extension of the ventral mesogastrium, leaving it with a tenuous blood supply. At surgery, one sees a red or purple, wedge-shaped area in the right lateral dependent border of the greater omentum. The pathologic findings in resected surgical specimens include venous thrombosis and a hemorrhagic inflammatory infiltrate with fat necrosis. Depending on the time course, there may be varying degrees of organizing fibroblastic reaction within the fatty lesion.

The characteristic clinical signs and symptoms associated with segmental omental infarction include acute right upper

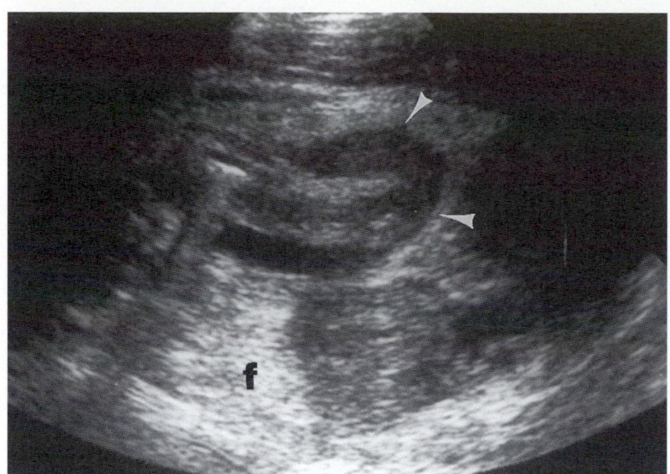

FIGURE 92–4. Acute appendicitis with associated infiltration of mesenteric fat. Longitudinal view through the right lower abdomen demonstrates an enlarged, noncompressible appendix (*arrowheads*) with surrounding infiltration of the mesenteric fat (f).

quadrant pain, low-grade fever, and leukocytosis. Additional symptoms include nausea, diarrhea, and constipation. On physical examination, an abdominal mass can often be palpated in children, but rarely in adults. Occasionally there is exquisite, point tenderness caused by local peritoneal irritation just over the site of the omental infarction. The symptom complex may suggest one of the more common diagnoses of cholecystitis, diverticulitis, or appendicitis, depending upon the location of the pain and the age of the patient.

The characteristic sonographic finding associated with segmental omental infarction is an ovoid or cakelike, diffusely hyperechoic mass in the anterior aspect of the peritoneal cavity to the right and slightly above the umbilicus (Fig. 92-2). Evaluation with a high-frequency linear transducer may show heterogeneity within the mass (Fig. 92-3). The echogenicity of the mass is typically greater than that of the surrounding peritoneal fat or solid viscera. The mass may be adherent to the peritoneum. It is usually noted at the point of maximum tenderness. It often demonstrates mass effect on adjacent organs, such as the liver. Typically, the mass is not compressible when pressure is applied with the transducer. Segmental omental infarction may secondarily involve the bowel, gallbladder, or appendix.

The sonographic finding of focally increased echogenicity is nonspecific and simply implies infiltration of fluid or inflammatory cells within the mesenteric or omental fat. This may be associated with a variety of infectious, inflammatory, or neoplastic processes, including acute appendicitis and pancreatitits. Sonography can distinguish secondary inflammatory changes from primary omental infarction by identifying the associated pathology in one or more intraabdominal organs. For example, acute appendicitis is frequently associated with inflammatory changes in the surrounding small-bowel mesentery. Thus, echogenic fat may be noted surrounding an enlarged, noncompressible appendix in acute appendicitis (Fig. 92-4). The identification of appendiceal enlargement establishes that the abnormality of mesenteric fat is a secondary finding.

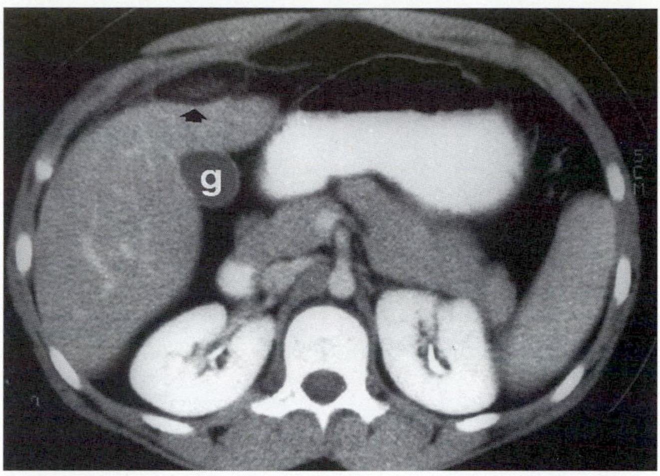

A

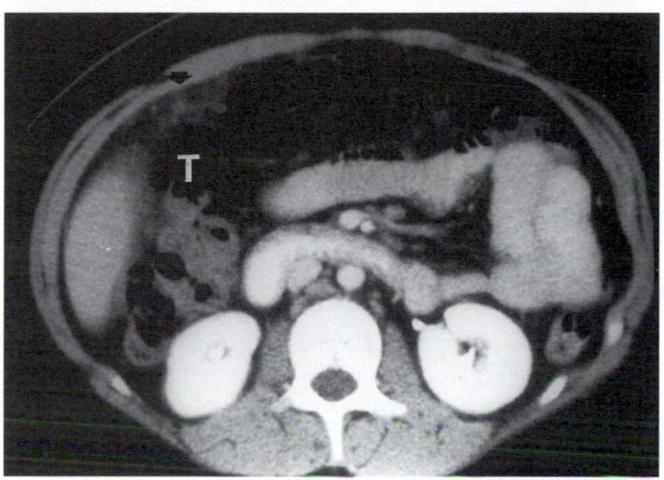

B

FIGURE 92–5. Segmental omental infarction. ***A.*** Contrast-enhanced computed tomography (CT) through the upper abdomen in the same child as in Fig. 92-1 demonstrates an oval-shaped mass in the omental fat (*arrow*) anterior to the liver, associated with inflammatory stranding. ***B.*** A CT section 2 cm below *A* shows stranding within the omental fat (*arrow*) anterior to the liver and transverse colon (T).

Computed tomography (CT) may be utilized to better demonstrate the extent of disease and exclude other pathology. The characteristic CT appearance of segmental omental infarction includes an ill-defined mass of fat attenuation adjacent to the anterior peritoneum, with strands of soft tissue attenuation coursing through the lesion (Fig. 92-5). The stranding indicates inflammatory changes within the omental fat. Again, adjacent organs are typically not involved.

The differential diagnosis of a fat-containing omental mass includes fatty tumors of the mesentery, such as lipoblastoma in children and liposarcoma in older individuals. These neoplasms may be difficult to differentiate from segmental omental infarction on the basis of their initial appearance on sonography or CT. However, differentiation can usually be made on the basis of clinical presentation and clin-

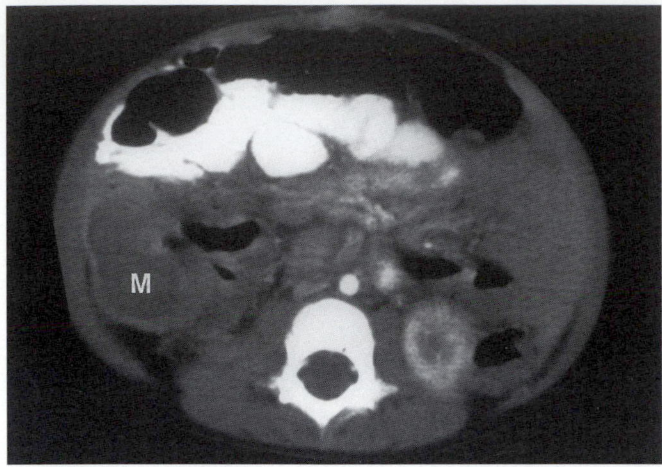

FIGURE 92–6. Segmental omental infarction with associated omental abscess. Contrast-enhanced computed tomography scan through the lower abdomen demonstrates a well-defined mass of mixed attenuation, with rim enhancement (M) lateral to the cecum. The surgical specimen showed necrotic fatty tissue with purulent exudate.

ical and imaging follow-up. The clinical signs and symptoms and imaging abnormalities associated with segmental omental infarction are seen to gradually resolve over a period of several weeks.

In the past, segmental omental infarction was treated surgically. However, recent reports indicate that most children can successfully be managed nonoperatively. Occasionally, adhesions or abscess formation complicates segmental omental infarction, and these complications require surgical intervention (Fig. 92-6). The usual clinical course of patients with uncomplicated omental infarction is gradual, spontaneous resolution of the symptoms. Serial evaluation with sonography demonstrates a gradual decrease in the size of the mass.

References

Balthazar EJ, Lefkowitz RA: Left-sided omental infarction with associated omental abscess: CT diagnosis. *J Comput Assist Tomogr* 17:379–381, 1993.

Borushok KF, Jeffrey RB, Laing FC, Townsend RR: Sonographic diagnosis of perforation in patients with acute appendicitis. *AJR* 154:275–278, 1990.

Crofoot DC: Spontaneous segmental infarction of the greater omentum. *Am J Surg* 139:262–264, 1980.

Epstein LI, Lempke RE: Primary idiopathic segmental infarction of the greater omentum: Case report and collective review of the literature. *Ann Surg* 167:437–443, 1968.

Myers MT, Grisoni E, Sivit CJ: Omental infarction in a nine year old girl. *Emerg Radiol* 2:112–114, 1997.

Noordzij J, Puylaert JB, Smithuis RH, Langezaal OA: Rightsided segmental infarction of the omentum. *Eur J Surg* 160:703–705, 1994.

Puylaert JBCM: Right-sided segmental infarction of the omentum: Clinical, US, and CT findings. *Radiology* 185:169–172, 1992.

Schnur PL, McIlrath DC, Carney JA, Whittaker LD: Segmental infarction of the greater omentum. *Mayo Clin Proc* 47:751–755, 1972.

Section H
GYNECOLOGIC TRACT

93

It's Friday afternoon, and you are leaving your department. You get an emergency call to evaluate a newborn female with prominent labia. Someone has performed an ultrasound (US) and has diagnosed a pelvic mass. There is great clinical concern. You are shown Fig. 93-1. What is the diagnosis? What imaging action should be done next? If ambiguous genitalia were the clinical concern, would this have been an appropriate time to image the child's pelvis?

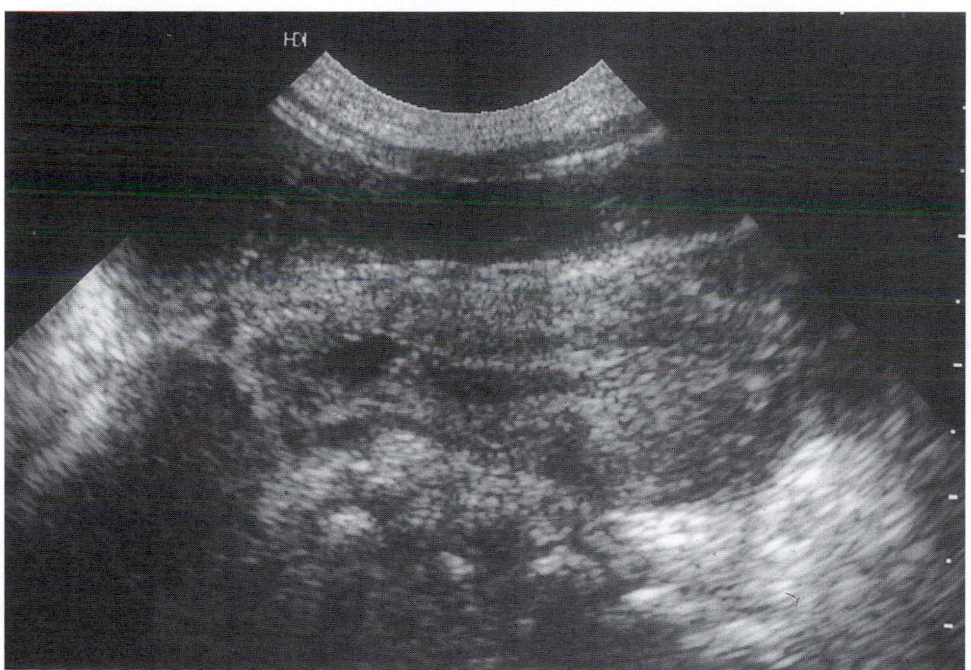

FIGURE 93–1. Pelvis. Ultrasound. Longitudinal plane.

CHAPTER 93

Normal Uterus in the Newborn

HARRIS L. COHEN

AND MARYANNE RUGGIERO-DELLITURRI

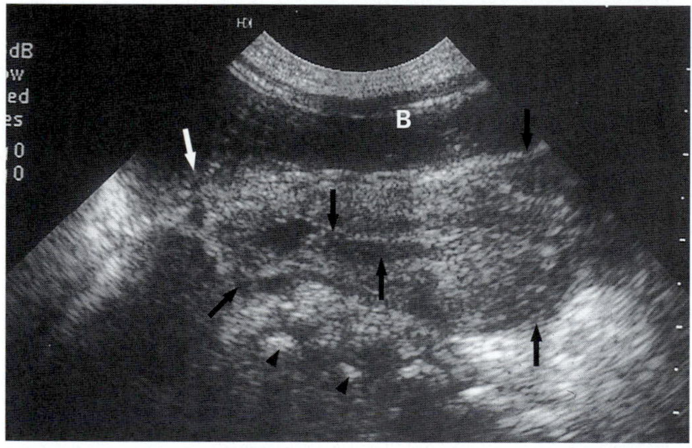

FIGURE 93–2. Annotated version of Fig. 93-1. Normal neonatal uterus. Pelvis. Ultrasound. Longitudinal plane. A spade-shaped structure (*arrows*) is noted posterior to the fluid-filled bladder (B) and anterior to the echogenic (air-filled) rectum. The shape is due to the prominence of the cervix compared to the fundus in newborns. High gonadotropin levels of the newborn are responsible for both the evident endometrial stripe (*small arrows*), not usually seen in older children until puberty, and the small amount of echoless fluid seen in the superior endometrial cavity. This can be related to the occasional vaginal bleeding of the newborn. Arrowheads point to echogenic vertebral bodies.

Figure 93-2, the annotated version of Fig. 93-1, shows a spade-shaped mass posterior to the bladder and anterior to the gas-filled rectum. It has a small amount of central fluid superiorly and a central echogenic line within much of its midline. It is the normal neonatal uterus. Clinical concern was assuaged. The uterus of the newborn is more prominent than that of the older child. This is an excellent time to image the uterus and prove its presence on US.

THE EMBRYOLOGY OF THE FEMALE GENITAL SYSTEM

As an introduction to many of the cases in the gynecology section of this book, it pays to review, briefly, some information on the embryology of the female genital system. The primitive gonad differentiates into a testis at 7 weeks of fetal life only in the presence of the H-Y antigen, found on the Y chromosome. If there is no Y chromosome, differentiation into an ovary will begin at 17 weeks gestation if two X chromosomes are present.

The development of the urinary system is closely associated with that of the genital system. Urogenital ridges develop from the intermediate mesoderm and are situated on each side of the primitive aorta. They give rise to parts of the genital and urinary systems. The association of uterine and renal abnormalities is quite common, and when there is a gynecologic anomaly, one should evaluate the renal bed to rule out ectopia or agenesis (Fig. 93-3). Both sexes develop two different pairs of genital ducts. Under the influence of testosterone, parts of the wolffian or mesonephric duct system develop into the epididymis, vas deferens, and seminal vesicles. By 6 weeks, a müllerian (paramesonephric) duct has developed lateral to each ipsilateral wolffian (mesonephric) duct. In the female, the müllerian duct system (MDS) develops into the fallopian tubes, uterus, and upper two-thirds of the vagina, and the wolffian system degenerates. External genital development proceeds along female lines except in the presence of androgens. If the MDS is dysgenetic, the uterus or vagina may be absent or rudimentary, as in the Mayer-Rokitansky-Küster-Hauser syndrome. Such patients have normal karyotypes and normal secondary sex development but have associated renal (50 percent) and skeletal (12 per-

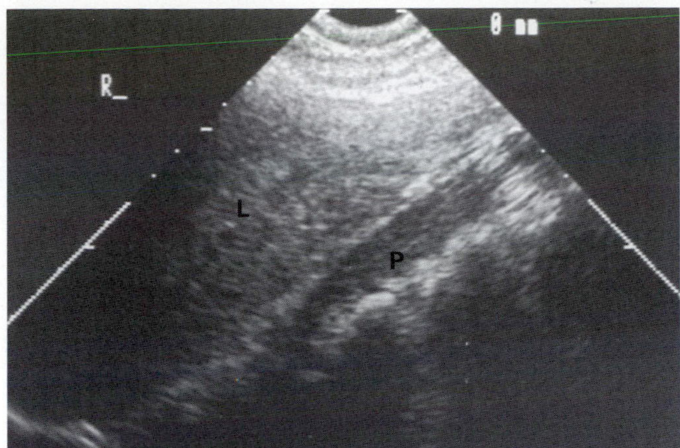

FIGURE 93–3. Renal agenesis. Right upper quadrant. Longitudinal plane. The liver (L) and psoas (P) muscles are seen. No kidney is seen in the normal renal bed. A nuclear medicine examination proved that the right kidney was not in an ectopic location. This patient had a congenitally anomalous (bicornuate) uterus. When a gynecologic anomaly is discovered, the kidneys should routinely be imaged because of the known association of anomalies of the genital and urinary tracts.

cent) anomalies. By 11 weeks, a Y-shaped uterovaginal primordium has developed into the two fallopian tubes, and with fusion of a large portion of the MDS of both sides, a single uterus and upper two-thirds of the vagina results. This occurs in the presence or absence of ovaries, as long as there are no testes or high levels of androgens present. The testes produce testosterone, a masculinizing hormone, and müllerian inhibition factor (MIF), which suppresses the further development of the paramesonephric ducts.

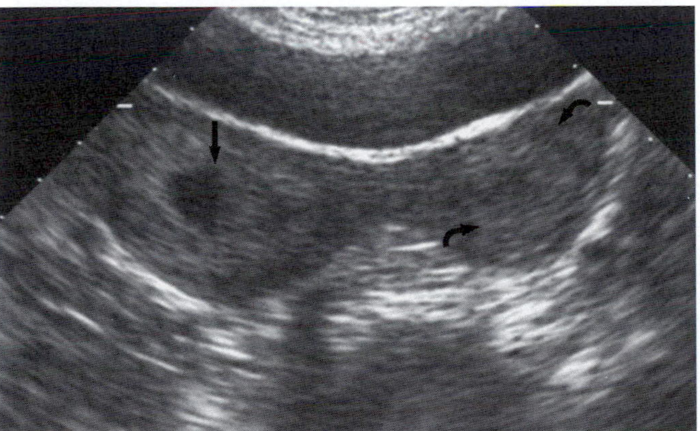

FIGURE 93–4. Bicornuate uterus. Transverse plane. The external contour of the uterus is concave. This is because the fundus is divided into two horns; there is a bicornuate uterus due to partial fusion of the müllerian ducts embryologically. In the right horn is a gestational sac (*arrow*). In the left horn, there is some increased echogenicity (*curved arrows*) because of the hormonal influence of the pregnancy on this portion of the uterus, which has its own functional endometrial cavity but no pregnancy. (*From Ruggierro M, Awobuluyi M, Cohen H, Zinn D: Imaging the pediatric pelvis: Role of ultrasound.* Radiologist *4:155–170, 1997, with permission.*)

In females, nonfusion or incomplete fusion of the MDS can lead to a wide spectrum of anomalies. Complete nonfusion results in a didelphys uterus, with two vaginas, two cervices, and two uterine bodies. Various anomalies are associated with incomplete müllerian duct fusion. Partial fusion of only the caudal ends of the MDS results in a bicornuate uterus, in which there is variable nonfusion of the cranial portion of the uterus, resulting in paired and variably separated uterine horns at the fundus that communicate with a correctly fused and therefore single uterine body, cervix, and vagina. The bicornuate uterus results in a wider than normal uterus that may be diagnosed on physical examination by an anterior uterine depression or by US when two endometrial cavities are imaged. This is best imaged either during the luteal phase of the menstrual cycle or during pregnancy (Fig. 93-4). Where the müllerian system joins the urogenital sinus, the lower one-third of the vagina develops by elongation of the primitive vaginal plate into a core of tissue that canalizes by week 20. The wolffian system degenerates in the normal female. Until late in fetal life the lumen of the vagina is separated from its vestibule by a hymenal membrane. The hymen usually ruptures in the perinatal period, remaining as a thin fold of mucous membrane around the vaginal entry.

THE NORMAL UTERUS OF THE NEWBORN, CHILD, AND ADOLESCENT

The normal uterus is rarely imaged antenatally. Perhaps this is because it gets lost amid echogenic bowel. This also results from limitations of imaging, particularly due to fetal positioning in late pregnancy. In addition, the increase in gonadotropin in neonates occurs after separation from the placenta. Uterine size and shape are affected in the first months by the temporarily high gonadotropin levels that develop from this separation. Neonatal findings of, e.g., an echogenic central endometrial cavity echo, a hypoechoic halo around the endometrial cavity echo (29 percent) (Figs. 93-2 and 93-5), or endometrial cavity fluid (23 percent) (Fig. 93-2), more typical of the adult uterus under the cyclical hormonal influences of postmenarchal life, can be noted; if seen, they are evidence of potential future changes with estrogenization in postmenarchal life.

The uterus of the newborn has a mean length of 3.5 cm. The length decreases to 2.6 to 3.0 cm by the fourth month of life. The shape of the newborn's uterus has been described as resembling a spade, with the anteroposterior (AP) measurement of the cervix greater than that of the fundus and the cervical length twice as great as the fundal length. My problem with this statement in the imaging literature is that it is difficult to figure out where the cervical length ends and the fundal length begins. Nussbaum et al noted that the uterus of infant girls was spade-shaped in 58 percent of cases and tube-shaped (AP measurement of the cervix equal to that of the fundus) in 32 percent. Only 10 percent of their premenarchal patients showed the classic adult pear-shaped uterus (Fig. 93-6), with its fundus wider than the cervix. After the first

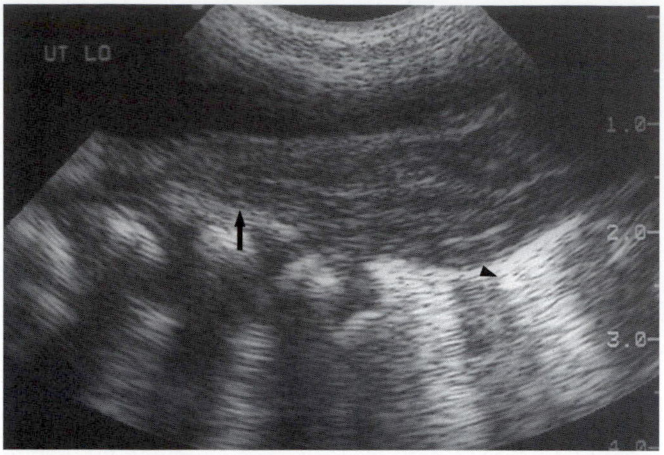

A

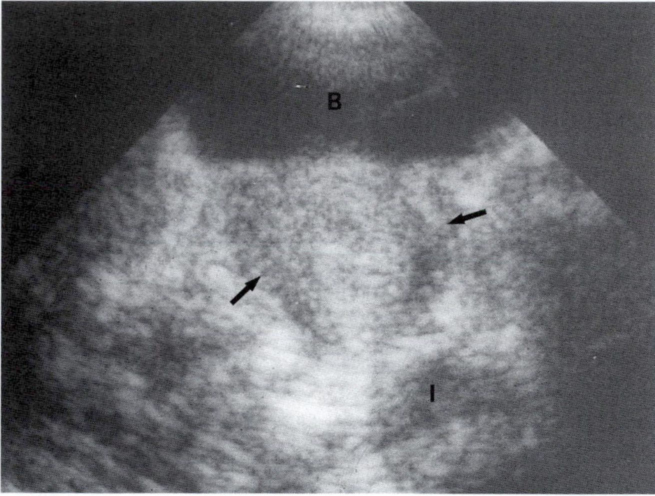

B

FIGURE 93–5. Normal neonatal uterus. ***A.*** Longitudinal plane. This is another normal neonatal uterus; it is perhaps even more typical than Fig. 93-2, in that there is no endometrial fluid, the uterine position is obviously neutral (i.e., not anteverted or retroverted), and there is no contained endometrial fluid. The fundus (*arrow*) is less wide than the cervix (*arrowhead*). ***B.*** Transverse plane. A prominent soft tissue mass (*arrows*) is seen posterior to the bladder in the cervical region of this neonate's uterus. Only in a neonate would one see this prominent a uterus on a transverse image of the pelvis. Someone unfamiliar with images of the uterus in the newborn, might suspect a pathologic mass. B = bladder. I = bowel.

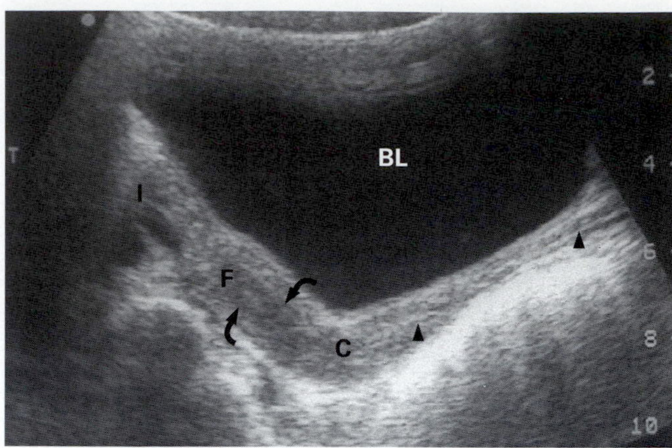

FIGURE 93–6. Normal adolescent uterus—pear shape. Longitudinal plane. The uterus of an adolescent is imaged. She is postmenarchal. The width of her uterine fundus (F) is wider than that of her cervix (C). A small amount of echogenicity is seen in her endometrial cavity. This is usually seen in individuals with estrogen activity. The echopenic area around her endometrial cavity (*curved arrow*) has been considered the equivalent to the normal junctional zone on magnetic resonance imaging. Some bowel (I) is noted superior to the uterine fundus. At times one may see a normal ovary at this site. Arrowheads point to the echogenic line in her vagina, consistent with mucosa. BL = bladder.

year of life, the tube shape (Fig. 93-7) predominates for the next several years of childhood. Uterine lengths increase gradually between 3 and 8 years of age, with the mean measurement for the premenarchal child being 4.3 cm. Orsini et al believe that this change in size, the change to a pear shape, and the reversal of the ratio of corpus to cervical length are due not only to increasing estradiol levels, but also to two independent variables: patient age and size. There is a moderate (r = 0.69) correlation of uterine length to weight in childhood.

After puberty, the typical uterus measures 5 to 8 cm in length. It descends deeper in the pelvis and no longer maintains the typical neutral position of the premenarchal years but may be anteverted or retroverted.

Information on the uterus is particularly important, since the identification of the uterus and determination of its size are key pieces of diagnostic information in several pediatric/adolescent gynecologic workups.

Whereas US can aid in the diagnosis of various MDS anomalies, particularly the bicornuate uterus and a uterus with partial or complete obstruction, magnetic resonance imaging (MRI) and its multiplanar imaging has been used successfully in the global analysis of several of these anomalies.

WHAT WOULD A UTERINE MASS LOOK LIKE IN A CHILD?

The image in Fig. 93-1 suggested a mass to the initial examiners. How would such a mass look? How common would such an occurrence be? An enlarged uterus in a child is uncommon. Müllerian duct anomalies—e.g., the bicornuate uterus, which may appear enlarged on the physical exam of a pregnant adult—are rarely discovered in children. The most common cause for an enlarged uterus is an obstructed uterus. An unusual cause is a tumor. Primary tumors of the uterus and vagina are rare in childhood. If they do occur, they are usually malignant.

Rhabdomyosarcomas (sarcoma botryoides) may arise from urogenital remnants in boys or girls. The most common site of involvement in the girl is the vagina, usually in the anterior wall near the cervix. Uterine tumors are usually sec-

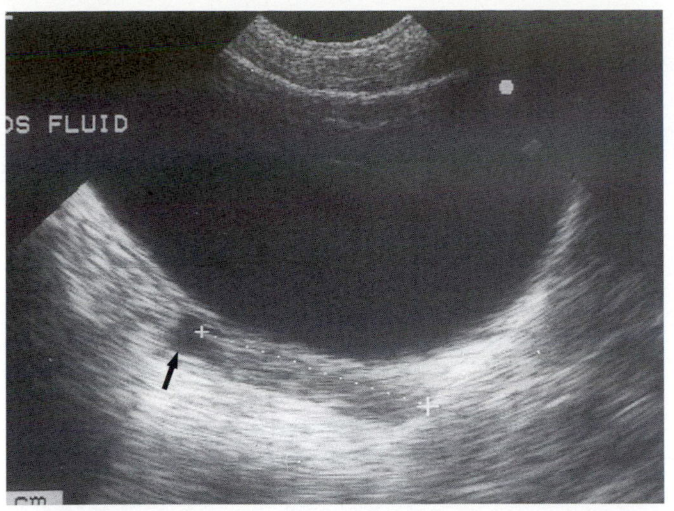

A

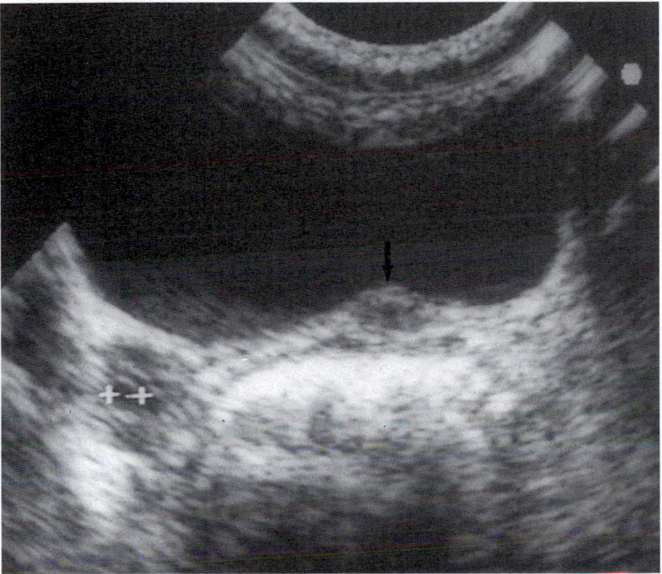

B

FIGURE 93–7. Normal uterus of a child—tubular shape. *A.* This normal child's uterus is tubelike in that the cervix and fundus are of equal width. Neither is particularly wide, as opposed to the cervix of the neonate or the fundus of the postmenarchal patient. There is an incidental small amount of fluid (*arrow*) around the fundus. This is the second most common place to find incidental free fluid, often due to ruptured physiologic cysts. The most common is in the cul de sac, posterior to the uterus. *B.* Transverse plane. Level of cervix. This image is shown to give the reader a feel for the normal child's uterus on transverse view. An arrow points to the uterus. Crosses mark off a few cysts in the right adnexa, which appears wider than the uterus. Note that the transverse uterus of the child is smaller than that of the neonate 93-5*B*.

ondary to vaginal spread but may occur primarily as well. The patient often presents with a pelvic mass and bloody vaginal discharge. A polypoid mass protruding from the vagina or introitus may be noted. Ultrasound may show an enlarged, inhomogeneous solid mass, which may be connected to the vagina (Fig. 93-8).

In summary, one of my classic axiomatic statements is that one must know what normal and its variations look like

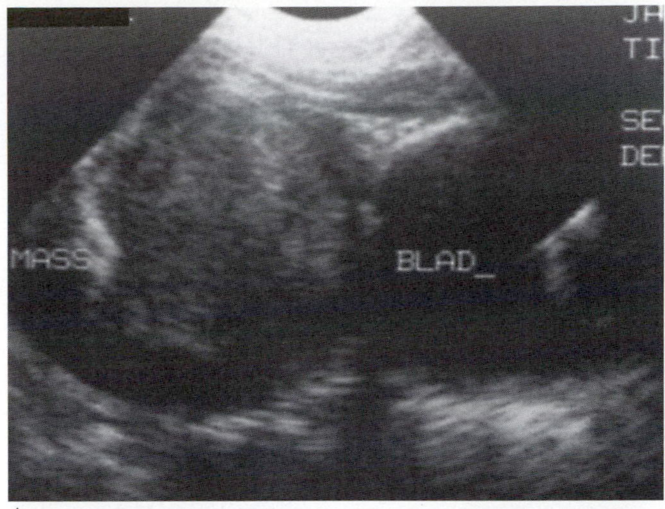

A

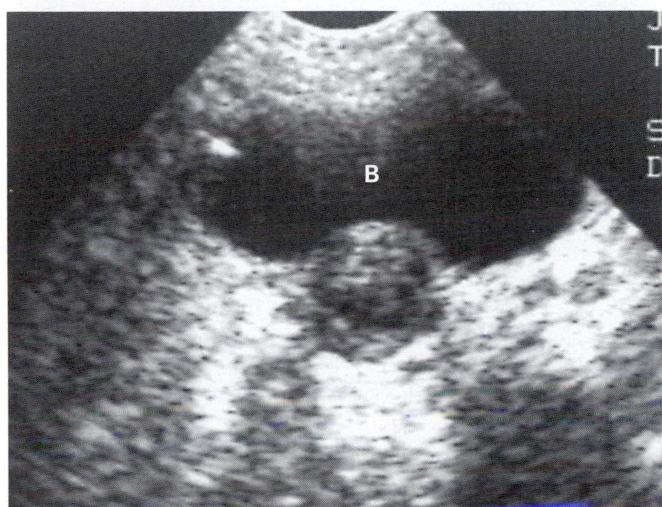

B

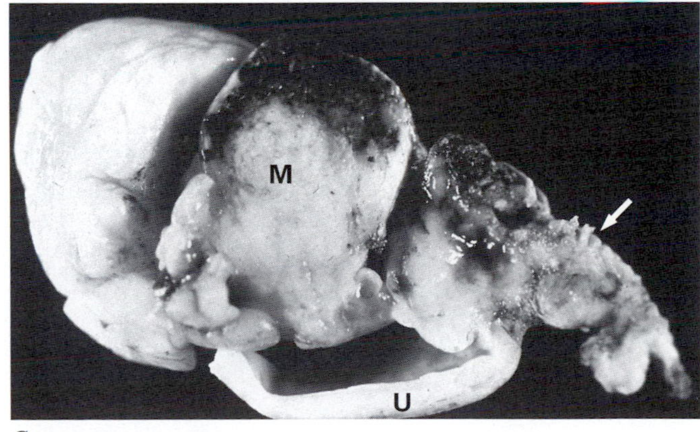

C

FIGURE 93–8. Uterine rhabdomyosarcoma. *A.* Longitudinal plane. A large solid mass (MASS) is seen superior to the bladder (BLAD). This 11-month girl presented with vaginal bleeding and a pelvic mass. *B.* Transverse plane. Level of cervix. The mass was followed to its origin in the lower uterine/cervical region. This view of the cervix shows the cervix to be only somewhat larger than normal. B = bladder. *C.* Pathology specimen. Longitudinal plane. A mass (M) is noted within the uterus (U). This mass, which proved to be a rhabdomyosarcoma, arose from the lower uterine segment and extended out of the cervix (*arrow*). (*From Cohen HL, Haller JO: Pediatric and adolescent genital abnormalities.* Clin Diagn Ultrasound *24:187–216, 1988, with permission.*)

in order to analyze and discover true abnormality. This is particularly true in fetal and pediatric work, where what is normal changes with age, growth, and changing hormonal environments. This case shows the variations in the normal uterus of the child as she grows. It highlights the prominent uterus of newborn life. If you didn't know the image before this case, you know it now. Its recognition will prevent concern similar to that evoked when the patient in Fig. 93-1 was first imaged.

References

Carrington B, Hricak H, Nuruddin R, et al: Mullerian duct anomalies: MR imaging evaluation. *Radiology* 176:715–720, 1990.

Cohen HL: The female pelvis, in *Syllabus: Current Concepts: A Categorical Course in Pediatric Radiology,* Siebert J (ed). Chicago, RSNA Publications, 1994:65–72.

Cohen HL: Evaluation of the adolescent and young adult with amenorrhea: Role of US, in *A Special Course in Ultrasound: Clinical Questions, Practical Answers,* Bluth E, Arger P, Hertzberg B, Middleton W (eds). Oak Brook, IL, RSNA Publications, 1996:171–184.

Cohen HL, Bober S, Bow S: Imaging the pediatric pelvis: The normal and abnormal genital system and simulators of its diseases. *Urol Radiol* 14:273–283, 1992.

Cohen HL, Haller JO: Pediatric and adolescent genital abnormalities. *Clin Diagn Ultrasound* 24:187–216, 1988.

Deutsch A, Gosink B: Normal female pelvic anatomy. *Semin Roentgenol* 17:241–250, 1982.

Forrest T, Elyaderani M, Muilenburg M, et al: Cyclic endometrial changes: US assessment with histologic correlation. *Radiology* 167:233–237, 1988.

Goldman H, Eaton D: Pediatric uroradiology, in *Radiology of the Urinary System,* Elkin M (ed). Boston, Little, Brown, 1980: 1034–1109.

Grimes C, Rosenbaum D, Kirkpatrick J Jr: Pediatric gynecologic radiology. *Semin Roentgenol* 17:284–301, 1982.

Moore K: *Before We Are Born: Basic Embryology and Birth Defects,* 3d ed. Philadelphia, Saunders, 1989:180–201.

Nussbaum AR, Sanders RC, Jones MD: Neonatal uterine morphology as seen on real-time US. *Radiology* 160:641–643, 1986.

Orsini L, Salardi S, Pilu G, et al: Pelvic organs in premenarchal girls: Real-time ultrasonography. *Radiology* 153:113–116, 1984.

Popovich M, Hricak H: Magnetic resonance imaging in the evaluation of gynecologic disease, in *Ultrasonography in Obstetrics and Gynecology*, 3d ed, Callen P (ed). Philadelphia, Saunders, 1994:660–688.

Reid R: Amenorrhea, in *Textbook of Gynecology,* Copeland L (ed). Philadelphia, Saunders, 1993:367–387.

Rosenberg H, Sherman N, Tarry W, et al: Mayer-Rokitansky-Kuster-Hauser syndrome: US aid to diagnosis. *Radiology* 161: 815–819, 1986.

Ruggierro M, Awobuluyi M, Cohen H, Zinn D: Imaging the pediatric pelvis: Role of ultrasound. *Radiologist* 4:155–170, 1997.

94

A 13-day-old female was referred for investigation of an interlabial mass. Ultrasound images of the pelvis (Fig. 94-1) were obtained. What do you see? What is the diagnosis?

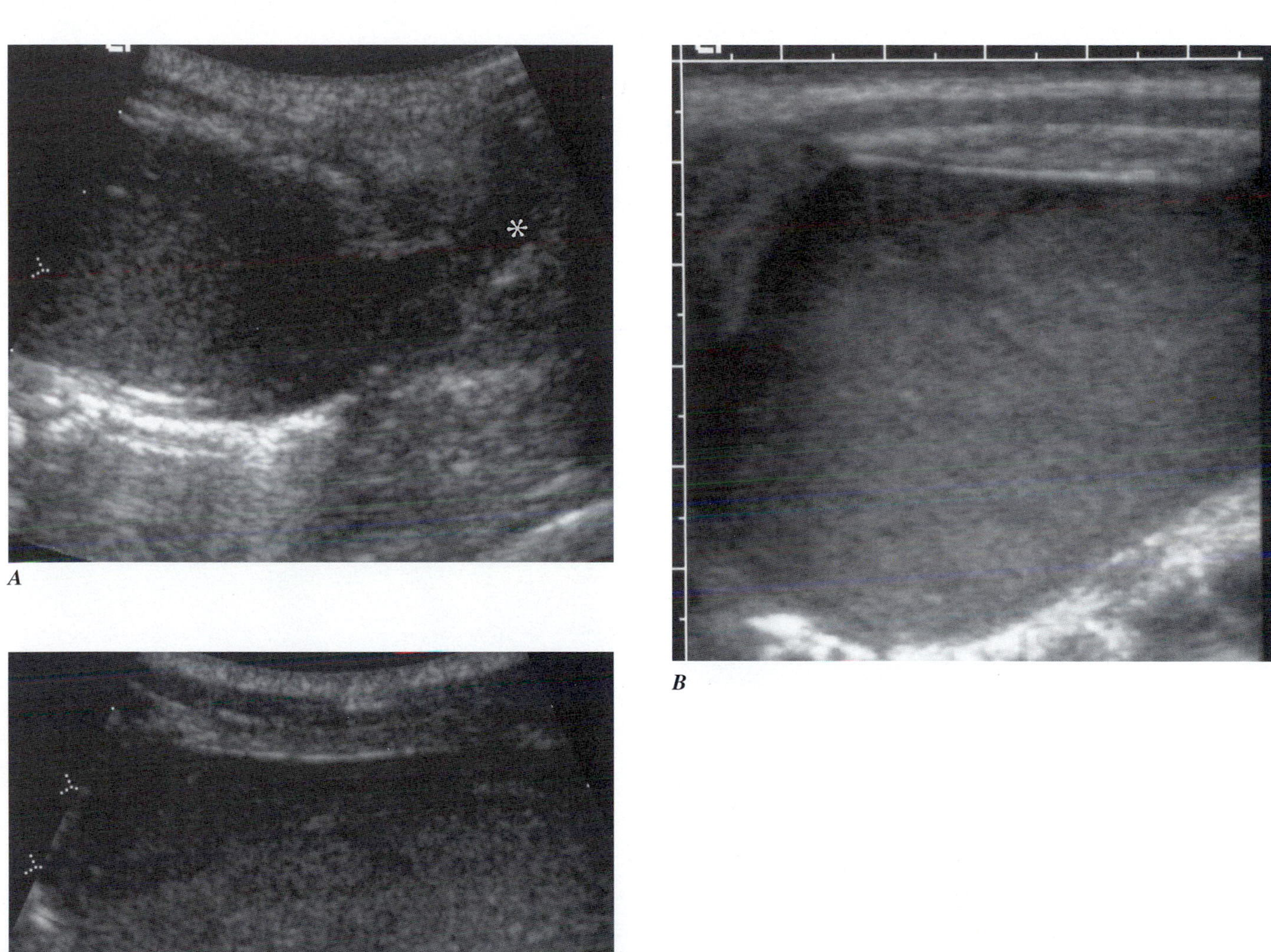

FIGURE 94–1. *A.* Lower pelvis. Longitudinal plane. Midline. Asterisk = bladder. *B.* Upper pelvis. Longitudinal plane. Midline. *C.* Upper pelvis. Transverse plane.

CHAPTER 94

Neonatal Hydrocolpos

HARRIET J. PALTIEL

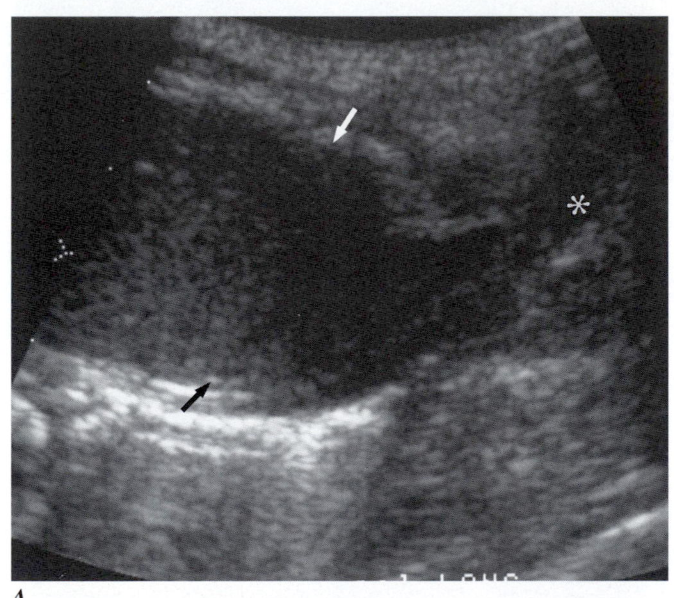

A

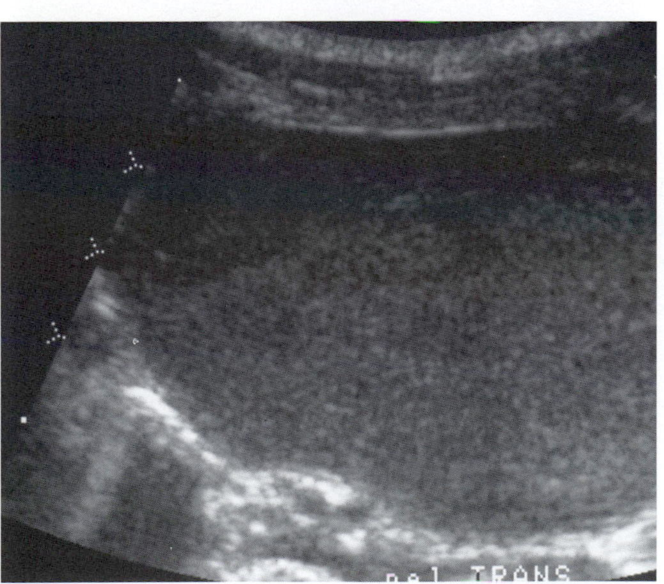

C

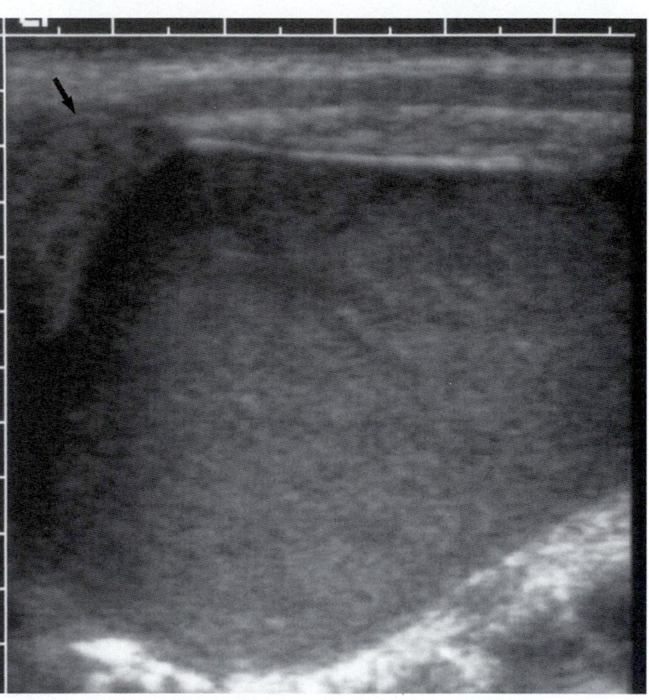

B

FIGURE 94–2. Imperforate hymen. Neonate. ***A.*** Lower pelvis. Longitudinal plane. Midline. Echogenic material filling a markedly enlarged vagina (*arrows*). The bladder (*asterisk*) is almost empty. ***B.*** Upper pelvis. Longitudinal plane. Midline. There is massive distention of the upper vagina. Nonvisualization of a thick wall at the periphery rules out the possibility of this being a distended uterus. The uterus (*arrow*) is actually seen superior to the anterior half of the vagina. It is not distended. ***C.*** Upper pelvis. Transverse plane. The vagina is very dilated in the transverse plane. Echogenic debris within its contained fluid is consistent with hemorrhagic fluid, highly proteinaceous fluid, or a combination of the two.

Figure 94-2*A* to *C* (the annotated version of Fig. 94-1) demonstrates a massively distended vagina filled with echogenic material. The uterus (Fig. 94-2*B*) and kidneys (not shown) appear normal. On physical examination, there was a bulging hymen without a detectable orifice (Fig. 94-3; see

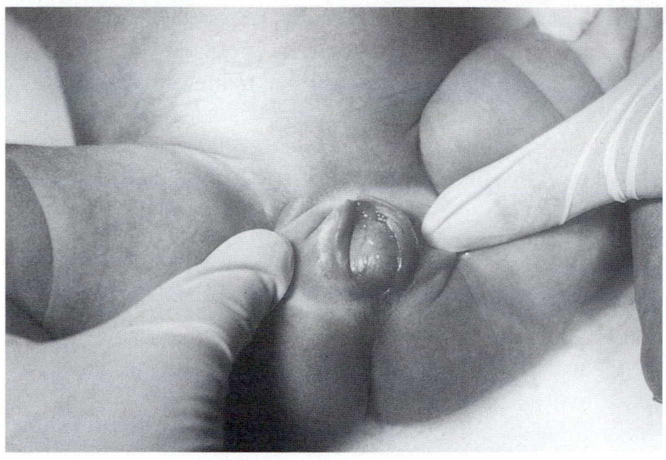

FIGURE 94–3. Neonatal hydrocolpos. Clinical image. There is a large interlabial mass that proved to be due to accumulated secretions proximal to the imperforate hymen. *(Reprinted with permission from Emans SJ: Vulvovaginal problems in the prepubertal child, in* Pediatric and Adolescent Gynecology, *4th ed., Emans SJ, Laufer MR, Goldstein DP (eds). Philadelphia, Lippincott-Raven, 1998:100, Fig. 11.)* (See Color Plate 24.)

also Color Plate 24). At surgery, the imperforate hymen was incised. There was drainage of approximately 250 mL of white mucoid material. The patient had neonatal hydrocolpos due to an imperforate hymen.

WHAT IS HYDROCOLPOS?

Hydrocolpos is a dilated, fluid-filled vagina. If the uterus is also dilated, the condition is called hydrometrocolpos. Hydrocolpos in the neonate usually occurs as a result of vaginal obstruction. There are two major forms of vaginal obstruction. In the first type, obstruction is due to an imperforate hymen (Fig. 94-4), a transverse vaginal septum (Fig. 94-5), or segmental vaginal atresia (Fig. 94-6). In the second type, vaginal obstruction occurs in association with a urogenital sinus or cloacal malformation. The communication of the distal vagina with the urogenital sinus may be stenotic (Fig. 94-7), resulting in a distended, fluid-filled vagina, or the urogenital sinus itself may be narrow, leading to obstruction of both the bladder and the vagina (Fig. 94-8). In girls with the cloacal malformation, the bladder, vagina, and rectum have a single perineal opening (Fig. 94-9). The cloacal channel is short and often obstructed, resulting in severe hydrocolpos.

WHAT IS AN IMPERFORATE HYMEN?

An imperforate hymen is probably the most common obstructive anomaly of the female reproductive tract. Until late in fetal life, the vaginal lumen is separated from the cavity of the urogenital sinus by the hymen, which usually ruptures during the perinatal period and remains as a fold of mucous membrane around the entrance to the vagina. Failure of this membrane to rupture results in an imperforate hymen. Because of the vaginal outflow obstruction, there is the poten-

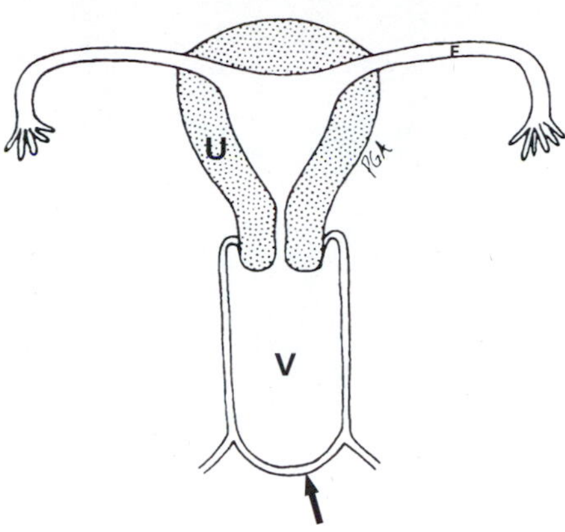

FIGURE 94–4. Imperforate hymen. Schematic drawing. Coronal plane. U = uterus, F = fallopian tube, V = vagina. Arrow points to imperforate hymen. *(Modified from The American Fertility Society. Classifications of adnexal adhesions, distal tubal occlusion, tubal occlusion secondary to tubal ligation, tubal pregnancies, Müllerian anomalies and intrauterine adhesions.* Fertil Steril *49:944–955, 1988, with permission.)*

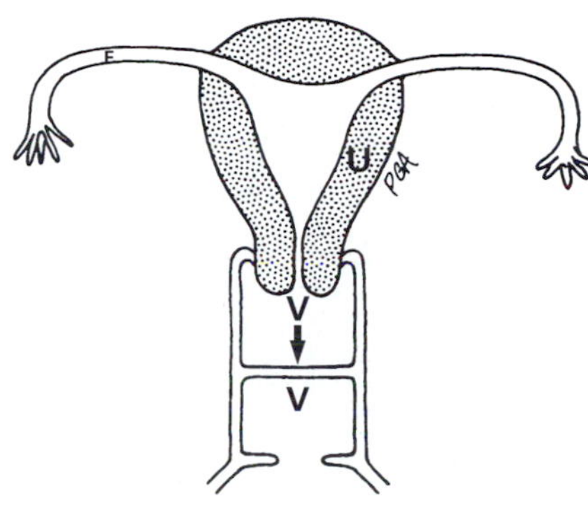

FIGURE 94–5. Transverse vaginal septum. Schematic drawing. Coronal plane. U = uterus, F = fallopian tube, V = vagina. Arrow points to transverse vaginal septum. *(Modified from The American Fertility Society. Classifications of adnexal adhesions, distal tubal occlusion, tubal occlusion secondary to tubal ligation, tubal pregnancies, Müllerian anomalies and intrauterine adhesi*

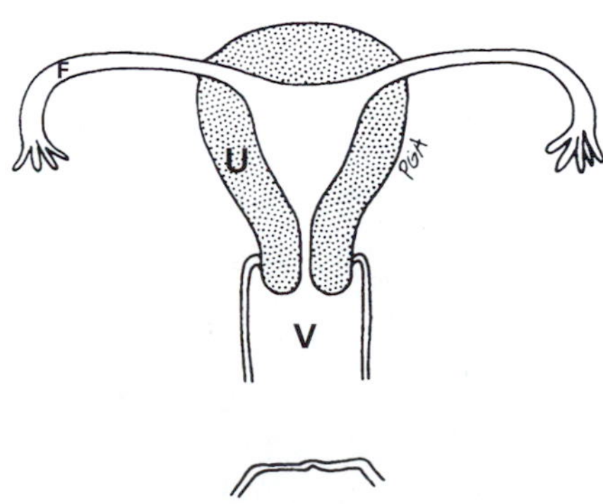

FIGURE 94–6. Lower vaginal atresia. Schematic drawing. Coronal plane. U = uterus, F = fallopian tube, V = vagina. No lower vagina is seen because it is atretic. *(Modified from The American Fertility Society. Classifications of adnexal adhesions, distal tubal occlusion, tubal occlusion secondary to tubal ligation, tubal pregnancies, Müllerian anomalies and intrauterine adhesions.* Fertil Steril *49:944–955, 1988, with permission.)*

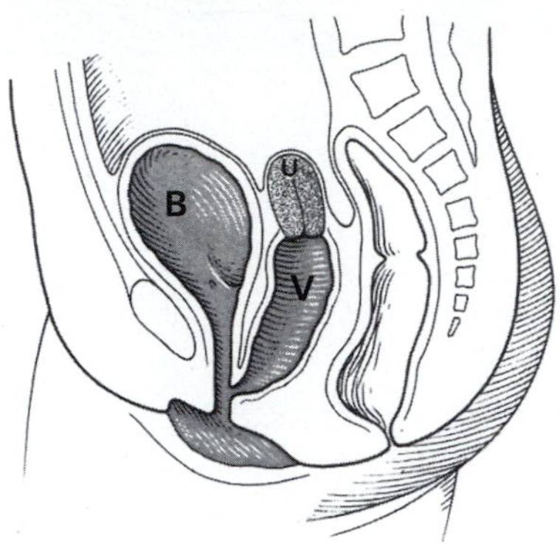

FIGURE 94–7. Urogenital sinus with stenotic vaginal orifice. Schematic drawing. Longitudinal plane. The vagina (V) communicates with the urethra as a urogenital sinus. Stenosis of the vaginal orifice is responsible for vaginal distention due to relative obstruction. B = bladder, U = uterus. (*From Williams D: Urogenital sinus abnormalities, in* Surgical Pediatric Urology, *Eckstein H, Hohenfellner R, Williams D (eds). Philadelphia, Saunders, 1977:441–442, with permission.*)

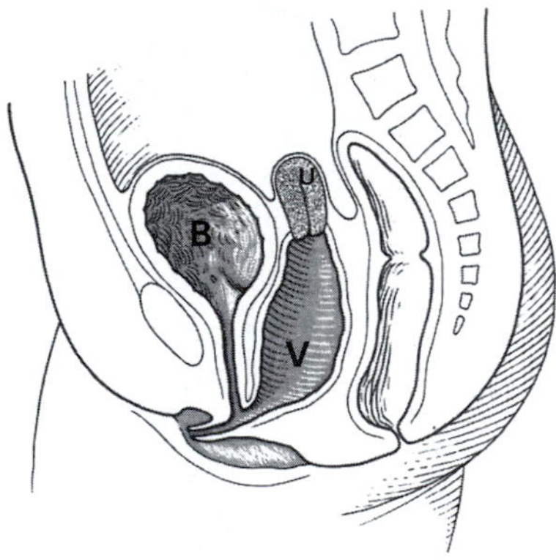

FIGURE 94–8. Urogenital sinus with vulval obstruction and pseudopenis. Schematic drawing. Longitudinal plane. The vaginal (V) dilatation is due to an obstruction at the vulva, beyond the confluence of the vaginal and urethral components of the urogenital sinus. B = bladder, U = uterus. (*From Williams D: Urogenital sinus abnormalities, in* Surgical Pediatric Urology, *Eckstein H, Hohenfellner R, Williams D (eds). Philadelphia, Saunders, 1977:441–442, with permission.*)

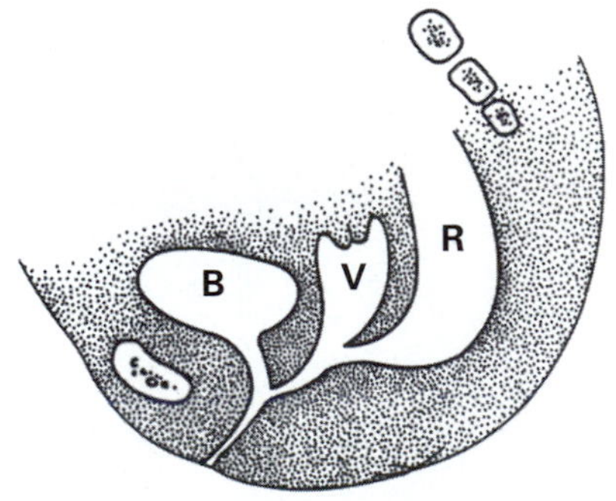

FIGURE 94–9. Cloacal malformation. Schematic drawing. Longitudinal plane. In girls with the cloacal malformation, the bladder (B), vagina (V), and rectum (R) have a single perineal opening. The cloacal channel is short and often obstructed, resulting in severe hydrocolpos. (*From Jaramillo D, Lebowitz RL, Hendren H: The cloacal malformation: Radiologic findings and imaging recommendations.* Radiology, *177:442, 1990, with permission.*)

tial for significant accumulation of fetal cervical and vaginal secretions, which are stimulated by circulating maternal estrogens. The diagnosis of imperforate hymen may be made at birth. Several reports in the literature have also described prenatal sonographic diagnosis of this disorder. If the condition is undiagnosed, the vaginal secretions resorb, and the patient will be asymptomatic until puberty, when menstrual blood will redistend the vagina. An imperforate hymen is almost always an isolated finding.

Ultrasonographic evaluation of the pelvis is performed to assess vaginal and uterine size, to detect anomalies of the uterus or kidneys, and to document the presence of any associated hydronephrosis. The bladder is frequently empty, presumably because of compression by the distended vagina, or because the vagina is more distensible than the bladder and fills preferentially. Transperineal sonography may be used to differentiate an imperforate hymen from a low vaginal septum. Serial postoperative sonographic studies are useful to assess the response to treatment. Long-term clinical follow-up is essential, as the distended, hypertrophied vagina and uterus tend to develop intercurrent infection during their slow return to normal. In patients with an accumulation of mucus or blood, antibiotics are routinely prescribed to prevent infection.

DIFFERENTIAL DIAGNOSIS OF INTERLABIAL MASS

The differential diagnosis of an interlabial mass includes prolapsed ectopic ureterocele, prolapsed urethra, paraurethral cyst, and vaginal rhabdomyosarcoma. These entities can usually be distinguished on the basis of gross appearance, location, and relationship to the urethra.

References

The American Fertility Society. Classifications of adnexal adhesions, distal tubal occlusion, tubal occlusion secondary to tubal ligation, tubal pregnancies, Müllerian anomalies and intrauterine adhesions. *Fertil Steril* 49:944–955, 1988.

Bartholomew TH, Gonzales ET Jr: Urologic management in cloacal dysgenesis. *Urology* 11:549–557, 1978.

Blask AR, Sanders RC, Gearhart JP: Obstructed uterovaginal anomalies: Demonstration with sonography. Part I. Neonates and infants. *Radiology* 179:79–83, 1991.

Cohen HL, Bober SE, Bow SN: Imaging the pediatric pelvis: The normal and abnormal genital tract and simulators of its diseases. *Urol Radiol* 14:273–283, 1992.

Emans SJH, Laufer MR, Goldstein DP (eds): *Pediatric and Adolescent Gynecology,* 4th ed. Philadelphia, Lippincott Raven, 1998:100, 322–323.

Marshall FF, Jeffs RD, Sarafyan WK: Urogenital sinus abnormalities in the female patient. *J Urol* 122:568–572, 1979.

Moore KL, Persaud TVN: The urogenital system, in *The Developing Human: Clinically Oriented Embryology,* 6th ed., Moore KL, Persaud TVN (eds). Philadelphia, Saunders, 1998:303–347.

Nussbaum AR, Lebowitz RL: Interlabial masses in little girls: Review and imaging recommendations. *AJR* 141:65–71, 1983.

Reed MH, Griscom NT: Hydrometrocolpos in infancy. *AJR* 118: 1–13, 1973.

Sawhney S, Gupta R, Berry M, Bhatnagar V: Hydrometrocolpos: Diagnosis and follow-up by ultrasound—a case report. *Australas Radiol* 34:93–94, 1990.

Scanlan KA, Pozniak MA, Fagerholm M, Shapiro S: Value of transperineal sonography in the assessment of vaginal atresia. *AJR* 154:545–548, 1990.

Taybi H: Pseudoneoplastic masses (pseudotumors) in children. Part two: Pseudotumors of abdomen, skeleton, and soft tissue. *Med Radiogr Photogr* 54:41–71, 1978.

Westerhout FC, Hodgman JE, Anderson GV, Sack RA: Congenital hydrocolpos. *Am J Obstet Gynecol* 89:957–961, 1964.

Williams D: Urogenital sinus abnormalities, in *Surgical Pediatric Urology,* Eckstein H, Hohenfellner R, Williams D (eds). Philadelphia, Saunders, 1977:441–442.

Wilson DA, Stacy TM, Smith EI: Ultrasound diagnosis of hydrocolpos and hydrometrocolpos. *Radiology* 128:451–454, 1978.

Winderl LM, Silverman RK: Prenatal diagnosis of congenital imperforate hymen. *Obstet Gynecol* 85:857–860, 1995.

95

A newborn was thought to have a right pelvic mass on physical examination. A uterus was seen and was normal. Figure 95-1 was obtained on a pelvic ultrasound (US) exam at the site of the palpated mass. What do you see? What is the diagnosis? Should anything be done?

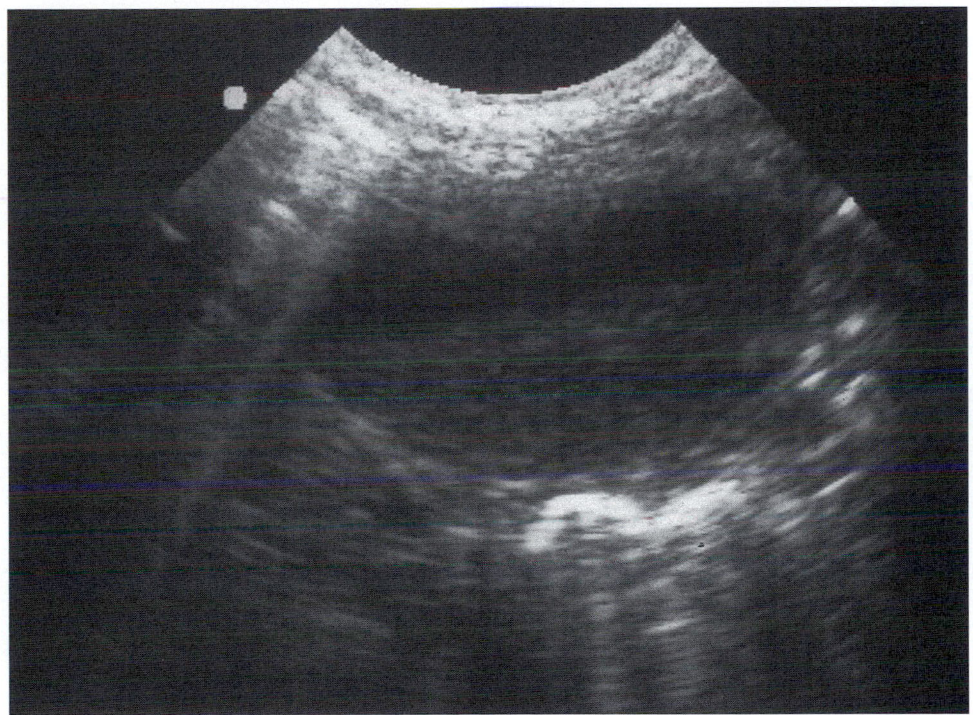

FIGURE 95–1. Pelvis. Right side. Longitudinal plane.

CHAPTER 95

Neonatal Ovarian Torsion

HARRIS L. COHEN AND BRIAN GALE

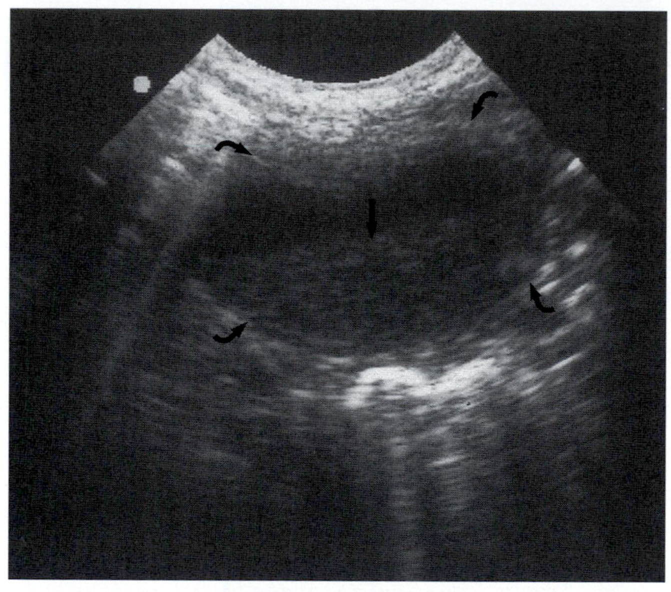

FIGURE 95–2. Annotated version of Fig. 95-1. Ovarian torsion in neonate. Pelvis. Right side. Longitudinal plane. A cystic mass (*curved arrows*) with a fluid debris level (*arrow*) consistent with a settling hemorrhagic cyst is seen in this newborn. In a female, such a mass is assumed to be of ovarian origin until disproven. Hemorrhagic adenexal cystic masses in newborns suggest ovarian torsion. Patients with possible ovarian torsion are operated on. This patient's ovary was torsed and surgically removed.

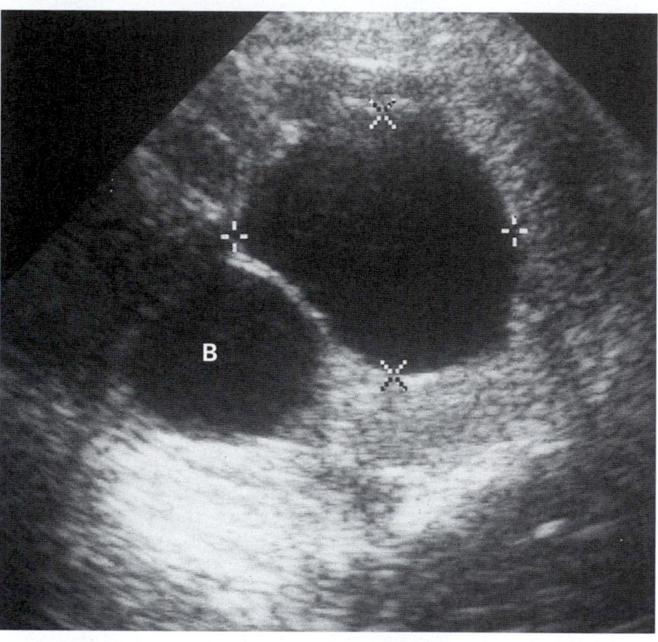

FIGURE 95–3. Fetal ovarian cyst. Area of fetal bladder. Transverse oblique plane. The bladder (B) was imaged with a second larger cystic mass (*crosses*) near it. One might consider a bowel duplication cyst, but in a female fetus a cystic ovary must be considered first. That is what this proved to be. After birth, the cyst involuted with time.

Figure 95-2, the annotated version of Fig. 95-1, shows a cystic mass that measured 2 by 3.8 cm. This is enlarged for normal newborn adnexa. In addition, it has an atypical echogenicity pattern. It contains a fluid level with a dependent echogenic area and a superior echoless area. The findings are consistent with settling of hemorrhage, with the lighter and more echoless superior fluid layer composed of serum. Although a hemorrhagic cyst may be a relatively innocuous finding and cause of pain in the adolescent, it is not an innocent finding in the neonate. In the neonate, this is one of a few findings suggesting ovarian torsion. This patient underwent an operation that confirmed this diagnosis. The torsed ovary was removed.

THE NEONATAL OVARY—WHAT IS NORMAL?

Small follicular cysts are very common in the newborn. They are of no clinical concern. What is of concern is a cystic mass so prominent that it is either imaged in fetal life (Fig. 95-3) or palpated on examination of the newborn. The cause may sim-

TABLE 95-1
Ovarian Measurements in the First Two Years of Life

Age Group	Patient #	Imaged Ovaries	Mean Ovarian Volume (cm^3)%	Volume (95% Confidence Interval)	% with Cysts
1 day–3 months	34	34	1.06	0.03–3.56	82
4–12 months	21	34	1.05	0.18–2.71	88
13–24 months	22	30	0.67	0.15–1.68	80

SOURCE: *Cohen HL, Shapiro M, Mandel F, Shapiro M: Normal ovaries in neonates and infants: A sonographic study of 77 patients 1 day to 24 months old.* AJR *160:583–586, 1993.*

ply be related to noninvoluted physiologic cysts that were the result of maternal hormone stimulation as a fetus or high gonadotropin levels in the neonate. Gonadotropin [follicle-stimulating hormone (FSH)] levels rise abruptly at birth because of the decrease in circulating estrogen and progesterone levels that occurs as a result of separation of the fetus from the placenta and the mother's hormonal environment. Gonadotropin levels are greatest in the first 3 months of life. Gonadotropins stimulate the development of ovarian cysts in terms of both number and size. I believe some individuals have ovaries that are more sensitive to such FSH stimulation, whether it occurs in neonatal life or in later peripubertal times, during the menstrual cycle or during pregnancy.

We have shown (Table 95-1) that in the first 3 months of life, normal ovaries have a mean volume of 1.06 cm^3 (Cohen et al, 1993). That is not a remarkable measurement compared to what has been reported in the literature. However, what is important to note is that volumes can range from 0.03 to as high as 3.56 cm^3, often, in part, because of contained cysts. This upper confidence interval for volume decreases with age over the first 2 years of life, probably reflecting decreased gonadotropin levels and decreased numbers of cysts. We noted that 82 percent of 34 imaged ovaries in the 0- to 3-month-old age group had imaged ovarian cysts. (The actual percentage of ovaries with cysts and the size of the largest cyst in each ovary did not vary much between 1 day and 2 years of life, despite decreasing gonadotropin levels). Finding a cystic neonatal ovary (Fig. 95-4) is not abnormal or unusual. The problem arises when there is evidence, as in this case, of hemorrhage within the ovary, suggesting ovarian torsion.

FETAL AND NEONATAL CYSTIC OVARIAN MASS

A cystic fetal ovary, usually due to a larger noninvoluted follicular cyst, may, on occasion, be noted near the fluid-filled bladder (Fig. 95-3). Normally the ovary is not seen in fetal life, probably because it is obscured by the surrounding small bowel. The uterus is also not typically seen in antenatal life. Because the normal fetal and neonatal pelves are small, masses within them may extend into the abdomen, and the position of an ovarian mass may then make its pelvic origin difficult to determine. These cysts are almost universally benign. They are usually unilocular. If the ovary is pedunculated and therefore at greater risk for torsion, its position will change from exam to exam, e.g., it will be in the left lower quadrant on one exam and in the left upper quadrant on another.

After birth, these cysts may produce symptoms in the neonate from torsion, rupture, or purportedly, when large, intestinal obstruction or respiratory compromise. Symptomatic cysts and their ovaries are studied surgically. Controversy has existed as to what to do with large cysts that are asymptomatic. One author claimed a 60 percent incidence of early torsion among these ovaries and therefore believes their disappearance to be due to torsion of the ovary, perhaps because of the heaviness of the cyst, rather than involution of a physiologic cyst. However, other groups, including our own, who have followed such ovaries with the better US equipment of today have been able to satisfy the clinicians by showing them that the cysts may be followed to involution, with the ovary eventually attaining, within weeks to months, a more normal appearance. Many surgeons now follow asympto-

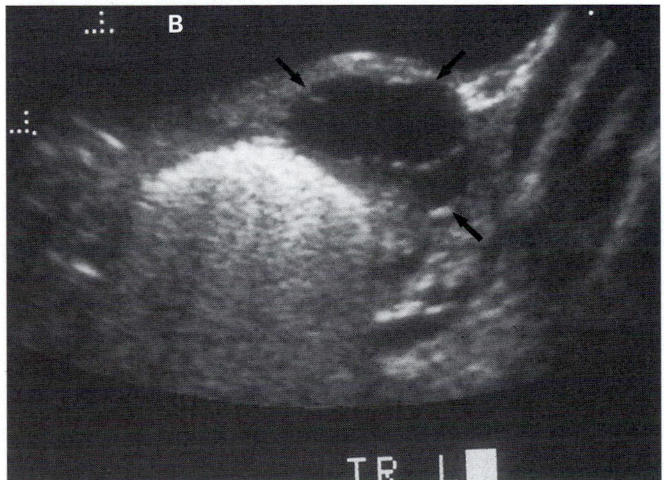

FIGURE 95-4. Cystic adnexa in newborn. Left pelvis. Transverse plane. A cystic left adnexa (*arrows*) is noted. When there is no contained hemorrhage, it is currently thought of as just a stimulated or hyperstimulated ovary and followed over time. Most return to a normal ovarian image within weeks. Using "tincture of time" for an asymptomatic newborn may save the patient from an operation.

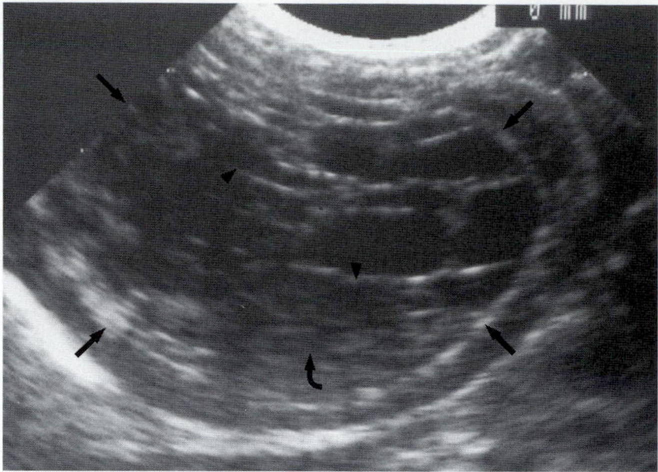

FIGURE 95–5. Ovarian torsion. Longitudinal plane. A large, multiseptated (*arrowheads*) ovary (*arrows*) with an area of echogenicity in its dependent area consistent with hemorrhage (*curved arrow*) was noted in this symptomatic newborn. The patient was operated on as a probable case of ovarian torsion, which was proven at surgery. (*From Cohen HL: The female pelvis, in* Syllabus: Current Concepts: A Categorical Course in Pediatric Radiology, *Siebert J (ed). Chicago, RSNA Publications, 1994:65–72, with permission.*)

matic newborns with simple small ovarian cystic masses or an enlarged ovary containing several cysts, conservatively.

Clinical concern, as stated, is greater when the cysts show evidence of pedunculation and therefore the potential to torse, or evidence of torsion having occurred [the finding of a fluid debris (hemorrhage) level, a contained retracting clot, or multiple septations (Fig. 95-5)].

NEONATAL OVARIAN TORSION—SOME CLINICAL FACTS

Neonatal ovarian torsion is uncommon; it is said to occur in 1 in 2500 live births. Torsion compromises first lymphatic, then venous, and finally the arterial supply to the ovary. This can cause congestion and hemorrhagic infarction. When infarction and necrosis occur, pathologic evaluation generally does not reveal any residual ovarian tissue. Torsion can involve the ovary and/or the fallopian tube. Neonates can present with pain, fever (either low- or high-grade), and leukocytosis. Alternatively, the clinical presentation can be subtle, with abdominal fullness the only presenting symptom. The finding at surgery of unilaterally absent ovaries suggests the possibility of a chronic asymptomatic ovarian torsion with resultant necrosis and amputation rather than congenital ovarian agenesis. This is particularly true when there is no associated genitourinary system anomaly.

TABLE 95-2
Ultrasound Imaging Findings Suspicious for Neonatal Ovarian Torsion

1. Change in ovary position from exam to exam (pedunculated)
2. Hemorrhage fluid level in cystic mass
3. Clot or clot retraction
4. Multiseptated (be wary to separate this from an ovary with several cyst walls)

PERINATAL COMPLEX OVARIAN CYSTS AND OVARIAN TORSION—SOME TREATMENT FACTS

Several published series indicate that when fetal or neonatal ovarian cysts measure ≥4 cm, the risk of torsion or other symptoms rises. Spontaneous resolution of cyst is most common in those <5 cm. Those 10 cm or greater are at risk of rupture.

Treatment of ovarian torsion is surgical and is aimed at preserving the torsed ovary and avoiding complications. At laparotomy, an ovary that does not appear to be irreversibly damaged can be detorsed. Complex ovarian cysts are also treated surgically. Treatment of ovarian cysts diagnosed in either the fetus or the neonate is aimed at preventing torsion, rupture, or hemorrhage. Options include conservative observation, excision, needle aspiration, and/or biopsy. The choice of treatment is guided by the size of the lesion. Cysts measuring less than 4 to 5 cm tend to be treated conservatively. Most authors recommend excision of cysts measuring ≥5 cm, preserving ovarian parenchyma whenever possible. In their group of patients with ovarian cysts measuring <5 cm, Suita et al found no cases of torsion or rupture. Large neonatal ovarian cysts are increasingly being treated with percutaneous needle aspiration. Some authors advocate aspiration of large antenatal ovarian cysts.

PLEASE NOTE

Table 95-2 reviews the US findings that should make the examiner consider the diagnosis of a neonatal or perinatal ovarian torsion.

References

Alrabeeah A, Galliani CA, Giacomantonio M, et al: Neonatal ovarian torsion: Report of three cases and review of the literature. *Pediatr Pathol* 8:143–149, 1988.

Amodio J, Abramson S, Berdon W, et al: Postnatal resolution of large ovarian cysts detected in utero. Report of two cases. *Pediatr Radiol* 17:467–469, 1987.

Avni E, Godart S, Israel C, Schmitz C: Ovarian torsion cyst presenting as a wandering tumor in a newborn: Antenatal diagnosis and postnatal assessment. *Pediatr Radiol* 13:169–171, 1983.

Cohen HL: The female pelvis, in *Syllabus: Current Concepts: A Categorical Course in Pediatric Radiology,* Siebert J (ed). Chicago, RSNA Publications, 1994:65–72.

Cohen HL, Bober S, Bow S: Imaging the pediatric pelvis: The normal and abnormal genital tract and simulators of its diseases. *Urol Radiol* 14:273–283, 1992.

Cohen HL, Shapiro M, Mandel F, Shapiro M: Normal ovaries in neonates and infants: A sonographic study of 77 patients 1 day to 24 months old. *AJR* 160:583–586, 1993.

Comstock C: Fetal masses: Ultrasound diagnosis and evaluation. *Ultrasound Quart* 6:229–256, 1988.

Graif M, Itzchak Y: Sonographic evaluation of ovarian torsion in childhood and adolescence. *AJR* 150:647–649, 1988.

Katz VL, McCoy MC, Kuller JA, et al: Fetal ovarian torsion appearing as a solid abdominal mass. *J Perinatol* 16:302–304, 1996.

Montagne J: Postnatal resolution of large ovarian cysts detected in utero; letter to the editor. *Pediatr Radiol* 18:248, 1988.

Mordehai J, Mares AJ, Barki Y, et al: Torsion of uterine adnexa in neonates and children: A report of 20 cases. *J Pediatr Surg* 26:1195–1199, 1991.

Nussbaum A, Sanders R, Hartman D, et al: Neonatal ovarian cysts. Sonographic-pathologic correlation. *Radiology* 168:817–821, 1988.

Sherer D, Shah Y, Eggers P, Woods J: Prenatal sonographic diagnosis and subsequent management of fetal adnexal torsion. *J Ultrasound Med* 9:161–163, 1990.

Suita S, Sakaguchi T, Ikeda K, Nakano H: Therapeutic dilemmas associated with antenatally detected ovarian cysts. *Surg Gynecol Obstet* 171:502–508, 1990.

96

A 16-year-old girl is being studied for secondary amenorrhea. Figure 96-1 is a transverse view of her pelvis. What is the diagnosis? What other diagnoses should be considered in the workup of a teenager with amenorrhea?

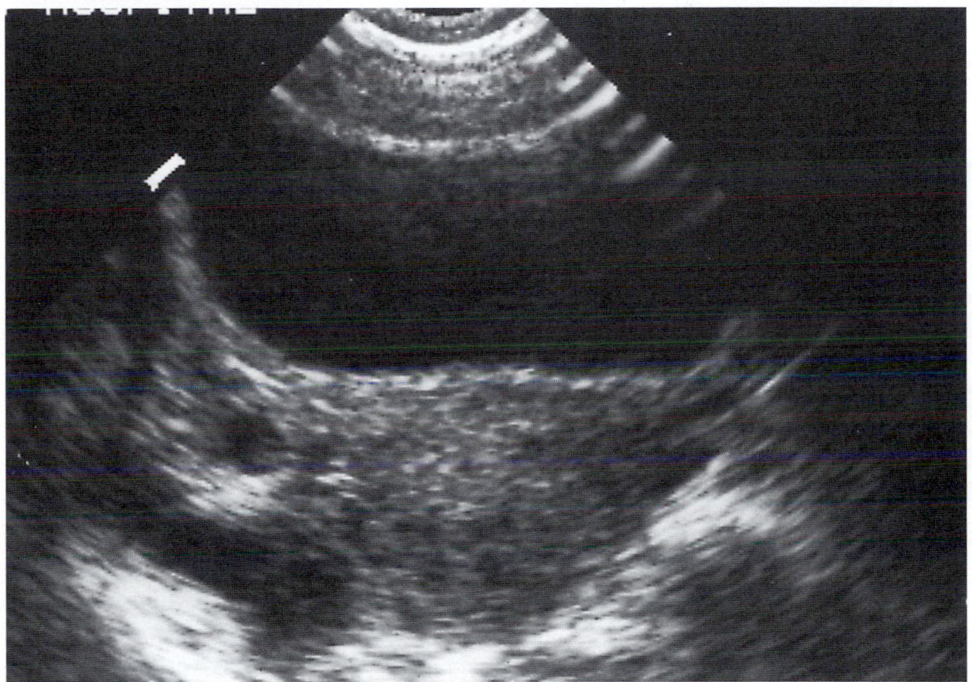

FIGURE 96–1. Pelvic ultrasound. Transverse plane.

CHAPTER 96

Ectopic Pregnancy Causing Amenorrhea

HARRIS L. COHEN AND DANIEL L. ZINN

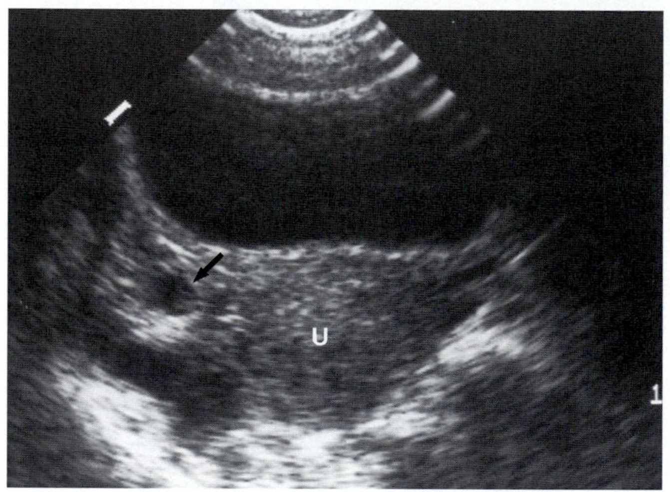

FIGURE 96–2. Annotated version of Fig. 96-1. Pelvic ultrasound. Transverse plane. A cystic area with a contained echogenicity (*arrow*) is seen to the right of the uterus (U) in the adnexal region. No intrauterine gestational sac is seen. The contained echogenicity within the adnexal area showed fetal heart motion, consistent with a diagnosis of a live ectopic pregnancy. Without evident heart motion, one might have to consider the possibilty that the echogenicity was due to a clot within a functional cyst. Other views confirmed that this was an ectopic pregnancy.

Figure 96-2, the annotated version of Fig. 96-1, shows the uterus posterior to the bladder. The uterus in this transverse image is of normal adult shape and size. To the right of the uterus, in the adnexal region, is a cystic structure with a contained echogenicity. Without the history of amenorrhea, one might consider a functional adnexal cyst with an unusual contained clot. The history, a positive β human chorionic gonadotropin (hCG) level in the blood, and fetal heart motion on real-time examination helped confirm that the right adnexal area cyst was a gestational sac with a contained fetal pole. Pregnancy, whether a normal intrauterine one (Fig. 96-3) or one in an ectopic location (Fig. 96-4; see also Color Plate 25), as in this case, is the major concern and the most likely physiologic condition to consider in a normal teenager with secondary amenorrhea. The most common pathology causing secondary amenorrhea is polycystic ovary syndrome (PCOS).

WHAT IS AMENORRHEA?

The complaint of amenorrhea is a key indication of the need to analyze a teenager's pelvis, in particular her gynecologic tract. Primary amenorrhea is defined as a lack of menses by age 16. Secondary amenorrhea is defined as the cessation of menses at any point in time after menarche and prior to menopause. A variety of normal physiologic changes (e.g., pregnancy) as well as various embryologic, genetic, and/or endocrinologic abnormalities may lead to disruption of menses. The radiologist must use the patient's and clinician's historical, physical, and laboratory findings as tools to aid in an accurate imaging assessment and, if possible, a diagnosis. Causes of amenorrhea may include problems involving the components of the hypothalamic–pituitary–ovarian–uterine (vaginal) (HPOU) axis that are responsible for normal menses. Computed tomography (CT) and magnetic resonance imaging (MRI) are used for the analysis of the hypothalamus and pituitary. Ultrasound (US) is the key tool in assessing the ovaries, uterus, and vagina.

THE MENSTRUAL CYCLE—A BRIEF REVIEW

Menstruation is defined as the periodic vaginal bleeding that is the end result, when there is no pregnancy, of the cyclical stimulation of ovarian follicles and the associated buildup and eventual shedding of uterine mucosa. The shedding of the mucosa is the menses. In humans, there is, on average, a 28-day cycle between one menses and the next. The menstrual cycle is divided into follicular, ovulatory, and secretory phases. The first day of the cycle (day 1) is arbitrarily defined as the first day of periodic bleeding. The follicular (also known as the proliferative or preovulatory) phase of the cycle occurs between the 5th and 14th days. Several primordial ovarian follicles are stimulated, enlarge, and are surrounded by follicular fluid. Pulsatile release of gonadotropin-releasing hormone (GnRH) from the hypothalamus stimulates the secretion of luteinizing hormone (LH) and follicle-stimulating hormone (FSH) by the pituitary. One follicle becomes dominant by day 6 of the cycle, and the others become atretic. Under the influence of LH and FSH, this maturing ovarian (graafian) follicle continues to grow, eventually producing estrogen from its theca interna as well as granulosa cells. Under the influence of estrogens (estradiol) from the developing follicles, the endometrium increases in thickness, with increases in the numbers of its glandular cells and stroma. By the midfollicular phase, FSH levels begin to decline. At day 14, or midcycle, the distended follicle ruptures following a surge of LH, and ovulation, the release of an ovum into the abdominal cavity, occurs. The ovulatory and secretory (or luteal) phases of the cycle then begin. The ovum enters the fallopian tubes and either eventually implants in the uterus after fertilization or passes through the uterus and out of the body through the vagina. The ruptured graafian follicle becomes hemorrhagic (corpus hemorrhagicum). The clotted blood is replaced by lipid-rich luteal cells and, as the corpus luteum, the follicle produces estrogen and progesterone. Under the influence of increases in estrogen and progesterone levels, the endometrium "matures" in preparation for possible implantation. This occurs within 8 to 9 days of ovulation. The endometrium becomes highly vascularized and slightly edematous, with associated thickening of its mucosa and increases in glandular length. Progesterone is responsible, among other things, for the endometrial production of prostaglandins. The secretory phase of the cycle is remarkably constant at 14 days. The temporal variability of the menstrual cycle among patients is usually related to the length of the follicular/proliferative phase.

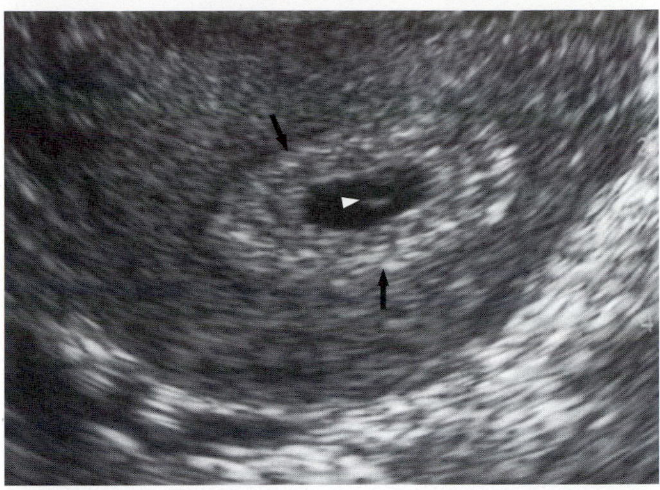

A

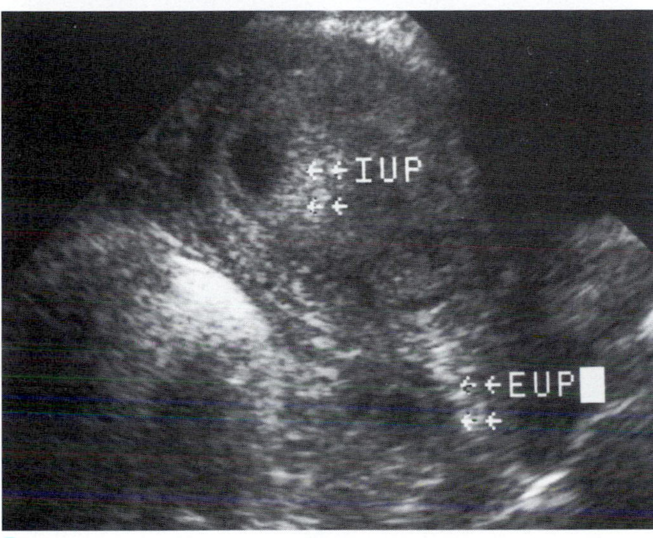

B

FIGURE 96–3. Intrauterine pregnancy. Pelvic ultrasound. ***A.*** Transvaginal examination. Longitudinal plane. An echogenic rind (*arrows*), consistent with trophoblastic tissue, surrounds a cystic area that is the gestational sac within the uterus. The gestational sac is completely surrounded by uterine tissue, confirming that it is intrauterine and excluding the possibility of a cornual ectopic pregnancy. A yolk sac (*arrowhead*) is seen within the sac. ***B.*** Heterotopic pregnancy. Transabdominal examination. Longitudinal plane. An intrauterine gestational sac (*IUP arrows*) is seen within the uterus. A subtler cystic area is also seen posterior to the cervix (*EUP arrows*). Fetal poles, each with heart motion, were seen in both sacs on other views. Even though they are not usual, heterotopic pregnancies, ones in which there are concurrent intrauterine *and* extrauterine pregnancies, occur at a rate of 1 in 4000 to 1 in 6500 pregnancies, with the rate as high as 1 in 100 pregnancies in infertility patients treated with assisted reproductive technologies.

ENDOMETRIAL BREAKDOWN—MENSES

If a pregnancy occurs, the corpus luteum persists, and no period occurs until after delivery. If fertilization does not occur, the corpus luteum degenerates, and the blood levels of estrogen and progesterone fall. With decreasing hormonal support, the endometrium thins, and there is increased coiling of its spiral arteries. Foci of necrosis appear in the endometrium and coalesce. Lysosome breakdown in necrotic endometrial cells releases enzymes involved in prostaglandin formation. Prostaglandins cause vasospasm, leading to spiral artery wall necrosis and initially spotty and then more confluent menstrual bleeding. The superficial two-thirds of the endometrium, the stratum functionale, fed by the long, coiled spiral arteries, is shed. The deepest third, the stratum basale, supplied by short, straight basilar arteries, remains intact and serves as a regenerative layer for new endometrial proliferation.

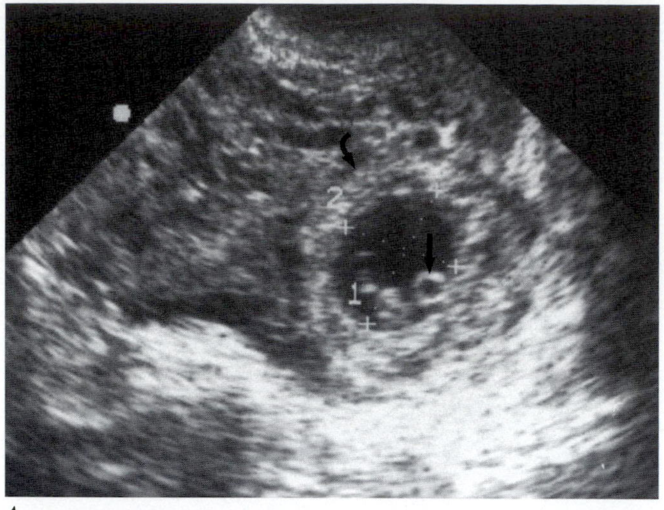

A

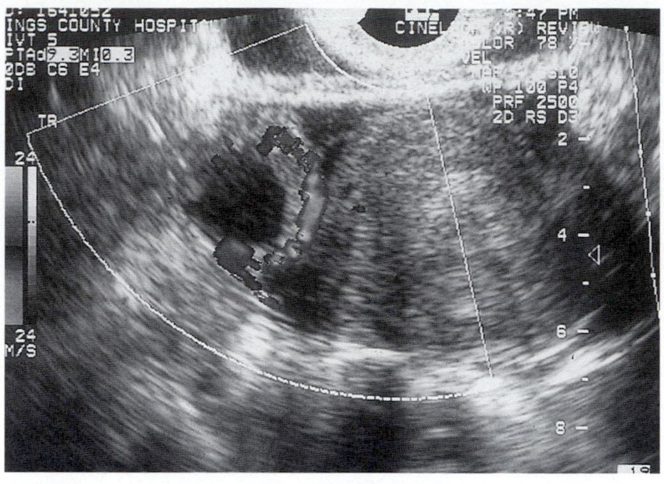

B

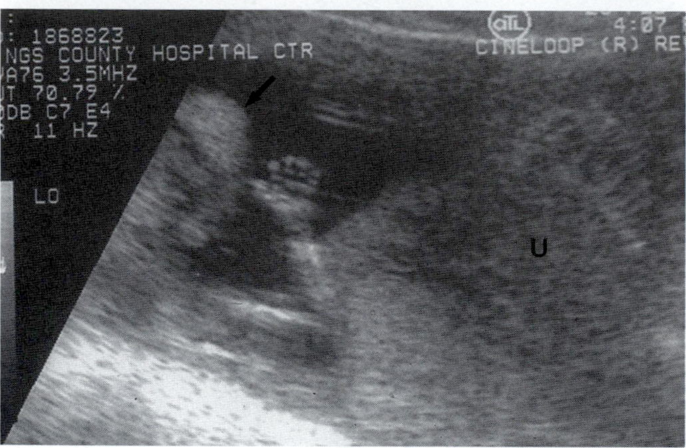

C

FIGURE 96–4. Ectopic pregnancy. ***A.*** Transvaginal examination. Transducer pointing toward left adnexa. Longitudinal oblique plane. The inner dimensions of an ectopic gestational sac are marked off. A yolk sac (*arrow*) and adjacent fetal pole are imaged within the sac. The echogenic rind (*curved arrow*) about the sac is trophoblastic tissue. This ectopic pregnancy was found to be in the left fallopian tube of a teenager who presented with vague abdominal pain and amenorrhea. ***B.*** Transvaginal examination. Transverse plane. Transducer pointing toward the right adnexa. Color Doppler examination. Color surrounds a mass with a contained cyst in the right adnexal region. No cyst or intrauterine pregnancy is seen in the uterus of this pregnant teenager. Ectopic pregnancies may have bright vascular flow noted within their trophoblastic periphery, as in this case. However, this may also be noted in the tissue peripheral to a corpus luteal cyst of pregnancy. Other views proved the adnexal area cystic "mass" to be a gestational sac with a contained fetal pole. (See Color Plate 25.) ***C.*** Transabdominal examination. Abdominal pregnancy. A waving fetus and an empty uterus (U). This fetus was not surrounded by evident trophoblastic tissue. The fetus was bigger than could be supported within an unruptured fallopian tube (usually no greater than 9 to 12 weeks). It was not partially surrounded by uterine tissue, as would be seen in a case of a cornual ectopic pregnancy. A fetus can grow as long as 20 weeks before the cornu is at risk for rupture. This was an unusual abdominal pregnancy. Ultrasound was unable to note the placental connection to the maternal intestine. Arrow points to fetal forehead.

PHYSIOLOGIC CHANGES AT PUBERTY AND THE NORMAL OVULATORY MENSTRUAL CYCLE

All the components necessary for menstruation can be found in the normal female at the time of birth. This is evidenced by the occasional neonatal withdrawal bleeding. Ordinarily, until the age of at least 8 years, an unknown "central restraining mechanism" prevents the pulsatile release of GnRH from the hypothalamus that is necessary for ovulation and corpus luteal development. In early puberty, the pulsatile GnRH release is maximal only at night, but with time, the typical adult pattern of continuous pulsatile secretion occurs.

Unopposed estrogen production leads to progressive uterine growth and endometrial proliferation. There is breast budding, physiologic leukorrhea, and accelerated linear growth of the girl. Axillary and pubic hair development are the result of ovarian and adrenal gland androgen production. The HPOU continues to mature. Over an approximately 2-year span, cycles with subnormal progesterone production and shortened intermenstrual intervals are replaced by normal corpus luteal function and fertile cycles. Improved nutrition and living conditions are thought to be responsible for the gradual fall in mean menarchal ages over the last century. In North America, the mean menarchal age is currently 12.4 years, with a range of 9 to 17 years. Menarche usually occurs 2 to 5 years after breast bud development.

THE NORMAL PEDIATRIC AND ADOLESCENT UTERUS

Much of the diagnostic guidance provided by US in the analysis of amenorrhea is related to the identification of the uterus and the determination of its shape and size as being premenarchal (infantile) or postmenarchal (adult). As we saw in Chap. 93, the shape and size of the uterus change during pediatric life. After the first months to year of life, the child's uterus is typically tube-shaped, with the anteroposterior di-

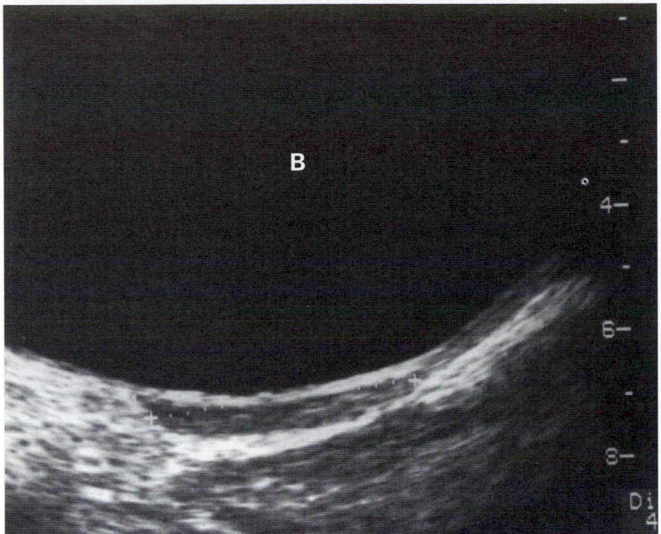

FIGURE 96–5. Infantile uterus in a patient with chronic disease (Crohn's). The uterus is marked off by crosses. It is 4 cm long and tubular in shape. This is normal in a child but is abnormal in a 16-year-old. The patient suffered from amenorrhea and retarded sexual development. She had been suffering with Crohn's disease for many years. B = bladder.

mensions of the cervix and the fundus being similar. The newborn's uterus has a mean length of 3.5 cm. This decreases to 2.6 to 3.0 cm by the fourth month of life. Uterine lengths increase gradually between 3 and 8 years of age. The mean measurement for the premenarchal child is 4.3 cm. After puberty, the uterus measures 5 to 8 cm in length. It descends deeper in the pelvis and no longer maintains the typical neutral position of the premenarchal years but may be anteverted or retroverted. With estrogenization, the endometrial cavity lining appears echogenic and thick on US exam.

AMENORRHEA: CLINICAL AND LABORATORY ASSESSMENT

Indications for the US evaluation of the teenage pelvis include amenorrhea (primary or secondary), delayed or retarded sexual development, lower abdominal pain, and pelvic mass. Any of these complaints or a combination may be the presentation of a patient with amenorrhea. There is overlapping of presentations, causes, and images among patients with amenorrhea. Many of the factors that cause pubertal delay may cause primary or secondary amenorrhea. Primary amenorrhea has many causes involving several systems. It may be seen in adolescents with normal pubertal development as well as in those with delayed sexual development, those with delayed menarche with some pubertal development, and those with delayed menarche plus virilization.

Lack of pubertal development by 13 years is 2 standard deviations beyond normal and should be worked up. Workups may be delayed for a year if there is a known debilitating illness or if the patient is involved in a competitive or endurance activity such as ballet or track. Any halt in pubertal development is a cause for concern and an endocrinologic workup. Only 0.3 percent of patients without menarche by 15.5 years will eventually develop it.

A careful medical history should include neonatal history (e.g., maternal hormone ingestion or androgen-producing tumor may account for virilization; neonatal hypoglycemia may suggest hypopituitarism); patient history, including growth data as well as previous surgery, irradiation, or chemotherapy or a history of an eating disorder or other psychological difficulty; and family history [ages of menarche; histories of abnormalities such as congenital adrenocortical hyperplasia (CAD), ovarian tumors, or thyroiditis]. Physical examination should rule out a visual field disturbance or other neurologic problem that may suggest pituitary or other central nervous system disease. Among patients with pubertal development, laboratory evaluation should include a pregnancy test whenever pregnancy is a possible cause of amenorrhea.

AMENORRHEA: DIFFERENTIAL DIAGNOSTIC CONCERNS AND THE IMAGING WORKUP

Amenorrhea has many causes involving several systems. Patients with amenorrhea can be divided into several groups.

Amenorrhea with delayed sexual development. There is a wide age variation in the onset of adolescence. Sexual development is considered to be delayed if there is no breast budding by age 13. These hypoestrogenic patients typically have an infantile (Fig. 96-5) rather than an adult uterus. The diagnosis may be categorized on the basis of levels of gonadotropin (i.e., FSH and LH) production. Hypogonadotropic hypogonadism (low to normal LH and FSH levels) is usually due to hypothalamic or pituitary dysfunction with varied causes, including tumors, chronic illness (such as cystic fibrosis, Crohn's disease, and other causes of poor nutritional intake, increased caloric need, or malabsorption), endocrinopathy, head trauma, or irradiation. Hypergonadotropic (high FSH and LH levels) hypogonadism patients have amenorrhea because of ovarian failure, whether linked to karyotype abnormalities (e.g., Turner's syndrome or XY gonadal dysgenesis), due to irradiation (usually greater than 800 rads to the pelvis) or chemotherapy, or on an autoimmune basis (autoimmune oophoritis).

Amenorrhea due to male intersex. Male pseudohermaphrodites are often not recognized as such until adolescence, when they present with primary amenorrhea. Inadequate or delayed (after the time of maximal fetal sexual structure sensitivity) androgen production leads to incomplete production of müllerian inhibition factor (MIF) and only partially masculinized genitalia. A vagina, uterus, and/or fallopian tubes may develop. Testicular feminization syndrome (Fig. 96-6) is a form of male intersex. In its com-

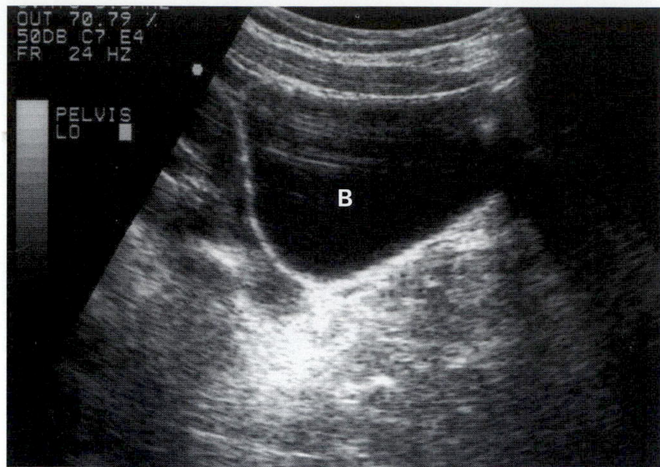

FIGURE 96–6. Testicular feminization syndrome. Transabdominal examination. Longitudinal midline plane. No uterus is seen posterior to the fluid-filled bladder (B). This teenager was brought up as a female and was discovered to be karyotypically male during a workup for primary amenorrhea at age 17.

plete form, affected patients have a normal male karyotype and testes that produce androgens and, in particular, MIF, which causes ipsilateral müllerian duct involution and prevents uterine, fallopian tube, and (upper) vaginal development. End-organ insensitivity, however, allows the development of a phenotypically normal female, often presenting at puberty with primary amenorrhea and/or inguinal masses (undescended testes). These patients have normal breast development and a peculiar lack of body hair. Ultrasound examination will show neither a uterus nor ovaries.

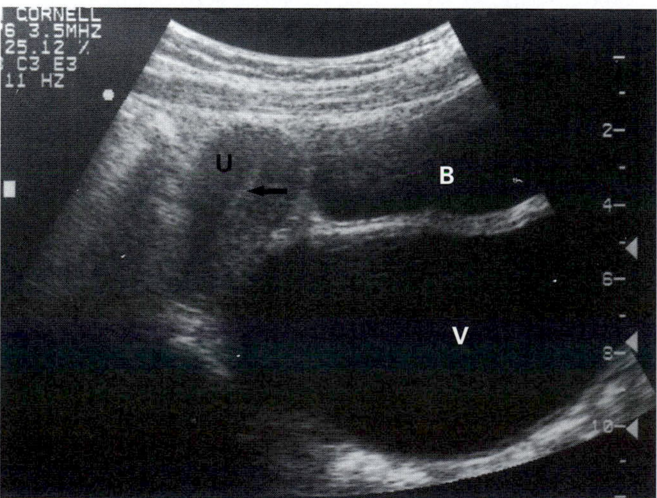

FIGURE 96–7. Hematocolpos. Transabdominal examination. Longitudinal plane. A large, fluid-filled structure with relatively thin walls is noted posterior to the fluid-filled bladder (B). The uterus (U) is normal, and its endometrial cavity (*arrow*) is not dilated. This patient is a 13-year-old with a short history of recurrent monthly pain. An imperforate hymen is the cause of her vaginal obstruction. Despite the fact that this was hemorrhagic fluid, it is not echogenic. The hemorrhagic material may have lysed during her cycle, and she was not having active hemorrhage (her period) at this time.

Amenorrhea due to virilization. Virilized patients may present with primary or, more commonly in the case of PCOS, secondary amenorrhea. Increased free testosterone due to adrenal or ovarian tumors (rare) and other causes leads to virilization, with voice deepening, clitorimegaly, increased muscle mass, and temporal balding. Marked androgen production, particularly from rapidly growing tumors, results in defeminization, with amenorrhea, vaginal mucosal atrophy, and decreased breast size as well as virilization. Ultrasound of virilizing tumors usually shows a unilaterally enlarged solid ovarian mass with abnormal echogenicity. Most hyperandrogenic adolescents will be found to have PCOS. These patients have hyperestrogenic hyperandrogenic chronic ovulation and often suffer from obesity (31 percent), hirsutism (62 percent), and menstrual irregularities (80 percent). The US of PCOS patients shows high numbers of subcapsular follicles in enlarged and echodense (from stromal hypertrophy) ovaries.

Amenorrhea due to uterine or vaginal obstruction. These patients have normally developed secondary sexual characteristics and normal estrogenization. Ultrasound allows the diagnosis of uterine (metro) or vaginal (colpo) dilatation due to obstruction that prevents the egress of the products of menses. Patients may present with a mass, a history of monthly abdominal pain, or, occasionally, difficulty with micturition. Ultrasound will typically show a distended midline tubular structure between the bladder and the rectum, containing fluid with variable echogenicity. The uterus will have a thick wall; the distended vagina will have a thin wall. Scattered echoes in the fluid are due to cellular debris, mucoid material (muco), and/or blood (hemato) proximal to the obstruction. Hematocolpos (Fig. 96-7) or hematoretrocolpos occurs in 1 in 1000 to 2000 teenagers and is usually due to an imperforate hymen (the most common congenital anomaly of the female genital tract) or a transverse vaginal septum. When only hematometra is present, one must consider a more unusual abnormality, such as cervical dysgenesis. A more difficult diagnostic picture is presented by the rarer obstructions of portions of an anomalous genital system, e.g., one uterine horn of a bicornuate system. Ultrasound or MR imaging of the vagina, cervix, and uterus helps provide presurgical anatomic information. Transverse perineal US may define the thickness of the obstruction for the surgeon (Fig. 96-8).

Amenorrhea due to uterine aplasia or hypoplasia. This category is said to be the cause of 15 percent of primary amenorrhea cases; the diagnosis is suggested by total absence of the uterus in the presence of normal ovaries. Mayer-Rokitansky-Küster-Hauser syndrome patients, for example, have amenorrhea due to vaginal atresia with associated and variable uterine abnormalities. These patients are karyotypically normal and have normal secondary sexual characteristics. Their fallopian tubes and ovaries are

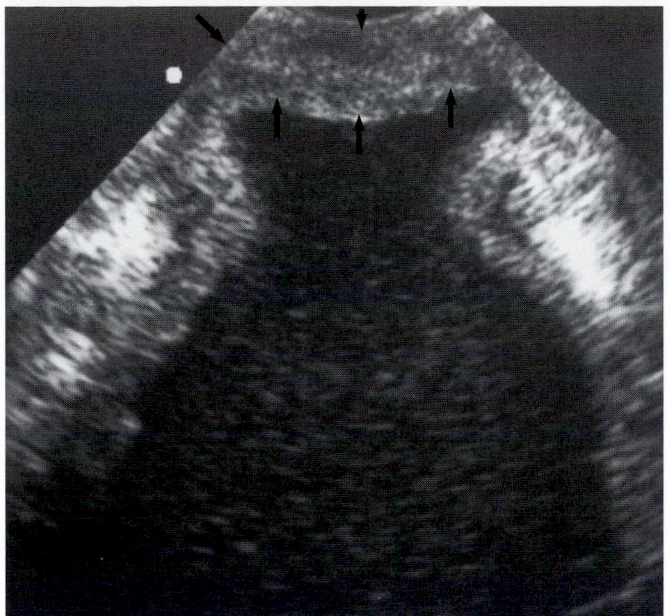

FIGURE 96–8. Imperforate hymen. Transperineal examination. Longitudinal plane. The high-frequency transducer used to image this teenager's thickened hymen (*arrows*) does not allow enough far-field penetration to note the concurrent hematometra. On this image, we can see echogenic material consistent with hemorrhage in the dilated distal portion of the vagina (hematopolpos). Her surgeon requested this image to determine the thickness of the obstruction he would have to deal with at surgery.

normal. These patients have a high incidence of associated renal (50 percent) and skeletal (12 percent) abnormalities.

SECONDARY AMENORRHEA

All causes of delayed puberty and primary amenorrhea may also be causes of secondary amenorrhea. The main pathologic cause of secondary amenorrhea is PCOS. Pregnancy is the most common physiologic cause of secondary amenorrhea in girls over 9 years. Adolescents may deny having had intercourse. As little as a 2- to 3-week delay in menses should cause clinical concern and a pregnancy test. Transvaginal (TV) US (Fig. 96-4) has allowed earlier and more accurate diagnosis of pregnancy, whether intrauterine or extrauterine (ectopic) in location.

The increased incidence of ectopic pregnancy in teenagers is due to the increasing incidence of pelvic inflammatory disease (PID) and partially treated PID in this population. The majority of ectopic pregnancies occur in a fallopian tube. About 97 percent occur in the isthmic or ampullary end of the tube. Less than 0.1 percent occur free in the abdomen (Fig. 96-4*C*). When the pregnancy grows beyond the ability of the fallopian tube to be distended (usually by 8 to 12 weeks), the tube may rupture and an abdominal crisis that may lead to death occur. A more difficult form of ectopic pregnancy to pick up is the cornual ectopic, which should be diagnosed if a gestation is incompletely surrounded by uterine tissue. Consider a cornual ectopic if a gestational sac is at the cornua, i.e., the periphery of the uterus. This may be best noted in the transverse plane and simulated only by pregnancy in a congenitally anomalous uterus (e.g., pregnancy in one horn of a difficult-to-diagnose bicornuate uterus) or in a uterus with multiple leiomyomas. Because cornual ectopics are partially within the uterus, they can grow for a greater number of weeks (i.e., to about 20 weeks gestational age) and the consequences of their rupture are more severe, causing more significant emergent clinical problems to the mother.

Ectopic pregnancy is the leading cause of first-trimester maternal deaths and is the cause of 6 to 11 percent of all maternal deaths. The diagnosis is readily made when an extrauterine gestational sac, proven by a contained yolk sac or fetal pole, is seen. It should be considered if two masses, one the normal adnexa, are seen on the same side of the uterus in a pregnant patient without evidence of an intrauterine pregnancy (IUP). Serum β hCG levels help make the diagnosis, but they can be decreased in a nonviable pregnancy. High β hCG levels require continued consideration of an ectopic unless there has been a recent abortion or there is a proven IUP. Significant cul de sac fluid, particularly if echogenic due to hemorrhage, can help suggest the diagnosis. Use of transvaginal transducers has helped the diagnosis with better near-field resolution, but transabdominal (TA) imaging has allowed the diagnosis when the ectopic gestational sac is higher up in the pelvis/abdomen. We start our exam with a global TA view and then use TV for improved imaging of an area of concern. Imaging of an intrauterine pregnancy suggests a lesser likelihood of ectopic pregnancy, but the two can occur together at a rate of about 1 in 5000 pregnancies. At one point, there was hope that noting a "ring of fire" (Fig. 96-4*B*)—i.e., significant (low-resistance) vascular flow around an ectopic gestational sac—would help diagnosis. However, similar flow may occur about a normal corpus luteal cyst. The US diagnosis of ectopic pregnancy requires abnormal gray-scale images before it can be made with confidence.

References

Bullough V: Age at menarche. A misunderstanding. *Science* 213:365–366, 1981.

Cohen HL: Evaluation of the adolescent and young adult with amenorrhea: Role of US, in *Syllabus: A Special Course in Ultrasound: Clinical Questions, Practical Answers*, Bluth E, Arger P, Hertzberg B, Middleton W (eds). Oak Brook, IL, RSNA Publications, 1996:171–184.

Cohen HL, Bober S, Bow S: Imaging the pediatric pelvis: The normal and abnormal genital system and simulators of its diseases. *Urol Radiol* 14:273–283, 1992.

Emans S, Goldstein D: The physiology of puberty, in *Pediatric and Adolescent Gynecology,* 3d ed, Emans S, Goldstein D (eds). Boston, Little, Brown, 1990:95–124.

Emans S, Goldstein D: Delayed puberty and menstrual irregularities, in *Pediatric and Adolescent Gynecology,* 3d ed, Emans S, Goldstein D (eds). Boston, Little, Brown, 1990:149–242.

Falsetti L, Pasinetti E, Mazzani M, Gastaldi A: Weight loss and menstrual cycle: Clinical and endocrinological evaluation. *Gynecol Endocrinol* 6:49–56, 1992.

Pellerito J, Taylor K, Quedens-Case C, et al: Ectopic pregnancy: Evaluation with endovaginal color imaging. *Radiology* 183: 407–411, 1992.

Ruggiero-Delituri M, Awobuluyi M, Cohen HL, Zinn D: Imaging the pediatric pelvis. Role of ultrasound. *Radiologist* 4:155–170, 1997.

Scanlan K, Pozniak M, Fagerholm M, Shapiro S: Value of transperineal sonography in the assessment of vaginal atresia. *AJR* 154:545–548, 1990.

Shah R, Woolley M, Costin G: Testicular feminization syndrome: The androgen insensitivity syndrome. *J Pediatr Surg* 27: 757–760, 1992.

Shawker T, Garra B, Loriaux D, et al: Ultrasonography of Turner's syndrome. *J Ultrasound Med* 5:125–129, 1986.

Zinn H, Cohen HL, Zinn D: Ultrasound diagnosis of ectopic pregnancy: Importance of transabdominal imaging. *J Ultrasound Med* 16:603–608, 1997.

97

A somewhat obese 18-year-old with a long history of menstrual irregularity is sent to you for evaluation. She appears mildly hirsute. Figure 97-1 is a pelvic ultrasound image. What diagnosis can you suggest? Should the discovery of ovarian follicles or small (e.g., less than 15 mm) cysts be considered unusual in children and adolescents?

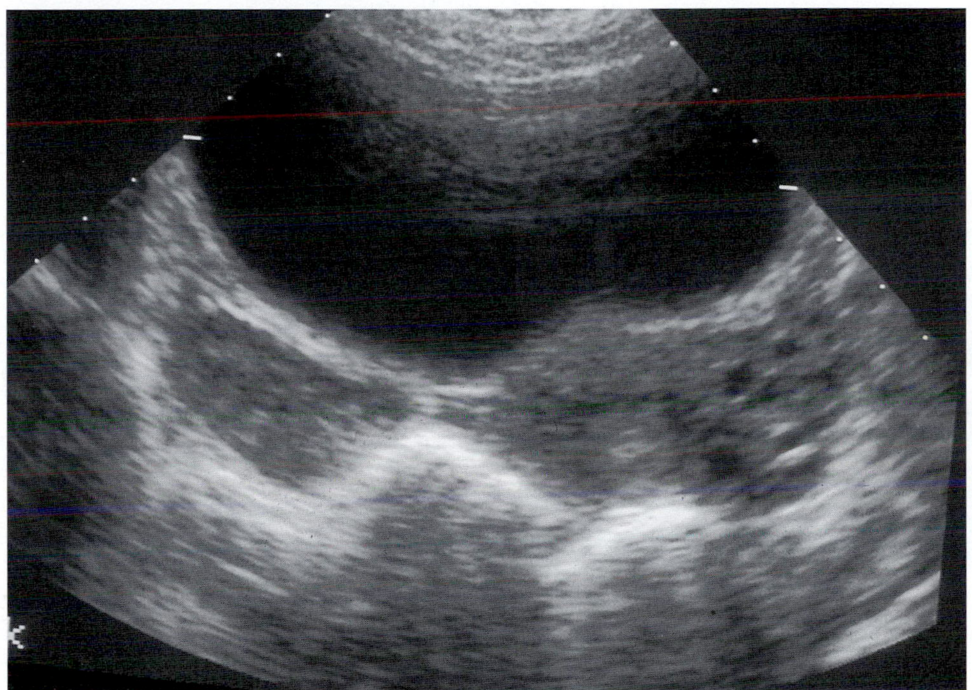

FIGURE 97–1. Pelvic ultrasound. Transabdominal technique. Transverse plane.

CHAPTER 97

Polycystic Ovary Syndrome

HARRIS L. COHEN

AND MARYANNE RUGGIERO-DELLITURRI

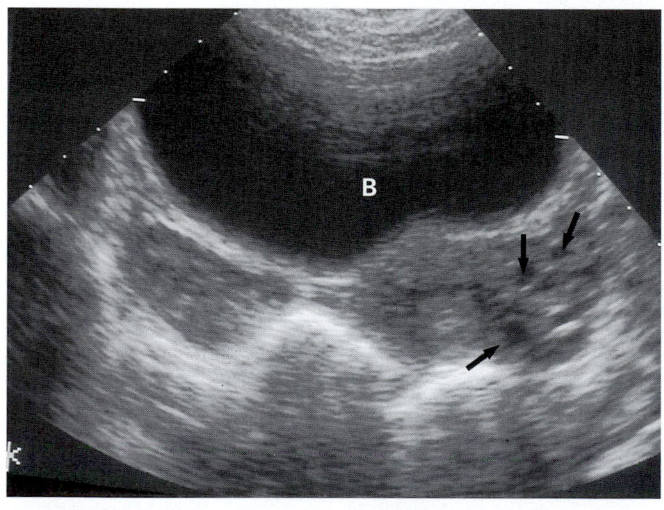

FIGURE 97–2. Annotated version of Fig. 97-1. Polycystic ovary syndrome. Pelvic ultrasound. Transabdominal technique. Transverse plane. Both adnexa are upper limits of normal to enlarged in size. Each has a determined volume of 19 cm^3. Multiple follicles (*arrows*) are seen in the left adnexa. They are less well seen on the right in this image, but the image highlights the increased echogenicity of the adnexa, which is best seen on the right. None of the follicles in either adnexa is larger than 10 mm. The left adnexa appears adherent or adjacent to the uterus. When enlarged, an adnexa that is adjacent to the uterus may simulate adherence, an indicator of past inflammatory disease. Adherence may also be simulated by normal adnexa at the side of a retroverted uterus. B = bladder.

Figure 97-2, the annotated version of Fig. 97-1, shows two enlarged adnexa. Both contained multiple small follicles, with those in the left adnexa being more apparent in this image. Both ovaries were more echogenic than normal. This is best seen in the right adnexa of this image. A history of menstrual irregularity in an adolescent coupled with obesity or hirsutism suggests the need to consider polycystic ovary syndrome (PCOS). The image's enlarged ovary and multiple small follicles, none larger than 10 mm, suggest the diagnosis of PCOS. Increased echogenicity within the ovary (Fig. 97-3) can be seen in many PCOS patients. Laboratory findings are necessary to confirm the diagnosis.

The imaging diagnosis is not always straightforward. Certainly the presence of follicles or cysts in the ovary of the normal adolescent or normal child is not uncommon. One can have the symptoms of obesity, menstrual irregularity, and hirsutism, individually or in combination, in normal patients as well as in those with other abnormalities. There are patients with familial hirsutism. Many young teenagers take a while for their cycles to become regular. Many individuals are obese. If signs of virilization are found, a workup to rule out a virilizing adrenal or ovarian tumor is required. Certainly if a unilateral ovarian mass, usually solid, is imaged, an endocrinologically active ovarian tumor must be considered. Androgen excess may also occur in cases of idiopathic hirsutism, late-onset forms of congenital adrenal hyperplasia, exaggerated adrenarche, Cushing's disease, hyperprolactinemia, and acromegaly. Most hyperandrogenic adolescents are found to have PCOS.

WHAT IS POLYCYSTIC OVARY SYNDROME?

Polycystic ovary syndrome (also known as Stein-Leventhal syndrome) is a hyperandrogenic state with resultant peripheral conversion of larger than normal amounts of estrogen.

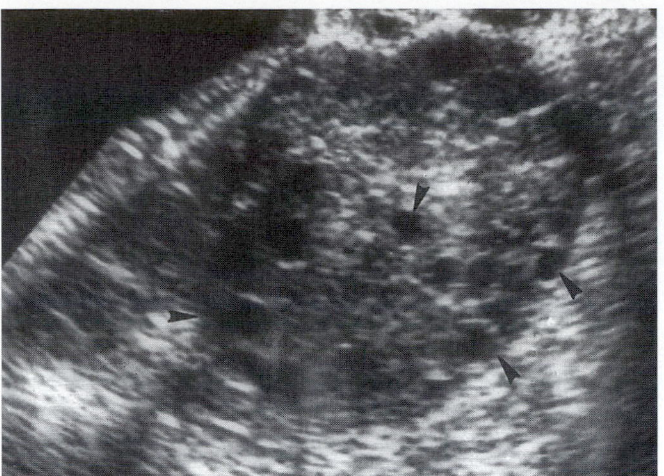

FIGURE 97–3. Polycystic ovary syndrome. Transvaginal image through right ovary. Longitudinal plane. The ovary was enlarged—greater than 20 cm^3. There is bright echogenicity seen within the ovary, consistent with stromal hypertrophy. Multiple small follicles (*arrows*), none greater than 10 mm and therefore consistent with a state of anovulation, are seen in this obese and hirsute teen with a history of menstrual irregularities who was proven to have PCOS. (*From Cohen HL, Eisenberg P, Mandel F, Haller J: Ovarian cysts are common in premenarchal girls: A sonographic study of 101 children 2–12 years old.* AJR *159:89–91, 1992, with permission.*)

The chronic hyperestrogenic hyperandrogenic stimulation leads to chronic anovulation and is responsible for the classic bilaterally enlarged ovaries, which may be asymmetric and usually contain multiple cysts. Polycystic ovary syndrome is the most common pathologic cause of amenorrhea, usually secondary, in the adolescent and young adult. Patients often, but far from always, suffer from the classic triad of obesity (31 percent), hirsutism (62 percent), and amenorrhea (80 percent). Laboratory diagnosis is made by noting increased luteinizing hormone (LH)/follicle-stimulating hormone (FSH) ratios and elevated androstenedione levels.

WHAT ARE THE ULTRASOUND FINDINGS OF POLYCYSTIC OVARY SYNDROME?

There are continuing attempts to pin down what are the abnormal ultrasound (US) findings in PCOS. There is an overlap between normal US findings and those considered consistent with PCOS and those actually found in PCOS patients. This is true whether patients are examined with transabdominal (TA) or transvaginal (TV) US. One must be aware of the fact that TVUS will show increased numbers of ovarian cysts in both normal and PCOS patients compared to TA examinations. Patients with PCOS have large numbers of subcapsular follicles in enlarged and more echodense ovaries. One group from Brazil suggested that ovarian volumes of greater than 10 cm^3 in adolescent girls with menstrual disorders and/or hirsutism suggest PCOS. A Japanese group noted mean ovarian volumes of 10.3 cm^3 in 47 affected patients, significantly greater than those in a control group. Among their PCOS patients, 94 percent had either an ovarian volume >6.2 cm^3 or more than 10 follicles of 2 to 8 mm diameter (Fig. 97-4), while 6 percent had normal volumes and numbers of follicles. There are, however, many normal adolescents with ovarian volumes greater than 6.2 cm^3. Our US laboratory uses 15 to 20 cm^3 as a gray zone for ovarian enlargement and a figure of 20 cm^3 or greater as evidence of definitive enlargement in adults and older adolescents. The increased ovarian echogenicity (Fig. 97-3) found in the ovaries of patients with PCOS is a helpful diagnostic finding. It has been linked to pathologically proven ovarian stromal hypertrophy. Increased ovarian stroma is considered evidence of hyperandrogenism. One group found such PCOS ovaries to have greater volumes and their vessels lower-resistance flow than normal ovaries. Androstenedione levels are linked to higher uterine artery resistance. We have not studied our PCOS patients with Doppler to prove or disprove these points.

Not all polycystic ovaries are due to hyperandrogenism. Unopposed estrogen stimulation from any source can result in polycystic ovaries. Genetic deficiencies of the enzymes 21-hydroxylase, 3β-hydroxysteroid dehydrogenase, and 11β-hydroxylase have all been associated with polycystic ovary development.

THE NORMAL PEDIATRIC OVARY—CYSTS ARE COMMON

Several dogmatic statements regarding the US of pediatric ovaries have fallen by the wayside over the last decade, perhaps because of improved US technology. At one time, imaging the pediatric ovary was thought to be difficult. However, ovaries of neonates and older pediatric patients *can be* imaged and quite often are. We have reported imaging (in three dimensions) 64 percent of the ovaries of 77 newborn to

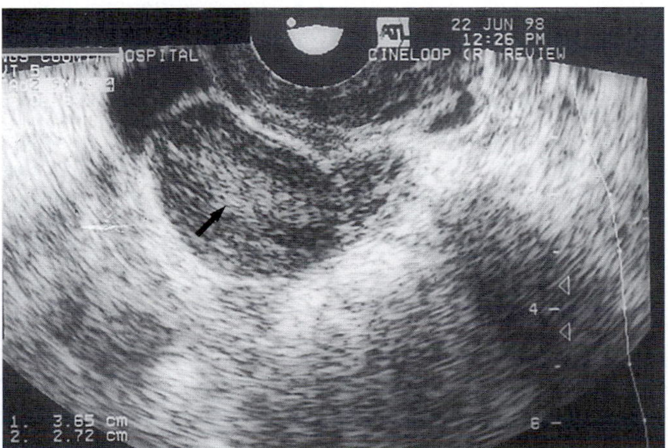

FIGURE 97–4. Polycystic ovary syndrome. Transvaginal image through right ovary. This patient has prominent echogenicity (*arrow*) within a 23-cm^3 (enlarged) ovary whose cysts were not well imaged.

2-year-old patients, and 78 percent of the ovaries of 101 premenarchal girls between 2 and 12 years. Ovaries are often found posterior or lateral to the uterus. They should be looked for in transverse US imaging at the side of the uterus while angulating the transducer in a superior-inferior direction and in parasagittal scanning, medial and anterior to the iliac vessels. I often seek the uterine cornua on transverse section to see if I can follow a hint of fallopian tube (not truly seen unless obstructed) or other adnexa peripherally to a less readily imaged ovary. Ovaries may be present anywhere along their embryologic course from the kidney's inferior border to the level of the broad ligament, where they are usually found. The true absence of an ovary is rare. The discovery at surgery of absence of an ovary and its ipsilateral fallopian tube suggests an antenatal torsion with secondary necrosis.

Our concepts of what represent normal ovarian volumes and echogenicity pattern have evolved over the last decade. At one time, normal mean volume for children below 10 years was considered to be as low as 0.7 cm^3. Reported mean volumes for premenarchal girls range between 0.75 and 4.18 cm^3. Statistically significant ovarian volume differences exist among children with Tanner 3 and greater classifications of pubertal development. There is a volume of greater than 3 cm^3 among those with Tanner 3; 4 to 4.6 cm^3 with Tanner 4; and 5 to 7.5 cm^3 with Tanner 5. One study found the normal postpubertal ovarian volume to be 5.2 cm^3 with a standard deviation of 2.7 cm^3. One group noted a mean volume in the second decade of 7.8 cm^3.

The typical premenarchal ovary is no longer considered to be homogeneously solid in echogenicity, but rather is heterogeneous, i.e., containing follicles/physiologic cysts, whether seen in the neonate or older child (Fig. 97-5). The significance of this for the analysis of clinical problems is that the presence of follicles or cysts cannot be used to intimate precocious puberty or to suggest menarche or near menarche. Follicular cysts can be imaged throughout childhood. Microcysts (9 mm or less) were imaged in as many as 72 percent of 81 imaged ovaries in a 2- to 6-year-old group and in 68 percent of 56 imaged ovaries in a 7- to 10-year-old group of normal children. Even macrocysts (those >9 mm) were seen, but to a far lesser extent in both groups. These findings, although reported in the US literature over the last decade, are consistent with pathology literature reports (as far back as Rokitansky in 1861) noting that cystic follicles are common in the autopsied ovaries of fetuses, neonates, and children. Ovarian follicles begin maturing at or before birth.

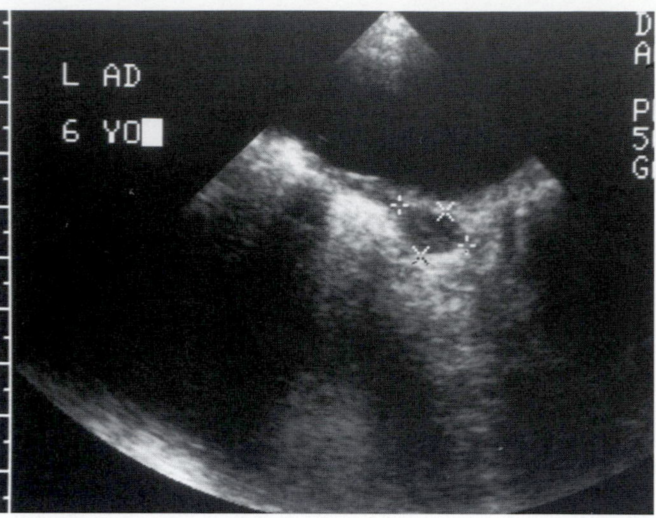

FIGURE 97–5. Normal ovary with follicles. Transabdominal image through left ovary. A normal ovary in a 6-year-old is seen to contain several small follicles/cysts (*arrow*). A heterogeneous echogenicity is most typical for the ovary throughout the pediatric age range.

KEY POINTS

Bilaterally enlarged ovaries with increased contained echogenicity suggest PCOS in patients with some combination of menstrual irregularity, obesity, and hirsutism. Cysts of patients with PCOS should not be large; they are typically less than 10 mm in diameter. Ovarian follicles and cysts are normally seen throughout childhood.

References

Battaglia C, Artini P, D'Ambrogio G, et al: The role of color Doppler imaging in the diagnosis of polycystic ovary syndrome. *Am J Obstet Gynecol* 172:108–113, 1995.

Cohen HL: Evaluation of the adolescent and young adult with amenorrhea: Role of US, in *Syllabus: A Special Course in Ultrasound: Clinical Questions, Practical Answers*, Bluth E, Arger P, Hertzberg B, Middleton W (eds). Oak Brook, IL, RSNA Publications, 1996:171–184.

Cohen HL, Haller JO: Pediatric and adolescent genital abnormalities. *Clin Diagn Ultrasound* 24:187–216, 1988.

Cohen HL, Eisenberg P, Mandel F, Haller J: Ovarian cysts are common in premenarchal girls: A sonographic study of 101 children 2–12 years old. *AJR* 159:89–91, 1992.

Cohen HL, Shapiro M, Mandel F, Shapiro M: Normal ovaries in neonates and infants: A sonographic study of 77 patients 1 day to 24 months old. *AJR* 160:583–586, 1993.

Cohen HL, Tice H, Mandel F: Ovarian volumes measured by US: Bigger than we think. *Radiology* 177:189–192, 1990.

Emans S, Goldstein D: Delayed puberty and menstrual irregularities, in *Pediatric and Adolescent Gynecology,* 3d ed, Emans S, Goldstein D (eds). Boston, Little, Brown, 1990:149–242.

Goldzieher J, Green J: The polycystic ovary: I. Clinical and histologic features. *J Clin Endocrinol Metab* 22:325–338, 1962.

Herter L, Magalnaes J, Spritzer P: Association of ovarian volume and serum LH levels in adolescent patients with menstrual disorders and/or hirsutism. *Braz J Med Biol Res* 26:1041–1046, 1993.

Orsini L, Salardi S, Pilu G, et al: Pelvic organs in premenarchal girls: Real-time ultrasonography. *Radiology* 153:113–116, 1984.

Polhemus D: Ovarian maturation and cyst formation in children. *Pediatrics* 11:588–594, 1953.

Salardi S, Orsini L, Cacciari E, et al: Pelvic ultrasonography in premenarchal girls: Relation to puberty and sex hormone concentrations. *Arch Dis Child* 60:120–125, 1985.

Takahashi K, Okada M, Ozaki T, et al: Transvaginal ultrasonographic morphology in polycystic ovarian syndrome. *Gynecol Obstet Invest* 39:201–206, 1995.

98

An afebrile 13-year-old complains of left pelvic pain for 2 days. She has no sexual history. Figure 98-1 shows the ultrasound (US) examination's main finding. What do you see? What is the most likely diagnosis? What other abnormalities should be considered?

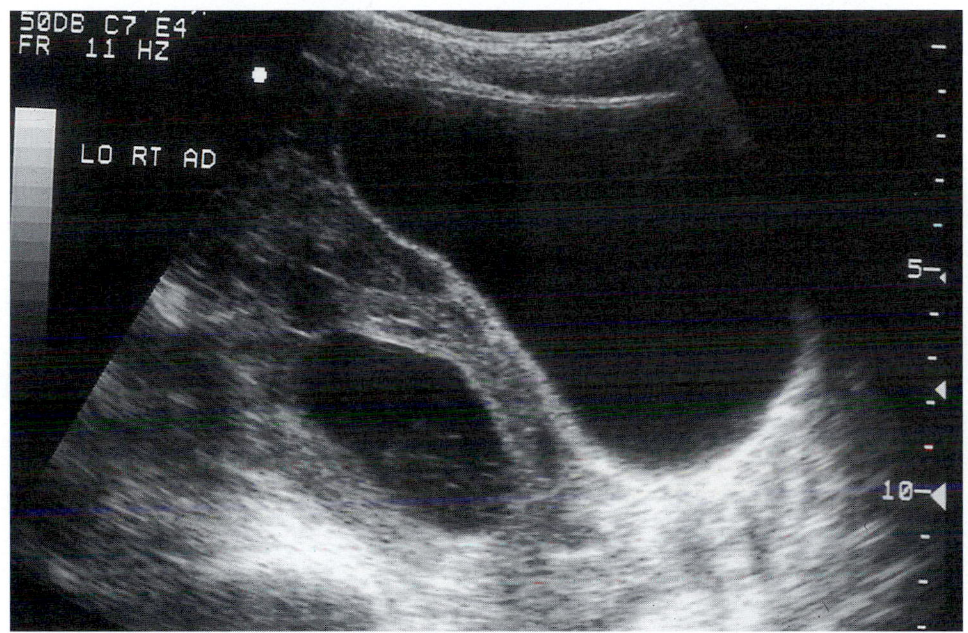

FIGURE 98–1. Pelvic ultrasound. Longitudinal plane through right ovary.

CHAPTER 98

Hemorrhagic Ovarian Cysts

BRIAN GALE AND HARRIS L. COHEN

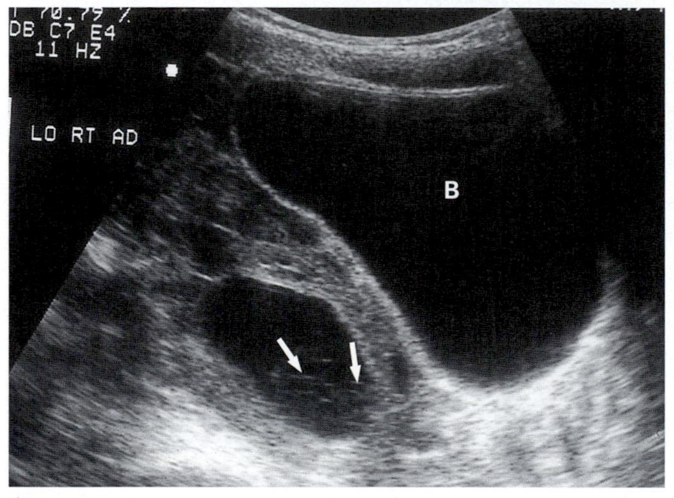

A

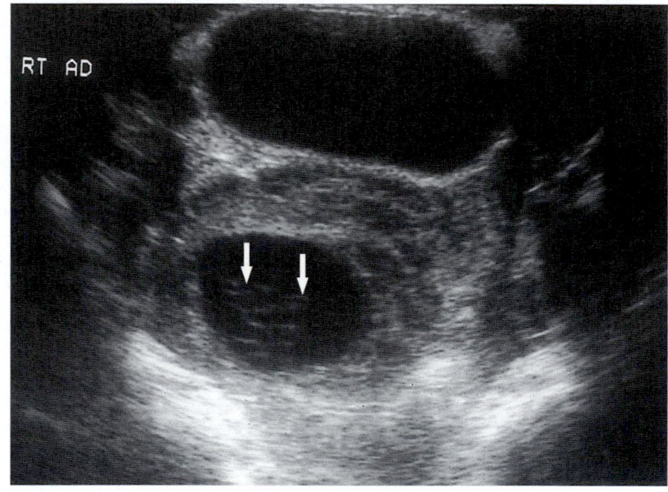

B

FIGURE 98–2. Hemorrhagic cyst. Pelvic ultrasound. ***A.*** Annotated version of Fig. 98-1. Longitudinal plane through right ovary. The right adnexa is enlarged because of a contained predominantly echoless area. Within the large echoless area's dependent portion are linear echoes (*arrows*), consistent with hemorrhage. B = bladder. ***B.*** Transverse plane through right adnexal mass. This orthogonal view again shows bright linear echogenicities (*arrows*), consistent with fibrin deposition in this right adnexa's hemorrhagic cyst.

Figure 98-2*A*, the annotated version of Fig. 98-1, shows a right adnexa containing a large echoless area with contained echogenic debris that appears somewhat dependent. Figure 98-2*B* is an orthogonal (transverse) view. The contained echogenicity is most consistent with a hemorrhagic ovarian cyst. However, endometriomas and tuboovarian abscesses can appear quite similar. All three possibilities usually have more contained echogenicity than is seen in Fig. 98-2.

DIFFERENTIAL DIAGNOSTIC POSSIBILITIES

An endometrioma, the "chocolate" (i.e., hemorrhagic) cystic mass associated with endometriosis (Fig. 98-3), usually is a concern in patients with unusually painful periods and a history of infertility. It is usually not a problem of adolescence. The discovery of a normal ovary on the ipsilateral side of the mass might suggest this diagnosis. The ovary itself, however,

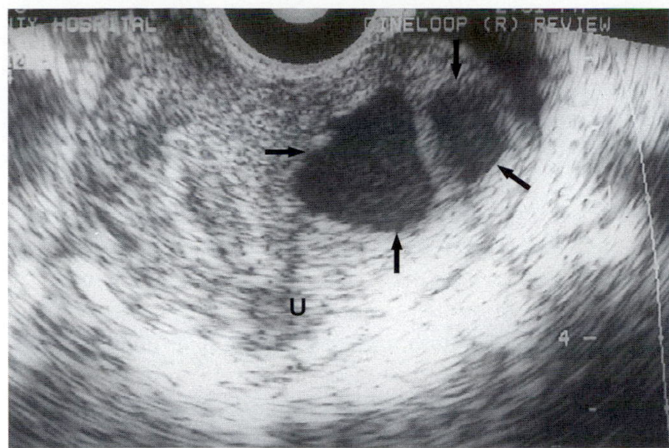

FIGURE 98–3. Endometrioma. Transvaginal examination. Transverse oblique plane through the uterus. An echopenic mass (*arrows*) with a single septation and filled with contained debris is hard to separate from the uterus (U) of this adult patient with a history of painful periods and infertility. This was proven surgically to be an endometrioma. Its contained hemorrhage can certainly simulate the contained hemorrhage in a functional cyst (i.e., a hemorrhagic cyst).

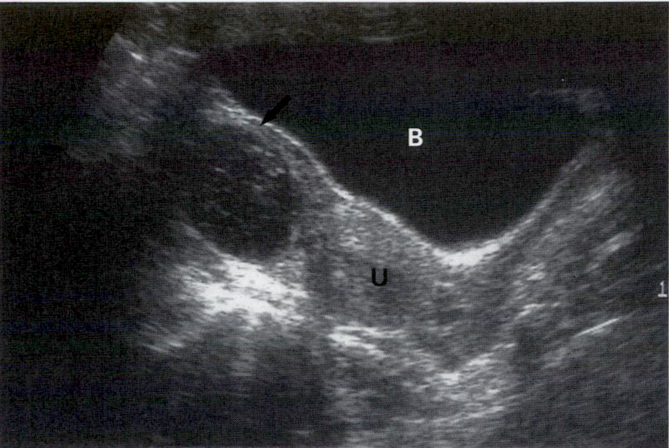

FIGURE 98–4. Tuboovarian abscess simulating a hemorrhagic cyst. ***A.*** Transabdominal examination. Longitudinal plane through the midline. An echopenic mass (*arrow*) is seen in the right adnexal area superior to the uterus (U). Despite looking like a classic hemorrhagic cyst with contained echogenic debris, it proved to be a simulator—a tuboovarian abscess. B = bladder.

may be involved. The US diagnosis of endometriosis (ectopic and extrauterine endometrial tissue) is difficult when there is no focal mass, i.e., no endometrioma.

The tuboovarian abscess (TOA) can look dramatically similar (Fig. 98-4) to the hemorrhagic cyst. A history consistent with sexual contact and pelvic inflammatory disease, including fever and cervical motion tenderness, will suggest this diagnosis.

OVARIAN CYSTS IN CHILDREN AND ADOLESCENTS

The normal pediatric ovary and its adnexa are not felt on physical examination. Nonneoplastic cysts of follicular origin—i.e., functional ovarian cysts—are the most common cause of enlargement. The diagnosis of such cysts becomes more difficult when they are hemorrhagic and lose their classic US characteristics (echoless, sharp posterior wall, and strong posterior acoustic enhancement). Such cysts may contain diffuse homogeneous or complex internal echoes (Fig. 98-5) or fluid debris levels with decreased through transmission—i.e., posterior enhancement—allowing confusion with other masses, including neoplasms. Hemorrhagic cysts are a not uncommon reason for a teenager to present with lower abdominal or pelvic pain. Once a hemorrhagic cyst is diagnosed, resolution of pain and confirmation of a stable hematocrit allow conservative management and the use of "tincture of time," with the hemorrhagic cyst followed by US to resolution. Such resolution includes the disappearance of or change in the cyst's echogenic hemorrhagic contents as a result of clot lysis or complete disappearance of the cyst itself. In one study, imaging allowed a ready diagnosis; only 11 of 102 hemorrhagic ovarian cysts required surgery for diagnosis.

WHAT ARE FUNCTIONAL OVARIAN CYSTS?

As we have noted elsewhere in this text, follicles are seen throughout childhood. In the menstruating adolescent female, cysts are classified as physiologic (usually less than 3 cm), functional (retention cyst), or neoplastic. Hemorrhagic ovarian cysts (HOC) represent a complication that arises in physiologic/functional ovarian cysts. Functional ovarian cysts occur as a result of the failure of a normal maturing follicle to involute. The cyst continues to enlarge, usually because of a temporary or persistent hormonal imbalance. This is usually a process that begins around menarche, which explains its not uncommon occurrence in adolescence. Hemorrhagic ovarian cysts can develop in ovarian follicles at any stage in

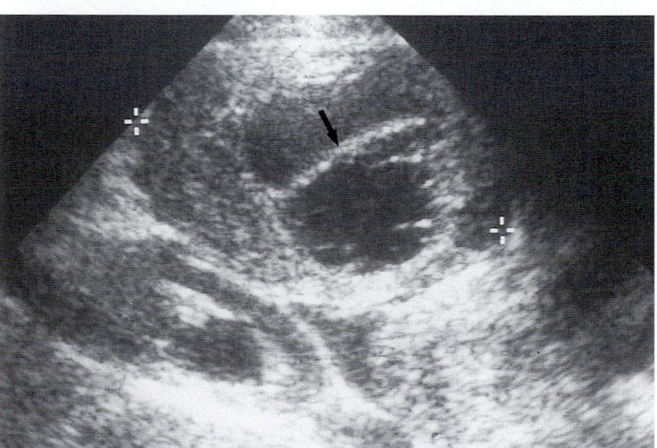

FIGURE 98–5. Hemorrhagic cyst. Transabdominal examination. Longitudinal plane through right adnexa. A moderately thick septum (*arrow*) separates two echopenic areas with a small amount of contained debris, within an otherwise prominent but normal-appearing ovary. Note the similarity with Fig. 98–3.

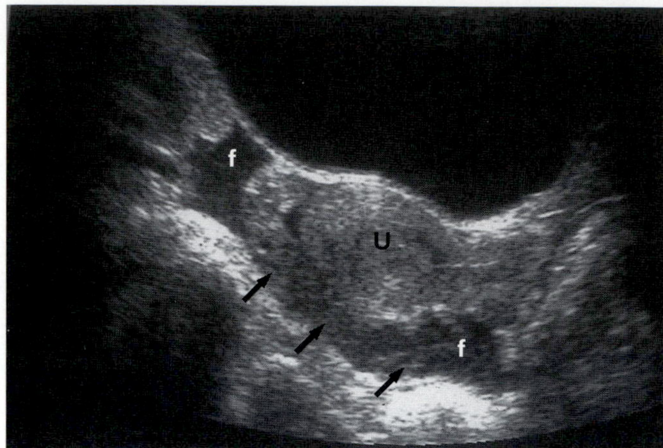

FIGURE 98–6. Echogenic cul de sac fluid due to ruptured hemorrhagic cyst. Transabdominal examination. Longitudinal plane through the uterus. Echogenic debris is seen in fluid (f) posterior to the uterus (U) (*arrows*), within the cul de sac, and extending superior to the uterus. This patient's hemorrhagic cyst ruptured. The debris is greater in the more dependent area in fluid (f).

their maturation, including as they undergo atresia. They may develop in the corpus luteum, the residua of the dominant or graafian follicle, after ovulation. They may be seen antenatally or in newborns. Their occurrence in the fetus is thought to be the result of ovarian stimulation by maternal hormones. The majority of functional ovarian cysts are treated conservatively—i.e., watched clinically—and resolve spontaneously. Rarely, they can be complicated. The most common complication is ovarian torsion, which occurs more often in ovaries with large cysts or masses. Functional cysts may rupture and result in free cul de sac fluid (Fig. 98-6), which may be echogenic, or even more significant amounts of peritoneal fluid.

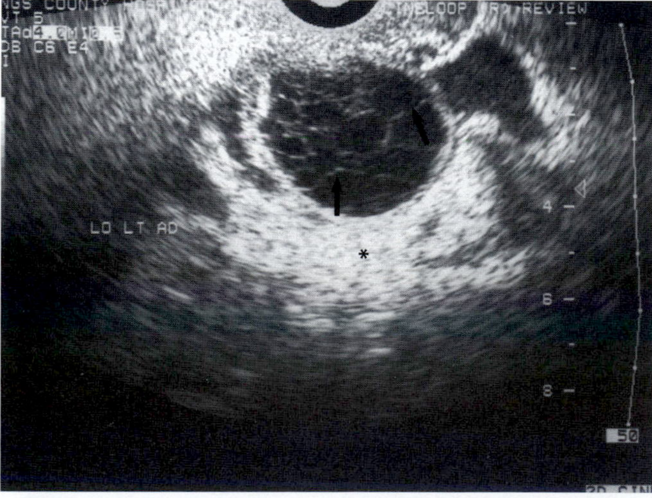

FIGURE 98–7. Hemorrhagic cyst. Transvaginal examination. Transverse plane through left adnexa. Multiple thin echogenic strands are seen crisscrossing a predominantly cystic mass (*arrows*) with excellent through transmission (*). This is a typical image of a hemorrhagic cyst, whether seen on transvaginal or transabdominal examination. Again, it may look similar to an endometrioma or a tuboovarian abscess. (*Reprinted from Ruggiero-Dellitturri M, Awobuluyi M, Cohen HL, Zinn D: Imaging the pediatric pelvis: Role of ultrasound.* Radiologist *4:155–170, 1997, with permission.*)

WHAT ARE HEMORRHAGIC CYSTS?

Functional cysts may also develop internal hemorrhage. Hemorrhagic ovarian cysts occur when theca interna vessels rupture into the cyst cavity. The typical clinical presentation is either that of sudden, severe, transient lower abdominal pain of 1 to 3 h duration, or that of lower abdominal pain and palpable mass. The pain is thought to result from sudden distention of the ovarian cyst from hemorrhage. Among 70 adolescent and adult patients with HOC studied by Baltarowich et al, only 4 percent were asymptomatic. Some 26 percent of the patients in this series had prior, concurrent, or subsequent simple ovarian cysts or HOCs. It may be that just as some individuals have a greater tendency to produce functional cysts, some individuals may also have a greater tendency to develop hemorrhagic cysts in particular hormonal environments. In the majority of cases, the clot hemolyzes and is gradually absorbed.

ULTRASONOGRAPHIC FINDINGS OF THE HEMORRHAGIC OVARIAN CYST

Hemorrhagic ovarian cysts tend to be clearly separable from the uterus. Their size ranges widely, with one study noting a size range of 2.5 to 14 cm in length. The HOC may vary in image echogenicity, ranging from anechoic to hyperechoic and from homogeneous to heterogeneous. The majority are heterogeneous in echogenicity. According to one study of 15 HOCs, 93 percent will either have hypoechoic and hyperechoic areas separated by a thin or thick septum-like echo (Fig. 98-5) or else be hypoechoic and contain lamellar thin to thick echoes (Figs. 98-2 and 98-7) in various orientations. They may, however, be anechoic and contain hypoechoic material or contain a round hyperechoic mass, representing a blood clot. The clot can appear as a small mass within an anechoic cavity or can fill the cavity. When clot fills the HOC cavity, it can be confused with a solid mass. The fundamental sonographic feature that indicates the cystic nature of the mass despite its contained echogenicity is increased through transmission. A changing US appearance can help make the diagnosis of HOC. Image change is expected, since hemorrhage changes its US appearance with time. The initial bright echogenicity of acute hemorrhage, which results from fibrin deposition, becomes less bright and eventually fluid-like as the fibrin dissolves and as the clot lyses.

Technically, a transvaginal (TV) examination using a higher-frequency transducer (e.g., 6.5 MHz) can help improve evaluation of the contents of any complex cystic mass that lies low in the pelvis and close to the transducer. One group suggests that TV exams always be performed in such cases. We don't find this to be necessary: We find the HOC image, similar at times to that of a TOA, easy to diagnose, with the appropriate accompanying history, on transabdominal (TA) examination. We would use TV if we had a concern about possible dilatation of a fallopian tube, which would help point the diagnosis to pelvic inflammatory disease or TOA. However, such situations are unusual. We do *not* perform TV exams on virginal patients.

THE DIFFERENTIAL DIAGNOSIS OF THE HEMORRHAGIC OVARIAN CYST—OTHER CONSIDERATIONS

Beyond the possibilities of its true imaging simulators, TOA and endometrioma, a "strict" differential diagnosis of the HOC would include the differential diagnosis of complex ovarian masses. One may consider a benign cystic teratoma (if it does not have a significant solid component), an ectopic pregnancy (but it would have to be chronic or complicated so as not to look like a gestational sac with a contained fetal pole), a torsed ovary (but ovarian torsion, which can occur to an ovary with an HOC, is usually very large, with volumes between 150 and 400 cm^3), and an appendiceal abscess (but an ipsilateral adnexa could not be imaged).

KEY POINT

Tuboovarian abscesses can look like hemorrhagic cysts, and vice versa. Histories and physical exam findings, including your own if you are using a TA or a TV probe, can help you make the correct diagnosis.

References

Baltarowich OH, Kurtz A, Pasto M, et al: The spectrum of sonographic findings in hemorrhagic ovarian cysts. *AJR* 148:901–905, 1987.

Bass IS, Haller JO, Friedman AP, et al: The sonographic appearance of the hemorrhagic ovarian cyst in adolescents. *J Ultrasound Med* 3:509–513, 1984.

Case records of the Massachusetts General Hospital: Weekly clinicopathological exercises. Case 6-1995. A one-month-old girl with an intraabdominal mass found on prenatal ultrasonographic examination [clinical conference]. *N Engl J Med* 23:522–527, 1995.

Cohen HL: The female pelvis, in *Syllabus: Current Concepts: A Categorical Course in Pediatric Radiology,* Siebert J (ed). Chicago, RSNA Publications, 1994:65–72.

Cohen HL, Bober S, Bow S: Imaging the pediatric pelvis: The normal and abnormal genital system and simulators of its diseases. *Urol Radiol* 14:273–283, 1992.

Ishihara K, Nemoto Y: Sonographic appearance of hemorrhagic ovarian cyst with acute abdomen by transvaginal scan. *Nippon Ika Daigaku Zasshi* 64:411–415, 1997.

Kayaba H, Tamura H, Shirayama K, et al: Hemorrhagic ovarian cyst in childhood: A case report. *J Pediatr Surg* 31:978–979, 1996.

Nussbaum AR, Sanders RC, Hartman DS, et al: Neonatal ovarian cysts: Sonographic-pathologic correlation. *Radiology* 168:817–821, 1988.

O'Brien PM, DiMichele DM, Walterhouse DO: Management of an acute hemorrhagic ovarian cyst in a female patient with hemophilia A. *J Pediatr Hematol Oncol* 18:233–236, 1996.

Ruggiero-Delituri M, Awobuluyi M, Cohen HL, Zinn D: Imaging the pediatric pelvis: Role of ultrasound. *Radiologist* 4:155–170, 1997.

Sarihan H, Unal M, Ozoran YS: Massive haemoperitoneum due to spontaneous rupture of ovarian cyst in children. A report of 2 cases. *S Afr J Surg* 34:44–46, 1996.

Surratt J, Siegel M: Imaging of pediatric ovarian masses. *Radiographics* 11:533–548, 1991.

Yoffe N, Bronshtein M, Brandes J, Blumenfeld Z: Hemorrhagic ovarian cyst detection by transvaginal sonography: The great imitator. *Gynecol Endocrinol* 5:123–129, 1991.

99

A 15-year-old patient is being evaluated for a urinary tract infection. Figure 99-1 was obtained during the ultrasound evaluation of the pelvis. Abnormality was noted. What is the diagnosis?

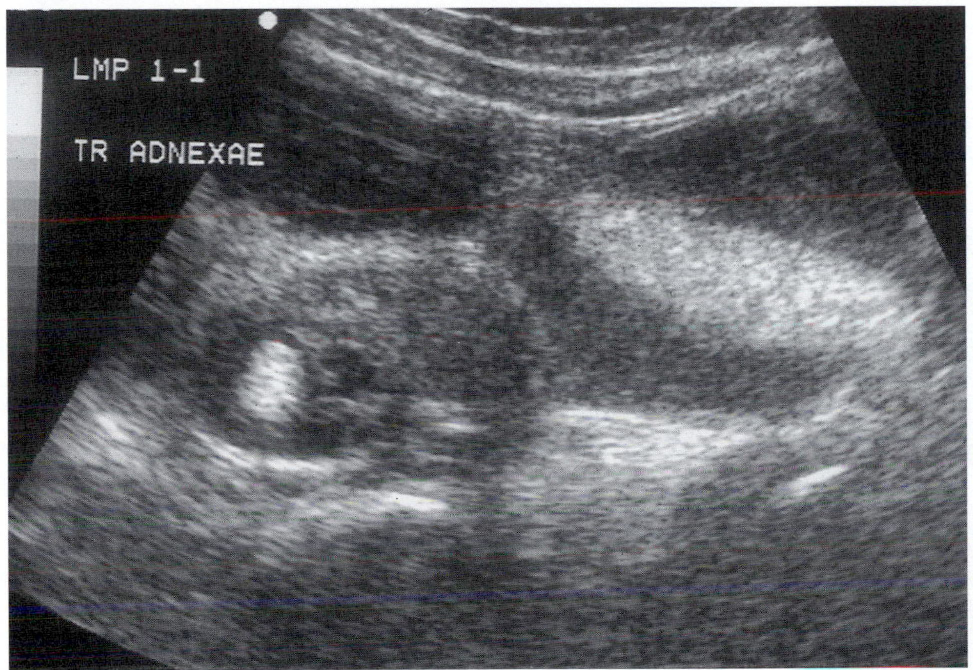

FIGURE 99–1. Pelvis. Transverse plane.

CHAPTER 99

Benign Cystic Teratomas of the Ovary

HARRIS L. COHEN AND YAIR I. SAFRIEL

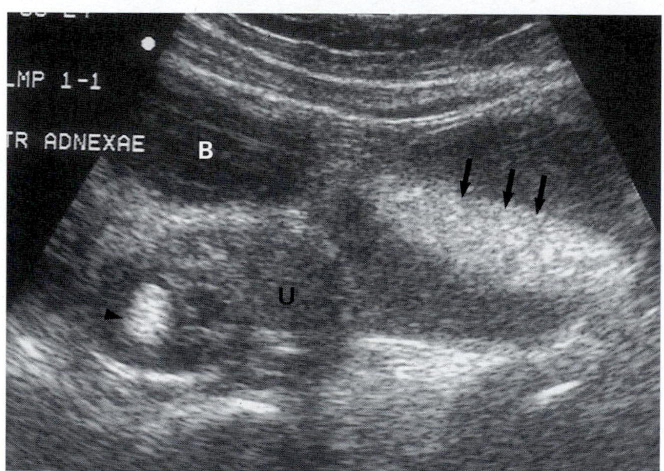

FIGURE 99–2. Annotated version of Fig. 99-1. Bilateral ovarian teratomas. Pelvis. Transverse plane. A fluid debris level (*arrows*) is seen in the left adnexa. The image is due to echogenic material made up of particulate debris having sunk to below the lighter cystic component and therefore becoming the dependent portion of a left ovarian teratoma. A smaller, highly echogenic area (*arrowhead*) is seen in the right adnexa. This is an intraovarian teratoma. The uterus (U), which looks similar in echogenicity to a portion of the left teratoma, separates the adnexa. B = bladder.

Figure 99-2, the annotated version of Fig. 99-1, shows a large left adnexal teratoma, indicated by a fluid level with dependent highly echogenic material and less echogenic and lighter material floating in its upper portion. The right ovary shows a small, highly echogenic area within it. Although this might be simulated, particularly if smaller, by acute hemorrhage in a cyst, it too is a teratoma, albeit intraovarian and without an evident cystic component. Most authorities do not recommend surgery for teratomas that are completely within an ovary's parenchyma. This patient's left adnexal teratoma was surgically removed.

BENIGN CYSTIC TERATOMAS—CLINICAL FACTORS

Ovarian neoplasms are uncommon in children. When they are noted, the majority (67 percent) are of germ cell origin, predominantly mature ovarian teratomas or dermoid cysts. The majority of adult ovarian tumors are not of germ cell origin, but rather epithelial in origin (i.e., mucinous and serous cystadenomas and cystadenocarcinomas). Teratomas are therefore more typical of the adolescent or young adult population. Although the two tumor types are talked about almost interchangeably, dermoids, by definition, contain two cell layers, mesoderm and ectoderm, while teratomas are made up of elements from all three germ cell layers, including the endoderm. Almost all dermoids and teratomas are benign. Malignancy is found in 2 to 10 percent of cases or less.

Teratomas can be found in children. They are usually asymptomatic, and this may be why the exact numbers in older females who have not needed an ultrasound (US) exam of the pelvis may be underestimated. However, at least one-third of cases present with symptomatology. Of teratomas diagnosed in children because of symptoms, the usual history is that of a 6- to 11-year-old with an abdominal mass (65 to 70 percent) or pain secondary to torsion of or hemorrhage within the cyst. Teratomas are most often discovered by chance in pelvic US exams performed in adolescents for amenorrhea, bladder infection, pelvic inflammatory disease (PID), or pregnancy workups. One-fourth of ovarian teratomas are bilateral.

ULTRASOUND CHARACTERISTICS OF MATURE OVARIAN TERATOMAS

The US appearance of teratomas is highly variable as a result of the varied contents of such masses. The classic US appear-

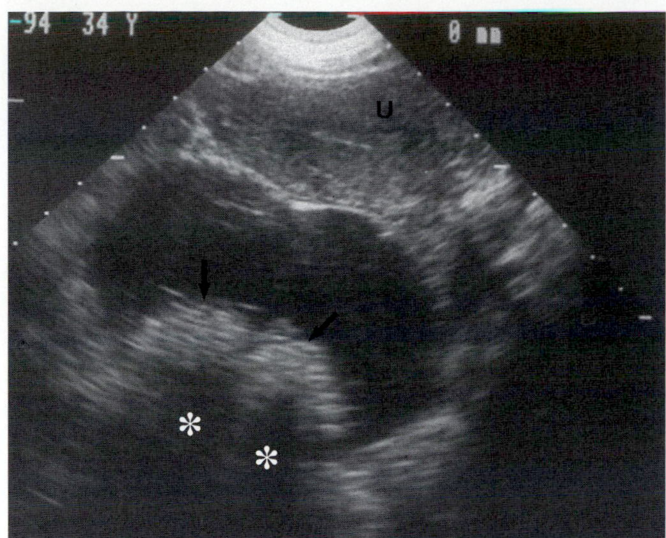

FIGURE 99–3. Ovarian teratoma. Pelvis. Transabdominal examination. Transverse plane. The uterus (U) is seen anteriorly, with its contained endometrial cavity echogenicity. Posterior and to the right of the uterus is a mass that is predominantly cystic and contains a bilobed, highly echogenic component (*arrows*) with posterior shadowing (asterisk). The classic ultrasound image of a teratoma is one in which there is a cystic mass with at least one highly echogenic mural nodule (also known as a dermoid plug). Contained teeth were responsible for this teratoma's mass with shadowing. The shadowing is a good example of how some of the teratoma's contents may obscure other portions of the mass.

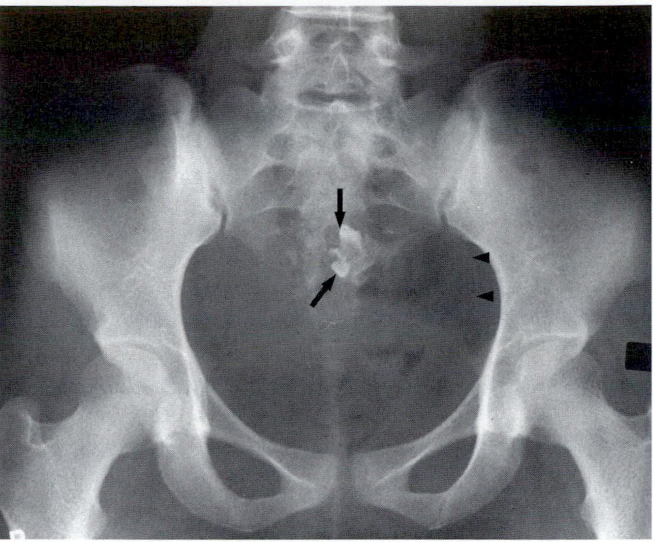

FIGURE 99–4. Ovarian teratoma containing teeth. Plain film of the pelvis. Teeth (*arrows*) are seen overlying a teenager's sacrum. This is pathognomonic for teratoma, if the child hasn't swallowed teeth recently. The radiolucent area (*arrowhead*) lateral to the teeth helps denote the fatty contents of the teratoma and confirm the diagnosis. It may, however, be simulated by air within bowel. (*From Cohen HL, Haller JO: Pediatric and adolescent genital abnormalities.* Clin Diagn Ultrasound *24:187–216, 1988, with permission.*)

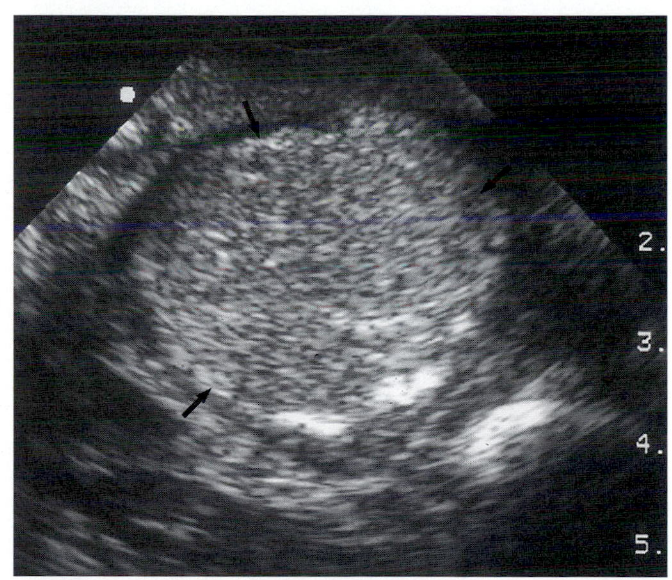

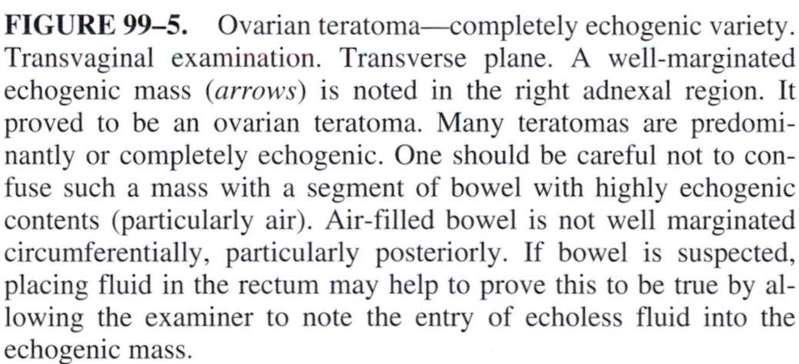

FIGURE 99–5. Ovarian teratoma—completely echogenic variety. Transvaginal examination. Transverse plane. A well-marginated echogenic mass (*arrows*) is noted in the right adnexal region. It proved to be an ovarian teratoma. Many teratomas are predominantly or completely echogenic. One should be careful not to confuse such a mass with a segment of bowel with highly echogenic contents (particularly air). Air-filled bowel is not well marginated circumferentially, particularly posteriorly. If bowel is suspected, placing fluid in the rectum may help to prove this to be true by allowing the examiner to note the entry of echoless fluid into the echogenic mass.

ance shows a prominent cystic component (Fig. 99-3) and at least one contained mural nodule (dermoid plug), which is often echogenic due to contained fat, hair, sebum, or calcium (e.g., teeth or bone). The contained teeth (Fig. 99-4) and bone and perhaps other components may cause posterior shadowing of the sound beam. The shadowing may obscure deeper portions of the mass. This phenomenon has been termed the "tip of the iceberg" sign. The anechoic component of teratomas is made up of serous fluid or sebum, which is in a fluid state when at body temperature. Fat–fluid levels and hair–fluid levels may be seen as part of the cystic component of the mass. Echogenic fat may float on top of the cystic component, or, as in Fig. 99-1, echogenic particulate matter may be the dependent component of a fluid debris level.

Two-thirds of teratomas are sonographically complex cysts, with anechoic, hypoechoic, and echogenic components. It is claimed that one-third of cases are either purely echoless (perhaps because the solid component is at the mass's periphery and not imaged) or purely echogenic (Fig. 99-5). We have seen many purely echogenic ovarian teratomas but none, as yet, that were purely cystic. Occasionally, the cystic component of a teratoma may be so large or

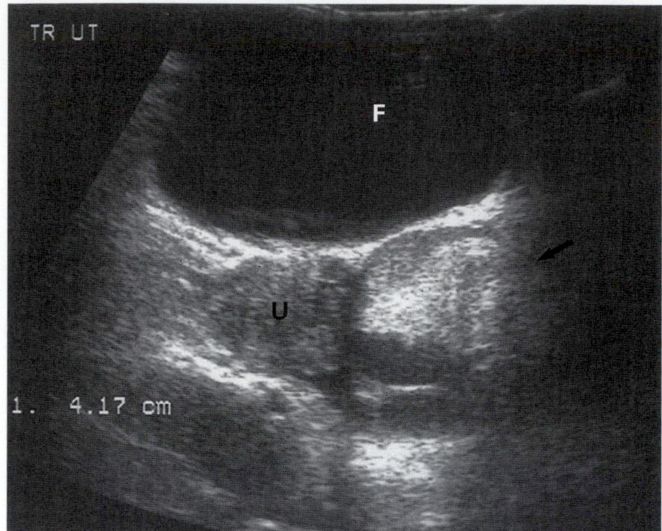

FIGURE 99–6. Ovarian teratoma—cystic component simulating bladder. Transabdominal examination. Transverse plane. A highly echogenic mass (*arrow*) is seen to the left of the uterus (U). A teratoma was diagnosed, apparently posterior to a fluid-filled (F) bladder. However, physical examination revealed an adolescent who appeared pregnant. What appeared to be bladder proved to be a small portion of a 17-cm-long ovarian teratoma's cystic component.

so positioned that it may simulate the bladder (Fig. 99-6), or may extend beyond the pelvis and have its size underestimated or its contained echogenic components missed. Correct US diagnosis requires knowledge of the variable appearance of the teratoma and knowledge of possible pitfalls in diagnosis, including imaging simulators.

A Turkish study of 943 women with 1095 adnexal masses, including 147 pathologically proven dermoids, found US to be 94 percent sensitive, 98 percent accurate, and 99 percent specific for differentiating mature and benign teratomas from other adnexal masses. The US findings used for the accurate diagnosis of teratomas were an echogenic mass with or without acoustic enhancement (consistent with sebum with lipophilic contaminants or hair), a dermoid plug (Fig. 99-3), layered lines, a fat–fluid level (Fig. 99-2), isolated bright echoes with acoustic shadowing within a complex mass, hair in low-viscosity fluid (Fig. 99-7; see also Color Plate 26), contained teeth or bone fragments, or an intraovarian echogenic mass (Fig. 99-2) with or without shadowing or enhancement (evidence of an intraovarian dermoid cyst).

Classic benign teratomas do not look like malignant teratomas. In analyzing ovarian masses for malignancy, noting an ovarian mass that is purely cystic or one that has a markedly echogenic component suggests that it is benign. A lack of ascites helps assure this.

TECHNICAL ASPECTS OF OVARIAN TERATOMA DIAGNOSIS BY ULTRASOUND

As for any pelvic mass, routine transabdominal imaging in orthogonal planes should be performed. Follow the cystic component to its most superior extent. Evaluate the contents at the periphery of the mass. Occasionally transvaginal (TV) examinations will help better evaluate the echogenic components of a teratoma. The TV exam may denote individual bright linear echogenicities within the echogenic component of the mass, denoting individual hairs or groups of hair strands (Fig. 99-7).

Doppler evaluation has not been needed for the diagnosis. One group noted that ovarian teratomas have no internal blood flow, but one-fourth of cases have evident flow to the teratoma's periphery/capsule. This group warns examiners to be concerned about malignancy when vascularized soft tissue is found within a cystic teratoma.

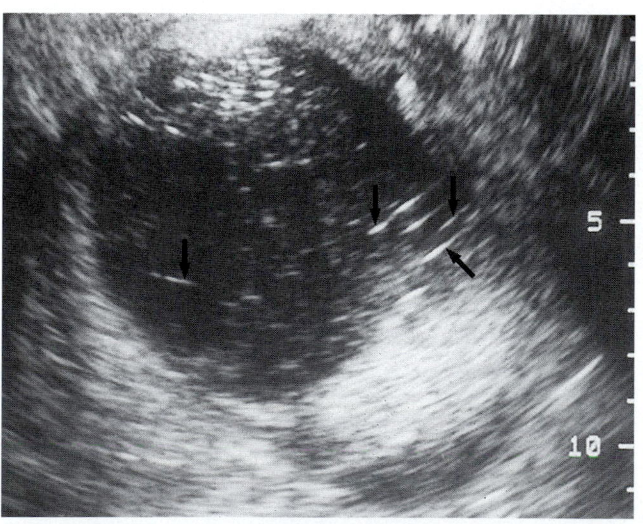

A

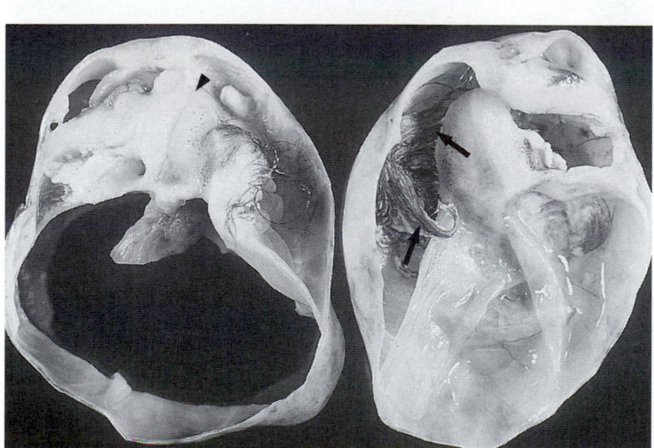

B

FIGURE 99–7. Ovarian teratoma containing hair. ***A.*** Transvaginal examination. Longitudinal plane. A mass with highly echogenic and cystic components typical of cystic teratoma is seen. Bright linear echogenicities (*arrows*) within the mass are consistent with individual strands of hair. Hair, as a component of a teratoma, can be seen on transabdominal examination as well, but its separation from the other components of the echogenic portion of the mass is sometimes improved with the transvaginal technique. ***B.*** Pathology specimen. This is the cut specimen of an adolescent's teratoma. Hair (*arrows*) is noted within it, as are solid tissue (which proved to be cerebellar in histologic type) and sebaceous material (*arrowhead*). One can see how US could image individual hair strands. At least half of this mass is cystic. (See Color Plate 26.)

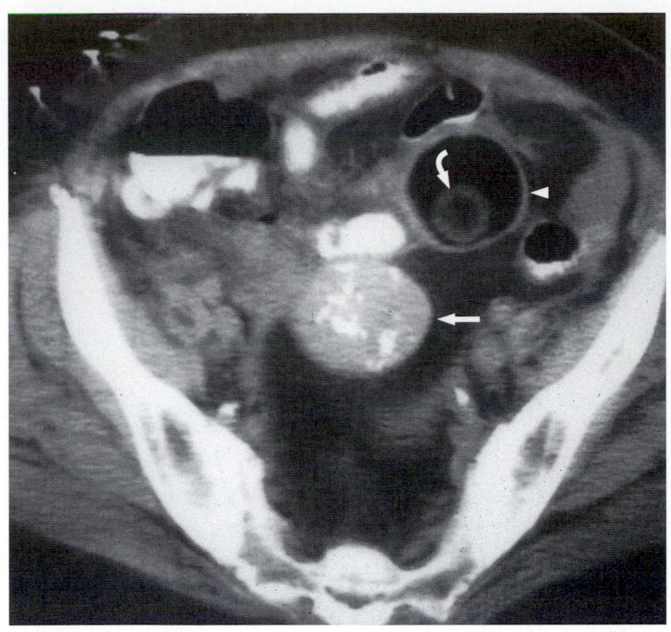

FIGURE 99–8. Ovarian teratoma. Computed tomography examination. Transverse plane through upper pelvis. A calcified myoma (*arrow*) is seen in this young adult's pelvis. A teratoma (*arrowhead*) containing fat (which appears black on this image, consistent with a density almost as low as that of nearby bowel gas) and a contained mural nodule (*curved arrow*) are noted. The fat content of the mass was confirmed by very negative Hounsfield unit numbers (i.e., –600).

DO TERATOMAS IN CHILDREN DIFFER FROM THOSE IN ADOLESCENTS AND YOUNG ADULTS?

One report noted that dermoids in postpubertal girls contain more mural nodules than those in younger girls (70 percent vs. 40 percent) and produce more shadowing (70 percent vs. 15 percent). This might suggest that these are different tumors. However, it is known that teratomas that have not been operated on can change their appearance over time, e.g., two teeth that were bicuspid-like in one decade may appear as molars a decade later. The reported difference between the prepubertal and postpubertal groups may simply be due to the evolving nature of the neoplasm based on its contained germ-cell-layer components.

THE USE OF OTHER MODALITIES IN THE DIAGNOSIS OF OVARIAN TERATOMA

Years ago, when the US images of ovarian teratomas were less well known, we would often order a plain film to cement our diagnosis, looking for either the radiolucency of contained fat or the radiodensity of contained calcification (bone or teeth) (Fig. 99-4). That is no longer necessary in our US laboratory. However, it is a useful option to have if necessary. Computed tomography (CT) (Fig. 99-8) can certainly detect the classic presence of fat within a dermoid. The imaging diagnosis of the teratoma by CT or magnetic resonance imaging (MRI) can be based on the presence of a dermoid plug (or Rokitansky protuberance) with contained fat or calcium within the teratoma's cystic component. This finding is better made by CT than by MRI, which has difficulty imaging calcification. The imaging diagnosis is best made by US.

SIMULATORS OF THE ULTRASOUND IMAGE OF OVARIAN TERATOMAS

Hemorrhagic cysts may initially be so echogenic as to simulate the echogenic component of a teratoma or create a simulating fluid/fluid layer. "Tincture of time" (a 6-week follow-up) will help denote the difference. The dermoid will not change over those 6 weeks. A teratoma may be simulated by echogenic bowel in the posterior pelvis. Homogeneously echogenic teratomas are sharply marginated around their entire periphery, while the posterior border of air-filled echogenic bowel is usually not sharp because of its contained air and its reflection and refraction of sound.

References

Brown DL, Doubilet PM, Miller FH, et al: Benign and malignant *ovarian* masses: Selection of the most discriminating gray-scale and Doppler sonographic features. *Radiology* 208:103–110, 1998.

Caspi B, Appelman Z, Rabinerson D, et al: The growth pattern of ovarian dermoid cysts: A prospective study in premenopausal and postmenopausal women. *Fertil Steril* 68:501–505, 1997.

Cohen HL, Bober S, Bow S: Imaging the pediatric pelvis: The normal and abnormal genital tract and simulators of its diseases. *Urol Radiol* 14:273–283, 1992.

Cohen HL, Haller JO: Pediatric and adolescent genital abnormalities. *Clin Diagn Ultrasound* 24:187–216, 1988.

Ekici E, Soysal M, Kara S, et al: The efficiency of ultrasonography in the diagnosis of dermoid cysts. *Zentralbl Gynakol* 118: 136–141, 1996.

Guinet C, Ghossain M, Buy JN, et al: Mature cystic teratomas of the ovary: CT and MR findings. *Eur J Radiol* 20:137–143, 1995.

Hertzberg B, Kliewer M: Sonography of benign cystic teratoma of the ovary: Pitfalls in diagnosis. *AJR* 167:1127–1133, 1996.

Kurjak A, Kupesic S, Babic MM, et al: Preoperative evaluation of cystic teratoma: What does color Doppler add? *JCU* 25: 309–316, 1997.

Ruggiero-Dellliturri M, Awobuluyi M, Cohen HL, Zinn D: Imaging the pediatric pelvis: Role of ultrasound. *Radiologist* 4:155–170, 1997.

Siegel M: Female pelvis, in *Pediatric Sonography,* 2d ed, Siegel M (ed). New York, Raven, 1995:446–449.

Sisler C, Siegel M: Ovarian teratomas: A comparison of the sonographic appearance in prepubertal and postpubertal girls. *AJR* 154:139–141, 1990.

Zalel Y, Caspi B, Tepper R: Doppler flow characteristics of dermoid cysts: Unique appearance of struma ovarii. *J Ultrasound Med* 16:355–358, 1997.

100

A 23-month-old girl presented with signs of precocious puberty and lower abdominal pain and was sent for ultrasound (US) evaluation. Figures 100-1 and 100-2 were obtained during that study. What do you see? What is the diagnosis?

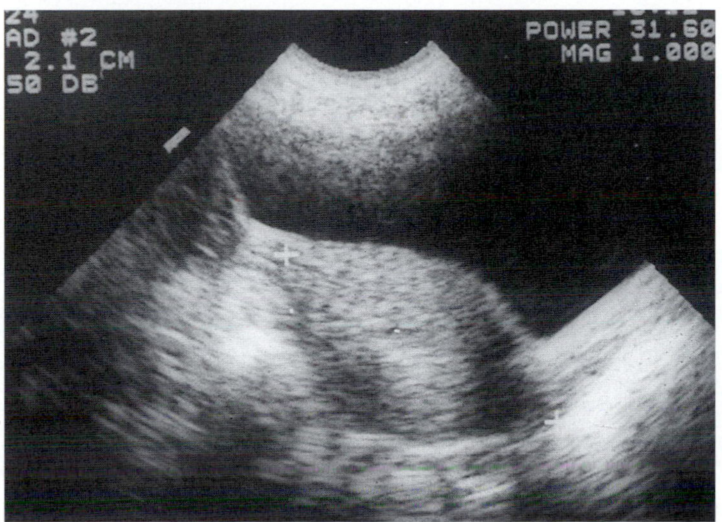

FIGURE 100–1. Pelvis. Longitudinal plane through midline.

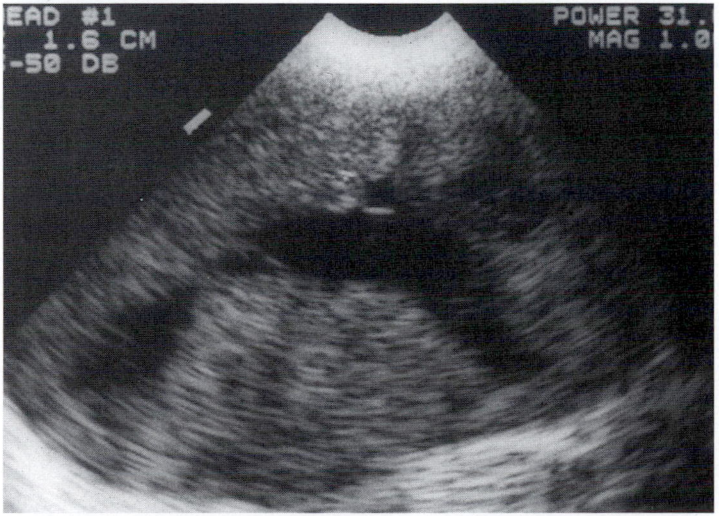

FIGURE 100–2. Pelvis. Longitudinal plane through right adnexal region.

CHAPTER 100

Granulosa Cell Tumor of the Ovary

HARRIS L. COHEN AND DAVID L. WELLS

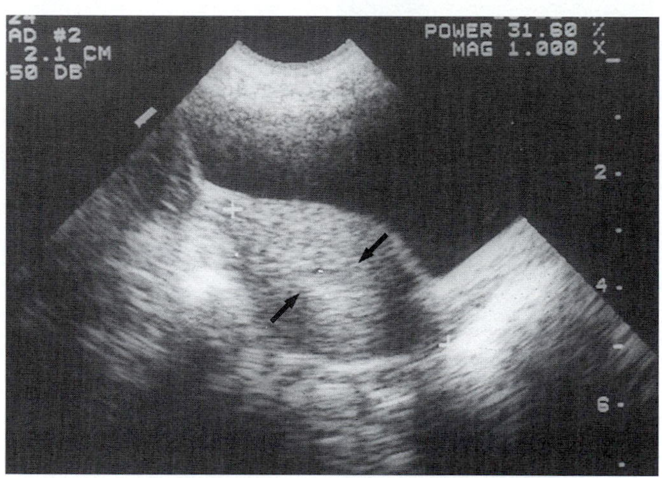

FIGURE 100–3. Annotated version of Fig. 100-1. Enlarged, adult-shaped uterus. Pelvis. Longitudinal plane through midline. A wide and long (4.2 cm) uterus is abnormal for a child. A prominent endometrial cavity (*arrows*) is not sharply defined on this image. These findings were consistent with the significant estrogenization and precocious puberty noted in this 23-month-old girl, who had a granulosa cell tumor of the ovary.

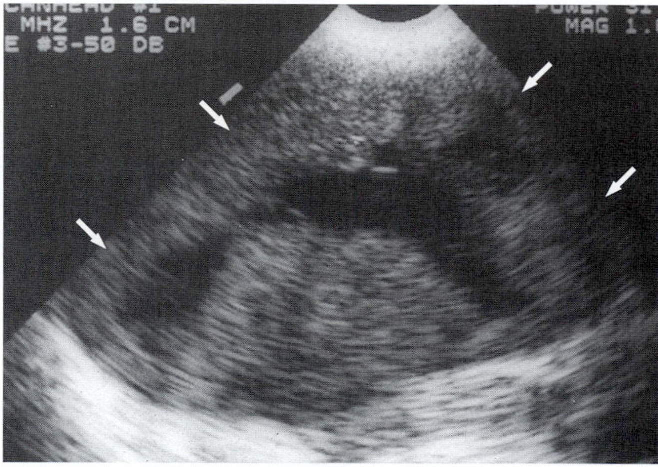

FIGURE 100–4. Annotated version of Fig. 100-2. Pelvis. Longitudinal plane through right adnexal region. A large solid tumor (*arrows*) with echopenic central areas due to necrosis is seen. This is the granulosa cell tumor. It was much larger than the normal-sized left adnexa.

Figure 100-3, the annotated version of Fig. 100-1, shows an adult-shaped uterus in a child. Figure 100-4, the annotated version of Fig. 100-2, shows a heterogeneous, predominantly solid ovarian mass. The ovarian tumor most likely to cause precocious puberty and estrogenization in a girl is the granulosa cell tumor, which this proved to be. It was malignant.

OVARIAN TUMORS IN CHILDREN

In children, a unilaterally enlarged ovary without contained cysts may represent a neoplasm. Ovarian tumors are uncommon in children. Some 60 percent are of germ cell origin. Of the germ cell tumors, 70 percent are teratomas, 25 percent are dysgerminomas, and 5 percent are endodermal sinus (Fig. 100-5) or yolk sac tumors. One-fifth of pediatric ovarian tumors are epithelial cell in origin, including cystadenoma (80 percent) and cystadenocarcinoma (10 percent). The final 10 percent of pediatric ovarian tumors are sex cord tumors or tumors of stromal/mesenchymal origin. Of those, 15 percent are arrhenoblastomas and 75 percent are granulosa theca cell tumors. Granulosa theca cell tumors are the most common ovarian cause of isosexual precocious puberty.

Overall, one-third of ovarian neoplasms in children are malignant. This percentage, however, decreases as a child's age increases. A greater percentage, as many as half, of hor-

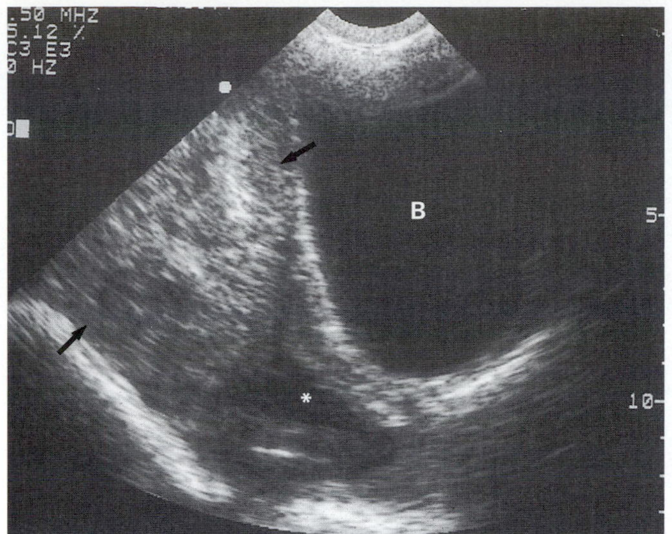

FIGURE 100–5. Endodermal sinus tumor. Pelvis. Longitudinal plane. There was some free fluid in the peritoneum (*asterisk*) of this teenager with a large solid but heterogeneous mass whose lowermost portion is seen posterior to the bladder (*arrows*). The mass was malignant. B = bladder.

monally active tumors, often granulosa cell tumors, are malignant. Of the malignant lesions, 85 percent are germ cell tumors (dysgerminoma, immature teratoma, endodermal sinus tumor, embryonal cell carcinoma, and choriocarcinoma), 10 percent are stromal (Sertoli-Leydig cell, granulosa theca cell, and undifferentiated neoplasms), and 5 percent are epithelial cell tumors (serous and mucinous adenocarcinoma).

Noting the uncommonness of ovarian tumors compared to other causes of a noncystic ovarian mass, Wu and Siegel, in a review of 70 such masses in girls ranging in age from neonate to late adolescence, found 18 complex masses, of which 7 were hemorrhagic cysts (3 predominantly cystic and 4 predominantly solid in appearance), 5 were teratomas, 5 were tuboovarian abscesses, and only 1 was a malignant dysgerminoma. Of solid-appearing adnexal masses, 2 were torsed ovaries, 3 were echo-filled hemorrhagic cysts, and 3 were neoplasms (2 teratomas and 1 dysgerminoma).

ULTRASOUND IMAGING OF PEDIATRIC OVARIAN TUMORS—WHAT SHOULD I WORRY ABOUT?

In order to diagnose a solitary enlarged adnexa that may be due to pelvic inflammatory disease (salpingo-oophoritis) or neoplasm, one can readily compare the ovary of concern to its contralateral mate. If the contralateral ovary is not imaged or if one is worried about an ovary's size, one must again remember that previous reports that the mean volume of the normal adult ovary is 3 cm^3 have been replaced by the knowledge that normal ovarian volume ranges between 0.2 and 4.9 cm^3 in the first decade of life, and between 1.7 and 18.5 cm^3 in the second decade. Menstruating females have a 95 percent confidence interval for ovarian volumes of between 2.5 and 21.9 cm^3. Again, we begin to be concerned enough to follow an ovary at 15 cm^3, and we consider ovaries enlarged at 20 cm^3 or greater.

Malignant tumors in postpubertal girls are usually large in size, often as great as or greater than 15 cm in longest length by the time they are discovered. On US imaging, they are predominantly solid, with contained areas of necrosis. While coarse calcifications are typical of the malignant teratoma, stippled calcifications can be seen in the dysgerminoma. Endodermal sinus tumors typically have both echogenic and hypoechoic components. They grow rapidly, and patients often present because of abdominal pain, occasionally including pain due to torsion or rupture of the tumor. When predominantly cystic masses are imaged, contained papillary projections or signs of capsular invasion are worrisome as indicators of malignancy. Serous cystadenocarcinoma, a more common adult ovarian malignant neoplasm, with its typically multiseptated cystic appearance, is rarely noted before puberty and is uncommon in adolescence. Malignant ovarian tumors may metastasize by direct extension to adjacent structures or by hematogenous or lymphangitic spread to more distant locations. Findings beyond the ovary—i.e., significant ascites, pelvic fixation, or distant metastases—can underline concern that a given ovarian mass is malignant and probably metastatic. Computed tomography (CT) and magnetic resonance imaging (MRI) provide a more global analysis of the mass and its relationship to its surrounding tissues. Both CT and MRI are superior to US for tumor staging and allow a global view for lymphadenopathy, as well as peritoneal (Fig. 100-6) and omental metastases, all indicators of malignancy. Common sites for distal parenchymal metastases are the liver and lung.

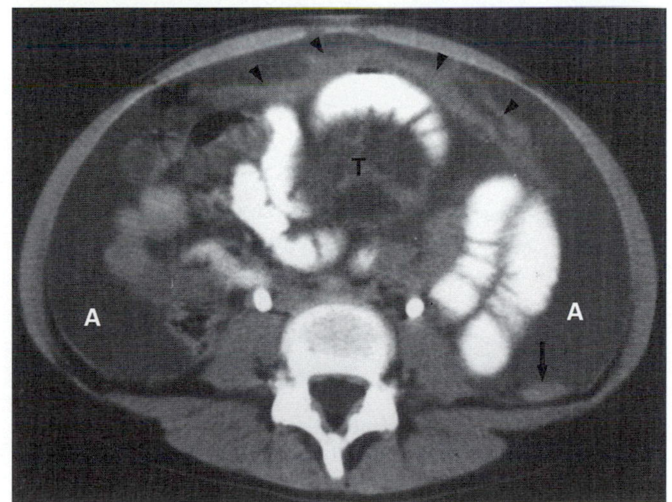

FIGURE 100–6. Endodermal sinus tumor with metastatic spread. Computed tomography. Transverse plane, lower abdomen. The most superior extension of the endodermal sinus tumor (T) of Fig. 100-5 is seen. There is significant ascites (A), omental caking (*arrowheads*), and a peritoneal metastatic nodule (*arrow*). Findings were consistent with significant metastatic spread of tumor in an 8-year-old girl. (*From Cohen HL, Bober S, Bow S: Imaging the pediatric pelvis: The normal and abnormal genital tract and simulators of its diseases.* Urol Radiol *14:273–283, 1992, with permission.*)

TUMORS ASSOCIATED WITH ENDOCRINE FUNCTION—A POSSIBLE CAUSE OF AMENORRHEA

Only 1 in 20 ovarian tumors has functional endocrine activity. Testosterone is the most potent of the circulating androgens. It is produced in normal females by the adrenal (25 percent) and the ovary (25 percent) and by peripheral conversion of Δ^4-androstenedione (50 percent). Only 1 percent is typically free and biologically active. Excess androgen production will cause virilization, resulting in voice deepening, clitoromegaly, increased muscle mass, and temporal balding. Increased free testosterone may be seen in virilizing tumors of the adolescent ovary, usually due to Sertoli-Leydig cell tumors (once known as androblastomas or arrhenoblastomas) or hilar cell tumors. The marked androgen production of these solid, most predominantly unilateral, and rapidly growing tumors results in defeminization, with amenorrhea, vaginal mucosal atrophy, and decreased breast size as well as virilization. Ultrasound will show unilateral enlargement, with abnormal adnexal echogenicity. This is a rare cause of amenorrhea.

The most common malignant tumor is the estrogen-producing granulosa cell tumor (Fig. 100-7). These tumors grow rapidly and often disrupt the normal menstrual cycles of adolescents, producing amenorrhea or menorrhagia. Thecomas, which account for 2 to 3 percent of all ovarian tumors, can also produce significant amounts of estrogen.

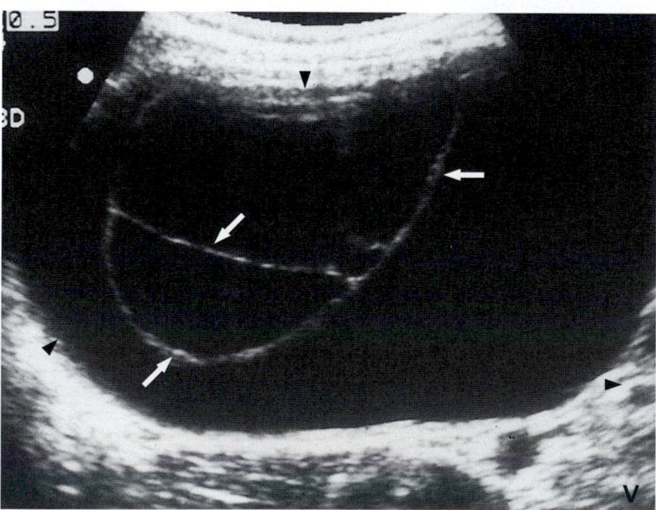

FIGURE 100–7. Granulosa theca cell tumor. Abdomen. Transverse plane. A large, predominantly cystic mass (*arrowheads*) with contained septations (*arrows*), more typical of a cystadenoma, was seen extending from the pelvis and into the abdomen of this adolescent. When tumors are large, their area of origin may not be clearly defined. This teenager had a granulosa cell tumor of the ovary. The tumor was hormonally active (estrogen-producing), and the patient presented with both a mass and secondary amenorrhea. V = vertebral body. (*From Ruggiero-Dellitурri M, Awobuluyi M, Cohen HL, Zinn D: Imaging the pediatric pelvis: Role of ultrasound.* Radiologist *4:155–170, 1997, with permission.*)

TWO OTHER TUMORS TO BE AWARE OF

Rare solid ovarian fibromas may be associated with ascites or pleural effusion in Meigs' syndrome. The US image is variable, from anechoic to solid and calcified. If the mass is bilateral and calcified, the ovarian involvement may be part of the basal cell nevus syndrome, with its associated multiple basal cell carcinomas, as well as mandibular cyst and rib anomalies.

Ovarian enlargement, symmetric or asymmetric, in a child with a history of leukemia may reflect leukemic infiltration of the ovary. With better treatment of the central nervous system and bone marrow sanctuary sites in leukemia, the gonads (ovary or testes) have become a key site of potential leukemic recurrence.

References

Athey P, Malone R: Sonography of ovarian fibromas/thecomas. *J Ultrasound Med* 6:431–436, 1987.

Cohen HL: The female pelvis, in *Syllabus: Current Concepts: A Categorical Course in Pediatric Radiology,* Siebert J (ed). Chicago, RSNA Publications, 1994:65–72.

Cohen HL: Evaluation of the adolescent and young adult with amenorrhea: Role of US, in *Syllabus: A Special Course in Ultrasound: Clinical Questions, Practical Answers*, Bluth E, Arger P, Hertzberg B, Middleton W (eds). Oak Brook, IL, RSNA Publications, 1996:171–184.

Cohen HL, Haller JO: Pediatric and adolescent genital abnormalities. *Clin Diagn Ultrasound* 24:187–216, 1988.

Cohen HL, Tice H, Mandel F: Ovarian volumes measured by US: Bigger than we think. *Radiology* 177:189–192, 1990.

Comstock C: Fetal masses: Ultrasound diagnosis and evaluation. *Ultrasound Quart* 6:229–256, 1988.

Emans S, Goldstein D: Delayed puberty and menstrual irregularities, in *Pediatric and Adolescent Gynecology,* 3d ed, Emans S, Goldstein D (eds). Boston, Little, Brown, 1990:149–242.

Grimes C, Rosenbaum D, Kirkpatrick J Jr: Pediatric gynecologic radiology. *Semin Roentgenol* 17:284–301, 1982.

Lane D, Birdwell R: Ovarian leukemia detected by pelvic sonography. A case report. *Cancer* 58:2338–2342, 1986.

Larsen W, Felmar E, Wallace M, Frieder R: Sertoli-Leydig cell tumor of the ovary: A rare cause of amenorrhea. *Obstet Gynecol* 79:831–833, 1992.

Levitin A, Haller K, Cohen HL, et al: Endodermal sinus tumor of the ovary: Imaging evaluation. *AJR* 167:791–793, 1996.

Ruggiero-Delliturri M, Awobuluyi M, Cohen HL, Zinn D: Imaging the pediatric pelvis: Role of ultrasound. *Radiologist* 4:155–170, 1997.

Siegel M, Surratt J: Pediatric gynecologic imaging. *Obstet Gynecol Clin North Am* 19:103–127, 1992.

Surratt J, Siegel M: Imaging of pediatric ovarian masses. *Radiographics* 11:533–548, 1991.

Wu A, Siegel M: Sonography of pelvic masses in children: Diagnostic predictability. *AJR* 148:1199–1202, 1987.

101

A 13-year-old awoke suddenly with left lower quadrant pain. An emergency ultrasound (US) exam revealed the cause. Figure 101-1 is one of the study's images. She is not pregnant. What does she have? Would Doppler help?

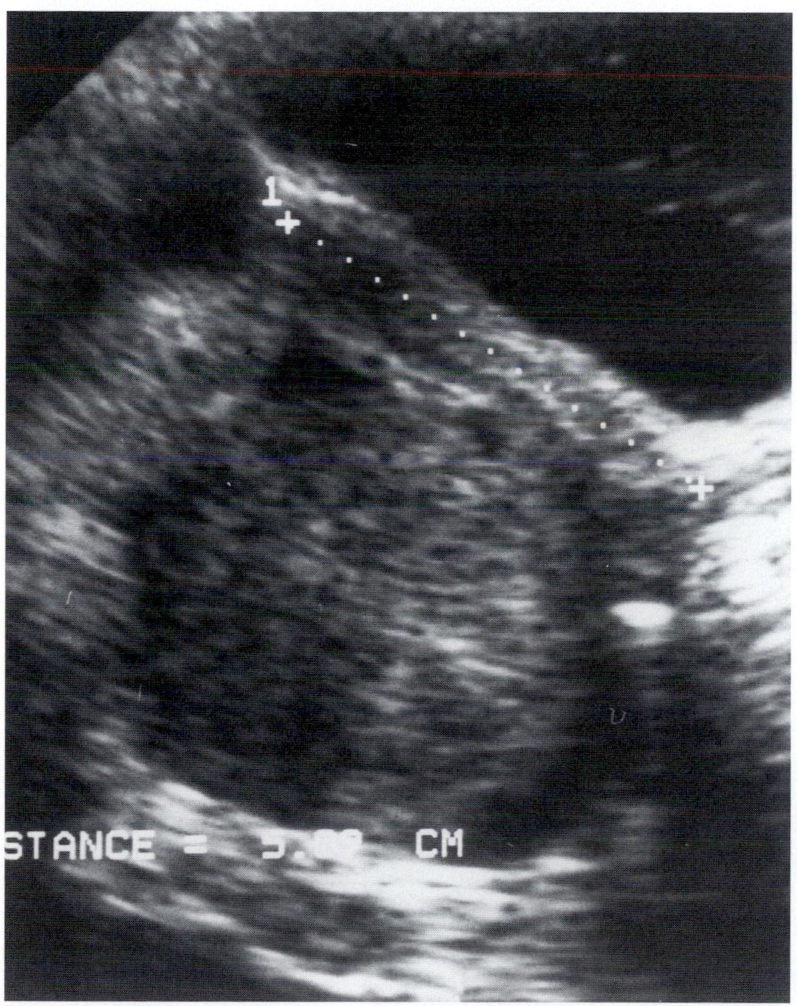

FIGURE 101–1. Pelvis. Longitudinal plane. The uterus is marked off by measurement points.

CHAPTER 101

Ovarian Torsion

HARRIS L. COHEN AND YAIR I. SAFRIEL

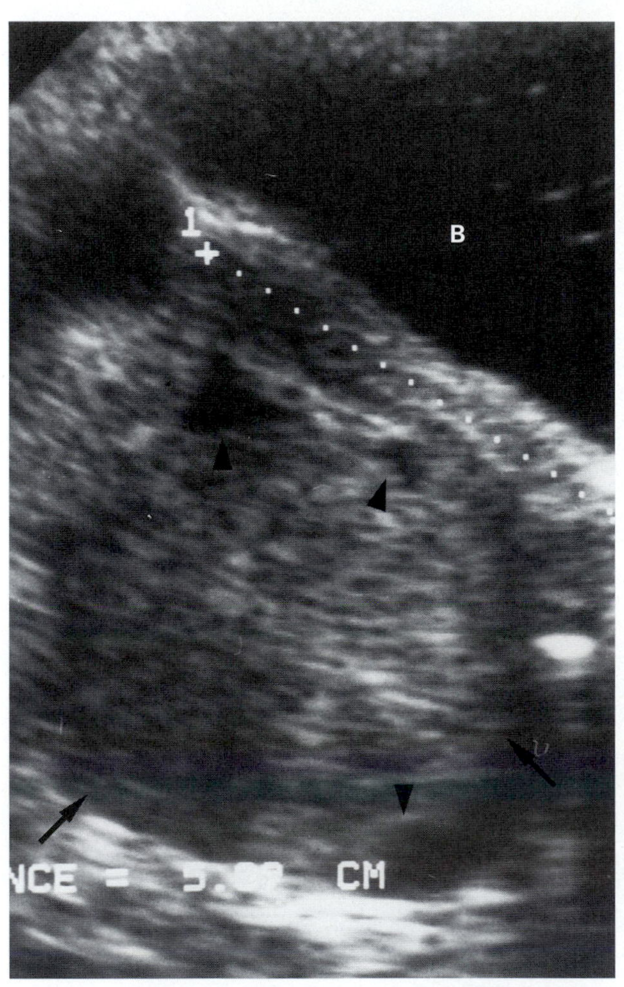

FIGURE 101–2. Annotated version of Fig. 101-1. Ovarian torsion. Pelvis. Longitudinal plane. The uterus is marked off by measurement points. It is 5 cm in length. Posterior to it is a large solid mass (*arrows*) with a few peripheral cysts (*arrowheads*). This is a relatively classic image for ovarian torsion, although the echogenicity of the ultrasound image is related to the variable internal contents of the torsed ovary. This mass, which is the patient's torsed left adnexa, was much larger than the patient's normal right adnexa. B = bladder.

Figure 101-2, the annotated version of Fig. 101-1, shows an enlarged solid mass posterior to the uterus. Its volume was noted to be greater than 100 cm^3. Some peripheral cysts are seen within it. More were seen on other views. The patient's right ovary was normal in size. No left adnexa other than this mass was imaged. This mass, particularly in light of the history, is a torsed ovary.

WHAT IS OVARIAN TORSION? CLINICAL INFORMATION

Ovarian torsion is an uncommon but important cause of abdominal pain in the first three decades of life. It is caused by partial or complete rotation of the ovary on its pedicle, compromising first lymphatic, then venous, and finally arterial flow. It is rare before menarche but common in the immediate postmenarchal years. It is more common in patients with cysts (Fig. 101-3) or other ovarian or paraovarian masses (Fig. 101-4). Historically, the diagnosis has been made surgically. The affected patients' symptoms may simulate gastroenteritis, appendicitis, intussusception, or any other acute abdominal disorder in the child or adolescent. There is often acute pain. The patient may be awakened from sleep. Associated complaints of nausea, vomiting, or constipation may occur and mislead the clinician. Fever is rare. This fact can help differentiate right-sided torsion from classical cases of appendicitis. In contrast to appendicitis, the pain is sharp and localized immediately. At least half of affected patients claim prior bouts of such pain. Prompt diagnosis and surgical detorsion can help avoid irreversible damage to the ovary.

Ovaries involved in torsion have a variable appearance that is related to the degree of internal hemorrhage, stromal edema, and infarction. The ovaries may appear cystic (Fig. 101-5), cystic with septations, cystic with a debris layer (Fig. 101-6), or complex with mixed solid and cystic components, as well as solid (Fig. 101-2). Each of these images may suggest its own list of differential diagnostic considerations. One

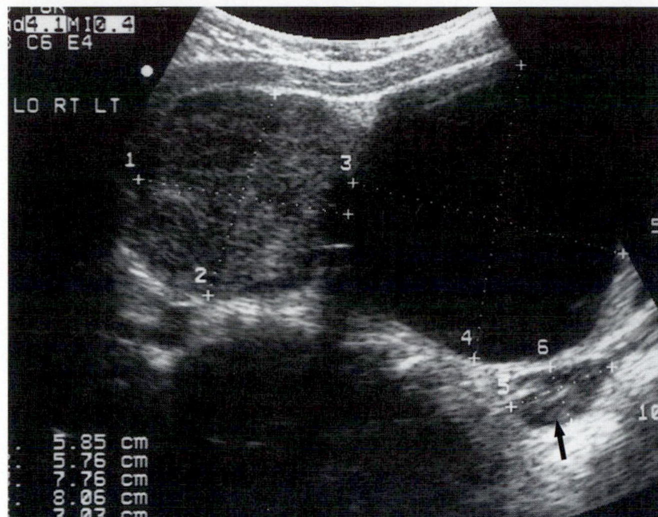

FIGURE 101–3. Ovarian torsion—functional cyst. Transabdominal pelvic examination. Angled right parasagittal plane. A very large, surgically proven torsed right ovary is made up of a large solid component of ovarian parenchyma (measurements 1 and 2) and a large cystic component consisting of a physiologic cyst (measurements 3 and 4). The angulation required to obtain the entire image of the torsed right adnexa allows imaging of the normal contralateral left adnexa (measurements 5 and 6). The difference in size is obvious. (*From Ruggiero-Delliturri M, Awobuluyi M, Cohen HL, Zinn D: Imaging the pediatric pelvis: Role of ultrasound.* Radiologist *4:155–170, 1997, with permission.*)

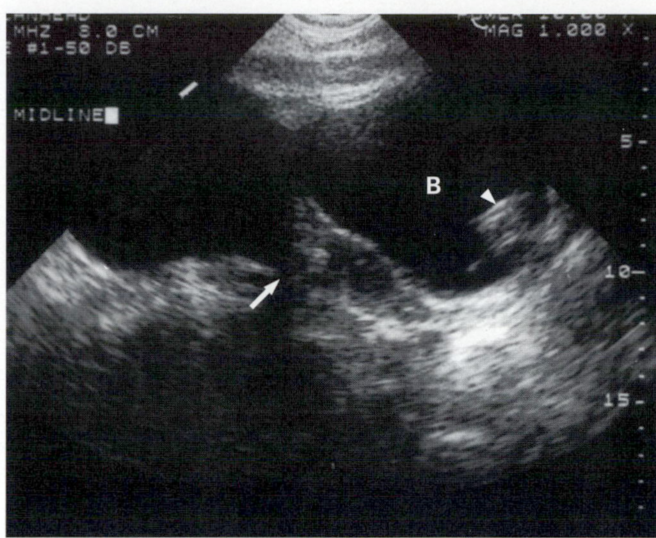

FIGURE 101–5. Ovarian torsion—functional cyst. Transabdominal pelvic ultrasound. Longitudinal midline plane. A cystic mass with a small amount of contained debris and a somewhat pointed inferior margin (*arrow*) was symptomatic and very large. The patient had a torsed noninvoluted functional cyst seen at surgery. B = Bladder with contained foley catheter (*arrowhead*).

relatively specific sonographic image noted in 7 of 11 cases reported by Graif and Itzchak showed a unilaterally enlarged solid ovary with multiple peripheral (i.e., cortical zone) follicles. Figure 101-1 is an example of this. An important point to remember is that a torsed ovary is *much* larger than a normal ovary. Ovarian volumes of 150 to 400 cm^3 are often measured. One group noted the volumes of the torsed ovaries to be 3.2 to 24 times greater than the volumes of the unaffected ovaries.

DOPPLER IN THE DIAGNOSIS OF OVARIAN TORSION—CAN IT HELP?

Historically, color Doppler was of limited reliability in the analysis of ovarian torsion. This is because Doppler signal may be difficult to obtain even in normal ovaries. Even when

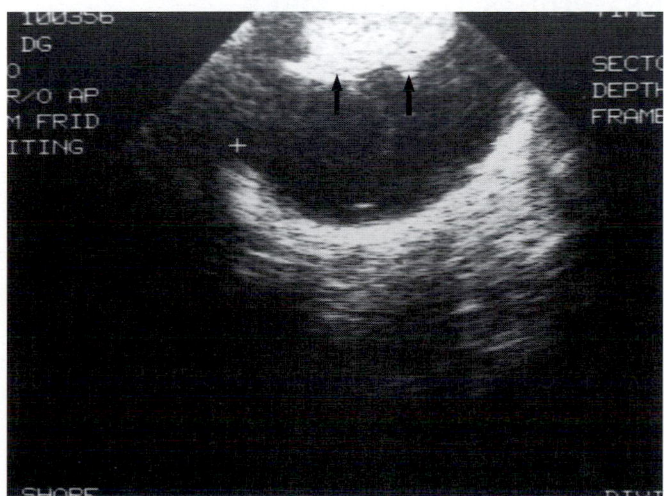

FIGURE 101–4. Ovarian torsion—teratoma. Transabdominal pelvic ultrasound. Longitudinal plane through right side. This patient was awakened from sleep by right lower quadrant pain, began vomiting, and was sent from the emergency room for US to "rule out appendicitis." A large solid mass is seen. The highly echogenic component seen superficially (*arrows*) within the mass is the echogenic fat of this torsed ovarian teratoma.

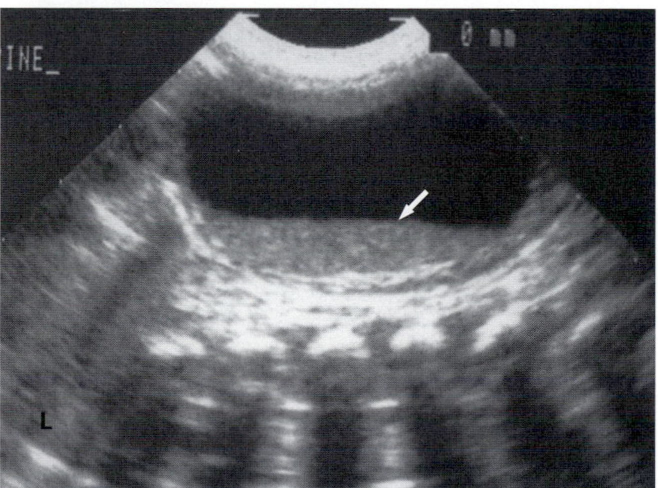

FIGURE 101–6. Torsed ovary, probably of fetal origin. Longitudinal plane through palpated right-sided abdominopelvic mass of a newborn. A hemorrhagic debris/fluid layer (*arrow*) is noted in the mass. Hemorrhage within the cystic mass, particularly in a newborn, suggests a torsion of the ovary that occurred in fetal life.

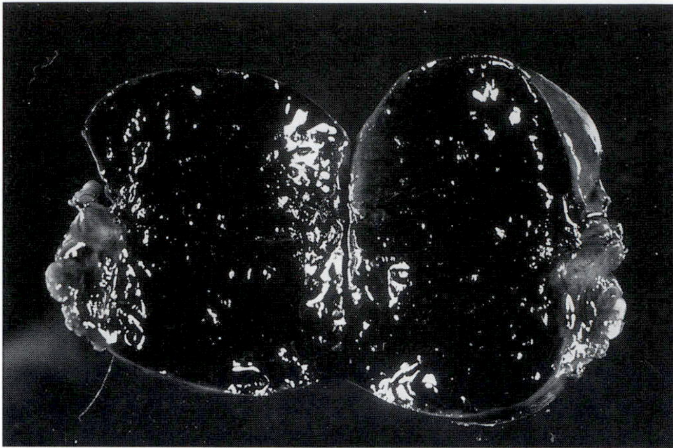

FIGURE 101–7. Necrotic ovary. Pathology specimen. The contents of this torsed ovary consist of clot. The parenchyma was necrotic. (*From Cohen HL, Haller JO: Pediatric and adolescent genital abnormalities.* Clin Diagn Ultrasound *24:187–216, 1988, with permission.*)

color flow is determined, there are well-documented cases of ovaries that have had peripheral and even central arterial flow found within them and yet have been proven to be torsed. Various groups have reported on their successes with color Doppler, particularly for determining ovarian viability. One group notes that an assurance of viability can be made by imaging only central *venous* flow in a torsed ovary. A Korean group reported an 87 percent diagnostic accuracy for determining viability by verifying blood flow changes at the twisted vascular pedicle itself. This may not be as simple as it sounds. Their patients with no blood flow at the twisted pedicle had necrotic ovaries (Fig. 101-7). Of 11 cases with flow at the twist, 10 were not necrotic. All 5 of that group's ovaries that were untwisted were saved.

Detorsion or removal of a mass (e.g., cystectomy) that causes a torsion will, it is hoped, save the gonad and preserve its function. The time from clinical complaint to diagnosis and therapy is a large factor in this, and US analysis with or without Doppler is certainly time-efficient.

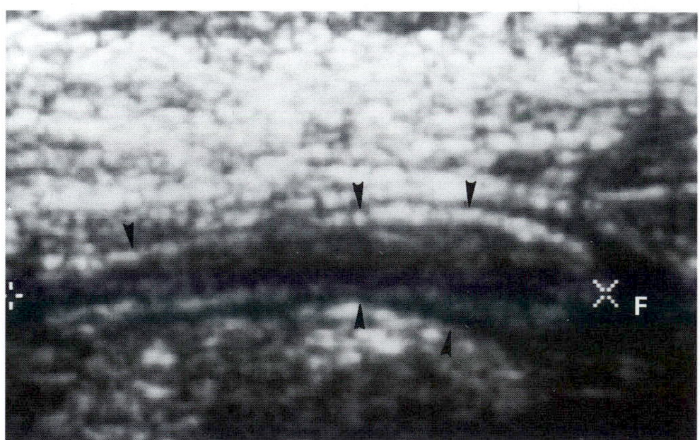

FIGURE 101–8. Appendicitis. Longitudinal plane through appendix. Compression sonography with linear array transducer. The appendix (*arrowheads*) is tubular in shape and ends blindly (X). Its diameter was greater than 6 mm, and it was noncompressible, suggesting a US diagnosis of nonperforative appendicitis. A small amount of peritoneal fluid (F) is seen surrounding the tip. (*From Cohen HL, Bober S, Bow S: Imaging the pediatric pelvis: The normal and abnormal genital system and simulators of its diseases.* Urol Radiol *14:273–283, 1992, with permission.*)

CLINICAL SIMULATORS: WHAT SHOULD YOU LOOK FOR?

Many causes of abdominal pain can simulate the pain or the perceived pain of ovarian torsion. In all cases of pelvic US to evaluate abdominal and pelvic pain, determine whether the patient is pregnant or not to rule out concern about an intrauterine or ectopic pregnancy. Evaluate the uterus in the nonpregnant patient for obstruction, and evaluate the ovaries of the pregnant or nonpregnant patient for abnormalities of size and echogenicity pattern. Unilaterally enlarged ovaries may be due to neoplasm or functional cyst, and there may be pain from torsion or hemorrhage. If both ovaries are enlarged and the patient is febrile and has a vaginal discharge, consider pelvic inflammatory disease, with or without tuboovarian abscesses. Thickened nearby bowel may suggest Crohn's disease or another localized bowel abnormality. Delayed secondary sexual characteristics can be seen in patients with chronic diseases such as Crohn's, and, as we have learned, the assessment of uterine size and shape (in adolescents, at least) may suggest grounds for concern. Certainly, one must always consider appendicitis, particularly nonperforative, when one images a blind-ending tubular structure that is noncompressible and has an outer wall–to–outer wall measurement of greater than 6 mm (Fig. 101-8).

KEY POINTS TO REMEMBER

The ovary in an ovarian torsion is *enlarged.* If no ovary can be seen in a given case that has been imaged well, there is probably no ovarian torsion. If both ovaries are similar in size, torsion is an unlikely diagnosis. Certainly, if color flow is noted in a normal ovary and not in an ovary of concern, one must consider torsion. But remember, arterial flow, and even central flow, can be seen in some proven cases. Look for venous flow. Compare it to that of the opposite side. If no flow is noted on either side (and even if it is), put significant reliance on the gray-scale image and the determined ovarian volumes.

References

Ben-Arie A, Lurie S, Graf G, Insler V: Adnexal torsion in adolescents: Prompt diagnosis and treatment may save the adnexa. *Eur J Obstet Gynecol Reprod Biol* 63:169–173, 1995.

Cohen HL: The female pelvis, in *Syllabus: Current Concepts: A Categorical Course in Pediatric Radiology,* Siebert J (ed). Chicago, RSNA Publications, 1994:65–72.

Cohen HL, Bober S, Bow S: Imaging the pediatric pelvis: The normal and abnormal genital system and simulators of its diseases. *Urol Radiol* 14:273–283, 1992.

Cohen HL, Haller JO: Pediatric and adolescent genital abnormalities. *Clin Diagn Ultrasound* 24:187–216, 1988.

Fleischer A, Stein S, Cullinan J, Warner M: Color Doppler sonography of adnexal torsion. *J Utrasound Med* 14:523–528, 1995.

Graif M, Itzchak Y: Sonographic evaluation of ovarian torsion in childhood and adolescence. *AJR* 150:647–649, 1988.

Lee E, Kwon H, Joo H, et al: Diagnosis of ovarian torsion with color Doppler sonography: Depiction of twisted vascular pedicle. *J Ultrasound Med* 17:83–89, 1998.

Ruggiero-Delliturri M, Awobuluyi M, Cohen HL, Zinn D: Imaging the pediatric pelvis: Role of ultrasound. *Radiologist* 4:155–170, 1997.

Quillin S, Siegel M: Color Doppler ultrasound of children with acute lower abdominal pain. *Radiographics* 13:293–310, 1993.

Surratt J, Siegel M: Imaging of pediatric ovarian masses. *Radiographics* 11:533–548, 1991.

Warner M, Fleischer A, Edell S, et al: Uterine adnexal torsion: Sonographic findings. *Radiology* 154:773–775, 1985.

Willms A, Schlund J, Meyer W: Endovaginal Doppler ultrasound in ovarian torsion: A case series. *Ultrasound Obstet Gynecol* 5:129–132, 1995.

102

A 16-year-old girl presents with acute pelvic pain and fever. Figure 102-1 represents a pelvic ultrasound obtained in a transverse plane through a fluid-filled bladder. What medical problem should you be worried about? Can this image be simulated by anything else?

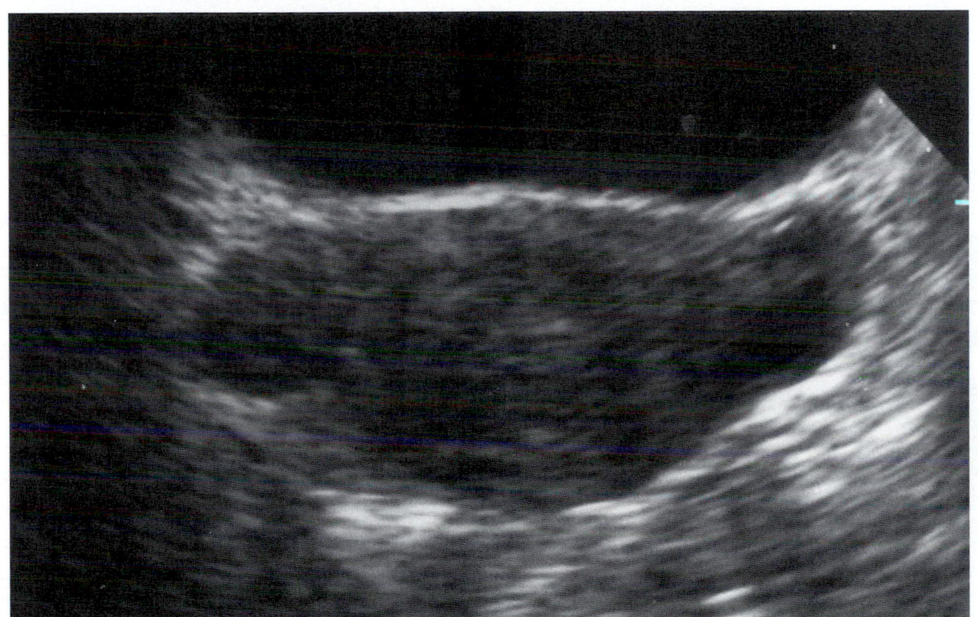

FIGURE 102–1. Pelvic ultrasound. Transverse plane through uterus.

CHAPTER 102

Salpingo-oophoritis—Pelvic Inflammatory Disease

KAREN K. MOELLER AND HARRIS L. COHEN

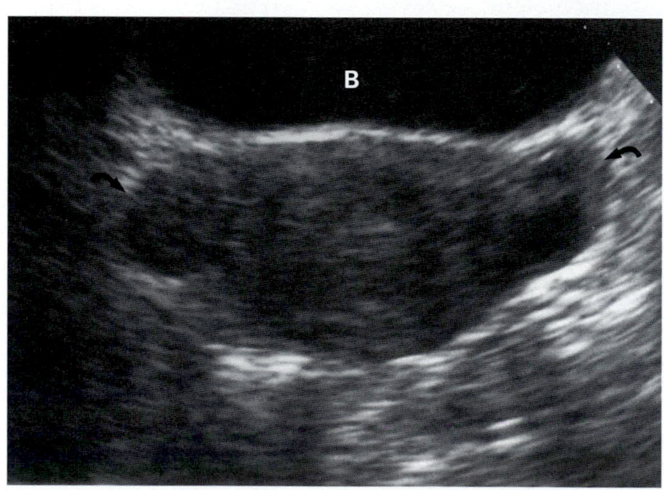

FIGURE 102–2. Annotated version of Fig. 102-1. Pelvic ultrasound. Transverse plane. The fluid-filled bladder (B) is seen anteriorly. The uterus is seen in the midline. Both ovaries (*curved arrows*) hug its borders. Each ovary contains a few follicles that appear unremarkable. Adherence suggests pelvic inflammatory disease of unknown age. The acute nature of this patient's clinical complaint suggested acute salpingo-oophoritis.

Figure 102-2 (the annotated version of Fig. 102-1) shows ovaries that are somewhat prominent and adherent to the teenager's uterus. This finding is one that we have often seen in cases of acute pelvic inflammatory disease (PID). It is usually seen in patients with salpingo-oophoritis. However, once ovaries are adherent, they remain so for years. The inflammatory cause of such ovarian adherence is usually PID, but adherence can occur with the inflammation associated with appendicitis, Crohn's disease, and other gastrointestinal conditions as well. This image of prominent adnexa adherent to the uterus, which we term the "koala bear" sign because of its resemblance to the face of a koala, can be simulated by the image of the ovaries in relationship to the uterus in cases of retroverted uterus (Fig. 102-3). Ovarian adherence can also be simulated by ovaries adjacent to an enlarged leiomyomatous uterus, a situation not commonly found in teenagers. Normally, ovaries are not adherent, although they can sometimes, when in a less than usual position, appear adjacent to the uterine walls. Because of the above, the diagnosis of PID hinges not only on the image of adherent and prominent adnexa, but also on the patient's clinical findings.

WHAT IS PELVIC INFLAMMATORY DISEASE?

Pelvic inflammatory disease includes a spectrum of abnormality that ranges from isolated endometritis to extension of infection into the tubes and ovaries, resulting in tuboovarian abscess (TOA), and even beyond and into the peritoneum, resulting in disseminated peritonitis. The causative organisms often represent a mixture of aerobes and anaerobes. *Chlamydia trachomatis* and *Neisseria gonorrhoeae* are isolated most frequently. Pelvic inflammatory disease typically is an ascending infection, with these organisms moving from the vagina into the "higher" portions of the gynecologic tract. The risk for PID is especially high in adolescents because of the high incidence of multiple sexual partners and the prevalence of gonorrhea and chlamydia in this age group. The long-term sequelae of PID can be detrimental to the teenager's remaining reproductive life, with future infertility,

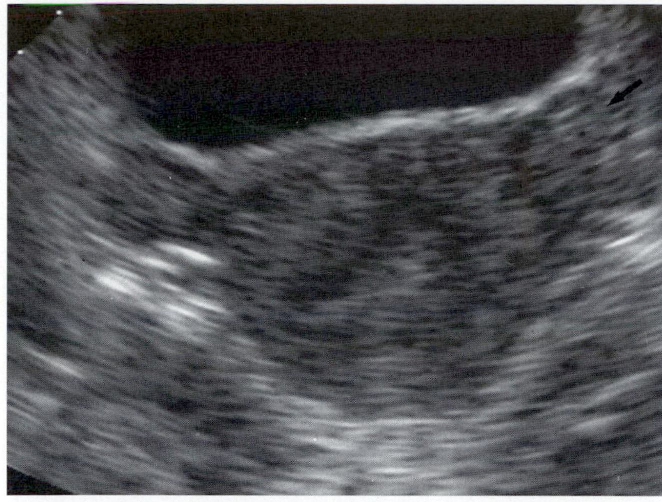

A

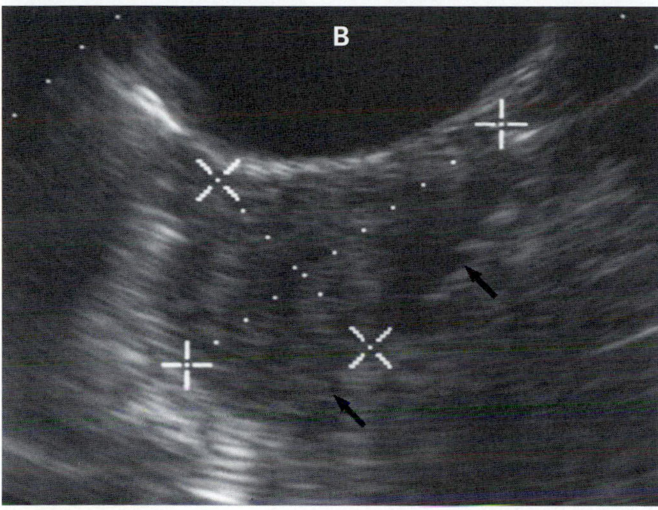

B

FIGURE 102–3. Retroverted uterus, a simulator of the "koala bear" sign of pelvic inflammatory disease (PID). Pelvic ultrasound. ***A.*** Transverse plane. Left adnexa (*arrow*) appear prominent and adherent. The patient did not have PID symptoms or signs. ***B.*** Sagittal plane. The finding of a retroverted uterus (*arrows*) helps explain the apparent "adherence" of the left adnexa. B = bladder.

increased incidence of ectopic pregnancy, and chronic pelvic pain all possibilities.

WHAT CLINICAL AND LABORATORY FINDINGS SHOULD SUGGEST PELVIC INFLAMMATORY DISEASE?

The most common symptoms of PID are pelvic pain and vaginal discharge. Findings on clinical exam include the cardinal features of lower abdominal tenderness, bilateral adnexal tenderness, and cervical motion tenderness. Additional features include an oral temperature of 38°C or greater, abnormal cervical or vaginal discharge, a white blood cell count of 10,000 or greater, and an erythrocyte sedimentation rate of 15 mm/h or greater.

It is important to note, however, that not all patients have an elevated temperature. Approximately 40 percent of patients with documented PID have normal laboratory values. Gram staining of cervical secretions to denote the causative organisms is often negative. Diagnosing PID on clinical and laboratory grounds alone, therefore, is often difficult. Strict adherence to diagnosing PID only in women with an elevated fever or white blood cell count will produce false negatives and allow some sufferers to escape diagnosis. It has also been established that diagnosis based on clinical findings alone is only 65 percent accurate.

ULTRASOUND TECHNIQUE FOR PELVIC INFLAMMATORY DISEASE DIAGNOSIS

The limitations of a strictly clinical diagnosis of PID and other causes of pelvic pain highlight the need for laboratory and imaging diagnostic criteria as well. Ultrasound can certainly help point to a diagnosis for pelvic pain. It can establish that there is an abnormality in the gynecologic tract or show that the cause of pelvic pain is from another source—e.g., gastrointestinal. Although laparoscopy has always been considered the gold standard for accurately defining PID, its use is limited because of its expense, its invasiveness, and the fact that it is not readily available. Sonography offers a noninvasive technique for confirming the presence and extent of disease. The examination can be accomplished by transabdominal (TA) and/or transvaginal (TV) techniques. Transabdominal imaging requires bladder filling, which takes time and may be uncomfortable. It gives a more global view of the pelvic contents, however. Transvaginal examinations allow excellent imaging via a higher-frequency (5- to 7.5-MHz) probe. The far field of view, however, is limited. The technique may not always be tolerated, particularly if there is significant cervical motion tenderness, even in a sexually active adolescent. We tend to evaluate each case individually and prefer to begin, in most instances, with the global view afforded by TA imaging.

WHAT ARE THE ULTRASOUND FINDINGS IN PELVIC INFLAMMATORY DISEASE?

Ultrasound findings in PID range from normal imaging exams, typically seen in cases of acute salpingitis, to cases in which there are large pelvic masses due to TOA(s), with or without associated hydrosalpinx. The uterine endometrial cavity may have prominent echogenicity or may be enlarged as a result of contained fluid. Most times it appears unremarkable. The uterus can appear prominent, with enlarged ovaries, as in our image of symmetrically adherent adnexa. The adherence need not be symmetric. The fallopian tubes, which are generally not seen by ultrasound when normal, can become distended with fluid (hydrosalpinx). These anechoic, sometimes tortuous tubular structures (Fig. 102-4) can sometimes be better assessed by TV examination. Although the

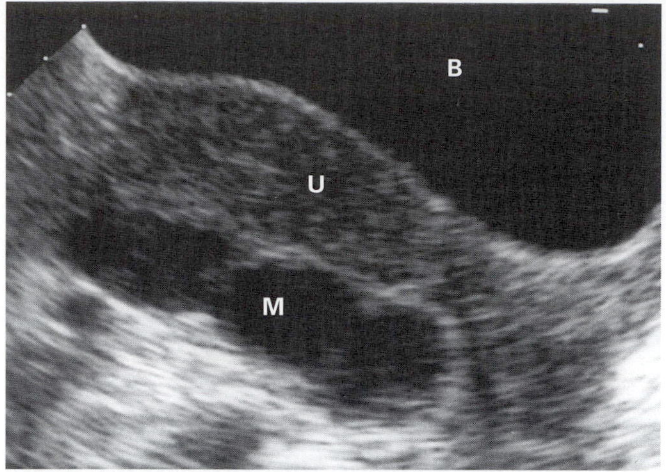

A

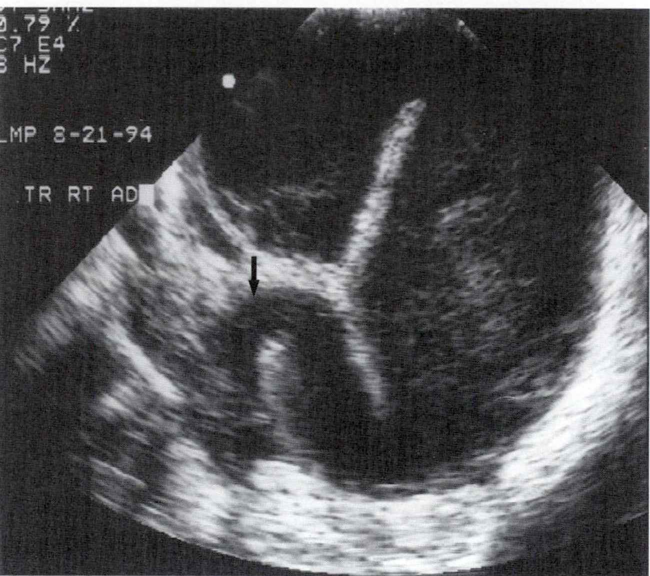

B

FIGURE 102–4. Pyosalpinx. Pelvic ultrasound. ***A.*** Midline longitudinal plane. The uterus (U) is posterior to the bladder on this magnified image. Posterior to the uterus, in the cul de sac, is a tubular cystic mass (M) with some contained echogenicity. In this teenager with symptoms of pelvic inflammatory disease, this is at least a hydrosalpinx. The contained echoes point to the greater but not exclusive possibility of pyosalpinx. ***B.*** Transvaginal exam. Region of right adnexa. This pyosalpinx was better imaged by higher-frequency transvaginal scanning, performed with the transducer very near the object of interest. The tubular nature of this relatively echoless, debris-filled mass can be readily recognized. An arrow points to a turn in the less dilated proximal end of the fallopian tube. This tube was noted on other views to extend from the uterine cornu. Its contained echogenicity suggests but does not confirm the presence of infected material, i.e., pus.

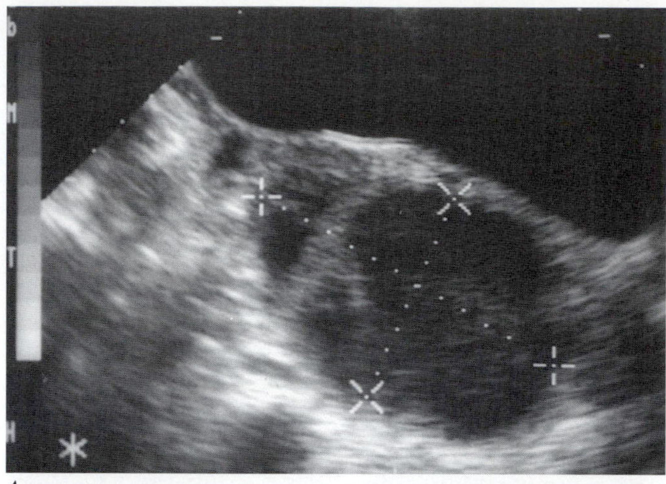

A

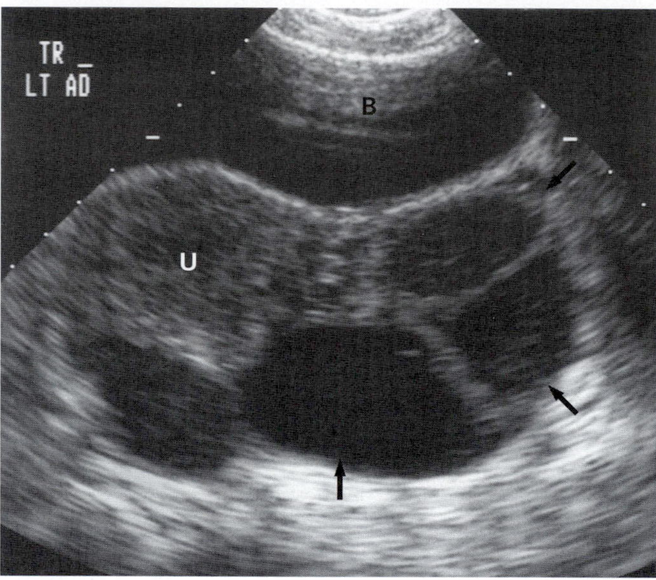

B

FIGURE 102–5. Tuboovarian abscess (TOA). Pelvic ultrasound. ***A.*** Longitudinal plane. Right adnexal region. Crosses mark off a predominantly echopenic mass that has replaced the ovary in this teenager. It was due to a TOA. ***B.*** Transverse plane. Midline and left adnexal region. A complex, predominantly cystic mass with echogenic debris in some of the cystic areas is noted in the left adnexal region of this young adult. It was due to a TOA.

tubular structures are said to be typically distended by echoless fluid in hydrosalpinx and by echo-filled fluid in pyosalpinx, these appearances can be reversed. In individual cases, proteinaceous but uninfected fluid may be echogenic, and infected fluid may be echoless. Other features that aid in diagnosing pyosalpinx include thickened tube walls and linear echoes protruding from the walls.

Ovaries affected by PID, as has been stated, may appear enlarged. We use a volume of 15 to 20 cm^3 as a gray zone for adnexal enlargement in the mature postmenarchal female, with volumes greater than 20 cm^3 being evidence of definitive enlargement. We have reported ovarian sizes of 11 cm^3 or greater in cases of PID, specifically salpingo-oophoritis reported in young teens with no prior history of gynecologic infection. Others have reported ovaries as enlarged at 14 cm^3 or greater. The US finding of fluid in the cul de sac can be seen in patients with PID, but not particularly often. It is a nonspecific finding, since it is often visualized as a normal physiologic finding in postmenarchal females, often due to rupture of a physiologic cyst.

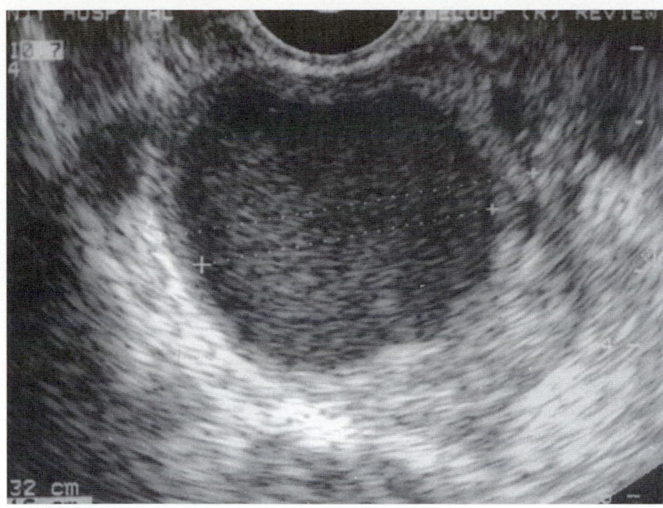

FIGURE 102–6. Tuboovarian abscess (TOA). Transvaginal image. A large mass marked off by crosses shows significant contained echogenicity. The debris in this TOA was not as well seen on the transvesicle examination.

A key finding suggestive of significant PID is the TOA. Tuboovarian abscesses are said to be present in approximately 14 to 38 percent of patients hospitalized for PID. A TOA represents further extension of the inflammation, with involvement of the fallopian tube and the ovary. With continued progression, there is total replacement of the normal structures by the inflammatory process. Its important to recognize the presence of a TOA, because patients with TOAs may require more aggressive treatment, including alternative antibiotic regimens or percutaneous drainage.

If there is progression to TOA, a complex, predominantly cystic mass (Fig. 102-5) is visualized on US examination. Frequently, the cystic mass demonstrates low-level internal echoes, produced by purulent material and cellular debris. At times, the cystic areas may appear more echoless on TA examination, whereas TV images will show that they are filled with echogenic material (Fig. 102-6). Cases of less significant salpingo-oophoritis may also contain cystic areas, but these are within a predominantly solid enlarged ovary and are more typical of, and usually are, functional cysts. Since these findings of PID are part of one spectrum, it may be hard, at times, to distinguish exactly when or if a structure has gone from an infected ovary with contained cysts to an ovary replaced by TOA. The TOA is located in the region of the adnexa, usually on either side of the uterus. Part of the cystic component of the TOA may be a dilated and infected fallopian tube. Ultrasound images, usually obtained in longitudinal plane, may help show the tubular shape of a portion of the TOA's echoless structure, suggesting that a dilated fallopian tube is part of the mass. A TOA mass may seem to incorporate the uterus and can be as large as 25 cm. As a helpful imaging point, a normal ovary is *not* detected on the same side as a tuboovarian abscess.

Tinkanen and Kujansuu examined TOAs utilizing TV Doppler sonography. The group found a low resistive waveform at the margin of the acute infectious complex and noted a resistive index (RI) of less than 0.5 in patients with acute PID. The RI values increased with resolving TOAs. The process of angioneogenesis during acute PID is thought to be responsible for these findings, as it is thought to be responsible for the low resistive indices in neoplasia. If this is true, this technique could potentially be useful in determining the effectiveness of treatment of a TOA.

DIFFERENTIAL DIAGNOSIS OF TOA

The differential diagnosis of TOA includes any complex cystic pelvic mass seen in adolescents. Pelvic abscesses from other etiologies such as appendicitis or Crohn's disease may look similar but usually are not intimately related to the uterus, are often located posterior to it, and are found beyond a normal ipsilateral ovary. A chronic ectopic pregnancy may simulate a TOA, although ectopic pregnancies tend to be more solid in appearance. Certainly, the clinical histories should differ. Endometriomas and hemorrhagic cysts can look exceptionally similar to TOAs on US. Again, correlation with history and clinical examination will help make the diagnosis.

As an aside, the ability to obtain accurate histories from adolescents, particularly about sexual subjects, varies with the examiner, the patient, and the surroundings (i.e., who is in the room when the questions are being asked). Obtaining a history is an art like any other in medicine. The US examination is the perfect place to obtain historical, clinical, and imaging correlation, sometimes all at the same time.

References

Bulas DI, Ahlstrom PA, Sivit CJ, et al: Pelvic inflammatory disease in the adolescent: Comparison of transabdominal and transvaginal sonographic evaluation. *Radiology* 183:435–439, 1992.

Eschenbach DA: Acute pelvic inflammatory disease. *Urol Clin North Am* 11:65–79, 1984.

Fried AM, Kenney CM, Stigers KB, et al: Benign pelvic masses. *Radiographics* 16:321–334, 1996.

Golden N, Cohen H, Genanari G, Neuhoff S: The use of pelvic ultrasonography in the evaluation of adolescents with pelvic inflammatory disease. *Am J Dis Child* 141:1235–1238, 1987.

Golden N, Neuhoff S, Cohen H: Pelvic inflammatory disease in adolescents. *J Pediatr* 114:138–143, 1989.

Jain KA, Jeffrey RB: Pictorial essay: Transabdominal and endovaginal sonography of adnexal masses. *Clin Imaging* 15: 245–252, 1991.

Jain KA, Jeffrey RB: Evaluation of pelvic masses with magnetic resonance imaging and ultrasonography. *J Ultrasound Med* 13:845–853, 1994.

Moore L, Wilson SR: Ultrasonography in obstetric and gynecologic emergencies. *Radiol Clin North Am* 32:1005–1022, 1994.

Patten RM, Vincent LM, Wolner-Hanssen P, et al: Pelvic inflammatory disease. Endovaginal sonography with laparoscopic correlation. *J Ultrasound Med* 9:681–689, 1990.

Taipale P, Tarjanne H, Ylostalo P: Transvaginal sonography in suspected pelvic inflammatory disease. *Ultrasound Obstet Gynecol* 6:430–434, 1995.

Teele RL, Share JC: Ultrasonography of the female pelvis in childhood and adolescence. *Radiol Clin North Am* 30:743–758, 1992.

Tinkanen H, Kujansuu E: Doppler ultrasound findings in tubo-ovarian complex. *JCU* 21:175–178, 1993.

Uhrich PC, Sanders RC: Ultrasonic characteristics of pelvic inflammatory masses. *JCU* 4:199–204, 1976.

COLOR PLATES*

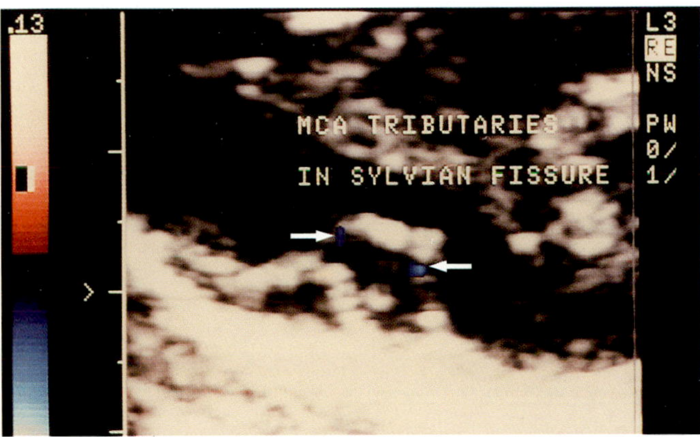

Plate 1 (Fig. 1-11*C*). Close-up of fetal brain periphery at an area similar to the echogenic structures at the periphery of the brain in ***B***. Color Doppler shows vascular flow (*arrows*) within these structures. This and their spectral patterns confirmed that they were middle cerebral artery tributaries in the Sylvian fissure.

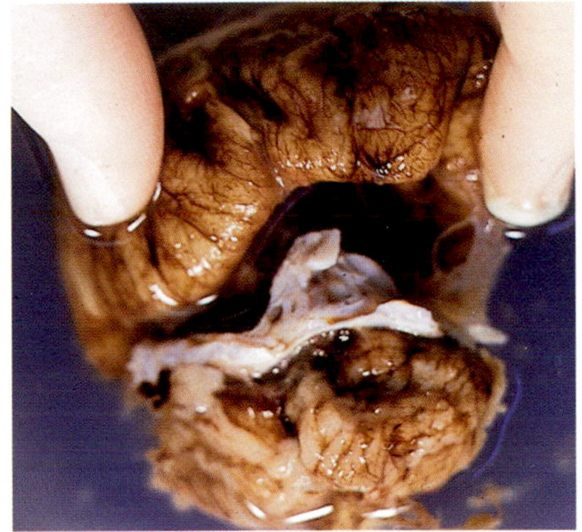

Plate 2 (Fig. 2–5). Monoventricle of holoprosencephaly. Pathology specimen. Coronal plane viewed from the back. The pathologist's fingers are at the boundaries of the brain surrounding the single ventricle, seen as the open space within the brain. The white material is the tentorium, and the cerebellum is seen below it.

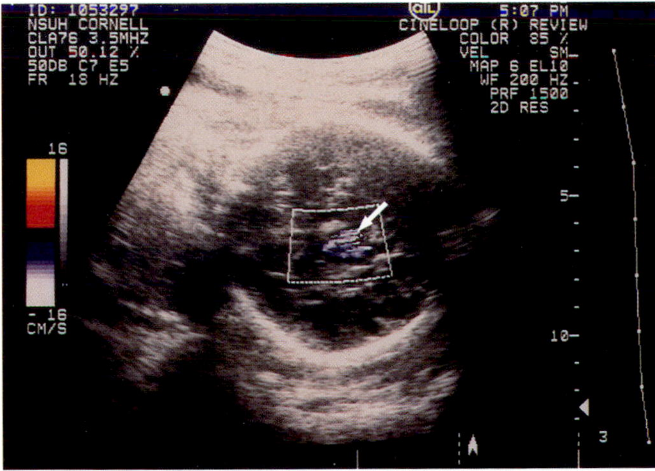

Plate 3 (Fig. 3–6). Fetal head. Color Doppler. Axial plane. The cystic area immediately filled with color (*arrow*), proving it to be vascular. The biphasic and irregular venous spectral pattern obtained showed it to be typical of a vein of Galen "aneurysm" or other arteriovenous malformation.

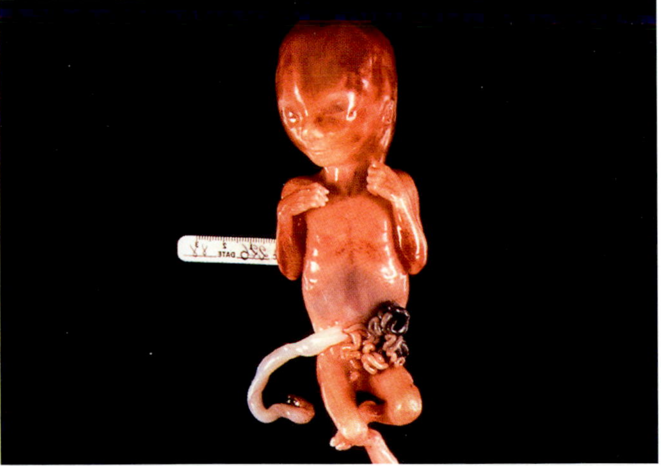

Plate 4 (Fig. 11–5*A*). Gastroschisis. Pathology specimen. ***A.*** Fetus with gastroschisis. Autopsy specimen. Frontal projection. The umbilical cord (*arrow*) is in its normal midline position. The mass extending from the left of the midline abdominal wall defect is small bowel.

**The figures in parentheses following the Plate numbers have been double-numbered in order to indicate the chapter in which they are discussed and the order of their citation therein.*

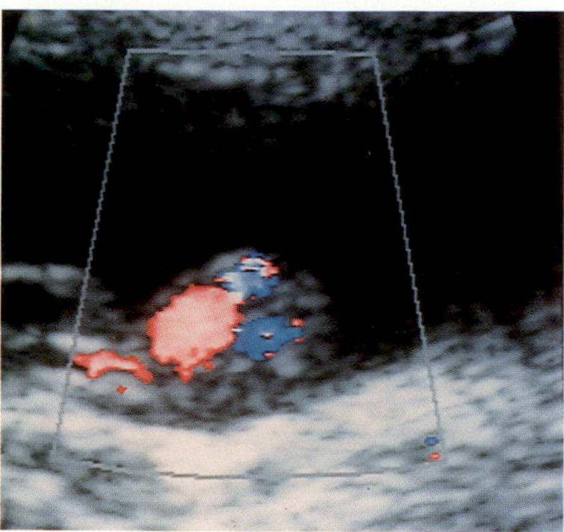

Plate 5 (Fig. 24–6). Normal umbilical cord. Axial plane through the cord. Using color Doppler, one can note that the direction of flow in the larger vessel, the vein, is pink/red, indicating flow in a direction opposite to the flow (blue) in the arteries. The spectral patterns of these vessels confirmed these facts.

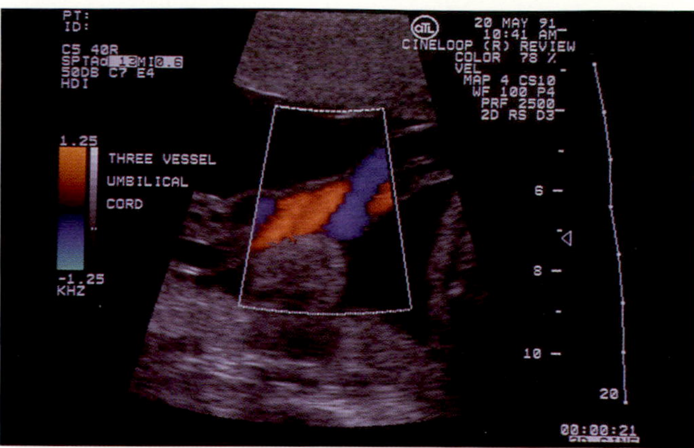

Plate 6 (Fig. 24–8). Normal umbilical braiding or coiling. Color Doppler image. Longitudinal oblique plane through umbilical cord. There is a normal three-vessel cord, with the two arteries (in red) coiled about the single umbilical vein (blue). This coiling or braiding of vessels about one another is not found in cases of SUA. *[Image used with permission of Advanced Technology Laboratories (ATL).*

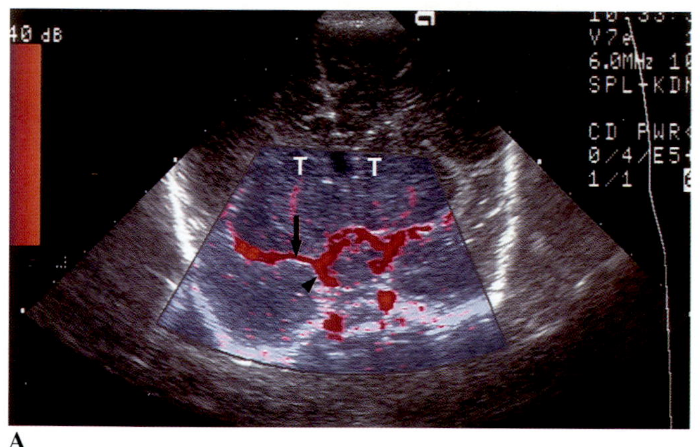

A

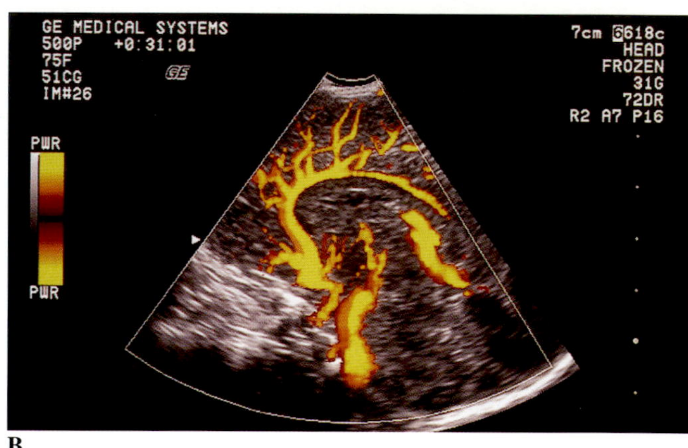

B

Plate 7 (Fig. 27–16*A* and *B*). Power Doppler used in neonatal neurosonography. ***A.*** Neonatal head. Coronal plane. Several of the vessels of the circle of Willis are noted. An arrow points to the right middle cerebral artery. An arrowhead points to the left posterior communicating artery. Tiny vessels in the area of the thalami (T) are thalamostriate arteries. These vessels may be difficult to image with routine color Doppler, which relies on Doppler frequency shift data. Power Doppler, which relies on the overall amplitude of the Doppler signal and has improved decibel sensitivity at the loss of directional information, readily shows these vessels. ***B.*** Neonatal head. Sagittal plane. Power Doppler readily shows various branches

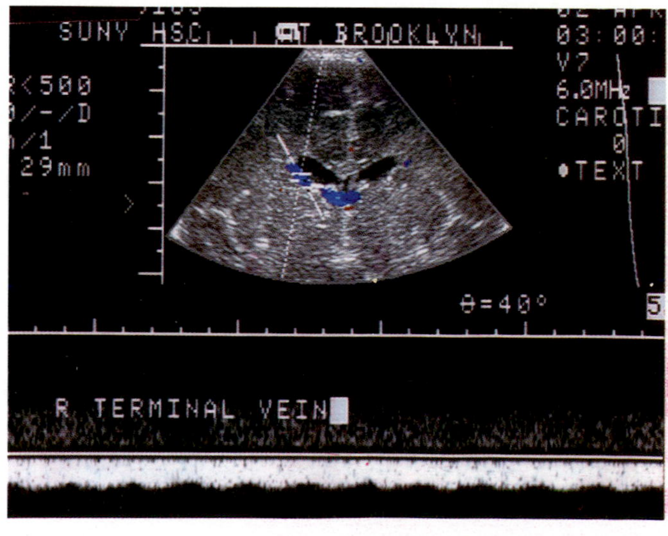

Plate 8 (Fig. 27–20). Normal terminal vein. Coronal plane. Color Doppler. This triplex (gray-scale image, color Doppler, and spectral pattern) image of the frontal horn area of a premature infant with known grade I SEH shows flow *(insonated blue line)* in the right terminal vein. A normal venous spectral pattern *(arrow)* showing a typical continuous sinusoid pattern (slight change in peak flow with respiratory motion) is seen. With slight angulation, a normal left terminal vein was noted on another image. This helped prove the terminal veins to be normal and unaffected by the grade I SEH (not seen on this image).

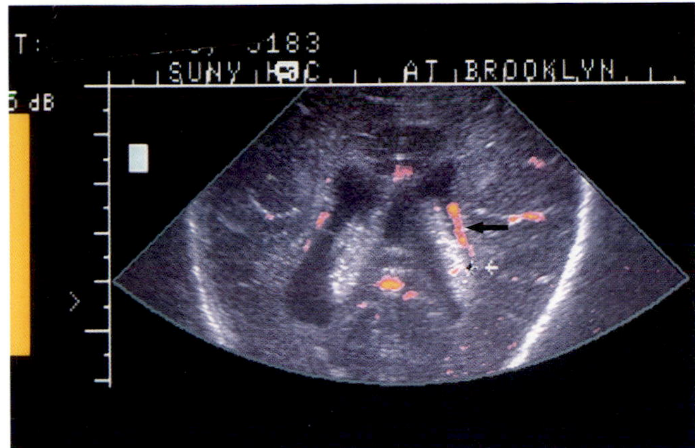

Plate 9 (Fig. 28–4). Color Doppler flow in choroid plexus. Head ultrasound. Coronal view. Power Doppler. Occasionally one may need to prove that an echogenic structure is the normal choroid rather than an acute clot. Only choroid has vascular flow within it. This is an image of flow (*arrow*) in a normal left choroid plexus.

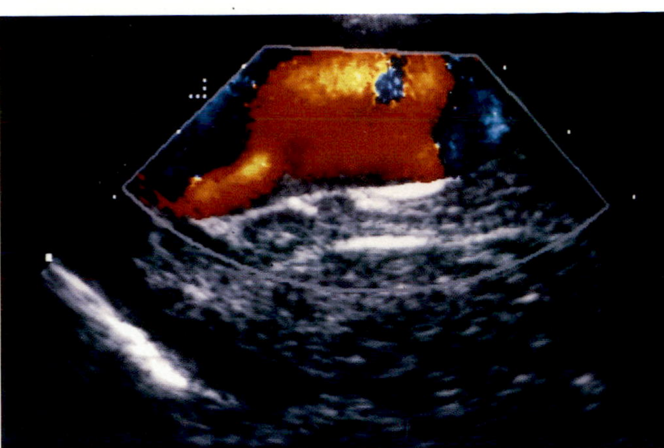

Plate 10 (Fig. 31–5*B*). Neonatal head ultrasound. Sagittal plane. This image concentrated on the echoless tubular structure at the rostrum of this neonate's head. Significant color Doppler flow is seen in this vessel. Turbulent and biphasic venous Doppler signal proved it to be part of a very large AVM.

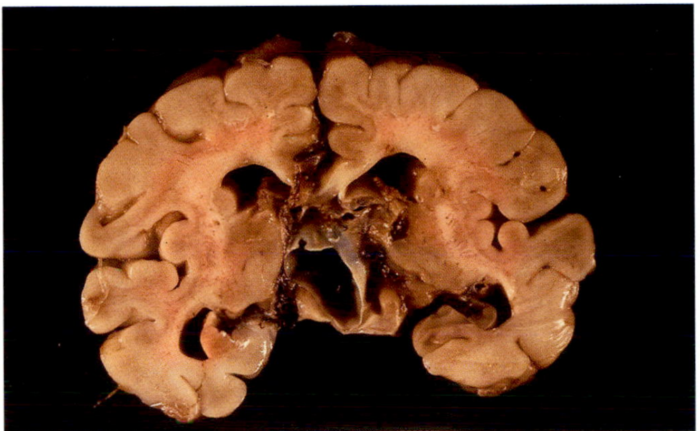

Plate 11 (Fig. 31–7*C*). Postmortem brain specimen. Coronal plane. This patient died soon after birth. Arrows point to the lateral ventricles of the specimen. They are more dilated than normal. They sit lateral to the dilated galenic AVM (*small arrows*). The AVM was the midline cystic mass noted on ultrasound, and its mass impression was responsible for the hydrocephalus.

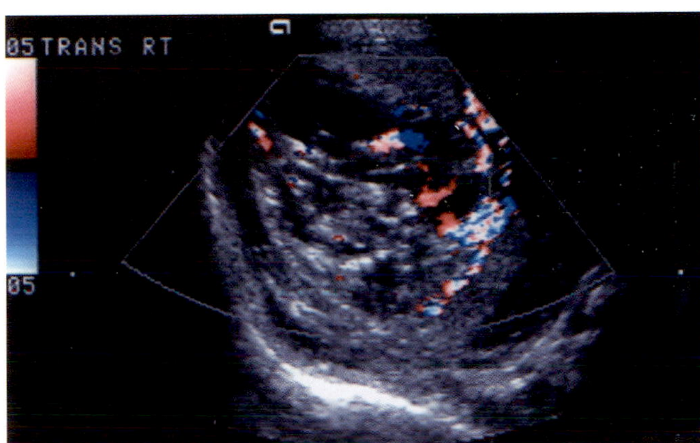

Plate 12 (Fig. 38–4). Hemangioendothelioma on color Doppler sonography. Transverse view through the liver in the same child as in Fig. 38-1 demonstrates increased blood flow within the hemangioendothelioma.

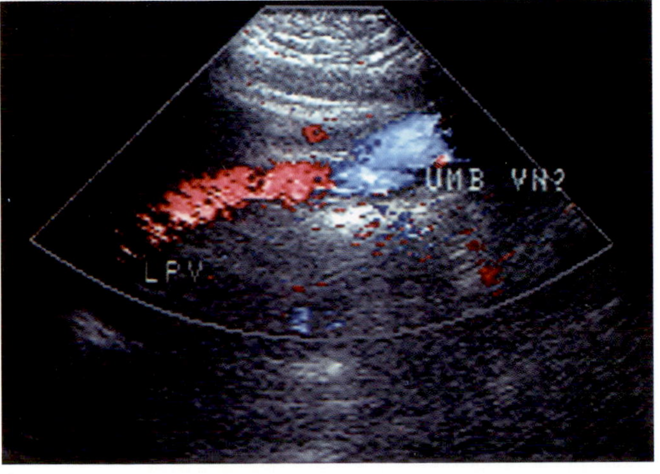

A

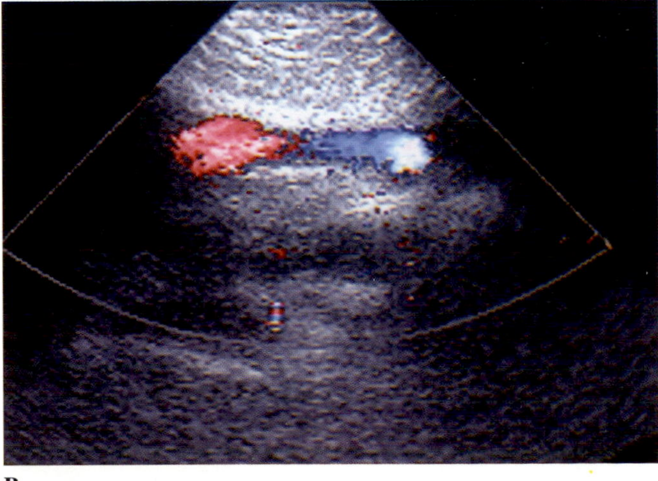

B

Plate 13 (Fig. 40–5*A* and *B*). Recanalized umbilical vein associated with portal hypertension. ***A.*** Longitudinal view through the left lobe of the liver in a child with portal hypertension demonstrates flow in the left portal vein (LPV), communicating with a recanalized umbilical vein (UMB VN). ***B.*** Longitudinal midline view through the abdomen in the same patient demonstrates flow in the recanalized umbilical vein.

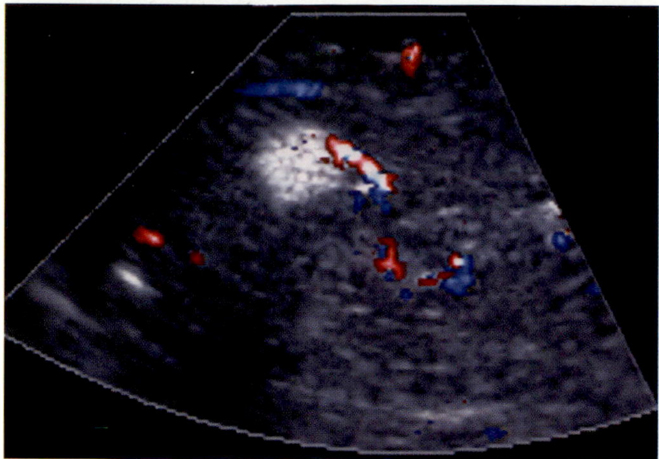

Plate 14 (Fig. 43–1*B*). Transverse *(A)* and longitudinal *(B)* views through the right lobe of the liver.

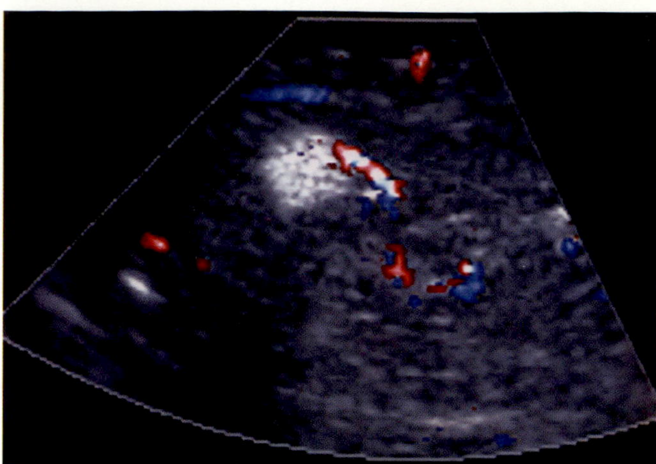

Plate 15 (Fig. 43–2*B*). Cavernous hemangioma of the liver. Transverse (*A*) and longitudinal (*B*) demonstrate increased vascularity within the focal hyperechoic hepatic lesion.

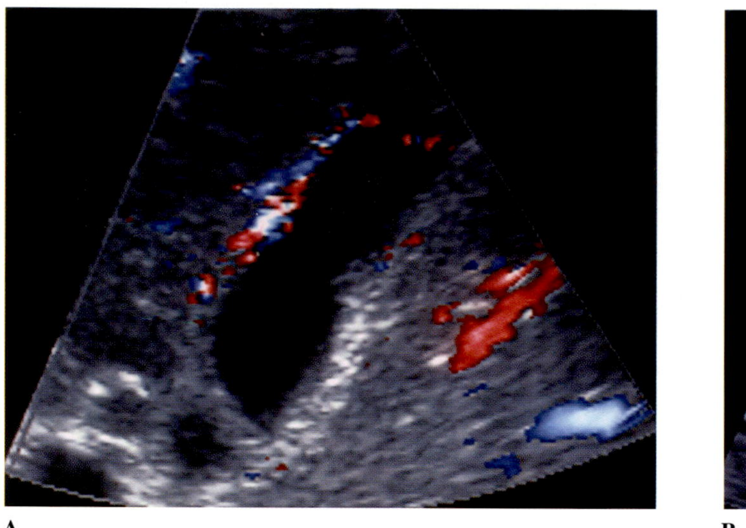

A

B

Plate 16 (Fig. 44–1*A* and *B*). Longitudinal *(A)* and transverse *(B)* views through the gallbladder with color Doppler sonography.

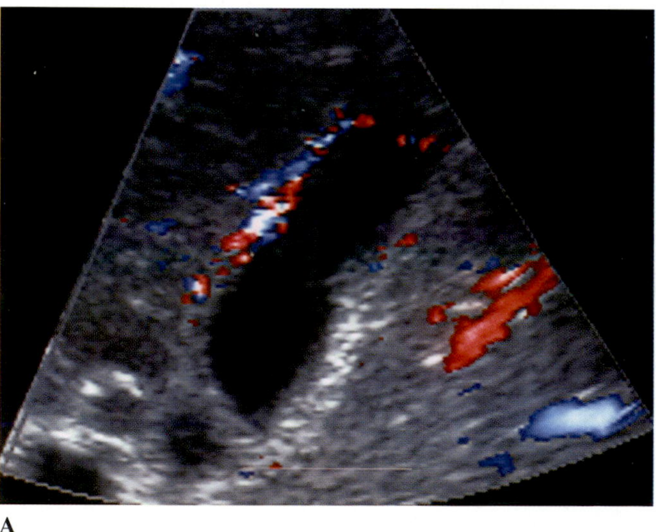

A

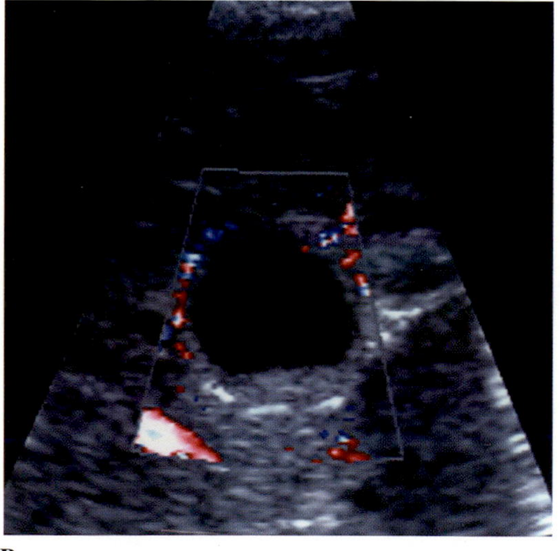

B

Plate 17 (Fig. 44–2*A* and *B*). Acute cholecystitis with hypervascularity of the gallbladder. Longitudinal *(A)* and transverse *(B)* views through the gallbladder demonstrate wall thickening and marked hyperemia on color Doppler.

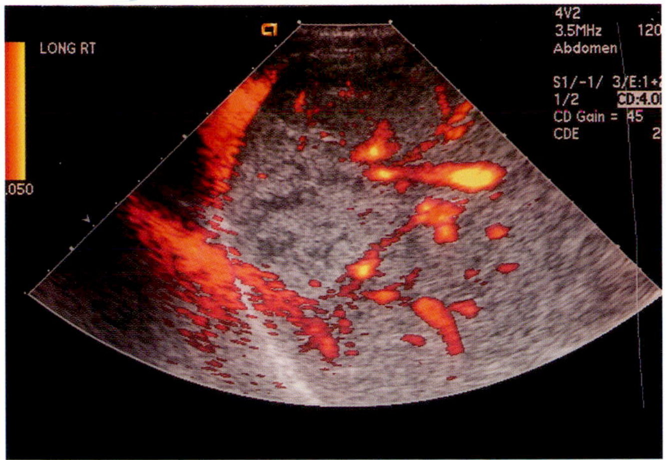

Plate 18 (Fig. 47–4). Color Doppler sonography demonstrating absence of flow in the region of an intraparenchymal hepatic hematoma. Longitudinal view through the liver with color Doppler sonography shows absence of blood flow at the site of the intraparenchymal hematoma.

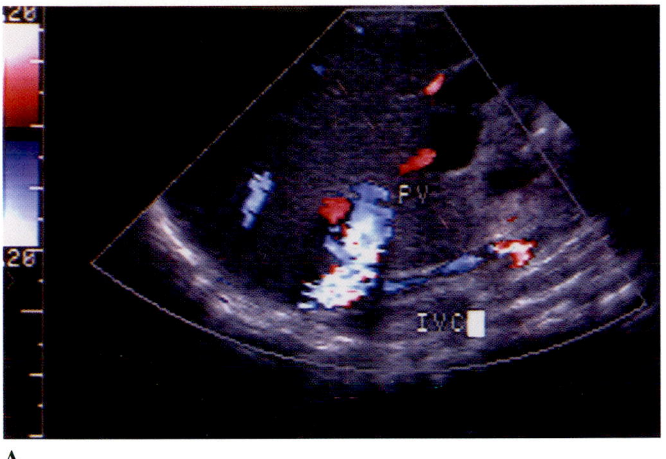

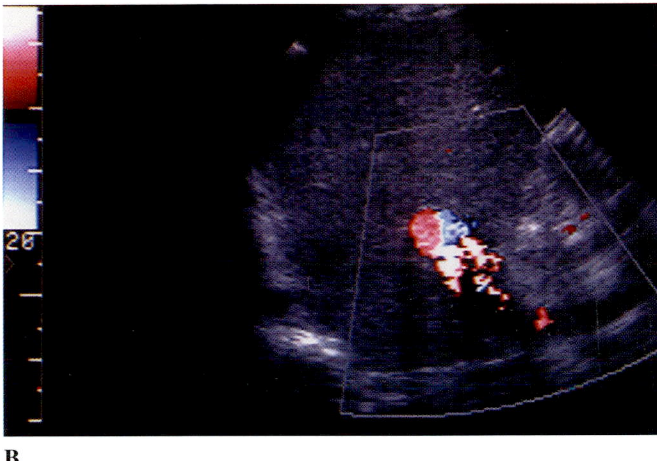

A

B

Plate 19 (Fig. 53–3*A* and *B*). ***A.*** Persistent ductus venosus. Longitudinal view through the liver in the same child as in Fig. 53-1 with color Doppler demonstrates normal hepatopedal flow (toward the liver) in the main portal vein. ***B.*** Persistent ductus venosus. Longitudinal view through the liver in the same child as in ***A*** shows that the direction of flow through the ductus venosus is from the left portal vein (PV) to the inferior vena cava (IVC).

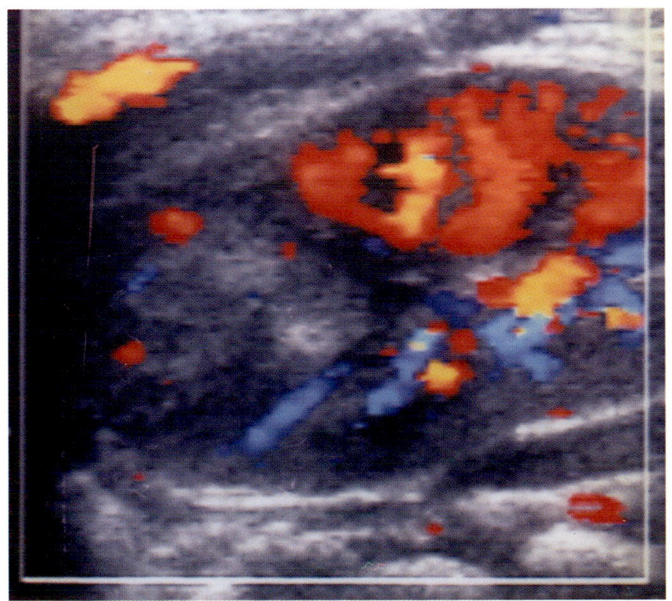

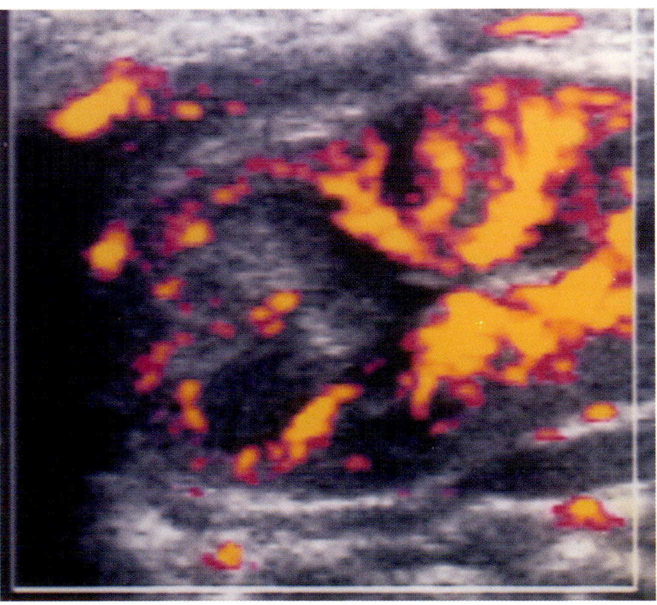

B

C

Plate 20 (Fig. 73–1*B* and *C*). Color Doppler sonography ***(B)*** and power color Doppler sonography ***(C)***.

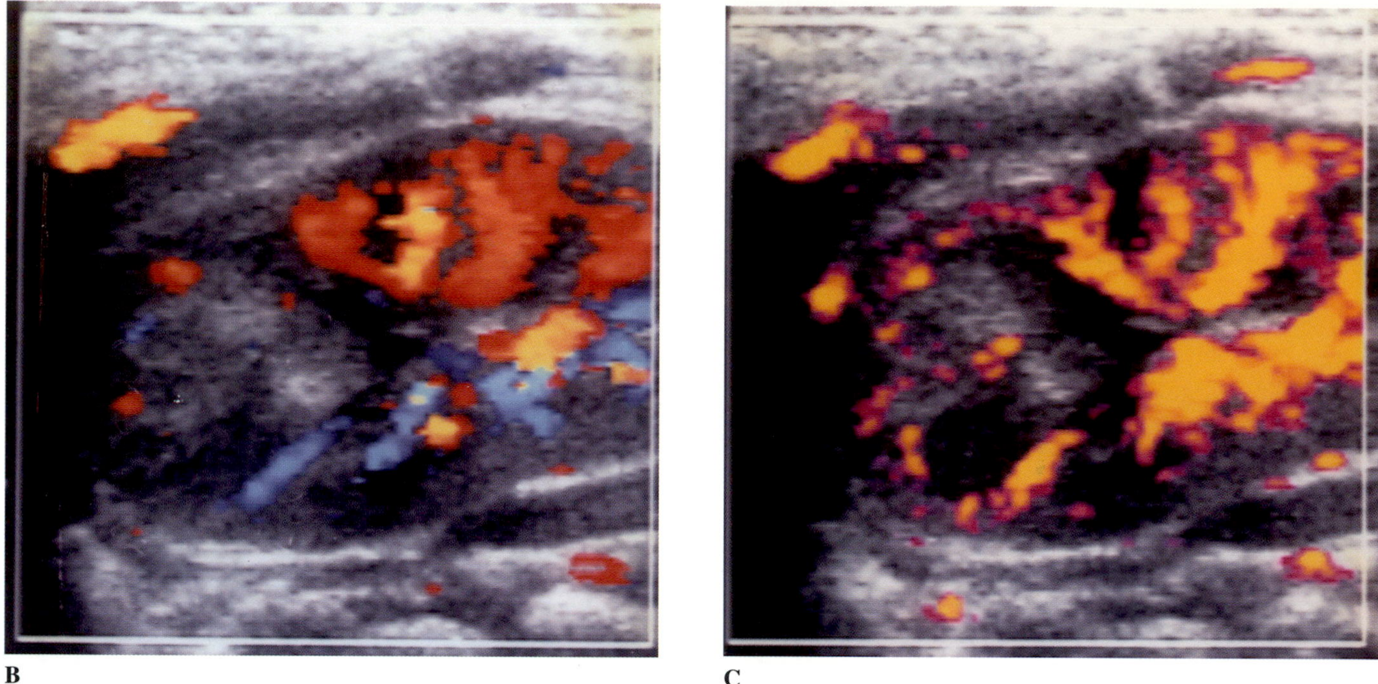

Plate 21 (Fig. 73–2*B* and *C*). Longitudinal view of the left kidney in the same patient with color Doppler shows decreased vascularity in the left upper pole ***(B)***. Longitudinal view of the left kidney in the same patient with power Doppler also shows decreased vascularity in the left upper pole, consistent with acute pyelonephritis ***(C)***.

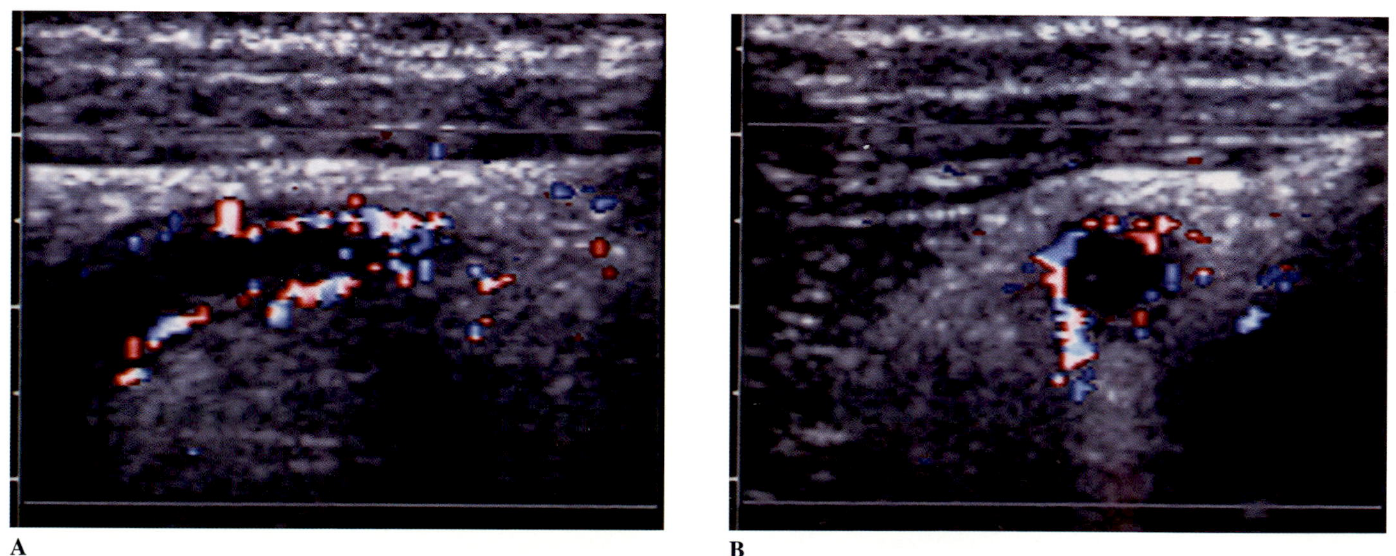

Plate 22 (Fig. 87–7*A* and *B*). Acute appendicitis on color Doppler sonography. ***A.*** Longitudinal view through the appendix with color Doppler sonography in a child with acute appendicitis demonstrates marked hyperemia in the appendiceal wall. ***B.*** Transverse view through the appendix in the same child as in ***A*** with color Doppler sonography again shows marked appendiceal hyperemia.

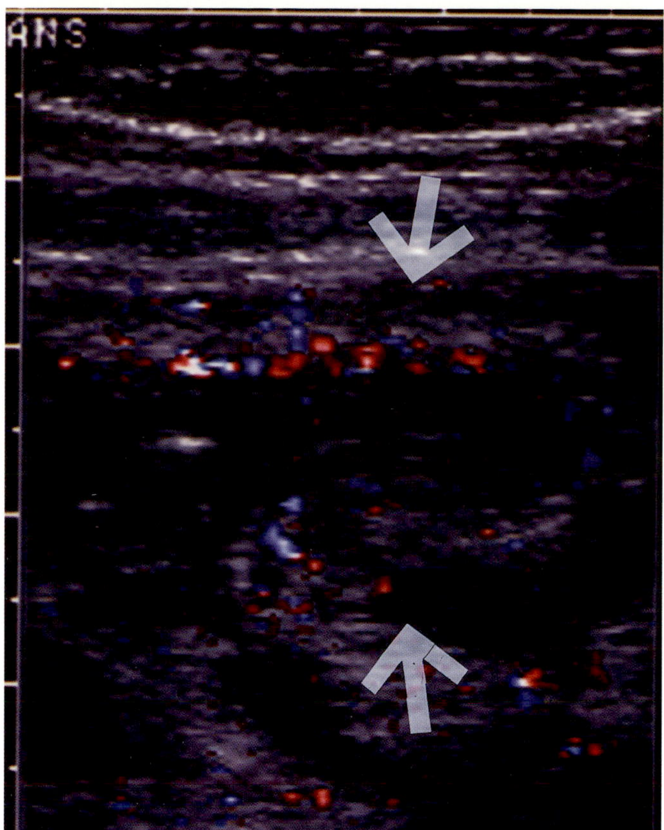

Plate 23 (Fig. 91–5). Neutropenic typhlitis with hyperemia demonstrated on color Doppler examination. Transverse view of the right lower quadrant in a child with neutropenic typhlitis after a bone marrow transplant shows cecal thickening (*arrows*) with pronounced bowel wall hyperemia by color Doppler. Note the thickened hyperechoic mucosal/submucosal layer and the hypoechoic muscularis layer.

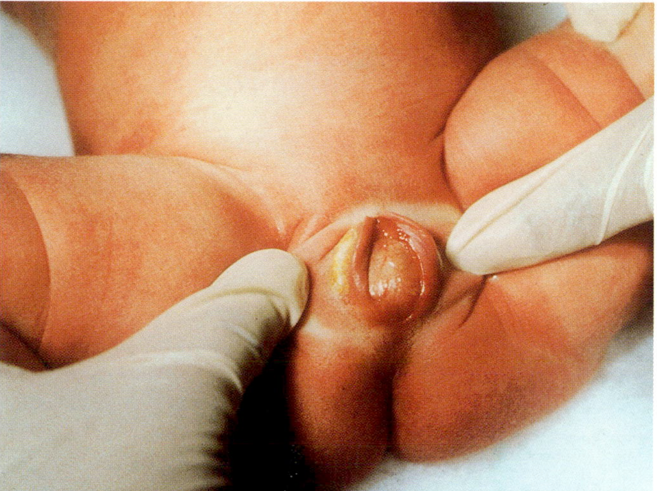

Plate 24 (Fig. 94–3). Neonatal hydrocolpos. Clinical image. There is a large interlabial mass that proved to be due to accumulated secretions proximal to the imperforate hymen. *(Reprinted with permission from Emans SJ: Vulvovaginal problems in the prepubertal child, in* Pediatric and Adolescent Gynecology, *4th ed., Emans SJ, Laufer MR, Goldstein DP (eds). Philadelphia, Lippincott-Raven, 1998:100, Fig. 11.)*

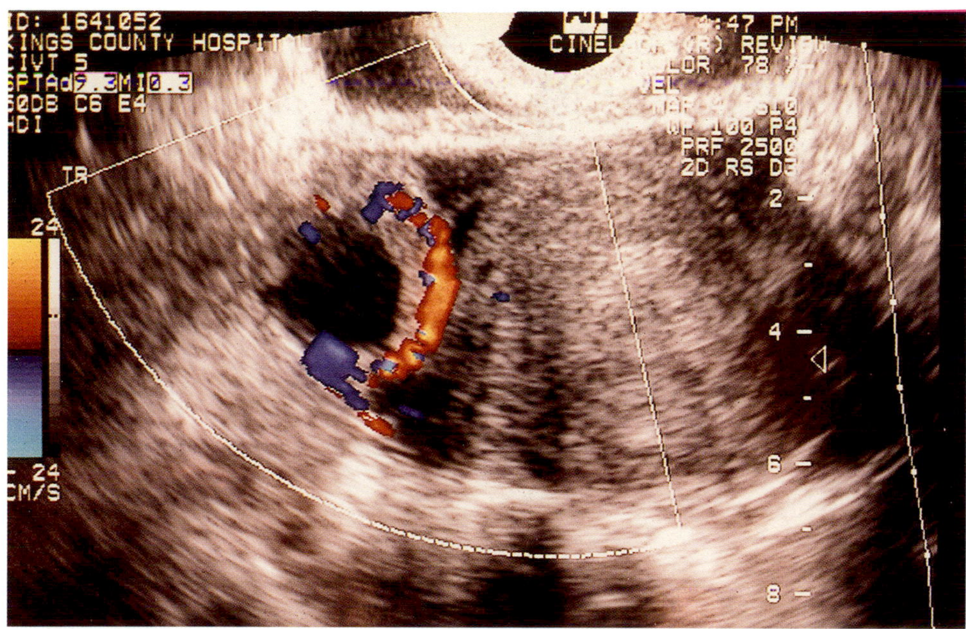

Plate 25 (Fig. 96–4*B*). Ectopic pregnancy. ***B.*** Transvaginal examination. Transverse plane. Transducer pointing toward the right adnexa. Color Doppler examination. Color surrounds a mass with a contained cyst in the right adnexal region. No cyst or intrauterine pregnancy is seen in the uterus of this pregnant teenager. Ectopic pregnancies may have bright vascular flow noted within their trophoblastic periphery, as in this case. However, this may also be noted in the tissue peripheral to a corpus luteal cyst of pregnancy. Other views proved the adnexal area cystic "mass" to be a gestational sac with a contained fetal pole.

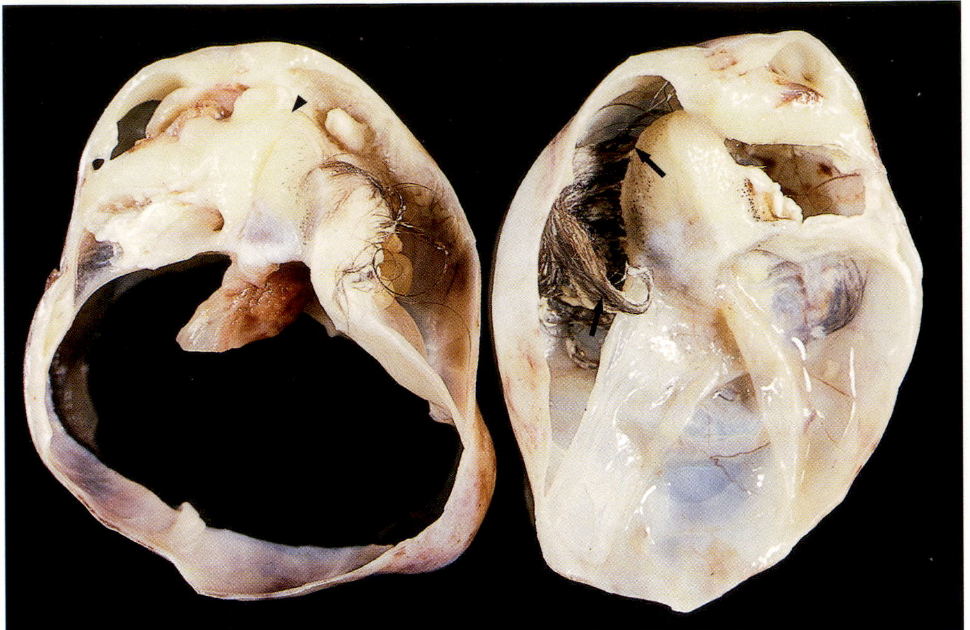

Plate 26 (Fig. 99–7*B*). Ovarian teratoma containing hair. ***B.*** Pathology specimen. This is the cut specimen of an adolescent's teratoma. Hair (*arrow*) is noted within it, as are solid tissue (which proved to be cerebellar in histologic type) and sebaceous material (*arrowhead*). One can see how US could image individual hair strands. At least half of this mass is cystic.

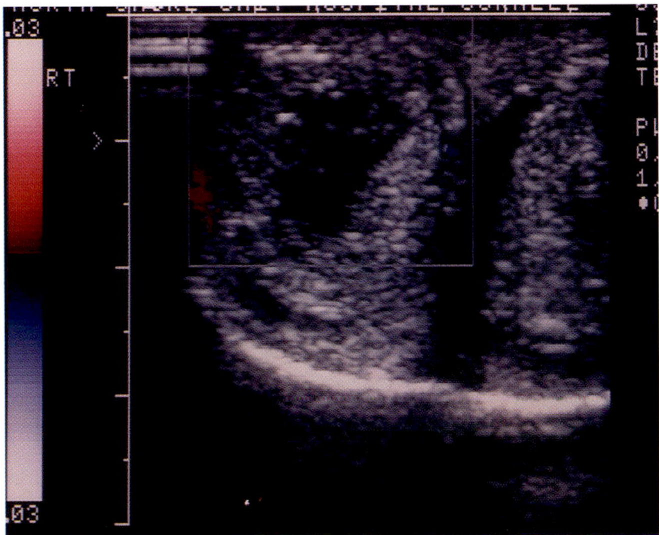

Plate 27 (Fig. 103–3). Torsed right testicle. Color Doppler exam. Transverse plane. The box within which color flow can be assessed is over the right testicle. No vascular flow was identified within it. (*From Gross BR, Cohen HL, Schlessel JS: Perinatal diagnosis of bilateral testicular torsion: Beware of torsions simulating hydroceles.* J Ultrasound Med *12:479–481, 1993, with permission.*)

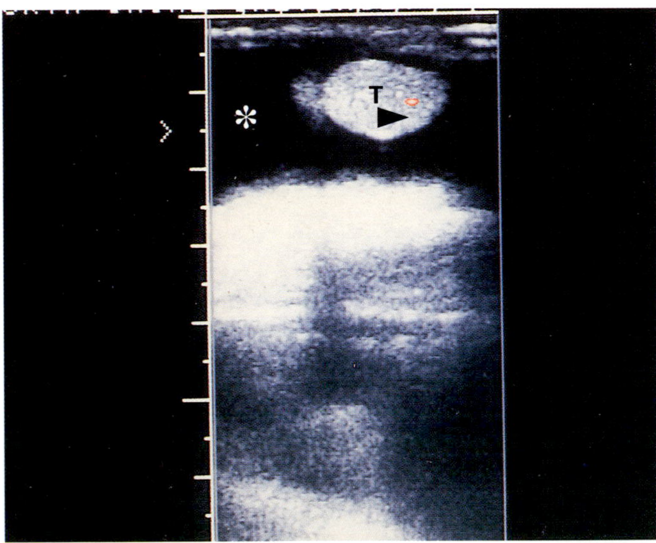

Plate 28 (Fig. 103–5). Large hydrocele, normal testicular echogenicity. Right testicle. Longitudinal plane. Color Doppler examination. The testicle of a newborn with a large hydrocele (*) is noted. The normal testis is of homogeneous echogenicity. Note that the echogenicity is greater than that in the previous images of cases of torsion. A small dot of color seen in the testicle was proven on spectral examination to be due to arterial flow.

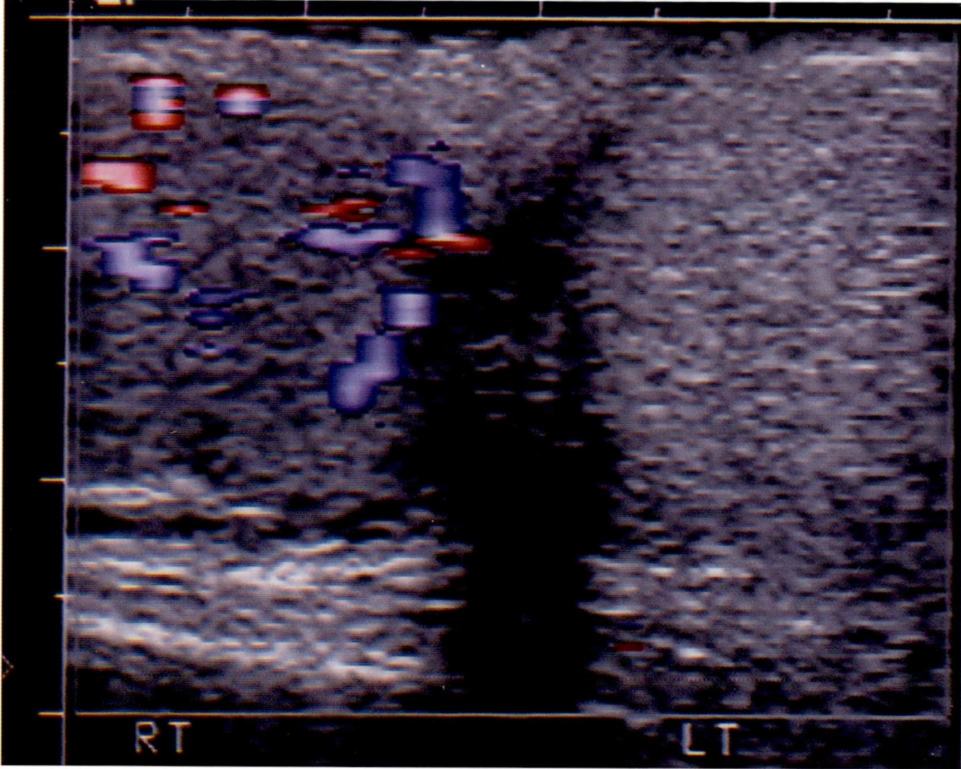

Plate 29 (Figs. 104–2 and 104–4*A*). **104–2** Scrotal ultrasound. Color Doppler. Transverse plane. **104–4*A*.** Annotated version of Fig. 104-2. Transverse plane through both testes. The color Doppler image of the scrotum demonstrates right testicular perfusion. The swollen left testis is not perfused. There is therefore left testicular torsion.

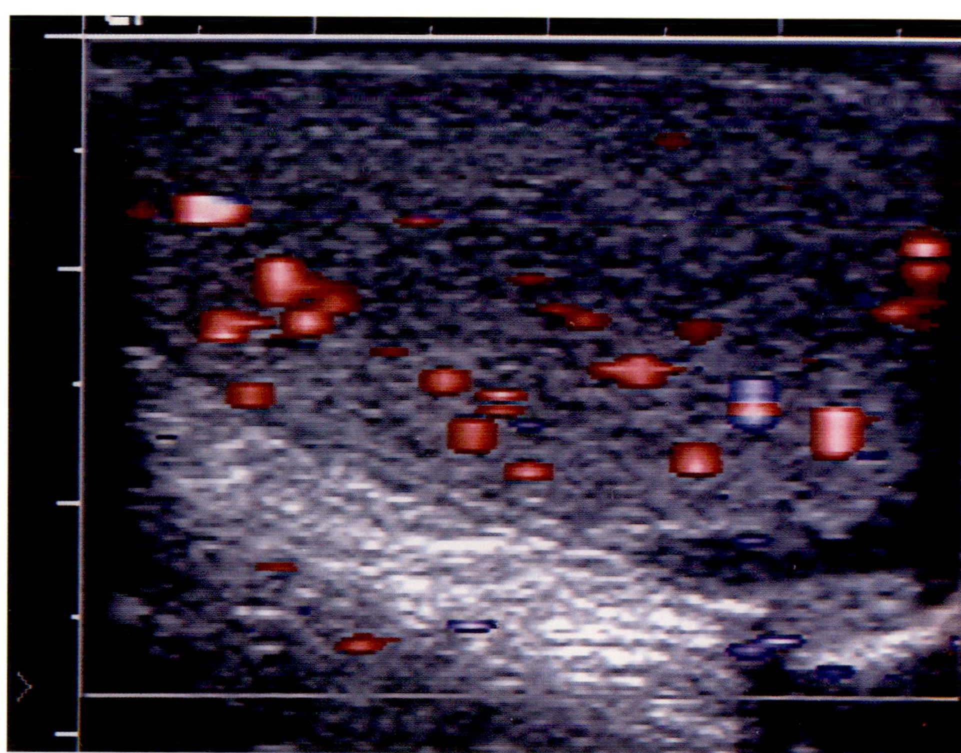

Plate 30 (Fig. 104–4*B*). Normal right testicle. Sagittal plane. This image confirms the finding of color flow in the normal right testicle.

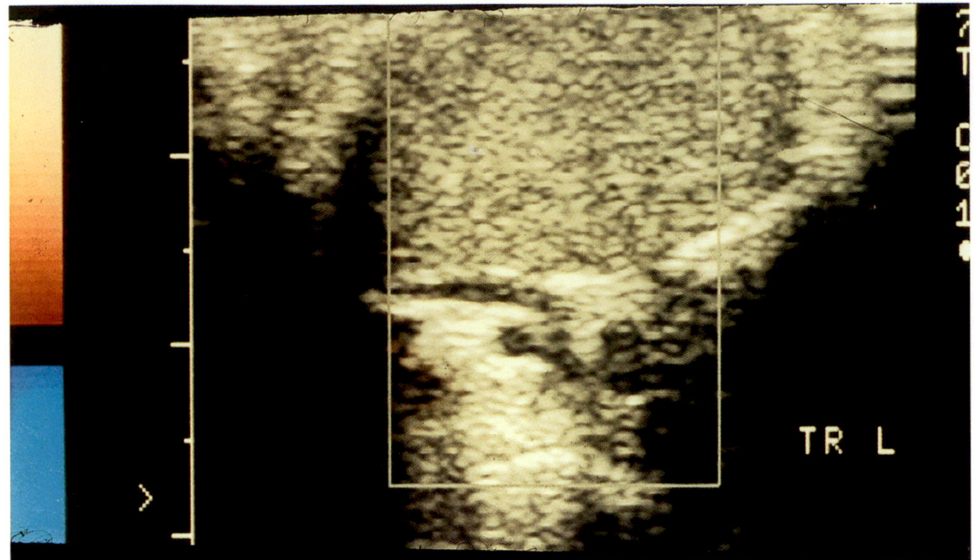

Plate 31 (Figs. 106–1*A* and 106–2*A*). 106–1*A*. Left hemiscrotum. Transverse plane. Color Doppler. **106–2*A*.** Annotated version of Fig. 106-1*A*. Varicocele. Left hemiscrotum. Transverse plane. Color Doppler. Patient at rest. Tubular and circular echopenic structures are seen posterior to the left testicle.

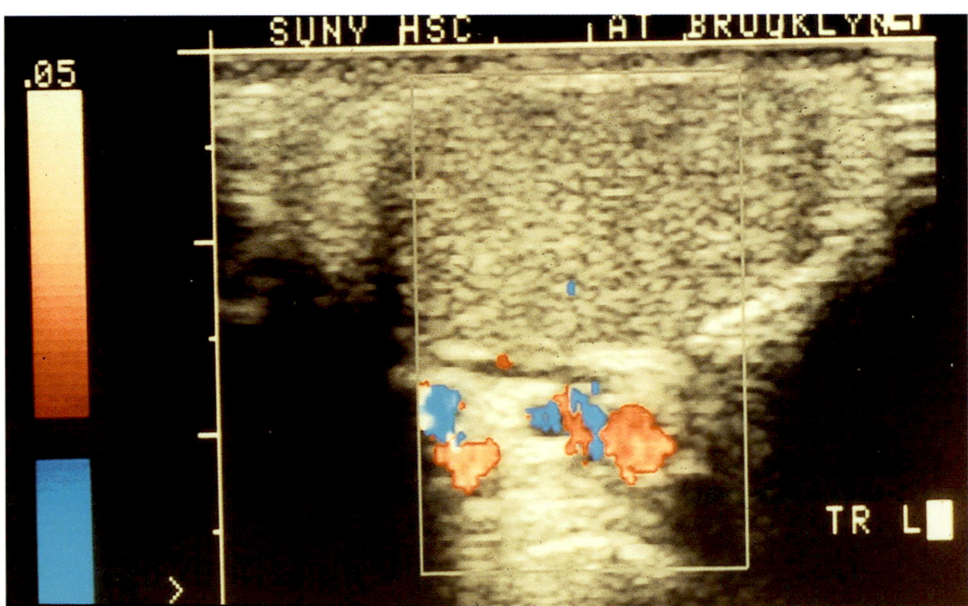

Plate 32 (Figs. 106–1*B* and 106–2*B*). 106–1*B*. Left hemiscrotum. Transverse plane. Color Doppler. **106–2*B*.** Annotated version of Fig. 106-1*B*. Varicocele. Left hemiscrotum. Transverse plane. Color Doppler. Patient bearing down. Color, consistent with vascular flow, is seen in the echopenic extratesticular structures within the Doppler's "color box." The spectral pattern was venous, proving the presence of a left varicocele in a patient with a known right varicocele.

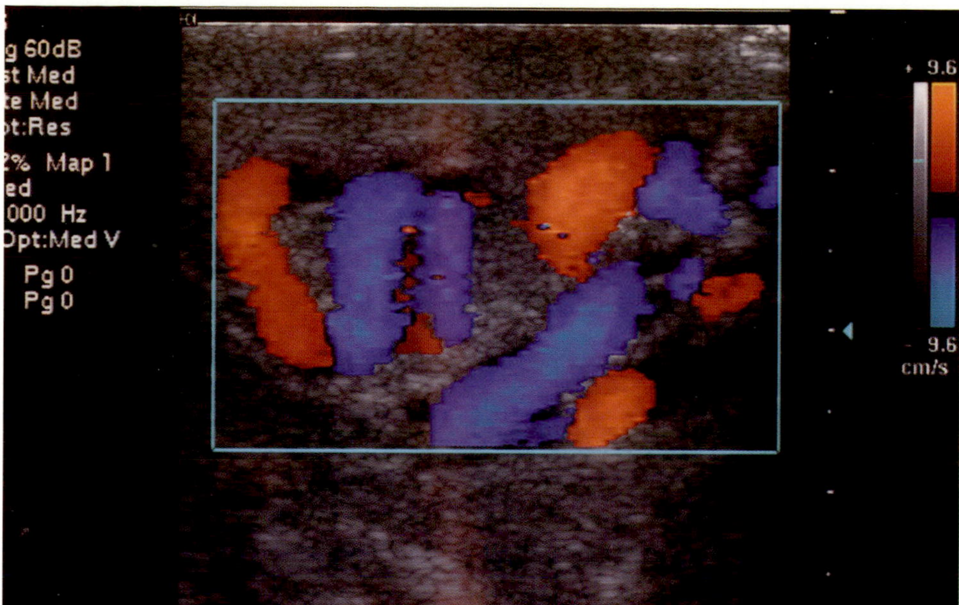

Plate 33 (Fig. 106–4). Grade II varicocele. Color Doppler. Longitudinal plane lateral to left testicle. Very large venous structures are imaged during a Valsalva maneuver. None were seen without bearing down. The vessels are 1 to 2 cm in diameter, consistent with Grade II varicocele.

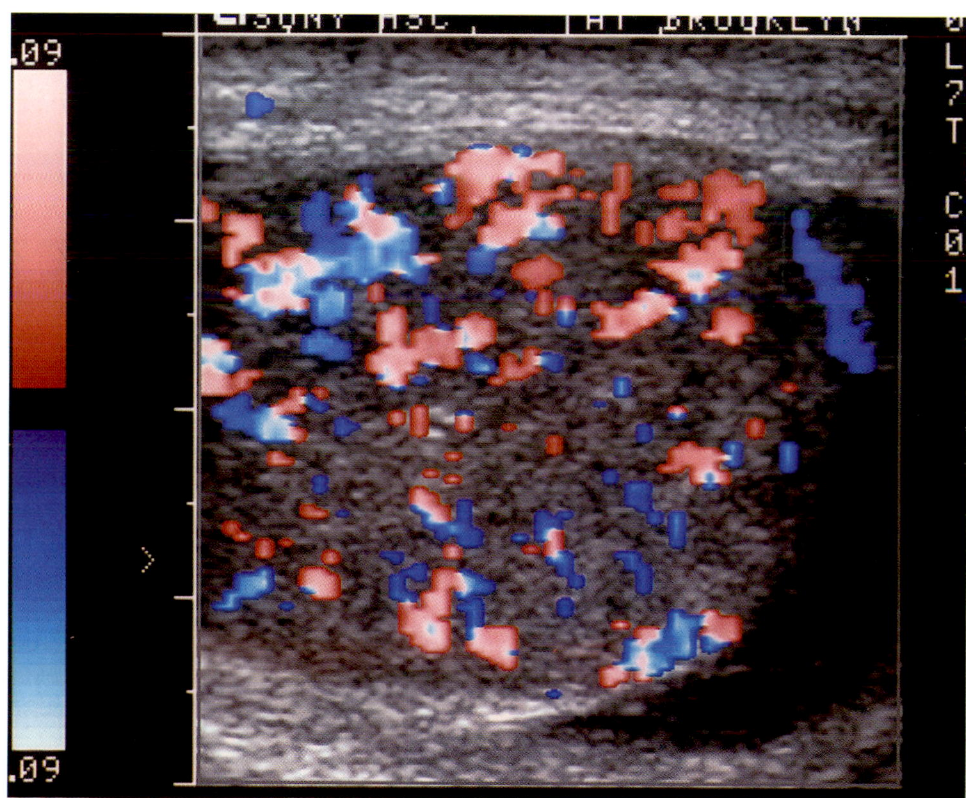

Plate 34 (Fig. 107–5). Orchitis. Right testicle. Longitudinal plane. Color Doppler examination. Hyperperfusion, predominantly of the superficial half of the testicle, noted by increased color Doppler signal, is seen in an area of the testicle noted on gray-scale examination to be echopenic. This adolescent had orchitis.

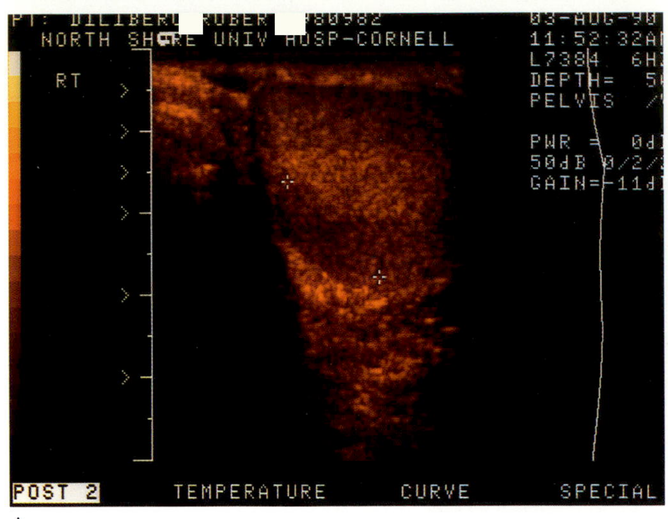

A

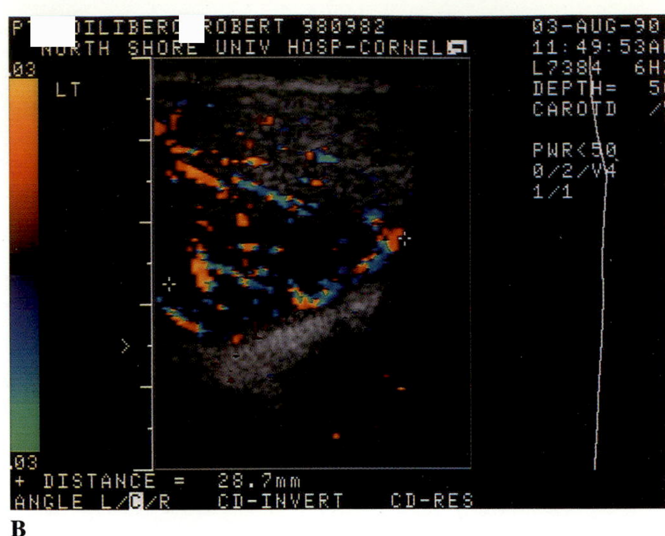

B

Plate 35 (Fig. 108–5*A* and *B*). Leukemic metastases/infiltration of testicle. ***A.*** Right testicle. Transverse plane. Color was used to highlight findings of the gray-scale image. The right testicle of this teenager with a history of leukemia in remission was enlarged and heterogeneous in echogenicity. Crosses are seen at the edges of one of the testicles' echopenic areas. Variable echogenicity of the testicle is nonspecific but suggests the need to rule out infiltrative disease. This is particularly true in a patient with leukemia. Similar findings may be seen with orchitis. ***B.*** Left testicle. Longitudinal oblique plane. Color Doppler. Significant increased color flow was noted in various areas of this heterogeneous left testicle. Both testes were enlarged and heterogeneous. The findings suggest infiltrative disease of the testicles. Although the increased vascular flow may have been simulated by an orchitis, the flow increase in a leukemic patient in remission may be the first imaging clue of recurrent leukemia with involvement of the testicular "sanctuary" site. That is what this case proved to be.

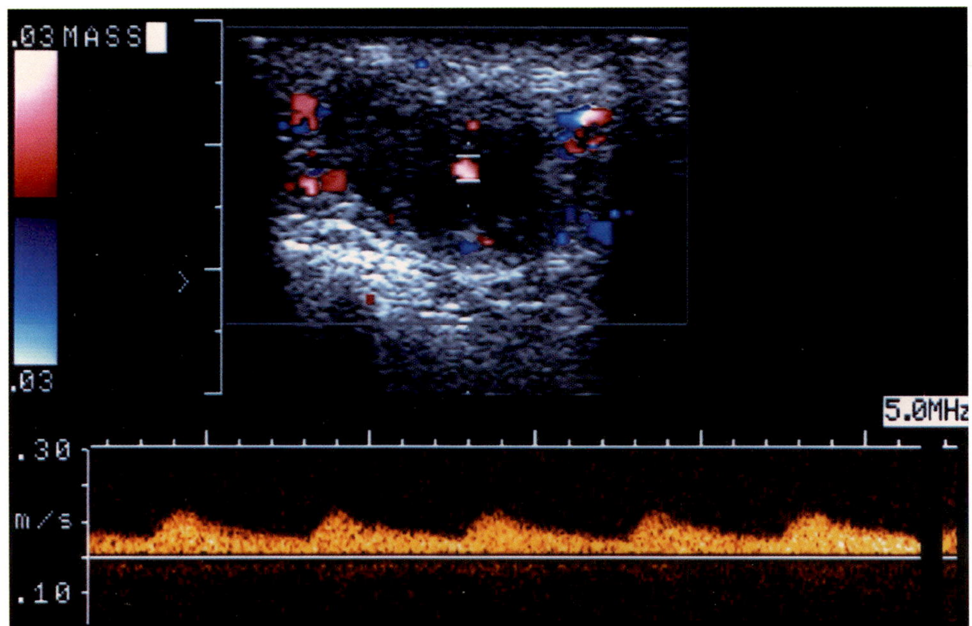

Plate 36 (Fig. 110–3). Color Doppler sonography of paratesticular rhabdomyosarcoma. Longitudinal view through the right scrotum in the same child as in Fig. 110-1 demonstrates hyperemia within the paratesticular mass.

Section J
TESTES

103

A newborn with an enlarged scrotum was sent to the ultrasound (US) laboratory for evaluation. Figure 103-1 is an image from that study. What is your concern? What is the diagnosis? Would Doppler help?

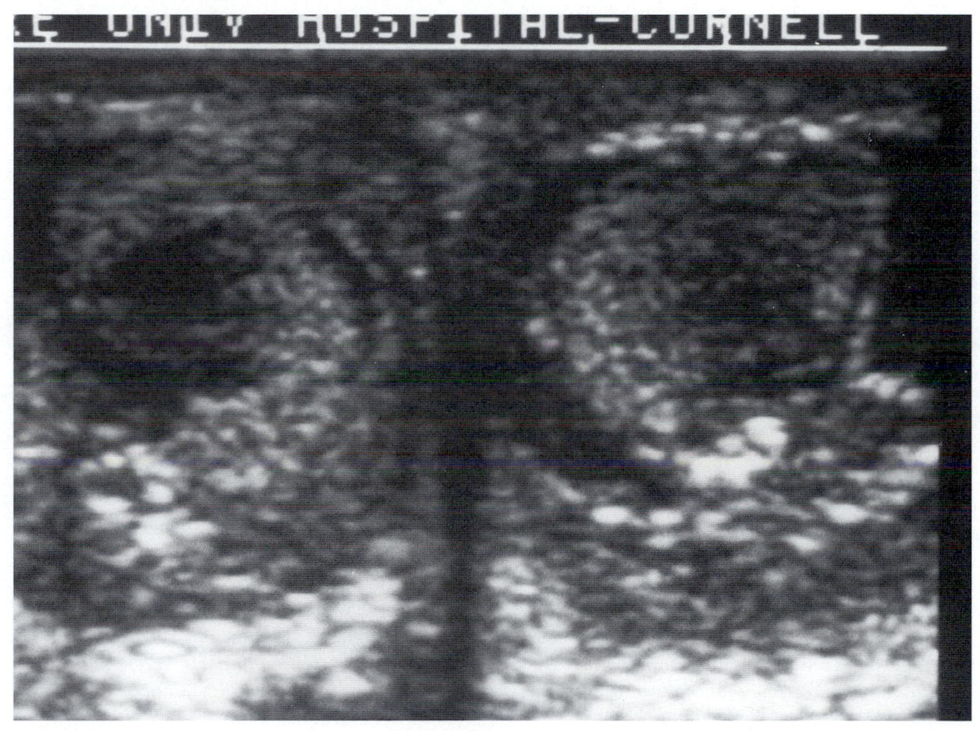

FIGURE 103–1. Scrotum. Transverse plane.

CHAPTER 103

Fetal and Neonatal Testicular Torsion

HARRY L. ZINN AND HARRIS L. COHEN

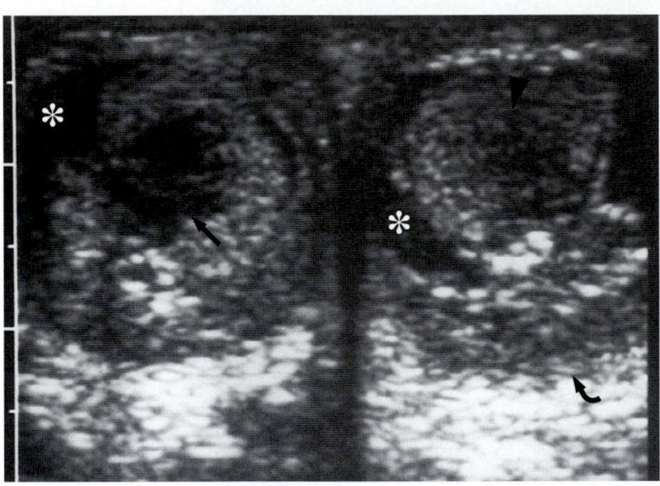

FIGURE 103–2. Annotated version of Fig. 103-1. Bilateral testicular torsion. Scrotum. Transverse plane. The right testicle is echopenic centrally (*arrow*), with only a small area of its periphery maintaining normal echogenicity. A smaller echopenic area (*arrowhead*) is noted in the left testicle. The scrotal wall (*curved arrows*) is thickened. Tiny right and larger left hydroceles (*) are present.

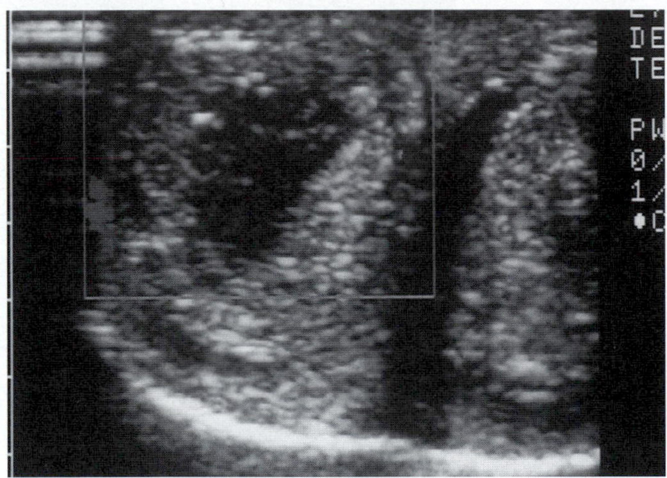

FIGURE 103–3. Torsed right testicle. Color Doppler exam. Transverse plane. The box within which color flow can be assessed is over the right testicle. No vascular flow was identified within it. (*From Gross BR, Cohen HL, Schlessel JS: Perinatal diagnosis of bilateral testicular torsion: Beware of torsions simulating hydroceles.* J Ultrasound Med *12:479–481, 1993, with permission.*) (See Color Plate 27.)

Figure 103-2, the annotated version of Fig. 103-1, shows the right testicle of the newborn to be echopenic except at its periphery. The left testicle also is echopenic centrally. The scrotal wall is thickened. There are a tiny right and a small left hydrocele. Echopenic testes, particularly in the fetus or newborn, suggest the likelihood of testicular torsion. Lack of vascular flow (Fig. 103-3; see also Color Plate 27), within the testes confirmed the diagnosis of torsion.

This neonate was actually imaged as a fetus (Fig. 103-4) and was noted by his examiners to have what appeared to be a large hydrocele. However, it was actually an enlarged echopenic testicle. The second testicle was more normal in size, but surrounded by hydrocele, and echopenic as well. The fact that echopenic testes were imaged antenatally indicates that the torsion had its origin in fetal life.

The testes of a fetus or of a newborn, just like those of any male, should be homogeneously echogenic (Fig. 103-5; see also Color Plate 28). Hydroceles are not uncommon in fetal and neonatal life.

TESTICULAR TORSION IN THE NEONATE AND FETUS

We know that testicular torsion occurs in adolescents. Testicular torsion can *also* be a significant source of morbidity in

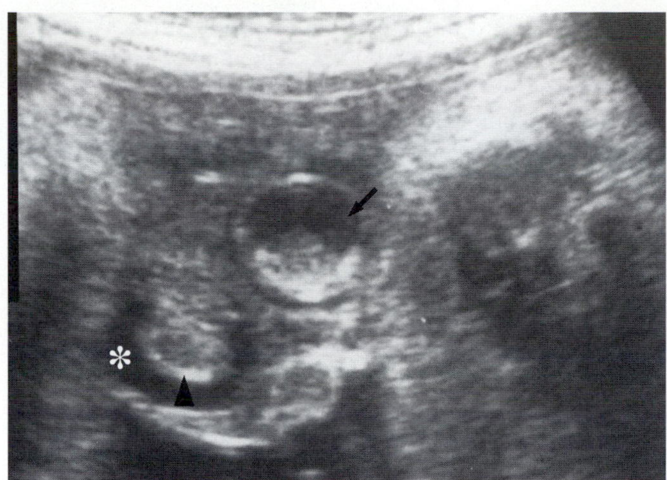

FIGURE 103–4. Bilateral torsion in fetal testes. Fetal scrotum. Coronal plane. The right testicle (*arrow*) of this 38-week fetus is on the reader's right. It is predominantly echopenic. A small peripheral hydrocele is seen. The left testicle (*arrowhead*) is smaller in size and also somewhat echopenic. It is surrounded by a moderate hydrocele (*) (*From Gross BR, Cohen HL, Schlessel JS: Perinatal diagnosis of bilateral testicular torsion: Beware of torsions simulating hydroceles.* J Ultrasound Med *12:479–481, 1993, with permission.*)

the neonate. Instances of testicular torsion peak in males during two age periods, the neonatal and the adolescent. The typical adolescent torsion is intravaginal and is the result of twisting of the spermatic cord while the testicles are suspended in the tunica vaginalis. Intravaginal torsion is associated with the "bell and clapper" deformity, which occurs when there is a complete investment of the testis and epididymis by the tunica vaginalis. Torsion during the neonatal period is usually extravaginal, with no bell and clapper deformity present. In extravaginal torsion, the spermatic cord and its adjacent tunica twist together as a unit. This is felt to be due to increased mobility of the entire vaginalis. Most cases of testicular torsion in newborns are believed to have occurred in utero. Torsion leads to hemorrhagic infarction and necrosis of the testicle.

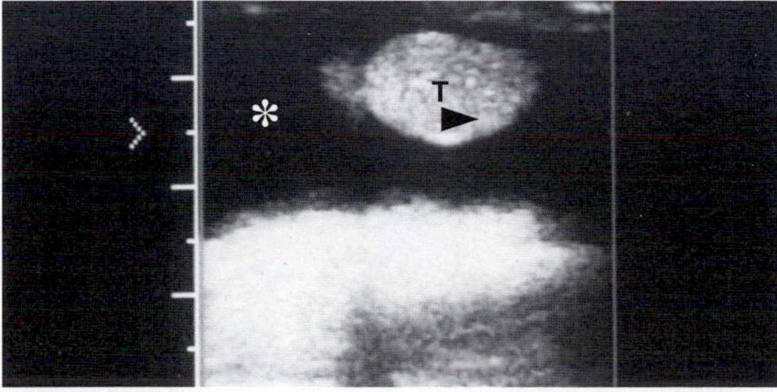

FIGURE 103–5. Large hydrocele, normal testicular echogenicity. Right testicle. Longitudinal plane. Color Doppler examination. The testicle of a newborn with a large hydrocele (*) is noted. The normal testis is of homogeneous echogenicity. Note that the echogenicity is greater than that in the previous images of cases of torsion. A small dot of color (*arrowhead*) seen in the testicle was proven on spectral examination to be due to arterial flow. (See Color Plate 28.)

Testicular salvage is more likely when surgical detorsion is performed early. The salvage rate can be as high as 80 to 100 percent if surgery is performed within 5 to 6 h of the onset of pain. The salvage rate drops to 70 percent if surgery is performed within 6 to 12 h and only 20 percent if surgery is performed after 12 h. Obviously, salvage is less likely if a torsion occurred much earlier during antenatal life.

PERINATAL TESTICULAR TORSION—ULTRASOUND FINDINGS

The usual sonographic appearance of testicular torsion in the newborn is that of an inhomogeneously hypoechoic testicle, perhaps with a brightly echogenic rim of normal parenchyma. There have been reported cases of testicular torsion in which the testicle appeared isoechoic or hyperechoic to the normal contralateral testicle. A study by Middleton et al of adolescent testicular torsion found that normal testicular echogenicity in the setting of testicular torsion correlated strongly with viability at surgery, whereas a hypoechoic or heterogeneous testicle was usually nonviable. A torsed testicle can appear larger than the normal contralateral testicle. Scrotal skin thickening, reactive hydrocele, and an enlarged, heterogeneous epididymis may also be seen.

USE OF DOPPLER IN TESTICULAR TORSION ANALYSIS

Color Doppler sonography has complemented gray-scale imaging for many conditions diagnosed by US. It has revolutionized the diagnosis of torsion of the testicles of adolescents, replacing scintigraphy as the first and usually only step taken to prove intratesticular vascular flow. When performed in combination with gray-scale imaging, color Doppler can also provide information that is helpful in diagnosing other conditions that clinically mimic acute testicular torsion. This is particularly true for epididymitis and epididymoorchitis. Infectious causes of acute testicular pain usually produce hyperemia and increased vascular flow. In contrast, the absence of color flow signal is diagnostic of acute testicular torsion. It is reported that 540° of torsion are required to cause total occlusion of blood flow. Lesser degrees of torsion can, at the very least, cause testicular ischemia, if not infarction. If there is only ischemia, flow may still be detected. Some loss of at least the diastolic component of the intratesticular arterial flow may help point to the abnormality (ischemia).

ULTRASOUND AND DOPPLER ANALYSIS OF ANTENATAL AND NEONATAL TESTICULAR TORSION

Antenatal and neonatal testicular torsion can be a more difficult diagnosis to make than torsion in an adolescent. The

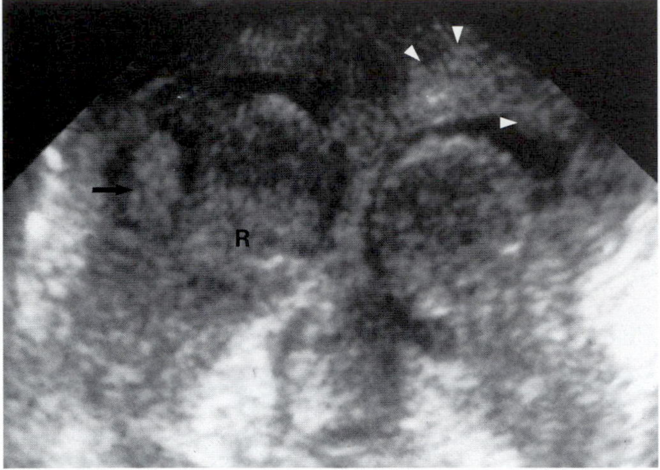

A

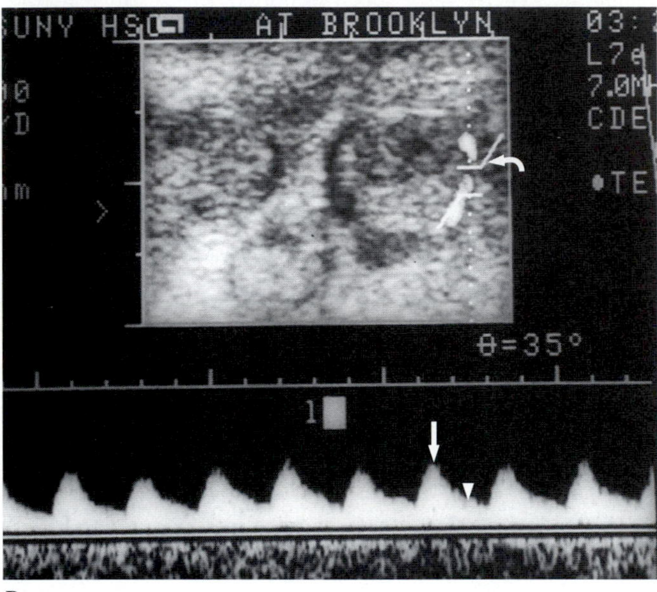

B

FIGURE 103–6. Bilateral testicular torsion in a newborn. ***A.*** Scrotum. Transverse plane. The scrotal wall is thickened (*arrowheads*). This actually aided ultrasound imaging of the scrotal contents by increasing the size of the scrotum and increasing the distance from transducer and skin surface to the testes themselves. Both testes are predominantly echopenic, suggesting probable torsion. R = right testicle. Incidentally noted is an oval mass (*arrow*) lateral to the right testicle due to a torsed appendix testes. ***B.*** Scrotum. Transverse plane. Triplex Doppler (image, spectra, and color flow) imaged in black and white. An insonated (white curved line at its periphery) left testicle shows an arterial spectrum with low-resistance systolic (*arrow*) and diastolic (*arrowhead*) flow. Whether the diastolic component is truly somewhat less than normal or whether this is due to technique is unknown. No signal could be obtained centrally, suggesting a poor prognosis for the testicle at surgery, which is what was discovered. Only power Doppler could image central flow in the contralateral right testicle, which was able to be saved. Interestingly, on a follow-up exam several months after surgery, the echopenic echogenicity pattern reverted to an almost homogeneous (normal pattern). (*From Zinn HL, Cohen HL, Horowitz M: Testicular torsion in neonates: The importance of power Doppler imaging.* J Ultrasound Med *17:385–388, with permission.*)

small "package" of the newborn scrotum makes analysis technically difficult. Stand-off pads are cumbersome and not useful given the neonate's scrotal size. At times, I will try to cup the scrotum with the proximal portion of my second through fourth fingers and guide the transducer with the thumb of that hand. Normal testicular blood flow during the antenatal period is low. The absence of color signal may indicate true torsion or may be technical in nature, reflecting the difficulty Doppler has in detecting normal but slow blood flow.

A helpful technological advance in recent years is power Doppler, with its greater sensitivity (at least 10 to 15 dB) to flow. Power Doppler sonography depends on the integrated power of the Doppler signal, as opposed to the reliance on mean frequency shift in conventional color Doppler. Using it, we have been able to detect flow in neonatal testicles that was too low to detect by conventional color Doppler (Fig. 103-6). Power Doppler can provide information on flow within the testicle independent of the angle of insonation. Color and duplex Doppler require imaging at a 60° angle or less to avoid errors in determination of peak systolic velocity within a vessel. This is, however, far less a concern in the analysis of testicular torsion. The main goal in analyzing cases of testicular torsion is to note whether or not there is central testicular arterial flow. The more sensitive an imaging device is in detecting flow, the better. The disadvantage that power Doppler is sensitive to nearby motion artifacts is not a problem in evaluating a patient with suspected testicular torsion because there is no motion artifact from nearby moving structures. Information about flow direction is not necessary. We reported a case several years ago of a fetus born with bilaterally echopenic testes suggestive of bilateral torsion beyond surgical help. Color flow showed only peripheral flow in the left testicle (Fig. 103-6*B*). This testicle was unable to be saved at surgery. The right testicle, which showed central flow only on power Doppler examination, was able to be saved. Preoperative information obtained by US and Doppler prepared the surgical team for what they would find.

Ultrasound helps decisions to be made regarding surgical management. Correct imaging diagnoses and the exclusion of other scrotal pathologic conditions allow the avoidance of surgery for those neonates who do not need it. When surgery is the treatment of choice, a correct US diagnosis allows timing of the surgery to be determined so as to best avoid the greater risks of surgery and anesthesia that do exist in the first days of life.

KEY POINTS

Testicular torsion can occur in perinatal life. Be concerned about abnormalities in testicular echogenicity. Use one testicle and its vascular flow noted by Doppler as a basis of comparison for the other. Unhappily, if there is bilateral abnormality, finding a lack of color flow in both testes and a normal echogenicity pattern leaves the examiner unable to know whether there is torsion or there is technical difficulty in denoting normal flow in small testes. Use of power Doppler or scintigraphy may help. Interestingly, the echogenicity pattern of one of our torsion cases, in which a single testicle was saved after surgery at birth, showed a reversal of the echopenic echogenicity within that testicle to an almost homogeneously echogenic image on a follow-up a few months later. One should probably consider echopenic echogenicity in torsion as evidence of, perhaps, edema, as it is in inflammation or in other conditions of the testes, and not only as evidence suggesting necrosis.

References

Atkinson GO, Patrick LE, Ball TI, et al: The normal and abnormal scrotum in children: Evaluation with color Doppler sonography. *AJR* 158:613–617, 1992.

Burks DD, Markey BJ, Burkhard TK, et al: Suspected testicular torsion and ischemia: Evaluation with color Doppler sonography. *Radiology* 175:815–821, 1990.

Chin DH, Miller EI: Generalized testicular hyperechogenicity in acute testicular torsion. *J Ultrasound Med* 4:495–496, 1985.

Cohen HL, Haller J: Scrotal ultrasound in the pediatric and adolescent patient. *Radiology Report* 2:276–290, 1990.

Gross BR, Cohen HL, Schlessel JS: Perinatal diagnosis of bilateral testicular torsion: Beware of torsions simulating hydroceles. *J Ultrasound Med* 12:479–481, 1993.

Hricak H, Lue T, Filly RA, et al: Experimental study of the sonographic diagnosis of testicular torsion. *J Ultrasound Med* 2:349–356, 1983.

Jerkins GR, Noe N, Hollabaugh RS, et al: Spermatic cord torsion in the neonate. *J Urol* 129:121–122, 1983.

Lee FT, Winter DB, Madsen FA, et al: Conventional color Doppler velocity sonography versus color Doppler energy sonography for the diagnosis of acute experimental torsion of the spermatic cord. *AJR* 167:785–790, 1996.

Middleton WD, Middleton MA, Dierks M, et al: Sonographic prediction of viability in testicular torsion: Preliminary observations. *J Ultrasound Med* 16:23–27, 1997.

Middleton WD, Siegel BA, Melson GL, et al: Acute scrotal disorders: Prospective comparison of color Doppler US and testicular scintigraphy. *Radiology* 7:177–181, 1990.

Rubin JM, Bude RO, Carson PL, et al: Power Doppler US: A potentially useful alternative to mean frequency-based color Doppler US. *Radiology* 190:853–856, 1994.

Stone K, Kass E, Cacciarelli A, Gibson D: Management of suspected antenatal torsion: What is the best strategy. *J Urol* 153:782–784.

Williamson RCN: Torsion of the testis and allied conditions. *Br J Surg* 63:465–476, 1994.

Zerin JM, DiPietro MA, Grignon A, Shea D: Testicular infarction in the newborn: Ultrasound findings. *Pediatr Radiol* 20:329–330, 1990.

Zinn HL, Cohen HL, Horowitz M: Testicular torsion in neonates: The importance of power Doppler imaging. *J Ultrasound Med* 17:385–388, 1998.

104

A 14-year-old boy was hit in the scrotum by a baseball one day prior to presentation. He was sent for sonographic evaluation with the complaint of severe left testicular pain. Ultrasonographic views of the right and left testicles (Figs. 104-1 and 104-2) were obtained. What is the diagnosis?

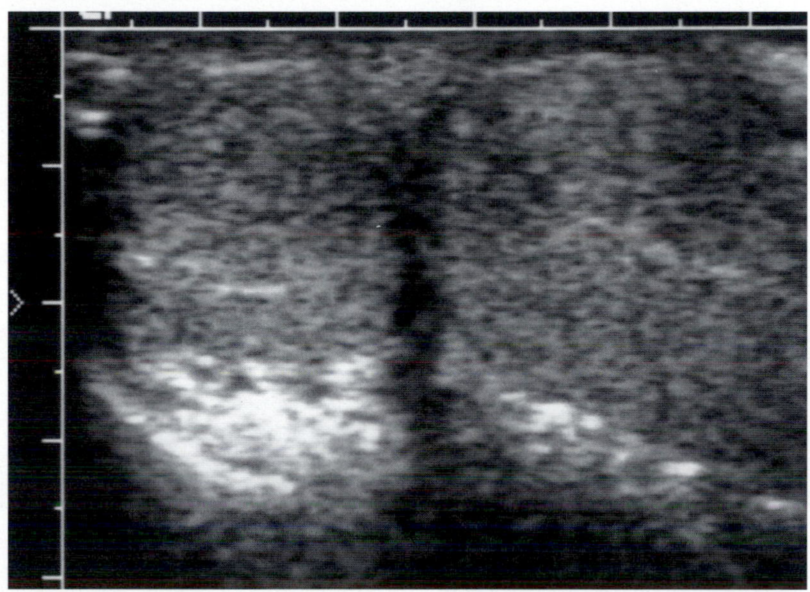

FIGURE 104–1. Scrotal ultrasound. Transverse plane. The right testicle is on the reader's left.

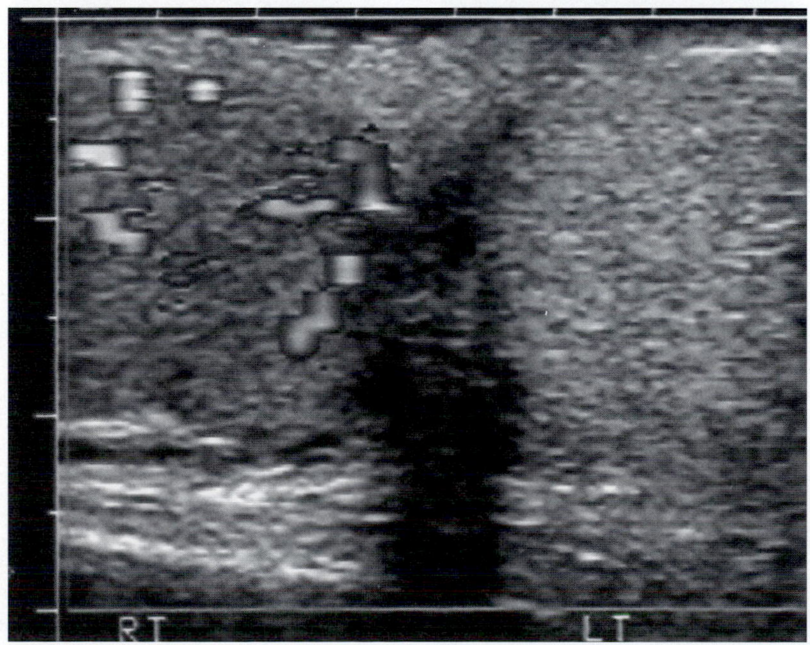

FIGURE 104–2. Scrotal ultrasound. Color Doppler. Transverse plane. (See Color Plate 29.)

CHAPTER 104

Acute Left Testicular Torsion in an Adolescent

HARRIET J. PALTIEL

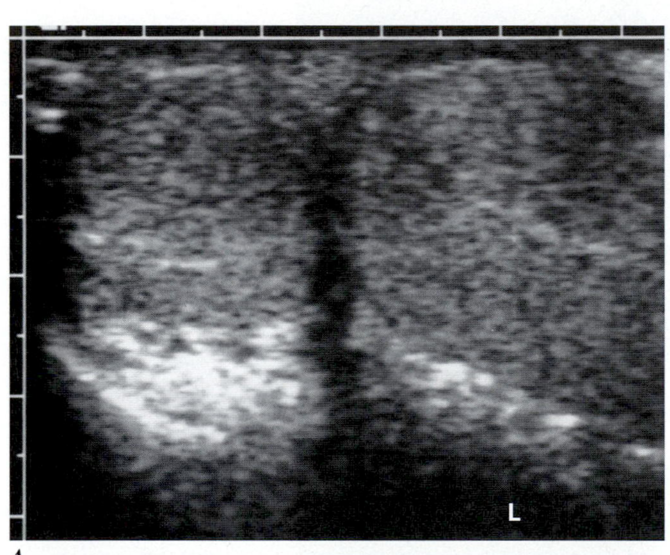

A

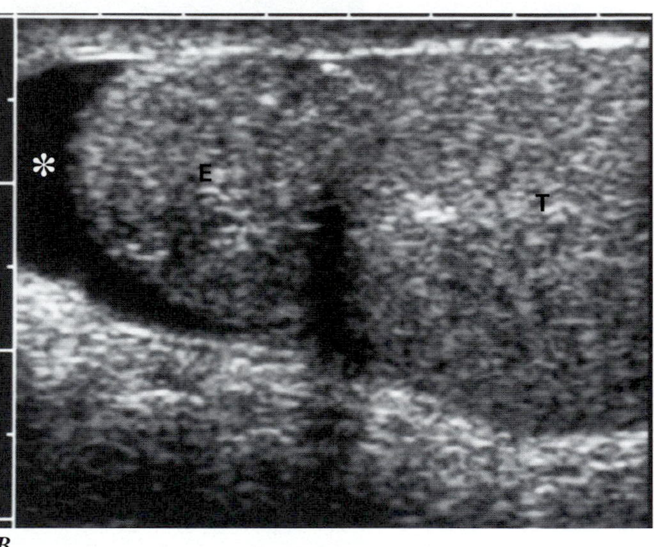

B

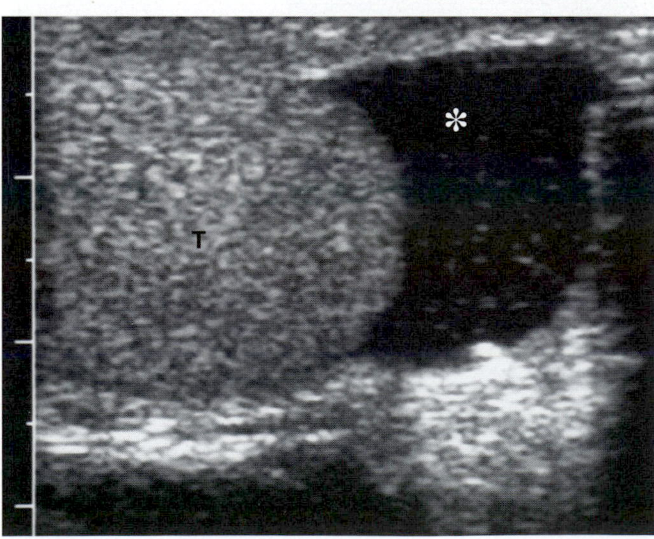

C

FIGURE 104–3. Testicular torsion—gray-scale findings. Scrotal ultrasound. ***A.*** Annotated version of Fig. 104-1. Transverse plane. The left testicle is larger than the right because of swelling. Such an image might be simulated by asymmetrically positioned testes due to torsion. The echogenicity of the left testis is comparable to that of the normal right testis. ***B.*** Sagittal plane through the left hemiscrotum. There is an enlarged epididymis. A small hydrocele is superior to the epididymis. E = epididymis, T = testis. ***C.*** Sagittal plane through left hemiscrotum. There is a hydrocele (*asterisk*) with contained echogenicity, possibly from hemorrhagic debris, although echogenicity can be commonly seen in chronic hydroceles and is thought to be due to the cholesterol content of the hydrocele. The hydrocele appears inferior to the testis. T = testis.

Figure 104-3*A,* the annotated version of Fig. 104-1, demonstrates a swollen left testis compared to the testicle on the right but no definitive difference in echogenicity. Figure 104-4*A* (see also Color Plate 29), the annotated version of Fig. 104-2, is a color Doppler image that shows normal right

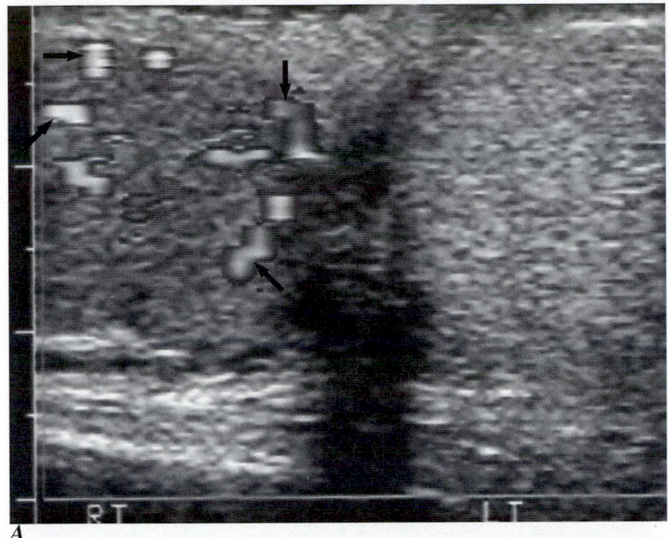

A

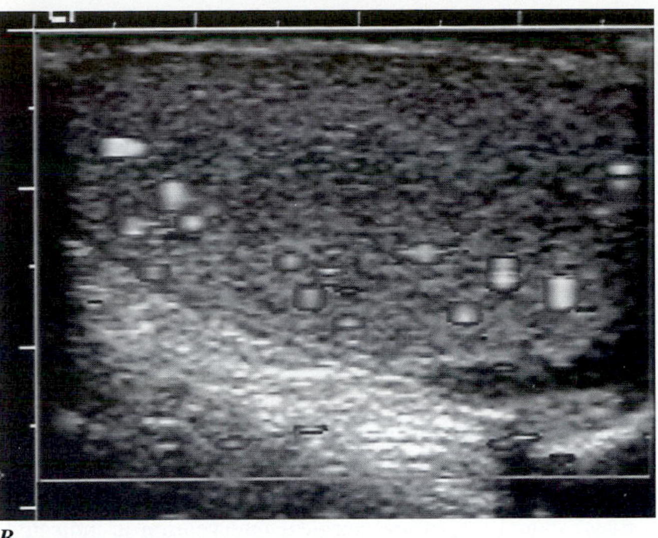

B

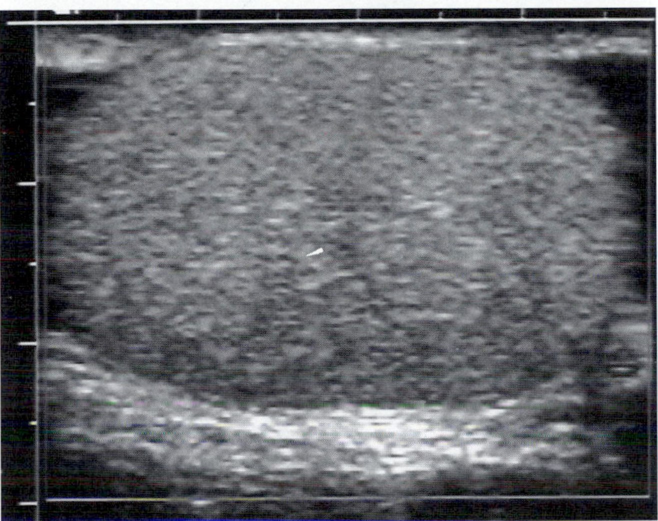

C

FIGURE 104–4. Testicular torsion—Doppler and gray-scale findings. Scrotal ultrasound. ***A.*** Annotated version of Fig. 104-2. Transverse plane through both testes. The color Doppler image of the scrotum demonstrates right testicular perfusion. The swollen left testis is not perfused. There is therefore left testicular torsion. (See Color Plate 29.) ***B.*** Normal right testicle. Sagittal plane. This image confirms the finding of color flow in the normal right testicle. (See Color Plate 30.) ***C.*** Torsive left testicle. Sagittal plane. Despite the presence of a color flow box around the entire left testicle and the use of the same technique that enabled flow to be seen on the right, no flow is noted in the left testicle. It is not perfused.

testicular perfusion but no left testicular perfusion (Fig. 104-4; see also Color Plate 30). The ultrasound (US) diagnosis is testicular torsion. Additional images of the left hemiscrotum show an enlarged epididymis (Fig. 104-3*B*) and an echogenic hydrocele (Fig. 104-3*C*).

On physical examination, this boy had an enlarged, indurated left testicle. He was taken to surgery following the positive US exam, at which time the left testis was detorsed and bilateral orchiopexies were performed. The left testis appeared marginally viable, with a slight improvement in perfusion following detorsion.

ACUTE SCROTAL PAIN IN BOYS

Treatment of a boy with acute scrotal symptoms is usually based on the clinical history and results of physical examination. If acute testicular torsion is likely, immediate surgical exploration is warranted. The rationale for this aggressive approach is that progressive ischemia will inevitably lead to testicular necrosis if surgical detorsion is not achieved within several hours. A vast majority of boys who present with acute scrotal pain and/or swelling have nonsurgical conditions, most often torsion of the appendix testis or epididymitis. Because the clinical appearances of these conditions are frequently indistinguishable from that of testicular torsion, imaging is often done to assist with the diagnosis and help avoid unnecessary surgery.

Although testicular torsion can occur at any age, it is more common in the newborn period and the early stages of puberty. Torsion of the testicular appendages usually occurs in prepubertal boys, while epididymitis is more frequent in adolescents and young adults with a history of sexual activity.

Associated symptoms, such as nausea and vomiting, are common with testicular torsion, whereas fever and voiding symptoms such as urgency, frequency, and dysuria are suggestive of epididymitis.

TESTICULAR TORSION

The underlying cause of testicular torsion in older children is called the "bell clapper" deformity because the testicles of those at risk for torsion lack a normal attachment (Fig. 104-5) to the tunica vaginalis; instead, they hang freely within it. This anatomic abnormality (Fig. 104-6) is usually bilateral. When torsion occurs, the spermatic cord twists within the tunica vaginalis, occluding the blood supply to the testicle and resulting in hemorrhagic infarction.

The typical clinical history of an adolescent with testicular torsion is one of the acute onset of severe testicular pain and tenderness. Torsion may occur while the patient is active, while the patient is at rest, or following scrotal trauma. Early in the course of testicular torsion, physical findings may also include a high-riding testicle with a transverse lie, scrotal erythema, and edema.

WHY TIME IS OF THE ESSENCE IN DIAGNOSING TORSION

Testicular salvage is usually possible only when the duration of torsion is less than 12 h. After 12 h, salvage rates are poor. When the history and clinical examination are strongly suggestive of testicular torsion, and symptoms have been present for less than 12 h, urgent surgical intervention is indicated. Imaging studies are not performed in definitive cases, since they may result in needless delay and thereby jeopardize testicular viability. When the duration of symptoms is longer than 12 h or the diagnosis is unclear, an imaging study may be useful in establishing the correct diagnosis.

IMAGING FOR TESTICULAR TORSION

At one time, examination of the testes with nuclear medicine agents to "rule out torsion" was the gold standard. Both scrotal scintigraphy and, more recently, color Doppler ultrasonography (US) have been shown to detect testicular perfusion with a high degree of diagnostic accuracy.

Scrotal scintigraphy is performed using technetium 99m pertechnetate. In patients with testicular torsion, little or no radioisotope reaches the testis (Fig. 104-7), whereas in patients with torsion of an appendage or epididymitis, blood flow is normal or increased. The examination usually takes between 20 to 30 min to perform. However, in many centers, the radioisotope may not be immediately available, resulting in a delay in diagnosis. This modality is also limited by its relatively poor spatial resolution and use of ionizing radiation.

Gray-scale US coupled with color Doppler imaging permits an assessment of intrascrotal contents as well as direct visualization of intratesticular vessels. It is usually readily available and rapidly performed. Torsion is diagnosed when blood flow to the symptomatic testicle is diminished or absent. When normal or increased blood flow is documented, testicular torsion is excluded. Surgery is performed to detorse the affected testicle and to anchor the other testicle in order to prevent future torsion. When the torsive testis is obviously necrotic, it is removed.

EDITOR'S COMMENT

Color Doppler, particularly with improvements in sensitivity to flow, has been a great tool for making the diagnosis of testicular torsion. Power Doppler has improved the analysis of

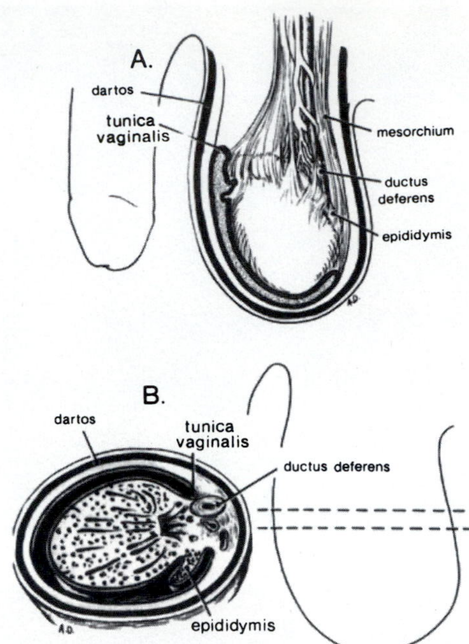

FIGURE 104–5. Normal scrotal anatomy. Schematic drawing. ***A.*** A longitudinal image through one testicle shows normal anatomy, in which the tunica vaginalis *does not* cover the posterior epididymis. ***B.*** A cross section of the scrotum at the level of the superior third of the testis shows the uncovered epididymis approximated to the scrotal wall. This attachment precludes testicular rotation. (*From Holder LE, Martine JR, Holmes ER III, Wagner HN Jr: Testicular radionuclide angiography and static imaging: Anatomy, scintigraphic interpretation, and clinical indications.* Radiology *125:739–752, 1977, with permission.*)

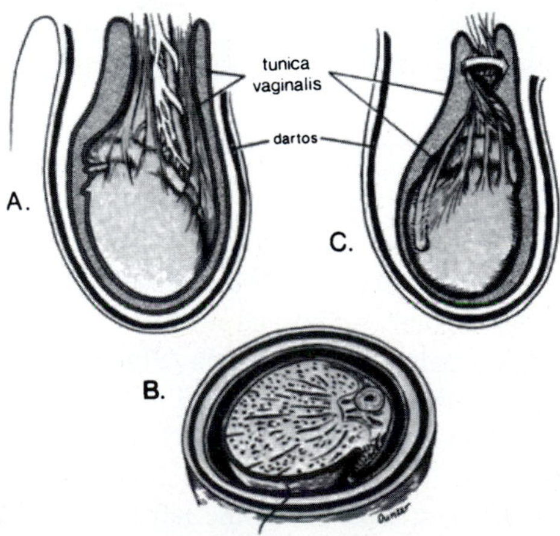

FIGURE 104–6. Congenital variation in anatomy leading to possible testicular torsion. Schematic drawing. ***A.*** A longitudinal image through one testicle shows that the tunica vaginalis completely surrounds the testis and epididymis, so that they resemble a "clapper in a bell." ***B.*** A cross section of the scrotum at the level of the superior third of the testis shows the tunica vaginalis (*curved black line*) interposed between the epididymis and the scrotal wall. This prevention of attachment allows the possibility of testicular torsion. ***C.*** Equivalent to ***A*** after testicular torsion. A white arrow, seen superiorly, indicates the site and axis of the testicular torsion. (*From Holder LE, Martine JR, Holmes ER III, Wagner HN Jr: Testicular radionuclide angiography and static imaging: Anatomy, scintigraphic interpretation, and clinical indications.* Radiology *125: 739–752, 1977, with permission.*)

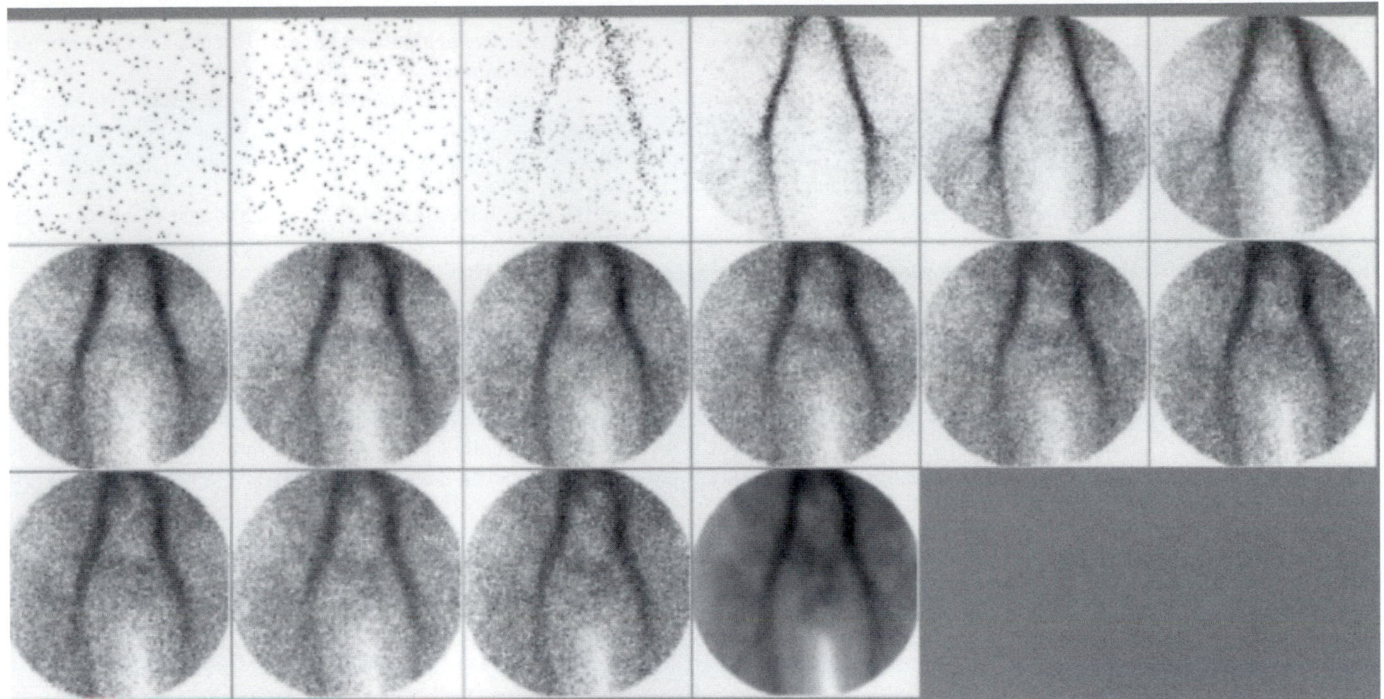

A

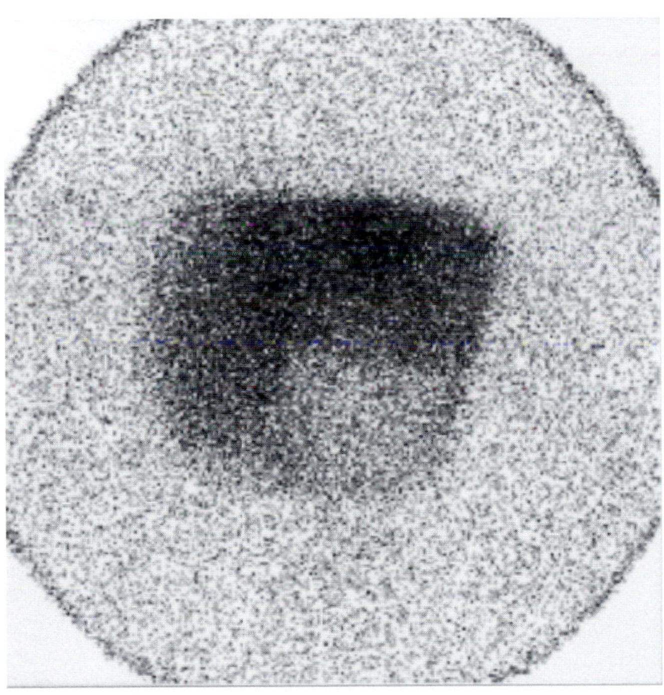

B

FIGURE 104–7. Testicular torsion—diagnosis by nuclear scintigraphy. ***A.*** Radionuclide angiography. The patient is facing the reader, and the right hemiscrotum is on the reader's left. The immediate angiographic phase images are normal. However, the last image, the immediate tissue phase, suggests an asymmetry of tracer amount in the scrotum. There is increased tracer uptake in the upper region of the left hemiscrotum *(arrow)* and less tracer uptake inferiorly. ***B.*** Pinhole magnification. This magnified image reveals decreased tracer uptake in the left hemiscrotum in the area of the testicle (*arrow*), consistent with acute testicular torsion. (*Courtesy of S. Ted Treves, M.D.*)

flow even more, particularly in the assessment of the smaller, and therefore technically more difficult, scrotum of the child. Nothing, however, is straightforward. We have seen flow change during an exam with torsion and detorsion. We use the assessment of testicular echogenicity as an aid in the diagnosis. An older torsed testis (i.e., one where there has been a delay in diagnosis) usually is more echopenic than the contralateral side. We used to think that that indicated irreversible infarction. This is not necessarily always true. In this case, edema may account for the homogeneous echogenicity of the torsed testicle (Fig. 104-4) that makes it appear more "normal" than the other. Flow analysis with Doppler, as long as one can technically obtain flow on the normal side, is the final judge.

Testicular torsion can occur from trauma. This case is probably an example. Obviously the trauma acted as a catalyst for the occurrence of torsion in an anatomically abnormal scrotum, i.e., one in which each testis hangs like a clapper in a bell, without attachment to the scrotal wall and at risk for a twist that may seal its fate.

References

Bader TR, Kammerhuber F, Herneth AM: Testicular blood flow in boys as assessed at color Doppler and power Doppler sonography. *Radiology* 202:559–564, 1997.

Barth RA, Shortliffe LD: Normal pediatric testis: Comparison of power Doppler and color Doppler US in the detection of blood flow. *Radiology* 204:389–393, 1997.

Cass AS, Cass BP, Veerarhgavan K: Immediate exploration of the unilateral acute scrotum in young male subjects. *J Urol* 124:829–832, 1980.

Chen DCP, Holder LE, Kaplan GN: Correlation of radionuclide imaging and diagnostic ultrasound in scrotal diseases. *J Nucl Med* 27:1774–1781, 1986.

Cohen HL, Shapiro MA, Haller JO, Glassberg K: Torsion of the testicular appendage. Sonographic diagnosis. *J Ultrasound Med* 11:81–83, 1992.

Gelfand MJ, Williams PJ, Rosenkrantz JG: Pinhole imaging: Utility in testicular imaging in children. *Clin Nucl Med* 5:237–240, 1980.

Holder LE, Martine JR, Holmes ER III, Wagner HN Jr: Testicular radionuclide angiography and static imaging: Anatomy, scintigraphic interpretation, and clinical indications. *Radiology* 125:739–752, 1977.

Kass EJ, Stone KT, Cacciarelli AA, Mitchell B: Do all children with an acute scrotum require exploration? *J Urol* 150:667–669, 1993.

Lewis AG, Bukowski TP, Jarvis PD, et al: Evaluation of acute scrotum in the emergency department. *J Pediatr Surg* 30:277–282, 1995.

Middleton WD, Siegel BA, Melson GL, et al: Acute scrotal disorders: Prospective comparison of color Doppler US and testicular scintigraphy. *Radiology* 177:177–181, 1990.

Paltiel HJ, Connolly LP, Atala A, et al: Acute scrotal symptoms in boys with an indeterminate clinical presentation: Comparison of color Doppler sonography and scintigraphy. *Radiology* 207: 223–231, 1998.

Paltiel HJ, Rupich RC, Babcock DS: Maturational changes in arterial impedance of the normal testis in boys: Doppler sonographic study. *AJR* 163:1189–1193, 1994.

Patriquin HB, Yazbeck S, Trinh B, et al: Testicular torsion in infants and children: Diagnosis with Doppler sonography. *Radiology* 188:781–785, 1993.

Stage KH, Schoenvogel R, Lewis S: Testicular scanning: Clinical experience with 72 patients. *J Urol* 125:334–337, 1981.

Taylor GA, Connolly LP, Treves ST: Scrotal scintigraphy, in *Pediatric Nuclear Medicine,* 2d ed, Treves ST (ed). New York, Springer-Verlag, 1995:400–410.

105

A 16-year-old has had an acutely enlarged scrotum since being kicked there by his sister the day before. He has has significant pain and has been sent for an ultrasound (US) to "rule out torsion." His Doppler examination was normal. Figure 105-1 is an image from his examination. What is the diagnosis? Can there be other causes? What should one look for on the US exam of the testicle?

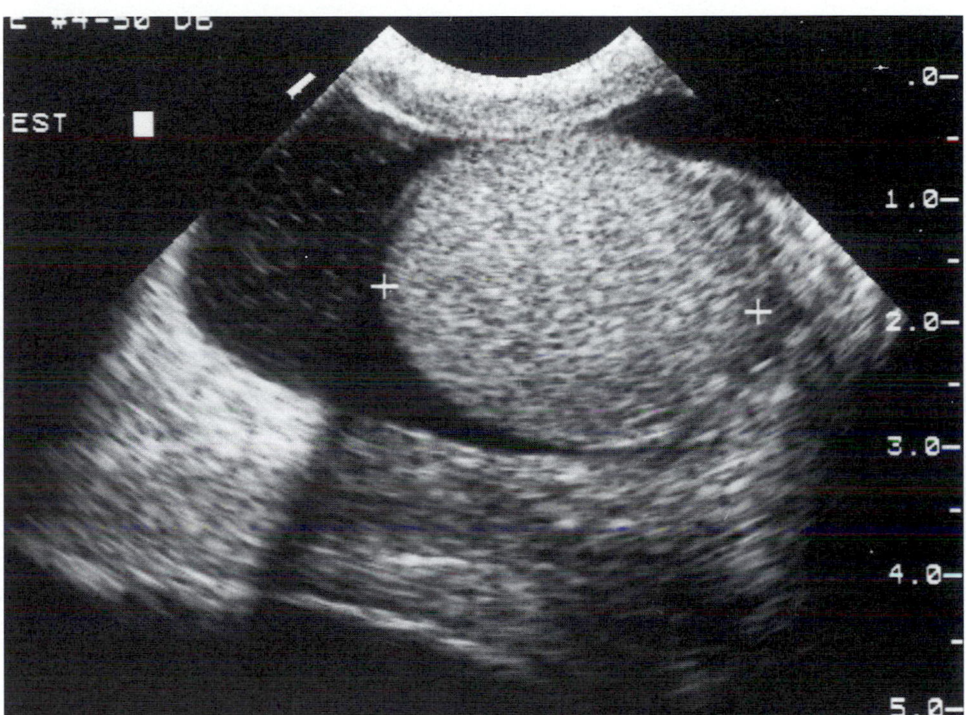

FIGURE 105–1. Right hemiscrotum. Longitudinal plane.

CHAPTER 105

Hematocele

HARRIS L. COHEN

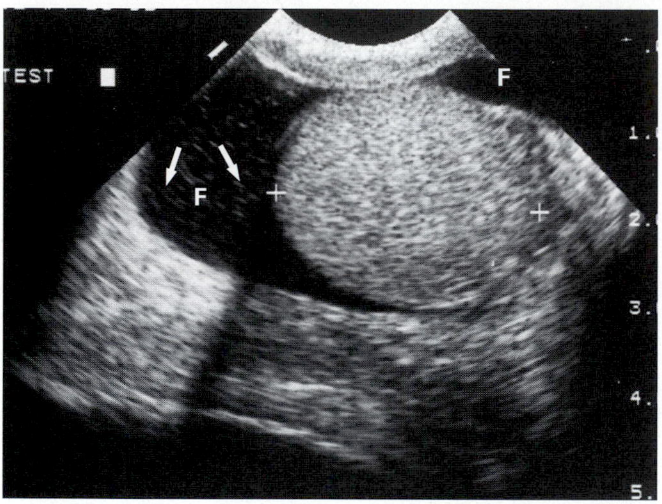

FIGURE 105–2. Annotated version of Fig. 105-1. Hematocele. Right hemiscrotum. Longitudinal plane. Bright echoes (*arrows*) are seen in fluid (F) surrounding, but predominantly superior to, a normal right testicle (*marked off by crosses*). This was due to hematocele from trauma that occurred the day prior to examination.

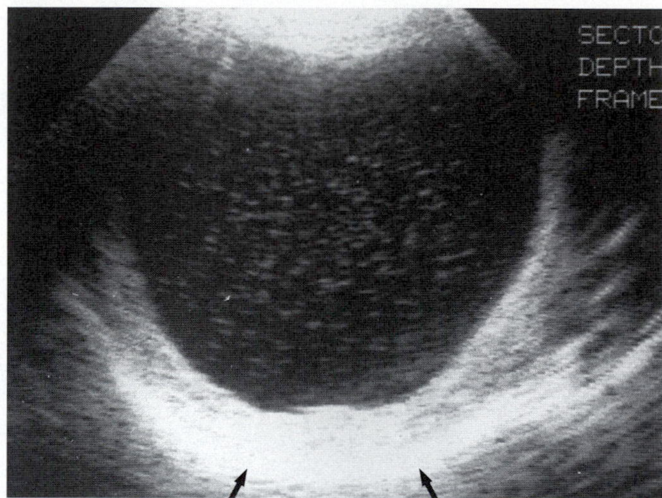

FIGURE 105–3. Hematocele. Transverse plane superior to testicle. Many echoes are seen in the large amount of fluid within the superior scrotum. Excellent through transmission (*arrows*) confirms the fluid nature of the hematocele.

Figure 105-2, the annotated version of Fig. 105-1, shows a testicle of normal size and echogenicity. It had normal flow noted by the reported normal Doppler evaluation. These findings go against the possibility of testicular torsion. What is seen is relatively echoless fluid surrounding much of the testicle, particularly superiorly. Figure 105-3 shows even more echo-filled fluid superior to the testicle. The patient has a large hematocele. A chronic hydrocele might simulate this image. In posttraumatic hematocele, the echogenic material is usually hemorrhagic debris, which, depending on the time of injury, may be from fibrin deposition and clot formation or from various stages of clot dissolution. In cases of chronic or subacute hydrocele, the echogenic material has been found to be cholesterol crystals contained within the fluid. If a hematocele is discovered, even if testicular echogenicity and vascular flow appear normal, the testicle should be studied for any contour abnormality (Fig. 105-4) that might suggest rupture of the strong, tight, and adherent covering of the testicle, the tunica albuginea, and the need to surgically repair it.

SOME NORMAL PEDIATRIC SCROTAL ANATOMY INFORMATION

The normal infant testicle is 1.5 cm long and 1 cm wide. It is said to be at its largest size (2 cm long and 1.2 cm wide) and volume (2 cm^3) for early childhood during the first several months of life because of the prominent gonadotropin levels and related androgen surge. There is a subsequent decline. By 6 months, the testicle is somewhat smaller in volume than at 2 months. Volume remain stable until about 6 years of age, then increases slowly until pubescence, when enlargement

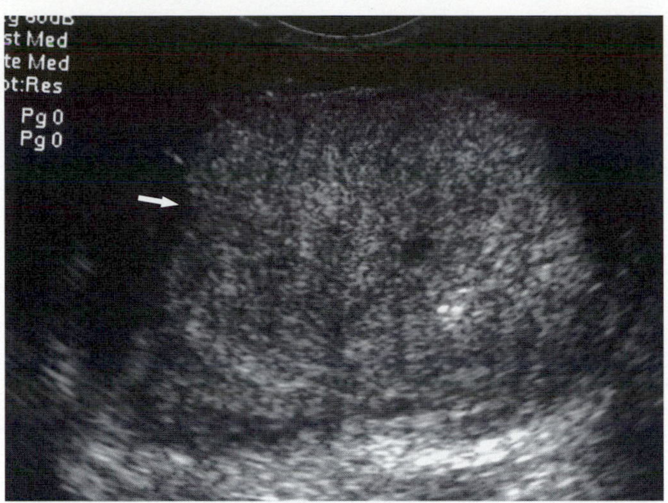

FIGURE 105–4. Testicular fracture—contour irregularity. Left testicle. Longitudinal plane. There is a contour irregularity (*arrow*) in the superior portion of the testicle, suggesting rupture of the tunica albuginea and a need for surgery to repair and salvage the testicle. Some 90 percent of ruptured testes can be salvaged if surgery is performed within 72 h. This 18-year-old's injury was due to a gunshot wound that went through the scrotum. Asymmetrical vascular flow within the testicle also suggested significant injury, which was confirmed at surgery.

again occurs with a rise in gonadotropins. A Swiss study showed normal volumes of 2 to 5 mL at 12 years, 5 to 10 mL at 13 years with the beginning of testicular growth in most of that population, and 15 to 30 mL after a rapid growth spurt at about 15 years. Testicular size is a good indicator of tubular function and spermatogenesis. The mature postpubescent tes-

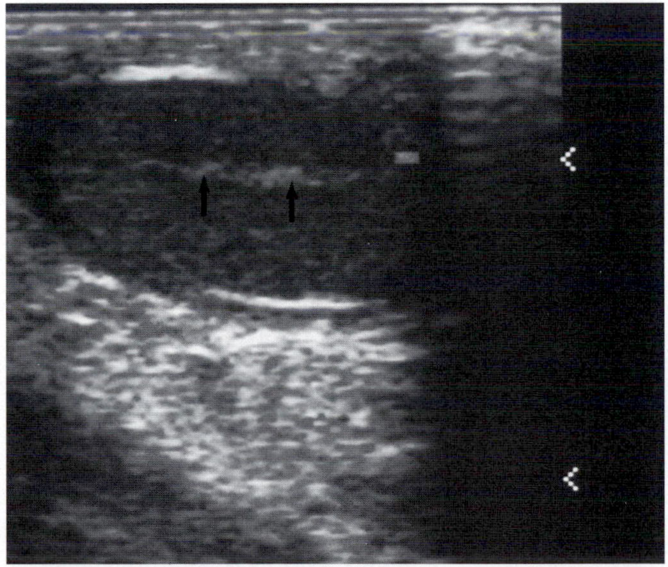

FIGURE 105–5. Mediastinum testis. Longitudinal oblique plane through the left testicle. The normal mediastinum testis (*arrows*) is seen as the linear echogenicity in this testicle. This highly echogenic normal structure is the inward extension of the tunica albuginea. Although not typically seen in the testes of young children, its presence within a soft tissue structure in an unusual location, e.g., the inguinal canal, can help suggest that the structure is a testicle.

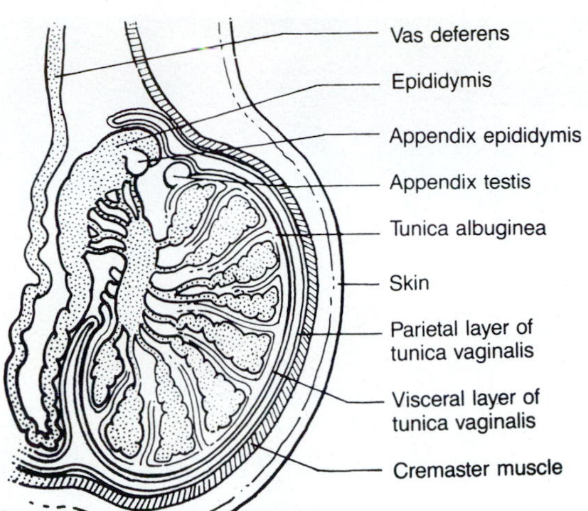

FIGURE 105–6. Normal scrotal anatomy—the tunica vaginalis. Diagram. One can see the potential space between the visceral and parietal layers of the tunica vaginalis in which hydrocele or hematocele may accumulate. These layers are predominantly anterior to the testicle. They do not surround the posterior superior aspect of the testicle. Anterior testicle is to the reader's right.

ticle is 3 to 5 cm long by 2 to 3 cm wide by 2 to 3 cm deep, is ovoid, and has a homogeneous middle-level echogenicity. Echognicity is said to increase beyond 8 years of age due to germ cell and tubular maturation. As US machines have improved, slight heterogeneity can be seen in many normal testes. Use of the contralateral testicle for comparison will allow notation of an echogenicity pattern that is unusual and of concern.

A highly echogenic central linear density (Fig. 105-5) may be seen posteriorly and superiorly. This is the mediastinum testis, which is the inward extension of the testicle's tunica albuginea. It is said not to be usually seen until age 15. Fibrous septae extending from the mediastinum divide the testes into more than 250 lobules. The spermatic cord, draining veins, lymphatics, nerves, the vas deferens, and a single testicular artery run through the mediastinum.

The scrotal wall should be between 3 and 6 mm thick. Beneath the scrotal wall are the two layers of the tunica vaginalis (Fig. 105-6), the outer (parietal) and the inner (visceral) layers, which are the residua of the processus vaginalis (the peritoneum that descended with the testicle from the abdomen). The visceral layer covers the testicle on its anterior border and is attached to the tunica albuginea. Between the tunica's inner visceral wall and the outer parietal surface is a potential space that may often normally contain 1 to 2 mL of fluid. It is here that the fluid of hematocele or hydrocele may accumulate.

WHAT IS A HEMATOCELE?

Hematoceles are complex extratesticular fluid collections filled with hemorrhagic material that separate the layers of the tunica vaginalis. Acutely, they are echogenic. With time, they become less echogenic and are imaged as fluid with

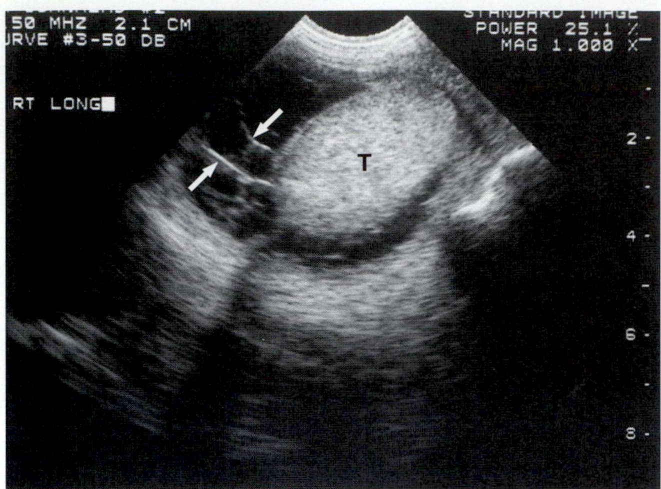

FIGURE 105–7. Septations in a chronic traumatic hydrocele. Longitudinal plane through right hemiscrotum. A normal right testicle is surrounded by fluid. Septations (*arrows*) are seen within the fluid superior to the testicle. This finding is consistent with the patient's history of old trauma and hematocele.

contained low-level echoes (similar to Figs. 105-2 and 105-3, despite their being about 1 day old) or as hydroceles with contained septations (Fig. 105-7). These findings can also be seen in individuals with infected hydroceles. Hematoceles may develop from intrascrotal trauma but may also accumulate from distal trauma (e.g., bleeding from an injured spleen) if there is continued patency of the processus vaginalis. When a hematocele is due to trauma, unless there is an associated break in the tunica albuginea or unless testicular blood flow is compromised, the presence of the hematocele or even a testicular fracture is not an indication for surgery.

HYDROCELE—WHAT IS IT? SHOULD I WORRY?

A hydrocele is the most common scrotal mass in a child. It is fluid within the layers of the tunica vaginalis, which, although predominantly anterior to the individual ipsilateral testicle, appears to surround the testicle except for the area at the epididymal head. The proximal portion of the processus vaginalis typically closes before 18 months of age. This prevents abdominal contents from entering the scrotum and the tunica vaginalis. Residual fluid from testicular descent is responsible for the very common noncommunicating hydroceles, which are found in at least 15 percent of male fetuses beyond 28 weeks of life and therefore are a relatively common third-trimester finding (Fig. 105-8) that usually is physiologic and resolves spontaneously. It is reported in at least 16 of every thousand newborns (Fig. 105-9). This fluid tends to be resorbed by 6 to 9 months of age. The processus is closed in 50 to 75 percent of individuals by the time they are born. The vast majority of the remainder close by the end of the first year of life. If the processus fails to close, a communicating hydrocele (or hematocele if a patient is status post abdominal trauma) can develop. One therefore must be wary of

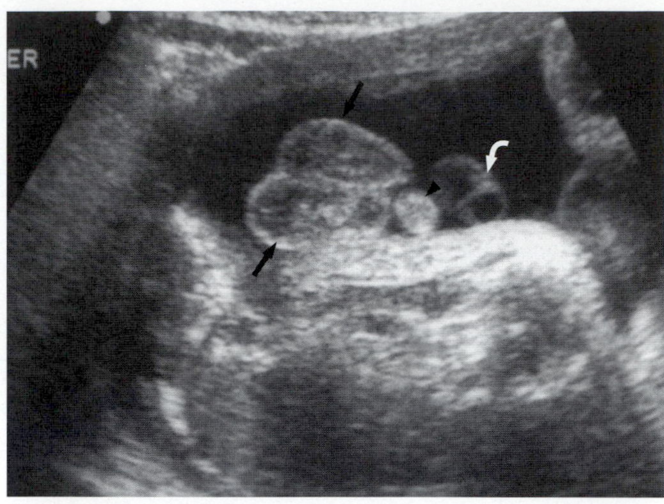

A

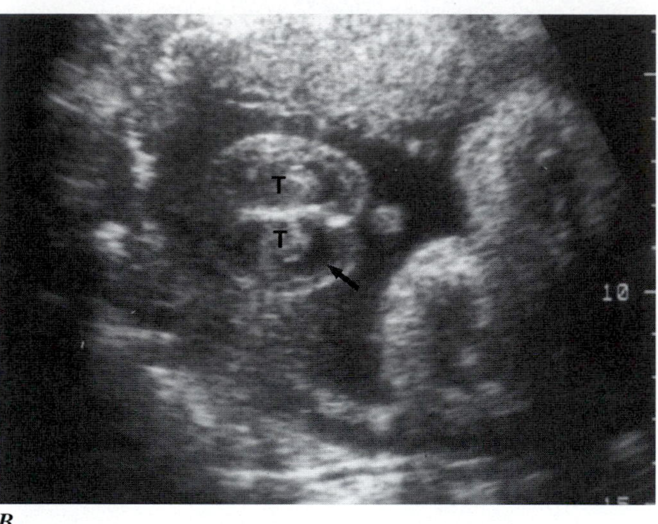

B

FIGURE 105–8. Fetal scrotum. ***A.*** Normal. Coronal plane through the scrotum. The scrotum (*arrows*) is imaged without contained fluid. This third-trimester fetus did not have a hydrocele. Arrowhead points to penis in cross section. ***B.*** Bilateral hydrocele. Coronal plane through the scrotum. Echoless fluid (*arrow*) is seen surrounding each of two testes (T) in a fetus. This is not an uncommon finding in a third-trimester fetus, as this one is. Curved arrow points to the umbilical cord, imaged in cross section in Fig. 105–8*A*.

increasing fluid in a pediatric hydrocele because it suggests a patent processus and therefore the possible presence of an associated inguinal hernia, sometimes denoted by bowel extending into the scrotum (Fig. 105-10). Intrascrotal hernias may obscure US analysis because of their contained air.

It is well known that the patent processus of fetal life allows the possible descent of meconium into the scrotum in cases of meconium peritonitis. This meconium would calcify and appear as a small echogenic mass or masses within the scrotum but beyond the testicle. Obviously, pus, air, urine, or cerebrospinal fluid (in patients with ventriculoperitoneal shunts) may also enter the scrotum if there is continued patency of the processus vaginalis.

In most instances in the child or adolescent, a hydrocele is idiopathic. As many as 50 percent are thought by some to be

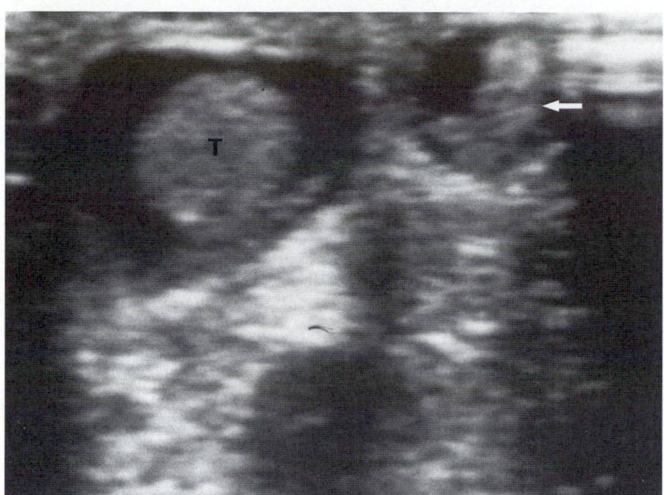

FIGURE 105–9. Bilateral hydrocele in newborn. Scrotum. Transverse plane. This image shows the right testicle (T) best. It is surrounded by the echoless fluid of a hydrocele. A hydrocele is also seen in the left hemiscrotum. The imaged soft tissue (*arrow*) is predominantly epididymis. This fluid was from a noncommunicating hydrocele and was apparently resorbed within a few weeks.

the result of trauma. Hydrocele may also accumulate as the result of epididymitis, epididymoorchitis, torsion, or neoplasm. Calcifications may occasionally develop within the scrotum of patients with chronic hydroceles and chronic inflammation, purportedly from shed cells and disturbed hydrocele resorption.

ABDOMINOSCROTAL HYDROCELES

Unusual cases of hydroceles have been reported in which a collection of fluid in the tunica vaginalis (i.e., a hydrocele)

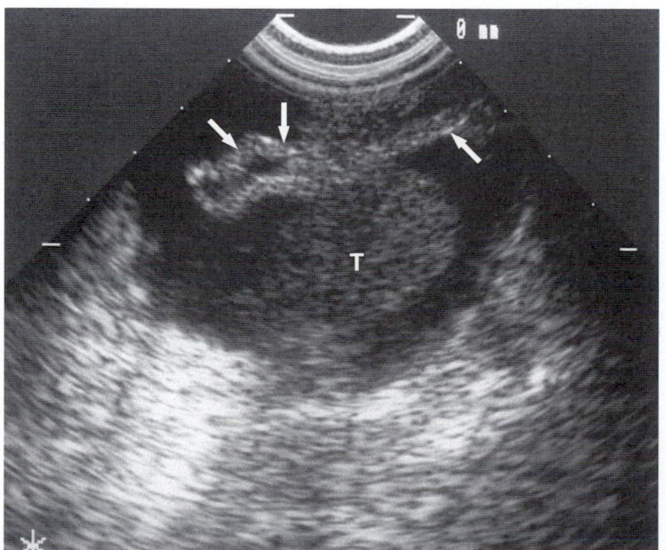

FIGURE 105–10. Herniated bowel within the scrotum. Right hemiscrotum. Transverse plane. Hydrocele surrounding a testicle (T). Within the scrotum, and imaged because of surrounding fluid, is a tubular structure (*arrows*) that is a loop of herniated bowel.

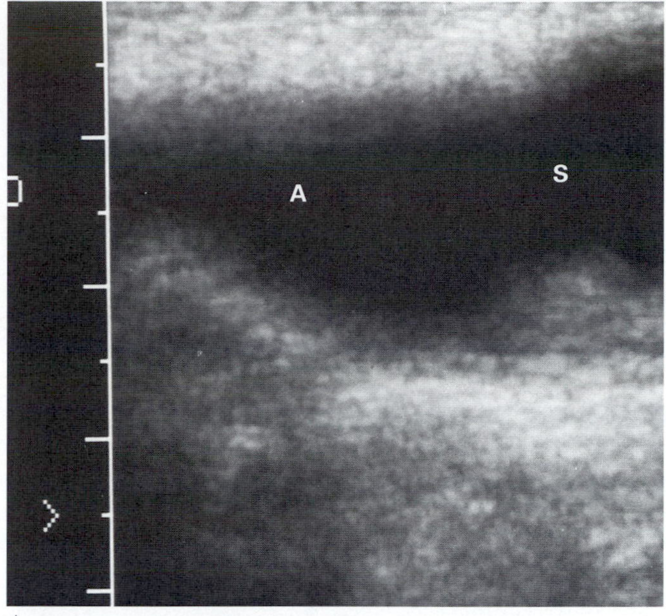

A

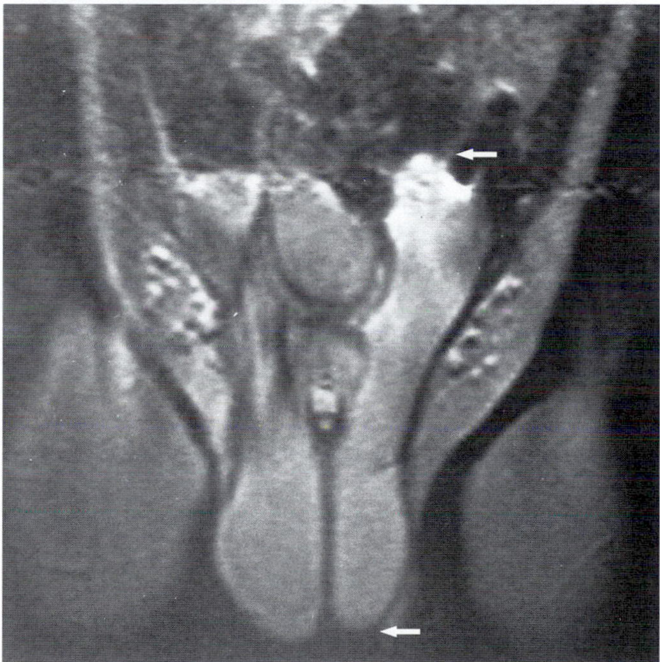

B

FIGURE 105–11. Abdominoscrotal hydrocele. This 4-year-old presented with bilateral lower abdominal masses. ***A.*** Ultrasound. Left hemiscrotum. Longitudinal plane through right hemiscrotum and right inguinal area. The intrascrotal ultrasound showed an obvious hydrocele. This longitudinal image shows fluid extending from the scrotum (S = upper scrotum) to the inguinal/abdominal region (A), proving this to be an abdominoscrotal hydrocele. ***B.*** Magnetic resonance imaging. Abdomen/pelvis. Coronal plane. T2-weighted image. Using this technique, water is white. Abdominoscrotal hydroceles extend from both sides of the scrotum up into the abdomen. The one on the left extends highest. Arrows points to the superior and inferior extents of the left abdominoscrotal hydrocele.

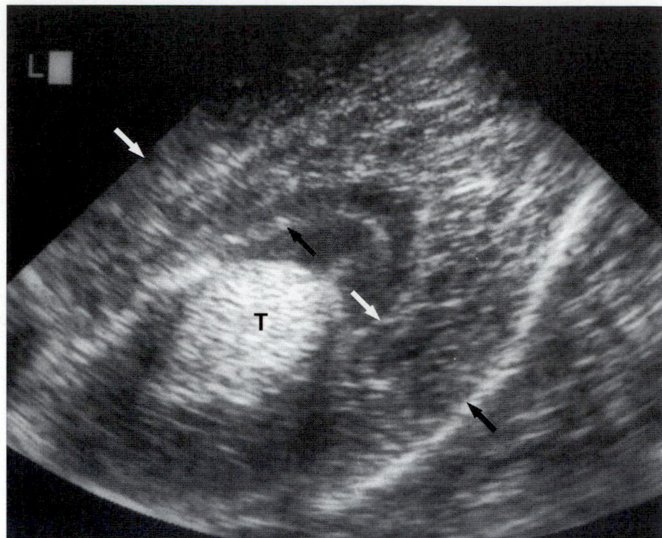

FIGURE 105–12. Scrotal wall edema. Ultrasound (US). Left hemiscrotum. Longitudinal plane. This patient presented with pain and scrotal enlargement. He was sent to US to rule out torsion and hydrocele. The patient's family forgot to tell the clinicians that the patient had nephrotic syndrome. The testicle (T) is normal. A small amount of fluid is noted around the testicle. However, the scrotal wall is severely thickened (*arrows*), which accounts for the large scrotal size.

extends along the spermatic cord and through the inguinal canal into the abdominal cavity. Such a hydrocele presents as an inguinal or intraabdominal mass and must be considered when evaluating inguinal and lower abdominal masses that occur in the first year of life. They are discovered at abdominal palpation in children with scrotal hydroceles or by noting that a hydrocele evaluated by US extends above the scrotum and into the inguinal region (Fig. 105-11) and/or abdomen. They are treated by total excision of the mass through an extensive inguinal incision.

As a final point, not all scrotal enlargement is due to contained fluid. In older adults, massive scrotal enlargement often has a prominent component of scrotal thickening. This is less common in children. One may however, come across a child with nephrotic syndrome who may present with an enlarged scrotum made up predominantly of an edematous and therefore thickened scrotal wall (Fig. 105-12).

KEY POINTS TO REMEMBER

Hydroceles are common in the fetus and young child. Be wary if they grow in size, suggesting a communicating hydrocele. Hematoceles may develop from local or distant trauma.

References

Booth J: Abdominoscrotal hydrocele. *J Pediatr Surg* 22:177–178, 1987.

Burgues P, Alvarez J, Hernandez L, Texidor J: Abdominoscrotal hydrocele. *J Pediatr Surg* 21:987–988, 1986.

Cassorla F, Golden S, Johnsonbaugh R, et al: Testicular volume during early infancy. *J Pediatr* 99:742–743, 1981.

Cohen HL, Haller J: Scrotal ultrasound in the pediatric and adolescent patient. *Radiology Report* 2:276–290, 1990.

Gooding G, Leonhardt W, Marshall G, et al: Cholesterol crystals in hydroceles: Sonographic detection. *AJR* 169:527–529, 1997.

Han B: Uncommon causes of scrotal and inguinal swelling in children: Sonographic appearance. *JCU* 14:421–427, 1986.

Krone K, Carrol B: Scrotal ultrasound. *Radiol Clin North Am* 23:121–139, 1985.

Namjoshi S: Calculi in hydroceles: Sonographic diagnosis and significance. *JCU* 25:437–441, 1997.

Prader A: Testicular size: Assessment and clinical importance. *Triangle* 7:240–243, 1966.

Pretorius D, Halsted M, Abels W, et al: Hydroceles identified prenatally: Common physiologic phenomenon? *J Ultrasound Med* 17:49–52, 1998.

Siegel M: The acute scrotum. *Radiol Clin North Am* 35:959–976, 1997.

Skoog S, Belman A: The communicating hematocele: An unusual presentation of blunt splenic trauma. *J Urol* 136:1092–1093, 1986.

Spier L, Cohen H, Kenigsberg K: Bilateral abdominoscrotal hydroceles: A case report. *J Pediatr Surg* 30:1382–1383, 1995.

Sujka S, Evans E, Nigam A: Delayed rupture of the spleen presenting as a scrotal hematoma. *J Trauma* 26:85–86, 1986.

106

A teenager with an obvious right-sided varicocele on physical examination is sent for evaluation of his testes by ultrasound (US). Figure 106-1*A* (see also Color Plate 31) and *B* (see also Color Plate 32) was obtained as part of that study. Is there an abnormality on the left? What is it? Is this good or bad news for the patient?

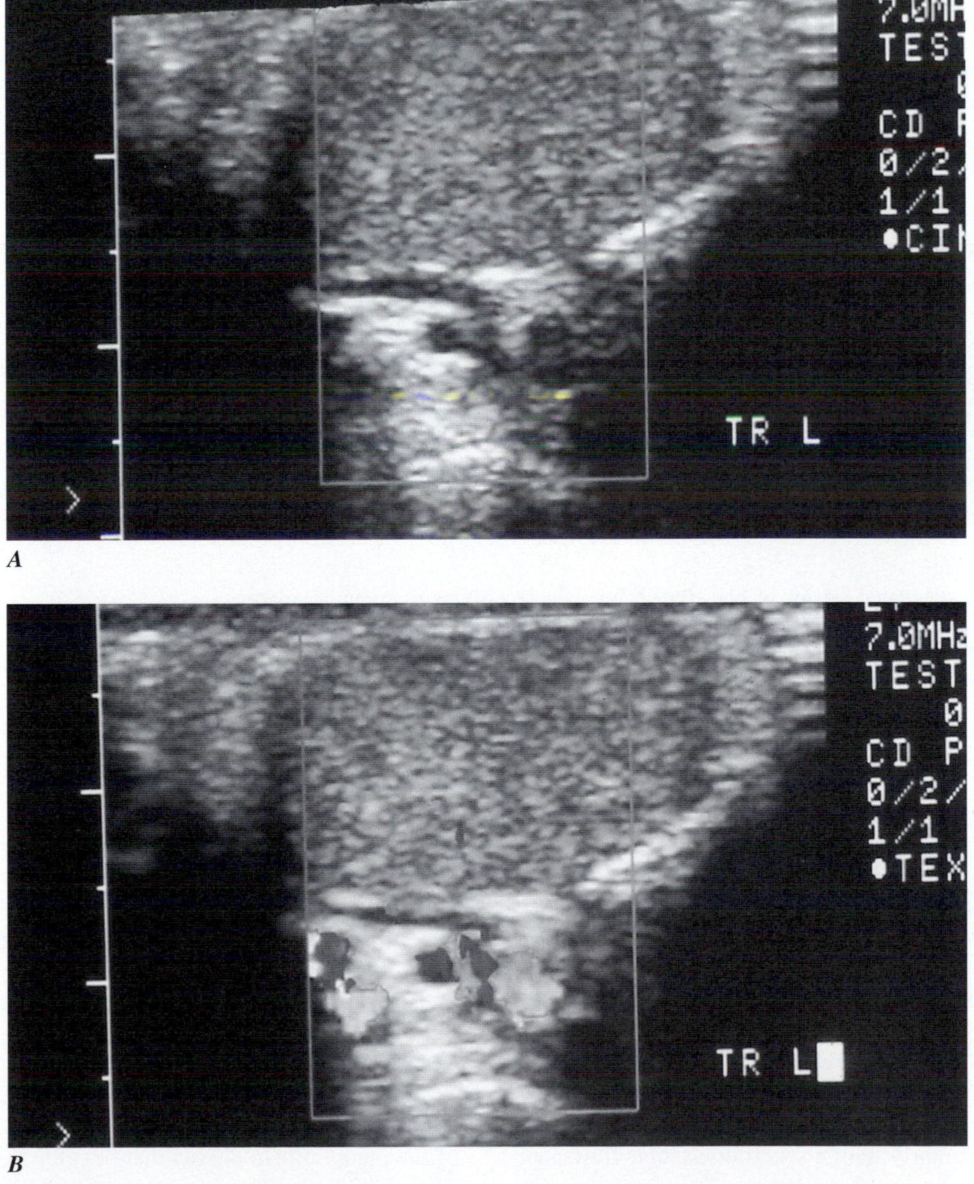

FIGURE 106–1. ***A.*** Left hemiscrotum. Transverse plane. Color Doppler. ***B.*** Left hemiscrotum. Transverse plane. Color Doppler. (See Color Plate 32.)

CHAPTER 106

Varicocele

HARRIS L. COHEN AND DANIEL L. ZINN

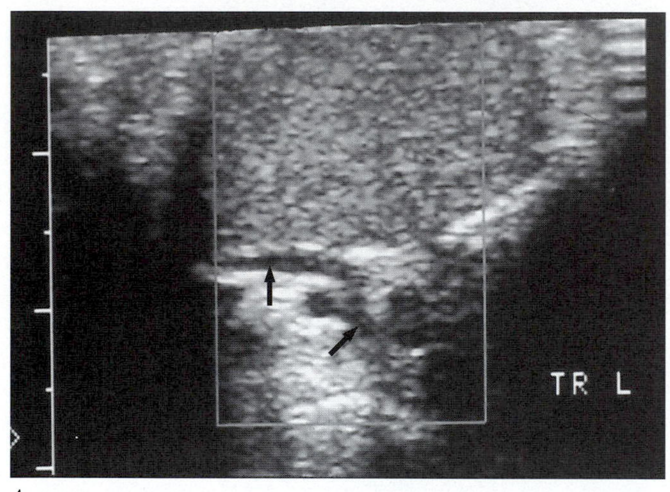

A

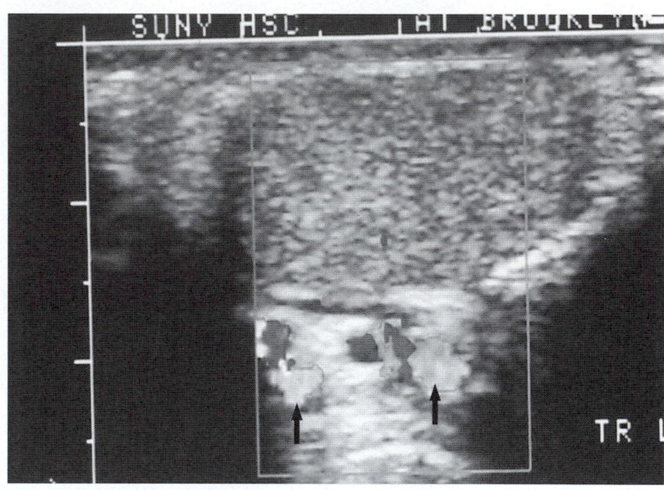

B

FIGURE 106–2. ***A.*** Annotated version of Fig. 106-1*A*. Varicocele. Left hemiscrotum. Transverse plane. Color Doppler. Patient at rest. Tubular and circular echopenic structures (*arrows*) are seen posterior to the left testicle (T). (See Color Plate 31.) ***B.*** Annotated version of Fig. 106-1*B*. Varicocele. Left hemiscrotum. Transverse plane. Color Doppler. Patient bearing down. Color, consistent with vascular flow, is seen in the echopenic extratesticular structures within the Doppler's "color box." The spectral pattern was venous, proving the presence of a left varicocele in a patient with a known right varicocele. (See Color Plate 32.)

Figure 106-2*A* (see also Color Plate 31) and *B* (see also Color Plate 32), the annotated version of Fig. 106-1, shows a normal testicle. Posterior to the testicle on Fig. 106-2*A* are tubular and cystic echopenic structures. They are probably vascular and are suggestive of varicocele, but no flow is seen despite the use of color Doppler. Figure 106-2*A* was obtained after the patient began bearing down. With this maneuver, color flow is seen in the tubular echopenic structures and varicocele is proven, particularly with a spectral vascular flow pattern showing venous signal (Fig. 106-3). The presence of a solitary varicocele only on the right side would have been of concern to the clinician, as it suggests a possible intraabdominal mass pressing on the inferior vena cava as the cause. However, with the finding of a left varicocele, this is of far less concern. This would therefore be good news for the patient.

WHAT ARE VARICOCELES?

Varicoceles are dilated (exceeding 2 mm in diameter) veins of the pampiniform plexus that develop because of incompetence of the internal spermatic vein. When large (exceeding 2 cm in diameter), they feel and look like a bag of worms in the scrotum. On ultrasound examination, they are tortuous, tubular, echo-free structures situated superior, lateral, and/or

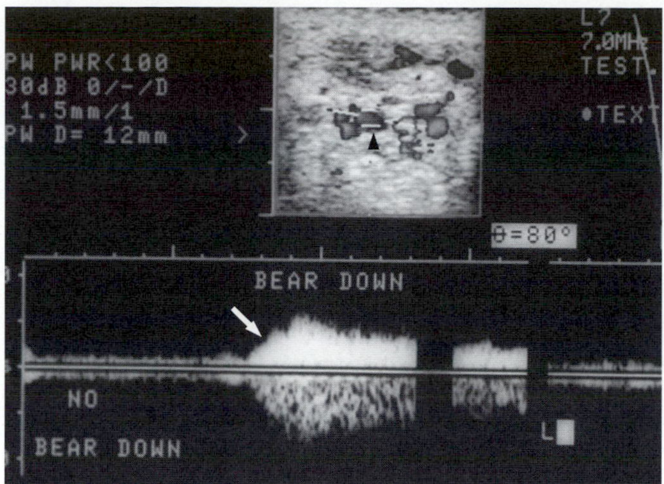

FIGURE 106–3. Varicocele—identification by Doppler spectral analysis. Left hemiscrotum at periphery. Longitudinal plane. Triplex Doppler. The top half of the image shows vessels within the scrotum of a teenager. One of the vessels was insonated (*arrowhead*). The bottom half of the image shows the Doppler spectrum. Venous flow of low velocity is seen when the patient was not bearing down. There is an increase in venous flow velocity (*arrow*) at the point in time where the patient bears down (BEAR DOWN). With relaxation, flow velocity decreases again.

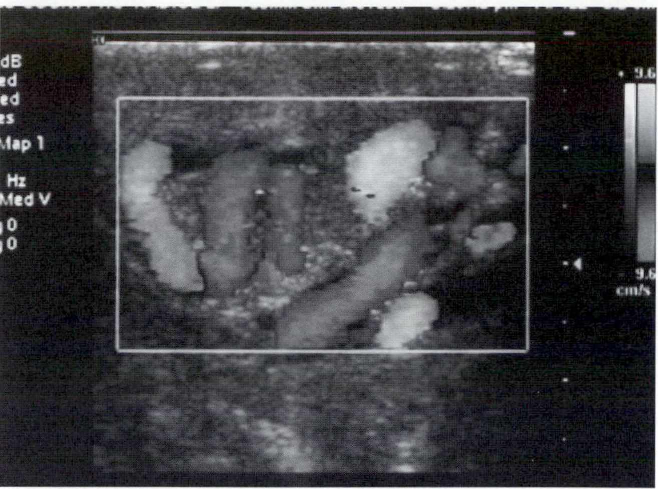

FIGURE 106–4. Grade II varicocele. Color Doppler. Longitudinal plane lateral to left testicle. Very large venous structures are imaged during a Valsalva maneuver. None were seen without bearing down. The vessels are 1 to 2 cm in diameter, consistent with Grade II varicocele. (See Color Plate 33.)

posterior to the testicle. Doppler examination, especially color Doppler (Fig. 106-2), can confirm the vascular nature of these structures.

VARICOCELES—CLINICAL FINDINGS AND CONCERNS

The diagnosis of a varicocele is of significance because of the association of varicoceles with infertility in the adult male. As many as 39 percent of infertile men are said to have varicoceles. There has also been some concern in the medical literature about a possible gonadotoxic effect of varicoceles on the testes over time. I have no cases to prove this, and I have found many incidental varicoceles in men evaluated for conditions other than fertility or testicular size differential. It is said that 10 percent of the general male population has varicoceles, and this does not include a probably larger group with subclinical cases. Prominent varicoceles can lead to decreased growth and atrophy of the ipsilateral testicle. This is the greatest clinical concern for the physicians of young adolescents with this problem. Patients are usually asymptomatic, although those with larger masses may complain of a pulling or dragging sensation in the scrotum or of testicular pain.

In a large Danish study involving 1072 boys and men, no varicoceles were found in any child between 6 and 9 years of age. Varicoceles are typically first discovered in adolescence. The 15 percent incidence among the 10- to 15-year-old Danes was similar to that in their adult population.

Varicoceles are graded according to their size. Some 65 percent are grade I—small, palpated with difficulty, and usually appearing as only mild thickening of the cord on physical examination of the standing adolescent. Another 24 percent are grade II—moderate in size (Fig. 106-4; see also Color Plate 33), easily diagnosed on physical examination, and consisting of a mass of veins 1 to 2 cm in diameter. Another 10 percent of cases are grade III—large in size and greater than 2 cm in diameter, looking like a "bag of worms."

SOLITARY RIGHT VARICOCELES ARE OF CONCERN

At least 10 percent of varicoceles are bilateral. Some say that as many as 70 percent may be bilateral. When varicoceles are unilateral, almost all (98 percent) of them are left-sided. Theoretically, this is a result of increased pressure on the left renal vein, with concomitant increased pressure and retrograde flow into its branch (the left spermatic vein), caused either by compression between the aorta and the superior mesenteric artery (the "nutcracker" phenomenon) or by incompetent or absent valves in the internal spermatic vein. The right spermatic vein comes off the inferior vena cava, and therefore right-sided varicoceles are extremely uncommon, especially in young men. The presence of an isolated right-sided varicocele may indicate neoplasm or another intraabdominal mass causing pampiniform plexus dilatation through proximal compression on the inferior vena cava.

ULTRASOUND EXAMINATION TIPS

As with all scrotal evaluations, we use a high-frequency transducer and set our system to be sensitive to low flow signal. Varicoceles may disappear on supine examination. Thus, physical examination and ultrasound examination performed in a standing position are often necessary in order to make the diagnosis. This is usually the last step of our examination

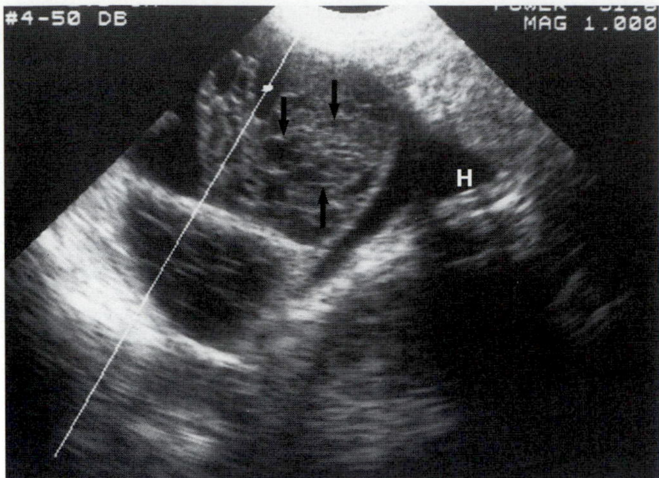

FIGURE 106–5. Intratesticular varicocele. Left hemiscrotum. Longitudinal plane. Duplex Doppler. Tubular cystic areas are the predominant structures within the left testicle (*arrows*) of this patient. There is hydrocele (H), and there was varicocele beyond the testicle. Doppler proved the tubular structures to have venous flow, consistent with a rare varicocele of the testicle itself.

if we have no answer. When we examine a patient in supine position on US, we ask the patient to bear down during the exam in order to increase blood flow in echoless structures suspected of being these dilated veins. We will see this on color flow imaging and prove it by obtaining a typical venous spectral pattern on insonation. The Valsalva maneuver will cause increased spectral velocity (Fig. 106-3). Rarely, the flow prominence will occur not with bearing down, but rather with the end of the Valsalva maneuver. We look at all areas surrounding the testicle as well as superior to the testicle in the area of the spermatic cord. We look with gray-scale, spectral, and color Doppler. Rare cases have been reported of dilated intratesticular varicoceles occurring in association with extratesticular varicoceles. We have seen one such case (Fig. 106-5). Doppler helps rule out simulation of varicocele by nonvascular tubular ectasia.

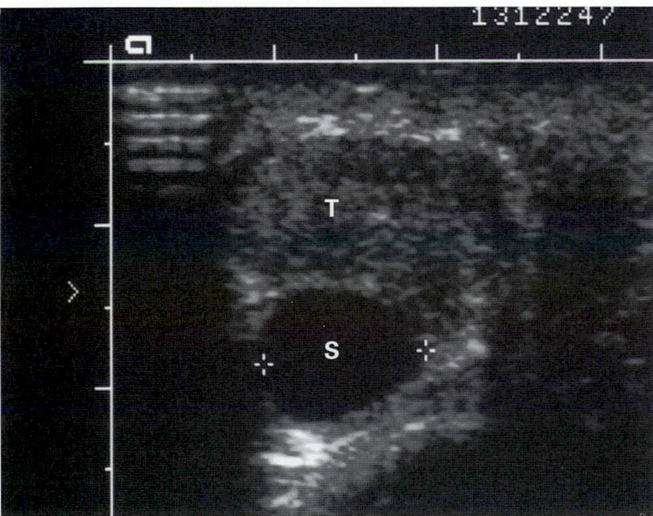

FIGURE 106–6. Spermatocele. Left testicle. Transverse plane. A cystic mass (S) is seen posterior to the left testicle (T) and within the area of the epididymis. It had no vascular flow within it. It is a spermatocele.

TREATMENT OF VARICOCELE

In adolescents, surgical ligation of the varicocele is recommended in cases of ipsilateral testicular volume loss (greater than 2 mL difference in testicular volume). Biopsies of such testicles have shown various degrees of decreased spermatogenesis, tubal hypoplasia, focal fibrosis, and arrest of germ cell maturation. Kass et al operated on 20 grade II to III patients with left varicocele and testicular volume loss and showed that 80 percent had an increase in their left testicular volume on follow-up after ligation.

DIFFERENTIAL DIAGNOSTIC CONSIDERATION

Cystic masses in the epididymis, known as spermatoceles when they are large and as epididymal cysts when they are small, can simulate a varicocele on cross section. They represent a confluence of dilated efferent ductules of the testis filled with seminal plasma. Most are idiopathic, although they can occur in patients with chronic epididymitis and have been reported in patients whose mothers were exposed to diethylstilbestrol (DES). On ultrasound examination, spermatoceles (Fig. 106-6) typically appear as solitary, echo-free masses that may or may not be be septated.

References

Brosman S: Male genital tract, in *Clinical Pediatric Urology,* 2d ed, Kelalis P, King L, Belman A (eds). Philadelphia, Saunders, 1985:1202–1219.

Cohen HL, Haller J: Scrotal ultrasound in the pediatric and adolescent patient. *Radiology Report* 2:276–290, 1990.

Dambro T, Stewart R, Carroll B: The scrotum, in *Diagnostic Ultrasound,* 2d ed, Rumack C, Wilson S, Charboneau J (eds). St Louis, Mosby–Year Book, 1998:809–810.

Kass E: Adolescent varicocele: Current concepts. *Semin Urol* 6:140–145, 1988.

Kass E, Chandra R, Bellman A: Testicular histology in the adolescent with a varicocele. *Pediatrics* 79:996–998, 1987.

Kurtz A, Middleton W: *Ultrasound. The Requisites.* St. Louis, Mosby, 1996:446–448.

McClure R, Hricak H: Scrotal ultrasound in the infertile man: Detection of subclinical unilateral and bilateral varicoceles. *J Urol* 135:711–714, 1986.

Ozcan H, Aytac S, Yagci C, et al: Color Doppler ultrasonographic findings in intratesticular varicocele. *JCU* 25:325–329, 1997.

Rogers W, Ralls P, Boswell W: Obstruction of the inferior vena cava by seminoma. *J Urol* 124:613–614, 1980.

Siegel M: Male genital tract, in *Pediatric Sonography,* 2d ed, Siegel M (ed). New York, Raven, 1995:479–512.

Weiss A, Kellman G, Middleton W, Kirkemo A: Intratesticular varicocele: Sonographic findings in two patients. *AJR* 158: 1061–1063, 1992.

107

A 13-year-old presents with a history of acute left scrotal pain. Figure 107-1*A* is a view of the scrotum in transverse plane without color Doppler. The echogenicity of the right testicle is normal. What is a major clinical consideration? Figure 107-1*B* is the same view obtained using color Doppler. Has your diagnosis changed? Mine did. What is the diagnosis?

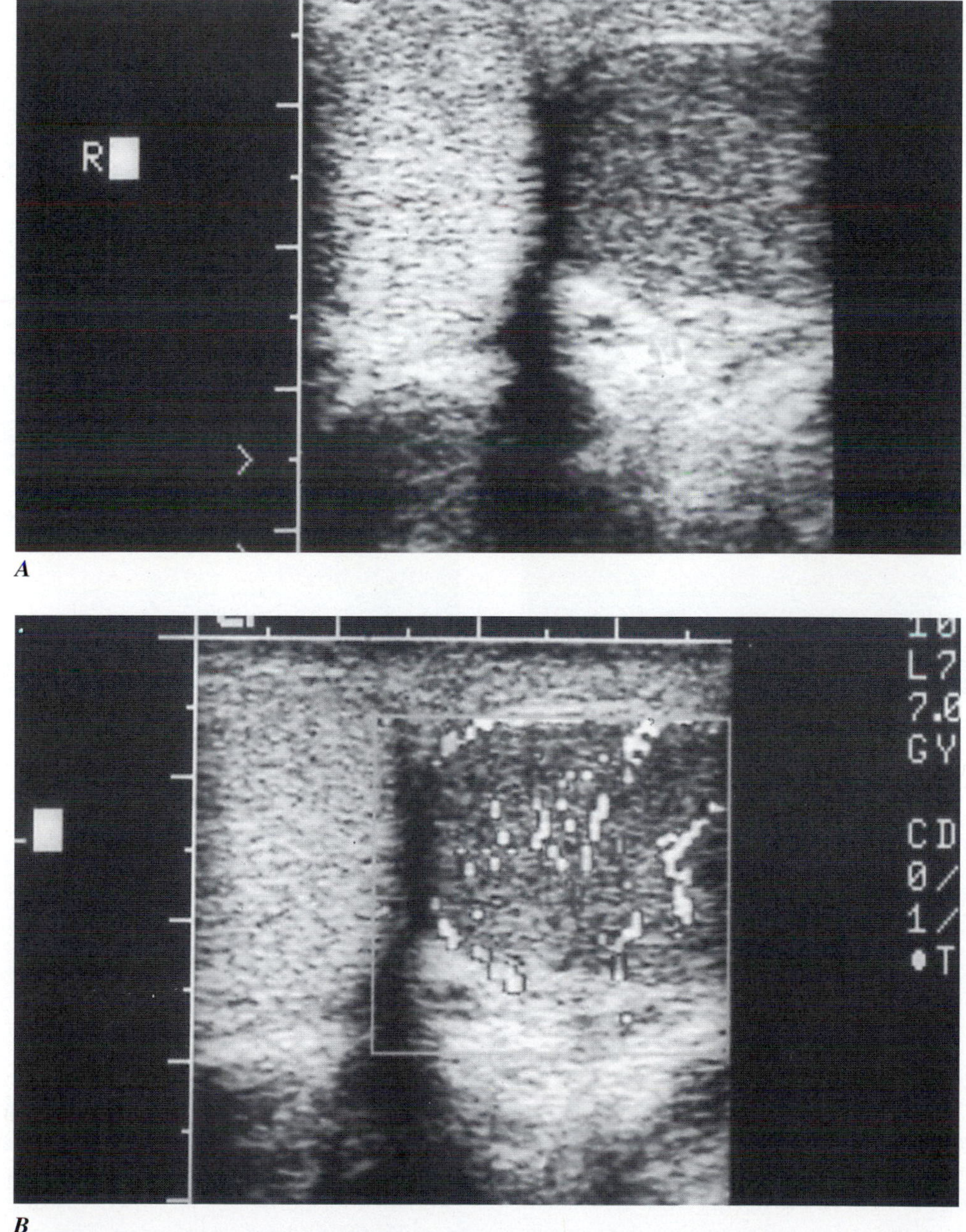

FIGURE 107–1. Scrotal ultrasound. Transverse plane. ***A.*** Without the use of color Doppler (image reproduced in black and white). ***B.*** Using color Doppler (image reproduced in black and white).

CHAPTER 107

Testicular Infection—Orchitis

HARRIS L. COHEN AND GEORGE KHORIATY

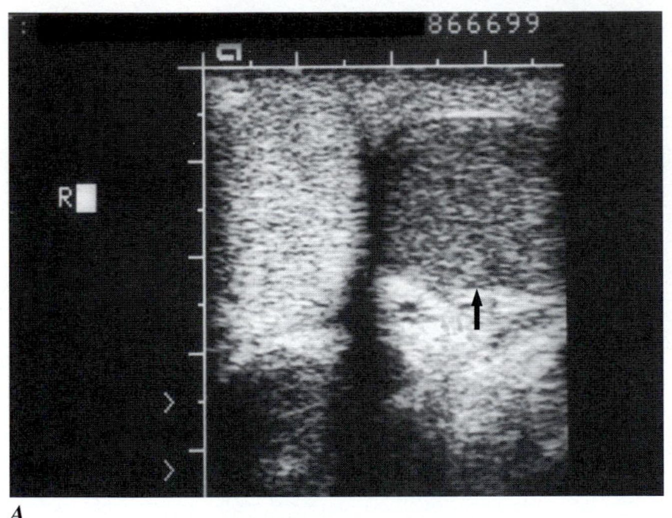

A

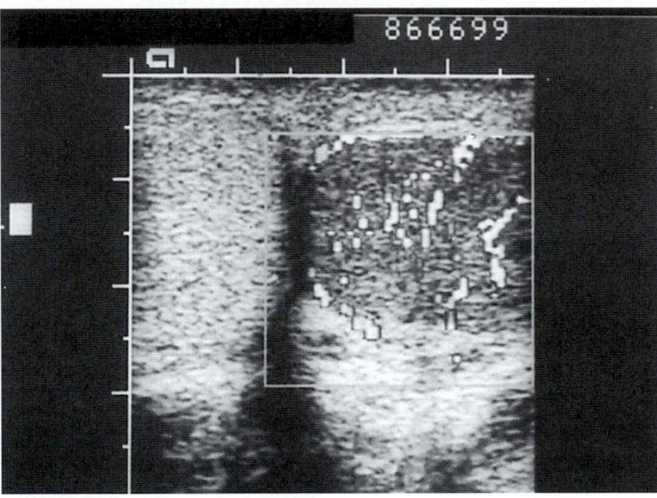

B

FIGURE 107–2. Annotated version of Fig. 107-1. Left testicular orchitis. Scrotal ultrasound. Transverse plane. ***A.*** Without the use of color Doppler (image reproduced in black and white). The left testicle (*arrow*) is far more echopenic than the right testicle. No focal mass, which may suggest tumor, is seen in either testicle. ***B.*** Using color Doppler (image reproduced in black and white). Prominent color flow, seen as linear white streaks, is seen throughout the left testicle. A similar view of the right testicle showed far less vascular flow. Increased flow from inflammation, consistent with the patient's proven orchitis, was correctly suggested.

Figure 107-2*A*, the annotated version of Fig. 107-1*A*, shows the left testicle as echopenic compared to the normal echogenicity pattern of the right testicle. There is no focal mass in either testicle. In light of the history of acute testicular pain, a left testicular torsion with a delayed diagnosis would be the first ultrasound (US) diagnostic consideration. However, color Doppler shows prominent testicular flow, including central flow. Although occasional testicular torsions with evident central flow have been reported, by the time the torsed testicle is echopenic, this confusing possibility is far less likely. The combination of an echopenic testicle with prominent or normal or increased vascular flow suggests the possibility of edema or infection. This was a case of viral orchitis. Many cases of infection of the testicle originate in the epididymis and extend into the adjacent testicle as an epididymoorchitis (Fig. 107-3).

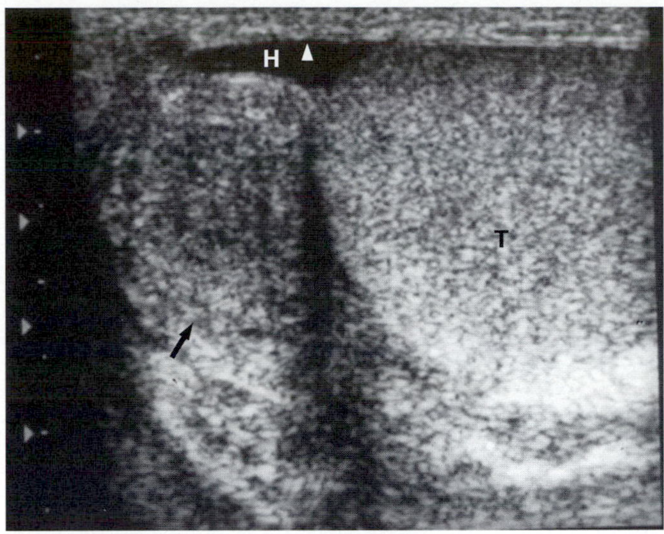

A

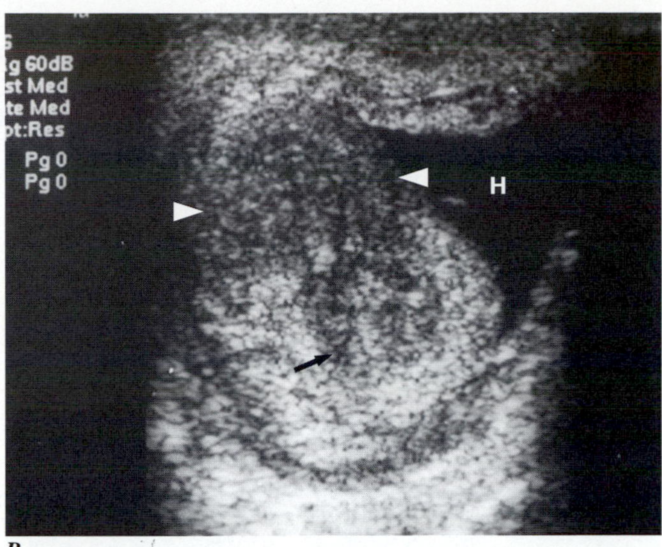

B

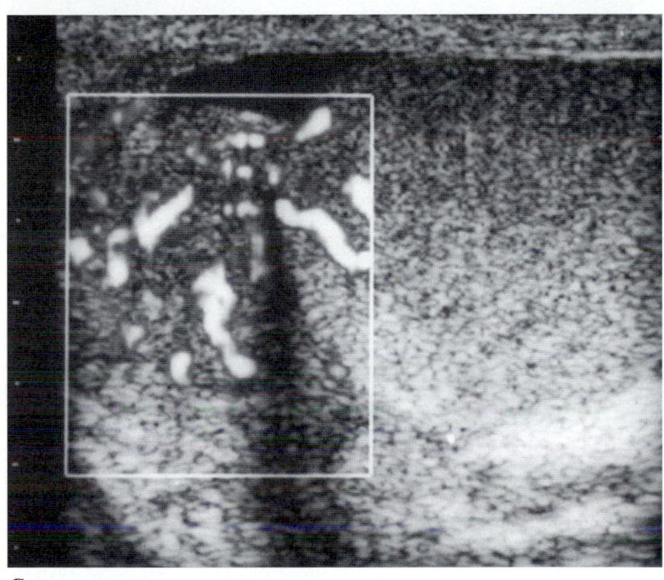

C

FIGURE 107–3. Left epidymoorchitis. Left hemiscrotum. ***A.*** Longitudinal plane. Superior is to the reader's left. The epididymis (*arrow*) is enlarged. It has an echopenic center, probably on the basis of edema. In this plane, the testicle (T) does not appear involved. The scrotal wall (*arrowheads*) is thicker than normal. This is a common finding in epididymoorchitis, as is the hydrocele (H). ***B.*** Transverse plane with inferior angulation. The epididymis (*arrowheads*) is echopenic from edema and the echopenic area of involvement extends into the testicle (*arrow*). H = hydrocele. ***C.*** Longitudinal plane. Color Doppler exam. This black-and-white image of a color Doppler examination of the epididymis and upper testicle shows prominent flow, indicated by linear echogenicities of vascular flow, in the epididymis and the superior testicle. This is despite the fact that the testicle appeared of normal echogenicity on this view. Other views showed the echopenic portion of the testicle to have very significant flow and the areas of normal echogenicity far less, but normal, vascular flow.

WHAT ARE EPIDIDYMITIS AND EPIDIDYMOORCHITIS?

The epididymis (Fig. 107-4) is a tortuous tubular structure lying along the posterolateral aspect of the testicle. The triangular head of the epididymis is seen just superior to the top of the testicle. The head is continuous with the body and tail, which travel inferiorly along the posterolateral margin of the testis. The head is about 3 to 4 times the diameter of the body and tail and is usually more echogenic. The epididymis is equal to or slightly greater than the testis in echogenicity.

Epididymitis, inflammation of the epididymis, is the most common cause of an acute painful scrotum in the postpubescent male. The cause is usually infectious, and these infections are usually bacterial, although in pediatric and adolescent patients epididymitis may be viral (e.g., caused by mumps). Interventional procedures may also cause such infections. Voiding dysfunction with elevated bladder pressures has been linked to the development of epididymitis in older children. In children younger than 5 years of age, structural anomalies may be the cause, and voiding cystourethrography and renal ultrasound are included in the workup in search of such anomalies. In the patient under 20 years of age, the ratio of epididymitis to torsion cases is 3:2, but after age 20, and with increasing sexual activity, it is 9:1. There are cases of epididymitis that are noninfectious in origin. Such cases may be due to trauma or to the reflux of sterile urine. Extension of epididymal infection into the testicle as epididymorchitis is said to occur in 20 percent of cases of adult epididymitis. The involvement is usually focal. The occurrence of a resultant abscess is rare.

Although typically the pain of epididymitis develops over 1 to 2 days, as opposed to suddenly, the clinical picture may simulate torsion. Unlike patients with torsion, patients with epididymitis are often febrile, and at least one-half of such patients complain of dysuria.

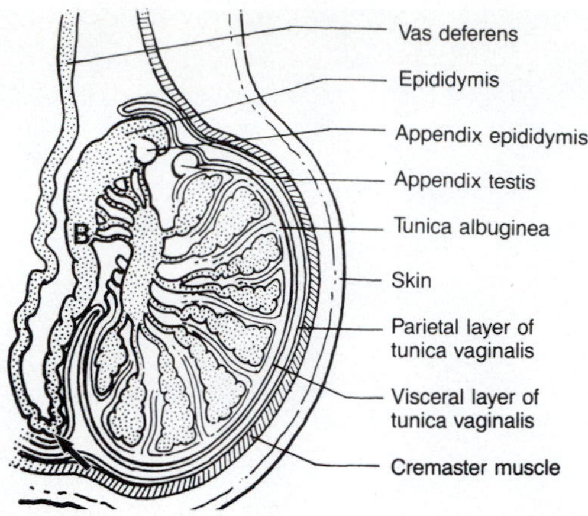

A

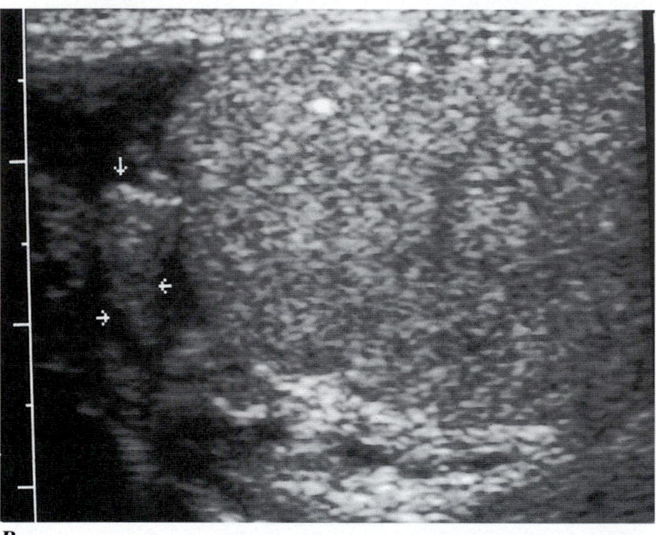

B

FIGURE 107–4. Normal epididymis. ***A.*** Schematic drawing. Longitudinal plane. Posterior is to the reader's left. The epididymis runs from its head, which lies superior to the testicle, along the posterior aspect of the testicle as the body (B) of the epididymis and ends as the tail (*arrow*) of the epididymis at the inferior aspect of the testicle. Note also the appendix testis and appendix epididymis, two of the three major normal appendages found off the epididymis or testicle that may torse and cause an acutely painful scrotum. ***B.*** Longitudinal plane through right testicle. A triangular structure (*arrows*) represents the normal head of the epididymis in this teenager whose contralateral side had enlargement due to epididymoorchitis.

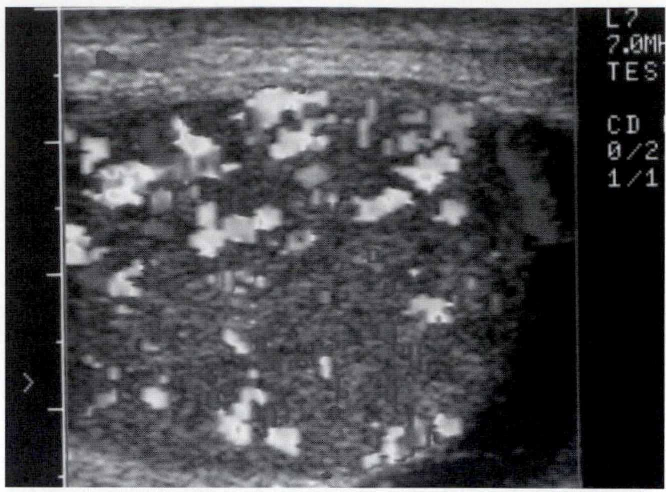

FIGURE 107–5. Orchitis. Right testicle. Longitudinal plane. Color Doppler examination. Hyperperfusion, predominantly of the superficial half of the testicle, noted by increased color Doppler signal, is seen in an area of the testicle noted on gray-scale examination to be echopenic. This adolescent had orchitis. (See Color Plate 34.)

ULTRASOUND FINDINGS OF EPIDIDYMITIS AND EPIDIDYMOORCHITIS

The most common finding in epididymitis is enlargement of the epididymis. Usually this occurs at the head of the epididymis, but it can occur anywhere along its course. A reactive hyrocele is usually present. The affected and enlarged epididymis (Fig. 107-3) may be of normal, increased, or decreased echogenicity. In chronic epididymitis, the echogenicity is increased.

Epididymoorchitis leads to enlargement of the testicle. It may be difficult to visually separate the involved testicle from the inflamed epididymis. Orchitis may be diffuse but is most easily noted on US when it is imaged as a focal hypoechoic area in the portion of testicle adjacent to the epididymitis. Although orchitis can occur as a result of the spread of organisms by lymphatic or hematogenous routes, it is usually caused by direct spread from the epididymis. Testicular ischemia may play a role in causing orchitis or may be a less than usual end result of epididymitis. This is because the inflamed and edematous epididymis compresses terminal branches of the spermatic vessels (making these ischemic peripheral areas more susceptible to bacterial invasion). The testicular mass of focal orchitis may simulate tumor on US examinations, but the clinical presentation, the association with an enlarged epididymis, and its resolution in weeks with appropriate antibiotic therapy and "tincture of time" help make the precise diagnosis. Most cases, regardless of etiology, have a similar US image. Unusual cases of tuberculous epididymitis and epididymoorchitis may be suggested by the presence of sinus tracts and the imaging of extratesticular calcification.

Color Doppler can show the involved epididymal and testicular areas (Fig. 107-5; see also Color Plate 34) of epididymoorchitis to both have increased vascular flow. However, in rare instances, blood flow in the testicle may be decreased or absent when it is compromised by the edema of epididymitis. In such cases, differentiation of epididymitis from testicular torsion by US may be impossible. It has been said that scintigraphy will show diffusely increased activity in the involved hemiscrotum of such patients, but such an image can also be obtained with recent spermatic cord detorsion or torsion of the testicular or epipidymal appendages.

TORSION OF A TESTICULAR OR EPIDIDYMAL APPENDAGE—WHAT IS THAT?

In evaluating the acute painful scrotum in a child or adolescent, one must consider testicular torsion and epididymitis,

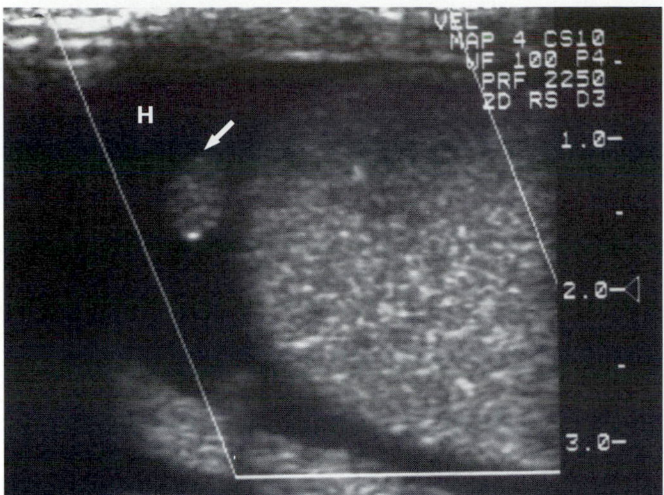

FIGURE 107–6. Normal appendix testis. Right testicle. Longitudinal plane. Surrounding hydrocele (H) allows imaging of a small echogenic structure (*arrow*) that came off the testicle and is a normal appendix testis.

entities we have already discussed. A simulator of these that is not clinically uncommon but is of far less concern than the other two conditions is torsion of one of the epididymal or testicular appendages (Fig. 107-5*A*). It usually occurs in children between 6 and 12 years of age. In one series, appendage torsion accounted for 35 percent of the cases of acute scrotal pain in children, whereas 45 percent of the cases were due to testicular torsion and 15 percent were due to epididymitis. The appendages are persistent vestigial remnants of the mesonephric and müllerian duct systems. There are three major ones: the appendix testis (Fig. 107-6) (a remnant of the müllerian duct), attached to the testicle's upper pole (and the most common one to torse); the appendix epididymis (a remnant of the mesonephron), attached to the head of the epididymis; and the vas aberrans (a remnant of the mesonephron), attached to the epididymis at the junction of its body and tail. Torsion of any of these can result in scrotal pain and swelling and local erythema, clinical complaints and findings similar to those in testicular torsion. More specific complaints of localized pain in the upper scrotum or the palpation of a firm, tender relatively mobile pea-sized nodule in the upper scrotum atttached to the epididymis or testis can help make the exact diagnosis and avoid surgery. Transillumination of the scrotum may show a small bluish or black body at the upper testicular pole, the "blue dot" sign. Ultrasound can certainly image the torsed appendage (Fig. 107-7) and perhaps show that it lacks vascular flow, but, more importantly, it can prove that there is normal vascular flow in the testes and thereby rule out testicular torsion. We have imaged torsed appendices as echogenic or echopenic with a thick or thin echogenic rind. Imaging a normal-sized epididymis will help rule out epididymitis.

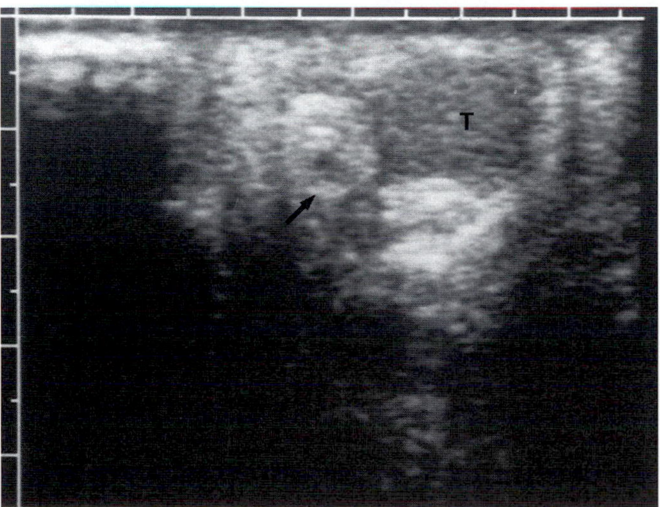

FIGURE 107–7. Torsed appendix testis. Right superior hemiscrotum. Transverse plane. A normal upper right testicle (T) is seen. Medial to it is an echogenic mass (*arrow*) that is a torsed appendix testis. This child presented with an acute scrotum but had a normal appendix and a normal testicle. (*From Cohen HL, Haller J: Scrotal ultrasound in the pediatric and adolescent patient.* Radiology Report *2:276–290, 1990, with permission.*)

TAKE HOME POINT

The sonologist can be of great help in analyzing the acute scrotum for epididymitis or epididymoorchitis vs. testicular torsion. Remember to consider simulation of these entities by torsion of a testicular or epididymal appendage.

References

Anderson P, Giacomantonio J: The acutely painful scrotum in children: Review of 113 consecutive cases. *Can Med Assoc J* 132:1153–1155, 1985.

Bukowski T, Lewis A, Reeves D, et al: Epididymitis in older boys: Dysfunctional voiding as an etiology. *J Urol* 154:762–765, 1995.

Chung J, Kim M-J, Lee T, et al: Sonographic findings in tuberculous epididymitis and epididymo-orchitis. *JCU* 25:390–394, 1997.

Cohen HL, Haller J: Scrotal ultrasound in the pediatric and adolescent patient. *Radiology Report* 2:276–290, 1990.

Cohen HL, Shapiro M, Haller J, Glassberg K: Torsion of the testicular appendage. Sonographic diagnosis. *J Ultrasound Med* 11:81–83, 1992.

Finkelstein M, Rosenberg H, Snyder H, Duckett J: Ultrasound evaluation of scrotum in pediatrics. *Urology* 27:1–9, 1986.

Frush D, Sheldon C: Diagnostic imaging for pediatric scrotal disorders. *Radiographics* 18:969–985, 1998.

Lentini J, Benson C, Richie J: Sonography of focal orchitis. *J Ultrasound Med* 8:361–366, 1989.

Paltiel H, Connolly L, Atala A, et al: Acute scrotal symptoms in boys with an indeterminate clinical presentation: Comparison of color sonography and scintigraphy. *Radiology* 207:223–231, 1998.

Rifkin M, Jurtz A, Goldberg B: Epididymitis examined by ultrasound: Correlation with pathology. *Radiology* 151:187–190, 1984.

Siegel M: Male genital tract, in *Pediatric Sonography,* 2d ed, Siegel M (ed). New York, Raven, 1995:479–512.

Siegel M: The acute scrotum. *Radiol Clin North Am* 35:959–976, 1997.

Skoglund R, McRoberts J, Radge H: Torsion of testicular appendages: Presentation of 43 new cases and a collective review. *J Urol* 104:598–604, 1970.

Strauss S, Faingold R, Manor H: Torsion of the testicular appendages: Sonographic appearance. *J Ultrasound Med* 16: 189–192, 1997.

108

A 10-year-old boy presented with isosexual precocious puberty. Figure 108-1 is an ultrasound (US) image of his scrotum. What do you see? What is the most likely diagnosis?

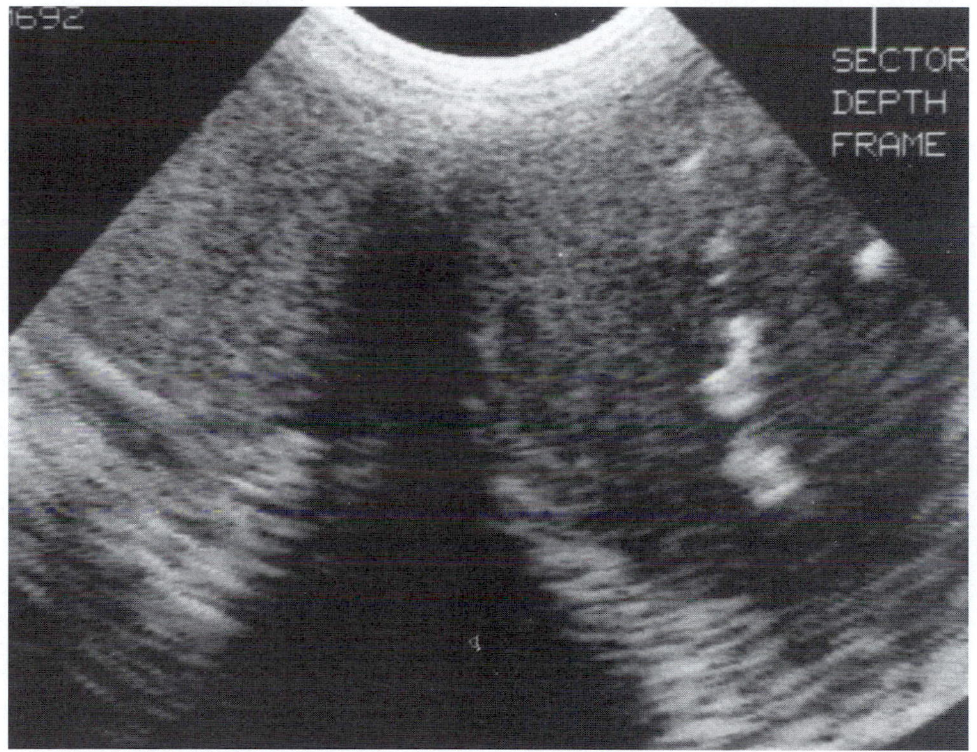

FIGURE 108–1. Scrotal ultrasound. Transverse plane.

CHAPTER 108

Leydig Cell Tumor of the Testicle

HARRIS L. COHEN AND JEAN TORRISI

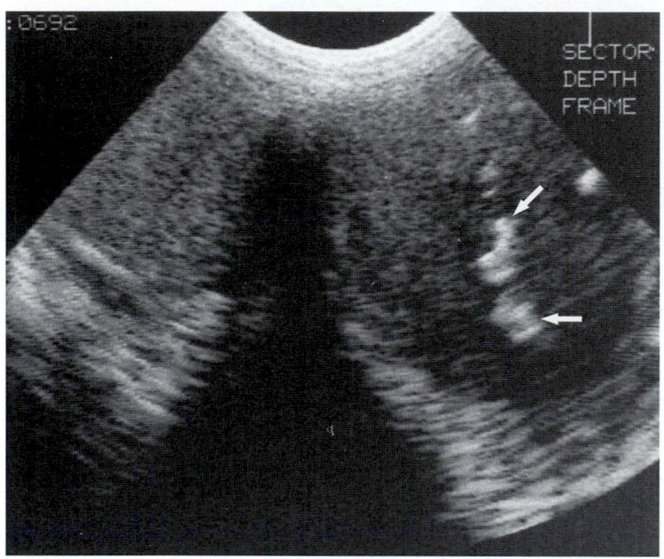

FIGURE 108–2. Annotated version of Fig. 108-1. Left Leydig cell tumor. Scrotal ultrasound. Transverse plane. The left testicle is larger than the right (R) testicle. It contains scattered calcifications (*arrows*). Its enlargement and contained calcifications suggest a testicular tumor. The history of isosexual precocious puberty suggests that the tumor is a Sertoli cell or Leydig cell tumor, which this proved to be.

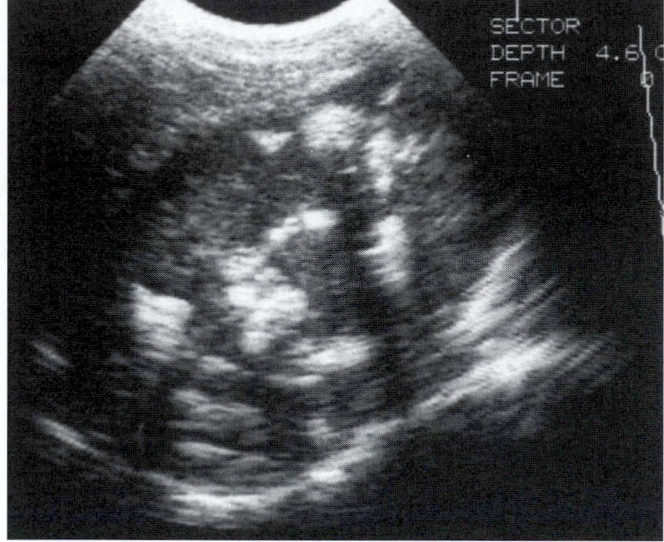

FIGURE 108–3. Leydig cell tumor. Longitudinal plane. This is the orthogonal projection of Fig. 108-2. The diffuse presence of calcifications is more easily noted.

Figure 108-2, the annotated version of Fig. 108-1, shows an enlarged left testicle compared to the right testicle. The enlarged testicle contained scattered calcifications (Fig. 108-3). Calcifications within a scrotum might suggest residua from meconium peritonitis that occurred when the child was a fetus. Calcified loose bodies found between the membranes of the tunica vaginalis (thought to be due to residua from tunica inflammation or torsion of testicular or epididymal appendages) as well as phleboliths and calcified hematomas may account for extratesticular calcification. The tiny seminiferous tubule calcifications of testicular microlithiasis, seen in normal individuals as well as in those with Down's or Klinefelter's syndrome and often suggesting the presence of a testicular germ cell neoplasm, are much smaller than those in this case. Prominent calcifications found within a testicle may be postinflammatory (sarcoid, tuberculosis), postinfarctive, or neoplastic, whether a "burned out" germ cell tumor or an acute testicular teratoma or teratocarcinoma. In this case, the combination of unilateral testicular enlargement with contained large calcifications suggests that this is a testicular

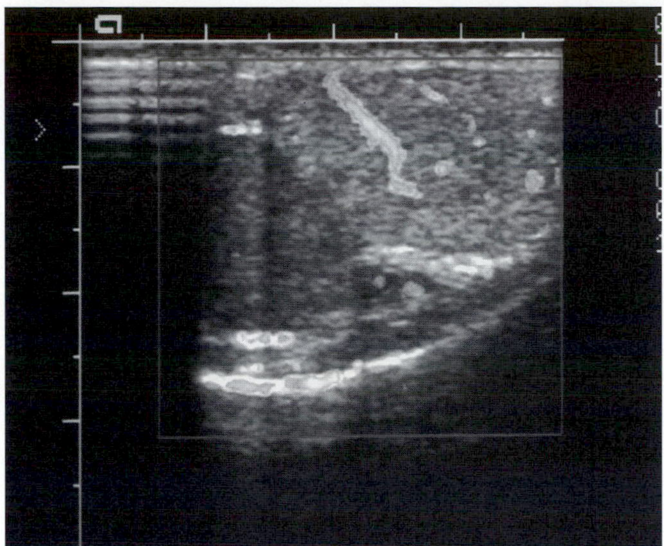

FIGURE 108–4. Bilobed testicle. Longitudinal plane. A young child with one lobulated mass in his scrotum was found to have a bilobed testicle, probably on the basis of a transverse testicular ectopia. The lower portion of the testicle was more echogenic and had more apparent flow on color Doppler. This testicle is being followed closely by clinical and US exams.

tumor. The history of isosexual precocious puberty suggests a Sertoli or Leydig cell tumor of the testicle. This case proved to be a Leydig cell tumor.

ENLARGED TESTES IN CHILDREN AND ADOLESCENTS

Benign causes of asymptomatic testicular enlargement may be idiopathic or be the result of such conditions as juvenile hypothyroidism with precocious puberty, X-linked megalotestis syndrome, and congenital adrenal hyperplasia. Patients with unilateral cryptorchidism may develop compensatory enlargement of the intrascrotal testis. Transverse testicular ectopia, an anomaly in which both testes migrate into the same hemiscrotum, may lead to the development of a bilobed and therefore enlarged testicle (Fig. 108-4), suggesting the false possibility of neoplasm. There is a higher incidence of testicular tumors developing in such testes.

TESTICULAR TUMORS IN CHILDREN

Although primary testicular tumors represent the most common solid tumors of 20- to 35-year-old men, they are uncommon before age 15, representing 1 percent of all childhood malignant tumors and 3 percent of all testicular tumors. Most testicular tumors present with testicular enlargement. Pain is usually secondary to torsion or intratumoral hemorrhage. Testicular tumors are divided into germ cell and non-germ cell types. Most testicular tumors are echopenic on US, although focal increased echogenicity may be seen with subacute hemorrhage or with scarring in burnt out tumors and metastases.

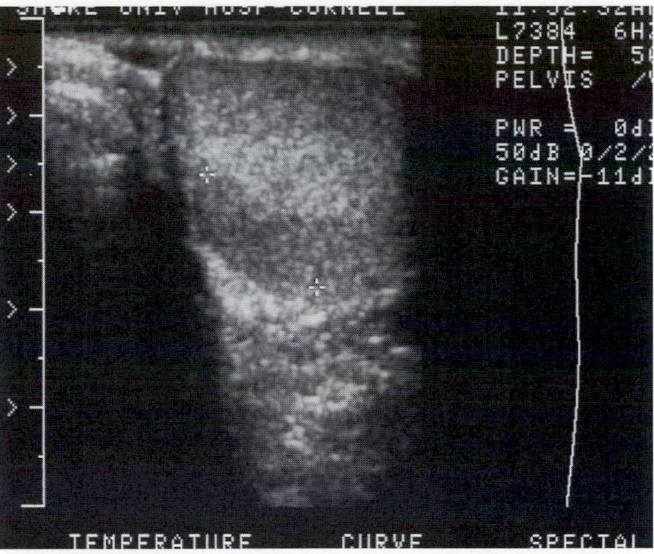

A

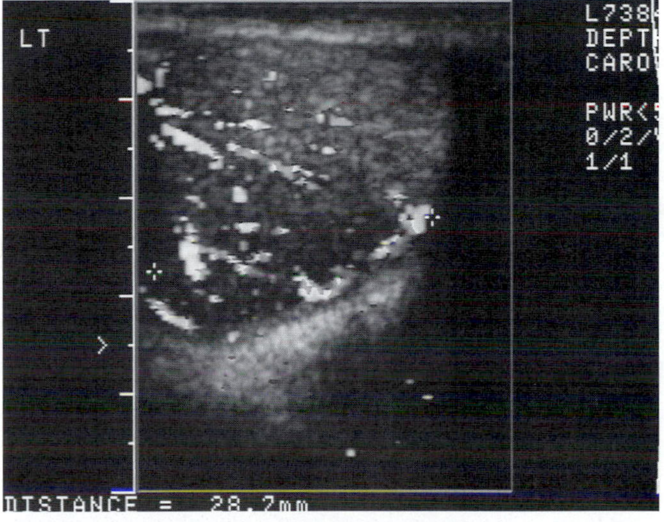

B

FIGURE 108–5. Leukemic metastases/infiltation of testicle. ***A.*** Right testicle. Transverse plane. Color was used to highlight findings of the gray-scale image. The right testicle of this teenager with a history of leukemia in remission was enlarged and heterogeneous in echogenicity. Crosses are seen at the edges of one of the testicles' echopenic areas. Variable echogenicity of the testicle is nonspecific but suggests the need to rule out infiltrative disease. This is particularly true in a patient with leukemia. Similar findings may be seen with orchitis. ***B.*** Left testicle. Longitudinal oblique plane. Color Doppler. Significant increased color flow was noted in various areas of this heterogeneous left testicle. Both testes were enlarged and heterogeneous. The findings suggest infiltrative disease of the testicles. Although the increased vascular flow may have been simulated by an orchitis, the flow increase in a leukemic patient "in remission" may be the first imaging clue of recurrent leukemia with involvement of the testicular "sanctuary" site. That is what this case proved to be. (See Color Plate 35.)

An echopenic intratesticular US image is nonspecific and may be simulated by infarcts, granulomas, and focal orchitis. Testicular metastases are rare in children, representing 0.06 percent of testicular tumors. Leukemia and lymphoma are the most common causes (Fig. 108-5; see also Color Plate 35).

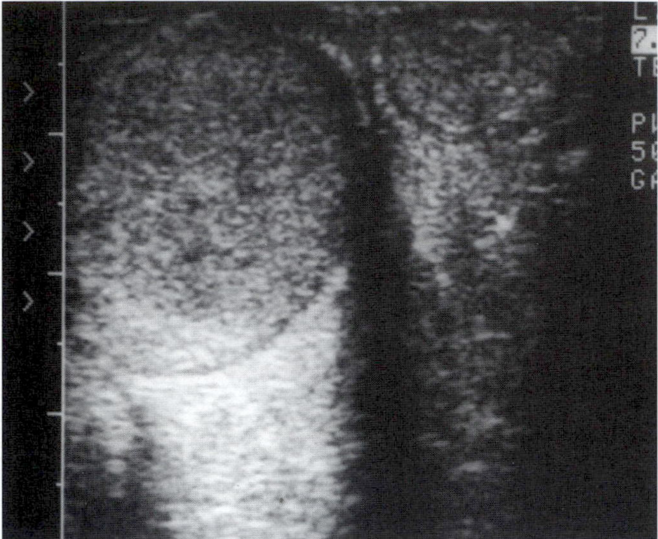

FIGURE 108–6. Endodermal sinus tumor of the testicle. Scrotal ultrasound. Transverse plane. The left testicle (*arrow*) is normal in size. The right testicle appears similar in echogenicity, but was much larger. The right testicle of this young child proved to contain an isoechoic endodermal sinus tumor.

Most (65 to 75 percent) of the primary testicular tumors in childhood are germinal cell (choriocarcinoma, seminoma, teratocarcinoma, yolk cell, embryonal carcinoma) in type. Embryonal cell carcinomas are common in adults but rare in children. Some 80 percent of pediatric testicular tumors are endodermal sinus or yolk cell carcinomas. Most (75 percent) of these tumors are diagnosed by 24 months of age and present as painless testicular enlargement (Fig. 108-6). They may be aggressive and invade the tunica, distorting the testicular contour. Frequent hemorrhage is responsible, particularly after clot dissolution, for contained echopenic areas. The tumors are typically at least somewhat well-circumscribed masses. Yolk sac testicular tumors may produce alpha fetoprotein (AFP), which is said to always be elevated in affected infants and can be used as a tumor marker for follow-up.

Teratomas represent 10 to 15 percent of childhood germ cell tumors, usually developing in children between 3 months and 5 years of age. Typically, they appear on US as complex masses with cystic and solid components. They may contain cartilage, bony spicules, keratin, or adipose tissue that causes areas of significantly increased echogenicity, which may shadow. They were once thought benign, but at least one-third of adults with this tumor will show metastases within 5 years of diagnosis. The course is more benign in children unless there are malignant yolk sac elements within the teratoma or it is histologically immature. Treatment varies from the transinguinal testicular isolation and enucleation done for a benign teratoma to the more aggressive radical inguinal orchiectomy performed for immature teratomas or cases with high AFP levels.

Some 25 to 30 percent of childhood testicular tumors are of nongerminal cell type—i.e., tumors of the gonadal stroma. Almost half (45 percent) are Leydig cell tumors, which have

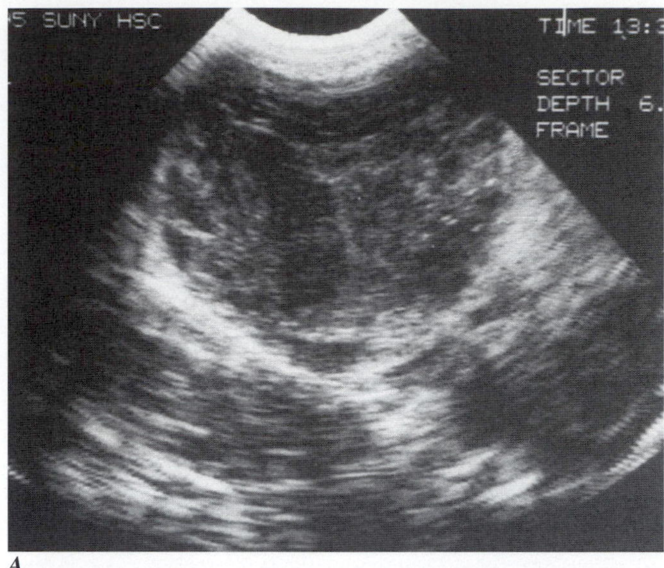

A

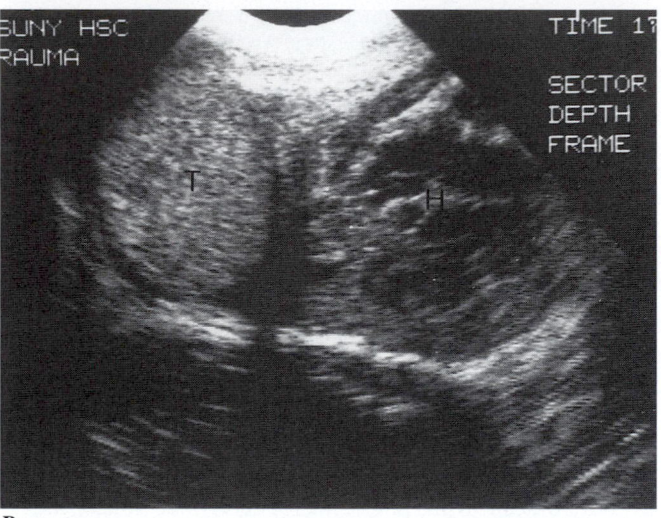

B

FIGURE 108–7. Intrascrotal hematoma. Scrotal ultrasound. ***A.*** Transverse plane. A heterogeneous, predominantly echopenic mass was seen in the lower two-thirds of the scrotum. It suggested a fractured testicle to the covering house officer. ***B.*** Longitudinal plane. Fortunately, for this patient, the orthogonal plane showed that the testicle (T) had been pushed superiorly by the large heterogeneous intrascrotal hematoma (H). Surgery was avoided. (*From Cohen HL, Shapiro M, Haller J, Glassberg K: Sonography of intrascrotal hematomas simulating testicular rupture in adolescents.* Pediatr Radiol *22:296–297, 1992, with permission.*)

a peak incidence at 4 years of age and are the most common testicular malignancy in black children. They are usually diagnosed between 2 and 9 years and are painless but commonly present with endocrine disturbances and sexual precocity. Precocious puberty or gynecomastia may occur if there is androgen or estrogen production by the tumor. Sertoli cell tumors, which represent 20 percent of the nongerminal cell tumors, are diagnosed at about 6 months of age. Gynecomastia caused by estrogen production may also occur.

Enlarged testes caused by leukemic or lymphomatous infiltration are uncommon but may be the primary manifestation (Fig. 108-5*A*) of these diseases. Some 8 percent of patients with acute lymphocytic leukemia have evident testicular involvement during the course of their disease. There is a 92 percent incidence noted among autopsy specimens. These enlarged testicles may have have focal or diffuse areas of decreased echogenicity. Areas of hemorrhage appear echogenic, and lymphatic obstruction may lead to hydrocele. Color Doppler may show increased vascular flow (Fig 108-5*B*) within the affected testes. It is said that as better treatment to prevent recurrence of central nervous system leukemia has developed, the incidence of the testes being a sanctuary for malignant cells in patients undergoing chemotherapy has increased. Periodic survey of the testes in such patients is important. Other metastatic tumors of the testes in children include Wilm's tumor, neuroblastoma, histiocytosis X, sinus histiocytosis, retinoblastoma, and rhabdomyosarcoma.

TRAUMA AND INTRASCROTAL HEMATOMA—A POSSIBLE SIMULATOR OF TESTICULAR TUMOR

Testicular tumors may be discovered because of pain after testicular trauma of various degrees. Testicular tumors may predispose a testis to rupture even with insignificant trauma. The main imaging goal in cases of testicular trauma is to note whether the testicle is normal or fractured. The presence of a break in the tunica albuginea, noted on US by irregularity of testicular contour, requires that the testicle be surgically repaired. The second goal is to make sure that the testicle does not contain a tumor. At times, intrascrotal and extratesticular hematomas may be so large as to displace the testicle superiorly and simulate the testicle itself. The heterogeneity of the intrascrotal hematoma might then be quite disturbing, suggesting a testicular tumor or fracture (Fig. 108-7) unless the testicle itself can be imaged and proven normal.

References

Cassie G: Rupture of the testis. Seminoma. *Br J Urol* 28:283–287, 1956.

Cohen HL, Haller J: Scrotal ultrasound in the pediatric and adolescent patient. *Radiology Report* 2:276–290, 1990.

Cohen HL, Shapiro M, Haller J, Glassberg K: Sonography of intrascrotal hematomas simulating testicular rupture in adolescents. *Pediatr Radiol* 22:296–297, 1992.

Dambro T, Stewart R, Carroll B: The scrotum, in *Diagnostic Ultrasound,* Rumack C, Wilson S, Charboneau J (eds). St Louis, Mosby, 1998:791–821.

Frush D, Sheldon C: Diagnostic imaging for pediatric scrotal disorders. *Radiographics* 18:969–985, 1998.

Kirsch A, Bastian W, Cohen HL, Glassberg K: Precocious puberty in a child with unilateral leydig cell tumor of the testis following orchiopexy. *J Urol* 150:1483–1485, 1993.

Jeffrey R, Laing F, Hricak H, McAninch J: Sonography of testicular trauma. *AJR* 141:993–995, 1983.

La Quaglia M: Genitourinary tract cancer in childhood. *Semin Pediatr Surg* 5:49–65, 1996.

Lupetin A, King W, Rich P, Lederman R: Ultrasound diagnosis of testicular leukemia. *Radiology* 146:171–172, 1983.

McAlister WH, Sisler CL: Scrotal sonography in infants and children. *Curr Probl Diagn Radiol* 19:207–241, 1990.

Saiontz H, Gilchrist G, Smithson W: Testicular relapse in childhood leukemia. *Mayo Clin Proc* 53:212–216, 1978.

Siegel M: Male genital tract, in *Pediatric Sonography,* 2d ed, Siegel M (ed). New York, Raven, 1995:479–512.

Sujka S, Evans E, Nigam A: Delayed rupture of the spleen presenting as a scrotal hematoma. *J Trauma* 26:85–86, 1986.

109

Figure 109-1 shows a 14-year-old boy with an asymmetrically enlarged right testicle. What are the findings? With what are the findings associated?

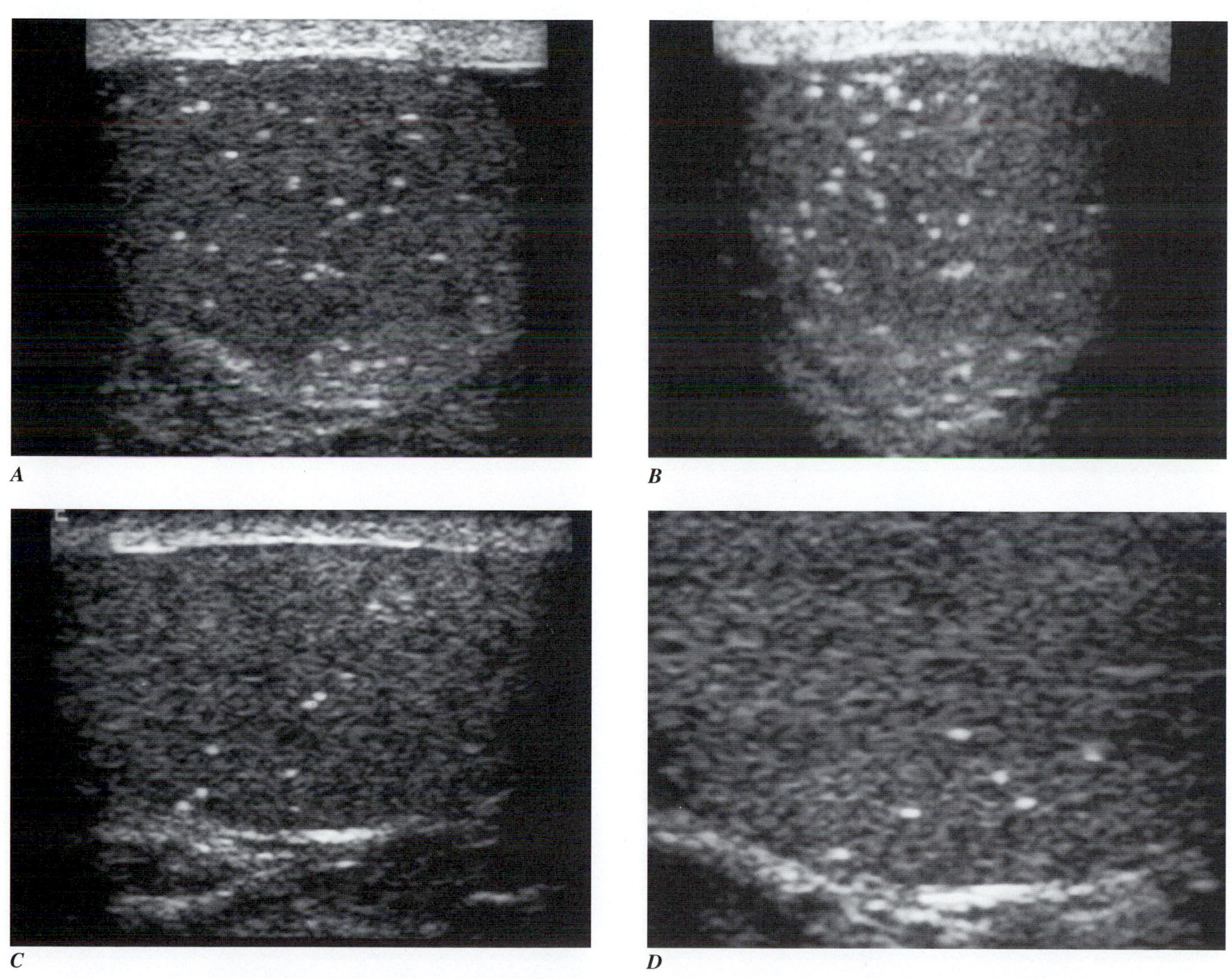

FIGURE 109–1. Longitudinal *(A)* and transverse *(B)* views through the right testis. Longitudinal *(C)* and transverse *(D)* views through the left testis.

CHAPTER 109

Testicular Microlithiasis

SHEILA C. BERLIN

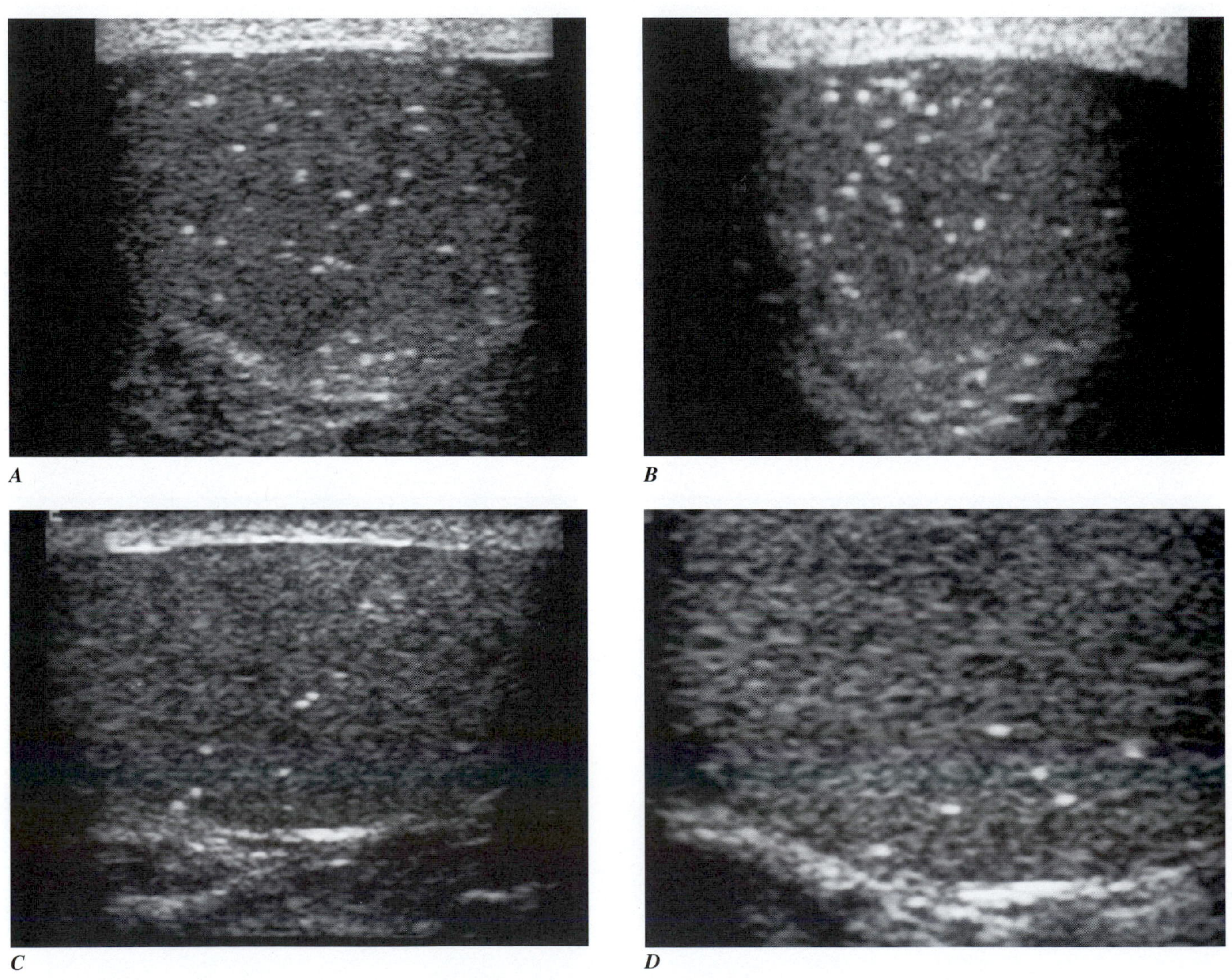

FIGURE 109–2. Testicular microlithiasis. Longitudinal *(A)* and transverse *(B)* views through the right testis and longitudinal *(C)* and transverse *(D)* views through the left testis demonstrate numerous bilateral, nonshadowing, punctate, hyperechoic foci consistent with testicular microlithiasis. Note the assymetric distribution with the microliths more densely concentrated in the right testis.

Testicular microlithiasis is a rare abnormality that is usually discovered as an incidental finding during scrotal sonography. It has been associated with a variety of clinical entities, including cryptorchidism, Klinefelter syndrome, male pseudohermaphrodism, infertility, and pulmonary alveolar and central nervous system microlithiasis. It has also been reported in conjunction with testicular tumors, varicocele, epididymitis, testicular trauma, testicular torsion, and primary testicular tumors. Its prevalence in the general population is not known. It has been reported in 0.05 percent of boys in autopsy studies.

Recent reports have highlighted the relationship between testicular microlithiasis and testicular germ cell neoplasms. The actual risk of developing a primary testicular malignancy in association with testicular microlithiasis remains unclear. The prevalence of associated testicular germ cell tumors is as high as 40 percent in one series. The time interval between the detection of testicular microlithiasis on sonography and tumor development has yet to be defined. However, there are reports of cases where over 10 years elapsed before overt tumor was recognized.

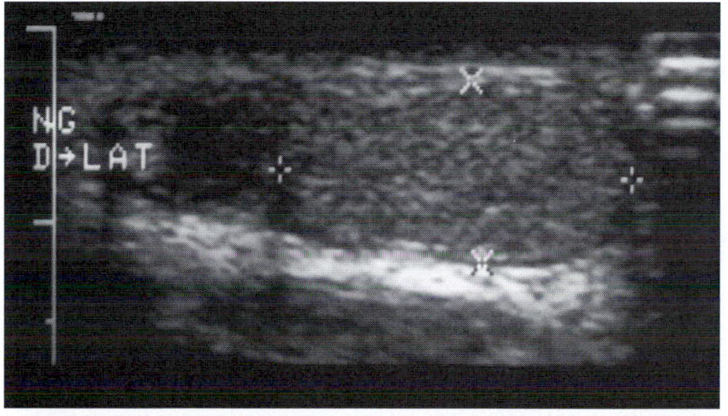

A

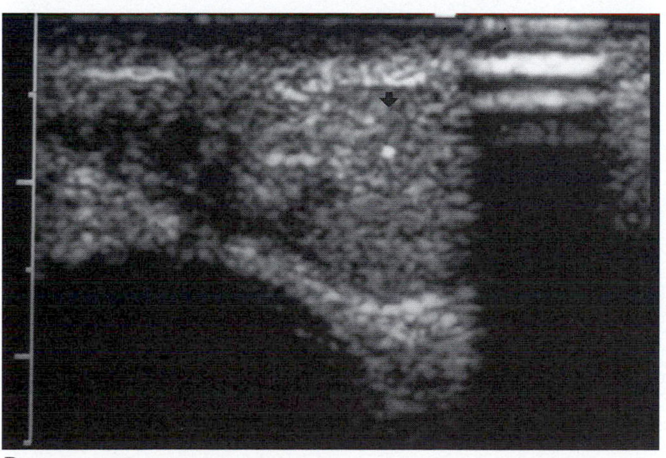

B

FIGURE. 109–3. Unilateral testicular microlithiasis in a repaired cryptorchid testis. ***A.*** Longitudinal view through the right testis in a child who previously underwent repair of an undescended testis demonstrates small testicular size. Note that the testis otherwise appears normal. ***B.*** Longitudinal view through the right testis in the same child now demonstrates testicular microlithiasis (*arrow*). The left testis was normal.

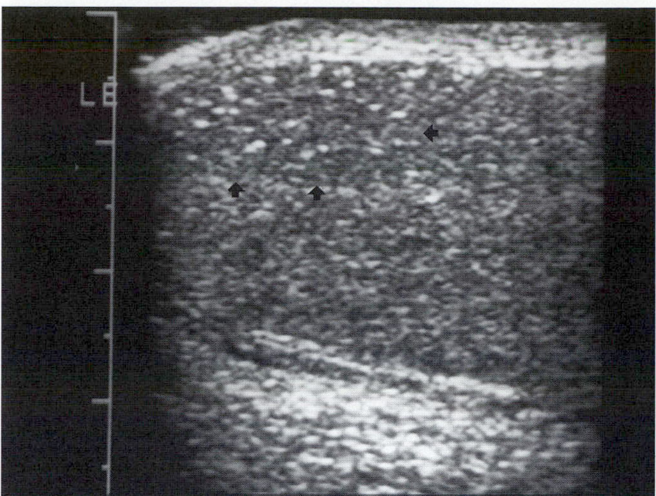

FIGURE 109–4. Peripheral distribution of testicular microlithiasis. Longitudinal view through the right testis of a 10-year-old boy with testicular microlithiasis demonstrates clustering of the microliths in the periphery of the testis (*arrows*).

Testicular microlithiasis is caused by the deposition of concretions within degenerating seminiferous tubules. Some 30 to 60 percent of the tubules can be obstructed by concretions formed from degenerating tubular epithelial cells that slough into the lumina. Calcium is present only within the central core of the lesion. The surrounding concentric laminations consist of collagen fibers. Individual microliths can measure from 50 to 350 μm in diameter.

The sonographic appearance of testicular microlithiasis is distinctive; therefore, biopsy is unnecessary to establish the diagnosis. Multiple punctate, echogenic foci 1 to 3 mm in diameter are noted scattered throughout otherwise normal-appearing testicular parenchyma (Fig. 109-2). These echogenic foci rarely cast acoustic shadows. This pattern has been likened to that of a snowstorm. The epididymis typically appears normal. The distribution of microliths may show considerable variation. Diffuse, bilateral involvement of both testes is most commonly seen. However, the process may be asymmetric (Fig. 109-2) or unilateral (Fig. 109-3), or the microliths may cluster in the peripheral testicular parenchyma (Fig. 109-4). Unilateral testicular microlithiasis is uncommon (Fig. 109-3). It has been reported only in association with unilateral cryptorchidism or intratesticular germ cell neoplasia.

Testicular microlithiasis should not be confused with testicular calcifications associated with testicular germ cell neoplasms. Microcalcifications have been reported in association with testicular germ cell neoplasms on histologic examination, particularly at sites of burned-out tumors. Differentiation of testicular microlithiasis from dystrophic calcifications within testicular tumors can usually be readily made on sonography. The punctate foci of testicular microlithiasis differ from the larger, coarse calcifications that may be associated with primary testicular tumors (Fig. 109-5). In cases of testicular microlithiasis associated with primary testicular tumor, there may be an increase in the microlith concentration at the primary tumor site.

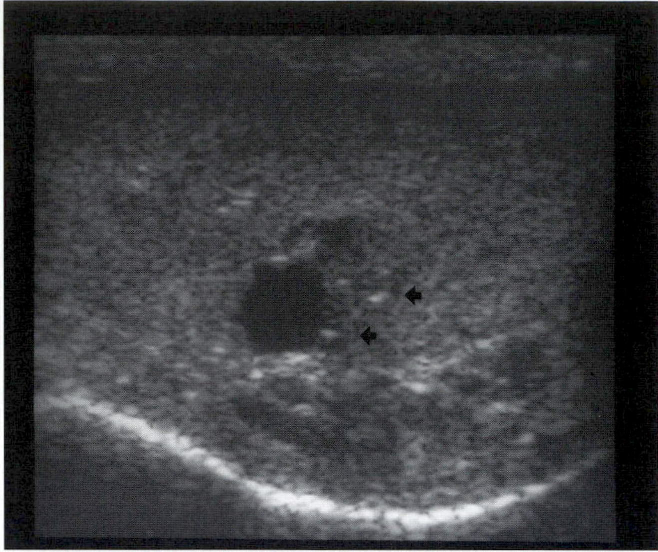

FIGURE 109–5. Dystrophic calcifications in a previously treated testicular germ cell neoplasm. Longitudinal view through the right testis demonstrates an intratesticular lesion (*straight arrow*) with heterogeneous echotexture, including solid regions that are hypoechoic relative to normal testis and a cystic region. The mass also contains several coarse hyperechoic foci representing dystrophic calcifications (*curved arrow*).

Because of the increased risk for primary testicular neoplasms associated with testicular microlithiasis, self-examination and follow-up scrotal sonography are recommended in this patient population. The interval and duration of sonographic follow-up have not been clearly defined. Typically children are followed by sonography at 6- to 12-month intervals.

References

Aizenstein RI, Hibbeln JF, Sagireddy B, et al: Klinefelter's Syndrome associated with testicular microlithiasis and mediastinal germ-cell neoplasm. *JCU* 25:508–510, 1997.

Backus ML, Mack LA, Middleton WD, et al: Testicular microlithiasis: Imaging appearances and pathologic correlation. *Radiology* 192:781–785, 1994.

Frush DP, Kliewer MA, Madden JF: Testicular microlithiasis and subequent development of metastatic germ cell tumor. *AJR* 167:889–890, 1996.

Gooding GA: Detection of testicular microlithiasis by sonography. *AJR* 168:281–282, 1997.

Jantzen DL: Testicular microlithiasis and seminoma. *Clin Radiol* 48:219–220, 1993.

Kessaris DN, Mellinger BC: Incidence and implication of testicular microlithiasis detected by scrotal duplex sonography in a select group of infertile men. *J Urol* 152:1560–1561, 1994.

Kwan DJ, Kirsch AJ, Chang DT, et al: Testicular microlithiasis in a child with torsion of the appendix testis. *J Urol* 153:183–184, 1995.

Miller RL, Wissman R, White S, et al: Testicular microlithiasis: A benign condition with a malignant association. *JCU* 24:197–202, 1996.

Taskinen S, Lehtinen A, Hovatta O, et al: Ultrasound and colour Doppler flow in the testes of adult patients after treatment of cryptorchidism. *Br J Urol* 78:248–251, 1996.

Vrachliotis TG, Neal DE: Unilateral testicular microlithiasis associated with a seminoma. *JCU* 25:505–507.

110

Figure 110-1 shows a 5-year-old boy with a painless scrotal mass. What are the findings? What is the differential diagnosis of a mass in this location?

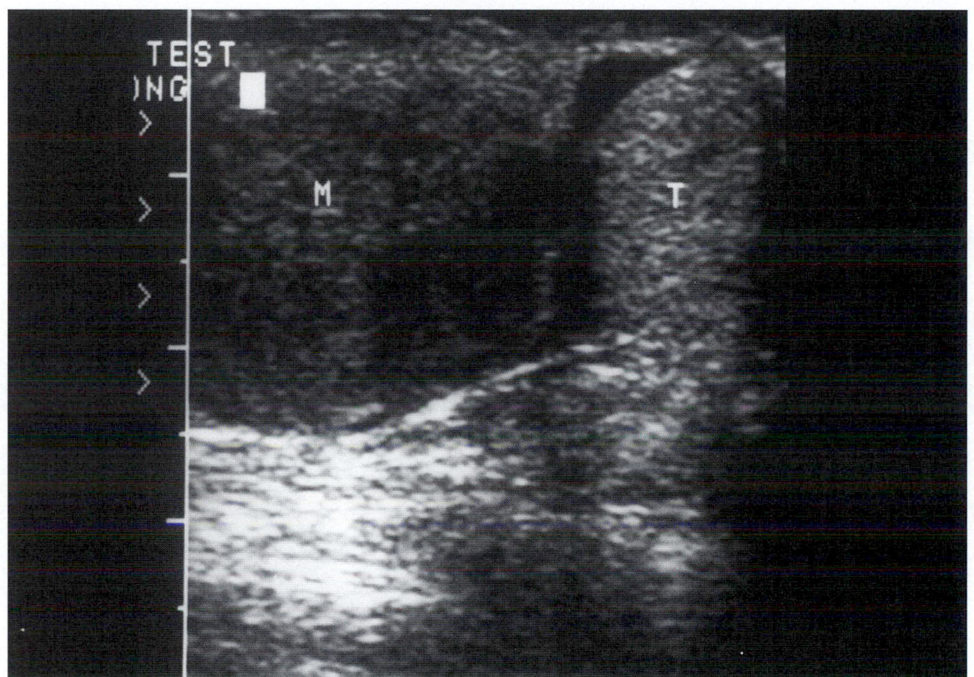

FIGURE 110–1. Longitudinal view through the right scrotum.

CHAPTER 110

Paratesticular Rhabdomyosarcoma

SHEILA C. BERLIN

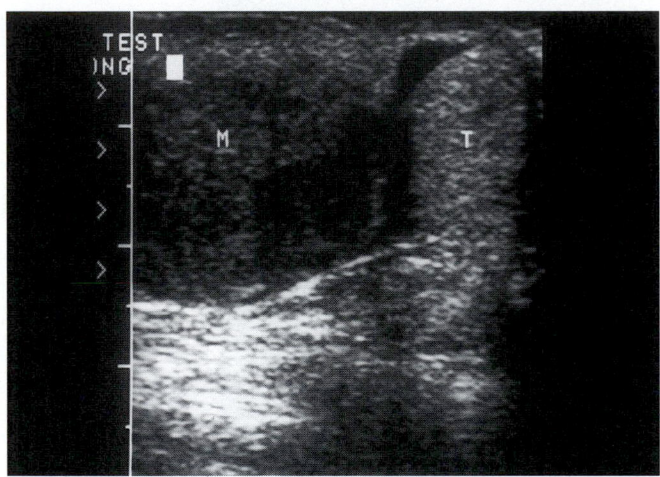

FIGURE 110–2. Paratesticular rhabdomyosarcoma. Longitudinal view through the right scrotum demonstrates a large, solid, predominantly hypoechoic paratesticular mass (M) that displaces the testis (T) inferiorly. No peristalsis was evident within the mass.

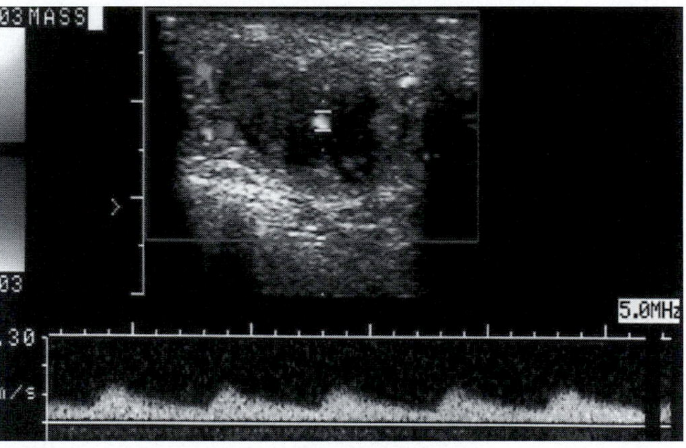

FIGURE 110–3. Color Doppler sonography of paratesticular rhabdomyosarcoma. Longitudinal view through the right scrotum in the same child as in Fig. 110-1 demonstrates hyperemia within the paratesticular mass. (See Color Plate 36.)

Paratesticular tumors can originate from the spermatic cord, epididymis, appendix testis, and tunica testis. Some 75 percent of these masses are benign. The majority are adenomatoid tumors. Additional less common benign neoplasms include fibroma, lipoma, and other mesenchymal tumors. Rhabdomyosarcoma is the most common paratesticular malignant tumor. It can arise from the spermatic cord, testis, or epididymis. Paratesticular rhabdomyosarcoma typically presents as a painless, rapidly enlarging scrotal mass in children under 5 years of age. Paratesticular rhabdomyosarcomas represent about 7 percent of all childhood rhabdomyosarcomas. The tumor has a good prognosis, with a 3-year survival rate of approximately 90 percent. Other paratesticular malignancies include metastatic neuroblastoma, lymphoma, leiomyosarcoma, and fibrosarcoma. Resection of the spermatic cord and testis by an inguinal approach is the favored treatment for these masses, as this surgery is associated with a lower rate of recurrence compared with a transscrotal approach.

The typical sonographic appearance of paratesticular rhabdomyosarcoma includes a solid paratesticular mass of variable echotexture that may compress or invade the adjacent testis (Fig. 110-2). Color Doppler usually shows hyperemia within the mass (Fig. 110-3; see also Color Plate 36). The tumors can reach a large size. Additionally, they may be infiltrative in nature, with poorly defined borders. Therefore, it may be difficult to definitively establish the site of origin

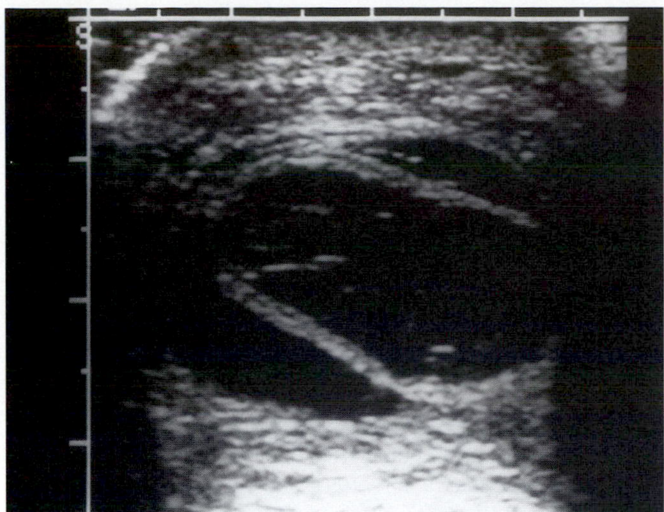

FIGURE 110–4. Complex hydrocele. Longitudinal view through the right scrotum in a 5-year-old boy with acute scrotal tenderness shows a large, complex cystic collection consistent with a large hydrocele.

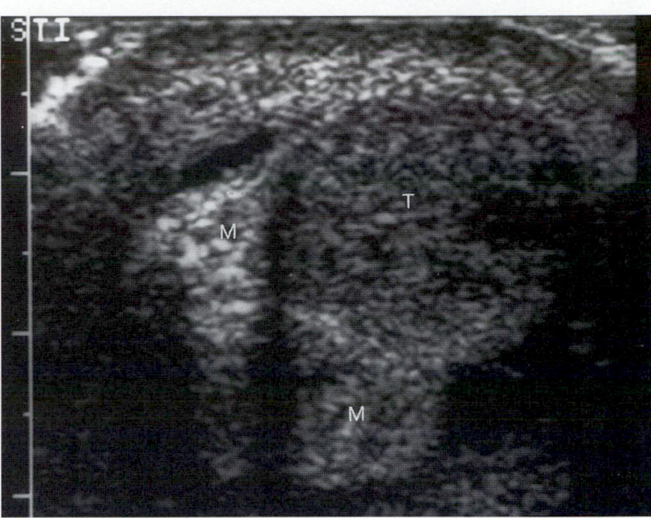

FIGURE 110–6. Extratesticular hematoma. Transverse view through the left scrotum in an 8-year-old boy with an acute history of testicular trauma shows multiple paratesticular masses (M). Note that the masses are primarily hyperechoic relative to the testis (T).

as external to the testis. Surgical exploration is usually required to make a definitive diagnosis.

The most common nonneoplastic paratesticular masses that may be seen on sonography include hydrocele, varicocele, spermatocele, epididymal cyst, hematoma, and hernia. The hydrocele is the most common scrotal mass in infants and children. It is a collection of fluid in the tunica vaginalis of the testicle. The typical sonographic appearance of a hydrocele is that of a thin-walled, anechoic fluid collection. Low-level echoes or septations may be present in cases complicated by infection or hemorrhage (Fig. 110-4). A varicocele consists of dilated veins draining the testis, usually in the pampiniform plexus, which provides the principal venous drainage of the testis. The characteristic appearance of a varicocele on sonography is that of multiple, anechoic, serpigenous vascular structures immediately above the testis. The venous varices increase in size and show augmented flow with the Valsalva maneuver. A varicocele is usually a unilateral lesion and occurs more frequently on the right. Spermatoceles and epididymal cysts appear as hypoechoic or anechoic lesions within the epididymis. Spermatoceles usually represent retention cysts of the small tubules of the head

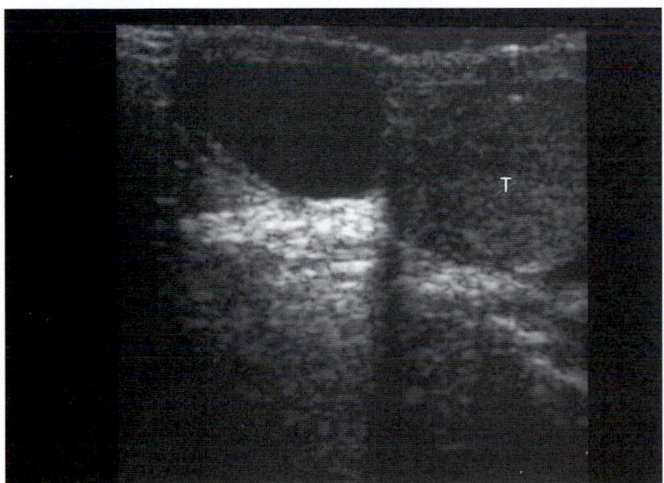

FIGURE 110–5. Epididymal cyst. Longitudinal view through the right scrotum in a 7-year-old boy with new onset of scrotal tenderness demonstrates a large epididymal cyst. T = testis.

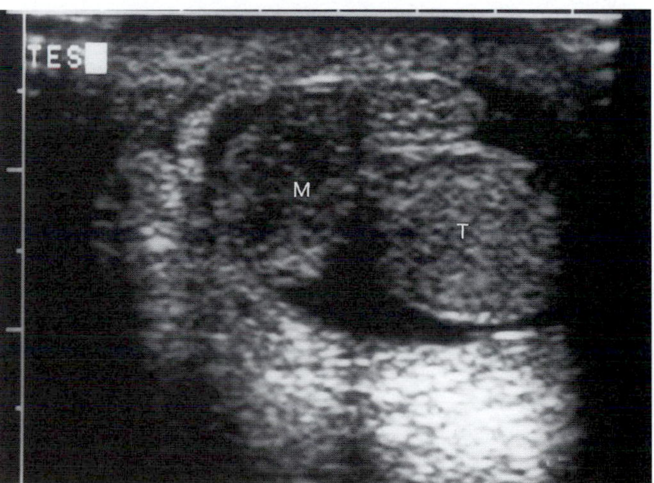

FIGURE 110–7. Paratesticular hernia. Transverse view through the right scrotum in a 3-year-old boy who presented with a painless scrotal mass. A paratesticular mass (M) displacing the right testis (T) is noted. The mass was noted to peristalse during real-time examination, indicative of bowel loops associated with a paratesticular hernia. Also note the associated hydrocele.

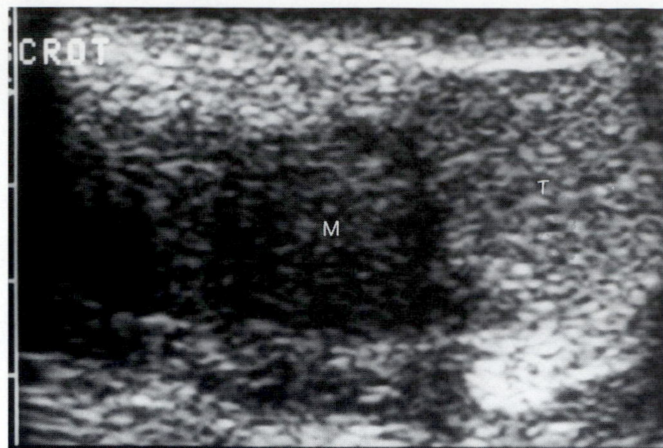

FIGURE 110–8. Paratesticular mass secondary to polyarteritis nodosa. Longitudinal view through the right scrotum in a 13-year-old boy who presented with a painless, firm scrotal mass demonstrates a hypoechoic paratesticular mass (M). At biopsy, the diagnosis of polyarteritis nodosa was made. T = testis.

of the epididymis while epididymal cysts represent dilatation of tubules within the epididymis. They appear on sonography as thin-walled cysts demonstrating acoustic enhancement posteriorly (Fig. 110-5). Internal echoes are occasionally noted due to cellular debris. An acute extratesticular hematoma appears as a heterogeneous mass (Fig. 110-6). Hyperechoic areas are commonly noted acutely. The lesion becomes increasingly hypoechoic with liquification and retraction. A large hematoma may make identification of the testis and epididymis difficult. A scrotal hernia is usually associated with a patent processus vaginalis containing bowel and/or omentum. The bowel loops and omentum in the scrotum may mimic a mass lesion (Fig. 110-7). On sonography, identification of peristalsing bowel loops confirms the diagnosis. If the bowel loops are fluid-filled and nonperistalsing, the lesion may mimic a hydrocele. Additional uncommon paratesticular lesions in children may be seen in association with sarcoidosis, tuberculosis, and polyarteritis nodosa (Fig. 110-8).

References

Argons GA, Wagner BJ, Lonergan GL, et al: Genitourinary rhabdomyosarcoma in children: Radiologic-pathologic correlation. *Radiographics* 17:919–937, 1997.

Benge BN, Byrd RL, Bergevin M, et al: Scrotal recurrence of paratesticular rhabdomyosarcoma in a previously undescended testicle 5 years after orchiectomy. *J Urol* 152:2117–2118, 1994.

LaQuaglia M: Genitourinary rhabdomyosarcoma in children. *Urol Clin North Am* 18:575–580, 1991.

Olney LE, Narayana A, Loening S, et al: Intrascrotal rhabdomyosarcoma. *Urology* 14:113–125, 1979.

Perselin ST, Menke DM: Isolated polyarteritis nodosa of the male reproductive system. *J Rheumatol* 19:985–988, 1992.

Ryan DM, Lesser BA, Crumley LA, et al: Epididymal sarcoidosis. *J Urol* 149:134–136, 1993.

Tessler FN, Tublin ME, Rifkin MD: Ultrasound assessment of testicular and paratesticular masses. *JCU* 24:423–436, 1996.

Wood A, Dewbury KC: Case report: Paratesticular rhabdomyosarcoma—color doppler appearances. *Clin Radiol* 50:130–131, 1995.

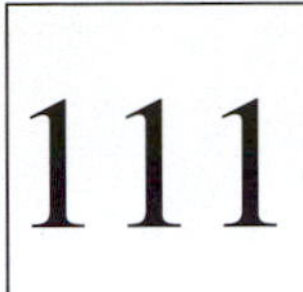

111

Figure 111-1 shows a 12-year-old boy with short stature. What do you see? What are the diagnostic considerations?

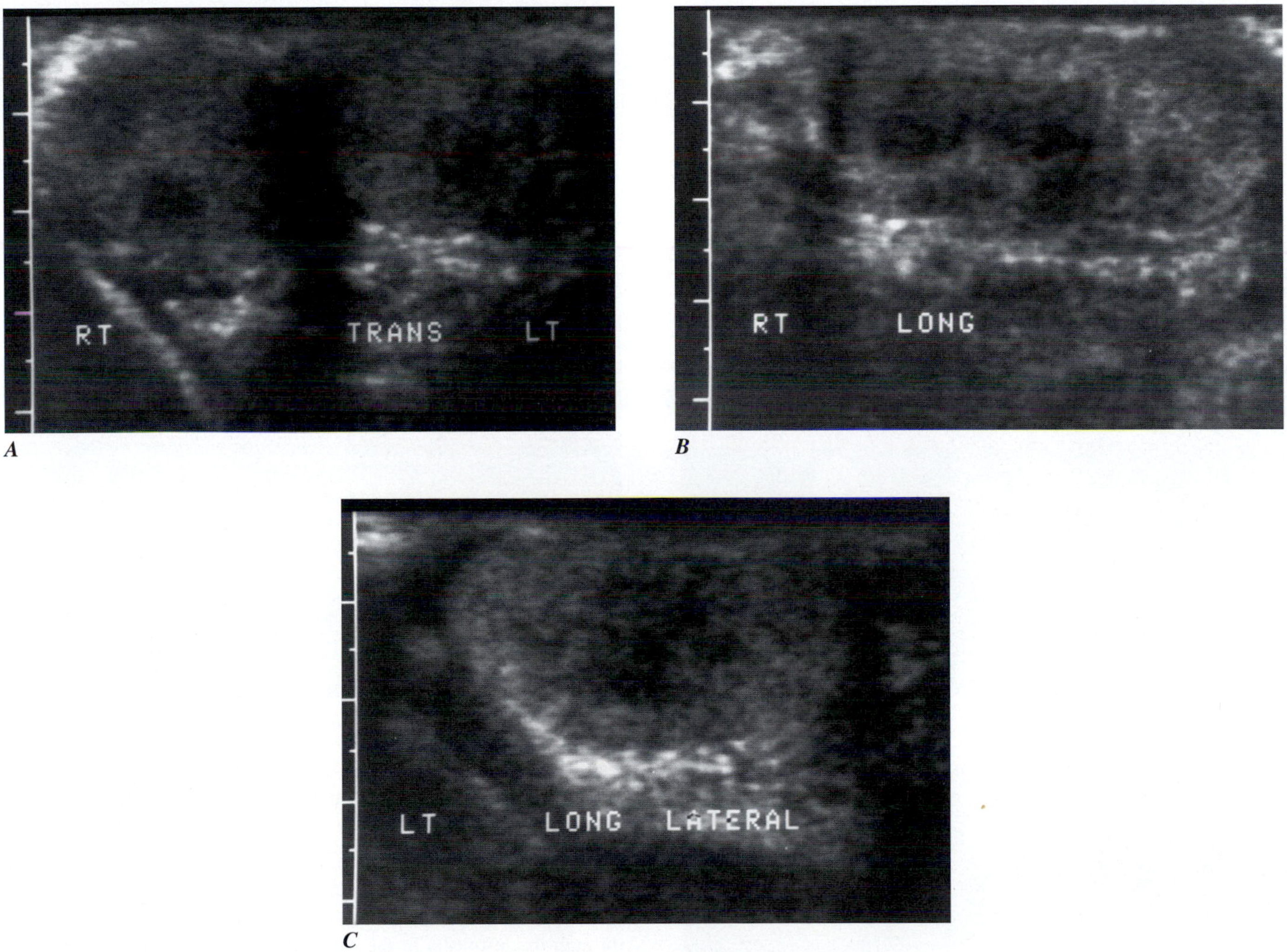

A

B

C

FIGURE 111–1. Transverse *(A)* and longitudinal (*B* and *C*) views through the scrotum.

CHAPTER 111

Testicular Adrenal Rest Tissue in Congenital Adrenal Hyperplasia

CARLOS J. SIVIT

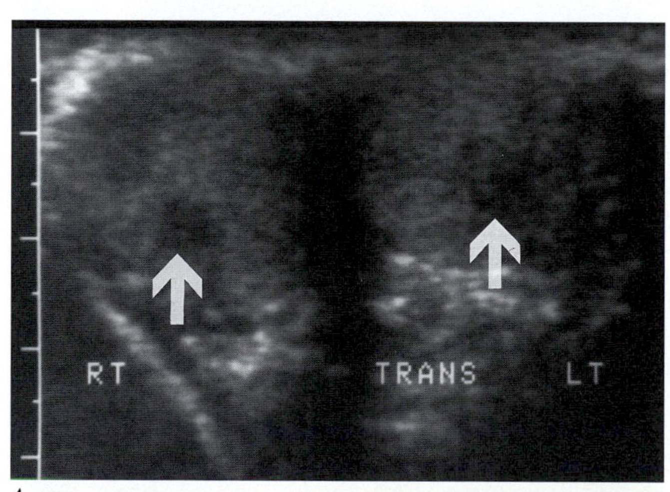

A

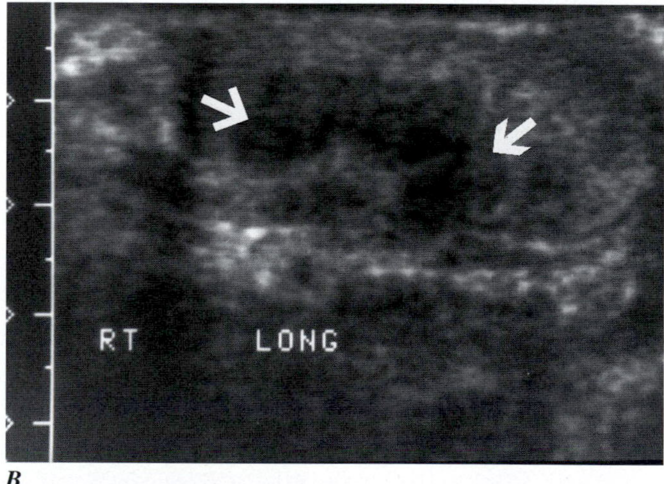

B

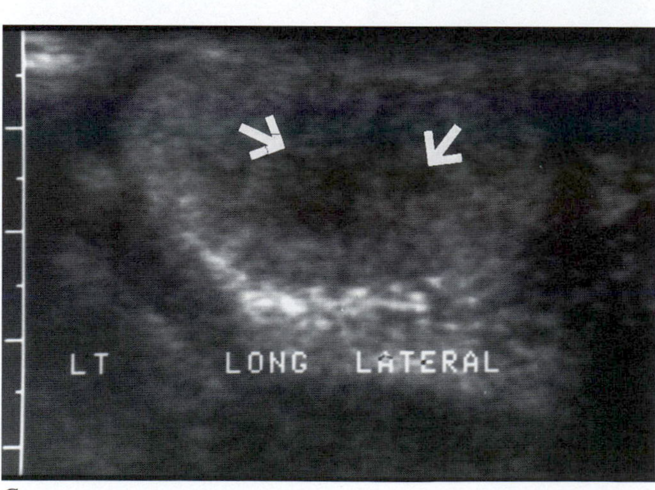

C

FIGURE 111–2. Testicular adrenal rest tissue in congenital adrenal hyperplasia. ***A.*** Transverse view through both testes in this child who has congenital adrenal hyperplasia (CAH) demonstrates multiple rounded, well-circumscribed, hypoechoic lesions (*arrows*). ***B.*** Longitudinal view through the right testis in the same child shows focal hypoechoic masses (*arrows*). Note that there is absence of disruption of the outer testicular contour. ***C.*** Longitudinal view through the left testis in the same child shows another central hypoechoic mass (*arrow*). This lesion is less well circumscribed than the others.

Congenital adrenal hyperplasia (CAH) results from an enzymatic defect in the biosynthetic pathway of adrenal steroids (Fig. 111-2). This deficiency results in deficient production of cortisol and the accumulation of hormonal precursors, some of which produce androgenic effects. The clinical man-

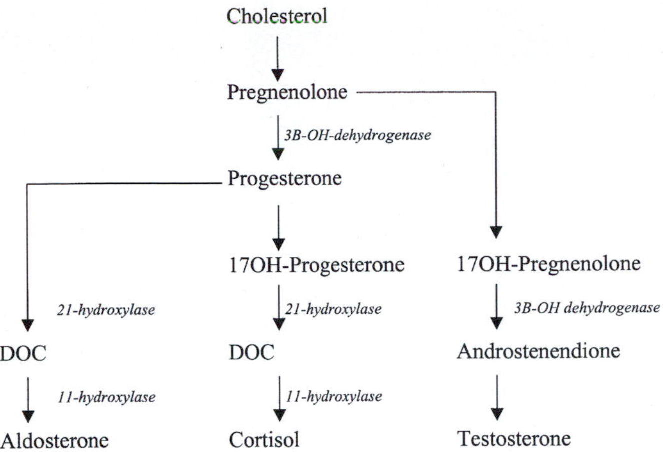

FIGURE 111–3. Metabolic pathway of aldosterone and cortisol biosynthesis and associated enzymatic defects resulting in congenital adrenal hyperplasia.

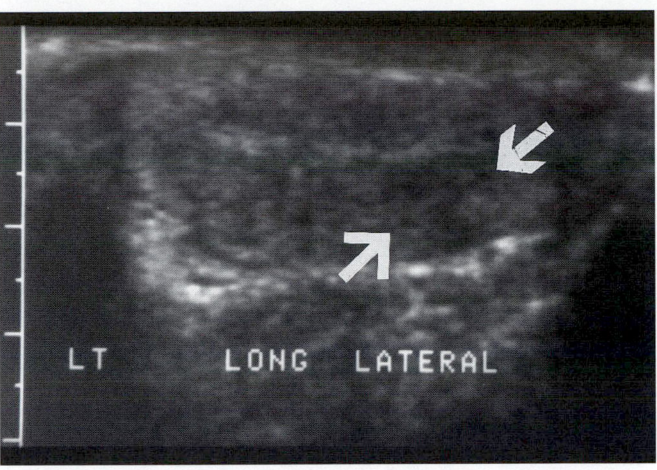

FIGURE 111–4. Preservation of the echogenic stripe of the mediastinum testes in a child with testicular adrenal rest tissue. Longitudinal view through the left testes in a child with congenital adrenal hyperplasia shows several ill-defined, hypoechoic nodules (*arrows*), representing testicular adrenal rests. Note that the echogenic stripe of the mediastinum testes is clearly seen and not distorted.

ifestations depend on the severity of the enzyme deficiency and its position in the enzymatic pathway. The most common enzymatic defect is a deficiency of 21-hydroxylase, which occurs in approximately 90 percent of cases (Fig. 111-3). Other observed enzymatic defects reported include 11-hydroxylase, 17-hydroxylase, and 3β-hydroxysteroid dehydrogenase deficiencies. Children with 21-hydroxylase deficiency may present during the neonatal period with virilization and salt wasting, may develop symptoms later in life, or may remain asymptomatic. The other enzymatic defects associated with CAH typically do not result in virilization.

Some male children with unrecognized or poorly controlled CAH may develop testicular masses representing adrenal rest tissue at puberty or following puberty. Ectopic adrenal rest tissue has been identified in various sites, including the celiac plexus region, the broad ligaments, and the testes. The sustained elevation of adrenocorticotropic hormones (ACTH) in CAH has been postulated to cause adrenal rest cells present in the testes to grow and become functionally active adrenal rest masses. These testicular masses are biochemically identical to the hyperplastic adrenal cortex. The tissue is endocrinologically active and hypertrophies when there are elevated levels of ACTH. Similar lesions may be found in patients with other conditions characterized by elevated levels of adrenocorticotropic hormone, such as Addison disease and Cushing syndrome. They typically atrophy following the administration of high doses of glucocorticoids. Thus, these testicular lesions signal poor hormonal control and indicate the need for more aggressive treatment.

The nodules associated with testicular adrenal rest tissue in children with CAH are typically multifocal throughout both testes. They may occur as a unilateral mass or masses in 25 percent of cases. Individual lesions are usually hypoechoic (Fig. 111-2), although there are occasional reports of solid hyperechoic lesions or of lesions that have a hyperechoic rim. The masses are minimally disruptive of surrounding testicular tissue. They typically do not distort the outer testicular contour. Additionally, when they are located near the mediastinum, the echogenic stripe of the mediastinum testes is still recognizable (Fig. 111-4). These features are useful in differentiating the masses from true testicular neoplasms. Calcifications within the lesions have not been reported. Some lesions may demonstrate increased vascularity on color Doppler examination. Peripheral vessels may be seen radiating toward the center of the mass. Since the presence of these masses is indicative of poorly controlled or unrecognized CAH, follow-up sonography is useful in monitoring response to therapy by showing a decrease in lesion size.

References

Avilla NA, Premkumar A, Shawker TH, et al: Testicular adrenal rest tissue in congenital adrenal hyperplasia: Findings at gray-scale and color doppler US. *Radiology* 198:99–104, 1996.

Seidenwurm D, Smathers RL, Kan P, et al: Intratesticular adrenal rests diagnosed by ultrasound. *Radiology* 155:479–481, 1985.

Shawker TH, Doppman JL, Choyke PL, et al: Intratesticular masses in association with abnormally functioning adrenal glands. *JCU* 20:51–58, 1992.

Vanzulli A, DelMaschio A, Paesano P, et al: Testicular masses in association with adrenogenital syndrome: US findings. *Radiology* 183:425–429, 1992.

Willi U, Atares M, Prader A, et al: Testicular adrenal-like tissue (TALT) in congenital adrenal hyperplasia: Detection by ultrasonography. *Pediatr Radiol* 21:284–287, 1991.

Section K

MISCELLANEOUS: NECK, CHEST, AND MUSCULOSKELETAL SYSTEM

112

Figure 112-1 shows a 6-week-old boy with torticollis. What do you see? What are the diagnostic considerations?

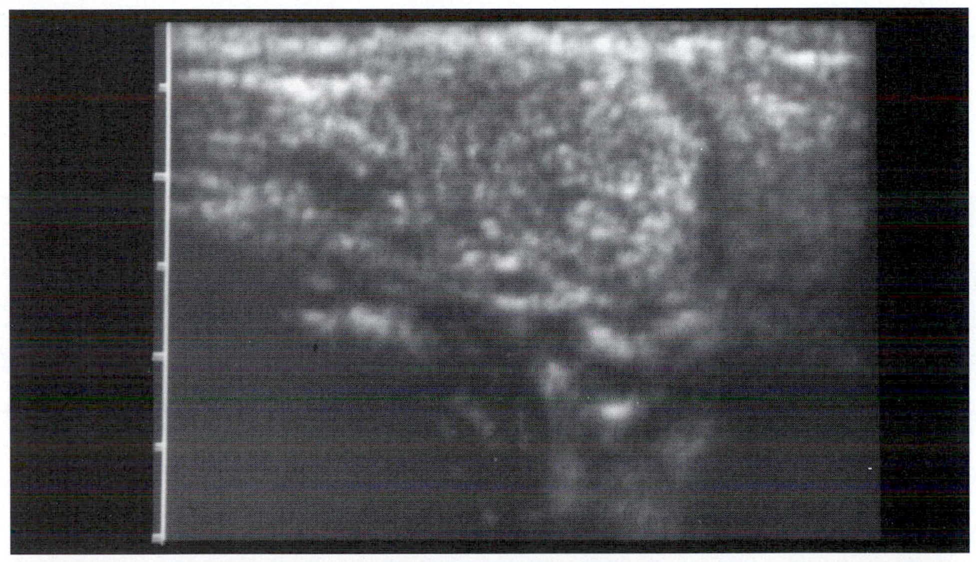

A

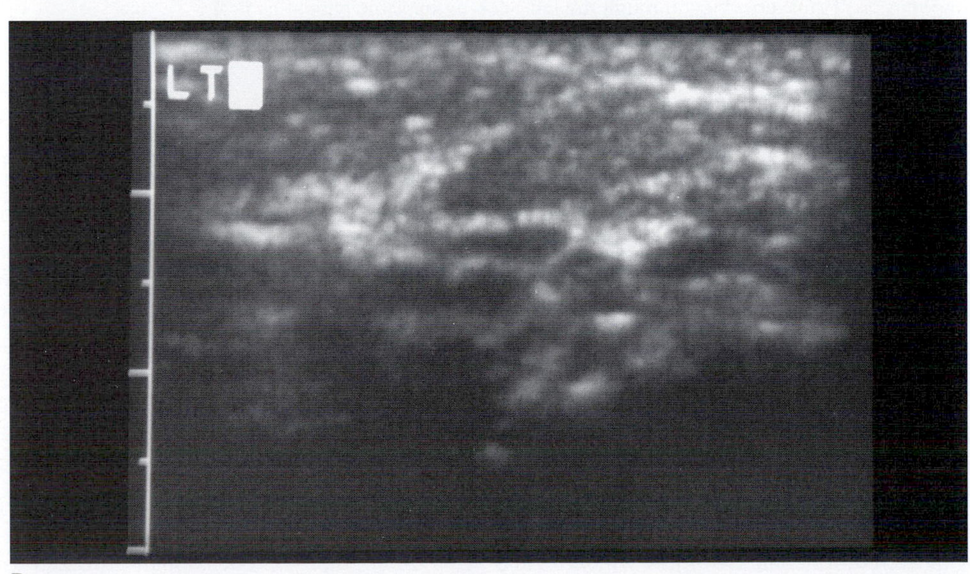

B

FIGURE 112–1. Transverse views through the right *(A)* and left *(B)* neck.

CHAPTER 112

Fibromatosis Colli

CARLOS J. SIVIT

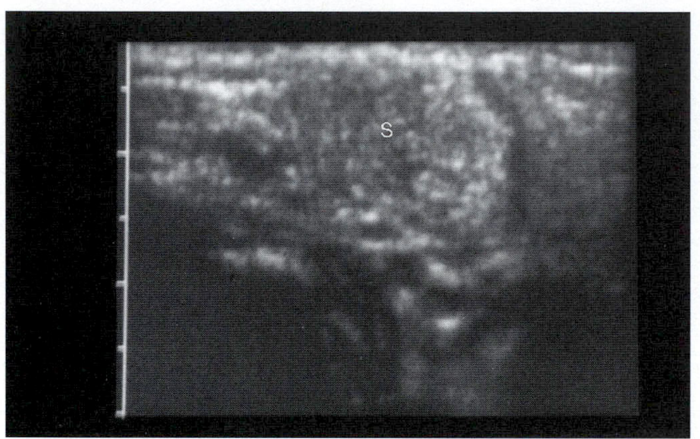

A

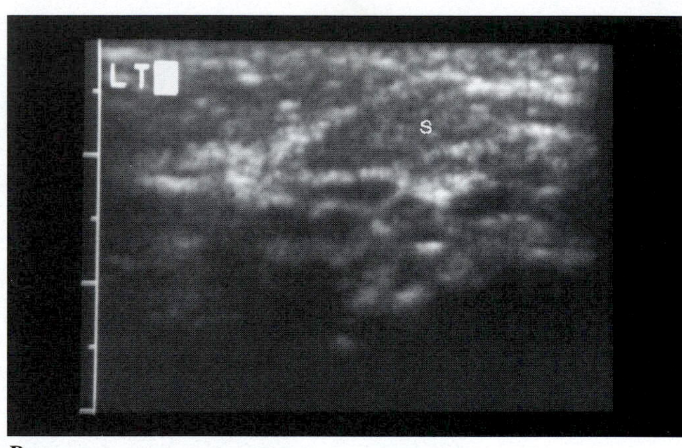

B

FIGURE 112–2. Fibromatosis colli. ***A.*** Transverse view through the right neck demonstrates diffuse enlargement of the right sternocleidomastoid muscle (S). The muscle is slightly hyperechoic relative to the adjacent musculature. Although having the appearance of a mass, the lesion is well circumscribed without extension outside of the muscle, consistent with fibromatosis colli. ***B.*** Normal sternocleidomastoid muscle. Transverse view through the left neck in the same patient as in ***A*** shows the normal left sternocleidomastoid muscle (S) for comparison. Note the size discrepancy between the right and left sternocleidomastoid muscles.

Fibromatosis colli is a benign lesion that is typically diagnosed in the first few months of life. It is usually observed in otherwise healthy infants. The infants most frequently present with a unilateral neck mass or with torticollis. The mass may be noted to enlarge over a period of several weeks. The majority of cases are unilateral. However, bilateral cases have been reported. Right-sided lesions are more common than left-sided lesions. This condition is the most common cause of torticollis in infancy.

Fibromatosis colli is felt to be related to birth trauma. Many cases are associated with difficult delivery, including breech position and forceps delivery. There are several proposed etiologies for this condition. The two most widely held theories are that it results from pressure necrosis followed by secondary fibrosis in the sternocleidomastoid muscle and that it is due to occlusion of venous outflow from the sternocleidomastoid muscle, resulting in edema, necrosis, and later fibrosis. Cytologic features associated with this condition include degenerated muscle cells and fibroblast proliferation.

The condition is usually treated nonoperatively. The therapeutic regime includes muscle-stretching exercises. There is usually gradual improvement after the institution of physical therapy, with increased range of motion over a period of 4 to 6 months. However, a small subset of children will not respond to physical therapy and require surgery for the correction of the condition.

Sonography is occasionally utilized to image infants with fibromatosis colli. The infant neck is best imaged with a

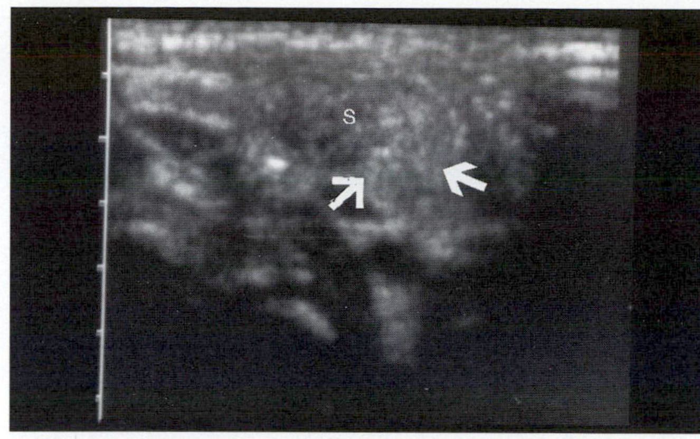

A

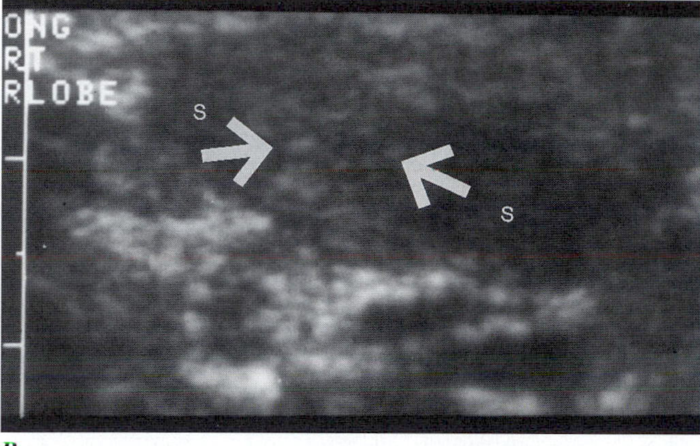

B

FIGURE 112–3. Fibromatosis colli with focal involvement of the sternocleidomastoid muscle. ***A.*** Transverse view through the right neck in a 3-month-old child who presented with torticollis demonstrates a focal mass (*arrows*) involving the medial half of the right sternocleidomastoid muscle. Note that the involved medial segment of the muscle is hyperechoic relative to the normal lateral half of the muscle (S). ***B.*** Fibromatosis colli with focal involvement of the sternocleidomastoid muscle. Longitudinal view through the right neck in the same patient as in Fig. 112-3*A* shows a focal mass (*arrows*) within the midaspect of the right sternocleidomastoid muscle. Note that the mass is hyperechoic relative to the normal upper and lower segments of the sternocleidomastoid muscle (S).

high-frequency (7-MHz) transducer. A linear array transducer is preferred in order to image a larger near field of view, since most structures of interest are relatively superficial. The sternocleidomastoid muscle is located anterior and lateral to the carotid artery and jugular vein and lateral to the thyroid gland. The normal muscle is hypoechoic relative to the thyroid gland.

The sonographic findings of fibromatosis colli include a well-circumscribed, solid mass within the sternocleidomastoid muscle in the anterior neck with variable echotexture (Fig. 112-2). Confirmation of the location of the mass within the sternocleidomastoid muscle can be made on real-time sonographic examination, as the mass is noted to move synchronously with the involved muscle. There may be focal (Fig. 112-3) or diffuse (Fig. 112-2) involvement of the sternocleidomastoid muscle. In cases of focal involvement, the lower two-thirds of the muscle is primarily involved. The echogenicity of the mass varies with the age of the lesion. The lesion may be hyperechoic, isoechoic, or hypoechoic relative to normal muscle. It typically is surrounded by a hypoechoic rim, which may represent normal adjacent muscle.

Computed tomography (CT) and magnetic resonance imaging (MRI) are also occasionally useful in the evaluation of infants with suspected fibromatosis colli in order to confirm the location of the lesion within the sternocleidomastoid muscle, to demonstrate clear surrounding fascial planes, and to show lack of associated lymphadenopathy, airway compression, vascular compression, or bone involvement. Both imaging modalities will show focal or diffuse enlargement of the involved sternocleidomastoid muscle. The mass is typically isodense to surrounding muscle on contrast-enhanced CT. The signal characteristics on MRI are variable. Both imaging modalities may show mass effect on the trachea or the carotid sheath associated with the sternocleidomastoid muscle enhargement. However, the mass should be localized to the sternocleidomastoid muscle without encasement of other structures.

The differential diagnosis of a neck mass in an infant includes malignant neoplasms, such as neuroblastoma, rhabdomyosarcoma, and lymphoma, and benign lesions, such as hemangioma and lymphangioma. The most useful imaging finding that suggests that the lesion is not fibromatosis colli is extension of the mass beyond the sternocleidomastoid muscle. Additionally, neuroblastoma and rhabdomyosarcoma characteristically have an infiltrative appearance, with irregular margins. They may also contain calcifications. Lymphoma is suggested by the presence of oval masses corresponding to enlarged lymph nodes along the cervical lymph node chain. A hemangioma can be identified on the basis of its pronounced vascularity on color Dopper. A lymphangioma has a variable echotexture but typically is predominantly cystic, although it may contain numerous septations.

References

Ablin DS, Jain K, Howell L, et al: Ultrasound and MR imaging of fibromatosis colli (sternocleidomastoid tumor of infancy). *Pediatr Radiol* 28:230–233, 1998.

Chan YL, Cheng JCY, Metreweli C: Ultrasonography of congenital muscular torticollis. *Pediatr Radiol* 22:356–360, 1992.

Crawford SC, Harnsberger HR, Johnson L, et al: Fibromatosis colli of infancy: CT and sonographic findings. *AJR* 151:1183–1184, 1988.

Eich GF, Hoeffel JC, Tschappeler H, et al: Fibrous tumours in children: Imaging features of a heterogenous group of disorders. *Pediatr Radiol* 28:500–509, 1998.

Freidman AP, Haller JO, Goodman JD, et al: Sonographic evaluation of non-inflammatory neck masses in children. *Radiology* 147:693–697, 1983.

Glasier CM, Seibert JJ, Williamson SL, et al: High resolution ultrasound characterization of soft tissue masses in children. *Pediatr Radiol* 17:233–237, 1987.

Kraus R, Bokyung KH, Babcock DS, et al: Sonography of neck masses in children. *AJR* 146:609–613, 1986.

Som PM, Sacher M, Lanzieri CF: Parenchymal cysts of the lower neck. *Radiology* 157:399–406, 1985.

Vasquez E, Enriquez G, Castellote A, et al: US, CT, and MR imaging of neck lesions in children. *Radiographics* 15:105–122, 1995.

113

Two young children had small masses seen in the anterior soft tissues of their necks. Both had masses that were not midline, but rather slightly off midline. Figure 113-1 is a transverse view of the soft tissues of the neck at the site of concern of one child. Figure 113-2 is a longitudinal view, slightly to the right of midline, from the other child. Both children had the same abnormality. What do you see? What do you think the abnormality is? Can these be thyroglossal duct cysts? Why not? If they were thyroglossal duct cysts, what would be the most important additional area to image?

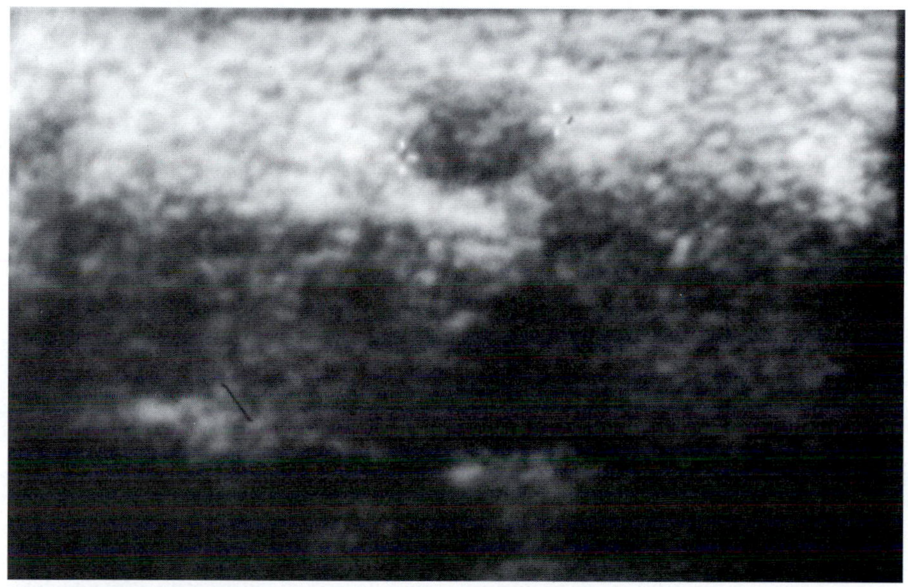

FIGURE 113–1. Pediatric anterior neck. Transverse plane.

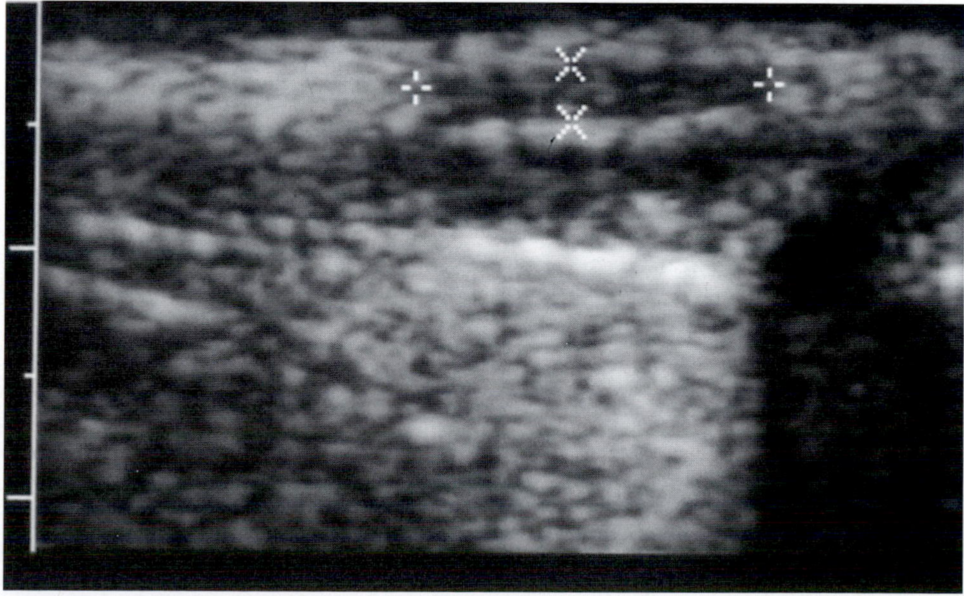

FIGURE 113–2. Pediatric anterior neck. Longitudinal plane, to the right of midline.

CHAPTER 113

Thyroglossal Duct Cyst

HARRIS L. COHEN

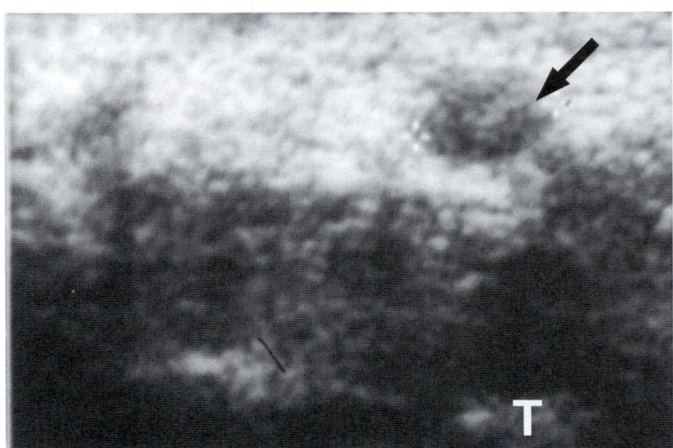

FIGURE 113–3. Annotated version of Fig. 113-1. Thyroglossal duct cyst. Anterior neck. Transverse plane. A circular echopenic structure (*arrow*) is seen. It is not cystic. It is slightly to the right of midline. Neither of these facts goes against thyroglossal duct cyst; in fact, they are very typical of it. The patient proved to have a thyroglossal duct cyst. T = trachea.

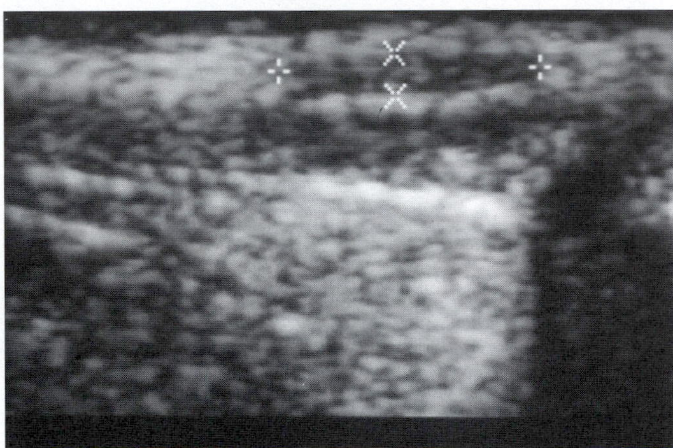

FIGURE 113–4. Annotated version of Fig. 113-2. Thyroglossal duct cyst. Anterior neck. Longitudinal plane, to the right of midline and through the mass. This is the equivalent of an orthogonal projection of Fig. 113-3, but it is in a different patient. The mass is 13.5 mm long and 2.6 mm wide. It proved to be a thyroglossal duct cyst.

Figure 113-3, the annotated version of Fig. 113-1, and Fig. 113-4, the annotated version of Fig. 113-3, are images of small, echopenic masses in the soft tissues of the anterior neck of two different children. The masses are not cystic and were both off the midline. Despite the fact that logically one might assume that such information would exclude consideration of a thyroglossal duct (TGD) cyst, it does not. In fact, in our and others' experience, an echopenic mass, rather than a classically cystic mass, and an off-midline position are very common imaging presentations for a TGD cyst. If a patient has a TGD cyst, as these two patients did, the most important next step is to prove that the patient has a normal thyroid gland.

The presence of an anatomically normal thyroid (Fig. 113-5) on ultrasound (US) examination is now considered sufficient evidence that there will be functioning thyroid tissue present *after* the surgical removal of the TGD cyst. Surgical removal of the cyst without proving the presence of thyroid tissue other than that which may be present in the TGD cyst may force an unfortunate patient into a lifetime of required thyroid hormone supplementation.

WHAT IS A THYROGLOSSAL DUCT CYST?

Thyroglossal duct cysts represent 70 percent of all the congenital anomalies of the neck discovered in postnatal life. The cyst usually presents as a painless swelling in the midline of the neck. The thyroid gland, the first endocrine gland to develop in the fetus, appears in the fourth week of antenatal life as a median thickening in the primitive pharyngeal floor. As it develops, it descends to its normal position in the neck as a downward growth known as the thyroid diverticulum. While descending, it maintains its connection to the

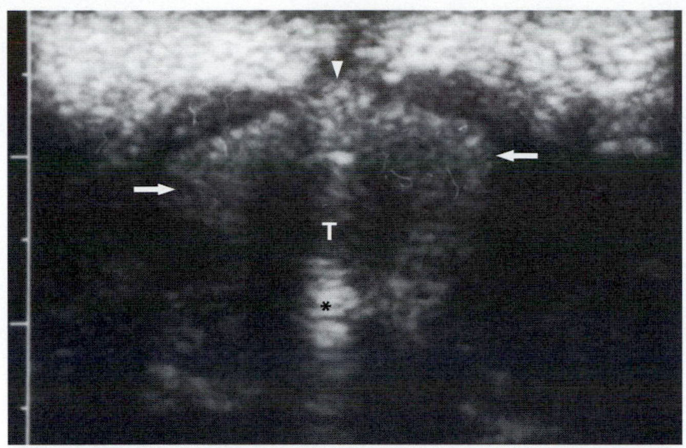

A

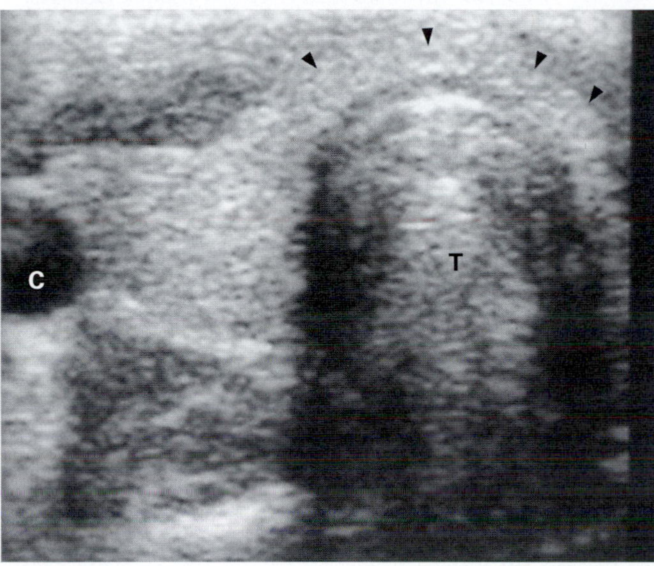

B

FIGURE 113–5. Normal thyroid. ***A.*** Anterior neck, caudal to the level of the mass (thyroglossal duct cyst). The lobes (*arrows*) are symmetric, and the thyroid's isthmus (*arrowhead*) is seen anterior to the trachea (T). Normal thyroid tissue is homogeneously echogenic. The echogenicity is greater than that of the surrounding soft tissue structures of the neck. Echogenicity within the trachea (*asterisk*) is due to "ring down" from contained air. ***B.*** Anterior neck, level of thyroid. This is the normal thyroid of another patient. The right lobe and isthmus (*arrow*) are noted. I show this image because it is a good example of the typical prominent echogenicity of the thyroid compared to the surrounding soft tissue structures of the neck. T = trachea, C = carotid artery. Arrowheads point to thyroid isthmus.

tongue by a thyroglossal duct whose opening in the tongue is known as the foramen cecum. By the seventh week of antenatal life, the thyroid should be in its normal position and the duct should disappear. Remnants of this duct may develop into cystic masses that present during childhood. These TGD cysts may be found anywhere from the tongue to the thyroid gland's isthmus. The majority (65 percent) are found below the hyoid bone, while 20 percent are suprahyoid and 15 percent are found at the level of the hyoid. They have been reported to have been imaged in fetal life.

Accessory thyroid tissue may exist in TGD remnants. Thyroid hormone may be produced in these ectopic glandular elements, but usually in quantities insufficient for normal function and development. More importantly, however, if the thyroid never fully developed and/or never descended below the cyst, the thyroid hormone production in the ectopic thyroid tissue of a TGD cyst may be all the patient has. It is of utmost importance to prove the existence of functioning thyroid tissue beyond the TGD cyst *before* performing the often cosmetic surgery to remove it. Several groups have noted that US imaging of normal thyroid parenchyma can exclude the need to confirm function by scintigraphy. In one recent reported case, a teenager had a TGD cyst removed and became hypothyroid because of a pseudothyroid appearance in the patient's neck area on US examination. This would be a worrisome case report but for the fact that the image reported as having a "pseudothyroid" appearance in no way resembles the classic homogeneously echogenic image of a thyroid. Rather, it is the image of more echopenic soft tissue of a neck without definitive thyroid tissue.

ULTRASOUND FINDINGS IN THYROGLOSSAL DUCT CYST

The TGD cyst may be variable in appearance. In one report of 12 children, aged 2 months to 16 years, who had confirmed TGD cysts, 9 had midline masses, while 2 had right of midline cysts and 1 a left of midline cyst. Only 5 of the masses were anechoic with a thin cyst wall denoting a classic cyst appearance; 7 of the masses were hypoechoic, 2 were homogeneously hypoechoic with thin walls, and 5 had some heterogeneity due to the echogenicity within them. Our 2 unknown cases would fit the latter pattern. Four of the masses were anechoic, but with a thick wall or internal debris. The masses ranged between 0.5 and 4 cm in diameter. Wadsworth and Siegel stated that wall thickness and contained internal echoes within such masses could not separate infected from noninfected TGD cysts.

ANY OTHER ANTERIOR NECK MASSES TO WORRY ABOUT?

Adenopathy

The differential diagnosis of anterior neck masses includes thyroid tumors, ectopic thyroid tissue, adenopathy, and abscess. Adenopathy is usually not midline. Abscess is usually painful. Tumors such as teratoma or neuroblastoma are not common at this site. Lymphomatous nodes and particularly metastatic nodes are far less common a problem in children than older adults, and also are not often anterior or midline.

Many of the neck masses we are asked to look at to rule out TGD cysts are small submental or anterolateral neck nodes. The differential diagnosis is easy if the masses are significantly off midline or if they contain the central echogenic fat typical of the hilum of a benign node (Fig. 113-6). How-

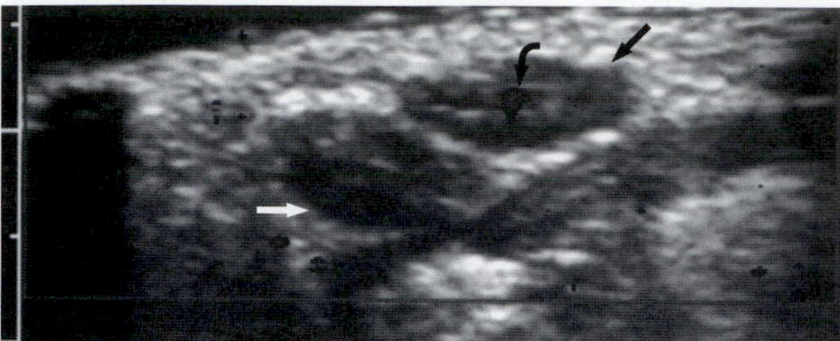

FIGURE 113–6. Prominent lymph nodes. Anterolateral neck, longitudinal plane. Two oval nodes (*arrows*) are noted in a child with left neck pain. The masses felt like inflamed benign nodes. They also look like them. They are oval in shape, and their more echogenic centers are typical of benign nodes. The central hilar echogenicity (from contained fat) is not as well seen on this image because of obscuring vascular flow on this black-and-white rendition of a color Doppler image. A curved arrow points to central flow within the hilum of one of the nodes. This single central hilar vessel is the classic flow pattern for a benign node.

ever, lymph nodes often lose their echogenic hilum when they become acutely infected or abscessed (Fig. 113-7), and their exact diagnosis becomes more difficult. Infected nodes are often painful. Obviously, most of our cases of infected nodes are predominantly masses of the lateral neck. In analyzing nodes by US, one group, using power Doppler, has reported three flow patterns among enlarged nodes. The finding of a single "vascular pole" (a single central hilar vessel) as in Fig. 113-6 is typical of inflammation and has been shown to be 85 percent sensitive and 90 percent specific for diagnosing a node as benign. The statistics are different for the two other Doppler flow patterns. Evidence of multiple central vessels, a large central vessel with prominent central feeders taking off from it, or the imaging of predominantly peripheral (and not central) flow forces the examiner to rule out the possibility of neoplasm. In all radiology modalities,

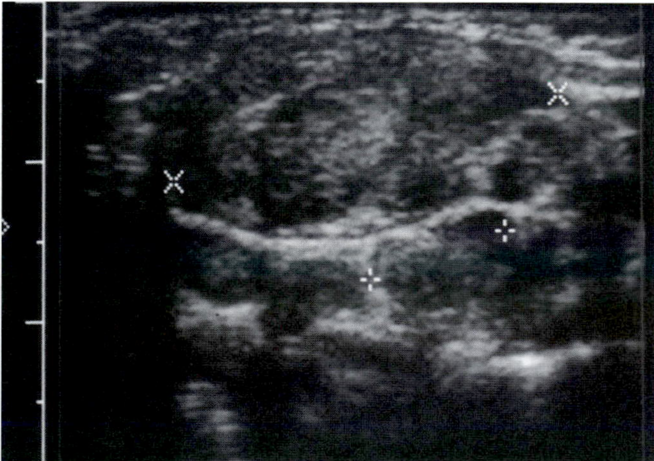

FIGURE 113–7. Enlarged nodes. Pediatric neck. Longitudinal plane. Many masses, none with central echogenic hila, are noted in the neck of this 3-month-old with scrofula. His mother was found to be PPD positive in the third month of pregnancy. The baby was 3 months old when he developed neck masses that proved to be infectious. Crosses mark off the bigger nodes. The largest is probably a coalescence of several nodes.

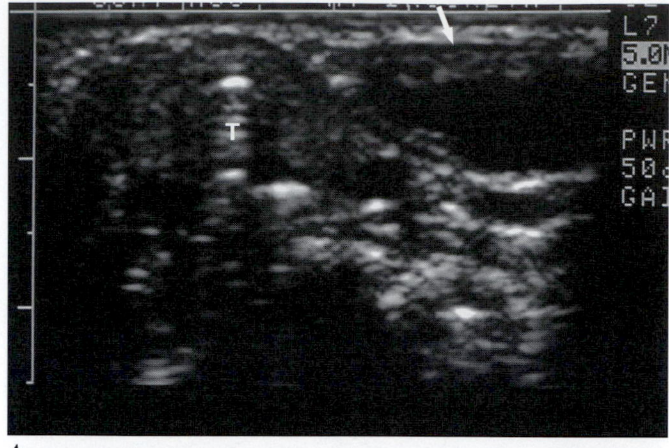

A

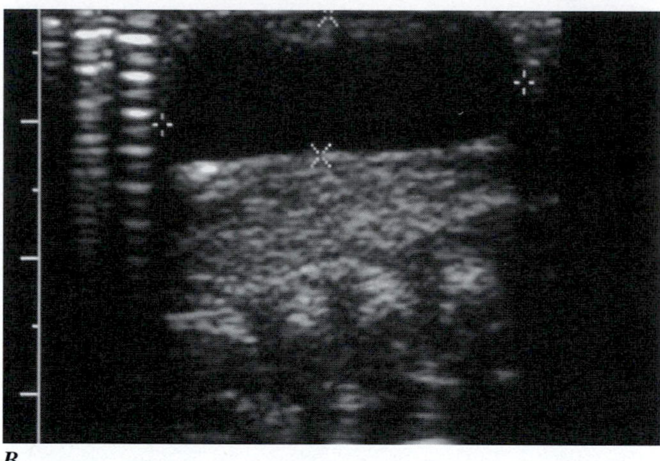

B

FIGURE 113–8. Branchial cleft cyst. Pediatric neck. ***A.*** Transverse plane. A normal thyroid surrounding the trachea (T) is seen on the reader's left. Lateral to the left thyroid lobe is a cystic mass (*arrow*) that has a somewhat thick wall. The patient presented at 13 hours of age because of leakage from two sinuses extending from this branchial cleft cyst onto the skin of the neck. ***B.*** Left neck. Longitudinal plane. The cystic mass, proven to be a branchial cleft cyst, is marked off by crosses.

however, vascular flow to areas of significant infection can often mimic flow to areas of neoplasm.

Branchial Cleft Cyst

The human head and neck develop from branchial (gill-like) structures known as the branchial apparatus. This apparatus includes branchial arches, pharyngeal pouches, branchial grooves, and branchial membranes. By the end of embryonic development, these structures have either developed into their adult derivatives or disappeared. Problems in the development and transformation of these embryonic structures lead to congenital anomalies of the head and neck. Many of these malformations are due to remnants of the branchial apparatus that did not disappear as they should have with embryonic growth and development. The third and fourth branchial arches are buried in the cervical sinus. Remnants of the cervical sinus or the second branchial groove may persist and form cysts. These branchial cleft cysts may be free in the neck, usually inferior to the mandible, but can develop anywhere anterior to the sternocleidomastoid muscle. Although they can develop anytime after birth, they are most often discovered in late childhood or early adulthood, manifesting as slowly enlarging painless masses. This is due to contained fluid and debris that has accumulated from desquamation of the cyst linings. Certainly if they have an associated draining sinus, they will be discovered sooner (Fig. 113-8).

ANY TECHNICAL TIPS?

Occasionally one may diagnose a mass as a thyroglossal duct cyst if it changes in position when the patient swallows or moves his tongue. Ultrasound imaging is best performed with a high-frequency (7.5 MHz or greater) linear array transducer. Occasionally a standoff pad may help; usually it does not. The TGD cyst is sometimes better seen if the child is examined sitting up, and occasionally better yet if the head is tilted back slightly when sitting. The transducer is placed directly on the visualized mass and evaluated in orthogonal projections. I then walk the transducer from high up at the tongue level to the thyroid level, looking for any other masses. This also helps remind me to image the thyroid gland. As with all pediatric procedures, personal techniques that improve one's rapport with a child (and mine vary with the child's age) and that enhance his or her desire to help with the study will allow better examinations. Then again, there will always be difficult days with limited patient cooperation. A steady hand and a quick exam (aided by cineloop techniques) usually will allow acceptable imaging.

As a final note, remember that thyroglossal duct cysts do not have to be midline or echoless. The majority of the TGD cysts I have examined have been at least slightly off midline. In the presence of a child with a thyroglossal duct cyst who is facing potential surgery, look for the thyroid and prove its presence.

References

Baatenburg de Jong RJ, Rongen RJ, Lameris JS, et al: Ultrasound characteristics of thyroglossal duct anomalies. *ORL J Otorhinolaryngology Relat Spec* 55:299–302, 1993.

Giovagnorio F, Caiazzo R, Avitto A: Evaluation of vascular patterns of cervical lymph nodes with power Doppler sonography. *JCU* 25:71–76, 1997.

Holland AJ, Sparnon AL, LeQuesne GW: Thyroglossal duct cyst or ectopic thyroid gland? *J Paediatr Child Health* 33:346–348, 1997.

Kraus R, Han B, Babcock D et al: Sonography of neck masses in children. *AJR* 146:609–613, 1986.

Lim-Dunham JE, Feinstein KA, Yousefzadeh DK, Ben-Ami T: Sonographic demonstration of a normal thyroid gland excludes ectopic thyroid in patients with thyroglossal duct cyst. *AJR* 164:1489–1491. 1995.

Moore K: *Before We Are Born. Basic Embryology and Birth Defects*, 3d ed. Philadelphia, Saunders, 1989:141–142.

Seibert J, Seibert R: Pediatric head and neck masses, in *Diagnostic Ultrasound,* 2d ed, Rumack C, Wilson S, Charboneau J (eds). St. Louis, Mosby–Year Book, 1998:1555–1587.

Siegel M: Neck, in *Pediatric Sonography,* 2d ed, Siegel M (ed). New York, Raven, 1995:103–137.

Suchet IB: Ultrasonography of the fetal neck in the second and third trimesters. Part 3. Anomalies of the anterior and anterolateral nuchal region. *Can Assoc Radiol J* 46:426–433, 1995.

Wadsworth DT, Siegel MJ: Thyroglossal duct cysts: Variability of sonographic findings. *AJR* 163:1475–1477, 1994.

114

An infant was born at term with respiratory distress secondary to meconium aspiration. Due to poor lung perfusion despite conventional ventilation with 100 percent oxygen as well as the intercurrent development of persistent pulmonary hypertension of the newborn, she was placed for several days in early life on extracorporeal membrane oxygenation (ECMO). Longitudinal (Fig. 114-1*A*) and transverse (Fig. 114-1*B*) sonograms of the right side of the neck were obtained at 1 year of age. Comparison views of the left side of the neck are shown in Fig. 114-2*A* and *B*. What do you see? What has happened to this patient?

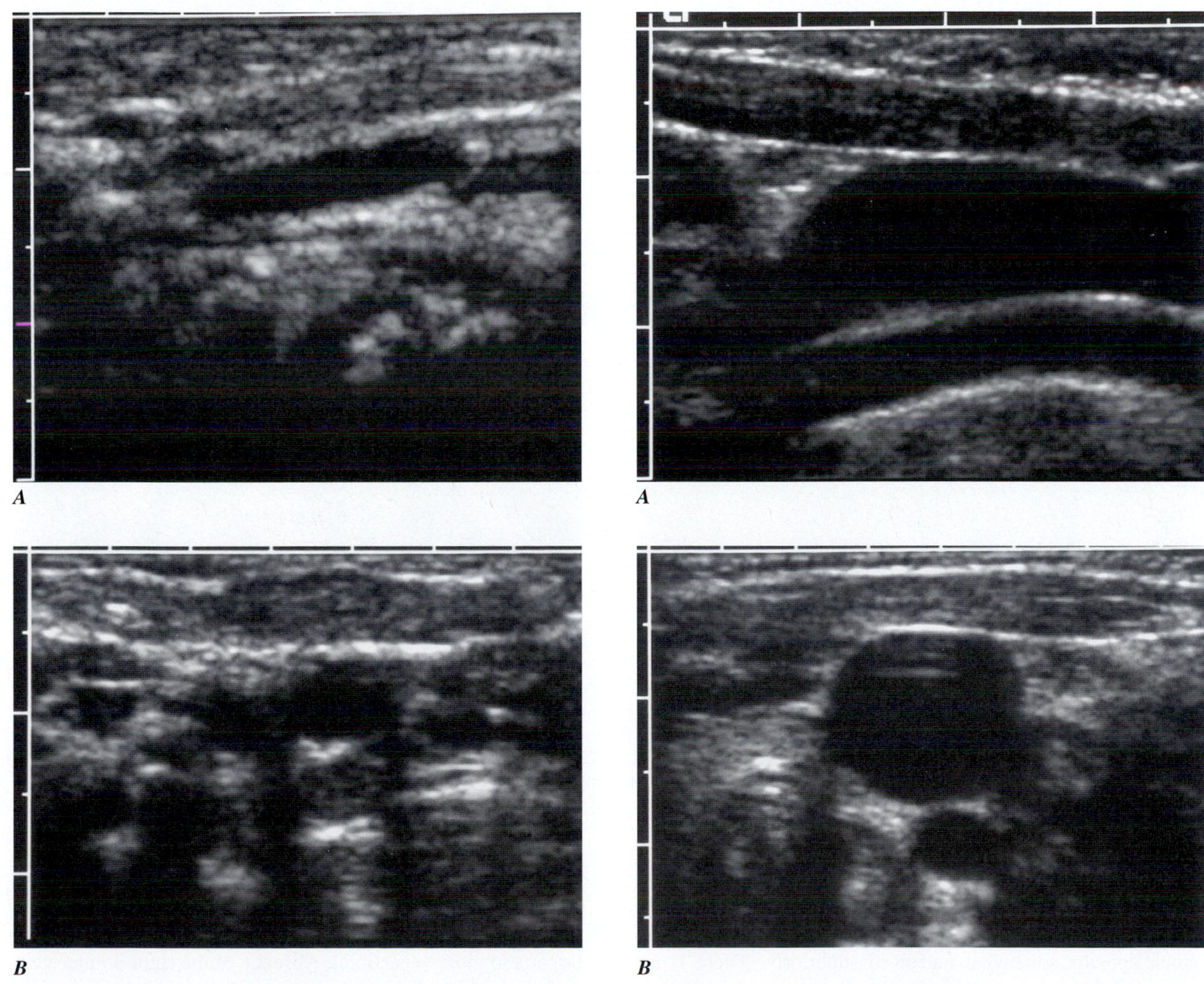

FIGURE 114–1. Pediatric neck. Ultrasound. Right side. ***A.*** Longitudinal plane. ***B.*** Transverse plane.

FIGURE 114–2. Pediatric neck. Ultrasound. Left side. ***A.*** Longitudinal plane. ***B.*** Transverse plane.

CHAPTER 114

Carotid Artery Reconstruction after ECMO

HARRIET J. PALTIEL

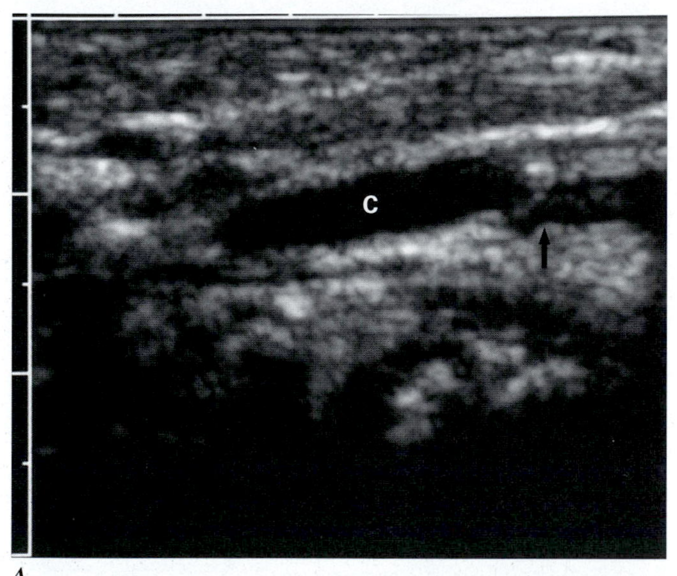

A

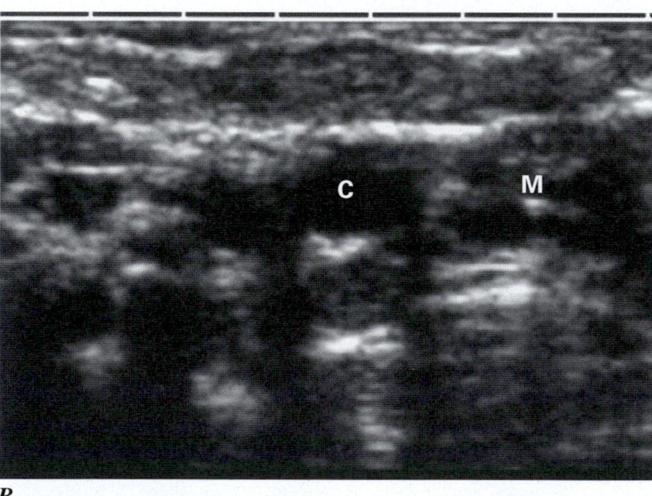

B

FIGURE 114–3. Annotated version of Fig. 114-1. Reconstructed carotid artery and absence of jugular vein. Pediatric neck. Ultrasound. Right side. ***A.*** There is irregularity to the margin (narrowing) of the carotid (C) artery at the site of repair (*arrow*) after ECMO and subsequent cannula removal, resection of the arteriotomy site, and an end-to-end anastomosis. There is no significant pre- or poststenotic dilatation. No jugular vein is seen, since it was ligated for ECMO and clotted off. ***B.*** Transverse plane. No jugular vein is seen. The carotid artery (C) is still patent. M = muscle.

Figure 114-3, the annotated version of Figure 114-1, shows an irregular margin to the right common carotid artery (RCCA) in its longitudinal plane (Fig. 114-3*A*). The arterial lumen appears somewhat narrowed superiorly. There is no evidence of a right jugular vein in either the longitudinal or the transverse plane (114-3*B*). These findings are in contrast to those of the normal left side of the patient's neck (Fig. 114-4, the annotated version of Fig. 114-2). In those images, the normal carotid walls parallel one another. Comparing the left carotid to the left jugular vein, the vein is imaged as larger and more superficial. Absence of the right jugular vein and irregularity of the right carotid wall and narrowing of its lumen suggests some external traumatic or iatrogenic insult. In this case, surgical reconstruction of the RCCA was re-

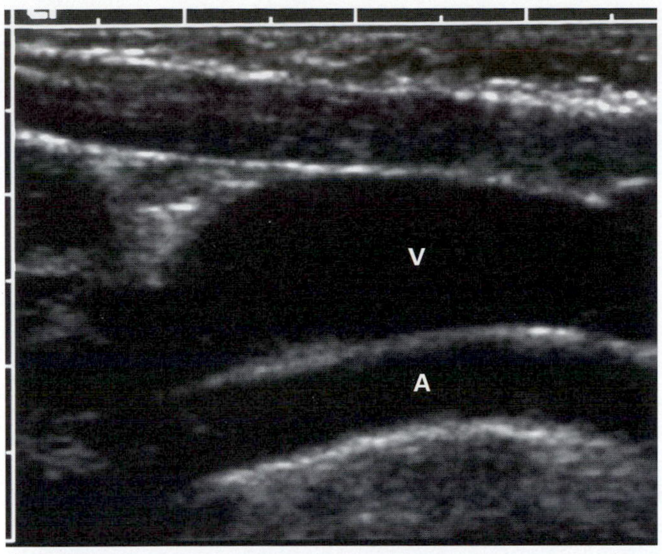

A

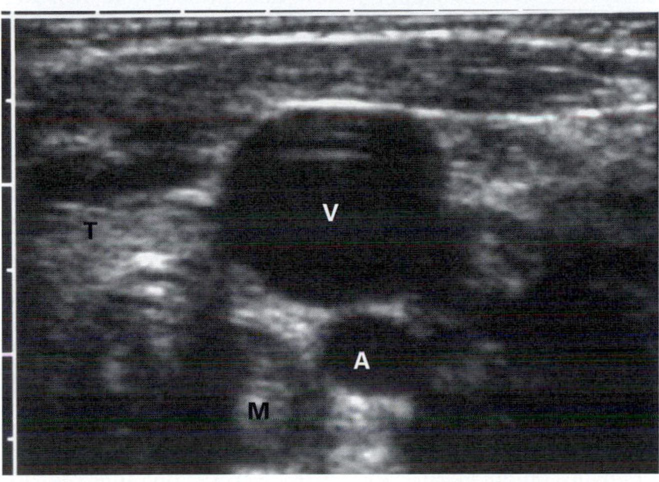

B

FIGURE 114–4. Annotated version of Fig. 114-2. Normal neck vessels in young child. Ultrasound. ***A.*** Longitudinal plane. The larger and more superficial neck vessel is the jugular vein (V). The carotid artery (A) is more tubular and has parallel walls. ***B.*** Transverse plane. The larger and more superficial vessel is the jugular vein (V). The smaller vessel is the common carotid artery (A), imaged proximal to its bifurcation. M = neck muscle, T = thyroid tissue.

sponsible for its irregular margins. Absence of the jugular vein was due to thrombosis after its ligation. This occurred in a patient who underwent ECMO and subsequent RCCA reconstruction.

WHAT IS ECMO?

Extracorporeal membrane oxygenation (ECMO) is a means of artificial pulmonary and cardiac life support used for newborn infants with life-threatening respiratory illnesses, usually caused by meconium aspiration syndrome, sepsis/pneumonia, persistent pulmonary hypertension, congenital diaphragmatic hernia, respiratory distress syndrome, or congenital heart disease. The technique most commonly employed is venoarterial (VA) cardiopulmonary bypass, in which both the right common carotid artery and the right internal jugular vein are cannulated (Fig. 114-5). After ECMO is discontinued, the arterial and venous cannulae are removed, and both vessels are usually permanently ligated. Reconstruction of the carotid artery at the time of decannulation is currently a technically feasible alternative to permanent ligation. It is thought that repair of this vessel may reduce the consequences of long-term decreased right hemispheric perfusion.

In patients who have undergone ECMO, the common carotid artery can be decannulated and controlled proximally and distally with a vascular clamp. The lumen is then inspected. The presence of internal dissection, flaps, thrombosis, or lack of free blood flow are contraindications to reconstruction. In the absence of these contraindications, the arteriotomy site is completely excised. The proximal and distal ends of the vessel are then assessed for ease of approximation. If tension on the anastomotic site is deemed excessive, reconstruction is abandoned and the vessel is doubly ligated. Otherwise, the carotid artery is reconstructed, usually in an end-to-end fashion.

MORE ON THIS PATIENT

A chest film of this infant obtained shortly after birth demonstrated hyperinflated lungs with extensive bilateral interstitial and airspace opacities due to meconium aspiration (Fig. 114-6*A*). Figure 114-6*B* shows the venous and arterial cannulae in place. After carotid artery reconstruction, a narrowing was noted at the site of the carotid artery anastomosis

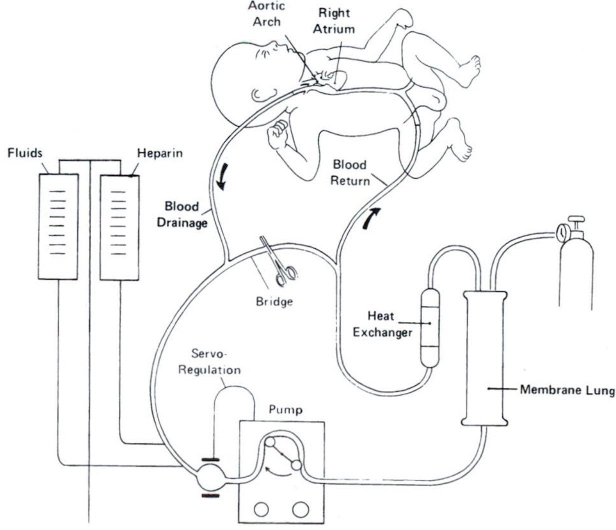

FIGURE 114–5. Circuit diagram for venoarterial extracorporeal membrane oxygenation. (*From Bartlett R, Andrews A, Toomasian J, et al: Extracorporeal membrane oxygenation for newborn respiratory failure: Forty-five cases.* Surgery *92:425–432, 1982, with permission.*)

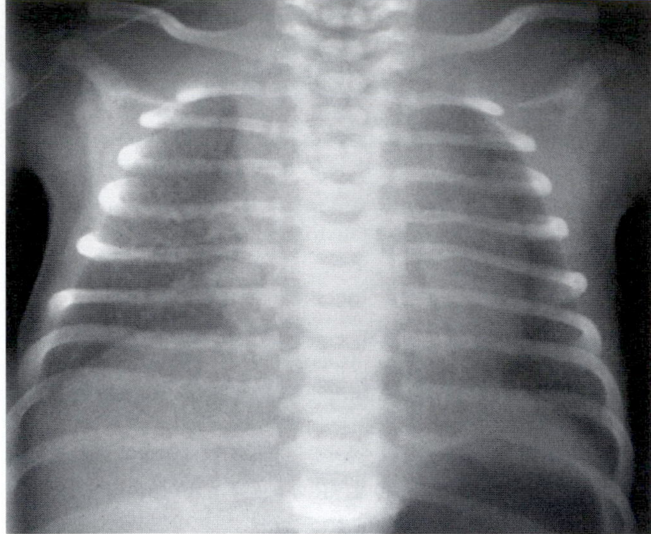

A

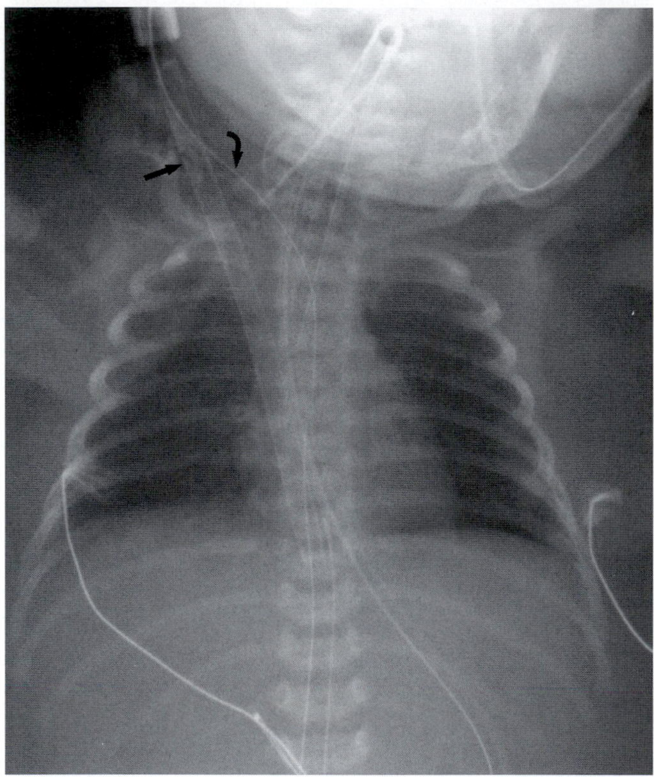

B

FIGURE 114–6. Anteroposterior chest films. ***A.*** Meconium aspiration syndrome. A chest film obtained shortly after birth demonstrates hyperinflated lungs with extensive bilateral (especially right-sided) interstitial and airspace opacities due to meconium aspiration. ***B.*** Extracorporeal membrane oxygenation (ECMO). The patient underwent ECMO. This image obtained following the procedure shows the venous (*arrow*) and arterial cannulae (*curved arrow*) in place.

(Fig 114-3*A*) without significant pre- or postanastomotic dilatation. Color Doppler imaging demonstrated patency of the vessel (Fig. 114-7*A*). Spectral waveform analysis revealed equivalent (ratio of 1.0) peak systolic velocities proximal (Fig. 114-7*B*) and distal (Fig. 114-7*C*) to the anastomosis.

CAROTID ARTERY EXAMINATION IN CHILDREN

As in adults, carotid artery examinations in children are performed with the patient supine, the neck slightly extended, and the head turned away from the side being studied. Linear 5- to 10-MHz transducers are used for gray-scale, color, and power Doppler imaging. Gray-scale examination may begin in the transverse or longitudinal plane. Transverse scans are obtained from the supraclavicular notch cephalad to the angle of the mandible. Blood flow velocities can be obtained and spectral analysis performed at any point along the vessel. The angle of insonation, θ, is the angle between the Doppler transducer's "line of sight" and the vessel. Ideally, spectral analysis is performed with an angle of near 0°, i.e., paralleling the insonated vessel. This angle of insonation is rarely achievable in a clinical setting. Insonation angles of up to 60° are considered acceptable and reliable for carotid spectral analysis. Errors in Doppler flow determination increase as the angle increases beyond 60° and toward 90°. At a 90° angle, no flow can be determined, since the Doppler equation relies on the cosine of θ, which at 90° is zero, rendering flow determination useless.

ECMO—SURVIVAL AND COMPLICATIONS

Over 9,000 newborn infants have been treated with ECMO, with an 81 percent overall survival rate. Approximately 80 percent of survivors are healthy children. The remaining 20 percent have some degree of pulmonary or neurologic impairment. Death or disability is caused by perinatal neurologic injury or pulmonary hypoplasia. Bleeding is the most frequent complication. Most of the adverse outcomes attributed to neonatal ECMO are secondary to either the effects of blood contacting a foreign surface in the ECMO circuit or altered blood flow patterns in the patient. The ultimate consequences of permanent ligation of the RCCA and the vascular, physiologic, and neurodevelopmental effects of these procedures in surviving infants are largely unknown. Although no adverse effects attributable to RCCA cannulation and subsequent permanent ligation are apparent in the majority of infants during or immediately after ECMO, some studies have reported infants who, on computed tomography (CT) scans obtained after decannulation from ECMO and prior to hospital discharge, had either right cerebral hemispheric ischemic abnormalities or contralateral hemorrhagic changes consistent with hyperperfusion of the left hemisphere. A 1991 metaanalysis suggested that vascular compromise resulting from RCCA ligation might have be responsible for these lateralized hemispheric lesions.

Several groups have attempted to analyze the effects of carotid reconstruction. Taylor et al calculated a velocity ratio (*A/B*) of the peak systolic velocity above the level of the anastomosis to the peak systolic velocity below the anastomosis to assess the degree of stenosis at the repair site. *A/B* ratios of 1.0 were normal. *A/B* ratios of 2.0 indicated at least a 50 percent obstruction to flow. Over a 1-year period, all the

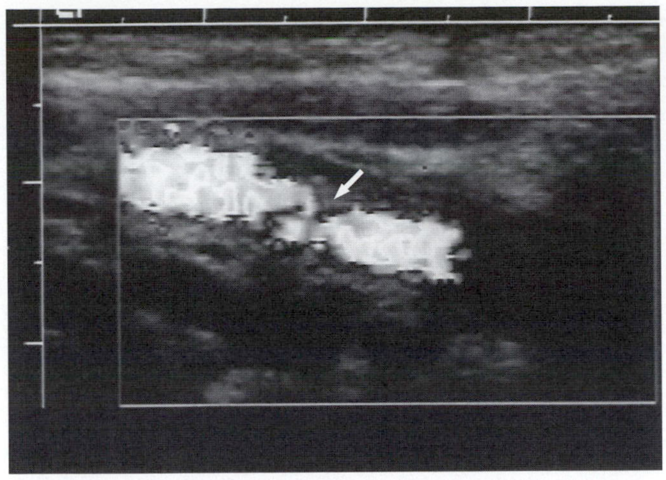

A

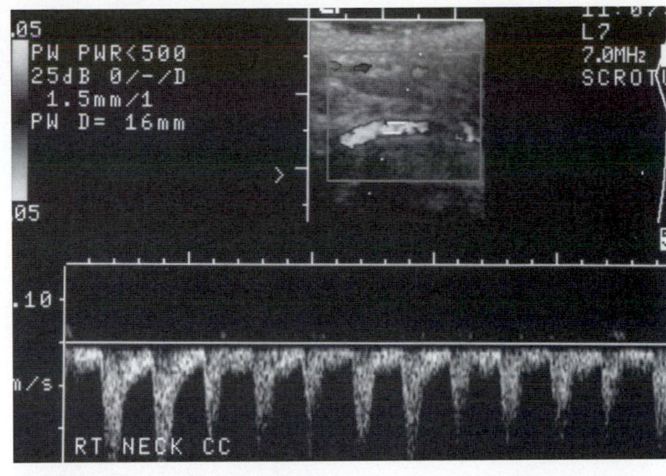

B

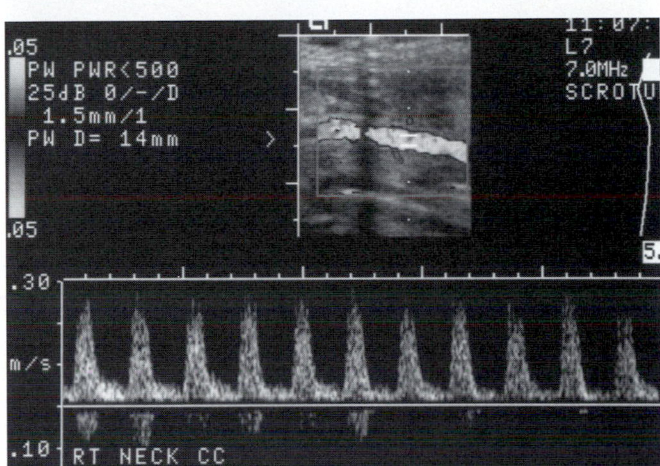

C

FIGURE 114–7. Color Doppler analysis of the right carotid artery. ***A.*** Longitudinal plane. There is patency of the reanastomosed common carotid artery, since vascular flow, evidenced by the contained color, is seen in the vessel, proximal to, at, and distal to the point of narrowing (*arrow*). ***B.*** Longitudinal plane. Triplex Doppler exam. Spectral waveform analysis. Spectral pattern was obtained in the distal right common carotid artery beyond the point of narrowing. ***C.*** Longitudinal plane. Triplex Doppler exam. Spectral waveform analysis. Spectral pattern was obtained in the distal right common carotid artery proximal to the point of common carotid narrowing. The ratio of peak systolic velocities below (in ***B***) and distal to (above) (in ***C***) the anastomosis was approximately 1.0 and suggests no flow abnormality. The change in flow direction, evidenced by a spectral pattern now below the baseline (*arrow*) is due to normal flow changing its direction in relationship to the transducer as it heads toward the transducer in ***B*** and away from the transducer (and therefore below baseline) when insonated in the more distal location.

infants they studied showed a marked improvement in *A/B* ratio and patency of the vessel. No infant had evidence of emboli to the right side of the brain by magnetic resonance imaging. Baumgart et al evaluated US, CT, and electroencephalogram (EEG) findings and neurodevelopmental outcome in 47 infants with carotid artery reconstruction and 93 without reconstruction. Color Doppler studies noted that carotid artery patency was usually attained after reconstruction and before hospital discharge. Right internal carotid and bilateral anterior and middle cerebral arterial blood flow velocities were generally higher in infants with reconstructed arteries. The distribution of flow in the brain appeared more symmetrical in this group. There were no significant differences in US, CT, or EEG findings for the reconstruction and the ligation groups early in their clinical courses. There was no evident differences in the incidence of developmental delays between the two groups in the first year of life.

Cheung et al studied 13 neonatal ECMO survivors who had carotid reconstruction over a 4-year period. Of 12 children with normal neonatal sonographic studies, narrowing developed in 7. Only 2 of the 7 children had hemodynamically significant stenosis (defined as a velocity ratio greater than 2.0). They saw no association between carotid US findings and ipsilateral or contralateral intracranial lesions on CT.

The advent of newer venovenous (VV) ECMO using a double-lumen catheter placed in the right atrium via the jugular vein precludes the need for carotid ligation. The use of this procedure is limited to those infants not requiring cardiac support. Increased future use of this form of ECMO may eliminate concern over the effects of arterial ligation.

EDITOR'S NOTE

Although this is an unusual case that is limited to centers with ECMO and sonologists/sonographers who see patients who have undergone it, knowledge of this cause of carotid narrowing should be borne in mind when imaging a child with such narrowing and no history of recent trauma or surgery.

Jugular vein clots are more often the result of long-term catheter placement (Fig. 114-8) than the result of the unusual history of ligation. Immediate (acute) clots may be echoless. They are echogenic with early fibrin deposition. They be-

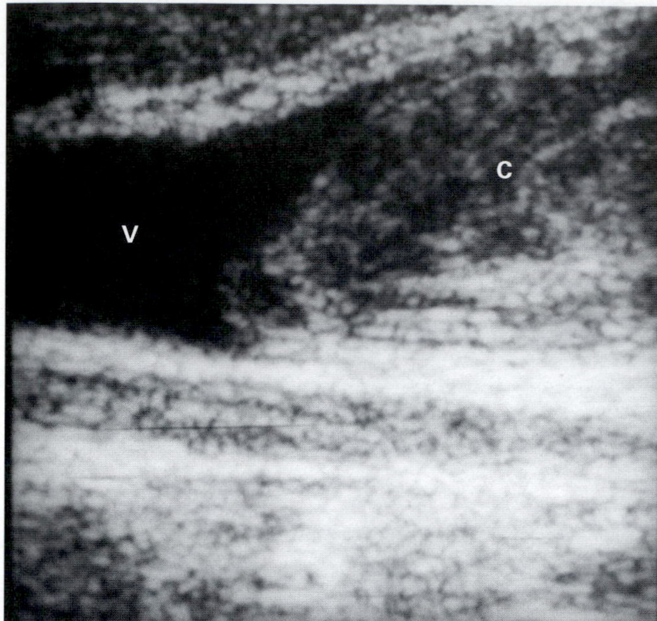

A

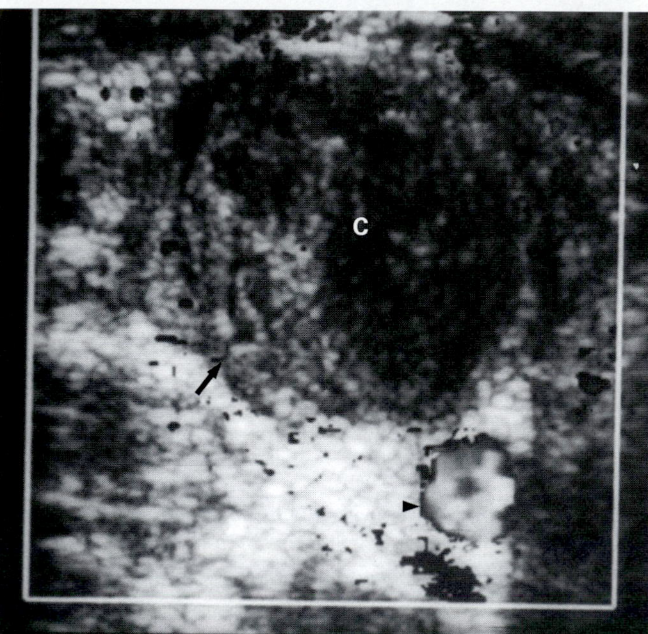

B

FIGURE 114–8. Right jugular vein clot. Ultrasound. ***A.*** Longitudinal plane. A heterogeneous clot (*arrow*) is seen in a somewhat distended right internal jugular vein that did not compress with transducer pressure. The heterogenity of the clot suggests that it is subacute to chronic in age. This patient was a teenager with leukemia who had long-term central venous catheterization. The exam was performed at the bedside after the patient was noted to have swelling of the neck and face. ***B.*** Transverse plane through proximal jugular vein. Color Doppler (image obtained in black and white). At this level, the clot (*arrows*) fills the venous lumen. The clot heterogeneity again suggests that it is not acute. The blood flow in the carotid artery (*arrowhead*) deep to the vein allows one to note how very large this clot-filled vein is.

come heterogeneous as the clot ages. They usually enlarge the affected vessel, and compression of a vein with a contained clot is abnormal and therefore difficult. Jugular venous clots, like other venous clots, may also develop in patients with vasculitides, trauma, local surgery, a nearby mass slowing vascular flow, or on medications or with disorders leading to a hypercoagulable state and resulting in increased clot formation.

References

Bartlett R, Andrews A, Toomasian J, et al: Extracorporeal membrane oxygenation for newborn respiratory failure: Forty-five cases. *Surgery* 92:425–432, 1982.

Baumgart S, Streletz LJ, Needleman L, et al: Right common carotid artery reconstitution after extracorporeal membrane oxygenation: Vascular imaging, cerebral circulation, electroencephalographic, and neurodevelopmental correlates to recovery. *J Pediatr* 125:295–304, 1994.

Cheung PY, Vickar DB, Hallgren RA, et al: Carotid artery reconstruction in neonates receiving extracorporeal membrane oxygenation: A 4 year follow up study. *J Pediatr Surg* 32:560–564, 1997.

DeAngelis GA, Mitchell DG, Merton DA, et al: Right common carotid artery reconstruction in neonates after extracorporeal membrane oxygenation: Color Doppler imaging. *Radiology* 182:521–525, 1992.

Ichiba S, Bartlett RH: Current status of extracorporeal membrane oxygenation for severe respiratory failure. *Artif Organs* 20:120–123, 1996.

Levy MS, Share JC, Fauza DO, Wilson JM: Fate of the reconstructed carotid artery after extracorporeal membrane oxygenation. *J Pediatr Surg* 30:1046–1049, 1995.

Mendoza JC, Shearer LL, Cook LN: Lateralization of brain lesions following ECMO. *Pediatrics* 88:1004–1009, 1991.

Schumacher RE: Extracorporeal membrane oxygenation. Will this therapy continue to be as efficacious in the future? *Pediatr Clin North Am* 40:1005–1017, 1993.

Schumacher RC, Roloff DW, Chapman R, Bartlett RH: Follow-up of infants treated with extracorporeal membrane oxygenation for newborn respiratory failure. *Pediatrics* 87:451–457, 1991.

Taylor BJ, Seibert JJ, Glasier CM, et al: Evaluation of the reconstructed carotid artery following extracorporeal membrane oxygenation. *Pediatrics* 90:568–572, 1992.

Wilson BG: Extracorporeal and intracorporeal techniques for the treatment of severe respiratory failure. *Respir Care* 41:306–317, 1996.

115

A febrile adolescent with sickle cell disease comes into the emergency room with right upper quadrant abdominal pain. She is sent to the ultrasound department for evaluation of her gallbladder. She has no gallstones. You, however, see a transverse view (Fig. 115-1) and a longitudinal view (Fig. 115-2) of her upper abdomen. What do you see? Where is the area of concern? What is the cause of her pain?

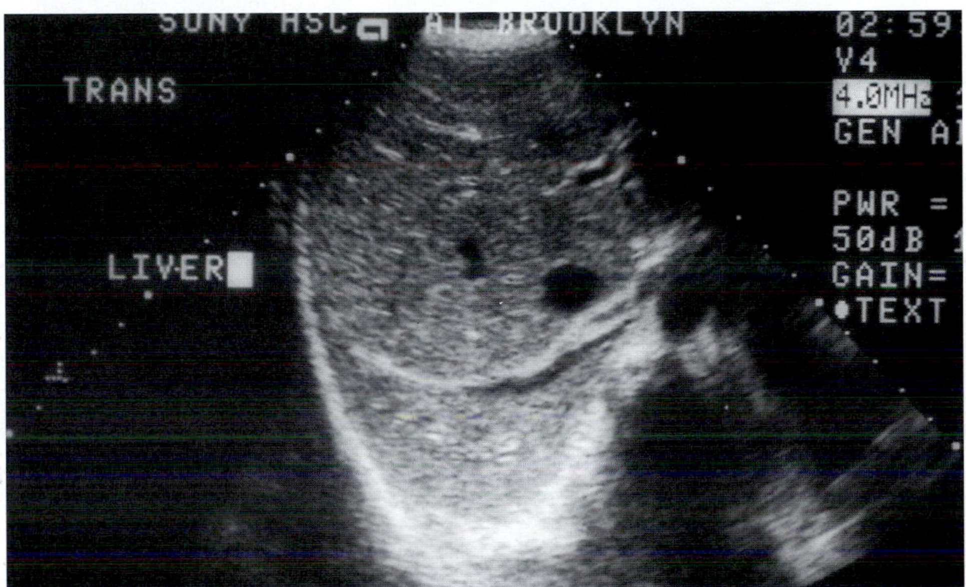

FIGURE 115–1. Ultrasound. Right upper quadrant. Transverse plane.

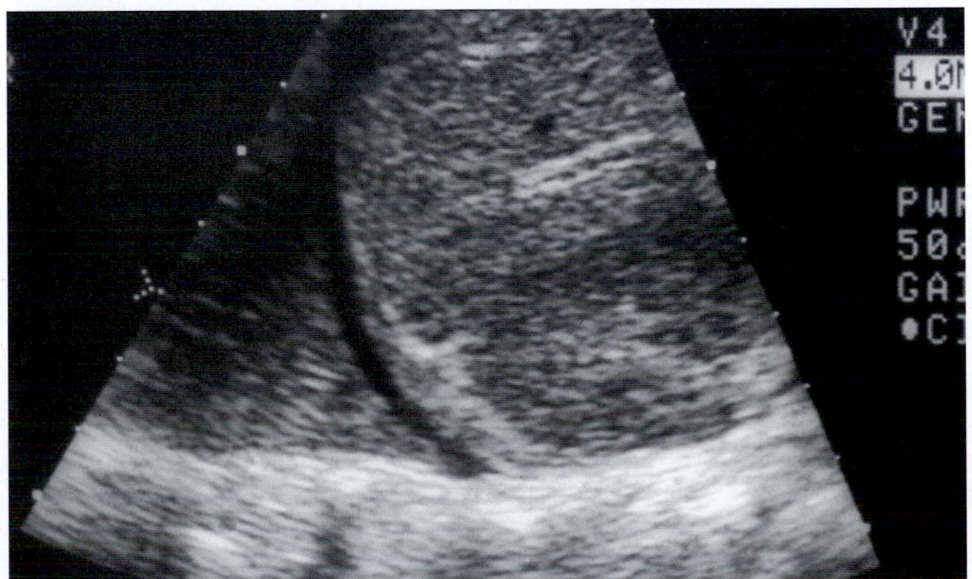

FIGURE 115–2. Ultrasound. Right upper quadrant. Longitudinal plane.

CHAPTER 115

Pneumonia/Atelectasis and Pleural Effusion

HARRIS L. COHEN AND MARLENA PURSNER

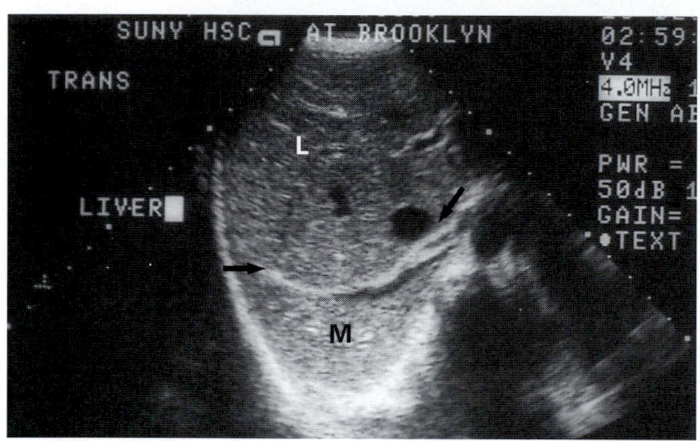

FIGURE 115–3. Annotated version of Fig. 115-1. Right lower lobe infiltrate and small pleural effusion. Ultrasound. Right upper quadrant. Transverse plane. An echogenic mass (M) is not a mirror image of the subdiaphragmatic liver (L) is seen posterior to the diaphragm (*arrows*), which is represented by a highly echogenic white line. A small sliver of echoless fluid is pleural effusion, seen between the diaphragm and the mass, which proved to be lung atelectasis/infiltrate. If the lung was normal and air-filled, it would not be able to be imaged.

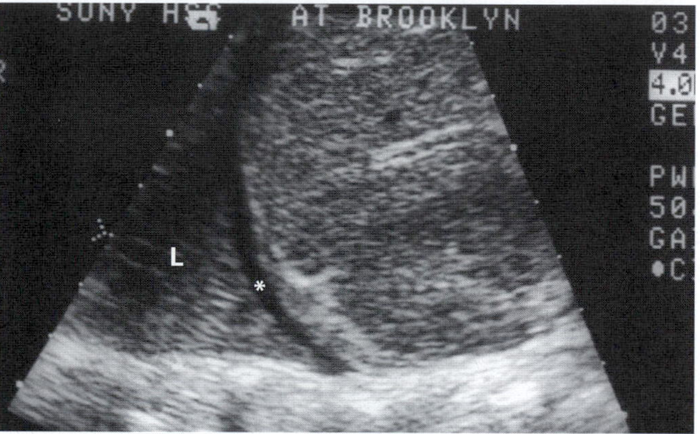

FIGURE 115–4. Annotated version of Fig. 115-2. Right lower lobe infiltrate and small pleural effusion. Ultrasound. Right upper quadrant. Longitudinal plane. Again noted is a mass, which is triangular and therefore more consistent with diseased (infected or atelectatic) lung (L) rather than neoplasm, above the diaphragm (*arrows*). The small amount of pleural effusion is represented by the echoless area (*) in the immediate supradiaphragmatic area.

Figures 115-3 and 115-4, the annotated versions of Figs. 115-1 and 115-2, show a mass above the diaphragm. It is triangular in shape (Fig. 115-4), which suggests that it is the lung itself. Analysis of the transverse image requires one to know that the posteroinferior lung—i.e., the base of the lower lobe—extends inferior to the dome of the diaphragm. This is well known to readers of lateral plain films. Because of this, pleural effusion or lung atelectasis/infiltrate will be seen posterior to the diaphragm on ultrasound (US) (Fig. 115-3), as it is on computed tomography (CT) images of the upper abdomen. We use the transverse image of the upper abdomen to rapidly survey for fluid in the pleural space (Fig. 115-5*A*). The analysis of the longitudinal image (Figs. 115-4 and 115-5*B*) is easier to comprehend because it shows the lung, as always superior to the diaphragm but posterior to its dome as it descends into the posterior costophrenic sulcus (costodiaphragmatic recess). The echoless sliver at the lung base of Figs. 115-3 and 115-4 is a small pleural effusion. This sickle cell patient was febrile and had clinical and follow-up findings consistent with pneumonia and atelectasis.

The image of the supradiaphragmatic mass in this case is not pathognomonic for pulmonary infiltrate, but because it maintains the normal shape of the lung, it is suggestive of an alveolar filling process rather than a pleural or other extrapulmonary mass. Alveolar filling processes are those in which the alveoli are filled with fluid and there is therefore no air to

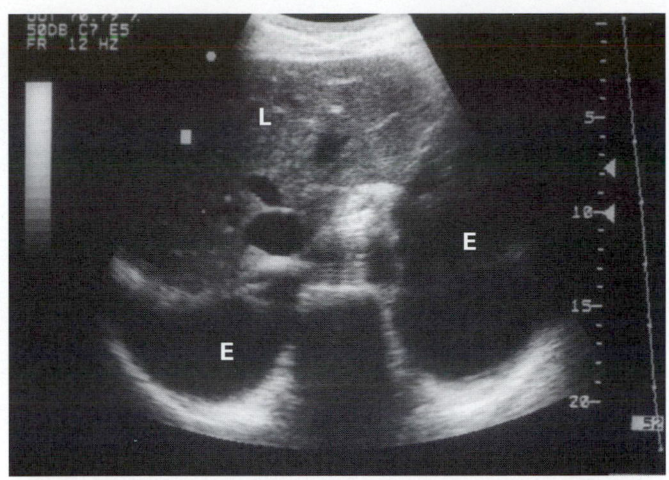

A

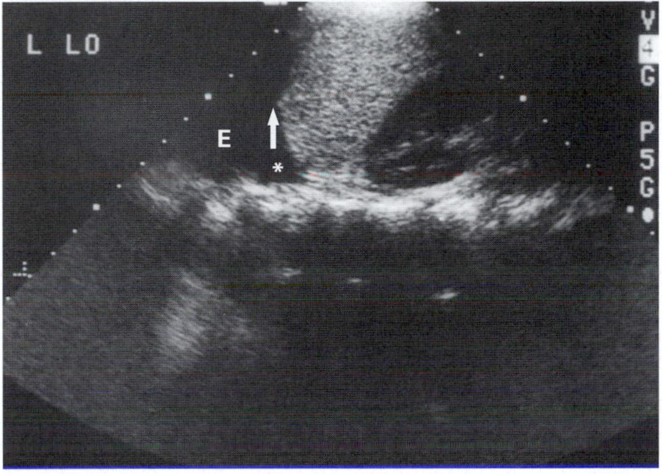

B

FIGURE 115–5. Pleural effusion. Ultrasound. ***A.*** Transverse plane through the upper abdomen. Large pleural effusions (E) are noted on the right and left sides of the abdomen. Liver (L) is seen anterior to the right pleural effusion. ***B.*** Longitudinal plane through the lung, liver, and right kidney. A large effusion (E) is seen above the liver. The posterior aspect of the effusion (*) as would be expected, anatomically, is inferior to the dome of the diaphragm (*arrow*).

interfere with ultrasound penetration or return to the transducer to create an image. The differential diagnostic possibilities for an alveolar filling process include cases in which clear fluid fills the alveoli (the transudate of congestive heart failure), bloody fluid fills the alveoli (pulmonary hemorrhage), and, as in this case, exudative fluid (with bacteria) from a (bacterial) pneumonia fills the alveoli. In children, particularly younger ones, the ability to differentiate between atelectasis and infiltrate, particularly on plain film (which is the method we follow for atelectasis/infiltrate), may be difficult and requires follow-up clinical examination and/or imaging. Rapid improvement of a pulmonary mass, with or without contained air bronchograms, suggests that the density was atelectatic lung, while a longer time period for the mass to disappear suggests an infiltrate. Many pediatric infiltrates may have an atelectatic component, and the term *atelectasis/infiltrate* is commonly used.

UPPER ABDOMINAL PAIN CAN ALSO BE DUE TO LUNG DISEASE

Besides the many abdominal causes of upper abdominal pain in the child, one must remember that pneumonia, whether in a sickle cell patient or a normal patient, may present with abdominal pain. Pleurisy or pleuropneumonia can cause abdominal pain, abdominal rigidity, and even vomiting. Clinical diagnosis is occasionally difficult, particularly when there is a delay in the appearance of thoracic signs. We always look at the lung base on US and on plain film examinations for upper abdominal pain.

I THOUGHT US WAS USELESS FOR EVALUATING THE LUNG

This case was used to highlight that, while the fact that sound waves are reflected by the bony thorax and reflected and refracted by air and aerated lung, effectively erasing any usable image of the intrathoracic contents, suggests that the lung is not an area to study by US, this is not always true. Knowledge of what information can be obtained and how various images in various planes may be interpreted can only make one a more complete sonologist/sonographer.

WHAT ARE THE INTRATHORACIC ABNORMALITIES THAT CAN BE NOTED?

Ultrasound provides a window to the nonaerated portions of the thorax and its contents. It can be used for the critically ill at the bedside. It is quite useful for assessing juxtadiaphragmatic and lateral densities noted on plain film. It can help with mediastinal lesions and diagnose rib fractures.

Ultrasound has been clearly shown to be helpful in denoting the presence, size, and distribution of pleural fluid. A US obtained in a supine position is considered more accurate than the plain film, even one taken in lateral decubitus position, for determining actual volumes of pleural effusion. In one study, a 20-mm-thick pleural collection on US evaluation was determined to be indicative of 380 ± 130 mL of fluid; 40-mm thickness is equivalent to 1000 ± 130 mL. Ultrasound allows for interventional treatment of infected and noninfected pleural fluid. Finding pleural nodules within an effusion may suggest that it is malignant.

ULTRASOUND OF THE LUNG—WHAT CAN BE SEEN?

The normal air-filled lung cannot be imaged by US. It will be imaged only if it is collapsed, fluid-filled as a result of any alveolar filling process, or surrounded by echoless pleural fluid (effusion) superior to the diaphragm. Lack of contained air is the reason why the fetal lung is well demonstrated in antenatal work. Ultrasound is of great help in differentiating between pleural effusion and consolidation. Collapsed lung

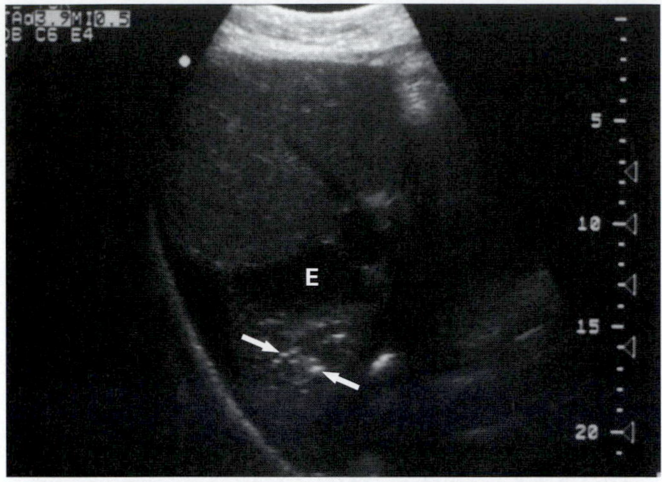

A

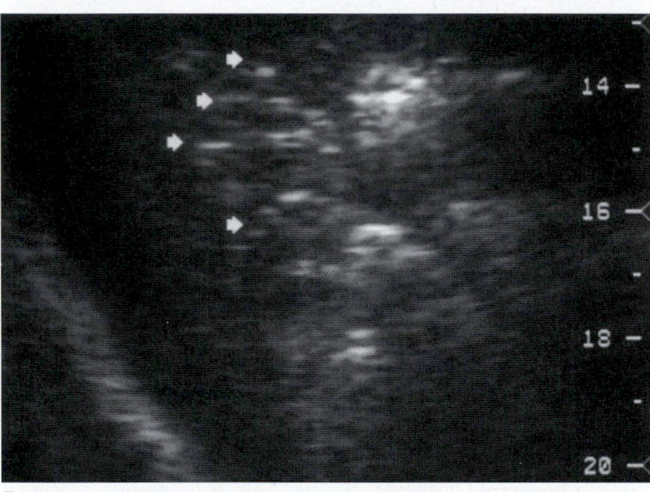

B

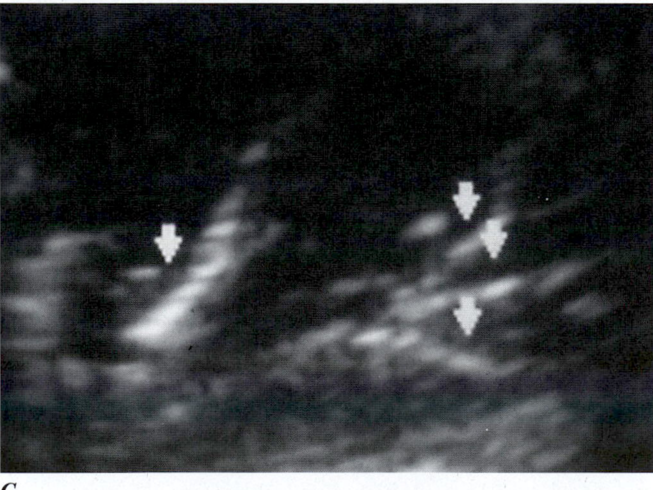

C

FIGURE 115–6. Air bronchograms in pneumonia. ***A.*** Pleural effusion and atelectatic lung. Upper abdominal ultrasound. Transverse plane. There is a large pleural effusion (E). Bright echoes (*arrows*) in the lung suggested air bronchograms. ***B.*** Close-up view of right lung. Transverse plane. The bright echoes proved to be echogenic air (*arrows*) in bronchi in a field of atelectatic lung of medium echogenicity. This could only have been seen with surrounding atelectatsis, i.e., "solid" lung. ***C.*** Left lung. Transverse plane. Much more readily identified branching pattern of air bronchograms (*arrows*) is noted in the left lung of another patient with pneumonia.

with residual air in the bronchi ("air bronchograms") is pathognomonic for atelectasis and/or infiltrate in plain film work. An equivalent image of air bronchograms can be seen on US (Fig. 115-6).

Obviously, as already noted, an intrathoracic mass in a child that is adjacent to lung and is either surrounded by fluid or at least not surrounded by aerated lung can also be seen. A key normal structure seen in the young child is the thymus (Fig. 115-7), which is anterior to the normal aerated lung and is a solid organ that is most prominent in early childhood. It is routinely homogeneous but less echogenic than the thyroid. It can be imaged for inhomogeneity, which may suggest abnormality, through ribs in an anterior chest approach or, better yet, from the midline at the suprasternal notch. As the child ages and the thymus becomes smaller and surrounded by air-filled lung in what then becomes the retrosternal "clear space" (clear because of contained air-filled lung), imaging of the thymus by US may no longer be possible.

THOUGHTS ABOUT THE DIAPHRAGM

As has been stated, in understanding the axial image of the upper abdomen, it is important to remember that the posterior lung extends inferior to the diaphragm within the posterior costophrenic sulcus. Another way of looking at this is to note the anatomic fact that the diaphragm's posterior attachment is considerably more inferior than its anterior attachment. Therefore, on a transverse image (Fig. 115-3), abnormality at the lung base would be seen posterior to the diaphragm. Again, this is true as well with axial images of the upper abdomen evaluated by computed tomography (CT).

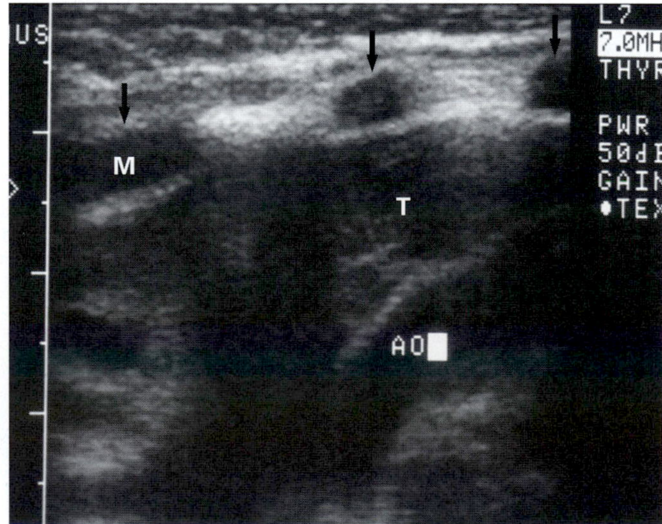

FIGURE 115–7. Normal thymus. Sagittal plane through upper chest. Suprasternal notch approach. Soft tissue consistent with normal thymus (T) is seen anterior to the echoless tubular aorta (AO). Echopenic bones of the sternum are seen (*arrows*) in the anterior chest wall. They are echopenic and allow through transmission because they are not well ossified early in life. This also allows easier imaging by ultrasound through the chest wall. This child is 3 months old. M = manubrium.

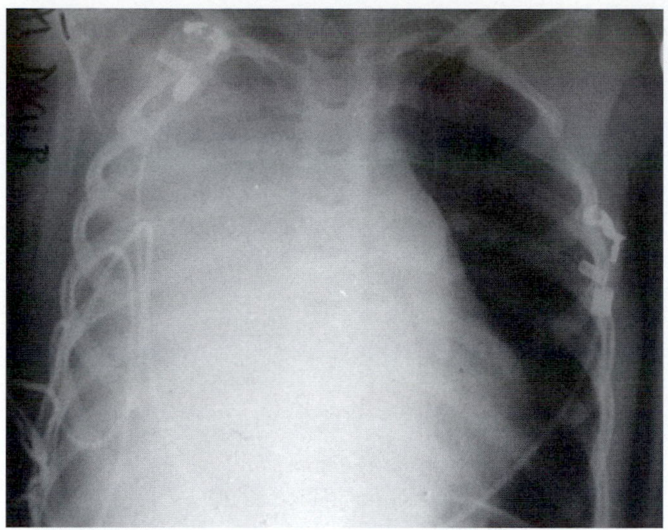

FIGURE 115–8. Large pleural effusion and atelectasis in patient with sickle cell disease. Chest film. Anteroposterior positioning. There is density creating "white-out" of the right lung. If this was all due to pleural effusion, the heart would have been pushed to the left. Since the enlarged heart of this sickle cell patient is predominantly on the right of the chest, there is obviously a component of atelectasis/infiltrate.

SICKLE CELL DISEASE AND THE LUNG—A FEW FACTS

Sickle cell disease is a chronic disorder resulting from a structural abnormality in hemoglobin. It occurs in several forms. It results in characteristic sickling of red blood cells. These rigid, deformed cells are easily damaged, resulting in a chronic hemolytic anemia. Infection may increase stress to these cells and their hemolysis. Hypoxemia and acidemia increase the tendency for these cells to sickle. The cells increase blood viscosity and compromise blood flow, leading to ischemia, thrombosis, and infarction. Clinical manifestations of sickle cell disease involve many organ systems. Sicklers undergo "crises," defined as acute changes in their clinical course. These may be anemic (hypoplastic and aplastic crises often are associated with viral infections, particularly parvovirus), hemolytic (with increasing jaundice), or vasoocclusive (the most common clinical complication, which can lead to, e.g., bone infarction, hand-foot syndrome in the very young, or lung infarction). The sickler's lungs are at risk for infarction with multiple emboli, infection, and atelectasis (infection, obstruction). In lung crises (Fig. 115-8), how much of the symptomatology is due to infarction, pleural effusion, or atelectasis/infiltrate is often difficult to determine. Patients often have abdominal pain from gallstones or parenchymal (liver or spleen) infarction, but as we have learned, abdominal pain may be referred from the lung base and pleura. Sicklers, particularly because of defective spleen function, are susceptible to infection. This is a major problem, particularly in the very young, before development of humoral immunity. Salmonella osteomyelitis is common in bones. Pneumococcal and streptococcal lung infections are common. Other lung infectious agents include *Haemophilus influenzae* and *Mycoplasma pneumoniae.*

A FINAL THOUGHT

You may not be able to normally see lung on US. Take a look anyway, particularly in patients with upper abdominal pain or a suspicion of effusion. We help clinicians daily with this practice. We note effusions they never suspected, often despite the chest x-rays.

References

Acunas B, Celik L, Acunas A: Chest sonography. Differentiation of pulmonary consolidation from pleural disease. *Acta Radiol* 30:273–275, 1989.

Cohen HL, Muller D, Zinn DL: Abnormal fetal chest, abdomen, pelvis, in *Diagnostic Medical Sonography. A Guide to Clinical Practice. Obstetrics and Gynecology,* 2d ed, Berman MC, Cohen HL (eds). Philadelphia, Lippincott, 1997:285–320.

Eibenberger KL, Dock WI, Ammann ME, et al: Quantification of pleural effusions: Sonography versus radiography. *Radiology* 191:681–684, 1994.

Gehmacher O, Mathis G, Kopf A, Scheier M: Ultrasound imaging of pneumonia. *Ultrasound Med Biol* 21:1119–1122, 1995.

Gorg C, Restrepo I, Schwerk WB: Sonography of malignant pleural effusion. *Eur Radiol* 7:1195–1198, 1997.

Henschke CI, Davis SD, Romano PM, Yankelevitz DF: Pleural effusions: Pathogenesis, radiologic evaluation, and therapy. *J Thorac Imaging* 4:49–60, 1989.

Herman T, McAlister W, Siegel M: Chest, in *Pediatric Sonography,* 2d ed, Siegel M (ed). New York, Raven, 1995:139–169.

Mathis G: Thoraxsonography—Part I: Chest wall and pleura. *Ultrasound Med Biol* 23:1131–1139, 1997.

Mentzer W: Sickle cell disease, in *Rudolph's Pediatrics*, 19th ed, Rudolph A (ed). Norwalk, CT, Appleton & Lange, 1991: 1123–1124.

Moore K: *Clinically Oriented Anatomy*, 3d ed. Baltimore, William & Wilkins, 1992:228–229.

Silen W: *Cope's Early Diagnosis of the Acute Abdomen,* 19th ed. New York, Oxford, 1996:276, 288–289.

Yang PC, Luh KT, Chang DB, et al: Value of sonography in determining the nature of pleural effusion: Analysis of 320 cases. *AJR* 159:329–331, 1992.

Yu C, Yang P, Chang D, Luh K: Diagnostic and therapeutic use of chest sonography: Value in critically ill patients. *AJR* 159: 695–701, 1992.

116

An asymptomatic newborn male was assessed because of an abnormal fetal ultrasound (US) of the chest. Figures 116-1 and 116-2 are now obtained in the left upper quadrant. What does the patient have? What technique could prove this to you?

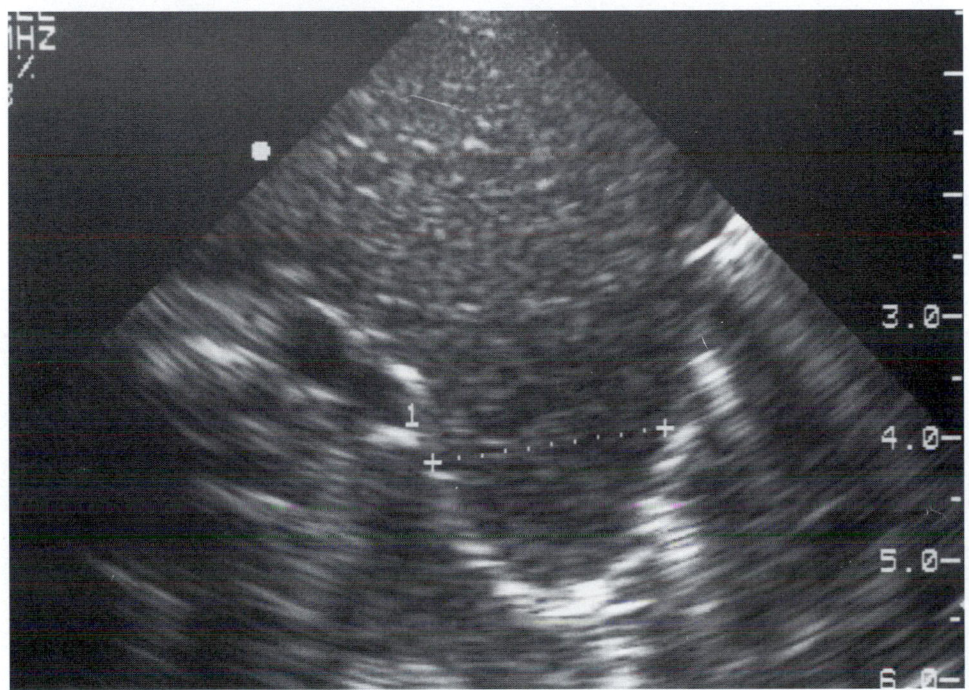

FIGURE 116–1. Ultrasound. Transverse plane through left upper abdomen, including spleen.

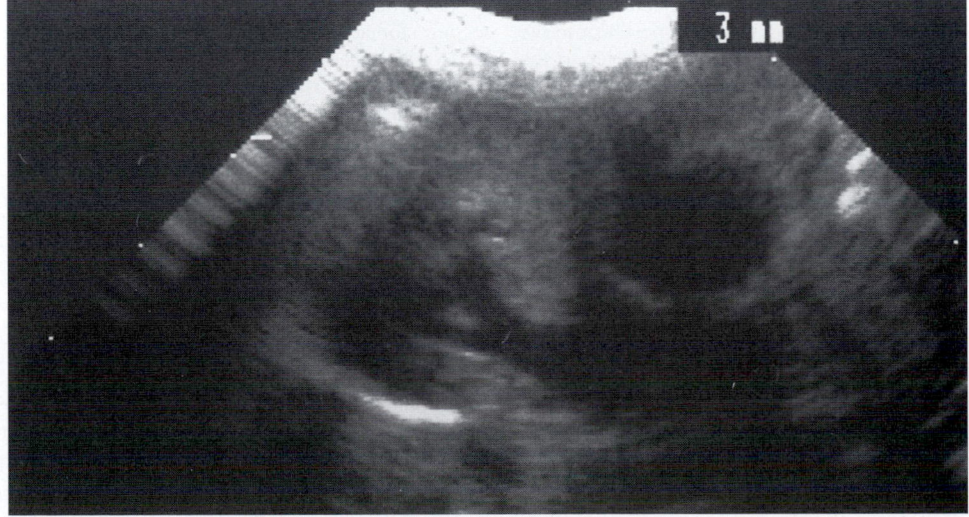

FIGURE 116–2. Ultrasound. Longitudinal plane through left upper quadrant including stomach.

CHAPTER 116

Pulmonary Sequestration

HARRIS L. COHEN

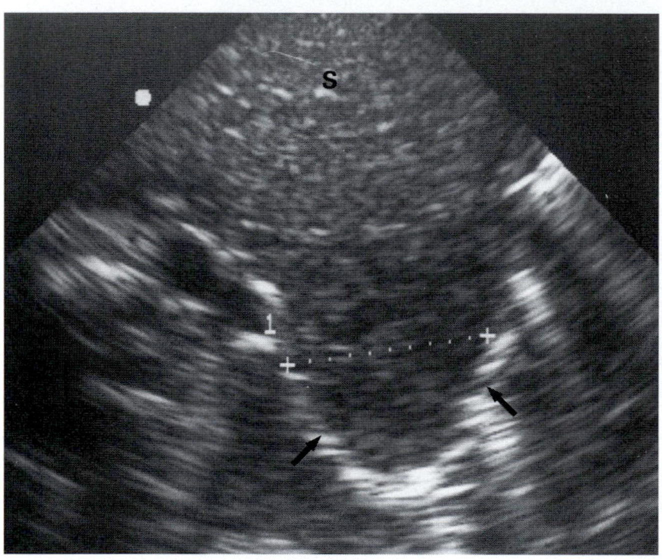

FIGURE 116–3. Annotated version of Fig. 116-1. Pulmonary sequestration. Ultrasound. Transverse plane through left upper abdomen. A solid mass, marked off by crosses, is seen posterior to the spleen (S). The echogenic diaphragm (*arrows*) is posterior to the mass, suggesting that the mass is within the abdomen.

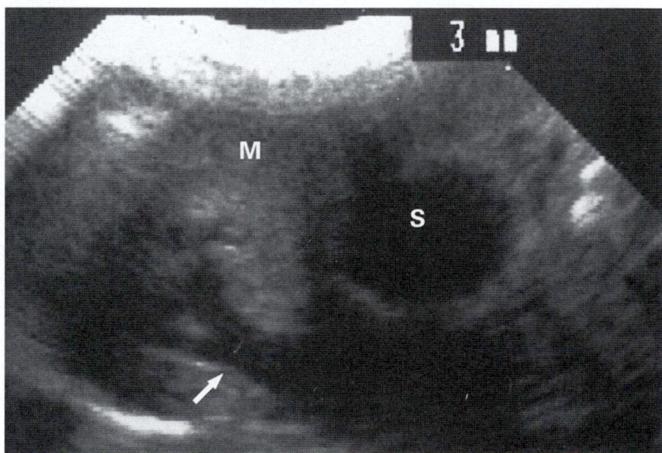

FIGURE 116–4. Annotated version of Fig. 116-2. Pulmonary sequestration. Longitudinal plane through left upper quadrant including stomach. The mass (M) is superior to the fluid-filled stomach (S). It appears to have a branching tubular structure within it that appears to be arising from lower in the abdomen. The branching nature suggests blood vessels.

Figures 116-3 and 116-4, the annotated versions of Figs. 116-1 and 116-2, show a solid subdiaphragmatic mass that is not the spleen, although it is of similar echogenicity to the spleen, and is superior to the stomach. Prominent branching tubular structures within it suggest blood vessels. A pulmonary sequestration was the key consideration. Color Doppler examination (Fig. 116-5) proved that these tubular structures were vessels and proved that the mass was a pulmonary sequestration by showing arterial flow entering the mass from branches of the abdominal aorta. The neonate did well and was followed clinically. The mass became smaller with time.

WHAT IS A PULMONARY SEQUESTRATION?

We have discussed pulmonary sequestration in the fetus in Chap. 9. The term *pulmonary sequestration* was first used in 1946 by Pryce to describe a mass of lung tissue without a normal connection to the tracheobronchial tree or the pulmonary artery. The mass is solid and nonfunctioning. It receives its blood supply from a systemic artery that theoretically is a systemic arterial connection to the base of the lung that failed to be obliterated with embryologic growth. Arterial flow into the sequestration is usually from

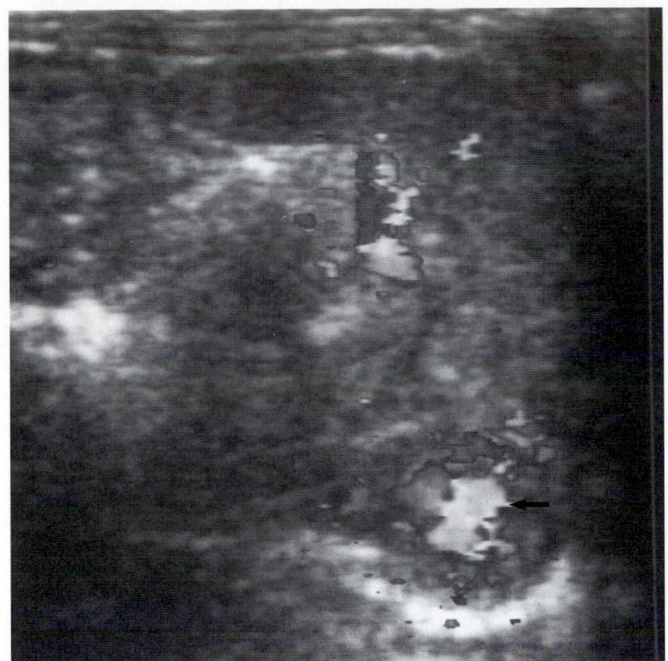

A

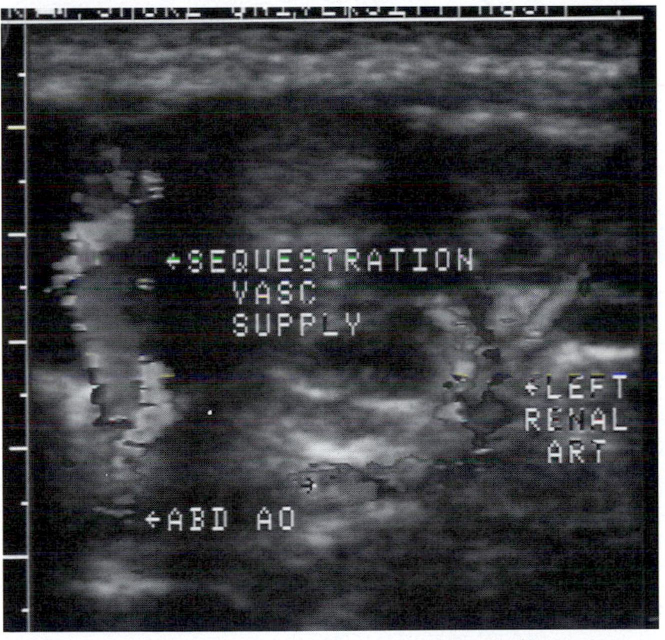

B

FIGURE 116–5. Pulmonary sequestration proven by color Doppler. ***A.*** Transverse plane. Image taken on black-and-white film. Blood flow is noted in the anterior parenchyma of the spleen. The posterior but subdiaphragmatic mass has significant flow (arrows) within it. ***B.*** Longitudinal plane. Color image. The abdominal aorta has branches feeding the left kidney (LEFT RENAL ART) as well as the solid, immediately subdiaphragmatic mass that proved to be a sequestration.

the thoracic or abdominal aorta, but flow from many different arteries, including the celiac, innominate, subclavian, and internal mammary arteries and even the ascending aorta and renal artery, has been identified on angiographic studies.

Pulmonary sequestrations are divided into two main types. The majority of sequestrations are *intralobar* in type. They are surrounded by visceral pleura and found in the posterior basal segment of the lower lobe. The majority (60 percent) involve the left lung. Venous drainage is via the normally expected route, the pulmonary veins. In the years prior to the development of high-resolution antenatal sonography and therefore the early identification of some cases, a diagnosis of intralobar pulmonary sequestration was rare in the first decade of life. Those who were diagnosed as such often presented with a history of recurrent infections.

The *extralobar* variety of pulmonary sequestration lies within its own pleura and has been labeled by some as an accessory lung or Rokitansky lobe. Unlike the equal gender distribution of the intralobar variety, the extralobar sequestration has a 4:1 male predominance. Some 90 percent of cases occur on the left side of the chest, but not as often in the lower lobes as with the intralobar variety. The arterial supply is from the aorta. Venous drainage is not into the pulmonary veins but into another vein, often the azygous, hemiazygous, or portal. Diagnosis is often made in early life. There is an association of extralobar pulmonary sequestration with diaphragmatic hernia. These sequestrations have been seen in the fetus and neonate as echogenic masses situated below the diaphragm. Many of the antenatal masses are seen as triangular. This is less easy to confirm by US postnatally because of the loss of US information at the chest periphery.

DIFFERENTIAL DIAGNOSTIC POSSIBILITIES

The imaging of abnormal vascular connections to a solid subdiaphragmatic mass identifies it as a pulmonary sequestration. Haddon and Bowen warn that the neovascularity of chronic lung infection may lead to a false diagnosis of pulmonary sequestration. This however, would be more of a consideration in an older patient with a significant pulmonary history. Solid sequestrations may appear to resemble type III cystic adenomatoid malformations. Morgagni and Bochdalek hernias containing solid parenchymal structures may also be considered.

IMAGING PULMONARY SEQUESTRATION

Obviously US, aided by Doppler, is the key method of diagnosis in fetal life. Hang et al reviewed the postnatal findings of a group of patients with pulmonary sequestration who were assessed with a variety of imaging modalities. These modalities helped make the diagnosis, preoperatively, in 87.5 percent of cases. Plain chest films demonstrated a solid mass in 14 patients and a cystic mass in 10. Bronchograms showed displacement of adjacent bronchi by a solid mass that did not fill with the injected contrast material. Of 4 cases diagnosed as sequestration by computed tomography (CT) 3 showed associated surrounding emphysema. Magnetic resonance imaging (MRI) readily showed anomalous arteries in all of the studied patients and abnormal venous drainage in fewer cases. Aortography demonstrated anomalous systemic arterial supply to the sequestrations of all studied patients. Nuclear scintigraphy has been used by some to make the diagnosis by noting a lack of perfusion in the mass during the pulmonary phase of a ventilation-perfusion technetium 99m pertechnetate scan followed by rapid perfusion during the systemic vascular phase of the study, denoting the sequestration's systemic vascular supply.

THE ULTRASOUND FINDINGS OF PULMONARY SEQUESTRATION

On US, the basilar masses of pulmonary sequestration are typically homogeneously solid and echogenic, with only entering or exiting vascular structures breaking up the homogeneity. Of 14 patients with pulmonary sequestration studied with US by Hang et al, 12 had completely solid masses and 2 had solid masses with contained cystic areas. Doppler proved vascular flow within 12 of the 14 cases studied. Masses of pulmonary sequestration remain solid as long as there is no bronchial communication. The only breaks in the homogeneously solid tissue are the cystic or tubular areas of feeding and draining blood vessels. If bronchial communication does develop, and it is said that this can occur after infection, bright echogenicities and reverberation, US evidence of the presence of air within any structure, will be seen and may confuse the diagnosis. As stated, Doppler, whether duplex, color, or power Doppler, can be used for rapid identification of the cystic areas as blood vessels.

PULMONARY SEQUESTRATIONS MAY DISAPPEAR

As with our case, it is known that pulmonary sequestrations may decrease in size over time. Sintzoff et al reported following a proven pulmonary sequestration in a premature baby boy who originally presented with respiratory distress and a right lower lobe opacity on chest x-ray. The mass decreased in size on follow-up examinations. Within 4 months the mass could no longer be demonstrated on plain film or US. Others have reported similar experiences of partial or total disappearance of pulmonary sequestration masses. These examples of "involutive pathology" would suggest that operative removal of these masses is not necessary. However, as with other pathologies that involute, such as the multicystic dysplastic kidney, time and imaging/clinical experience are necessary to note whether any negative consequences can occur as a result of leaving dysplastic tissue within the body.

A KEY POINT TO REMEMBER

When a solid mass is seen at the base of the lung or just below the diaphragm, think about pulmonary sequestration as a possibility. A quick color Doppler analysis may help male the diagnosis.

References

Cohen HL, Muller D, Zinn D: Abnormalities of the fetal chest, abdomen and pelvis, in *Diagnostic Medical Sonography. A Guide to Clinical Practice. Obstetrics and Gynecology,* 2d ed, Berman M, Cohen H (eds). Philadelphia, Lippincott, 1997: 285–319.

Eisenberg P, Cohen HL, Coren C: Color doppler in pulmonary sequestration diagnosis. *J Ultrasound Med* 11:175–176, 1992.

Luet'ic T, Crombleholme T, Semple J, D'Alton M: Early prenatal diagnosis of bronchopulmonary sequestration with associated diaphragmatic hernia. *J Ultrasound Med* 14:533–535, 1995.

Haddon M, Bowen AD: Bronchopulmonary and neurenteric forms of foregut anomalies. Imaging for the diagnosis and management. *Radiol Clin North Am* 29:241–254, 1991.

Hang JD, Guo QY, Chen CX, Chen LY: Imaging approach to the diagnosis of pulmonary sequestration. *Acta Radiol* 37:883–888, 1996.

MacGillivray T, Harrison M, Goldstein R, Adzick N: Disappearing fetal lung lesions. *J Pediatr Surg* 28:1321–1324, 1993.

Pryce D: Lower accessory pulmonary artery with intralobar sequestration of lung: A report of seven cases. *J Pathol* 58:457–467, 1946.

Sintzoff SA Jr, Avni EF, Rocmans P, et al: Pulmonary sequestration-like anomaly presenting as a spontaneously resolving mass. *Pediatr Radiol* 21:143–144, 1991.

West M, Donaldson J, Shkolnik A: Pulmonary sequestration. *J Ultrasound Med* 8:125–129, 1989.

117

A 16-year-old was sent to mammography for analysis of a mass in her areolar area that she had felt for several days. Mammography is avoided in her age group, and she was sent to ultrasound (US) for evaluation of the mass. Figures 117-1, an image of the mass in the longitudinal plane, and 117-2, an image of the mass in the transverse plane, are presented to you. What do you see? What would you recommend?

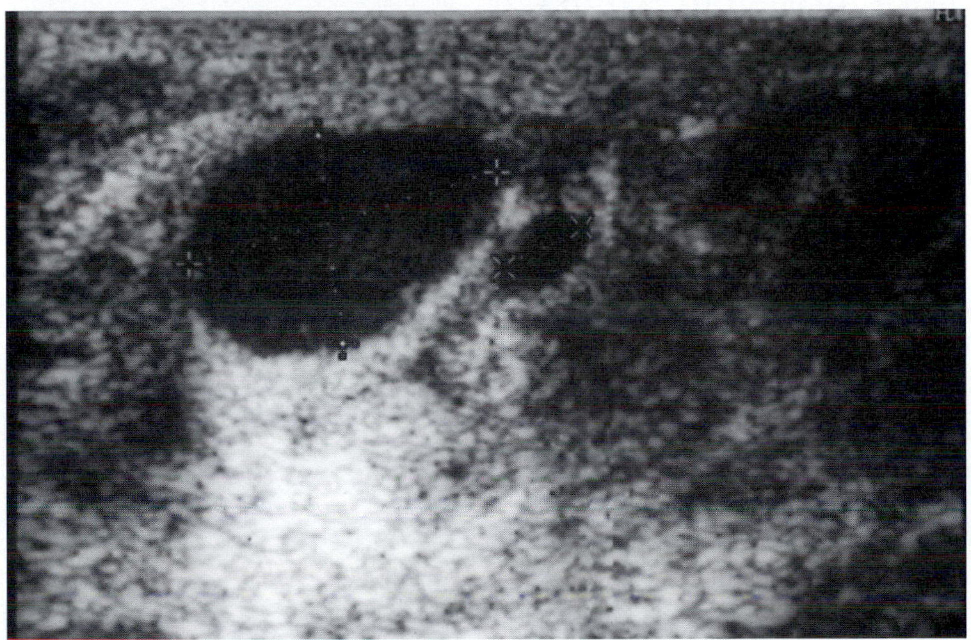

FIGURE 117–1. Breast. Ultrasound. Longitudinal plane through palpated mass.

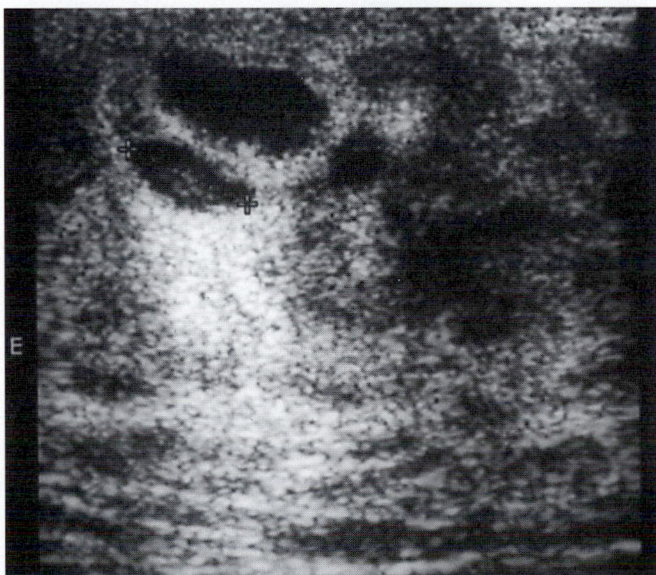

FIGURE 117–2. Breast ultrasound. Transverse plane through palpated mass.

CHAPTER 117

Complex Cysts in the Breast of an Adolescent

DAPHNE ROITBERG-MIZRAHI

AND HARRIS L. COHEN

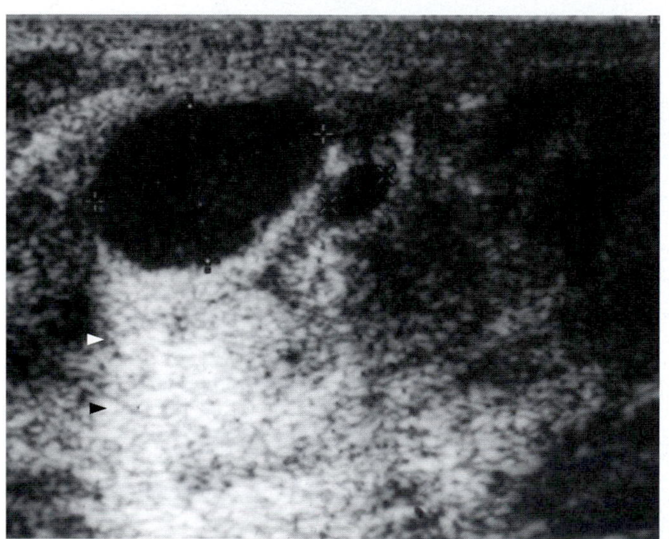

FIGURE 117–3. Annotated version of Fig. 117-1. Complex and simple breast cysts. Breast ultrasound. Longitudinal plane through palpated mass at 12 o'clock in areolar area. Two masses are seen on this image. The larger mass, marked off by arrows, measured 1.5 by 1.3 cm. Contained echoes within it negate a diagnosis of simple cyst. Excellent through transmission (*arrowheads*) suggests that it is probably a cyst. The smaller mass is a cyst and measures 4 mm in diameter.

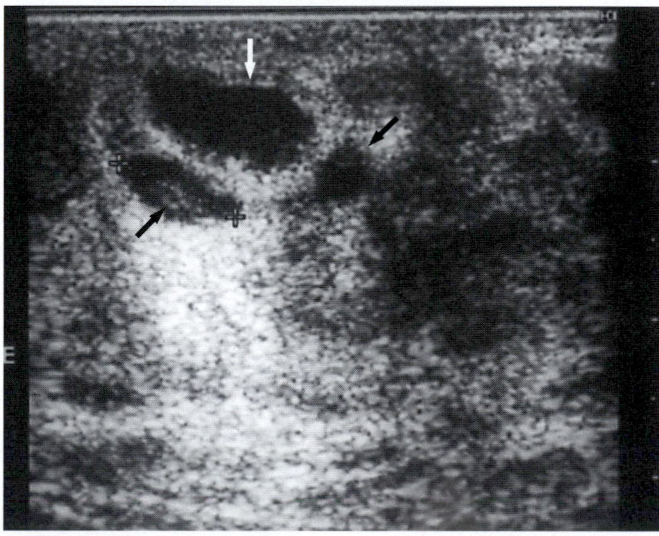

FIGURE 117–4. Annotated version of Fig. 117-2. Complex and simple breast cysts. Breast ultrasound. Transverse plane through palpated mass at 12 o'clock in areolar area. Three predominantly cystic masses are noted (*arrows*). Contained echoes within them define the cysts as complex.

Figures 117-3, the annotated version of Fig. 117-1, and 117-4, the annotated version of Fig. 117-2, show several relatively echoless masses, with the largest being 1.5 by 1.3 cm. They are not classic simple cysts because of contained low-level internal echoes. Excellent through transmission (posterior acoustic enhancement) suggested that they were cysts, but solid masses made up of multiple small cells (e.g., lymphomatous nodes) may appear echopenic and have good to excellent through transmission as well. If a simple cyst was discovered, the patient would be followed up clinically. Because the masses were complex, aspiration was performed to note their contents (and to send the material to the cytology or bacteriology lab if it appeared hemorrhagic or infected), as well as to relieve the patient's symptom of pain. Yellow fluid consistent with benign fibrocystic changes was aspirated from the cysts under US guidance. Nonhemorrhagic fluid is

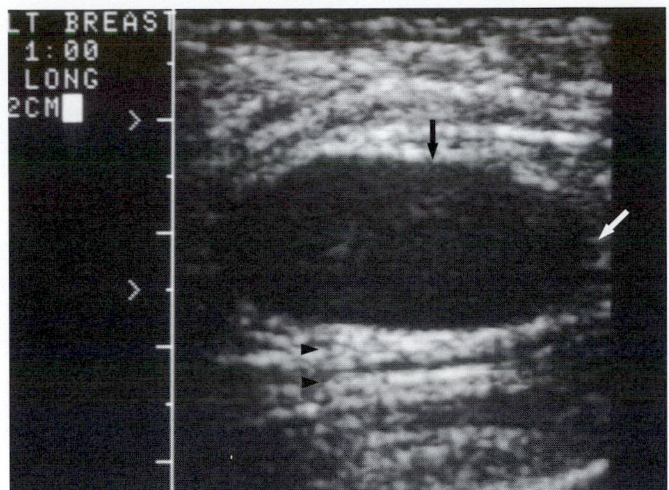

FIGURE 117–5. Fibroadenoma. Left breast ultrasound. Longitudinal plane through mass at 1 o'clock, 2 cm out from the nipple. An oval, homogeneously hypoechoic mass (*arrows*) with no more than medium through transmission (*arrowheads*) is seen in a 16-year-old girl who presented with a palpable mass. The through transmission is less than that seen with the complex cyst of Fig. 117-1. The border of the mass is smooth with slight lobularity. The mass is wider than it is tall, suggesting that it is benign. The ultrasound findings are consistent with a solid mass, a fibroadenoma, which this proved to be.

not considered suggestive for neoplasm. The patient was reassured and scheduled for a 6-month follow-up US examination.

PALPABLE BREAST LESIONS IN ADOLESCENTS

The most common mass seen in teenagers and in women under 30 years of age is a fibroadenoma (Fig. 117-5). Other causes of palpable lesions in the breasts of adolescents are normal but nodular breast tissue, cysts, and fibrosis. The risk-to-benefit ratio for mammography in teenagers with palpable breast lesions is considered too low to advocate its use as a front-line imaging modality. The breasts of women in this age group are more sensitive to the effects of radiation. Since breast cancer is decidedly rare in women under the age of 20, initial evaluation of palpable abnormalities is limited to US.

BREAST ULTRASOUND—GENERAL INFORMATION

Ultrasound is an established and valuable adjunct to mammography for both diagnosis and management in all age groups. Indications include the analyses of masses in the young patient and the differentiation between cystic and solid masses, as in this unknown case. Ultrasound can also be used to evaluate palpable abnormalities in pregnant and lactating women, to confirm and assess masses that are not completely imaged by mammography; to identify abscesses in patients with mastitis, and to evaluate the surgically altered breast. It can also be used to guide interventional procedures, such as the aspiration of the cysts in this case (Fig. 117-6). Breast US is not advocated for breast cancer screening.

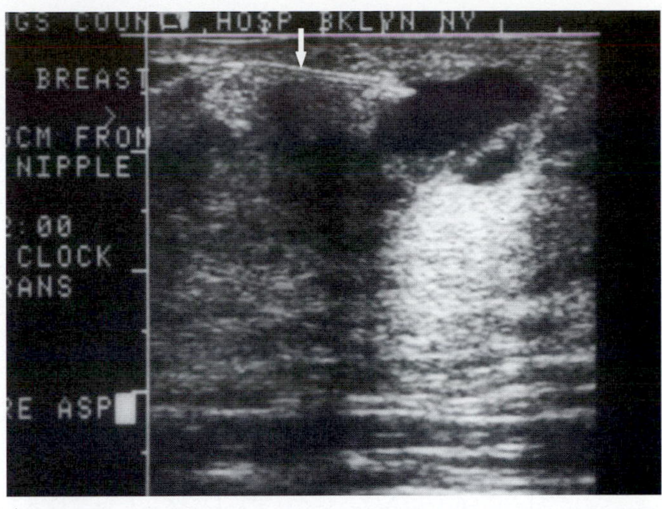

A

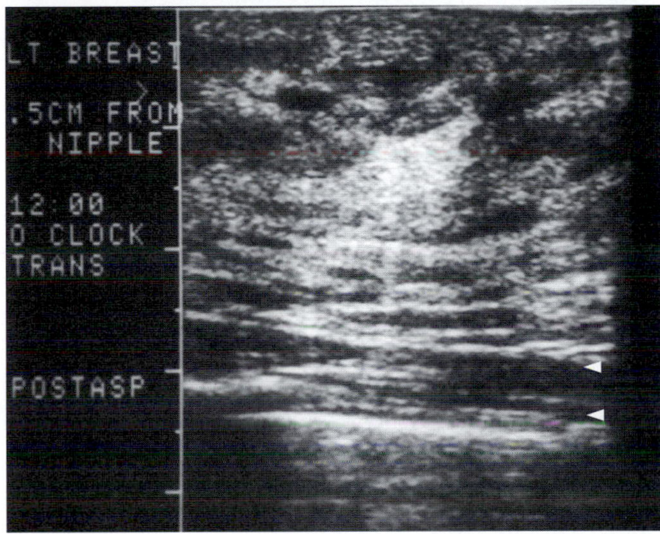

B

FIGURE 117–6. Ultrasound guidance of cyst aspiration. ***A.*** Preaspiration image. Longitudinal plane. The needle (*arrow*) is noted right at the entry border to the large, complex cyst. ***B.*** Postaspiration image. After aspiration of yellow viscous fluid to evacuate the cyst, the cyst is no longer visible. Note the echopenic chest wall muscles (*arrowheads*) deep to the breast.

TECHNICAL ASPECTS OF BREAST ULTRASONOGRAPHY

As with all exams requiring excellent near-field resolution, high-frequency transducers (usually 7.5 MHz and greater) that are linear array in type are used. Occasionally, stand-off pads may help the imaging of very superficial structures. In analyzing cysts, the focal zone should be positioned at the posterior margin of the lesion, to avoid artifactually created internal echoes.

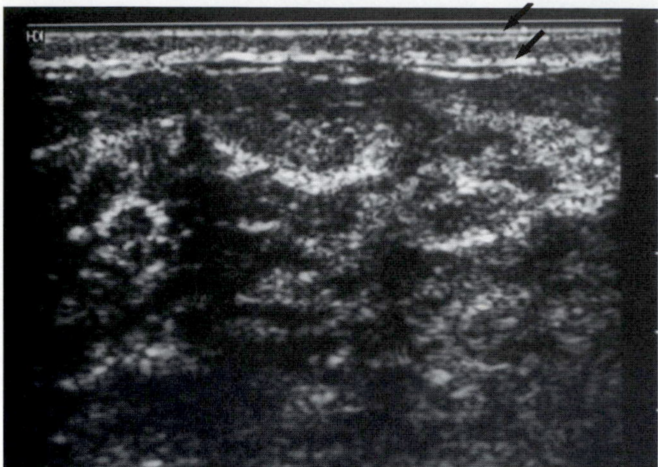

FIGURE 117–7. Normal breast parenchyma. Transverse plane. Normal lobules of breast tissue are noted. No cystic masses are seen in this normal area of breast. Note the classic appearance of the skin, superficially, as two echogenic lines (*arrows*) with a central echopenic area between them.

ULTRASONOGRAPHIC FEATURES OF NORMAL BREAST STRUCTURES

Breasts and their surrounding structures are composed of skin, ducts, adipose tissue, fibroglandular parenchyma, blood vessels, nipple areolar complex, retromammary muscle bundles, and lymph nodes. Each of these structures has a characteristic sonographic appearance. The skin appears as two thin echogenic lines sandwiching a hypoechoic zone, which represents the dermis (Fig. 117-7). Fat lobules are hypoechoic (despite the popular and false notion that all fat is echogenic using US) relative to the surrounding homogeneously echogenic glandular tissue. The nipple is of medium echogenicity and demonstrates posterior acoustic shadowing. The ribs are identified as hypoechoic, oval structures posterior to the pectoralis muscle. Lymph nodes, both axillary and intramammary, are seen as hypoechoic oval structures that frequently demonstrate central hilar echogenicity.

SONOGRAPHIC FINDINGS IN BREAST CYSTS AND MASSES

A simple cyst should be anechoic, should be sharply marginated (particularly at its better imaged posterior wall), and should demonstrate posterior acoustic enhancement on US evaluation. Pressure applied to a cyst with a transducer may alter the shape of the cyst, a feature not (usually) seen with solid lesions. When a simple breast cyst is diagnosed, no further action is required. Solid masses may be benign or malignant. Although only histologic analysis is absolutely definitive, several sonographic features have been described that can help in differentiating benign from malignant solid masses. Irregular or indistinct borders, posterior acoustic shadowing, ductal extension (branching pattern), an echogenic rim of variable thickness (probably representing reactive desmoplasia), orientation perpendicular to the skin ("taller than wide"), and the presence of microcalcifications suggest a malignant process. Mass orientation parallel to the skin, smooth or gentle marginal lobulations, an ellipsoid shape, intense homogeneous hyperechogenicity, and a thin echogenic capsule suggest a benign etiology.

Fibroadenomas are benign solid masses. They are classically oval, homogeneously hypoechoic relative to breast parenchyma, and isoechoic compared to fat lobules (Fig. 117-5). They have sharply defined macrolobulated borders and demonstrate medium acoustic attenuation properties.

CYST ASPIRATION USING ULTRASOUND GUIDANCE

Palpable cysts in symptomatic patients should be aspirated (Fig. 117-6). Aspiration is also indicated for symptomatic cysts and for cysts that do not fulfill all the criteria for a simple cyst, such as those that demonstrate internal echoes or septations. Nearly 30 percent of cysts are said to demonstrate low-level internal echoes. These echoes are more noticeable with higher-frequency transducers. Echoes within a cyst can be due to hemorrhage or to proteinaceous material within the cyst. They may, however, be due to an intracystic papilloma or an intracystic cancer.

Ultrasound is used to guide fine-needle aspirations as well as fine and large core-needle biopsies and presurgical needle localizations with needle hookwires. The freehand technique used in this case and associated with a low complication rate introduces the needle at a slight distance from the probe. The needle is kept perpendicular to the beam and parallel to the probe surface to maintain visualization of the complete needle and its course into the cyst. One hand is used to stabilize the probe while the other hand inserts the needle.

Remember: Ultrasound can help in evaluating breast masses in the adolescent, in whom mammography is to be avoided.

References

Adler DD: Ultrasound of benign breast conditions. *Semin Ultrasound CT MR* 10:106–118, 1989.

Bassett LW, Kimme-Smith C: Breast sonography: technique, equipment, and normal anatomy. *Semin Ultrasound CT MR* 10:82–89, 1989.

D'Orsi CJ, Mendelson EB: Interventional breast ultrasonography. *Semin Ultrasound CT MR* 10:132–138, 1989.

Evans WP: Breast masses. *Radiol Clin North Am* 33:1085–1108, 1995.

Feig SA: The role of ultrasound in a breast imaging center. *Semin Ultrasound CT MR* 10:90–105, 1989.

Fornage BD, Coan JD, David CL: Ultrasound guided needle biopsy of the breast and other interventional procedures. *Radiol Clin North Am* 30:167–185, 1992.

Jackson VP: Sonography of malignant breast diseases. *Semin Ultrasound CT MR* 10:119–131, 1989.

JacksonVP: The role of ultrasound in breast imaging. *Radiology* 177:305–311, 1990.

Jackson VP: The current role of ultrasonography in breast imaging. *Radiol Clin North Am* 33:1161–1170, 1995.

Kopans DB: *Breast Imaging.* Philadelphia, Lippincott-Raven, 1998:528–540.

Mendelson EB, The breast, in *Diagnostic Ultrasound,* Rumack CM, Wilson SR, Charboneau JW (eds). St. Louis, Mosby–Year Book, 1998:751–789.

Stavros AT, Thickman D, Rapp CL, et al: Solid breast nodules: Use of sonography to distinguish between benign and malignant lesions. *Radiology* 196:123–134, 1995.

118

This 5-day-old female infant was referred for evaluation because of abnormal hip findings on the newborn physical examination. Look at Fig. 118-1. What do you think?

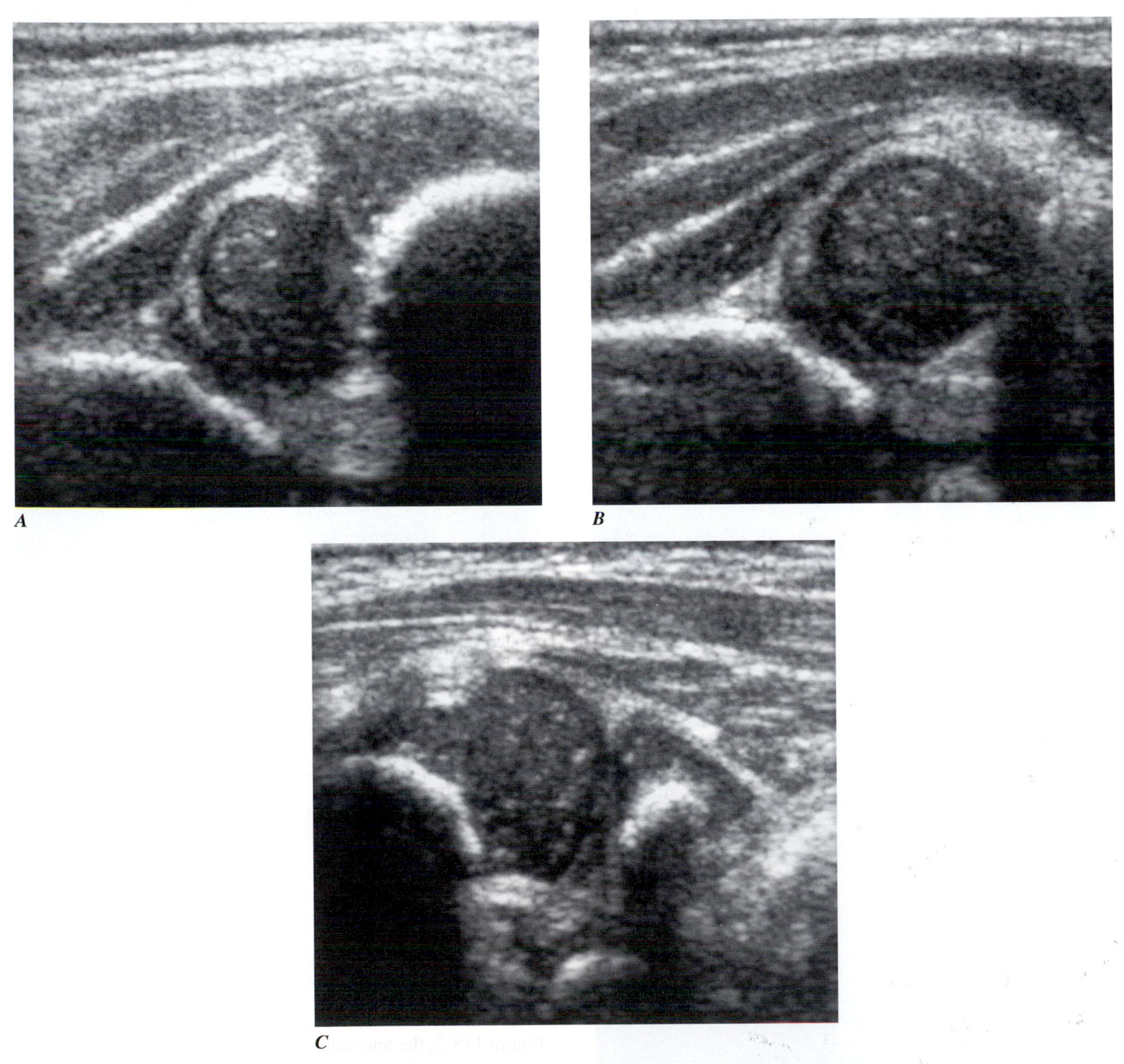

FIGURE 118–1. ***A.*** Coronal sonogram of the left hip, femur in neutral position. ***B.*** Coronal sonogram of the left hip, femur flexed 90°. ***C.*** Transverse sonogram of the left hip, femur flexed 90°.

In developmental dysplasia of the hip (DDH), formerly and incorrectly referred to as congenital dislocation of the hip, instability of the hip allows the femoral head to change position during the dynamic sonographic evaluation. Classically, flexion and adduction increase displacement of the femoral head and may provoke dislocation when posterior (downward, when the neonate is supine) stress is applied. Conversely, flexion and abduction improve position and may reduce a dislocated hip.

The Pavlik harness, a commonly used orthopedic splint device, holds the hip in flexion and abduction as treatment for DDH. Its purpose is to maintain reduction while instability resolves and the acetabulum forms correctly. This infant was maintained in a harness for 10 weeks. Periodic ultrasound exams confirmed complete reduction, return of stability, and development of the bony acetabulum. When this patient was 4 months of age, the sonographic examination was normal (Fig. 118-3).

EDITOR'S NOTE

As stated, hip dislocations may reduce with flexion and abduction. Certainly, they are often relocated in the frog leg lateral plain film view, limiting the effectiveness of this radiographic view for noting dislocation even when the femoral head is fully ossified. The images in Fig. 118-3 are good to look at to help in analyzing Fig. 118-1 and to learn what normal should look like.

Dr. Harcke has been one of the world's pioneers in US detection of DDH. The ACR Standard for the Performance of the Ultrasound for Detection of Developmental Dysplasia of the Hip, of which he was a principal author, further notes that

1. Ultrasound is an excellent method for imaging the immature—i.e., nonossified—hip. It allows ready imaging of cartilage, which it penetrates well. With hip ossification between 6 and 12 months, radiography becomes a more important tool. By the end of the first year of life, ossification of the femoral head is significant enough to prevent adequate sound beam penetration and further use of US to image the bones of the hip. (It is still used to detect joint effusions.)
2. Risk factors for DDH include abnormal physical exam findings (positive Ortolani or Barlow maneuvers), a family history of DDH, a breech presentation at birth, or evidence at birth of postural molding (e.g., torticollis or a foot deformity).
3. The basic exam, which should image in two orthogonal planes, includes (*a*) a coronal view at rest (taken through the lateral aspect of the hip in a longitudinal plane with the hip at rest at 15 to 20° of flexion), which is used to define the anatomy; (*b*) a coronal view with stress (the hip is adducted and the femoral shaft is flexed at 90° with stress directed posteriorly, the US equivalent of the pediatrician's Barlow maneuver, to note if the hip dislocates or subluxes; and (*c*) a transverse view (similar to a computed tomography axial view) with the hip flexed to note its position in relation to the acetabulum and any change in this position occurring with passive abduction and adduction of the infant's hip.

The infant is examined in supine position or alternatively held in a lateral side down position during the exam. Stress views obtained to note hip stability are not taken when examining the hips of an infant who is already undergoing treatment for DDH.

References

ACR Standard for the Performance of the Ultrasound for Detection of Developmental Dysplasia of the Hip. Reston, VA, ACR Publications, 1998.

Grissom LE, Harcke HT: The pediatric hip, in *Diagnostic Ultrasound,* 2d ed, Rumack CM, Wilson SR, Charboneau JW (eds). St. Louis, Mosby–Year Book, 1998:1799–1814.

Harcke HT, Grissom LE: Infant hip sonography: Current concepts. *Semin Ultrasound CT MRI* 15:256–263, 1994.

Harding MGB, Harcke HT, Bowen JR, et al: Ultrasound monitoring in the management of developmental dysplasia of the hip treated with the Pavlik harness. *J Pediatr Orthop* 17:189–198, 1997.

119

A 3-year-old girl presents with a history of 5 days of limp and fever and 1 day of refusing to walk. Sonographic images of both hips are shown in Fig. 119-1. Are these images normal, or are they indicative of abnormality? What is the abnormality?

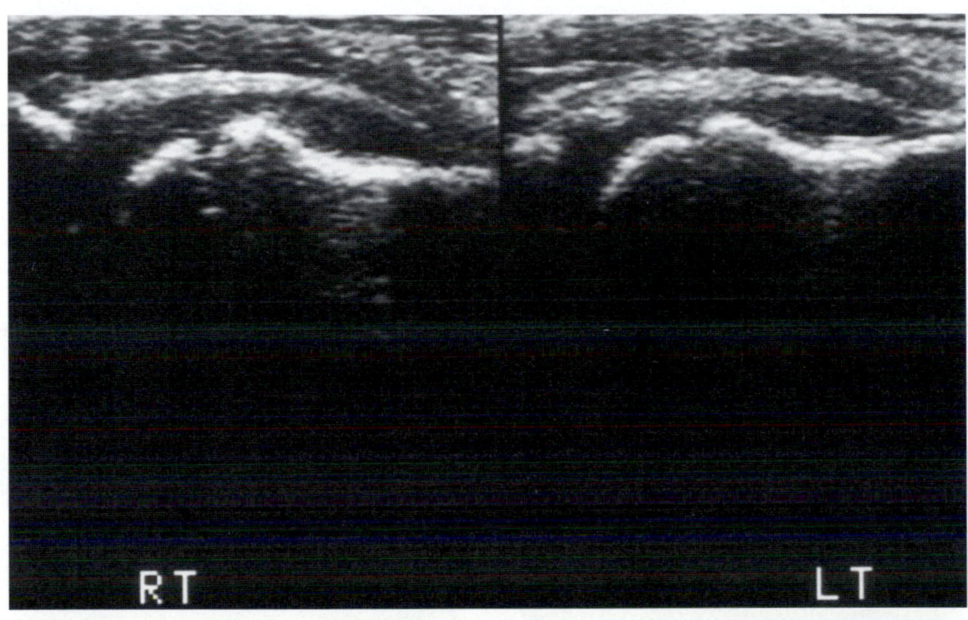

A

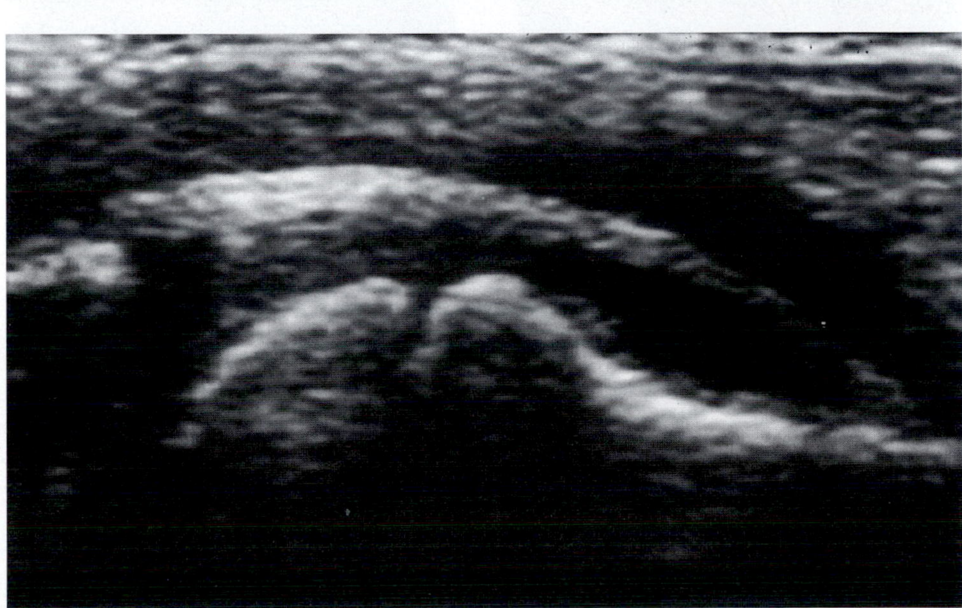

B

FIGURE 119–1. ***A.*** Right hip and left hip. Longitudinal plane. ***B.*** Right hip. Longitudinal plane. Magnified view.

CHAPTER 119

Bilateral Hip Joint Effusions

JAMES S. DONALDSON

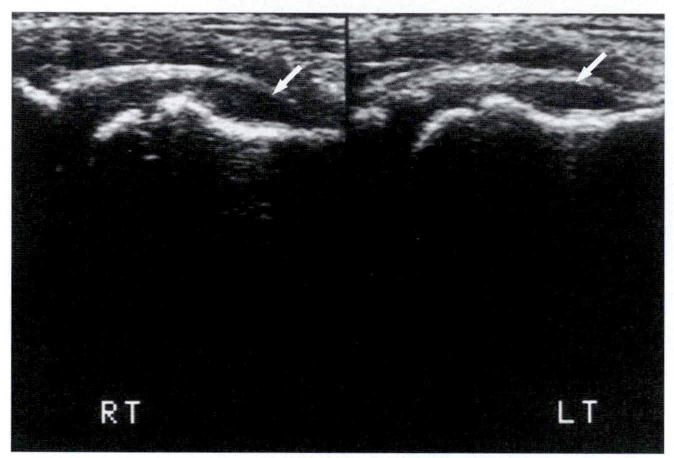

A

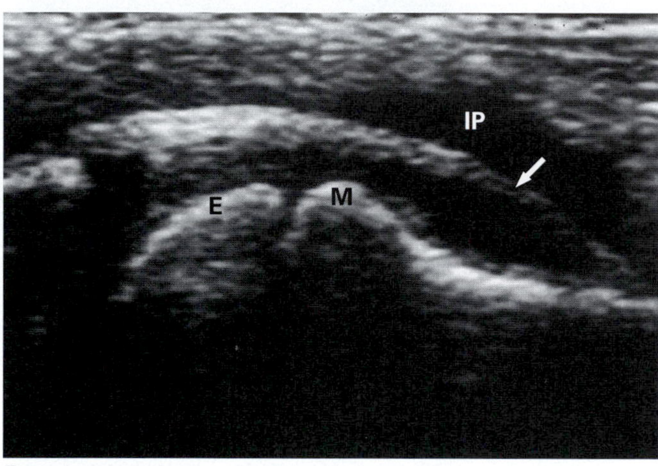

B

FIGURE 119–2. Bilateral hip effusions. ***A.*** Right hip and left hip. Longitudinal plane. Parasagittal US images demonstrate displacement of the joint capsules (*arrows*) of both right and left hips, indicating bilateral joint effusions. ***B.*** Right hip. Longitudinal plane. Magnified view. The joint capsule (*arrow*) is displaced by echoless fluid. E = epiphysis, M = femoral metaphysis, IP = iliopsoas muscle.

The ultrasound (US) images labeled right and left (Fig. 119-2, the annotated version of Fig. 119-1) were obtained from the anterior aspect of each hip sagittal to the femoral necks with the US transducer oriented oblique. Figure 119-3 is a schematic of the technique, Fig. 119-4 is a clinical image of the technique. The important findings are displacement of the anterior joint capsule of each hip caused by hypoechoic joint effusions, resulting in a convex shape of the joint space relative to the femoral neck (Fig. 119-2*B*). Note for comparison that on a normal hip (Fig. 119-5), the joint capsule (arrows) is concave and parallels the femoral neck.

The findings on the US images of this child are uncomplicated bilateral joint effusions. This was due to transient synovitis, or toxic synovitis. However, you can't make that specific diagnosis from the US alone. It requires either correlation with the clinical presentation or a hip aspiration, or it becomes a diagnosis of exclusion when other entities have been ruled out and the patient improves spontaneously. This child's temperature was 100.3°F, his white blood cell count was normal, and his erythrocyte sedimentation rate was not elevated. The joint was not aspirated. A radiograph was not obtained, and he improved in 3 days.

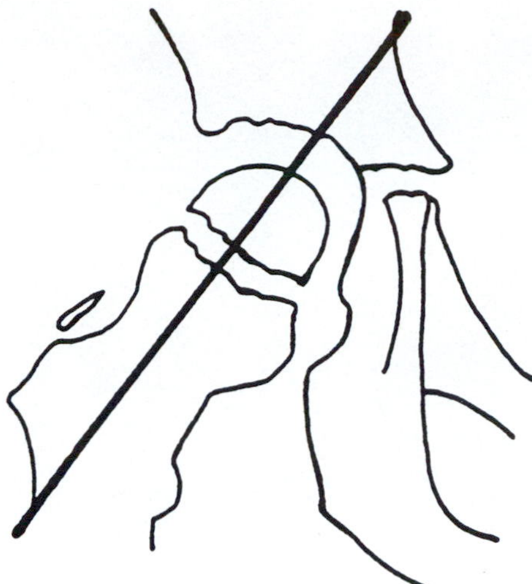

FIGURE 119–3. Ultrasound for hip effusion detection. Schematic drawing. The appropriate scanning plane (*thick black line*) to use is one that is parallel to the femoral neck. (*From Marchal GJ, Van Holsbeeck MT, Raes M, et al: Transient synovitis of the hip in children: Role of US.* Radiology *162:825–828, 1987, with permission.*)

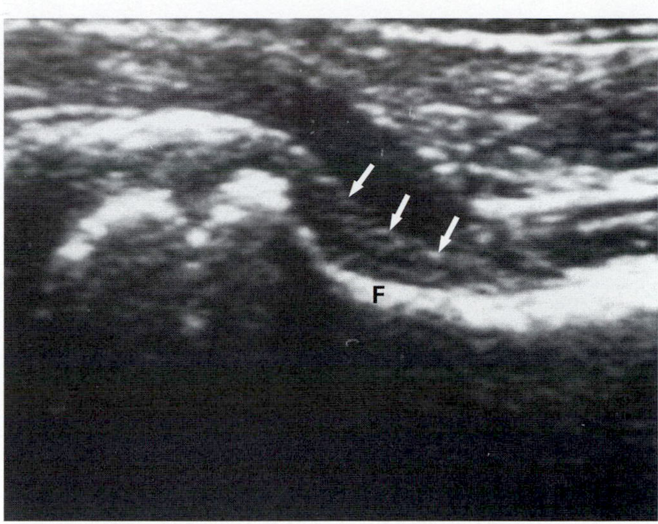

FIGURE 119–5. Normal right hip. The joint capsule (*arrows*) hugs the femoral surface. Lack of echoless fluid between the joint and the capsule proves that there is no effusion.

WHAT IS TRANSIENT SYNOVITIS?

Transient synovitis is the most common cause of painful hips in children. Three major etiologies have been proposed: viral infection, allergic reaction, and trauma. Evidence suggesting an infectious etiology includes a study by Spock, who noted that 70 percent of a group of patients with transient synovitis had an upper respiratory infection within the 2 weeks prior to presenting with their hip problem. Edwards has suggested that the etiology is allergic because most of the patients that he observed had a marked response to antihistamines. The third suspected cause is minor trauma, which is difficult to document or disprove in active 3-year-olds who fall down all the time.

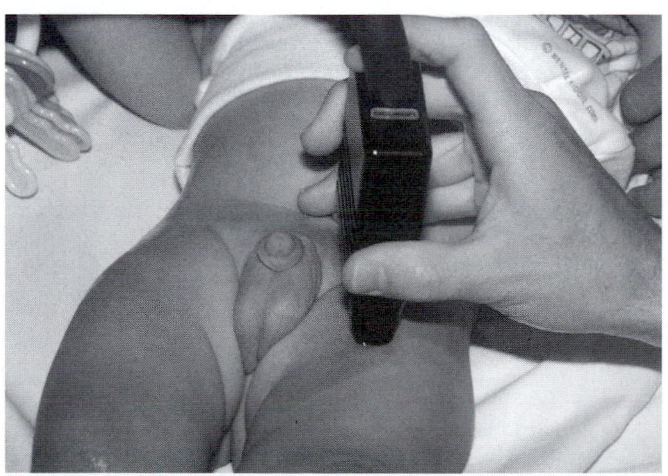

FIGURE 119–4. Ultrasound for hip effusion detection. Clinical photograph. Correct placement of the transducer on the left hip is seen in this image. Symmetric positioning of both thighs and legs is important for comparison views.

CLINICAL AND LABORATORY FINDINGS OF TRANSIENT SYNOVITIS

Clinical presentation includes muscle spasm about the hip, voluntary limitation of motion, and pain on attempted motion. The hip is usually externally rotated at rest. The patient usually has only a low-grade fever or no fever. Laboratory studies include a normal white count with a normal differential count and a sedimentation rate that is normal or only slightly elevated. If the hip is aspirated, serous sterile fluid is obtained.

OTHER CAUSES OF HIP EFFUSION AND REASONS TO USE THIS ULTRASOUND TECHNIQUE

Although transient synovitis may be the most common cause of hip effusion in the child, there are other causes. They include septic arthritis, rheumatoid arthritis, hemarthrosis, villonodular synovitis, osteoid osteoma, Legg-Calvé-Perthes disease, and slipped capital femoral epiphysis. Clinical and laboratory evaluation is often helpful but cannot differentiate among some of these entities. Certainly, if US is the first radiographic examination obtained, a hip effusion may be readily diagnosed using the simple technique used in this case. Clues to the diagnosis may also be present on US. Echogenic effusion, seen in Fig. 119-6 in a child with hemophilia, can confirm hemarthrosis. Irregularity of the epiphysis (Fig. 119-7) may suggest Legg-Calvé-Perthes disease. Debris within the joint (Fig. 119-8*A*) in a neonate with high fever leads to suspicion of a septic joint. Radiographs are often obtained and frequently can give additional clues to the diagnosis. In the patient with a septic joint, the left hip is noted to be dislo-

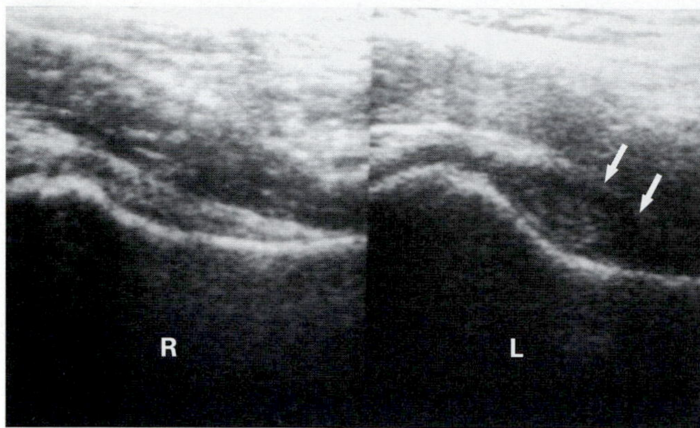

FIGURE 119–6. Echogenic effusion. Right (R) and left (L) hip joints. Parasagittal plane. The right side appears normal. The left side shows displacement of the joint capsule with echogenic material in the joint. This child was a known hemophiliac with new onset of hip pain.

cated on a plain film (Fig. 119-8*B*) consistent with the hip effusion. It is important to emphasize that a septic joint may contain debris-filled echogenic fluid, but it may also contain hypoechoic fluid, and so bacterial infection should be excluded by clinical criteria or joint aspiration.

EDITOR'S COMMENT

This is a simple technique. It is far simpler than the several maneuvers, all obtained through a lateral approach, that are required in the analysis of developmental dysplasia of the hip. In the case of effusion, one simply places the transducer parallel to the femoral neck and looks for convexity and fluid to suggest effusion and for concavity of the joint capsule or its paralleling of the bone to suggest normalcy. The information can help your clinician greatly. If you haven't tried it, please do.

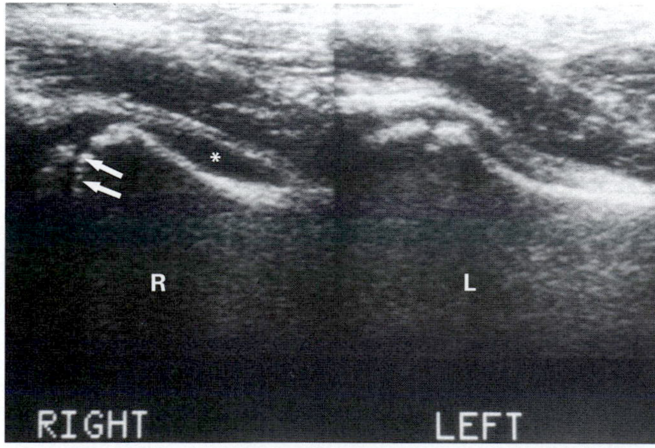

FIGURE 119–7. Small effusion associated with avascular necrosis. Right (R) and left (L) hip joints. Parasagittal plane. There is a right effusion (*). Note the irregular epiphysis (*arrows*) (when compared to the other hip) caused by avascular necrosis or Legg-Calvé-Perthes disease.

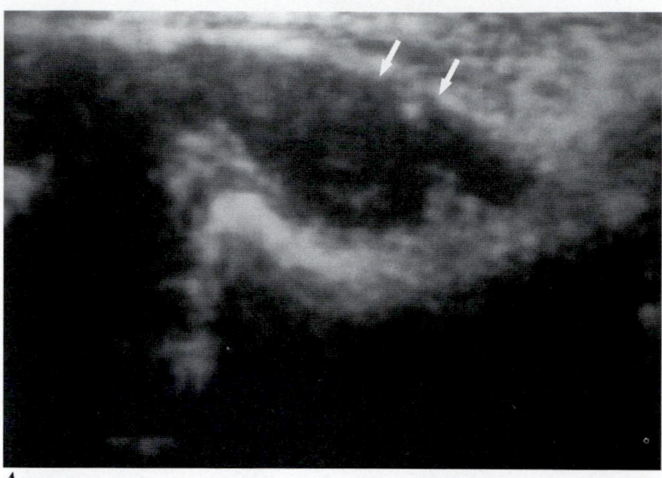

A

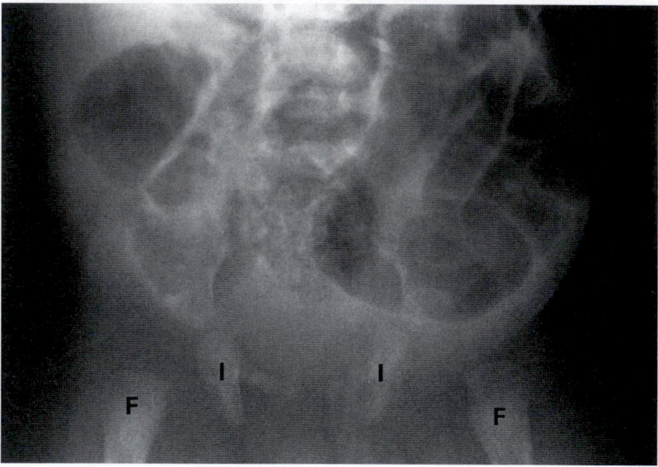

B

FIGURE 119–8. *A.* Septic joint. Ultrasound. Left hip. Longitudinal plane. There is displacement of the joint capsule (arrows). The material within the joint is echogenic. This suggests hemorrhagic or proteinaceous material. Certainly it is not typical of simple fluid. This febrile newborn was not moving his left leg and proved to have a septic joint with debris-filled effusion. ***B.*** Septic joint. Pelvis. Anteroposterior film. The left hip is displaced laterally. It is pushed out of the acetabulum by a large joint effusion, which turned out to be pus from a septic joint. Compare the distance between the femur (F) and the ischium (I) on each side to highlight the abnormality on the left. In order to state this with exactness, however, the film (and filming) of the hip must be done without patient rotation.

References

Alexander JE, Seibert JJ, Aronson J, et al: A protocol of plain radiographs, hip ultrasound, and triple phase bone scans in the evaluation of the painful pediatric hip. *Clin Pediatr* 27:175–181, 1988.

Edwards EG: Transient synovitis of the hip joint in children; report of 13 cases. *JAMA* 148:30–34, 1952.

Harcke HT: Hip in infants and children. *Clin Diagn Ultrasound* 30:179–199, 1995.

Marchal GJ, Van Holsbeeck MT, Raes M, et al: Transient synovitis of the hip in children: Role of US. *Radiology* 162:825–828, 1987.

Spock A: Transient synovitis of the hip joint in children. *Pediatrics* 24:1042–1049, 1959.

Terjesen T: Ultrasonography for diagnosis of slipped capital femoral epiphysis. Comparison with radiography in 9 cases. *Acta Orthop Scand* 63:653–657, 1992.

Terjesen T: Ultrasonography in the primary evaluation of patients with Perthes disease. *J Pediatr Orthop* 13:437–443, 1993.

Wirth T, LeQuesne GW, Paterson DC: Ultrasonography in Legg-Calve-Perthes disease. *Pediatr Radiol* 22:498–504, 1992.

Yousefzadeh DK, Ramilo JL: Normal hip in children: Correlation of US with anatomic and cryomicrotome sections. *Radiology* 165:647–655.

Zieger MM, Dorr U, Schulz RD: Ultrasonography of hip joint effusions. *Skeletal Radiol* 16:607–611, 1987.

120

A 13-year-old boy presented with acute pain and swelling of his left calf. Two images (Figs. 120-1 and 120-2) are presented to you. What is the diagnosis? What other diagnoses could be considered and evaluated via ultrasound (US)?

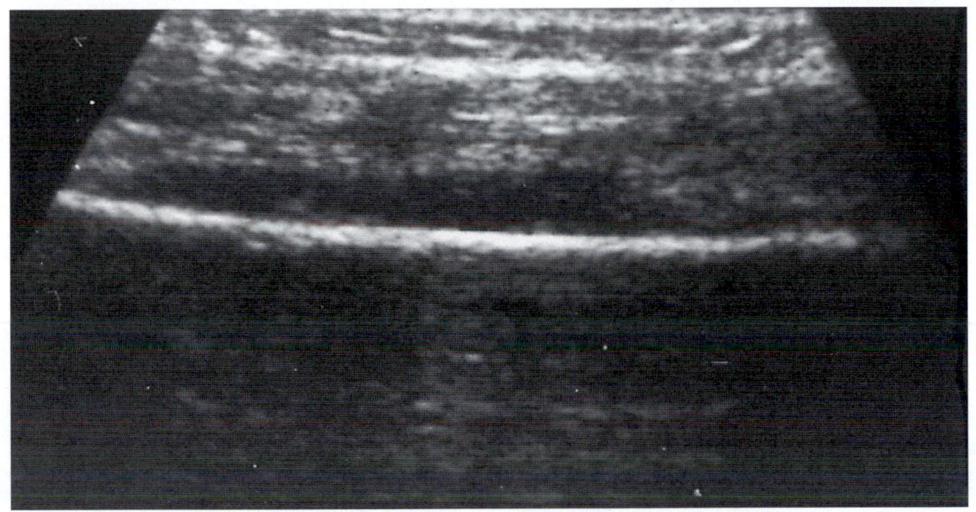

FIGURE 120–1. Ultrasound. Proximal fibula. Longitudinal plane.

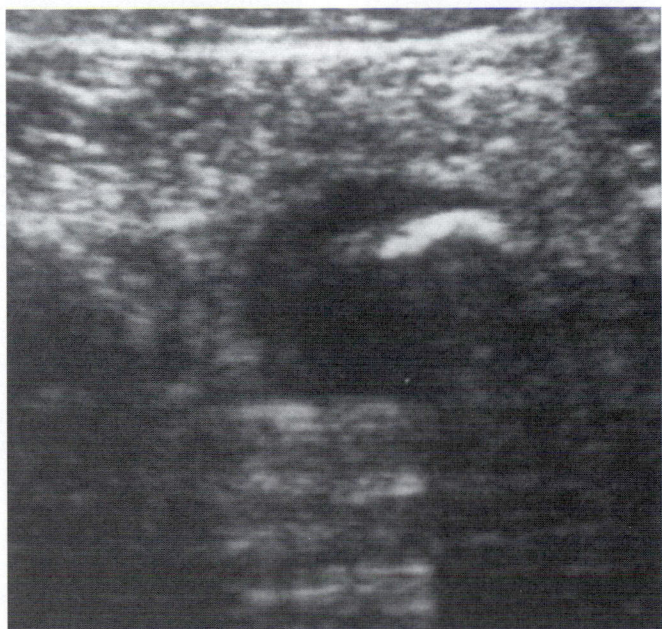

FIGURE 120–2. Ultrasound. Proximal fibula. Transverse plane.

CHAPTER 120

Osteomyelitis

MADHURI KIRPEKAR

AND HARRIS L. COHEN

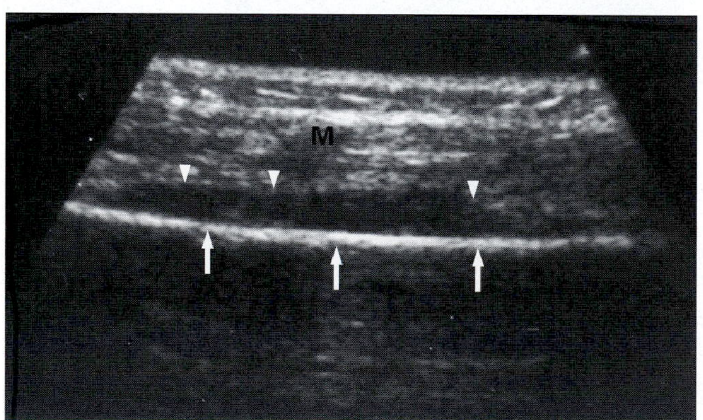

FIGURE 120–3. Annotated version of Fig. 120-1. Ultrasound of osteomyelitis. Proximal fibula. Longitudinal plane. The cortical bone (*arrows*) is the bright line at the bottom of the image. Between the cortical bone and the gray/white muscle (M) of the leg is an echopenic area (*arrowheads*) consistent with a collection. Arrows define the cortical bone of the fibula.

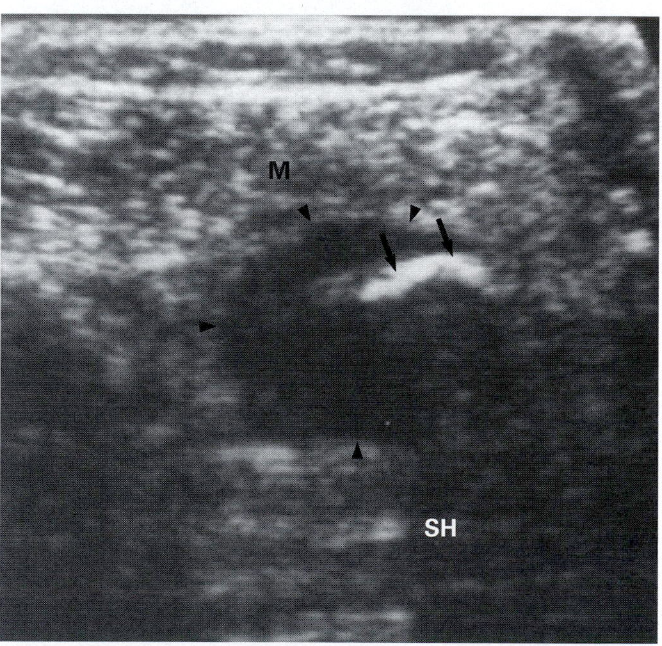

FIGURE 120–4. Annotated version of Fig. 120-2. Ultrasound of osteomyelitis. Proximal fibula. Transverse plane. The cortical bone (*arrows*) is the curvilinear area of bright echogenicity that is almost completely surrounded by anechopenic collection (*arrowheads*). The muscles (M) of the leg are of a heterogeneous solid echogenicity. They have good through transmission. As would be expected, there is shadowing (SH) posterior to the cortical bone.

This 13-year-old patient, as stated, had acute pain and swelling of the calf. On physical examination, the patient had calf swelling as well as erythema of the involved area. The patient had a concurrent low-grade fever. The clinical suspicion was that of venous thrombosis; on sonography, however, there was no evidence of a venous thrombosis. In Fig. 120-3, the annotated version of Fig. 120-1, a longitudinal view of the proximal fibula, there is a hypoechoic area around the bone. In Fig. 120-4, the annotated version of Fig. 120-2, which is a transverse view through the fibula, one can see periosseous fluid as it wraps almost completely around the fibula. In particular, note that there is no intervening soft tissue between the bone and the fluid. These US features are pathognomonic for the sonographic diagnosis of osteomyelitis. The periosseous fluid was thought to be an inflammatory exudate dissecting in a subperiosteal and/or

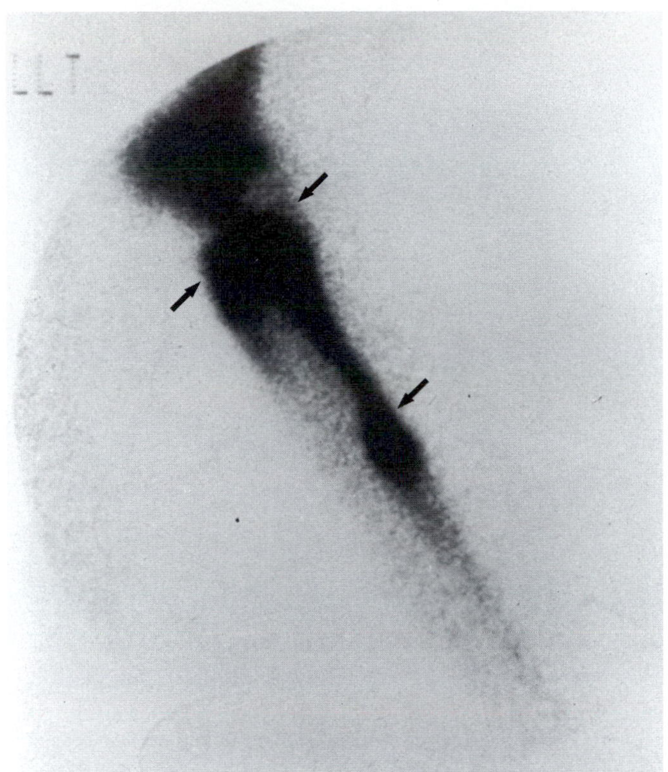

FIGURE 120–5. Osteomyelitis. Bone scan (late image). Left knee. There is marked increased tracer uptake in the proximal fibula (*arrows*).

extraperiosteal location. The periosseous fluid was aspirated, and appropriate antibiotic therapy was initiated. The patient did have a confirmatory bone scan (Fig. 120-5) and plain films (Fig. 120-6) that showed periosteal reaction.

DIFFERENTIAL DIAGNOSIS FOR LOWER-EXTREMITY PAIN AND SWELLING IN A CHILD

Most often, particularly in the adult patient, one would have to consider the possibility of a deep venous thrombosis (Fig. 120-7) of a leg vein. Deep venous thrombi do occur in children. This diagnosis was excluded in this case by evidence of normal venous compressibility as well as normal spectral augmentation with compression distal to the vessel being insonated. A normal vein will also show a decrease in venous flow in the lower extemities when a patient bears down or performs a Valsalva maneuver, indicating the absence of a complete venous obstruction between the insonated vessel and vessels that are more proximal to it along the way to the inferior vena cava.

Patients with swelling or mass behind the knee may have a popliteal or Baker's cyst (Fig. 120-8). Ultrasound can readily image this nonvascular cystic lesion in the soft tissues of the popliteal area. These possibilities may have been considered in this case, but not for long. The patient's physical findings and laboratory findings were different, and of course he had ultrasound images (Figs. 120-3 and 120-4) inconsistent with those diagnoses.

THE ULTRASOUND DIAGNOSIS OF OSTEOMYELITIS

Ultrasound is a frequently used modality for the evaluation of soft tissue abnormalities. Its use for the diagnosis of osteomyelitis and other musculoskeletal conditions is just becoming popular. In performing musculoskeletal sonography, we routinely use a high-frequency linear array transducer and scan in both longitudinal and transverse planes. If obvious skin ulcerations or openings are present, we can avoid direct contact with them by placing a transparent dressing over the involved area and then scanning. The most common clinical indication for US of an extremity is focal pain and swelling.

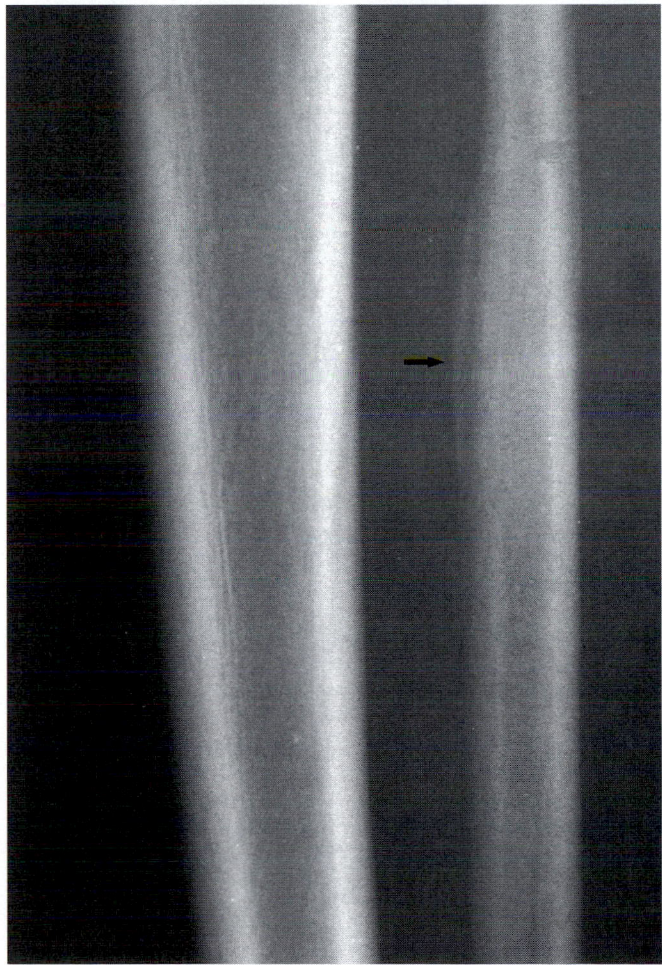

FIGURE 120–6. Osteomyelitis. Plain film. Proximal one-third to mid fibula and tibia. This film was obtained 2 days after the ultrasound diagnosis. It shows a normal tibia but periosteal elevation along the medial (*arrow*) and, to a lesser extent, the lateral aspect (*arrowhead*) of the proximal fibula. Periosteal reaction often develops within 10 days of a bout of osteomyelitis. The initial plain films of osteomyelitis are often normal. This is why nuclear medicine bone scans are performed when the clinician is concerned and plain films are negative.

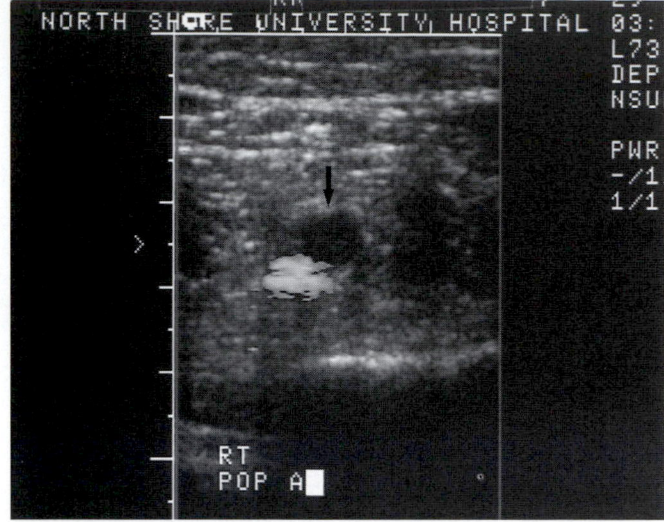

A

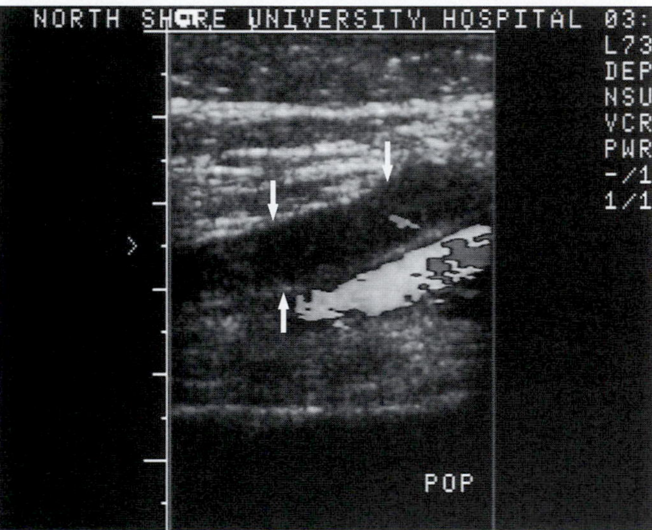

B

FIGURE 120–7. Deep venous thrombosis of the right popliteal vein. Color Doppler. Popliteal area. ***A.*** Transverse plane. Blood flow (*colored red*) is seen in the popliteal artery. No flow is seen in the adjacent vessel (*arrow*). Lack of flow and noncompressibility suggested a deep venous thrombosis involving the popliteal vein in an 18-year-old with systemic lupus erythematosus. ***B.*** Longitudinal plane. Tubular flow is seen in the popliteal artery. The spectral pattern and the quality of color flow in the vessel proved it to be the artery. A tubular echopenic area (*arrows*) superficial to the vascular flow was a popliteal vein filled with clot.

Sonography is frequently the first test to be performed, mostly to determine the integrity of the deep venous system. Subcutaneous fat usually appears homogenously echogenic or hypoechoic and can be recognized because of its location. Muscles typically appear as spindle-shaped hypoechoic structures containing fine linear striations. The cortex of the bone appears as a dense echogenic line with sharp acoustic shadowing or reverberation artifact posterior to it, allowing only the imaging of the near-field cortex of ossified bones.

The presence of fluid adjacent to the bone or within the soft tissues is always pathologic. The location of the fluid with respect to the bone is an important discriminating feature when trying to determine the primary pathologic process. A fluid collection contiguous to the bone is highly suggestive of osteomyelitis. A fluid collection separated from the bone by soft tissue is more likely of soft tissue origin—i.e., either an abscess or a hematoma (Fig. 120-9).

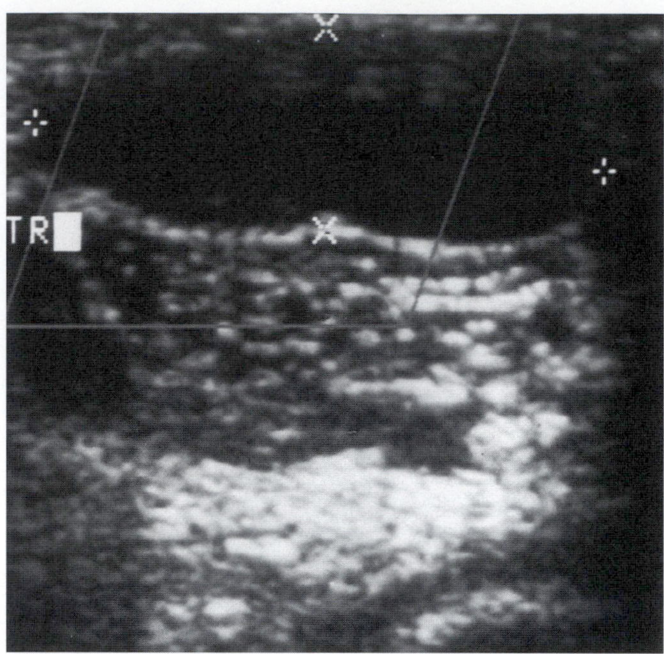

FIGURE 120–8. Baker's (popliteal) cyst. Ultrasound of popliteal area. Transverse plane. Color Doppler. A prominent cystic mass (*marked off by crosses*) is seen in the superficial popliteal area soft tissue of this 9-year-old female who presented with knee pain. No vascular flow was noted in the mass. Other images proved the presence of a normal popliteal vein and artery.

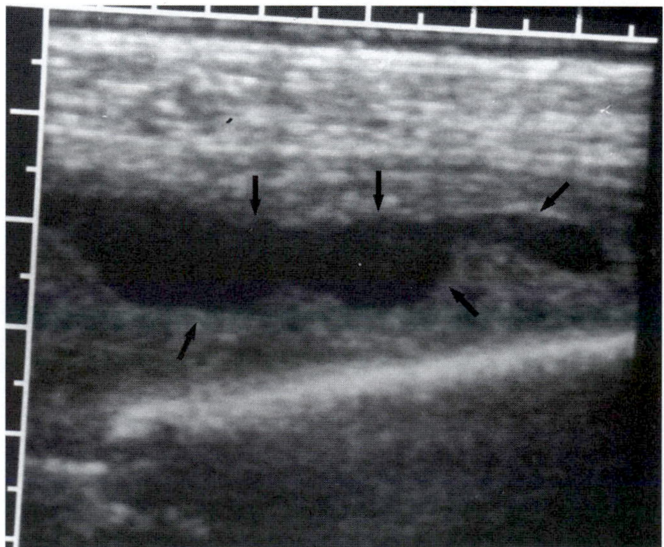

FIGURE 120–9. Soft tissue abscess. Longitudinal plane. This image was obtained in the midthigh of a 32-year-old with thigh pain and fever. Note that a fluid collection (*arrows*) is present but is not in direct contact with the bone. It, therefore, was not suggestive of osteomyelitis. Rather, it represented a soft tissue abscess.

The presence of periosseous fluid is felt to be a consequence of acute infection. Dissemination of organisms to the bone results in an acute inflammatory response. This results in vascular ischemia, edema, and bone necrosis. As intramedullary pressure increases, fluid permeates through the cortex, resulting in periosteal elevation and subperiosteal abscess formation in children. Since in adults the periosteum is firmly attached to the bone, the inflammatory debris may erode through the periosteum and produce extraperiosteal fluid and abscess collections. Patients with chronic osteomyelitis may have echogenic debris within the periosseous fluid that is in direct contact with the bone. Cortical disruption, sequestra, and sinus tracts, other features of chronic osteomyelitis, may be noted by US.

References

Abiri MM, DeAngelis GA, Kirpekar M, et al: Ultrasonic detection of osteomyelitis pathologic correlation in an animal model. *Invest Radiol* 27:111–113, 1992.

Abiri MM, Kirpekar M, Ablow RC: Osteomyelitis: Detection with US. *Radiology* 169:795–797, 1988.

Abiri MM, Kirpekar M, Ablow RC: Osteomyelitis: Detection with US. *Radiology* 172:509–511, 1989.

Boutin RD, Brossmann J, Sartoris DJ, et al: Update on imaging of orthopedic infections. *Orthop Clin North Am* 29:41–63, 1998.

Cleveland TJ, Peck RJ: Case report: Chronic osteomyelitis demonstrated by high resolution ultrasonography. *Clin Radiol* 49: 429–431, 1994.

Index

NOTE: Numbers in italics indicate pages which contain illustrations.

Table of Contents

ISBN 0-8385-8864-6
90000
9 780838 588642